# Women and Smoking

## A Report of the Surgeon General



2001

U.S. DEPARTMENT OF HEALTH AND HUMAN SERVICES
Public Health Service
Office of the Surgeon General
Rockville, MD

**National Library of Medicine Cataloging in Publication**

Women and smoking : a report of the Surgeon General.
Rockville, MD : U.S. Dept. of Health and Human Services,
Public Health Service, Office of the Surgeon General ;
Washington, D.C. : For sale by the Supt. Of Docs., U.S.
G.P.O., 2001.

1. Smoking – prevention & control. 2. Women's Health.
3. Tobacco – adverse effects. 4. Women – psychology.
5. Tobacco Use Disorder. I. United States. Public Health Service.
Office of the Surgeon General. II. Centers for Disease Control
and Prevention (U.S.) III. National Center for Chronic Disease
Prevention and Health Promotion (U.S.) IV. United States.
Office on Smoking and Health.

O2NLM: WM 290 W872 2001

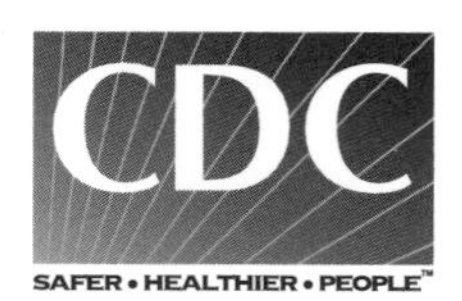


Centers for Disease Control and Prevention
National Center for Chronic Disease Prevention and Health Promotion
Office on Smoking and Health

This publication is available on the World Wide Web at
http://www.surgeongeneral.gov/library

For sale by the Superintendent of Documents, U.S. Government Printing Office,
Washington, D.C., 20402. ISBN 0-16-050751-0

# Message from Tommy G. Thompson

*Secretary of Health and Human Services*

Ever since the first Surgeon General's report on smoking in 1964, Americans have learned about the dangerous effects of smoking and how tragically this habit can end life. It is an irrefutable fact that smoking cigarettes and using other tobacco products causes cancer and often results in other debilitating illnesses and death. Our Nation, rightfully, remains on an important quest to raise public awareness of the dangers of smoking and to deter people from choosing this costly habit, particularly our young people.

Too often and for too long, however, smoking has been largely viewed in the context of men's health. But smoking wreaks a great and unique toll on the health of our women and teenage girls as well. The impact smoking is having on our Nation's women is alarming. Therefore, the work of Surgeon General David Satcher and the Centers for Disease Control and Prevention (CDC) in producing this report of the Surgeon General on women and smoking could not come at a better time. Frankly, this update and expansion of the 1980 Surgeon General's report, *The Health Consequences of Smoking for Women,* is long due. And we are all grateful for the time and hard work put into this report by the Surgeon General, his office, the Office of Women's Health, the CDC, the National Institutes of Health, and researchers and scientists from around the world.

This report shines a bright light on the devastating impact of smoking on women and the need for the Nation to come together and address this problem. Just look at a sample of the statistics summarized in this report.

- An estimated 27,000 more women died of lung cancer than of breast cancer in 2000.

- Three million women have died prematurely because of smoking since 1980, and on average, these women died 14 years prematurely.

- Twenty-two percent of women smoked cigarettes in 1998.

- And 30 percent of high school senior girls reported smoking in the past month, according to recent information.

The report goes well beyond just the statistical impacts of smoking to lay out specific health problems incurred by women who smoke. This report found that women who smoke have a lower bone density and experience a premature decline of lung function. These women also are at increased risk of conception delay and both primary and secondary infertility. For pregnant women who smoke, the risk is increased for low birth weight, perinatal mortality—both stillbirth and neonatal deaths—and sudden infant death syndrome after the child is born. Of course, there are the health dangers of smoking that most of us are familiar with but remain just as real and just as deadly for women: cancer, emphysema, heart disease, and stroke. Now, studies suggest that even exposure to environmental tobacco smoke has a causal link to cancer and heart disease.

If we are going to succeed in reducing the number of women who smoke in this country, we must first succeed in preventing our teenagers and young women from picking up the habit. Our antismoking efforts at the U.S. Department of Health and Human Services will focus intensively on keeping tobacco out of the hands of teenage girls and college-age women. These young women are greatly influenced by their peers and the glamor of smoking portrayed through magazines, television, and movies; we must be aggressive in educating them that smoking is very addictive, harmful, and lethal. These young women must know that once they start, it will be difficult to stop—and that the health risks are very real and costly.

All of society must engage in this endeavor, as well as the overall challenge of reducing smoking in this Nation, if we are to succeed. We must re-energize our efforts and commit time and resources—private and public—to the prevention of smoking initiation. We need to provide parents, teachers, and community leaders with tools and information that effectively convey the destructive message of cigarette use. And we need all aspects of the media to join the effort in addressing this societal problem. Our best defense against the dangers of smoking is a comprehensive approach to tobacco use prevention, which includes education that is accessible to all.

We must also strengthen the enforcement activities aimed at preventing youth smoking, including no marketing geared toward teenagers and absolutely no tobacco sales to minors. We must fully support law enforcement sting operations and other improved methods of ensuring that persons who purchase tobacco products are adults.

The cost of smoking is simply too high in this country. The impacts are a financial drain on our Nation's health care system, costing up to $73 billion annually. But more important, we are losing too many of our mothers and daughters prematurely as a result of smoking. We simply can't afford to lose any women to this harmful habit.

This Surgeon General's report provides an opportunity for America to focus on how damaging smoking is to the well-being of our women and girls. We must seize this opportunity to prevent smoking by women, and help those who do smoke to quit, which will improve the overall health of women in this country. And we must do this by working together as a Nation, for that is the only way we can truly succeed in addressing this devastating problem.

# Foreword

Women and girls in the United States are in the throes of an epidemic of tobacco-related diseases. Over time, the once-wide gender gap in smoking—and its health consequences—has narrowed considerably. Cigarette smoking was rare among women in the early part of this century, increased until the 1960s, and finally began to decline in the mid-1970s. During the past decade, however, reductions in smoking prevalence among adult women were minor, and tobacco use among teens increased markedly. By the late 1990s, more than one in five adult women was a regular smoker, and about 30 percent of high school senior girls reported having smoked within the past 30 days. Many of the tobacco-related diseases that have manifested today are the result of the cumulative effects of smoking initiated several decades ago. Unless we succeed in further curbing tobacco use among women and girls, the health effects of tobacco use will remain great for the foreseeable future.

This report reviews in detail what we know about smoking-related diseases among women, and documents that the toll of smoking on women's health is wide-ranging and staggering. Like their male counterparts who smoke, women smokers are at increased risk of cancer, cardiovascular disease, and pulmonary disease, but women also experience unique risks related to menstrual and reproductive function. In the face of so many strides that were made during the twentieth century to improve health outcomes for women, including enormous declines in maternal mortality, heart disease, and cervical cancer, to name but a few, it is tragic that an entirely preventable factor continues to claim so many women's lives.

Through its detailed examination of smoking patterns by demographic and other characteristics, this report confirms that it is often women who are more socioeconomically disadvantaged and girls who perform less well academically who are most likely to smoke in our society today. For example, the smoking prevalence in 1998 among women with 9 to 11 years of education was almost three times higher than that among women who had 16 or more years of education. Once a mark of sophistication among women in the social forefront, then adopted by middle-class women, smoking has increasingly become an addiction borne by women with the least resources in our society. The long history of tobacco marketing targeted to women is also chronicled here. The positive imagery in cigarette advertisements is greatly at odds with the negative health consequences suffered by so many women who smoke.

The importance of vigilance in our efforts to prevent initiation of smoking by girls and to promote cessation among female smokers of all ages is underscored by this report. To be successful, we know that a multipronged approach is necessary, including anti-tobacco media campaigns, increases in tobacco prices, promotion of nonsmoking in public places, curbs on tobacco advertising and promotion, enforcement of legislation to reduce youth's access to tobacco products, and effective tobacco use treatment programs. Women who smoke represent diverse subgroups of the population with unique issues and needs. An important subgroup is pregnant women, among whom smoking has declined in recent years but remains significant. Efforts to assist quitting among pregnant women (and their partners) can greatly impact not only their health but that of their infants and children. We must dramatically accelerate declines in smoking among both women and girls. Exciting models of new tobacco control programs in states show that this can be done. In Florida, where the Tobacco Pilot Program was begun in 1998, the prevalence of current smoking among middle school girls declined from 18.1 percent in 1998 to 10.9 percent in 2000—a 40-percent decline in just two years.

The challenge facing this Nation now is to establish effective tobacco control programs in every state and nationwide. No one who reads this report can help but recognize that combating smoking and the forces that promote it deserves to be among our very highest priorities for women's health.

Jeffrey P. Koplan, M.D., M.P.H.
Director
Centers for Disease Control and Prevention
and
Administrator
Agency for Toxic Substances and Disease Registry

# Preface

*from the Surgeon General,*
*U.S. Department of Health and Human Services*

Two decades have passed since the first Surgeon General's report on women and smoking was published in 1980. That report pointed out the first signs of an epidemic of smoking-related disease among women. This report documents that the epidemic became full-blown.

Cigarette smoking is the leading cause of preventable death in the United States, and women's share of tobacco-related disease has risen dramatically over the past half century. The point is underscored by the 600-percent increase since 1950 in women's death rates for lung cancer, a disease that is primarily attributable to smoking. Lung cancer accounted for only 3 percent of all female cancer deaths in 1950, whereas in 2000 it accounted for an estimated 25 percent. Already in 1987, lung cancer had surpassed breast cancer as the leading cause of cancer death in U.S. women, and in 2000 nearly 27,000 more women died of lung cancer (67,600) than breast cancer (40,800). In fact, more women are estimated to have died of lung cancer in the year 2000 than of cancers of the breast, uterus, and ovary combined. Of course, lung cancer is but one of the many diseases for which risk is greater among smokers than nonsmokers.

Despite these facts, 22.0 percent of U.S. adult women smoked in 1998. Moreover, between 1992 and 1997, the percentage of high school senior girls who reported smoking within the past 30 days increased from 26.1 percent to 35.2 percent before declining to 29.7 percent in 2000.

Since the first Surgeon General's report on women and smoking in 1980, thousands of studies have expanded both our knowledge of the effects of smoking on women's health and our understanding of the myriad factors that influence smoking initiation, maintenance, and cessation. The need for an updated compendium on women and smoking is great, and this report addresses that need.

Ironically, in the face of the overwhelmingly negative health effects of smoking, tobacco marketing has always used positive imagery and has attempted to capitalize on issues important to women and to exploit the women's movement. The same tobacco brand that for so long featured the slogan "You've come a long way, baby" more recently launched an advertising campaign with the theme "Find your voice." Tobacco advertisements suggest that women who smoke are liberated, sexually attractive, athletic, fun loving, and slim, whereas in reality women who smoke are often nicotine dependent, physically unhealthy, socioeconomically disadvantaged, or depressed. Tobacco companies also have tried to ingratiate themselves with women's causes, providing funding for women's sports, for women's professional organizations, and for anti-domestic violence programs and other issues of salience to women, not to mention providing huge sums in advertising revenues to women's magazines. Perhaps such support has contributed to the fact that women's lung cancer does not have a voice, in contrast to breast cancer, which has such a well-developed and effective advocacy community.

Although the *Healthy People 2000* objective of reducing the prevalence of current smoking among U.S. adult men and women to 15 percent is unlikely to be met, we should emphasize that nearly 80 percent of adult women in this country choose not to smoke. Nonsmoking is now by far the accepted norm. If the recommendations in this and previous reports were fully implemented, the *Healthy People 2010* objective to reduce the rate of tobacco use among girls and women in the country by more than 50 percent could be met.

Hopeful signs now exist that the lung cancer epidemic may have peaked among U.S. women. As this report goes to press, encouraging news comes from a report issued by the Centers for Disease Control and Prevention based on data from California and from the National Cancer Institute. In California, which has been at the forefront of tobacco control activities and where smoking prevalence has declined more rapidly than in the rest of the country, the lung cancer incidence rate among women has actually declined in recent years. Another report from California found that 33,300 fewer heart disease deaths occurred in the state between 1989 and 1997 among women and men combined than would have been expected during that time had earlier trends in heart disease mortality relative to the rest of the United States continued. California was the first state to implement a comprehensive statewide tobacco control program funded by a cigarette surtax that began in 1989. Today all states have enormous monetary settlement payments from the state lawsuits with the tobacco industry to recover the cost of smoking-related disease; unfortunately, few states have used these new resources to make the level of investments in the proven tobacco control strategies that could reduce the disease and death rates related to smoking.

Women in the United States and a number of other developed countries are less likely to be smokers than was the case 30 years ago. However, just the opposite trend is feared for women in many other parts of the world, particularly women in developing countries where smoking prevalence has traditionally been low but where the tobacco industry now recognizes tremendous market potential and is aggressively pursuing females. Thwarting increases in the use of tobacco among women around the world represents one of the greatest public health opportunities of our time.

David Satcher, M.D., Ph.D.
Surgeon General

## Acknowledgments

This report was prepared by the U.S. Department of Health and Human Services under the general direction of the Centers for Disease Control and Prevention, National Center for Chronic Disease Prevention and Health Promotion, Office on Smoking and Health.

David Satcher, M.D., Ph.D., Surgeon General, Office of Public Health and Science, Office of the Secretary, Washington, D.C.

Jeffrey P. Koplan, M.D., M.P.H., Director, Centers for Disease Control and Prevention, Atlanta, Georgia.

James S. Marks, M.D., M.P.H., Director, National Center for Chronic Disease Prevention and Health Promotion, Centers for Disease Control and Prevention, Atlanta, Georgia.

Lawrence W. Green, Dr.P.H., Acting Director, Office on Smoking and Health, National Center for Chronic Disease Prevention and Health Promotion, Centers for Disease Control and Prevention, Atlanta, Georgia.

Nicole Lurie, M.D., M.S.P.H., Principal Deputy Assistant Secretary for Health, Office of Public Health and Science, Office of the Secretary, Washington, D.C.

Beverly L. Malone, Ph.D., R.N., F.A.A.N., Deputy Assistant Secretary for Health, Office of Public Health and Science, Office of the Secretary, Washington, D.C.

Arthur Lawrence, Ph.D., R.Ph., Assistant Surgeon General, U.S. Public Health Service and Deputy Assistant Secretary for Health (Operations), Office of Public Health and Science, Office of the Secretary, Washington, D.C.

Kenneth Moritsugu, M.D., M.P.H., Deputy Surgeon General, U.S. Public Health Service, Office of the Surgeon General, Office of the Secretary, Washington, D.C.

Allan S. Noonan, M.D., M.P.H., CAPT, Senior Advisor, U.S. Public Health Service, Office of the Surgeon General, Office of the Secretary, Washington, D.C.

***Special thanks to***

Michael P. Eriksen, Sc.D., Centers for Disease Control and Prevention Assignee to the World Health Organization, Geneva, Switzerland.

Elizabeth Majestic, M.P.H., Associate Director for Planning, Evaluation, and Legislation, National Center for Chronic Disease Prevention and Health Promotion, Centers for Disease Control and Prevention, Atlanta, Georgia.

Terry F. Pechacek, Ph.D., Associate Director for Science, Office on Smoking and Health, National Center for Chronic Disease Prevention and Health Promotion, Centers for Disease Control and Prevention, Atlanta, Georgia.

***The editors of the report were***

Virginia L. Ernster, Ph.D., Senior Scientific Editor, Professor and Vice Chair, Department of Epidemiology and Biostatistics and Associate Director for Epidemiology, Prevention, and Control, UCSF Comprehensive Cancer Center, University of California, San Francisco, California.

Gayle Lloyd, M.A., Managing Editor, Office on Smoking and Health, National Center for Chronic Disease Prevention and Health Promotion, Centers for Disease Control and Prevention, Atlanta, Georgia.

Leslie A. Norman, Managing Editor, Office on Smoking and Health, National Center for Chronic Disease Prevention and Health Promotion, Centers for Disease Control and Prevention, Atlanta, Georgia.

Anne McCarthy, Technical Editor, Consultant to Palladian Partners, Inc., Silver Spring, Maryland.

Audrey L. Pinto, Technical Medical Writer and Editor, Consultant to Palladian Partners, Inc., Silver Spring, Maryland.

***Contributing editors were***

David G. Altman, Ph.D., Professor, Department of Public Health Sciences, Wake Forest University School of Medicine, Winston-Salem, North Carolina.

John A. Baron, M.D., Professor, Department of Medicine and Community and Family Medicine, Dartmouth Medical School, Hanover, New Hampshire.

Ellen R. Gritz, Ph.D., Professor and Chair, Frank T. McGraw Memorial Chair in the Study of Cancer, Department of Behavioral Science, The University of Texas, M. D. Anderson Cancer Center, Houston, Texas.

Corinne G. Husten, M.D., M.P.H., Chief, Epidemiology Branch, Office on Smoking and Health, National Center for Chronic Disease Prevention and Health Promotion, Centers for Disease Control and Prevention, Atlanta, Georgia.

Richard B. Rothenberg, M.D., M.P.H., Professor, Department of Family and Preventive Medicine, Emory University School of Medicine, Atlanta, Georgia.

Beti Thompson, Ph.D., Member, Fred Hutchinson Cancer Research Center, Seattle, Washington.

***Contributing authors were***

David G. Altman, Ph.D., Professor, Department of Public Health Sciences, Wake Forest University School of Medicine, Winston-Salem, North Carolina.

Amanda Amos, Ph.D., Senior Lecturer in Health Promotion, Public Health Sciences, Department of Community Health Sciences, University of Edinburgh Medical School, Edinburgh, United Kingdom.

John A. Baron, M.D., Professor, Department of Medicine and Community and Family Medicine, Dartmouth Medical School, Hanover, New Hampshire.

Neal Benowitz, M.D., Professor of Medicine, Psychiatry, and Biopharmaceutical Sciences, University of California, and Chief, Clinical Pharmacology, San Francisco General Hospital, San Francisco, California.

Lois Biener, Ph.D., Senior Research Fellow, Center for Survey Research, University of Massachusetts, Boston, Massachusetts.

William J. Blot, Ph.D., Chief Executive Officer, International Epidemiology Institute, Ltd., Rockville, Maryland.

Edward J. Boyko, M.D., M.P.H., Professor of Medicine, University of Washington and Director, Epidemiologic Research and Information Center, Veterans Affairs Puget Sound Health Care System, Seattle, Washington.

Louise A. Brinton, Ph.D., Chief, Environmental Epidemiology Branch, National Cancer Institute, Bethesda, Maryland.

David N. Burns, M.D., M.P.H., Medical Officer, Pediatric, Adolescent, and Maternal AIDS Branch, Center for Research for Mothers and Children, National Institute of Child Health and Human Development, Bethesda, Maryland.

Graham A. Colditz, M.D., Dr.P.H., Professor of Medicine, Channing Laboratory, School of Medicine, Harvard University, Boston, Massachusetts.

David B. Coultas, M.D., Professor of Internal Medicine and Chief, Division of Epidemiology and Preventive Medicine, School of Medicine, University of New Mexico, Albuquerque, New Mexico.

Alyssa N. Easton, Ph.D., M.P.H., Epidemiologist, Office on Smoking and Health, National Center for Chronic Disease Prevention and Health Promotion, Centers for Disease Control and Prevention, Atlanta, Georgia.

Brenda Eskenazi, Ph.D., Professor of Maternal and Child Health and Epidemiology Director, Center for Children's Environmental Health Research, School of Public Health, University of California, Berkeley, California.

Edwin B. Fisher, Ph.D., Professor of Psychology, Medicine, and Pediatrics and Head, Division of Health Behavior Research, Departments of Medicine and Pediatrics, Washington University, St. Louis, Missouri.

Brian R. Flay, D.Phil., Director, Health Research and Policy Centers, Chicago, Illinois.

Brian S. Flynn, Sc.D., Research Professor and Director, Office of Health Promotion Research, College of Medicine, University of Vermont, Burlington, Vermont.

Elizabeth T. Fontham, Dr.P.H., Professor and Chairman, Department of Public Health and Preventive Medicine, Louisiana State University Health Science Center, New Orleans, Louisiana.

Elizabeth A. Gilpin, M.S., Clinical Professor of Biostatistics and Director, Biostatistics Shared Resource, University of California at San Diego Cancer Center, La Jolla, California.

Deborah Grady, M.D., Professor and Vice Chair, Department of Epidemiology and Biostatistics and Department of Medicine, University of California, San Francisco, California.

Andrew Grandinetti, Ph.D., Assistant Researcher, Pacific Biomedical Research Center, University of Hawaii at Manoa, Honolulu, Hawaii.

Sharon M. Hall, Ph.D., Professor and Vice-Chair, Psychiatry, Department of Psychiatry, University of California, San Francisco, California.

Dorothy Hatsukami, Ph.D., Professor, Department of Psychiatry, University of Minnesota, Minneapolis, Minnesota.

S. Jane Henley, M.S.P.H., Epidemiologist, Department of Epidemiology and Surveillance Research, American Cancer Society, Atlanta, Georgia.

Frank B. Hu, M.D., Ph.D., Assistant Professor, Department of Nutrition, Harvard School of Public Health, Boston, Massachusetts.

Corinne G. Husten, M.D., M.P.H., Chief, Epidemiology Branch, Office on Smoking and Health, National Center for Chronic Disease Prevention and Health Promotion, Centers for Disease Control and Prevention, Atlanta, Georgia.

Nancy J. Kaufman, R.N., M.S., Vice President, The Robert Wood Johnson Foundation, Princeton, New Jersey.

Ichiro Kawachi, M.D., Ph.D., Assistant Professor of Medicine, Channing Laboratory, School of Medicine and Associate Professor of Health and Social Behavior, School of Public Health, Harvard University, Boston, Massachusetts.

Robert C. Klesges, Ph.D., Executive Director, University of Memphis Center for Community Health, University of Memphis, Memphis, Tennessee.

Edward Lichtenstein, Ph.D., Senior Research Scientist, Oregon Research Institute, Eugene, Oregon.

Alan D. Lopez, Ph.D., Epidemiologist, Prevention, Advocacy and Promotion, Programme on Substance Abuse, World Health Organization, Geneva, Switzerland.

Everly Macario, M.S., Ed.M., Associate Professor, Department of Health and Social Behavior, Harvard School of Public Health, Boston, Massachusetts.

Judith Mackay, MBE, FRCP (Edin), FRCP (Lon), FHKAM, Director, Asian Consultancy on Tobacco Control, Hong Kong, China.

Nejma Macklai, Epidemiologist, Tobacco-Free Initiative, World Health Organization, Geneva, Switzerland.

Ann M. Malarcher, Ph.D., Epidemiologist, Division of Chronic Disease Control and Community Intervention, National Center for Chronic Disease Prevention and Health Promotion, Centers for Disease Control and Prevention, Atlanta, Georgia.

Ruth E. Malone, R.N., Ph.D., Assistant Professor of Nursing and Health Policy, Institute for Health Policy Studies and Department of Physiological Nursing, University of California, San Francisco, California.

Joseph K. McLaughlin, Ph.D., President, International Epidemiology Institute, Ltd., Rockville, Maryland.

Deborah L. McLellan, M.H.S., Assistant Director, Center for Community Based Research, Division of Population Sciences, Dana-Farber Cancer Institute, Boston, Massachusetts.

Robert K. Merritt, M.A., Health Scientist, Division of Reproductive Health, National Center for Chronic Disease Prevention and Health Promotion, Centers for Disease Control and Prevention, Atlanta, Georgia.

Sherry L. Mills, M.D., M.P.H., Chief, Applied Sociocultural Research Branch, Behavioral Research Program, Division of Cancer Control and Population Studies, National Cancer Institute, Bethesda, Maryland.

Micah H. Milton, M.P.H., Behavioral Scientist, Office on Smoking and Health, National Center for Chronic Disease Prevention and Health Promotion, Centers for Disease Control and Prevention, Atlanta, Georgia.

Heidi L. Miracle-McMahill, M.S.P.H., Epidemiologist, Department of Epidemiology and Surveillance Research, American Cancer Society, Atlanta, Georgia.

Patricia Dolan Mullen, Dr.P.H., Professor of Behavioral Sciences and Health Education and Training Director, Center for Health Promotion and Prevention Research, University of Texas Science Center at Houston School of Public Health, Houston, Texas.

Judith K. Ockene, Ph.D., Professor of Medicine and Chief, Division of Preventive and Behavioral Medicine, Department of Medicine, University of Massachusetts Medical School, Worcester, Massachusetts.

C. Tracy Orleans, Ph.D., Senior Scientist, The Robert Wood Johnson Foundation, Princeton, New Jersey.

Kathyrn Osann, Ph.D., M.P.H., Associate Adjunct Professor, Division of Hematology and Oncology, Department of Medicine, College of Medicine, University of California, Irvine, California.

John Petraitis, Ph.D., Associate Professor, Department of Psychology, University of Alaska, Anchorage, Alaska.

Phyllis Pirie, Ph.D., Professor, Division of Epidemiology, School of Public Health, University of Minnesota, Minneapolis, Minnesota.

Richard W. Pollay, Ph.D., Professor of Marketing and Curator, History of Advertising Archives, Faculty of Commerce, University of British Columbia, Vancouver, British Columbia, Canada.

Cynthia S. Pomerleau, Ph.D., Senior Associate Research Scientist and Director, Nicotine Research Laboratory, Department of Psychiatry, University of Michigan, Ann Arbor, Michigan.

Alex V. Prokhorov, M.D., Ph.D., Associate Professor, Department of Behavioral Science, The University of Texas, M. D. Anderson Cancer Center, Houston, Texas.

Herbert H. Severson, Ph.D., Senior Research Scientist, Oregon Research Institute and Associate Professor of Counseling Psychology, College of Education, University of Oregon, Eugene, Oregon.

Dana M. Shelton, M.P.H., Assistant Director for Policy, Planning, and External Relations, Division of STD Prevention, National Center for HIV, STD, and TB Prevention, Centers for Disease Control and Prevention, Atlanta, Georgia.

Laura Solomon, Ph.D., Research Professor, Department of Psychology, University of Vermont, Burlington, Vermont.

Glorian Sorensen, Ph.D., M.P.H., Director, Community Based Research, Division of Cancer, Epidemiology, and Control, Dana-Farber Cancer Institute and Professor of Health and Social Behavior, Department of Health and Social Behavior, Harvard School of Public Health, Boston, Massachusetts.

Margaret Spitz, M.D., Chairman, Department of Epidemiology, The University of Texas, M. D. Anderson Cancer Center, Houston, Texas.

Beti Thompson, Ph.D., Member, Fred Hutchinson Cancer Research Center, Seattle, Washington.

Michael J. Thun, M.D., Vice President, Epidemiology and Surveillance Research, American Cancer Society, Atlanta, Georgia.

Suzanne Tyas, Ph.D., Postdoctoral Fellow, Centre on Aging, University of Manitoba, Winnipeg, Manitoba, Canada.

Kenneth D. Ward, Ph.D., Assistant Professor, University of Memphis Prevention Center, Memphis, Tennessee.

Elisabete Weiderpass, M.D., M.Sc., Ph.D., Associate Professor, Department of Medical Epidemiology, Karolinska Institutet, Stockholm, Sweden.

Gayle Windham, Ph.D., Senior Epidemiologist, Division of Environmental and Occupational Disease Control, California Department of Health Services, Oakland, California.

Anna H. Wu, Ph.D., Professor, Keck School of Medicine, Department of Preventive Medicine, Norris Comprehensive Cancer Center, University of Southern California, Los Angeles, California.

***Reviewers were***

Duane Alexander, M.D., Director, National Institute of Child Health and Human Development, National Institutes of Health, Bethesda, Maryland.

Robert Barbieri, M.D., Chairman, Department of Obstetrics and Gynecology, Brigham and Women's Hospital, Boston, Massachusetts.

Glen Bennett, M.P.H., Coordinator, Advanced Technologies Applications in Health Education, Office of Prevention, Education, and Control, National Heart, Lung, and Blood Institute, National Institutes of Health, Bethesda, Maryland.

Michelle Bloch, M.D., Ph.D., Medical Officer, Tobacco Control Research Branch, Division of Cancer Control and Population Sciences, National Cancer Institute, National Institutes of Health, Rockville, Maryland.

Gilbert J. Botvin, Ph.D., Professor and Director, Institute for Prevention Research, Department of Public Health, Cornell University Medical College, New York, New York.

Michael B. Bracken, Ph.D., Professor and Head, Division of Chronic Disease Epidemiology, Department of Epidemiology and Public Health, Yale University School of Medicine, New Haven, Connecticut.

David M. Burns, M.D., Professor of Medicine, Tobacco Control Policies Project, University of California, San Diego, California.

Olivia Carter-Pokras, Ph.D., Director, Division of Policy and Data, Office of Minority Health, Rockville, Maryland.

Jane A. Cauley, Dr.P.H., Associate Professor, Department of Epidemiology, University of Pittsburgh, Pittsburgh, Pennsylvania.

Sven Cnattingius, M.D., Ph.D., Professor, Department of Medical Epidemiology, Karolinska Institutet, Stockholm, Sweden.

Daniel W. Cramer, M.D., Sc.D., Professor of Obstetrics, Gynecology, and Reproductive Biology, Harvard University Medical School, Boston, Massachusetts.

Byron L. Cryer, M.D., Associate Professor of Medicine, University of Texas Southwestern Medical Center, Veterans Affairs Medical Center, Dallas, Texas.

K. Michael Cummings, Ph.D., M.P.H., Chairman and Senior Scientist, Department of Cancer Prevention, Epidemiology, and Biostatistics, Roswell Park Cancer Institute, Buffalo, New York.

Susan Curry, Ph.D., Director, Center for Health Studies, Group Health Cooperative, Seattle, Washington.

Ronald M. Davis, M.D., Director, Center for Health Promotion and Disease Prevention, Henry Ford Health System, Detroit, Michigan.

Andrew K. Diehl, M.D., M.Sc., Professor and Chief, Division of General Medicine, Department of Medicine, University of Texas Health Science Center, San Antonio, Texas.

Jeffrey L. Fellows, Ph.D., Health Economist, Office on Smoking and Health, National Center for Chronic Disease Prevention and Health Promotion, Centers for Disease Control and Prevention, Atlanta, Georgia.

David Felson, M.D., M.P.H., Professor of Medicine and Public Health, The Arthritis Center, School of Medicine, Boston University, Boston, Massachusetts.

Roberta G. Ferrence, Ph.D., Director, Ontario Tobacco Research Unit, University of Toronto, Toronto, Ontario, Canada.

Frederick L. Ferris III, M.D., Director, Division of Epidemiology and Clinical Research, Clinical Director, National Eye Institute, National Institutes of Health, Bethesda, Maryland.

Gary A. Giovino, Ph.D., M.S., Senior Research Scientist, Department of Cancer Prevention, Epidemiology, and Biostatistics, Roswell Park Cancer Institute, Buffalo, New York.

Alexander H. Glassman, M.D., Professor of Clinical Psychiatry, Department of Psychiatry, College of Physicians and Surgeons, Columbia University, New York, New York.

Thomas J. Glynn, Ph.D., Director, Cancer Science and Trends, American Cancer Society, Washington, D.C.

Amy Borenstein Graves, Ph.D., M.P.H., Associate Professor, Department of Epidemiology and Biostatistics, College of Public Health, University of South Florida, Tampa, Florida.

Lorraine Greaves, Ph.D., Executive Director, British Columbia Centre of Excellence for Women's Health, British Columbia Women's Hospital, Vancouver, British Columbia, Canada.

Betty Lee Hawks, M.A., Special Assistant to the Director, Office of Minority Health, U.S. Department of Health and Human Services, Rockville, Maryland.

Jack E. Henningfield, Ph.D., Associate Professor, Department of Psychiatry and Behavioral Sciences, The Johns Hopkins University School of Medicine, Bethesda, Maryland.

Marc C. Hochberg, M.D., M.P.H., Professor of Medicine and Epidemiology and Preventive Medicine, University of Maryland School of Medicine, Baltimore, Maryland.

John R. Hughes, M.D., Professor, Human Behavioral Pharmacology Laboratory, Department of Psychiatry, University of Vermont, Burlington, Vermont.

Wanda K. Jones, Dr.P.H., Deputy Assistant Secretary for Health (Women's Health), Office on Women's Health, Washington, D.C.

Donald Kadunce, M.D., Assistant Professor, Department of Dermatology, University of Utah, Salt Lake City, Utah.

Denise Kandel, Ph.D., Professor of Public Health in Psychiatry, Department of Psychiatry, College of Physicians and Surgeons of Columbia University and Chief, Department on the Epidemiology of Substance Abuse, New York State Psychiatric Institute, New York, New York.

Ichiro Kawachi, M.D., Ph.D., Assistant Professor of Medicine, Channing Laboratory, School of Medicine and Associate Professor of Health and Social Behavior, School of Public Health, Harvard University, Boston, Massachusetts.

Kay-Tee Khaw, Professor, Clinical Gerontology Unit, University of Cambridge, Cambridge, United Kingdom.

Douglas P. Kiel, M.D., M.P.H., Director for Medical Research, Hebrew Rehabilitation Center for Aged, Research and Training Institute and Associate Professor, Division on Aging, Harvard Medical School, Boston, Massachusetts.

Barbara Eden Kobrin Klein, M.D., M.P.H., Professor, Department of Ophthalmology and Visual Sciences, Department of Preventive Medicine, School of Medicine, University of Wisconsin, Madison, Wisconsin.

Lewis H. Kuller, M.D., Dr.P.H., University Professor of Public Health and Professor and Chair, Department of Epidemiology, Graduate School of Public Health, University of Pittsburgh, Pittsburgh, Pennsylvania.

John H. Kurata, Ph.D., M.P.H., Chief, Chronic Disease Epidemiology Section, California Department of Health Services, Sacramento, California.

Carlo La Vecchia, M.D., Laboratory of Epidemiology, Mario Negri Institute for Pharmacological Research and University of Milan, Milan, Italy.

Darwin R. Labarthe, M.D., Ph.D., James W. Rockwell Professor of Public Health, School of Public Health, The University of Texas-Houston, Health Science Center, Houston, Texas.

Harry A. Lando, Ph.D., Professor, Division of Epidemiology, School of Public Health, University of Minnesota, Minneapolis, Minnesota.

Douglas S. Lloyd, M.D., M.P.H., HRSA Senior Scholar, Association of Schools of Public Health, Washington, D.C.

Richard Logan, B.Sc., MBChB, M.Sc., MFPHM, FRCP, FRCPE, Professor of Clinical Epidemiology, Division of Public Health and Epidemiology, University of Nottingham, Queens Medical Centre, Nottingham, England.

Marc Manley, M.D., M.P.H., Special Assistant for Tobacco Policy, National Cancer Institute, National Institutes of Health, Rockville, Maryland.

Sonja M. McKinlay, Ph.D., President, New England Research Institutes, Inc., Watertown, Massachusetts.

Robin Mermelstein, Ph.D., Deputy Director, Health Research and Policy Centers and Department of Psychology, University of Illinois, Chicago, Illinois.

Linda D. Meyers, Ph.D., Deputy Director, Office of Disease Prevention and Health Promotion, Washington, D.C.

Kenneth Moritsugu, M.D., M.P.H., Deputy Surgeon General, U.S. Public Health Service, Office of the Surgeon General, Office of the Secretary, Washington, D.C.

Polly A. Newcomb, Ph.D., M.P.H., Member, Fred Hutchinson Cancer Research Center, Seattle, Washington, and Senior Scientist, University of Wisconsin, Madison, Wisconsin.

Patrick O'Malley, Ph.D., Research Scientist, Institute for Social Research, University of Michigan, Ann Arbor, Michigan.

Regina Otero-Sabogal, Ph.D., Associate Adjunct Professor, Institute for Health and Aging, University of California, San Francisco, California.

Nancy S. Padian, Ph.D., Co-Director, Center for Reproductive Health Research and Policy and Professor, Department of Obstetrics, Gynecology, and Reproductive Sciences, University of California, San Francisco, California.

Julie R. Palmer, Sc.D., Associate Professor, Slone Epidemiology Unit, Boston University School of Medicine, Brookline, Massachusetts.

Donald Maxwell Parkin, M.D., Chief, Unit of Descriptive Epidemiology, International Agency for Research on Cancer, Lyon, France.

Terry F. Pechacek, Ph.D., Associate Director for Science, Office on Smoking and Health, National Center for Chronic Disease Prevention and Health Promotion, Centers for Disease Control and Prevention, Atlanta, Georgia.

Linda L. Pederson, Ph.D., Visiting Scientist, Office on Smoking and Health, National Center for Chronic Disease Prevention and Health Promotion, Centers for Disease Control and Prevention, Atlanta, Georgia.

Cheryl L. Perry, Ph.D., Professor, Division of Epidemiology, School of Public Health, University of Minnesota, Minneapolis, Minnesota.

Göran Pershagen, M.D., Ph.D., Professor, Institute of Environmental Medicine, Karolinska Institutet, Stockholm, Sweden.

Richard Peto, FRS, Professor, University of Oxford, Clinical Trial Service Unit, Radcliffe Infirmary, Oxford, England.

Diana B. Pettiti, M.D., M.P.H., Director, Department of Research and Evaluation, Kaiser Permanente of Southern California, Pasadena, California.

John Pierce, Ph.D., Professor, Cancer Prevention and Control, University of California at San Diego, La Jolla, California.

Vivian Pinn, M.D., Associate Director for Research on Women's Health, National Institutes of Health, Bethesda, Maryland.

Ovide Pomerleau, Ph.D., Director, Behavioral Medicine Program, Department of Psychiatry, University of Michigan School of Medicine, Ann Arbor, Michigan.

Patrick L. Remington, M.D., M.P.H., Associate Professor, Department of Preventive Medicine, University of Wisconsin Medical School, Madison, Wisconsin.

Nancy A. Rigotti, M.D., Director, Tobacco Treatment and Research Center, Massachusetts General Hospital and Associate Professor of Medicine, Harvard Medical School, Boston, Massachusetts.

Barbara K. Rimer, Dr.P.H., Director, Division of Cancer Control and Population Sciences, National Cancer Institute, National Institutes of Health, Rockville, Maryland.

Thomas Rohan, M.D., Professor and Chairman, Department of Epidemiology and Social Medicine, Albert Einstein College of Medicine, Bronx, New York.

Elaine Ron, Ph.D., Chief, Radiation Epidemiology Branch, National Cancer Institute, National Institutes of Health, Bethesda, Maryland.

Lynn Rosenberg, Sc.D., Associate Director, Slone Epidemiology Unit, Brookline, Massachusetts, and Professor, School of Public Health, Boston University, Boston, Massachusetts.

Michael J. Rosenberg, M.D., M.P.H., President, Health Decisions, Inc., Chapel Hill, North Carolina.

Rosemary Rosso, J.D., Senior Attorney, Division of Advertising Practices, Federal Trade Commission, Washington, D.C.

Richard B. Rothenberg, M.D., M.P.H., Professor, Department of Family and Preventive Medicine, Emory University School of Medicine, Atlanta, Georgia.

Jonathan M. Samet, M.D., M.S., Professor and Chairman, Department of Epidemiology, School of Hygiene and Public Health, The Johns Hopkins University, Baltimore, Maryland.

Ulonda Shamwell, M.S.W., Associate Administrator for Women's Services, Substance Abuse and Mental Health Services Administration, Rockville, Maryland.

Donald R. Shopland, Coordinator, Smoking and Tobacco Control Program, National Cancer Institute, National Institutes of Health, Rockville, Maryland.

Nelson K. Steenland, Ph.D., Senior Epidemiologist, Division of Surveillance, Hazard Evaluations, and Field Studies, National Institute for Occupational Safety and Health, Centers for Disease Control and Prevention, Cincinnati, Ohio.

Robert S. Stern, M.D., Carl J. Herzog Professor of Dermatology, Harvard Medical School at Beth Israel Deaconess Medical Center, Boston, Massachusetts.

Scott L. Tomar, D.M.D., Dr.P.H., Epidemiologist, Division of Oral Health, National Center for Chronic Disease Prevention and Health Promotion, Centers for Disease Control and Prevention, Atlanta, Georgia.

Dimitrios Trichopoulos, M.D., Vincent L. Gregory Professor of Cancer Prevention and Professor of Epidemiology, School of Public Health, Harvard University, Boston, Massachusetts.

Jaylan Turkkan, Ph.D., Chief, Behavioral Sciences Research Branch, National Institute on Drug Abuse, National Institutes of Health, Rockville, Maryland.

K. M. Venkat Narayan, M.D., Chief, Epidemiology Section, Epidemiology and Statistics Branch, Division of Diabetes Translation, National Center for Chronic Disease Prevention and Health Promotion, Centers for Disease Control and Prevention, Atlanta, Georgia.

Ingrid Waldron, Ph.D., Professor of Biology, Department of Biology, University of Pennsylvania, Philadelphia, Pennsylvania.

Kenneth E. Warner, Ph.D., Richard D. Remington Collegiate Professor of Public Health, Department of Health Management and Policy, School of Public Health, University of Michigan and Director, University of Michigan Tobacco Research Network, Ann Arbor, Michigan.

Walter C. Willett, M.D., Dr.P.H., Professor of Epidemiology and Nutrition and Chair, Department of Nutrition, Harvard School of Public Health, Boston, Massachusetts.

Gayle Windham, Ph.D., Senior Epidemiologist, Division of Environmental and Occupational Disease Control, California Department of Health Services, Oakland, California.

Warren Winkelstein, Jr., M.D., M.P.H., Professor Emeritus of Epidemiology, Division of Public Health, Biology, and Epidemiology, School of Public Health, University of California, Berkeley, California.

Anna H. Wu, Ph.D., Professor, Keck School of Medicine, Department of Preventive Medicine, Norris Comprehensive Cancer Center, University of Southern California, Los Angeles, California.

Mitchell R. Zeller, J.D., Director, Office of Tobacco Programs, Food and Drug Administration, Rockville, Maryland.

***Other contributors were***

Kathleen Adams, Ph.D., Associate Professor, Rollins School of Public Health, Emory University and Health Economist, Division of Reproductive Health, National Center for Chronic Disease Prevention and Health Promotion, Centers for Disease Control and Prevention, Atlanta, Georgia.

Harmony Allison, M.P.H., Visiting Fellow, Office on Smoking and Health, National Center for Chronic Disease Prevention and Health Promotion, Centers for Disease Control and Prevention, Atlanta, Georgia.

Felicia M. Barlow, Project Coordinator, Palladian Partners, Inc., Silver Spring, Maryland.

Trudy Barnes, Project Coordinator, Palladian Partners, Inc., Silver Spring, Maryland.

Lara Boeck, Proofreader, Palladian Partners, Inc., Silver Spring, Maryland.

Alison Brown, Graphic Artist, Palladian Partners, Inc., Silver Spring, Maryland.

Tavian K. Cardwell, Graphic Artist, Palladian Partners, Inc., Silver Spring, Maryland.

Christine Choy, Administrative Assistant, Department of Epidemiology and Biostatistics, University of California, San Francisco, California.

Robyn Ertwine, Indexer, Palladian Partners, Inc., Silver Spring, Maryland.

Luis G. Escobedo, M.D., M.P.H., Border Health Epidemiologist, New Mexico Border Health Office, New Mexico Department of Health, Las Cruces, New Mexico.

Wanda Foster, Word Processing Specialist, Palladian Partners, Inc., Silver Spring, Maryland.

Sarah Gregory, Acting Managing Editor, Office on Smoking and Health, National Center for Chronic Disease Prevention and Health Promotion, Centers for Disease Control and Prevention, Atlanta, Georgia.

Barbara H. Hebb, Project Manager, SAIC, Oak Ridge, Tennessee.

Elizabeth L. Hess, E.L.S., Senior Technical Editor, Palladian Partners, Inc., Silver Spring, Maryland.

Lynn Hughley, Lead Graphic Artist, TRW, Inc., Atlanta, Georgia.

Yun Chen W. Lin, M.P.H., Technical Information Specialist, Office on Smoking and Health, National Center for Chronic Disease Prevention and Health Promotion, Centers for Disease Control and Prevention, Atlanta, Georgia.

William T. Marx, M.L.I.S., Technical Information Specialist, Office on Smoking and Health, National Center for Chronic Disease Prevention and Health Promotion, Centers for Disease Control and Prevention, Atlanta, Georgia.

Richard Mayeux, M.D., M.S.E., Gertrude H. Sergievsky Professor of Neurology, Psychiatry, and Public Health (Epidemiology), Gertrude H. Sergievsky Center, Columbia University, New York, New York.

Maribet McCarty, R.N., M.P.H., Technical Information Specialist, The Orkand Corporation, Atlanta, Georgia.

Cathy L. Melvin, Ph.D., M.P.H., Chief, Program Services and Development Branch, Division of Reproductive Health, National Center for Chronic Disease Prevention and Health Promotion, Centers for Disease Control and Prevention, Atlanta, Georgia.

Donald J. Sharp, M.D., Medical Epidemiologist, Office on Smoking and Health, National Center for Chronic Disease Prevention and Health Promotion, Centers for Disease Control and Prevention, Atlanta, Georgia.

Cate Timmerman, Co-President, Palladian Partners, Inc., Silver Spring, Maryland.

Angela Trosclair, M.S., Statistician, TRW, Inc., Atlanta, Georgia.

Lynne Wilcox, M.D., M.P.H., Director, Division of Reproductive Health, National Center for Chronic Disease Prevention and Health Promotion, Centers for Disease Control and Prevention, Atlanta, Georgia.

Peggy E. Williams, M.S., Writer-Editor, Analytical Sciences, Inc., Marietta, Georgia.

Trevor A. Woollery, Ph.D., Health Economist, Office on Smoking and Health, National Center for Chronic Disease Prevention and Health Promotion, Centers for Disease Control and Prevention, Atlanta, Georgia.

Derek Yach, M.D., Program Manager, Tobacco-Free Initiative, World Health Organization, Geneva, Switzerland.

# Women and Smoking

# Chapter 1. Introduction and Summary of Conclusions

# Introduction

This is the second report of the U.S. Surgeon General devoted to women and smoking. The first was published in 1980 (U.S. Department of Health and Human Services [USDHHS] 1980), 16 years after the initial landmark report on smoking and health of the Advisory Committee to the Surgeon General appeared in 1964 (U.S. Department of Health, Education, and Welfare [USDHEW] 1964). The 1964 report summarized the accumulated evidence that demonstrated that smoking was a cause of human cancer and other diseases. Most of the early evidence was based on men. For example, the report concluded, "Cigarette smoking is causally related to lung cancer in men.... The data for women, though less extensive, point in the same direction" (USDHEW 1964, p. 37). By the time of the 1980 report, the evidence clearly showed that women were also experiencing devastating health consequences from smoking and that "the first signs of an epidemic of smoking-related disease among women are now appearing" (USDHHS 1980, p. v). The evidence had solidified later among women than among men because smoking became commonplace among women about 25 years later than it had among men. However, it was still deemed necessary to include a section in the preface of the 1980 report titled "The Fallacy of Women's Immunity." In the two decades since, numerous studies have expanded the breadth and depth of what is known about the health consequences of smoking among women, about historical and contemporary patterns of smoking in demographic subgroups of the female population, about factors that affect initiation and maintenance of smoking among women (including advertising and marketing of tobacco products), and about interventions to assist women to quit smoking. The present report reviews the now massive body of evidence on women and smoking—evidence that taken together compels the Nation to make reducing and preventing smoking one of the highest contemporary priorities for women's health.

A report focused on women is greatly needed. No longer are the first signs of an epidemic of tobacco-related diseases among women being seen, as was the case when the 1980 report was written. Since 1980, hundreds of additional studies have expanded what is known about the health effects of smoking among women, and this report summarizes that knowledge. Today the Nation is in the midst of a full-blown epidemic. Lung cancer, once rare among women, has surpassed breast cancer as the leading cause of female cancer death in the United States, now accounting for 25 percent of all cancer deaths among women. Surveys have indicated that many women do not know this fact. And lung cancer is only one of myriad serious disease risks faced by women who smoke. Although women and men who smoke share excess risks for diseases such as cancer, heart disease, and emphysema, women also experience unique smoking-related disease risks related to pregnancy, oral contraceptive use, menstrual function, and cervical cancer. These risks deserve to be highlighted and broadly recognized. Moreover, much of what is known about the health effects of exposure to environmental tobacco smoke among nonsmokers comes from studies of women, because historically men were more likely than women to smoke and because many women who did not smoke were married to smokers.

In 1965, 51.9 percent of men were smokers, whereas 33.9 percent of women were smokers. By 1979, the percentage of women who smoked had declined somewhat, to 29.9 percent. However, the decline in smoking among men to 37.5 percent was much more dramatic. The gender gap in adult smoking prevalence continued to close after the 1980 report, but since the mid-1980s, the difference has been fairly stable at about 5 percentage points. In 1998, smoking prevalence was 22.0 percent among women and 26.4 percent among men. The gender difference in smoking prevalence among teens is smaller than that among adults. Smoking prevalence increased among both girls and boys in the 1990s. In 2000, 29.7 percent of high school senior girls and 32.8 percent of high school senior boys reported having smoked within the past 30 days (University of Michigan 2000).

In recent years, some research has suggested that the impact of a given amount of smoking on lung cancer risk might be even greater among women than among men, that exposure to environmental tobacco smoke might be associated with increased risk for breast cancer, and that women might be more susceptible than men to weight gain following smoking cessation. Other research indicated that persons with specific genetic polymorphisms may be especially susceptible to the effects of smoking and exposure to environmental tobacco smoke. These issues remain active areas of investigation, and no conclusions can be drawn about them at this time. Nonetheless, knowledge of the vast spectrum of smoking-related health effects continues to grow, as does knowledge that examination of gender-specific effects is important.

Smoking is one of the most studied of human behaviors and thousands of studies have documented its health consequences, yet certain questions and data needs exist with respect to women and smoking. For example, there is a need to better understand why smoking prevalence increased among teenage girls and young women in the 1990s despite the overwhelming data on adverse health effects; to identify interventions and policies that will prevent an epidemic of tobacco use among women whose smoking prevalence is currently low, including women in certain sociocultural groups within the United States and women in many developing countries throughout the world; to study the relationship of active smoking to diseases among women for which the evidence to date has been suggestive or inconsistent (e.g., risks for menstrual cycle irregularities, gallbladder disease, and systemic lupus erythematosus); to increase the data on the health effects of exposure to environmental tobacco smoke on diseases unique among women; to provide additional research on whether gender differences exist in susceptibility to nicotine addiction or in the magnitude of the effects of smoking on specific disease outcomes; and to determine whether gender differences exist in the modifying effects of genetic polymorphisms on disease risks associated with smoking. Many studies of smoking behavior and of the health consequences of smoking have included both females and males but have not reported results by gender. Investigators should be encouraged to report gender-specific results in the future.

## Preparation of the Report

This report of the Surgeon General was prepared by the Office on Smoking and Health, National Center for Chronic Disease Prevention and Health Promotion, Centers for Disease Control and Prevention, U.S. Department of Health and Human Services. It was produced with the assistance of experts in epidemiology, pharmacology, the behavioral sciences, medicine, and public health policy. Initial drafts were produced by more than 60 scientists who were selected because of their expertise and familiarity with the topics covered in this report. Their contributions were compiled into four major chapters that then underwent peer review by more than 80 experts, and the drafts were revised by the editors on the basis of the experts' feedback. Subsequently, the report was reviewed by various institutes and agencies within the Department of Health and Human Services, which resulted in final revisions to the report.

Because numerous experts contributed to this report, with varying preferences of terms to report outcome measures and statistical significance, the editors chose certain simplifying conventions to report research results. In particular, the term "relative risk" generally was adopted throughout the report for ratio measures of association—whether original study results were reported as relative risks, estimated relative risks, odds ratios, rate ratios, risk ratios, or other terms that express risk among one group of individuals (e.g., smokers) as a ratio of another (e.g., nonsmokers). Moreover, relative risks and confidence intervals were generally rounded to one decimal place, except when rounding could change a marginally statistically significant finding to an insignificant one. Thus, only when the original confidence limit was within 0.95 to 0.99 or within 1.01 to 1.04 were two decimal places retained in reporting the results.

Publication lags, even short ones, prevent an up-to-the-minute inclusion of all of the recently published articles and data. Therefore, by the time the public reads this report, some additional studies or data reports may have been published or released. The report has attempted to include the most up-to-date information available at the time of production.

## Organization of the Report

This report covers four major topics, each of which includes many subtopics: "Patterns of Tobacco Use Among Women and Girls" (Chapter 2), "Health Consequences of Tobacco Use Among Women" (Chapter 3), "Factors Influencing Tobacco Use Among Women" (Chapter 4), and "Efforts to Reduce Tobacco Use Among Women" (Chapter 5). The report concludes with "A Vision for the Future" (Chapter 6). Some subtopics covered are relevant to more than one section of the report and are discussed in more than one place and cross-referenced. This overlap is particularly true for the discussions of smoking and depression, weight, hormones, and pregnancy; some of these topics are discussed as correlates of smoking status in Chapter 2, as health effects of or physiologic influences on smoking in Chapter 3, and in relation to tailoring intervention and outcomes in Chapter 5. At the end of each chapter is a list of chapter conclusions, which are also included at the end of this chapter. The appendices describe the national surveys and other data sources used for the analyses of patterns of tobacco use over time presented in Chapter 2 and in Chapter 3. The major conclusions of the report were distilled from the chapter conclusions and appear below.

Other recent reports of the Surgeon General have been devoted to smoking and youth (USDHHS 1994), smoking and racial or ethnic minorities (USDHHS 1998), and interventions to reduce smoking (USDHHS 2000). The reader is encouraged to consult those reports for comprehensive reviews of the evidence on these topics. The present report focuses on data specific to women and girls and on comparisons of results by gender.

The reader will note that throughout the report the term "gender" is used with reference to results specific to females vs. males when it might reasonably be argued that the term "sex" is the appropriate term. In practice, the distinction is sometimes difficult to make, and usage across much of the literature reviewed here is inconsistent. Nonetheless, the editors and contributors to the report recognize the important distinction between purely biologic or physiologic differences of females and males, which technically constitute "sex" differences, and the more socially constructed roles for women and men, to which use of the term "gender" should arguably be limited (Fishman et al. 1999).

## Major Conclusions

1. Despite all that is known of the devastating health consequences of smoking, 22.0 percent of women smoked cigarettes in 1998. Cigarette smoking became prevalent among men before women, and smoking prevalence in the United States has always been lower among women than among men. However, the once-wide gender gap in smoking prevalence narrowed until the mid-1980s and has since remained fairly constant (Figure 1.1). Smoking prevalence today is nearly three times higher among women who have only 9 to 11 years of education (32.9 percent) than among women with 16 or more years of education (11.2 percent).
2. In 2000, 29.7 percent of high school senior girls reported having smoked within the past 30 days. Smoking prevalence among white girls declined from the mid-1970s to the early 1980s, followed by a decade of little change. Smoking prevalence then increased markedly in the early 1990s, and declined somewhat in the late 1990s. The increase dampened much of the earlier progress (Figure 1.2). Among black girls, smoking prevalence declined substantially from the mid-1970s to the early 1990s, followed by some increases until the mid-1990s. Data on long-term trends in smoking prevalence among high school seniors of other racial or ethnic groups are not available.
3. Since 1980, approximately 3 million U.S. women have died prematurely from smoking-related neoplastic, cardiovascular, respiratory, and pediatric diseases, as well as cigarette-caused burns. Each year during the 1990s, U.S. women lost an estimated 2.1 million years of life due to these smoking attributable premature deaths. Additionally, women who smoke experience gender-specific health consequences, including increased risk of various adverse reproductive outcomes.
4. Lung cancer is now the leading cause of cancer death among U.S. women; it surpassed breast cancer in 1987 (Figure 1.3). About 90 percent of all lung cancer deaths among women who continue to smoke are attributable to smoking.
5. Exposure to environmental tobacco smoke is a cause of lung cancer and coronary heart disease among women who are lifetime nonsmokers. Infants born to women exposed to environmental tobacco smoke during pregnancy have a small decrement in birth weight and a slightly increased risk of intrauterine growth retardation compared to infants of nonexposed women.
6. Women who stop smoking greatly reduce their risk of dying prematurely, and quitting smoking is beneficial at all ages. Although some clinical intervention studies suggest that women may have more difficulty quitting smoking than men, national survey data show that women are quitting at rates similar to or even higher than those for men. Prevention and cessation

interventions are generally of similar effectiveness for women and men and, to date, few gender differences in factors related to smoking initiation and successful quitting have been identified.

7. Smoking during pregnancy remains a major public health problem despite increased knowledge of the adverse health effects of smoking during pregnancy. Although the prevalence of smoking during pregnancy has declined steadily in recent years (Figure 1.4), substantial numbers of pregnant women continue to smoke, and only about one-third of women who stop smoking during pregnancy are still abstinent one year after the delivery.

8. Tobacco industry marketing is a factor influencing susceptibility to and initiation of smoking among girls, in the United States and overseas. Myriad examples of tobacco ads and promotions targeted to women indicate that such marketing is dominated by themes of social desirability and independence. These themes are conveyed through ads featuring slim, attractive, athletic models, images very much at odds with the serious health consequences experienced by so many women who smoke.

**Figure 1.1. Prevalence (%) of current smoking among adults aged 18 years or older, by gender, National Health Interview Survey, United States, 1965–1998**

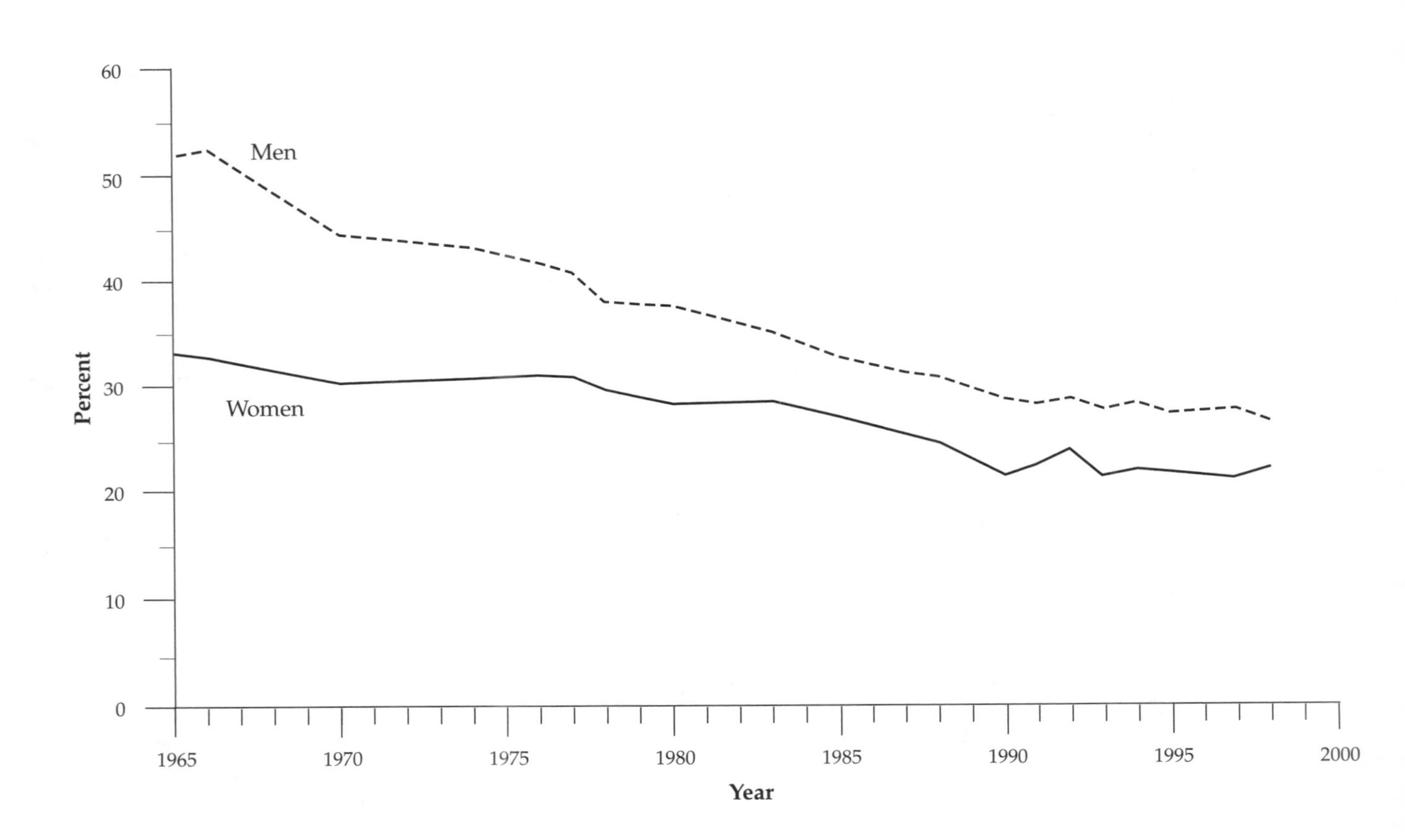


*Note:* Prevalence of current smoking is the percentage of all persons in each demographic category who reported smoking ≥ 100 cigarettes in their lifetime and who smoked at the time of the survey. Since 1992, estimates of current smoking explicitly include persons who smoked only on some days.

Sources: National Center for Health Statistics, public use data tapes, 1965–1998.

**Figure 1.2. Prevalence (%) of current smoking and daily smoking among high school senior girls, by race, Monitoring the Future Survey, United States, 1976–1997, aggregate data**

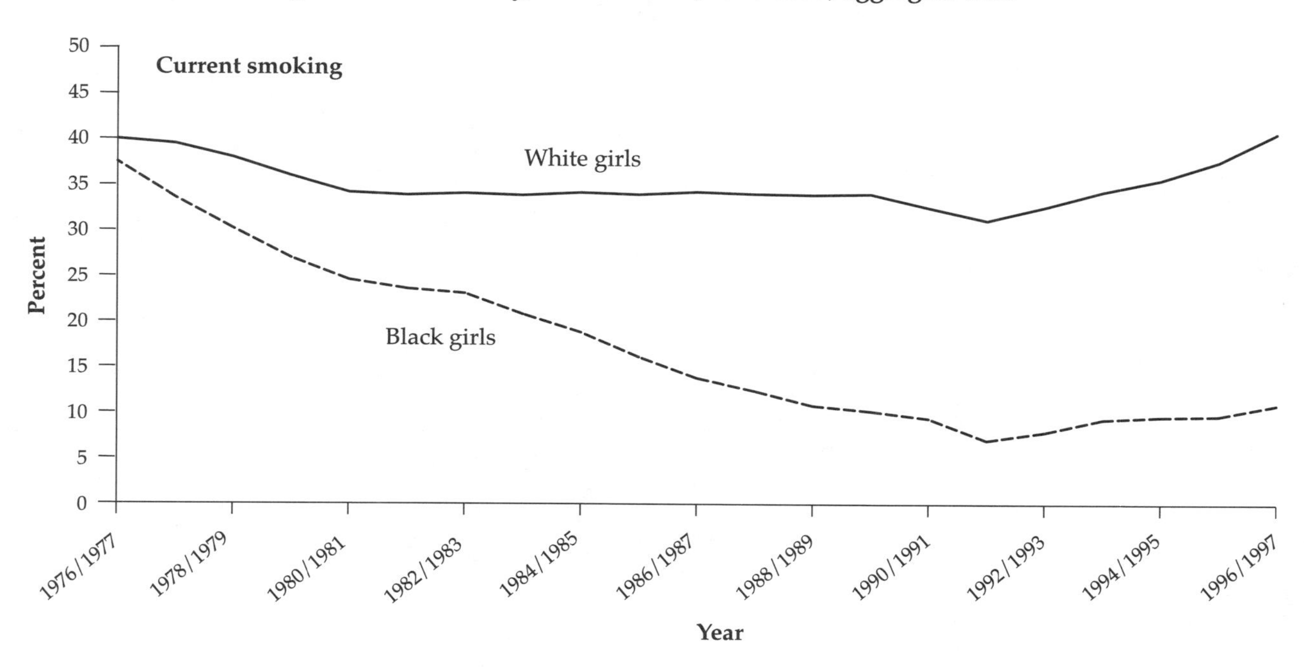


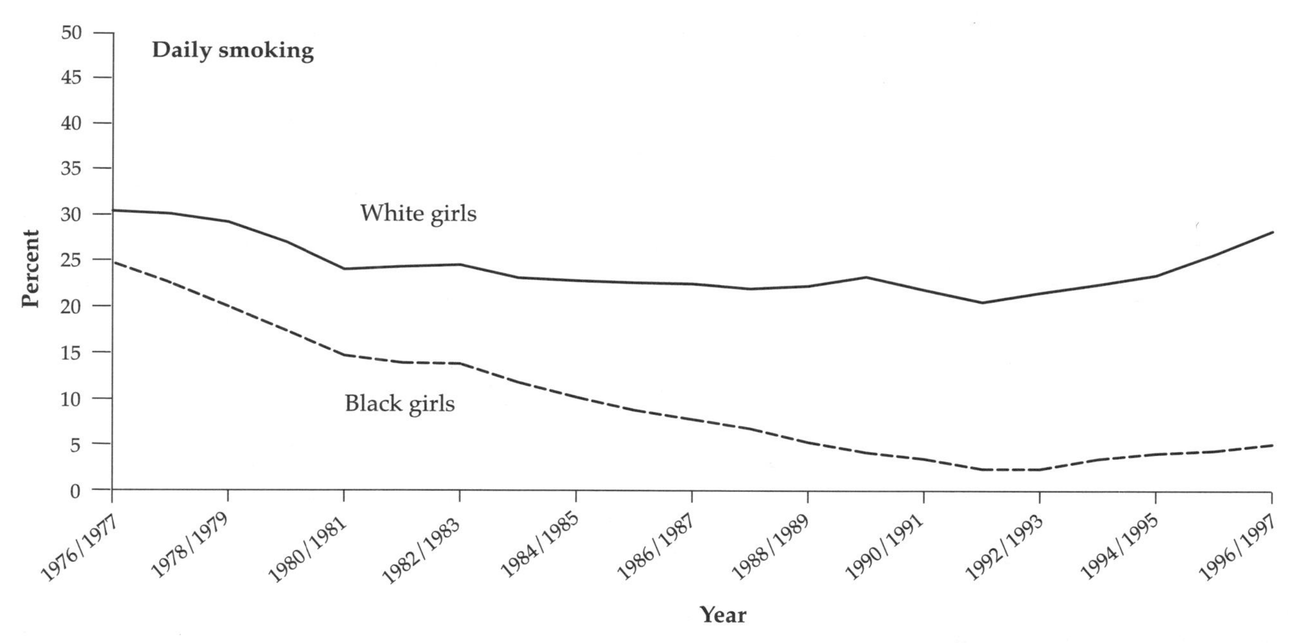


*Note:* Estimates are based on 2-year rolling averages, which are the percentages calculated by averaging data for specified year and previous year. Estimates for current smoking are based on responses to the question, "How frequently have you smoked cigarettes during the past 30 days?" Those reporting smoking ≥ 1 cigarette during the previous 30 days were classified as current smokers. Estimates for daily smoking were based on responses to the question, "How frequently have you smoked cigarettes in the past 30 days?" Those reporting smoking ≥ 1 cigarette/day during the previous 30 days were classified as daily smokers.
Sources: University of Michigan, Institute for Social Research, public use data tapes, 1976–1997.

**Figure 1.3. Age-adjusted death rates for lung cancer and breast cancer among women, United States, 1930–1997**

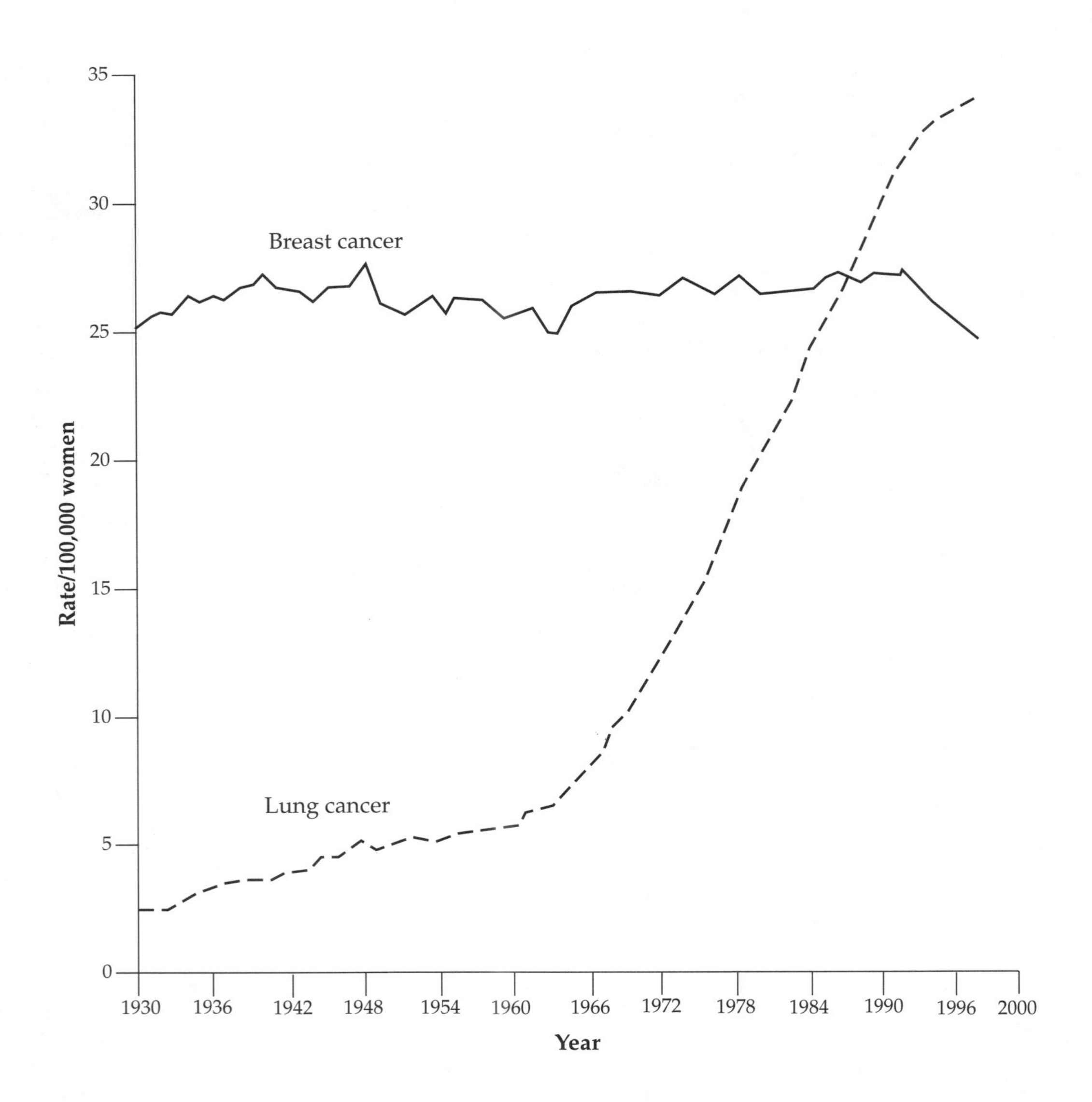


*Note:* Death rates are age adjusted to the 1970 population.
Sources: Parker et al. 1996; National Center for Health Statistics 1999; Ries et al. 2000; American Cancer Society, unpublished data.

**Figure 1.4. Prevalence (%) of cigarette smoking during pregnancy, 1989–1998**

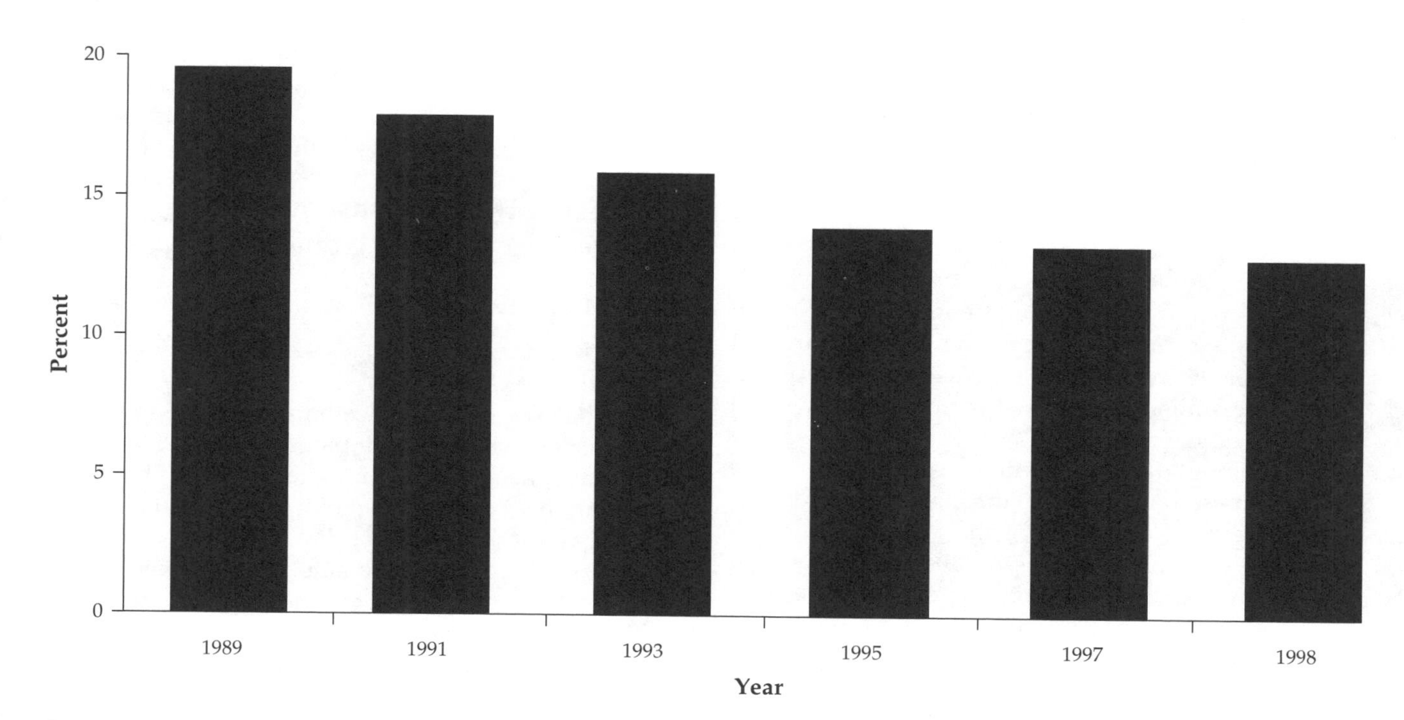


*Note:* Percentage excludes live births for mothers with unknown smoking status.
Sources: National Center for Health Statistics 1992, 1994; Ventura et al. 1995, 1997, 1999, 2000.

# Chapter Conclusions

Note that Chapter 1, which summarizes the report, and Chapter 6, which focuses on a vision for the future, do not have conclusions.

## Chapter 2. Patterns of Tobacco Use Among Women and Girls

1. Cigarette smoking became prevalent among women after it did among men, and smoking prevalence has always been lower among women than among men. The gender-specific difference in smoking prevalence narrowed between 1965 and 1985. Since 1985, the decline in prevalence has been comparable among women and men.
2. The prevalence of current smoking among women increased from less than 6 percent in 1924 to 34 percent in 1965, then declined to 22 to 23 percent in the late 1990s. In 1997–1998, smoking prevalence was highest among American Indian or Alaska Native women (34.5 percent), intermediate among white women (23.5 percent) and black women (21.9 percent), and lowest among Hispanic women (13.8 percent) and Asian or Pacific Islander women (11.2 percent). By educational level, smoking prevalence is nearly three times higher among women with 9 to 11 years of education (30.9 percent) than among women with 16 or more years of education (10.6 percent).
3. Much of the progress in reducing smoking prevalence among girls in the 1970s and 1980s was lost with the increase in prevalence in the 1990s:

current smoking among high school senior girls was the same in 2000 as in 1988. Although smoking prevalence was higher among high school senior girls than among high school senior boys in the 1970s and early 1980s, prevalence has been comparable since the mid-1980s.

4. Smoking declined substantially among black girls from the mid-1970s through the early 1990s; the decline among white girls for this same period was small. As adolescents age into young adulthood, these patterns are now being reflected in the racial and ethnic differences in smoking among young women. Data are not available on long-term trends in smoking prevalence among high school seniors of other racial and ethnic groups.
5. Smoking during pregnancy appears to have decreased from 1989 through 1998. Despite increased knowledge of the adverse health effects of smoking during pregnancy, estimates of women smoking during pregnancy range from 12 percent based on birth certificate data to as high as 22 percent based on survey data.
6. Historically, women started to smoke at a later age than did men, but beginning with the 1960 cohort, the mean age at smoking initiation has not differed by gender.
7. Nicotine dependence is strongly associated with the number of cigarettes smoked per day. Girls and women who smoke appear to be equally dependent on nicotine when results are stratified by number of cigarettes smoked per day. Few gender-specific differences have been found in indicators of nicotine dependence among adolescents, young adults, or adults overall.
8. The percentage of persons who have ever smoked and who have quit smoking is somewhat lower among women (46.2 percent) than among men (50.1 percent). This finding is probably because men began to stop smoking earlier in the twentieth century than did women and because these data do not take into account that men are more likely than women to switch to or to continue to use other tobacco products when they stop smoking cigarettes. Since the late 1970s or early 1980s, the probability of attempting to quit smoking and to succeed has been equally high among women and men.
9. Prevalence of the use of cigars, pipes, and smokeless tobacco among women is generally low, but recent data suggest that cigar smoking among women and girls is increasing.
10. Smoking prevalence among women varies markedly across countries; the percentages range from an estimated 7 percent in developing countries to 24 percent in developed countries. Thwarting further increases in tobacco use among women is one of the greatest disease prevention opportunities in the world today.

## Chapter 3. Health Consequences of Tobacco Use Among Women

### Total Mortality

1. Cigarette smoking plays a major role in the mortality of U.S. women.
2. The excess risk for death from all causes among current smokers compared with persons who have never smoked increases with both the number of years of smoking and the number of cigarettes smoked per day.
3. Among women who smoke, the percentage of deaths attributable to smoking has increased over the past several decades, largely because of increases in the quantity of cigarettes smoked and the duration of smoking.
4. Cohort studies with follow-up data analyzed in the 1980s show that the annual risk for death from all causes is 80 to 90 percent greater among women who smoke cigarettes than among women who have never smoked. A woman's annual risk for death more than doubles among continuing smokers compared with persons who have never smoked in every age group from 45 through 74 years.
5. In 1997, approximately 165,000 U.S. women died prematurely from a smoking-related disease. Since 1980, approximately three million U.S. women have died prematurely from a smoking-related disease.
6. U.S. females lost an estimated 2.1 million years of life each year during the 1990s as a result of smoking-related deaths due to neoplastic, cardiovascular, respiratory, and pediatric diseases as well as from burns caused by cigarettes. For every smoking attributable death, an average of 14 years of life was lost.
7. Women who stop smoking greatly reduce their risk for dying prematurely. The relative benefits of smoking cessation are greater when women stop smoking at younger ages, but smoking cessation is beneficial at all ages.

### Lung Cancer

8. Cigarette smoking is the major cause of lung cancer among women. About 90 percent of all lung cancer deaths among U.S. women smokers are attributable to smoking.
9. The risk for lung cancer increases with quantity, duration, and intensity of smoking. The risk for dying of lung cancer is 20 times higher among women who smoke two or more packs of cigarettes per day than among women who do not smoke.
10. Lung cancer mortality rates among U.S. women have increased about 600 percent since 1950. In 1987, lung cancer surpassed breast cancer to become the leading cause of cancer death among U.S. women. Overall age-adjusted incidence rates for lung cancer among women appear to have peaked in the mid-1990s.
11. In the past, men who smoked appeared to have a higher relative risk for lung cancer than did women who smoked, but recent data suggest that such differences have narrowed considerably. Earlier findings largely reflect past gender-specific differences in duration and amount of cigarette smoking.
12. Former smokers have a lower risk for lung cancer than do current smokers, and risk declines with the number of years of smoking cessation.

### International Trends in Female Lung Cancer

13. International lung cancer death rates among women vary dramatically. This variation reflects historical differences in the adoption of cigarette smoking by women in different countries. In 1990, lung cancer accounted for about 10 percent of all cancer deaths among women worldwide and more than 20 percent of cancer deaths among women in some developed countries.

### Female Cancers

14. The totality of the evidence does not support an association between smoking and risk for breast cancer.
15. Several studies suggest that exposure to environmental tobacco smoke is associated with an increased risk for breast cancer, but this association remains uncertain.
16. Current smoking is associated with a reduced risk for endometrial cancer, but the effect is probably limited to postmenopausal disease. The risk for this cancer among former smokers generally appears more similar to that of women who have never smoked.
17. Smoking does not appear to be associated with risk for ovarian cancer.
18. Smoking has been consistently associated with an increased risk for cervical cancer. The extent to which this association is independent of human papillomavirus infection is uncertain.
19. Smoking may be associated with an increased risk for vulvar cancer, but the extent to which the association is independent of human papillomavirus infection is uncertain.

### Other Cancers

20. Smoking is a major cause of cancers of the oropharynx and bladder among women. Evidence is also strong that women who smoke have increased risks for cancers of the pancreas and kidney. For cancers of the larynx and esophagus, evidence among women is more limited but consistent with large increases in risk.
21. Women who smoke may have increased risks for liver cancer and colorectal cancer.
22. Data on smoking and cancer of the stomach among women are inconsistent.
23. Smoking may be associated with an increased risk for acute myeloid leukemia among women but does not appear to be associated with other lymphoproliferative or hematologic cancers.
24. Women who smoke may have a decreased risk for thyroid cancer.
25. Women who use smokeless tobacco have an increased risk for oral cancer.

### Cardiovascular Disease

26. Smoking is a major cause of coronary heart disease among women. For women younger than 50 years, the majority of coronary heart disease is attributable to smoking. Risk increases with the number of cigarettes smoked and the duration of smoking.
27. The risk for coronary heart disease among women is substantially reduced within 1 or 2 years of smoking cessation. This immediate benefit is followed by a continuing but more gradual reduction in risk to that among nonsmokers by 10 to 15 or more years after cessation.
28. Women who use oral contraceptives have a particularly elevated risk of coronary heart disease if they smoke. Currently, evidence is conflicting as to whether the effect of hormone replacement

therapy on coronary heart disease risk differs between smokers and nonsmokers.

29. Women who smoke have an increased risk for ischemic stroke and subarachnoid hemorrhage. Evidence is inconsistent concerning the association between smoking and primary intracerebral hemorrhage.
30. In most studies that include women, the increased risk for stroke associated with smoking is reversible after smoking cessation; after 5 to 15 years of abstinence, the risk approaches that of women who have never smoked.
31. Conflicting evidence exists regarding the level of the risk for stroke among women who both smoke and use either the oral contraceptives commonly prescribed in the United States today or hormone replacement therapy.
32. Smoking is a strong predictor of the progression and severity of carotid atherosclerosis among women. Smoking cessation appears to slow the rate of progression of carotid atherosclerosis.
33. Women who are current smokers have an increased risk for peripheral vascular atherosclerosis. Smoking cessation is associated with improvements in symptoms, prognosis, and survival.
34. Women who smoke have an increased risk for death from ruptured abdominal aortic aneurysm.

**Chronic Obstructive Pulmonary Disease (COPD) and Lung Function**

35. Cigarette smoking is a primary cause of COPD among women, and the risk increases with the amount and duration of smoking. Approximately 90 percent of mortality from COPD among women in the United States can be attributed to cigarette smoking.
36. In utero exposure to maternal smoking is associated with reduced lung function among infants, and exposure to environmental tobacco smoke during childhood and adolescence may be associated with impaired lung function among girls.
37. Adolescent girls who smoke have reduced rates of lung growth, and adult women who smoke experience a premature decline of lung function.
38. The rate of decline in lung function is slower among women who stop smoking than among women who continue to smoke.
39. Mortality rates for COPD have increased among women over the past 20 to 30 years.
40. Although data for women are limited, former smokers appear to have a lower risk for dying from COPD than do current smokers.

**Sex Hormones, Thyroid Disease, and Diabetes Mellitus**

41. Women who smoke have an increased risk for estrogen-deficiency disorders and a decreased risk for estrogen-dependent disorders, but circulating levels of the major endogenous estrogens are not altered among women smokers.
42. Although consistent effects of smoking on thyroid hormone levels have not been noted, cigarette smokers may have an increased risk for Graves' ophthalmopathy, a thyroid-related disease.
43. Smoking appears to affect glucose regulation and related metabolic processes, but conflicting data exist on the relationship of smoking and the development of type 2 diabetes mellitus and gestational diabetes among women.

**Menstrual Function, Menopause, and Benign Gynecologic Conditions**

44. Some studies suggest that cigarette smoking may alter menstrual function by increasing the risks for dysmenorrhea (painful menstruation), secondary amenorrhea (lack of menses among women who ever had menstrual periods), and menstrual irregularity.
45. Women smokers have a younger age at natural menopause than do nonsmokers and may experience more menopausal symptoms.
46. Women who smoke may have decreased risk for uterine fibroids.

**Reproductive Outcomes**

47. Women who smoke have increased risks for conception delay and for both primary and secondary infertility.
48. Women who smoke may have a modest increase in risks for ectopic pregnancy and spontaneous abortion.
49. Smoking during pregnancy is associated with increased risks for preterm premature rupture of membranes, abruptio placentae, and placenta previa, and with a modest increase in risk for preterm delivery.
50. Women who smoke during pregnancy have a decreased risk for preeclampsia.

51. The risk for perinatal mortality—both stillbirth and neonatal deaths—and the risk for sudden infant death syndrome (SIDS) are increased among the offspring of women who smoke during pregnancy.
52. Infants born to women who smoke during pregnancy have a lower average birth weight and are more likely to be small for gestational age than are infants born to women who do not smoke.
53. Smoking does not appear to affect the overall risk for congenital malformations.
54. Women smokers are less likely to breastfeed their infants than are women nonsmokers.
55. Women who quit smoking before or during pregnancy reduce the risk for adverse reproductive outcomes, including conception delay, infertility, preterm premature rupture of membranes, preterm delivery, and low birth weight.

**Body Weight and Fat Distribution**

56. Initiation of cigarette smoking does not appear to be associated with weight loss, but smoking does appear to attenuate weight gain over time.
57. The average weight of women who are current smokers is modestly lower than that of women who have never smoked or who are long-term former smokers.
58. Smoking cessation among women typically is associated with a weight gain of about 6 to 12 pounds in the year after they quit smoking.
59. Women smokers have a more masculine pattern of body fat distribution (i.e., a higher waist-to-hip ratio) than do women who have never smoked.

**Bone Density and Fracture Risk**

60. Postmenopausal women who currently smoke have lower bone density than do women who do not smoke.
61. Women who currently smoke have an increased risk for hip fracture compared with women who do not smoke.
62. The relationship among women between smoking and the risk for bone fracture at sites other than the hip is not clear.

**Gastrointestinal Diseases**

63. Some studies suggest that women who smoke have an increased risk for gallbladder disease (gallstones and cholecystitis), but the evidence is inconsistent.
64. Women who smoke have an increased risk for peptic ulcers.
65. Women who currently smoke have a decreased risk for ulcerative colitis, but former smokers have an increased risk—possibly because smoking suppresses symptoms of the disease.
66. Women who smoke appear to have an increased risk for Crohn's disease, and smokers with Crohn's disease have a worse prognosis than do nonsmokers.

**Arthritis**

67. Some but not all studies suggest that women who smoke may have a modestly elevated risk for rheumatoid arthritis.
68. Women who smoke have a modestly reduced risk for osteoarthritis of the knee; data regarding osteoarthritis of the hip are inconsistent.
69. The data on the risk for systemic lupus erythematosus among women who smoke are inconsistent.

**Eye Disease**

70. Women who smoke have an increased risk for cataract.
71. Women who smoke may have an increased risk for age-related macular degeneration.
72. Studies show no consistent association between smoking and open-angle glaucoma.

**Human Immunodeficiency Virus (HIV) Disease**

73. Limited data suggest that women smokers may be at higher risk for HIV-1 infection than are nonsmokers.

**Facial Wrinkling**

74. Limited but consistent data suggest that women smokers have more facial wrinkling than do nonsmokers.

**Depression and Other Psychiatric Disorders**

75. Smokers are more likely to be depressed than are nonsmokers, a finding that may reflect an effect of smoking on the risk for depression, the use of smoking for self-medication, or the influence of common genetic or other factors on both smoking and depression. The association of smoking and depression is particularly important among women because they are more likely to be diagnosed with depression than are men.

76. The prevalence of smoking generally has been found to be higher among patients with anxiety disorders, bulimia, attention deficit disorder, and alcoholism than among individuals without these conditions; the mechanisms underlying these associations are not yet understood.
77. The prevalence of smoking is very high among patients with schizophrenia, but the mechanisms underlying this association are not yet understood.
78. Smoking may be used by some persons who would otherwise manifest psychiatric symptoms to manage those symptoms; for such persons, cessation of smoking may lead to the emergence of depression or other dysphoric mood states.

#### Neurologic Diseases

79. Women who smoke have a decreased risk for Parkinson's disease.
80. Data regarding the association between smoking and Alzheimer's disease are inconsistent.

#### Nicotine Pharmacology and Addiction

81. Nicotine pharmacology and the behavioral processes that determine nicotine addiction appear generally similar among women and men; when standardized for the number of cigarettes smoked, the blood concentration of cotinine (the main metabolite of nicotine) is similar among women and men.
82. Women's regulation of nicotine intake may be less precise than men's. Factors other than nicotine (e.g., sensory cues) may play a greater role in determining smoking behavior among women.

#### Environmental Tobacco Smoke (ETS) and Lung Cancer

83. Exposure to ETS is a cause of lung cancer among women who have never smoked.

#### ETS and Coronary Heart Disease

84. Epidemiologic and other data support a causal relationship between ETS exposure from the spouse and coronary heart disease mortality among women nonsmokers.

#### ETS and Reproductive Outcomes

85. Infants born to women who are exposed to ETS during pregnancy may have a small decrement in birth weight and a slightly increased risk for intrauterine growth retardation compared with infants born to women who are not exposed; both effects are quite variable across studies.
86. Studies of ETS exposure and the risks for delay in conception, spontaneous abortion, and perinatal mortality are few, and the results are inconsistent.

### Chapter 4. Factors Influencing Tobacco Use Among Women

1. Girls who initiate smoking are more likely than those who do not smoke to have parents or friends who smoke. They also tend to have weaker attachments to parents and family and stronger attachments to peers and friends. They perceive smoking prevalence to be higher than it actually is, are inclined to risk taking and rebelliousness, have a weaker commitment to school or religion, have less knowledge of the adverse consequences of smoking and the addictiveness of nicotine, believe that smoking can control weight and negative moods, and have a positive image of smokers. Although the strength of the association by gender differs across studies, most of these factors are associated with an increased risk for smoking among both girls and boys.
2. Girls appear to be more affected than boys by the desire to smoke for weight control and by the perception that smoking controls negative moods; girls may also be more influenced than boys to smoke by rebelliousness or a rejection of conventional values.
3. Women who continue to smoke and those who fail at attempts to stop smoking tend to have lower education and employment levels than do women who quit smoking. They also tend to be more addicted to cigarettes, as evidenced by the smoking of a higher number of cigarettes per day, to be cognitively less ready to stop smoking, to have less social support for stopping, and to be less confident in resisting temptations to smoke.
4. Women have been extensively targeted in tobacco marketing, and tobacco companies have produced brands specifically for women, both in the United States and overseas. Myriad examples of tobacco ads and promotions targeted to women indicate that such marketing is dominated by themes of both social desirability and independence, which are conveyed through ads

featuring slim, attractive, athletic models. Between 1995 and 1998, expenditures for domestic cigarette advertising and promotion increased 37.3 percent, from $4.90 billion to $6.73 billion.

5. Tobacco industry marketing, including product design, advertising, and promotional activities, is a factor influencing susceptibility to and initiation of smoking.
6. The dependence of the media on revenues from tobacco advertising oriented to women, coupled with tobacco company sponsorship of women's fashions and of artistic, athletic, political, and other events, has tended to stifle media coverage of the health consequences of smoking among women and to mute criticism of the tobacco industry by women public figures.

## Chapter 5. Efforts to Reduce Tobacco Use Among Women

1. Using evidence from studies that vary in design, sample characteristics, and intensity of the interventions studied, researchers to date have not found consistent gender-specific differences in the effectiveness of treatment intervention programs for tobacco use. Some clinical studies have shown lower cessation rates among women than among men, but others have not. Many studies have not reported cessation results by gender.
2. Among women, biopsychosocial factors such as pregnancy, fear of weight gain, depression, and the need for social support appear to be associated with smoking maintenance, cessation, or relapse.
3. A higher percentage of women stop smoking during pregnancy, both spontaneously and with assistance, than at other times in their lives. Using pregnancy-specific programs can increase smoking cessation rates, which benefits infant health and is cost effective. Only about one-third of women who stop smoking during pregnancy are still abstinent one year after the delivery.
4. Women fear weight gain during smoking cessation more than do men. However, few studies have found a relationship between weight concerns and smoking cessation among either women or men. Further, actual weight gain during cessation does not predict relapse to smoking.
5. Adolescent girls are more likely than adolescent boys to respond to smoking cessation programs that include social support from the family or their peer group.
6. Among persons who smoke heavily, women are more likely than men to report being dependent on cigarettes and to have lower expectations about stopping smoking, but it is not clear if such women are less likely to quit smoking.
7. Currently, no tobacco cessation method has proved to be any more or less successful among minority women than among white women in the same study, but research on smoking cessation among women of most racial and ethnic minorities has been scarce.
8. Women are more likely than men to affirm that they smoke less at work because of a worksite policy and are significantly more likely than men to attribute reduced amount of daily smoking to their worksite policy. Women also are more likely than men to support policies designed to prevent smoking initiation among adolescents, restrictions on youth access to tobacco products, and limits on tobacco advertising and promotion.
9. Successful interventions have been developed to prevent smoking among young people, but little systematic effort has been focused on developing and evaluating prevention interventions specifically for girls.

## Chapter 6. A Vision for the Future: What Is Needed to Reduce Smoking Among Women

Chapter 6 defines broad courses of action for reducing tobacco use among women. These five strategies for the future are as follows: Increase awareness of the impact of smoking on women's health and counter the tobacco industry's targeting of women. Support women's anti-tobacco advocacy efforts and publicize that most women are nonsmokers. Continue to build the science base on gender-specific outcomes and on how to reduce disparities among women. Act now: we know more than enough. Stop the epidemic of smoking and smoking-related diseases among women globally.

# References


Fishman JR, Wick JG, Koenig BA. The use of "sex" and "gender" to define and characterize meaningful differences between men and women. In: *Agenda for Research on Women's Health for the 21st Century*. Vol. 1. Bethesda (MD): National Institutes of Health, 1999:15–9. NIH Publication No. 99-4385.

National Center for Health Statistics. Advance report of new data from the 1989 birth certificate. *Monthly Vital Statistics Report* 1992:40(12 Suppl).

National Center for Health Statistics. Advance report of maternal and infant health data from the birth certificate, 1991. *Monthly Vital Statistics Report* 1994:42(11 Suppl).

National Center for Health Statistics. *Health, United States, 1999 with Health and Aging Chartbook*. Hyattsville (MD): U.S. Department of Health and Human Services, Centers for Disease Control and Prevention, National Center for Health Statistics, 1999. DHHS Publication No. (PHS) 99-1232-1.

Parker SL, Tong T, Bolden S, Wingo PA. Cancer statistics, 1996. *CA—A Cancer Journal for Clinicians* 1996;46(1):5–27.

Ries LAG, Eisner MP, Kosary CL, Hankey BF, Miller BA, Clegg L, Edwards BK, editors. *SEER Cancer Statistics Review, 1973–1997*. Bethesda (MD): National Cancer Institute, 2000.

University of Michigan. Cigarette use and smokeless tobacco use decline substantially among teens [press release]. Ann Arbor (MI): University of Michigan News and Information Services, 2000 Dec 14.

U.S. Department of Health, Education, and Welfare. *Smoking and Health. Report of the Advisory Committee to the Surgeon General of the Public Health Service*. U.S. Department of Health, Education, and Welfare, Public Health Service, Communicable Disease Center, 1964. DHEW Publication No. 1103.

U.S. Department of Health and Human Services. *The Health Consequences of Smoking for Women. A Report of the Surgeon General*. Washington: U.S. Department of Health and Human Services, Public Health Service, Office of the Assistant Secretary for Health, Office on Smoking and Health, 1980.

U.S. Department of Health and Human Services. *Preventing Tobacco Use Among Young People. A Report of the Surgeon General*. Atlanta: U.S. Department of Health and Human Services, Public Health Service, Centers for Disease Control and Prevention, National Center for Chronic Disease Prevention and Health Promotion, Office on Smoking and Health, 1994.

U.S. Department of Health and Human Services. *Tobacco Use Among U.S. Racial/Ethnic Minority Groups—African Americans, American Indians and Alaska Natives, Asian Americans and Pacific Islanders, and Hispanics. A Report of the Surgeon General*. Atlanta: U.S. Department of Health and Human Services, Centers for Disease Control and Prevention, National Center for Chronic Disease Prevention and Health Promotion, Office on Smoking and Health, 1998.

U.S. Department of Health and Human Services. *Reducing Tobacco Use. A Report of the Surgeon General*. Atlanta: U.S. Department of Health and Human Services, Centers for Disease Control and Prevention, National Center for Chronic Disease Prevention and Health Promotion, Office on Smoking and Health, 2000.

Ventura SJ, Martin JA, Curtin SC, Mathews TJ. Report of final natality statistics, 1995. *Monthly Vital Statistics Report* 1997;45(11 Suppl):1–57.

Ventura SJ, Martin JA, Curtin SC, Mathews TJ. Births: final data for 1997. *National Vital Statistics Report* 1999;47(18):1–96.

Ventura SJ, Martin JA, Curtin SC, Mathews TJ, Park MM. Births: final data for 1998. *National Vital Statistics Report* 2000;48(3):1–100.

Ventura SJ, Martin JA, Taffel SM, Mathews TJ, Clarke SC. Advance report of final natality statistics, 1993. *Monthly Vital Statistics Report* 1995;44(3 Suppl):1–83.

# Chapter 2. Patterns of Tobacco Use Among Women and Girls

# Introduction

This chapter summarizes trends and patterns of cigarette smoking and use of other tobacco products among women and girls and updates and expands the information in previous reports of the Surgeon General, particularly the 1980 report titled, *The Health Consequences of Smoking for Women* (U.S. Department of Health and Human Services [USDHHS] 1980). This report primarily uses U.S. national survey data, but where these data are sparse, particularly for racial and ethnic groups, regional surveys or other large surveys are used. In the case of international smoking patterns, data are provided by the World Health Organization (WHO) and international surveys. Gender-specific differences are discussed to the extent that data exist.

Sections of this chapter cover the prevalence of cigarette smoking among women and girls of different age groups; smoking during pregnancy; smoking initiation; nicotine dependence; smoking cessation; other tobacco use; exposure to environmental tobacco smoke; the relationship of smoking to body weight, other drug use, and mental health; and international trends in smoking prevalence. Young women and pregnant women are included in the estimates of smoking prevalence and cessation among women overall, but separate sections address smoking prevalence and cessation among these groups of women because they represent important populations for specific interventions.

National data from several sources were analyzed for this report. The data analyzed to assess smoking behavior among adults were obtained from the National Health Interview Surveys (NHIS) of 1965–1998, the 1992–1998 National Household Surveys on Drug Abuse (NHSDA), the 1999 Behavioral Risk Factor Survey (BRFS), the National Health and Nutrition Examination Survey III (NHANES III) (1988–1994), and the 1986 Adult Use of Tobacco Survey (AUTS). The sources used for analysis of data on children and adolescents were the Monitoring the Future (MTF) Surveys of 1976–1998, the NHSDA surveys of 1974–1998, the 1999 national Youth Risk Behavior Survey (YRBS), the Teenage Attitudes and Practices Survey I of 1989 (TAPS I), and the Teenage Attitudes and Practices Survey II of 1993 (TAPS II). Other sources were the National Teenage Tobacco Surveys (NTTS) of 1968, 1970, 1972, 1974, and 1979; the 1964, 1966, 1970, and 1975 AUTS; the Behavioral Risk Factor Surveillance System (BRFSS) for 1988–1997; the 1998 and 1999 MTF Surveys; and the 1999 National Youth Tobacco Survey (NYTS). Only published data from these surveys were used. These surveys use self-reported smoking status. Self-report is generally considered to be reliable except in certain situations, such as pregnancy or intensive treatment programs (see Appendix 3). Table 2.1 and Appendix 1 describe all years of data available for these data sources, but only selected years are used for this report. Appendix 2 defines the survey terms used in this report.

The following definitions and conventions are used in this chapter: "women" refers to females 18 years of age or older, and "girls" refers to females younger than 18 years of age. "Female" is used if the age range includes both women and girls. The terms "increase" and "decrease" are used to describe changes in an estimate only if the change is statistically significant at the 95 percent confidence interval (CI). If two estimates are not identical but have overlapping 95 percent CIs, the estimate is said to be "unchanged." For more precise estimates, combined years are used when sample sizes are small. The text or tables explicitly note the use of combined data.

# Cigarette Smoking Among Women

## Historical Trends in Smoking

Data on women's smoking before 1935 are anecdotal. *Fortune* magazine (*Fortune* 1935) conducted a national public opinion and consumer preference survey in the 1930s and a national Current Population Survey (Haenszel et al. 1956) was performed in 1955, but systematic surveillance of smoking behavior did

**Table 2.1. Sources of national survey data on tobacco use, United States**

| Survey | Years | Age or school grade of respondents | Type of survey |
|---|---|---|---|
| Adult Use of Tobacco Survey (AUTS) | 1964, 1966, 1970, 1975, 1986 | ≥ 21 years in 1964–1975<br>≥ 17 years in 1986 | Cross-sectional |
| Behavioral Risk Factor Surveillance System (BRFSS) | 1984–1999 | ≥ 18 years | Cross-sectional<br>State-specific estimates |
| Current Population Survey | 1955, 1966, 1967, 1985, 1989, 1992–1993, 1995–1996 | ≥ 15 years | Cross-sectional<br>Estimates by state and nation |
| Monitoring the Future (MTF) Survey | 1976–2000 | Grade 12<br>Grades 8 and 10 since 1991 | Cross-sectional with longitudinal component |
| National Health and Nutrition Examination Survey III (NHANES III) | 1988–1994 | ≥ 2 months | Cross-sectional |
| National Health Interview Survey (NHIS) | 1965, 1966, 1970, 1974, 1976, 1977, 1978, 1979, 1980, 1983, 1985, 1987, 1988, 1990, 1991, 1992, 1993, 1994, 1995, 1997, 1998 | ≥ 18 years | Cross-sectional |
| National Household Survey on Drug Abuse (NHSDA) | 1974, 1976, 1977, 1979, 1982, 1985, 1988, 1990, 1991, 1992, 1993, 1994, 1995, 1996, 1997, 1998 | ≥ 12 years | Cross-sectional |
| National Teenage Tobacco Survey (NTTS) | 1968, 1970, 1972, 1974, 1979 | 12–18 years | Cross-sectional with longitudinal component |
| National Youth Tobacco Survey (NYTS) | 1999 | Grades 6–12 | Cross-sectional |
| Teenage Attitudes and Practices Surveys (TAPS I, TAPS II) | 1989, 1993 | 12–18 years in 1989<br>10–22 years in 1993 | Cross-sectional with longitudinal component |
| Youth Risk Behavior Surveillance System (YRBSS) | 1991, 1993, 1995, 1997, 1999 | Grades 9–12 | Cross-sectional |

*Response rate, as defined by Council of American Survey Research Organizations, includes all calls made, even those that resulted in no answer or busy signal; does not include nonoperating or out-of-service numbers.

Sources: **AUTS:** U.S. Department of Health, Education, and Welfare (USDHEW) 1969, 1973, 1976; U.S. Department of Health and Human Services (USDHHS), public use data tape, 1986; USDHHS 1990a. **BRFSS:** Gentry et al. 1985; Remington et al. 1985; Frazier et al. 1992; Powell-Griner et al. 1997; Nelson et al. 1998; Centers for Disease Control and Prevention (CDC), Division of Adult and Community Health, public use data tape, 1999. **Current Population Survey:** U.S. Bureau of the Census 1995, 1996a,b; U.S. Bureau of the Census, National Cancer Institute supplement, public use data tape, 1995–1996. **MTF Survey:** University of Michigan, Institute for Social Research, public use data tapes, 1975–1998; Bachman et al. 1980a,b, 1981, 1984, 1985, 1987, 1991a, 1993a,b; Johnston et al. 1980a,b, 1982, 1984, 1986, 1991, 1992, 1993, 1994a,b, 1995a,b, 1996, 1997, 1999, 2000a;

| Mode of survey administration | Sample size | Response rate |
|---|---|---|
| Household interview in 1964 and 1966<br>Telephone interview in 1970 and later | 13,031 in 1986 | 74.3% in 1986 |
| Telephone interview | 1,248–7,543/state in 1999 | Median in 1999, 55.2%*<br>Range, 36.2–80.8% |
| Self-reported and proxy-reported household interview | 416,208 in 1995–1996 | 85.5% in 1995–1996 |
| Self-administered, school-based survey | 15,419–18,667/grade in 1998 | Students' rate, 86% in 1998<br>Range, 86–87% in 1991–1998<br>79–86% in 1977–1990<br>Schools' rate, 51% in 1998<br>Range, 51–60% in 1991–1998<br>59–72% in 1977–1990 |
| Household interview and physical examination | 30,100 | 74% (interview and physical examination) |
| In-person household and telephone interviews | 32,440 in 1998 | 73.9% in 1998<br>Average across survey years, 88% |
| In-person household interview<br>Beginning in 1994-B, self-administered answer sheet for responses to sensitive questions | 25,500 in 1998 | 77.0% in 1998<br>Average across survey years, 80% |
| Telephone interview in all surveys<br>In-person interview was also included in 1968 | 2,553–4,414 | Not available |
| Self-administered, school-based survey | 15,061 in 1999 | 84.2% in 1999 |
| Telephone interview, in-person interview, and mailed questionnaire | 9,965 in 1989<br>4,992 in 1993<br>7,960 in longitudinal component | 82.4% in 1989<br>89.3% in 1993<br>87.1% in longitudinal component |
| Self-administered, school-based survey | 15,349 in 1999 | 66% in 1999 |

University of Michigan 1999b, 2000. **NHANES III:** National Center for Health Statistics (NCHS), public use data tapes, 1988–1994; NCHS 1994b. **NHIS:** NCHS, public use data tapes, 1965–1998; NCHS 1975; Kovar and Poe 1985; Schoenborn 1988; Schoenborn and Marano 1988; Massey et al. 1989; USDHHS 1999a. **NHSDA:** Alcohol, Drug Abuse, and Mental Health Administration, public use data tapes, 1974–1991; Abelson and Atkinson 1975; Abelson and Fishburne 1976; Abelson et al. 1977; Miller et al. 1983; USDHHS 1988a, 1990b, 1991; Substance Abuse and Mental Health Services Administration (SAMHSA), public use data tapes, 1992–1998; SAMHSA 1993, 1995a,b, 1996, 1997, 1998a,b; 2000. **NTTS:** USDHEW 1972, 1979b. **NYTS:** CDC 2000b. **TAPS:** CDC, Office on Smoking and Health, public use data tapes, 1989, 1993; Allen et al. 1991, 1993; Moss et al. 1992; CDC 1994a,d. **YRBSS:** Kolbe 1990; CDC 1992; Kann et al. 1993, 1995, 1996, 1998, 2000; Kolbe et al. 1993; CDC, Division of Adolescent and School Health, public use data tape, 1999.

not begin in the United States until 1965. Other surveys before 1965 were often done for commercial purposes (Schuman 1977). For example, an annual marketing survey in Milwaukee, Wisconsin, was conducted by the *Milwaukee Journal*; the first survey of women was performed in 1935 (Burbank 1972; Howe 1984). Because smoking was more prevalent in urban areas than in rural areas, estimates of smoking prevalence among women in the Milwaukee surveys were higher than estimates that would have been obtained from a national population-based survey (*Fortune* 1935; Haenszel et al. 1956). This urban population was also probably younger, and younger women were more likely than older women to smoke during this period (Burbank 1972).

Women and girls in colonial New England and the wives of Presidents Andrew Jackson and Zachary Taylor reportedly smoked pipes (Gottsegen 1940; Robert 1952; Heimann 1960). Chewing tobacco, the primary form of tobacco used in the early 1800s, was used predominantly by men; women, however, did use snuff (Lander 1885; Gottsegen 1940; Robert 1952). Pipe use among women decreased before the Civil War (Heimann 1960). Cigarettes were introduced in the 1840s, and some use was reported among urban women (Brooks 1952; Robert 1952; Tennant 1971; Sobel 1978). Between the Civil War and World War I, men were the primary users of tobacco, but mountain women reportedly smoked pipes, factory women used snuff, Bohemian women smoked small cigars, and refined women smoked cigarettes (Robert 1952; Sobel 1978). In the 1800s, snuff was used by all classes in the South and by sophisticated New York women (Lander 1885). Many other women probably used tobacco secretly (e.g., in clandestine women's smoking clubs) (Lander 1885). The use of chewing tobacco declined in the United States after 1890 when strict laws were enacted that prohibited spitting. The introduction of blended and flue-cured cigarettes and the invention of an automated machine to produce cigarettes set the stage for widespread adoption of cigarette smoking (Wagner 1971).

In New York, a law was passed in 1908 making it illegal for women to smoke in public (Sullivan 1930; Sobel 1978). However, smoking among women began to increase, and some women smoked openly in the 1920s, as social and cultural changes lessened the taboos discouraging tobacco use by women (Sullivan 1930; Brooks 1952; Tennant 1971; Wagner 1971; Sobel 1978; Gritz 1980; USDHHS 1980; Ernster 1985; Waldron 1991). *Printers' Ink* noted in 1924 that World War I advanced the custom of smoking among women (Wessel 1924). Although Grace Coolidge is believed to have been the first First Lady to smoke cigarettes, Eleanor Roosevelt was the first to smoke publicly (Hoover 1934).

Estimates suggested that in 1924, women smoked about 5 percent of all cigarettes produced. By 1929, this proportion increased to 12 percent (Wills and Wills 1932). These data were used to derive estimates of smoking prevalence for women: 6 percent in 1924 and 16 percent in 1929 (USDHHS 1980). Burbank (1972) used data from the 1955 Current Population Survey to retrospectively determine smoking prevalence among women in 1930 and reported a considerably lower estimate (2 percent). The *Fortune* survey of 1935 (*Fortune* 1935) reported a national smoking prevalence of 26 percent among women younger than 40 years of age and 9 percent among women older than 40 years of age (18 percent overall). For women, the Milwaukee surveys showed a smoking prevalence of 20 percent in 1935 and 26 percent in 1940 (Figure 2.1) (*Milwaukee Journal* 1935, 1940). Other data also suggested that about 20 percent of women smoked between 1930 and 1945 (Burbank 1972).

During and after World War II, more women began smoking cigarettes (Schuman 1977). The Gallup Poll reported that 36 percent of women smoked in 1944 and 33 percent in 1949 (Gallup 1972a,b). According to the Milwaukee surveys, prevalence of current smoking among women was 38 percent in 1948 (Figure 2.1). Similarly, in the 1948 Framingham study, 40 percent of women were smokers (Gordon et al. 1975). Trade journal surveys in the late 1940s also estimated smoking prevalence among women to be 40 to 45 percent (Conover 1950). Early data are scarce for racial and ethnic groups, but data from the Mills and Porter (1953) 1947 household survey in Columbus, Ohio, indicated that 28 percent of white women and 36 percent of black women aged 20 years or older smoked cigarettes. A survey of 1,783 nonhospitalized persons in Texas in the early 1950s reported that 31 percent of both white women and black women smoked cigarettes (Kirchoff and Rigdon 1956).

The 1955 Current Population Survey was the first nationally representative survey of smoking prevalence; 32 percent of the women had ever smoked, and 24 percent were current smokers. The 1959 Cancer Prevention Study I (CPS-I), conducted by the American Cancer Society (ACS), was a survey of more than one million, primarily white, middle-class, well-educated adults aged 30 years or older from 25 states; 27 percent of the women were current smokers (Hammond and Garfinkel 1961; Stellman et al. 1988;

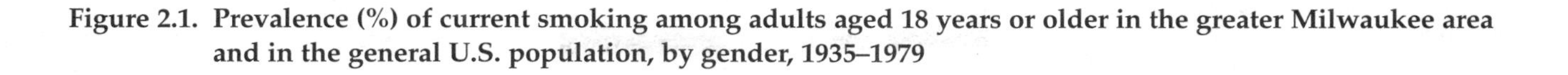

**Figure 2.1. Prevalence (%) of current smoking among adults aged 18 years or older in the greater Milwaukee area and in the general U.S. population, by gender, 1935–1979**

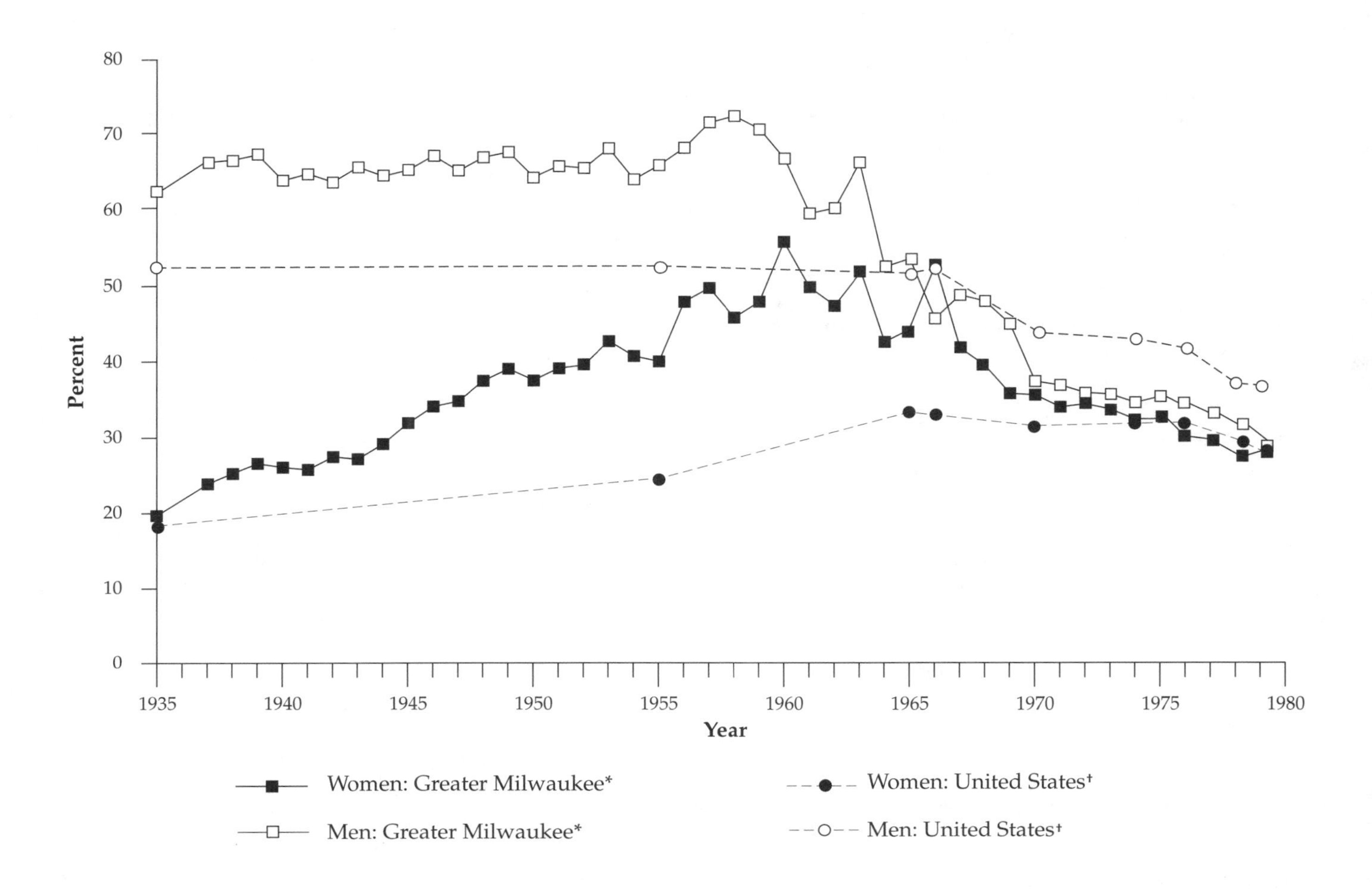


*Adapted from Howe 1984: *Milwaukee Journal,* Consumer analysis of the Greater Milwaukee market, 1924–1979. Before 1941, the wording of questions eliciting information on cigarette use and type of respondent are not recorded. In 1941–1954, men were asked, "Do you smoke cigarettes?" In 1955–1959, respondents were asked, "Do any men [women] in your household smoke cigarettes with [without] a filter tip?" In 1960–1965 and 1967, women and men were asked, "Have you bought, for your own use, cigarettes with [without] a filter tip in the past 30 days?" In 1966 and 1968–1979, women and men were asked, "Have you bought, for your own use, cigarettes with [without] a filter tip in the past 7 days?" Data since 1955 are based on the sum of the percentage of smokers who bought filter-tipped cigarettes and the percentage who bought nonfilter-tipped cigarettes in the past 30 days. Results overestimate smoking prevalence because respondents could answer "yes" to both questions. Data for women in 1976–1979 include only the percentage buying filter-tipped cigarettes; the question on the use of nonfilter-tipped cigarettes was dropped because of low response.

†Absence of data points from national surveys from 1935–1965 means these lines should not be interpreted as trends. The 1935 data are from the 1935 *Fortune* Survey III (*Fortune Magazine* 1935), the 1955 data are from the 1955 Current Population Survey (Haenszel et al. 1956), and the 1965–1979 data are from the National Health Interview Survey (Giovino et al. 1994).

Garfinkel and Silverberg 1990). Data from the Current Population Survey showed that prevalence of current smoking increased among women from 1955 through 1966 (National Center for Health Statistics [NCHS] 1970; Schuman 1977). In the Milwaukee surveys, smoking prevalence among women peaked in the early 1960s (Howe 1984). The 1964 AUTS, a nationally representative survey, reported that the prevalence of smoking was 31.5 percent among women 21 years of age or older (Centers for Disease Control [CDC] 1987b). Data from NHIS, first conducted in 1965, indicated that smoking prevalence among women was 33.9 percent in 1965 (Giovino et al. 1994). Prevalence decreased to 22.0 percent among women from 1965 through 1998. Most of this decline occurred from 1974 through 1990, but prevalence continued to decline from 1992 through 1998 (CDC 2000a).

Despite the variation in estimates of smoking prevalence across surveys, these data sources showed that the prevalence of smoking was consistently lower among women than among men. Prevalence was 18 percent among women and 52 percent among men in the *Fortune* survey (1935), 25 percent among women and 53 percent among men in the 1955 Current Population Survey (Haenszel et al. 1956), and 27 percent among women and 48 percent among men in the 1959 CPS-I (Garfinkel and Silverberg 1990).

## Smoking by Birth Cohort

Analyzing the smoking behavior of persons born during the same 5- to 10-year period (birth cohorts) provides an opportunity to examine when persons take up smoking and how smoking diffuses through a population over time. However, such analyses can underestimate smoking prevalence in early birth cohorts because smokers older than 40 years of age are more likely than nonsmokers to die (differential mortality). According to the 1959 CPS-I data for women aged 30 through 89 years, the estimated prevalence of current smoking among women increased from 1 percent in the 1870–1874 birth cohort to 43 percent in the 1925–1929 birth cohort (Hammond and Garfinkel 1968). On the basis of data from the 1965 follow-up survey of the same participants, the prevalence estimates for these cohorts of women were the same.

Using data from the 1978–1980 NHIS on the age at which regular cigarette use began and the age at complete smoking cessation, Harris (1983) reconstructed prevalence estimates for women and men born in 1880–1950. When he adjusted for differential mortality, he found that the effect was smaller for women than for men because the mortality differences between female smokers and nonsmokers in the earliest cohorts were small. Tolley and colleagues (1991) used NHIS data from 1970, 1978, 1979, 1980, and 1987 to reconstruct the prevalence of smoking in birth cohorts of whites and blacks by gender. They analyzed data on the age at which the respondent began smoking cigarettes fairly regularly, current smoking status, and time since the respondent last smoked regularly if the smoker had quit smoking. Although no adjustment was made for differential mortality, its effect was estimated at less than 1 percentage point for the earliest birth cohorts of women. Burns and others (1997) conducted the most recent analysis by birth cohort. They used NHIS data from 1970, 1978, 1979, 1980, 1987, and 1988 and adjusted the estimates for differential mortality. Current smoking prevalence was estimated for 5-year birth cohorts from 1885–1889 through 1965–1969. Results from all three of these analyses were consistent, and the estimates from Burns and coworkers are given here for white women and black women separately. To produce similar estimates for Hispanic women, NHIS data were used (NCHS, public use data tapes, 1978–1980, 1987, 1988), but no adjustment was made for differential mortality. Because of the smaller sample sizes, the estimates for Hispanic women are less precise than those for white women or black women, and because of the small sample sizes in earlier years, data are shown for blacks starting with the 1900–1904 cohort and for Hispanics starting with the 1910–1914 cohort.

According to NHIS data for white women, a dramatic increase in smoking prevalence occurred in the 1910–1914 birth cohort; for black women, a large increase occurred in the 1920–1924 birth cohort (Figure 2.2). For Hispanic women, the increase in smoking prevalence by cohort was gradual over time. For all three racial and ethnic groups, NHIS data showed a pattern of increased cigarette smoking among women in each successive birth cohort through the 1940–1944 birth cohort (Figure 2.2). The prevalence was low in the 1900–1904 birth cohort: a maximum prevalence of 24 percent among white women and 16 percent among black women. The sample size for Hispanic women was too small to assess the prevalence in this cohort. The highest prevalence among white women occurred in the 1925–1929 through 1940–1944 birth cohorts (49 percent) (Burns et al. 1997). Among black women, prevalence peaked in the 1935–1939 and 1940–1944 birth cohorts (51 percent) (Burns et al. 1997). Among Hispanic women, prevalence was highest in the 1920–1924 (31 percent) and 1940–1944 (29 percent) birth cohorts.

The Hispanic Health and Nutrition Examination Survey (HHANES) data showed that the pattern of smoking differed among subgroups of Hispanic women over time (Escobedo and Remington 1989). For example, among Mexican American women, prevalence peaked in the 1931–1940 birth cohort, but prevalence peaked among Puerto Rican American women in the most recent cohort studied, the 1951–1960 birth cohort.

Among whites, blacks, and Hispanics, smoking prevalence and the proportion of women who had ever smoked declined in cohorts of women born after 1944 (Figure 2.2). Escobedo and Peddicord (1996) suggested that this decline largely reflects smoking patterns among women with 12 or more years of education. Peak smoking among women with less than a high school education continued to increase for white women and for black women and remained stable for Hispanic women through the 1958–1967 birth cohort.

In all cohorts, smoking prevalence was lower among Hispanic women than among white women or black women (Figure 2.2). In the 1940–1944 birth cohort, smoking prevalence was comparable among white women and black women. In the last birth cohort presented in Figure 2.2 (1960–1964), the prevalence of smoking was higher among white women (40 percent) than among black women (37 percent). This cohort comprised women aged 19 through 23 years in 1988. In the last cohort studied (1965–1969) by Burns and coworkers (1997) (data not shown), the prevalence of smoking was higher among white women (34 percent) than among black women (26 percent). This finding is consistent with recent racial and ethnic trends in smoking prevalence among high school senior girls and young women (aged 18 through 24 years) (see "Cigarette Smoking Among Young Women" and "Cigarette Smoking Among Girls" later in this chapter).

The analyses by birth cohort showed that smoking became prevalent among men before it diffused to women (Figure 2.2). Among white men and black men, the dramatic increase in smoking prevalence occurred in the 1900–1904 birth cohort, and the prevalence of smoking was dramatically higher among men than among women in the earlier birth cohorts. For example, in the 1900–1904 birth cohort the peak prevalence of current smoking was 24 percent among white women and 75 percent among white men, and in the 1920–1924 birth cohort the peak prevalence was 46 percent among white women and 79 percent among white men. In Hispanic cohorts, smoking also became prevalent among men before it diffused to women (Escobedo and Remington 1989; Tolley et al. 1991; Burns et al. 1997). With each successive birth cohort, however, the patterns of cigarette smoking among women and men became increasingly similar. In the 1960–1969 cohorts of white adults, the peak smoking prevalence was comparable among women and men (McGinnis et al. 1987; Pierce et al. 1991b; Burns et al. 1997). This similarity by gender was also true for blacks (Burns et al. 1997), but for Hispanics, smoking prevalence remained lower among women than among men (Escobedo and Remington 1989; Escobedo et al. 1989).

Warner and Murt (1982) conducted a cohort analysis of the effect of the antismoking campaign on the prevalence of smoking from 1964 through the late 1970s. The investigators, assuming that well-established smoking patterns or trends would have persisted in the absence of the campaign, suggested that the prevalence among men had already been declining and that the campaign accelerated this trend. Among women, however, the prevalence of smoking was rising rapidly in the 1950s and 1960s and would have continued to rise into the 1970s were it not for the campaign. The antismoking campaign interrupted the diffusion of smoking among women, which caused the prevalence of current smoking to stabilize and then decline. The effect was substantial in all cohorts of women born between 1901 and 1960 but was greatest among women born between 1941 and 1950.

## Trends in Ever Smoking Among Women

Ever smoking is a measure of smoking during a person's lifetime. Table 2.2 presents NHIS data on trends in ever smoking among women, by intervals of approximately five years for 1965–1990, as determined by availability of data, and for 1992, 1995, and 1998. Ever smoking among women (≥ 18 years of age) is defined here as having smoked at least 100 cigarettes in one's lifetime. In 1965, the prevalence of ever smoking among women was 41.9 percent; it increased to 46.2 percent in 1985 and declined to 42.3 percent in 1990 (Table 2.2). The prevalence of ever smoking declined during 1990–1998 to 40.7 percent, but this decline was of borderline statistical significance. These data are consistent with AUTS data, which reported that the prevalence of ever smoking among women was 39 percent in 1964 and 43 percent in 1966 (U. S. Department of Health, Education, and Welfare [USDHEW] 1969).

**Figure 2.2. Prevalence (%) of current smoking for 5-year cohorts, by race and ethnicity, gender, and age, United States, 1890–1964**

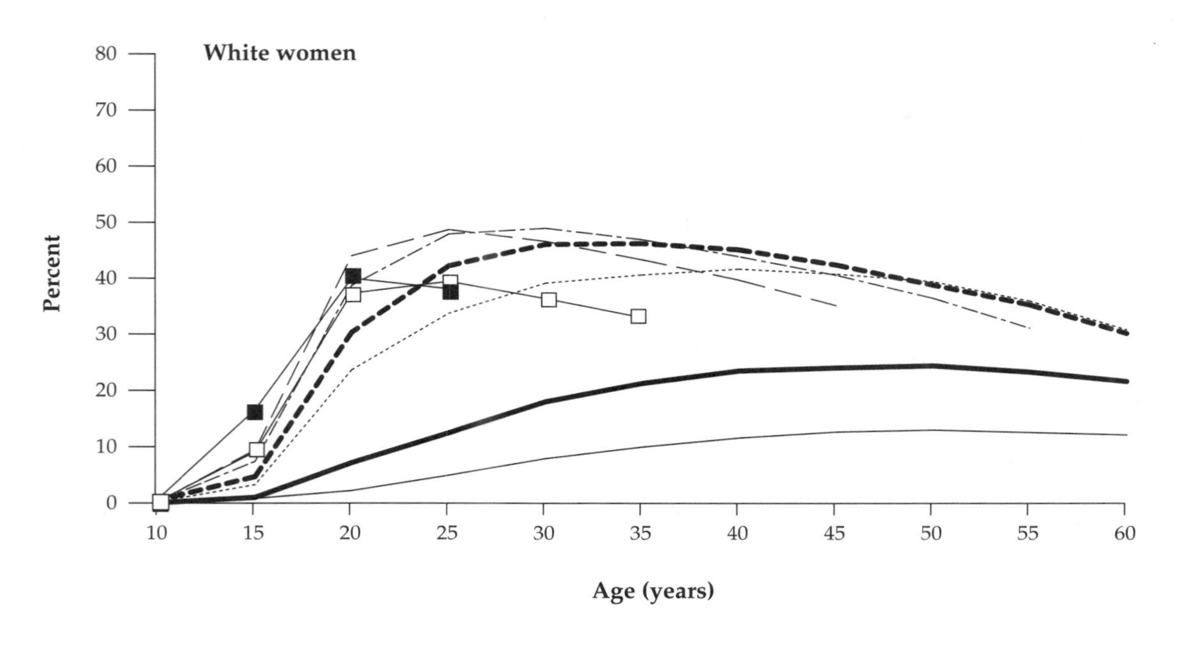


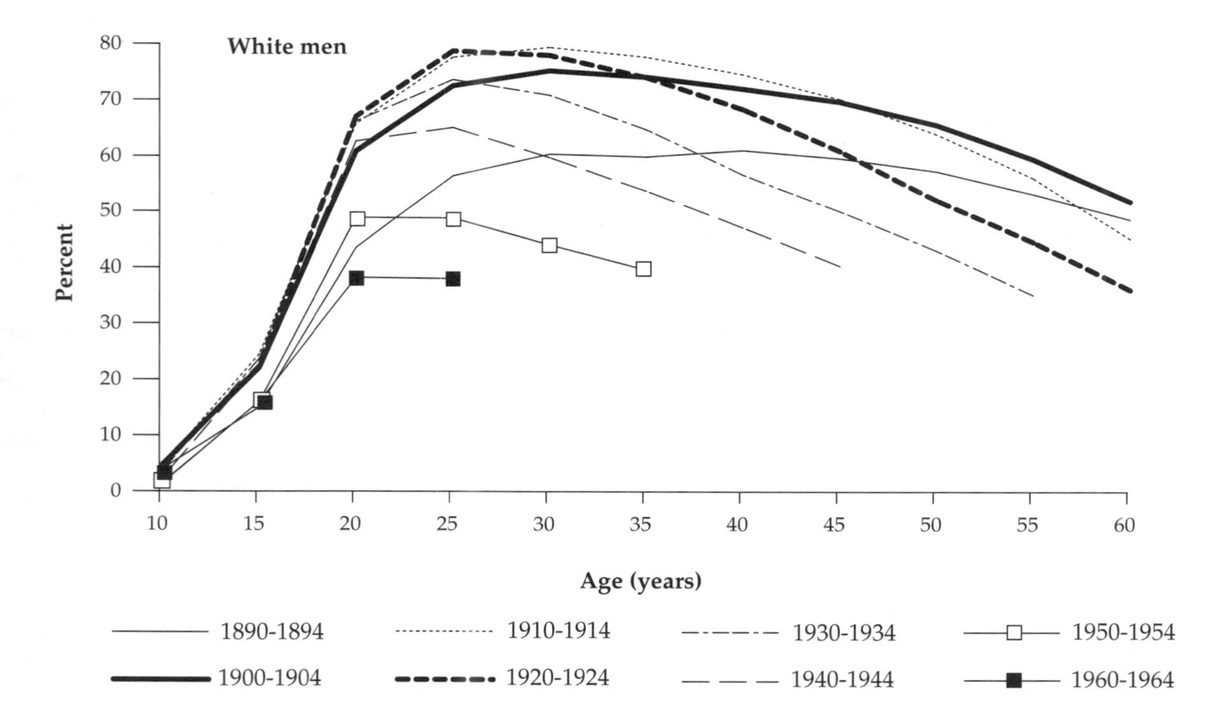


*Note:* Curves for prevalence of ever smoking, after adjusting for differential mortality, were used to estimate prevalence of current smoking for whites and blacks. No adjustment for differential mortality was used for Hispanics. Prevalence of current smoking is the percentage of the population that has initiated smoking by a given age, multiplied by the fraction of persons the same age who ever smoked who had stopped smoking. Data based on recalled age at initiation and recalled age at cessation from National Health Interview Surveys for 1978–1988.

Sources: National Center for Health Statistics, public use data tapes, 1978–1980, 1987, 1988; Burns et al. 1997.

**Figure 2.2. (Continued)**

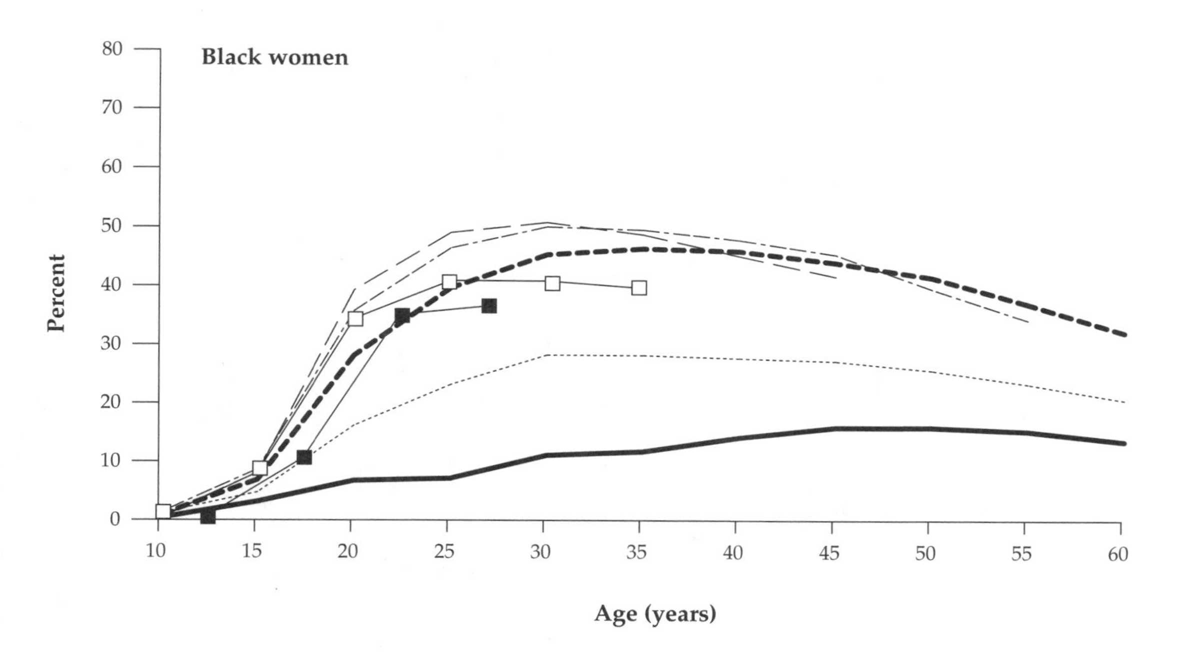


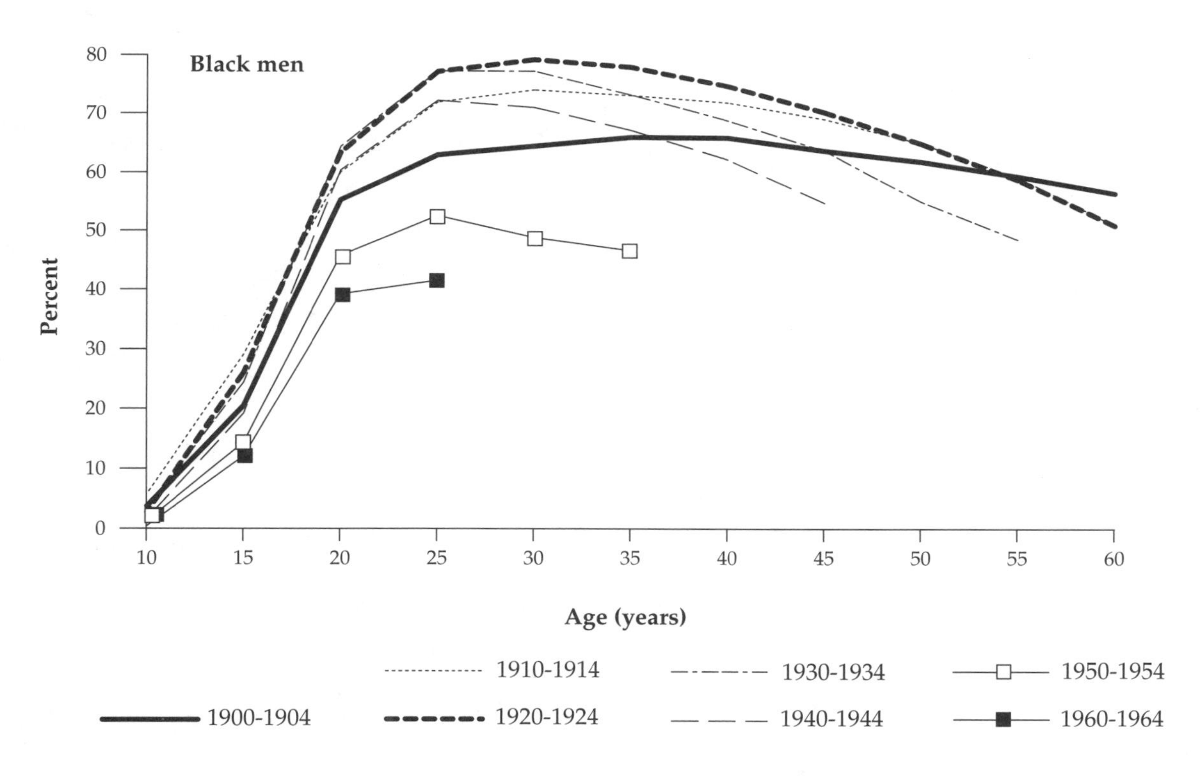

**Figure 2.2. (Continued)**

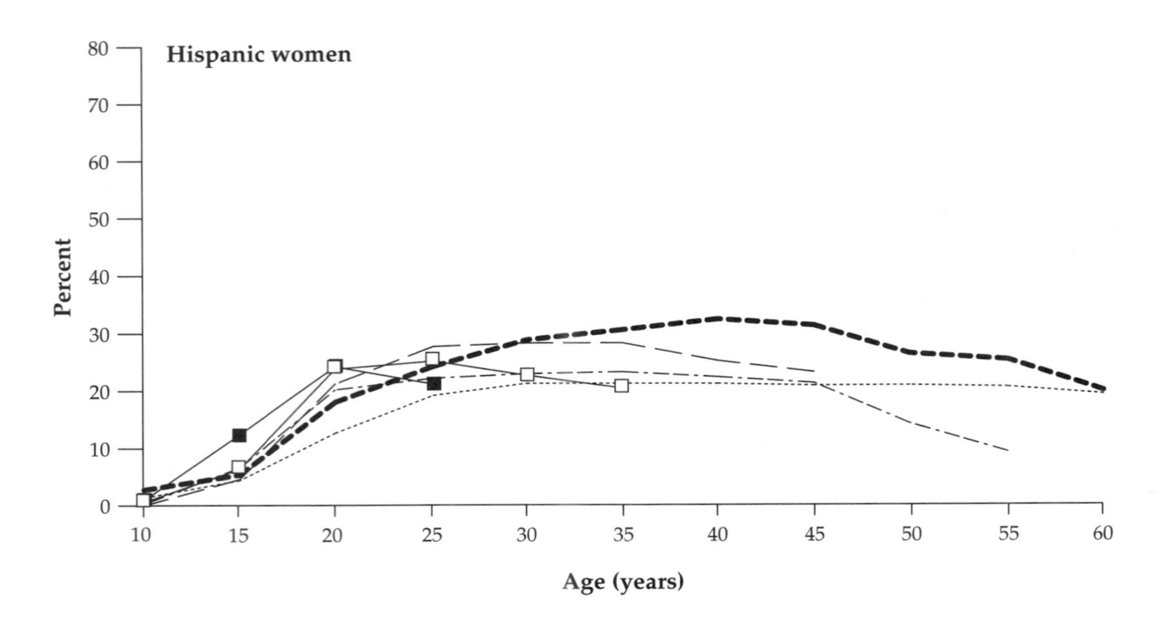


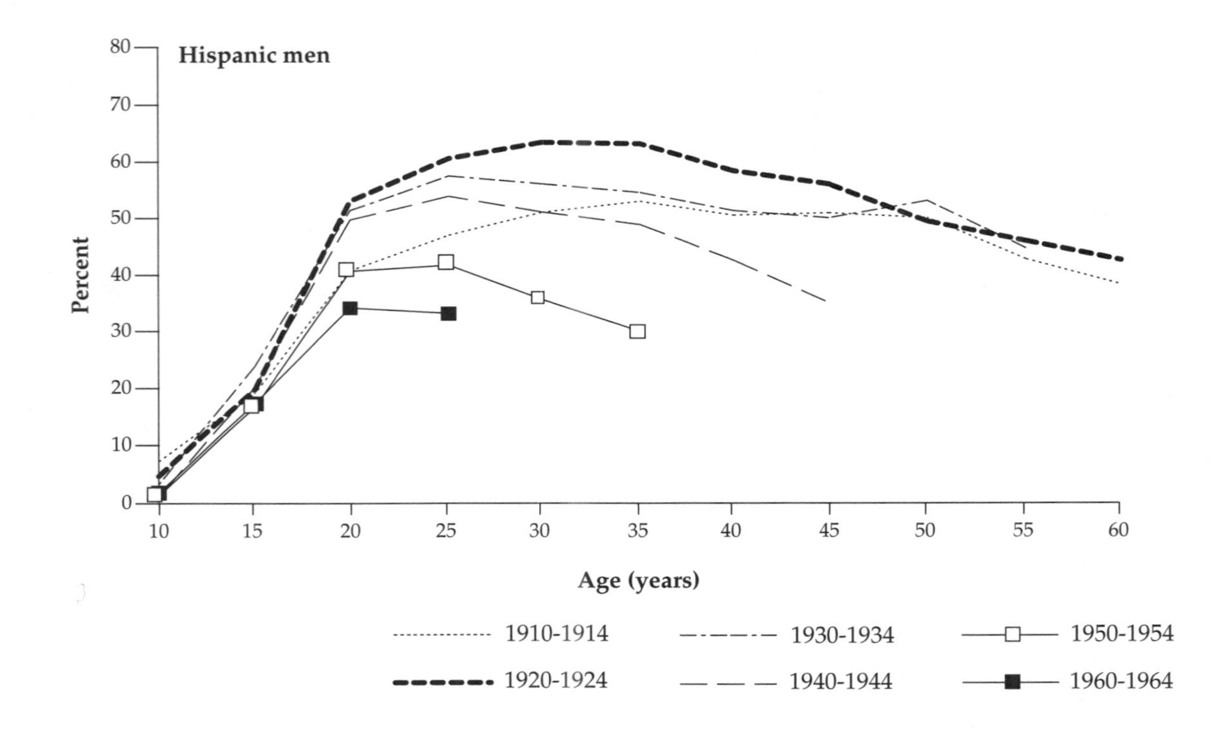

In 1965, the proportion of women who had ever smoked was highest among women aged 25 through 44 years; in 1998, it was highest among women aged 45 through 64 years (Table 2.2). This pattern reflects the aging of the cohorts of women born in the 1920s through 1940s, for whom the prevalence of smoking was the highest in this century (Tolley et al. 1991; Burns et al. 1997).

Ever smoking among white women increased significantly during 1965–1985 (Table 2.2). The prevalence was lower in 1990 but then remained unchanged through 1998; the prevalence in 1998 was essentially the same as that in 1965. Among black women, the prevalence of ever smoking also increased during 1965–1985. Although the increase was not statistically significant, the subsequent decrease during 1985–1998 was significant. Over time, a greater proportion of white women than black women has ever smoked. This difference was 1 percentage point (not statistically significant) in 1974 and 12.2 (95 percent CI for the difference, ± 2.5) percentage points in 1998 (Table 2.2). Ever smoking among Hispanic women, which decreased steadily from 1979 through 1998, was significantly lower than ever smoking among white women or black women for nearly all years. This finding is consistent with findings from other studies (Rogers and Crank 1988; Rogers 1991). Rogers (1991), for example, found that Mexican American women were more than twice as likely as white women or black women to have never smoked. During 1979–1998, inconsistent, nonsignificant fluctuations occurred in the prevalence of ever smoking for American Indian or Alaska Native women, probably because of small sample sizes (Table 2.2). For all years from 1965 through 1995, Asian or Pacific Islander women had the lowest prevalence of ever smoking among all racial and ethnic groups. Although a pattern of increasing prevalence of ever smoking was noted among Asian or Pacific Islander women from 1992 through 1998, this increase was not statistically significant.

In 1970, the prevalence of ever smoking was lower among women with 8 or fewer years of education and was comparable among women in other educational categories (Table 2.2). During 1970–1998, the decline in the prevalence of ever smoking was significant among women with 16 or more years of education but not among women with less education. Among women with fewer than 12 years of education, the prevalence of ever smoking increased significantly during 1970–1985 and then was unchanged from 1985 through 1998. Among women with 12 to 15 years of education, smoking prevalence was unchanged from 1970 through 1985, but then declined between 1985 and 1998. During 1985–1998, the prevalence of ever smoking decreased among women who lived at or above the poverty level but not among women who lived below the poverty level or who had unknown poverty status. The definition of poverty status, however, was different in 1998 than in previous years, making comparisons difficult. (See definition for "socioeconomic status" in Appendix 2.)

The prevalence of ever smoking peaked in 1985 for women (46.2 percent) and in 1965 for men (71.7 percent). For all years, the proportion of persons who had ever smoked was lower for women than for men, a finding noted by other researchers (Novotny et al. 1988; Covey et al. 1992).

## Ever Smoking Among Women by Demographic Characteristics

Ever smoking among women varies by age, race and ethnicity, and socioeconomic measures such as level of education and income (Table 2.2). In the 1998 NHIS data, the prevalence of ever smoking for women aged 18 years or older was 40.7 percent. The proportion of women who had ever smoked was significantly higher among women aged 45 through 64 years than among those in other age groups. The prevalence was lowest among Asian or Pacific Islander women and Hispanic women and highest among American Indian or Alaska Native women and white women. The prevalence of ever smoking was lowest among women having 8 or fewer, or 16 or more, years of education. The lower prevalence among women with 8 or fewer years of education is consistent with other reports: Zhu and colleagues (1996) found that this pattern held even after adjustment for age and other demographic variables. Similar patterns were seen in the 1997–1998 NHSDA (Substance Abuse and Mental Health Services Administration [SAMHSA], public use data tapes, 1997, 1998). Prevalence of ever smoking did not differ by poverty status (categorized as below the poverty level or at or above the poverty level). However, results from the 1990 NHIS suggested that the prevalence of ever smoking decreased for each category of annual income from $10,000 or more and that women in professional or technical occupations were less likely to have ever smoked (Metropolitan Insurance Companies 1992).

In the 1998 NHIS data, the prevalence of ever smoking was significantly lower among women (40.7 percent) than among men (53.8 percent) (Table 2.2). In all racial and ethnic groups except American Indians

**Table 2.2. Prevalence (% and 95% confidence interval) of ever smoking among women aged 18 years or older, by selected characteristics, National Health Interview Survey, United States, 1965–1998**

| Characteristic | 1965 | 1970 | 1974 |
|---|---|---|---|
| Women | 41.9 (±0.7) | 43.1 (±1.1) | 44.8 (±0.8) |
| Age (years) | | | |
| 18–24 | 44.3 (±1.9) | 40.7 (±1.5) | 41.8 (±2.1) |
| 25–44 | 53.4 (±1.3) | 53.4 (±1.4) | 53.4 (±1.3) |
| 45–64 | 40.6 (±1.2) | 45.2 (±1.7) | 48.4 (±1.5) |
| ≥ 65 | 14.1 (±1.4) | 18.6 (±1.4) | 22.6 (±1.6) |
| Race/ethnicity* | | | |
| White, non-Hispanic | 42.3 (±0.7) | 43.7 (±1.2) | 45.0 (±0.9) |
| Black, non-Hispanic | 39.4 (±2.2) | 39.5 (±2.4) | 44.0 (±3.0) |
| Hispanic | NA† | NA | NA |
| American Indian or Alaska Native | NA | NA | NA |
| Asian or Pacific Islander | NA | NA | NA |
| Education (number of years)§ | | | |
| ≤ 8 | NA | 30.3 (±1.1) | 31.9 (±2.1) |
| 9–11 | NA | 50.0 (±1.6) | 52.3 (±2.3) |
| 12 | NA | 47.9 (±1.5) | 48.9 (±1.4) |
| 13–15 | NA | 48.8 (±2.8) | 48.6 (±2.8) |
| ≥ 16 | NA | 46.7 (±2.6) | 48.1 (±3.2) |
| Socioeconomic status$^{\Delta}$ | | | |
| Below poverty level | NA | NA | NA |
| At or above poverty level | NA | NA | NA |
| Unknown | NA | NA | NA |
| Men | 71.7 (±0.7) | 70.4 (±0.6) | 70.8 (±1.0) |

*Note:* Prevalence of ever smoking is prevalence of all persons in each demographic category who reported smoking ≥ 100 cigarettes in their lifetime.
*Ethnicity was not determined in 1965, 1970, or 1974. Thus, estimates for whites and for blacks during these years likely include data for some persons of Hispanic origin.
†NA = Not available.

or Alaska Natives, women were less likely than men to have ever smoked (data not shown), a finding also noted by Rogers (1991).

## Trends in Current Smoking Among Women

Current smoking status is the most common measure used to assess trends in tobacco use. Data from the 1965–1998 NHIS on trends in current smoking among women are presented here. Current smoking is defined here as having ever smoked at least 100 cigarettes and smoking at the time of the survey. Since 1992, the definition of current smoking has explicitly included persons who smoke both every day or only on some days. The inclusion of these nondaily smokers increased the prevalence of current smoking among women aged 18 years or older by 0.9 percentage points, similar to the increase among adults overall (CDC 1994b). In NHIS data, the prevalence of current smoking among women decreased from 33.9 percent in 1965 to 22.0 percent in 1998 (Table 2.3). Most of this decline occurred during 1974–1990, but prevalence continued to decline from 1992 through 1998 (Giovino et al. 1994; CDC, 1994c, 1996, 1997c, 1999b, 2000a).

| 1979 | 1985 | 1990 | 1992 | 1995 | 1998 |
|---|---|---|---|---|---|
| 45.1 (±1.2) | 46.2 (±0.9) | 42.3 (±0.8) | 43.1 (±1.1) | 42.2 (±1.2) | 40.7 (±0.9) |
| | | | | | |
| 44.0 (±2.1) | 40.2 (±2.3) | 32.4 (±2.2) | 30.4 (±2.9) | 30.8 (±3.3) | 32.8 (±2.8) |
| 51.2 (±1.6) | 49.9 (±1.3) | 44.5 (±1.1) | 45.5 (±1.5) | 43.8 (±1.8) | 40.5 (±1.3) |
| 48.6 (±1.7) | 51.6 (±1.8) | 49.3 (±1.4) | 50.1 (±2.0) | 47.6 (±2.2) | 46.2 (±1.6) |
| 27.3 (±1.7) | 34.8 (±2.0) | 34.7 (±1.5) | 36.4 (±2.2) | 38.4 (±2.4) | 38.2 (±1.8) |
| | | | | | |
| 46.7 (±1.2) | 48.0 (±1.1) | 45.4 (±0.9) | 46.6 (±1.2) | 46.0 (±1.4) | 44.8 (±1.1) |
| 42.3 (±2.6) | 43.5 (±2.6) | 34.3 (±1.9) | 35.5 (±2.5) | 36.9 (±3.4) | 32.6 (±2.2) |
| 35.4 (±3.5) | 33.8 (±3.3) | 30.5 (±2.7) | 29.2 (±3.0) | 26.5 (±2.8) | 25.6 (±1.9) |
| 56.6 (±11.8)‡ | 47.8 (±13.8) | 54.6 (±11.4) | 56.0 (±12.5) | 53.0 (±14.7) | 57.7 (±11.3) |
| 24.3 (±8.1) | 20.0 (±6.5) | 13.9 (±3.9) | 12.0 (±4.2) | 13.8 (±4.1) | 16.8 (±4.6) |
| | | | | | |
| 33.1 (±2.3) | 36.4 (±2.7) | 32.2 (±2.4) | 33.5 (±3.0) | 34.2 (±3.8) | 33.0 (±2.9) |
| 52.2 (±2.5) | 54.9 (±2.3) | 53.0 (±2.2) | 52.7 (±3.0) | 54.4 (±3.5) | 51.5 (±2.6) |
| 47.4 (±1.9) | 49.3 (±1.6) | 47.4 (±1.2) | 48.6 (±1.7) | 47.6 (±2.0) | 45.0 (±1.6) |
| 50.5 (±2.8) | 49.6 (±2.2) | 44.7 (±1.7) | 47.3 (±2.3) | 45.9 (±2.8) | 45.7 (±1.8) |
| 43.8 (±2.0) | 41.7 (±2.2) | 35.8 (±1.7) | 35.9 (±2.2) | 34.1 (±2.6) | 31.3 (±1.7) |
| | | | | | |
| NA | 45.3 (±2.2) | 43.8 (±2.3) | 43.3 (±3.0) | 42.0 (±3.1) | 41.3 (±2.3) |
| NA | 46.9 (±1.0) | 42.5 (±0.9) | 43.5 (±1.1) | 42.8 (±1.4) | 41.2 (±1.1) |
| NA | 42.9 (±2.7) | 38.7 (±2.5) | 39.3 (±2.9) | 35.3 (±3.9) | 39.0 (±1.9) |
| 66.2 (±1.0) | 63.7 (±1.0) | 58.7 (±0.9) | 57.5 (±1.1) | 54.6 (±1.4) | 53.8 (±1.0) |

‡Estimate should be interpreted with caution because of the small number of respondents.
§For women aged ≥ 25 years. Data for five education categories not available for 1965.
ΔDefinition of poverty status changed in 1997. (See Appendix 2 for definitions.)
Sources: National Center for Health Statistics, public use data tapes, 1965, 1970, 1974, 1979, 1985, 1990, 1992, 1995, 1998.

During 1965–1998, the prevalence of current smoking was lowest among women aged 65 years or older (Table 2.3). The finding that, after age 25 years, the prevalence of smoking decreased as age increased was also seen in earlier studies: in the 1959 CPS-I, 41.7 percent of women aged 30 through 39 years, 26 percent of women aged 50 through 59 years, and 1 to 2 percent of women aged 80 years or older were current smokers (Hammond and Garfinkel 1961). Over time, smoking prevalence declined most among women of reproductive age (18 through 44 years): 13.6 (± 3.1) percentage points among women aged 18 through 24 years and 18.1 (± 1.7) percentage points among women aged 25 through 44 years (Table 2.3). Nevertheless, nearly 14 million women of reproductive age were smokers in 1998, and smoking prevalence in this group was higher (25.3 percent) than in the overall population of women aged 18 years or older (22.0 percent) (NCHS, public use data tape, 1998; CDC 1999b). Smoking prevalence was the same in 1965 and 1998 among women aged 65 years or older (Table 2.3), a finding noted in earlier studies (Novotny et al. 1990; CDC 2000a; Giovino et al. 1994).

In the NHIS data, smoking prevalence decreased among both white women and black women during 1965–1998 (Table 2.3). The prevalence of current smoking was generally comparable, but it was higher, and occasionally significantly so, among black women from 1970 through 1985 and higher among white women in 1990. Similar patterns were noted

**Table 2.3. Prevalence (% and 95% confidence interval) of current smoking among women aged 18 years or older, by selected characteristics, National Health Interview Survey, United States, 1965–1998**

| Characteristic | 1965 | 1970 | 1974 |
|---|---|---|---|
| Women | 33.9 (±0.6) | 31.5 (±0.8) | 32.1 (±0.8) |
| Age (years) | | | |
| 18–24 | 38.1 (±1.7) | 32.7 (±1.4) | 34.1 (±2.0) |
| 25–44 | 43.7 (±1.1) | 38.8 (±1.0) | 39.2 (±1.3) |
| 45–64 | 32.0 (±1.1) | 33.0 (±1.4) | 33.4 (±1.6) |
| ≥ 65 | 9.6 (±1.0) | 11.0 (±1.1) | 12.0 (±1.2) |
| Race/ethnicity* | | | |
| White, non-Hispanic | 34.0 (±0.7) | 31.6 (±0.9) | 31.7 (±0.8) |
| Black, non-Hispanic | 33.7 (±2.1) | 32.2 (±2.2) | 36.4 (±2.7) |
| Hispanic | NA[†] | NA | NA |
| American Indian or Alaska Native | NA | NA | NA |
| Asian or Pacific Islander | NA | NA | NA |
| Education (number of years)[§] | | | |
| ≤ 8 | NA | 22.3 (±1.0) | 22.5 (±1.8) |
| 9–11 | NA | 38.7 (±1.5) | 41.2 (±2.2) |
| 12 | NA | 34.2 (±1.3) | 34.5 (±1.4) |
| 13–15 | NA | 33.7 (±2.6) | 30.9 (±2.8) |
| ≥ 16 | NA | 26.7 (±1.9) | 26.6 (±2.8) |
| Socioeconomic status[Δ] | | | |
| Below poverty level | NA | NA | NA |
| At or above poverty level | NA | NA | NA |
| Unknown | NA | NA | NA |
| Men | 51.9 (±0.6) | 44.1 (±0.7) | 43.1 (±1.0) |

*Note:* Prevalence of current smoking is the percentage of all persons in each demographic category who reported smoking ≥ 100 cigarettes in their lifetime and who smoked at the time of the survey. Since 1992, estimates of current smoking explicitly include persons who smoked only on some days.

*Ethnicity was not determined in 1965, 1970, or 1974. Thus, estimates for whites and for blacks during these years likely include data for some persons of Hispanic origin.

among women of reproductive age, except that a significantly higher prevalence among white women was consistently noted since 1990 (data not shown). This pattern is probably due to recent racial and ethnic trends among young women (see "Cigarette Smoking Among Young Women" later in this chapter). These findings were also noted in other studies (McGinnis et al. 1987; Fiore et al. 1989; Hahn et al. 1990; USDHHS 1990b; Resnicow et al. 1991; CDC 2000a). Among Hispanic women, a decline in prevalence was noted during 1979–1998 (Table 2.3). Prevalence was also significantly lower among Hispanic women than among white women or black women during this period, and this finding is supported by other data (Holck et al. 1982; Marcus and Crane 1984, 1985; Markides et al. 1987; Fiore 1992). Using data from the Stanford Five-City Project, Winkleby and associates (1995) found that the difference in smoking prevalence between white women and Hispanic women decreased as education increased and that smoking prevalence was the same among white women and Hispanic women who were college graduates. The prevalence changed little during 1979–1998 among American Indian or Alaska Native women (Table 2.3). Among Asian or Pacific Islander women, prevalence decreased during 1979–1992 but then doubled from 1995 through 1998. However, the number of respondents in these racial and ethnic groups was

| 1979 | 1985 | 1990 | 1992 | 1995 | 1998 |
|---|---|---|---|---|---|
| 29.9 (±0.9) | 27.9 (±0.8) | 22.8 (±0.7) | 24.6 (±0.9) | 22.6 (±1.1) | 22.0 (±0.8) |
| | | | | | |
| 33.8 (±2.1) | 30.4 (±2.3) | 22.5 (±1.9) | 24.9 (±2.8) | 21.8 (±3.0) | 24.5 (±2.6) |
| 35.1 (±1.4) | 31.8 (±1.2) | 26.6 (±1.0) | 28.8 (±1.4) | 26.8 (±1.6) | 25.6 (±1.2) |
| 30.7 (±1.6) | 29.9 (±1.5) | 24.8 (±1.3) | 26.1 (±1.8) | 24.0 (±2.0) | 22.5 (±1.3) |
| 13.2 (±1.3) | 13.5 (±1.3) | 11.5 (±0.9) | 12.4 (±1.3) | 11.5 (±1.5) | 11.2 (±1.2) |
| | | | | | |
| 30.6 (±1.0) | 28.2 (±0.9) | 24.1 (±0.8) | 25.9 (±1.1) | 24.1 (±1.3) | 23.6 (±0.9) |
| 31.6 (±2.5) | 31.2 (±2.3) | 21.1 (±1.6) | 24.1 (±2.2) | 23.5 (±3.1) | 21.3 (±2.0) |
| 22.2 (±3.1) | 20.8 (±2.4) | 16.3 (±2.2) | 18.0 (±2.5) | 14.9 (±2.1) | 13.3 (±1.4) |
| 34.9 (±12.9)‡ | 28.4 (±10.0) | 37.8 (±11.9) | 39.8 (±12.4) | 35.4 (±13.9)‡ | 38.1 (±11.9) |
| 15.9 (±8.0)‡ | 11.0 (±4.9) | 5.9 (±2.3) | 4.0 (±2.3)‡ | 4.3 (±3.1)‡ | 9.9 (±4.2) |
| | | | | | |
| 21.1 (±1.7) | 21.1 (±1.9) | 16.6 (±1.9) | 18.7 (±2.6) | 17.8 (±2.8) | 16.7 (±2.4) |
| 38.0 (±2.2) | 37.2 (±2.5) | 33.9 (±2.2) | 32.2 (±2.7) | 33.7 (±3.5) | 32.9 (±2.5) |
| 31.1 (±1.5) | 30.4 (±1.3) | 26.6 (±1.1) | 28.7 (±1.5) | 26.2 (±1.8) | 25.2 (±1.4) |
| 30.9 (±2.3) | 27.0 (±1.8) | 21.6 (±1.3) | 24.1 (±1.9) | 22.5 (±2.2) | 22.8 (±1.5) |
| 22.2 (±1.9) | 16.6 (±1.6) | 12.7 (±1.1) | 14.5 (±1.6) | 13.7 (±1.8) | 11.2 (±1.2) |
| | | | | | |
| NA | 32.7 (±1.9) | 31.7 (±2.1) | 31.7 (±3.0) | 29.3 (±2.9) | 29.3 (±2.1) |
| NA | 27.4 (±0.9) | 21.7 (±0.7) | 23.8 (±1.0) | 21.8 (±1.1) | 21.3 (±0.9) |
| NA | 25.8 (±2.1) | 22.1 (±2.0) | 22.1 (±2.5) | 21.0 (±3.5) | 20.2 (±1.6) |
| | | | | | |
| 37.5 (±1.1) | 32.6 (±1.0) | 28.4 (±0.8) | 28.6 (±1.0) | 27.0 (±1.2) | 26.4 (±0.9) |

†NA = Not available.
‡Estimate should be interpreted with caution because of the small number of respondents.
§For women aged ≥ 25 years. Data for five education categories not available for 1965.
ΔDefinition of poverty status changed in 1997. (See Appendix 2 for definitions.)
Sources: National Center for Health Statistics, public use data tapes, 1965, 1970, 1974, 1979, 1985, 1990, 1992, 1995, 1998.

small and the increase was not statistically significant. In addition, procedural changes in the NHIS design and changes in the questions defining racial and ethnic groups occurred in 1997. Thus, these data must be interpreted with caution. Adjustment for age had little effect on the trends noted for racial and ethnic groups (USDHHS 1996a, 1998) (Figure 2.3). Similar patterns were also noted when the analysis was restricted to women of reproductive age (data not shown).

Data for 1959–1962 indicated the prevalence of current smoking was lowest among women with 8 or fewer years of education and highest among women with some college education (Hammond and Garfinkel 1964). However, in 1970–1998, the prevalence of smoking among women was highest among those with 9 to 11 years of education and lowest among those with 8 or fewer or 16 or more years of education (Table 2.3) (Green and Nemzer 1973; USDHEW 1976; Schuman 1977; Zhu et al. 1996). These educational patterns persist even after adjustment for demographic variables, including age (Remington et al. 1985; Zhu et al. 1996). This general pattern was also found in earlier surveys, such as the 1959 CPS-I (Hammond and Garfinkel 1961). NHIS data for 1970–1998 showed that the greatest decline in smoking prevalence occurred among women with 16 or more years of education (15.5 ± 2.3 percentage points),

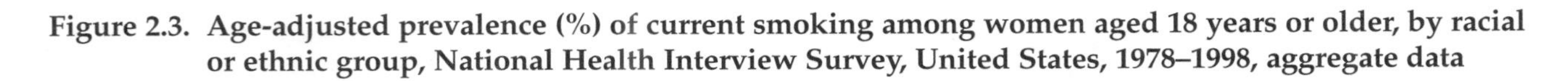

**Figure 2.3. Age-adjusted prevalence (%) of current smoking among women aged 18 years or older, by racial or ethnic group, National Health Interview Survey, United States, 1978–1998, aggregate data**

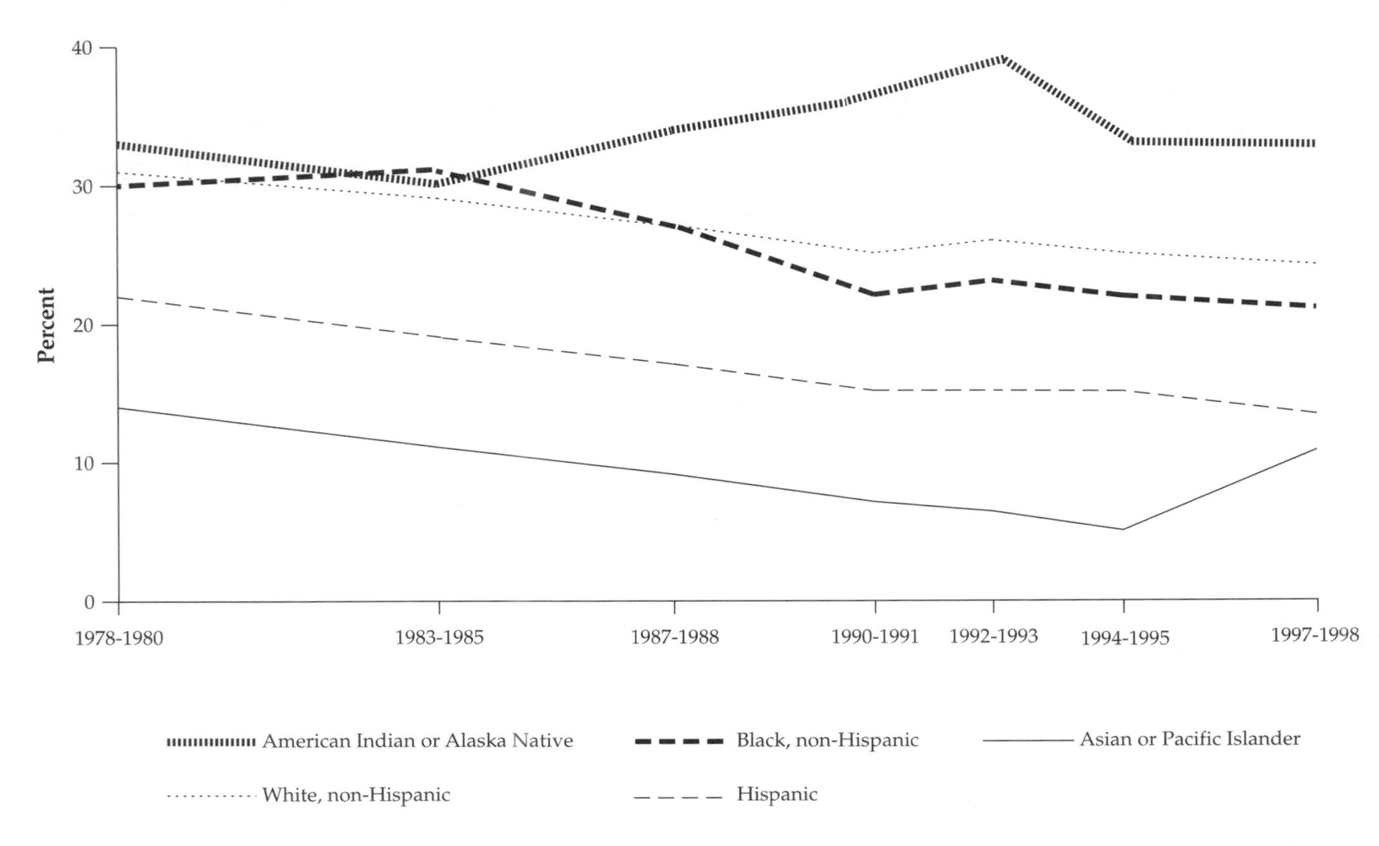


*Note:* Age-adjusted estimates were produced by using data aggregated for the following years: 1978, 1979, and 1980; 1983 and 1985; 1987 and 1988; 1990 and 1991; 1992 and 1993; 1994 and 1995; and 1997 and 1998. Data were adjusted to the 1990 National Health Interview Survey population. Prevalence of current smoking is the percentage of all persons in each demographic category who reported smoking ≥ 100 cigarettes in their lifetime and who smoked at the time of the survey. Since 1992, estimates of current smoking explicitly include persons who smoked only on some days.
Sources: National Center for Health Statistics, public use data tapes, 1978–1980, 1983, 1985, 1987, 1988, 1990–1995, 1997–1998.

a finding also noted by Giovino and colleagues (1994) (Table 2.3). Smoking prevalence among women with all levels of educational attainment decreased during 1970–1998. However, when the analysis was restricted to women of reproductive age, no decrease in smoking prevalence was noted among women with 12 years of education (NCHS, public use data tapes, 1970–1998) (data not shown). Other researchers found that education has become the most important demographic correlate of smoking status (Pierce et al. 1989a; Wagenknecht et al. 1990b; Berman and Gritz 1991; Fiore 1992).

For women, trends in smoking are more consistent for education than for income or occupation. Although education, income, and occupation are fairly well correlated as measures of socioeconomic status among men, the correlations among these measures are weaker among women (Coriell and Adler 1996).

The association between current smoking and income has changed over time among women. Studies conducted in 1964–1975 showed that the prevalence of smoking increased with income (USDHEW 1976; Schuman 1977). However, more recent NHIS data showed a decrease in prevalence with higher income (Metropolitan Insurance Companies 1992). In the NHIS data for 1985–1998, the prevalence of current smoking was higher among women living below the poverty level than among women living at or above the poverty level (Table 2.3). During this same period, prevalence decreased among women living at or above the poverty level. Among women of reproductive age, prevalence declined both for women living at or above the poverty level and for women living below the poverty level (data not shown).

No clear trends have emerged for the relationship between smoking prevalence among women and occupational status (Haenszel et al. 1956; Green and Nemzer 1973; Sterling and Weinkam 1976, 1978; USDHEW 1976; Schuman 1977; Waldron 1980; Stellman and Stellman 1981; Sorensen and Pechacek 1986; Brackbill et al. 1988; Schoenborn 1988; Waldron and Lye 1989; Ebi-Kryston et al. 1990; Wagenknecht et al. 1990b; Covey et al. 1992; Metropolitan Insurance Companies 1992). Some of the inconsistencies in trends result from differences in the definition of unemployment, such as whether housewives or others not in the labor force were included. Estimates from the 1987–1990 NHIS (Nelson et al. 1994) showed a smoking prevalence of 26.7 percent among employed women, 34.9 percent among unemployed women who were looking for work, and 22.1 percent among women not in the labor force (not employed and not looking for work).

Prevalence of smoking among military women aged 18 through 55 years (25.4 ± 1.2 percent) was no different from that in a comparison civilian population of women (26.6 ± 1.0 percent). The information on military women came from a Department of Defense Survey of Health Related Behaviors Among Military Personnel that was conducted in 1998. The final sample consisted of 17,264 active-duty military personnel from all branches of the military. Women in the Marines were more likely than civilian women to smoke, but women in the Army were less likely than civilian women to smoke (Bray et al. 1999). However, women military veterans were more likely than nonveterans to have ever smoked cigarettes (McKinney et al. 1997) or to be current smokers (Klevens et al. 1995; Whitlock et al. 1995).

Consistent with earlier reports (McGinnis et al. 1987; Fiore et al. 1989; Fiore 1992; Metropolitan Insurance Companies 1992), the decline in the prevalence of current smoking in the 1965–1998 NHIS data was greater among men (25.5 ± 1.0 percentage points) than among women (11.9 ± 1.0 percentage points) (Figure 2.4). However, during 1985–1998, the decline was comparable among women (5.9 ± 1.1 percentage points) and men (6.2 ± 1.3 percentage points). The prevalence of current smoking was lower among women than among men for all years during 1965–1998. This was true for all racial and ethnic groups except American Indians or Alaska Natives (Stellman and Garfinkel 1986; Rogers and Crank 1988; Resnicow et al. 1991; USDHHS 1998).

## Current Smoking Among Women by Demographic Characteristics

Current smoking among women varies by age, race and ethnicity, sexual orientation, and socioeconomic measures such as level of education and income. Estimates of the prevalence of current smoking among women by various demographic characteristics were obtained from the 1997–1998 NHIS and the 1997–1998 NHSDA. In NHIS data for 1997–1998, the prevalence of current smoking among women was 22.0 percent (CDC 2000a) (Table 2.4). Prevalence was highest among women aged 18 through 44 years (25–44 years in NHSDA) and lowest among women aged 65 years or older. Smoking prevalence was highest among American Indian or Alaska Native women (34.5 percent), intermediate among white women (23.5 percent) and black women (21.9 percent), and lowest among Hispanic women (13.8 percent) and Asian or Pacific Islander women (11.2 percent). Similar patterns were observed in the NHSDA, but the results were not statistically significant for American Indian or Alaska Native women.

National surveys are limited in their assessment of smoking behavior among racial and ethnic groups that constitute a small proportion of the U.S. population or that show variations in smoking prevalence by geographic location or subgroup. Therefore, results from other surveys are presented here for Hispanics, American Indians or Alaska Natives, and Asian or Pacific Islanders.

In the 1982–1983 HHANES, the age-adjusted smoking prevalence ranged from 24 percent among Mexican American women and Cuban American women to 30 percent among Puerto Rican American women (Escobedo and Remington 1989; Haynes et al. 1990). In contrast, NHIS data for the same period showed the prevalence of smoking among Hispanic women overall to be 20.4 percent. HHANES respondents were offered a choice of questionnaires in English or Spanish, so increased comprehension of the survey questions may account for the higher estimates of the prevalence in current smoking from HHANES. On the other hand, NHIS contains a wider range of Hispanic subgroups, some of which may have lower smoking prevalences (USDHHS 1998).

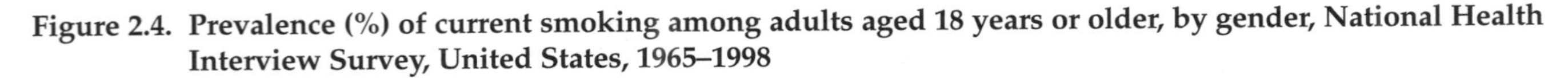

**Figure 2.4. Prevalence (%) of current smoking among adults aged 18 years or older, by gender, National Health Interview Survey, United States, 1965–1998**

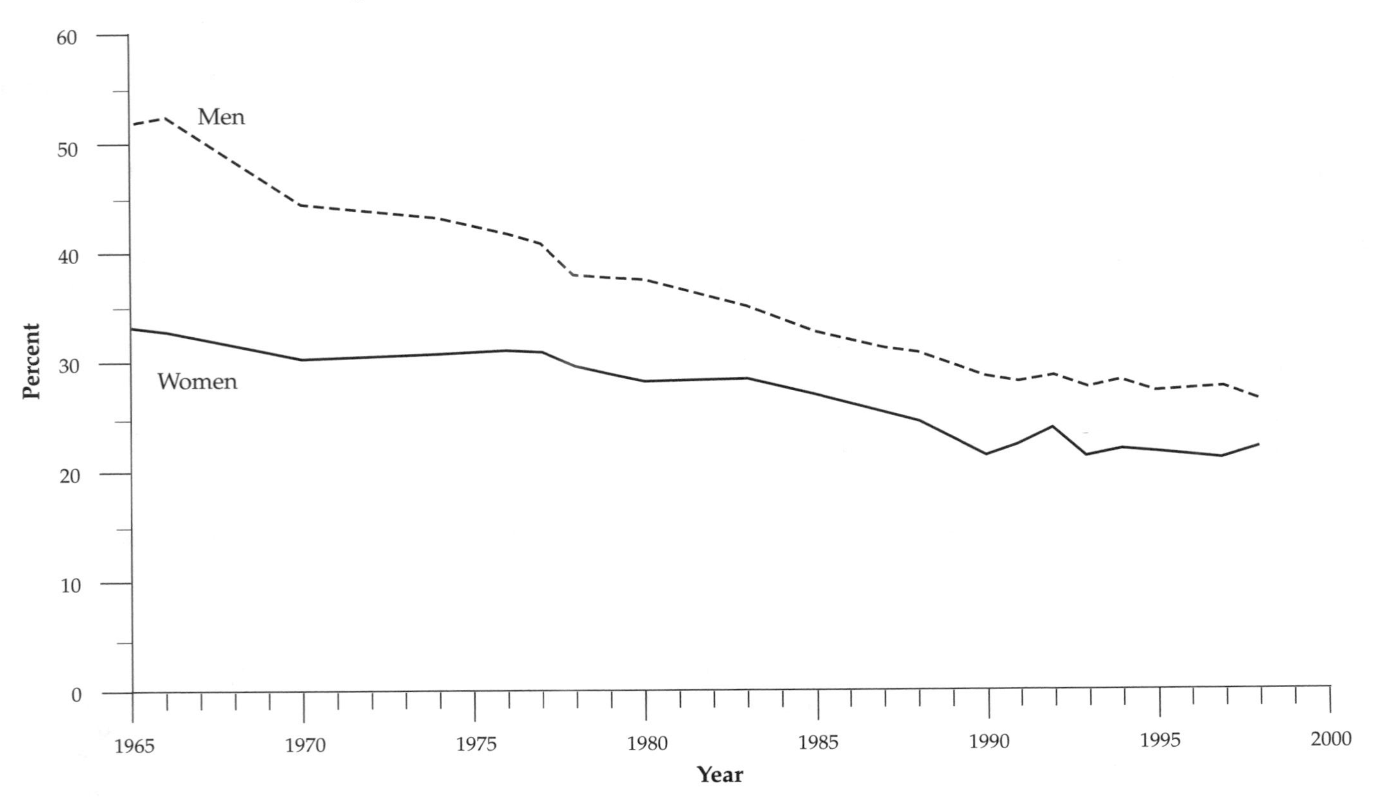


*Note:* Prevalence of current smoking is the percentage of all persons in each demographic category who reported smoking ≥ 100 cigarettes in their lifetime and who smoked at the time of the survey. Since 1992, estimates of current smoking explicitly include persons who smoked only on some days.
Sources: National Center for Health Statistics, public use data tapes, 1965–1998.

The 1987 Survey of American Indians and Alaska Natives of the National Medical Expenditure Survey (Lefkowitz and Underwood 1991) reported a smoking prevalence of 28.3 percent among women. This result is lower than the 1987–1988 NHIS estimate of 35.2 percent (USDHHS 1998). The difference was primarily due to different sampling frames and methods. In a 1989–1992 survey of 13 American Indian tribes (Welty et al. 1995), smoking prevalence among women was estimated at 29.3 percent, but it ranged from 12.9 percent among American Indian women in Arizona to 45.3 percent among American Indian women in North Dakota and South Dakota. Aggregated data from the 1988–1992 BRFSS showed that smoking prevalence among American Indian or Alaska Native women varied threefold by region—from 13.5 percent in the Southwest to 37.6 percent in the northern woodlands, 38.4 percent in the northern plains, and 41.7 percent in Alaska (USDHHS 1998). In BRFSS data for 1994–1996, similar patterns were noted. Prevalence was highest among American Indian or Alaska Native women living in the northern plains (43.5 percent) and in Alaska (40.6 percent), intermediate among women living in the East (33.4 percent) and on the Pacific coast (30.6 percent), and lowest among women living in the Southwest (18.6 percent). The prevalence among women in the Southwest was significantly lower than among women in the northern plains, Alaska, and the East (Denny and Holtzman 1999). In smaller studies, prevalence has been found to be low among Hopi women (5.4 percent) and Navajo women (4.0 percent) but high (45.2 percent) among American Indian women in Montana (Nelson et al. 1997; Strauss et al. 1997; Giuliano et al. 1998). Current Population Survey data for 1992–1993 showed a higher smoking prevalence among Alaska Native women (46 percent) than

**Table 2.4. Prevalence (% and 95% confidence interval) of current smoking among adults aged 18 years or older, by gender and selected characteristics, National Health Interview Survey (NHIS) and National Household Survey on Drug Abuse (NHSDA), United States, 1997–1998**

| Characteristic | NHIS, 1997–1998 | | NHSDA, 1997–1998 | |
|---|---|---|---|---|
| | Women | Men | Women | Men |
| Overall | 22.0 (±0.5) | 27.0 (±0.6) | 25.0 (±1.1) | 28.8 (±1.3) |
| Age (years) | | | | |
| 18–24 | 25.1 (±1.7) | 31.5 (±2.0) | 28.1 (±1.8) | 37.3 (±2.1) |
| 25–44 | 25.8 (±0.8) | 30.3 (±0.9) | 29.0 (±1.6) | 31.4 (±1.9) |
| 45–64 | 22.0 (±0.9) | 27.7 (±1.1) | 24.2 (±2.3) | 28.1 (±2.6) |
| ≥ 65 | 11.3 (±0.8) | 11.6 (±0.9) | 15.4 (±2.5) | 15.2 (±3.1) |
| Race/ethnicity | | | | |
| White, non-Hispanic | 23.5 (±0.6) | 27.0 (±0.7) | 26.7 (±1.3) | 28.8 (±1.6) |
| Black, non-Hispanic | 21.9 (±1.3) | 30.6 (±1.7) | 24.1 (±1.9) | 31.9 (±2.6) |
| Hispanic | 13.8 (±1.0) | 25.5 (±1.5) | 17.8 (±2.0) | 27.9 (±2.3) |
| American Indian or Alaska Native | 34.5 (±7.3) | 40.1 (±9.9) | 33.7 (±13.2) | 30.8 (±16.6) |
| Asian or Pacific Islander | 11.2 (±2.7) | 19.8 (±3.2) | 8.2 (±3.4) | 21.6 (±6.0) |
| Education (number of years)* | | | | |
| ≤ 8 | 15.9 (±1.6) | 28.9 (±2.1) | 18.5 (±3.9) | 28.7 (±4.8) |
| 9–11 | 30.9 (±1.6) | 39.3 (±2.0) | 36.2 (±4.0) | 46.1 (±4.8) |
| 12 | 26.1 (±1.0) | 33.2 (±1.2) | 30.1 (±2.3) | 32.4 (±2.7) |
| 13–15 | 22.9 (±1.0) | 27.0 (±1.2) | 25.7 (±2.4) | 27.1 (±3.0) |
| ≥ 16 | 10.6 (±0.8) | 12.2 (±0.9) | 11.9 (±1.8) | 15.2 (±2.3) |
| Socioeconomic status† | | | | |
| Below poverty level | 29.6 (±1.4) | 37.9 (±2.1) | NA‡ | NA |
| At or above poverty level | 21.6 (±0.6) | 26.5 (±0.7) | NA | NA |
| Unknown | 19.3 (±1.1) | 24.4 (±1.4) | NA | NA |

*Note:* Prevalence of current smoking in NHIS is the percentage of all persons in each demographic category who reported smoking ≥ 100 cigarettes in their lifetime and who smoked at the time of the survey. Estimates of current smoking explicitly include persons who smoked only on some days. Prevalence for NHSDA is the percentage of all persons in each demographic category who reported smoking ≥ 100 days in their lifetime and who smoked in the 30 days before the survey.

*For persons aged ≥ 25 years.

†See Appendix 2 for definition.

‡NA = Not available.

Sources: **NHIS:** National Center for Health Statistics, public use data tapes, 1997, 1998. **NHSDA:** Substance Abuse and Mental Health Services Administration, public use data tapes, 1997, 1998.

among American Indian women in the continental United States (35 percent) (Kaplan et al. 1997). Similarly, 1992–1995 combined BRFSS data from 15 states with substantial American Indian or Alaska Native populations showed that the age-standardized smoking prevalence was 30.1 percent among American Indian or Alaska Native women and 21.1 percent among white non-Hispanics in the same states (Denny and Taylor 1999).

Estimates from national surveys indicated that the prevalence of smoking among Asian or Pacific Islander women is lower than that among women in other racial and ethnic groups; data from California support these findings (Pierce et al. 1994a). However, state and local surveys showed that smoking prevalence varies dramatically among ethnic subgroups (USDHHS 1998). In a California survey, the prevalence among Asian women was highest among women of Japanese ancestry (14.9 percent) or Korean ancestry (13.6 percent) and lowest among women of Chinese ancestry (4.7 percent) (Burns and Pierce 1992). Similarly, in a survey of women enrolled in a prepaid health plan in California, 18.6 percent of Japanese American women and 7.3 percent of Chinese American women were current smokers (Klatsky and Armstrong 1991; USDHHS 1998).

Data on current smoking among lesbians and bisexual women are limited and have been based on convenience samples, which limits generalizability. The few existing studies strongly suggest that prevalence of smoking is higher than in the general population (Bradford et al. 1994; Skinner and Otis 1996; Valanis et al. 2000). A study of lesbians aged 17 years and older found the prevalence of current smoking in 1984–1985 to be 41 percent (Bradford et al. 1994). Another study in the late 1980s of lesbians aged 18 years and older yielded similar findings (Skinner and Otis 1996).

In the 1997–1998 NHIS data, smoking prevalence was highest among women with 9 to 11 years of education (30.9 percent) and lowest among those with 16 or more years of education (10.6 percent). This pattern was also seen for NHSDA (Table 2.4). The prevalence of smoking was higher among women living below the poverty level (29.6 percent) than among women living at or above the poverty level (21.6 percent), a pattern consistent with other data (Resnicow et al. 1991). In 1997–1998, smoking prevalence was 22.0 percent among women and 27.0 percent among men and was generally lower among women than among men across age, race, and socioeconomic groups.

BRFSS and the Current Population Survey both provide state-specific estimates of smoking prevalence. Although sample sizes are larger in the Current Population Survey, more recent data are available from BRFSS. Patterns in the two data sources were generally comparable (BRFSS, public use data tape, 1995–1996; CDC 1997b; Arday et al. 1997). Data from the 1999 BRFS indicated that the prevalence of smoking among women was highest in Nevada and Alaska and lowest in Utah and California (Figure 2.5). The prevalence of smoking was significantly lower among women than among men in one-third of the states (BRFSS, public use data tape, 1999).

## Trends in Quantity of Cigarettes Smoked

The quantity of cigarettes smoked is directly associated with addiction to nicotine and risk for numerous adverse health outcomes; it is inversely associated with success in smoking cessation (see "Nicotine Dependence Among Women and Girls" and "Smoking Cessation" later in this chapter) (Hammond and Garfinkel 1968; Gordon et al. 1975; McWhorter et al. 1990; Hellman et al. 1991; Coambs et al. 1992; Freund et al. 1992).

### Trends in Intermittent Smoking

NHIS data for intermittent smoking (smoking only on some days) for women 18 years of age or older showed no change from 1992 (14.8 ± 2.0 percent) through 1998 (16.9 ± 1.6 percent). Prevalence of intermittent smoking was higher among younger smokers, among blacks and Hispanics, and among persons with 16 or more years of education; no differences were noted by gender (NCHS, public use data tapes, 1992–1998). These patterns are consistent with previous findings (Husten et al. 1998).

### Trends in Heavy Smoking

Data from the Current Population Survey suggested that 8 to 9 percent of women who smoked consumed 21 or more cigarettes per day in 1955 and that 12 to 16 percent did so in 1966 (NCHS 1970). CPS data from 1959 (CPS-I) and 1982 (Cancer Prevention Study II [CPS-II]) showed that a far higher percentage of smokers smoked 20 or more cigarettes per day in CPS-II than in CPS-I; the absolute average difference was 20.6 percentage points (Hammond and Garfinkel 1961; Stellman and Garfinkel 1986; Garfinkel and Silverberg 1990; Burns et al. 1997).

For analysis of NHIS data, light smoking was defined as smoking fewer than 15 cigarettes per day, moderate smoking as smoking 15 to 24 cigarettes per day, and heavy smoking as smoking 25 or more cigarettes per day. The proportion of women smokers who were light smokers increased during 1965–1998, whereas the proportion who were moderate or heavy smokers was about the same in 1965 and 1998 (Table 2.5). However, the prevalence of heavy smoking increased from 13.8 percent of smokers in 1965 to 22.0 percent in 1979 and then decreased to 12.1 percent in 1998. Similarly, the mean number of cigarettes consumed per day by women who smoked was 7.0 in the 1934 *Milwaukee Journal* survey (USDHHS 1980), 13.0 in the 1955 Current Population Survey (Schuman 1977), 16.2 in the 1965 AUTS, and 17.0 in the 1970 AUTS (Green and Nemzer 1973). In NHIS data, the mean number of cigarettes smoked per day increased from 16.2 (no CI available) in 1965 to 17.6 (±0.2) in 1970 and 18.9 (±0.4) in 1979; it then declined to 15.0 (±0.4) in 1998 (NCHS, public use data tapes, 1965–1998). Increasing restrictions on where smoking is permitted and increases in the real price of cigarettes

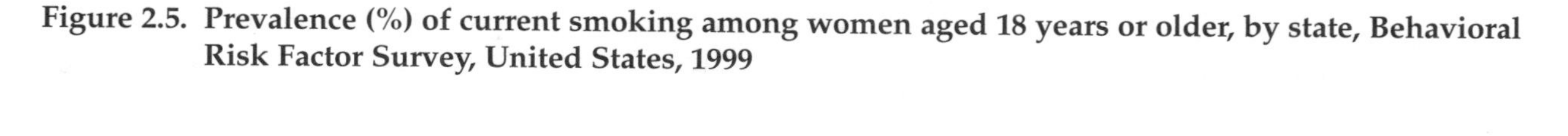

**Figure 2.5. Prevalence (%) of current smoking among women aged 18 years or older, by state, Behavioral Risk Factor Survey, United States, 1999**

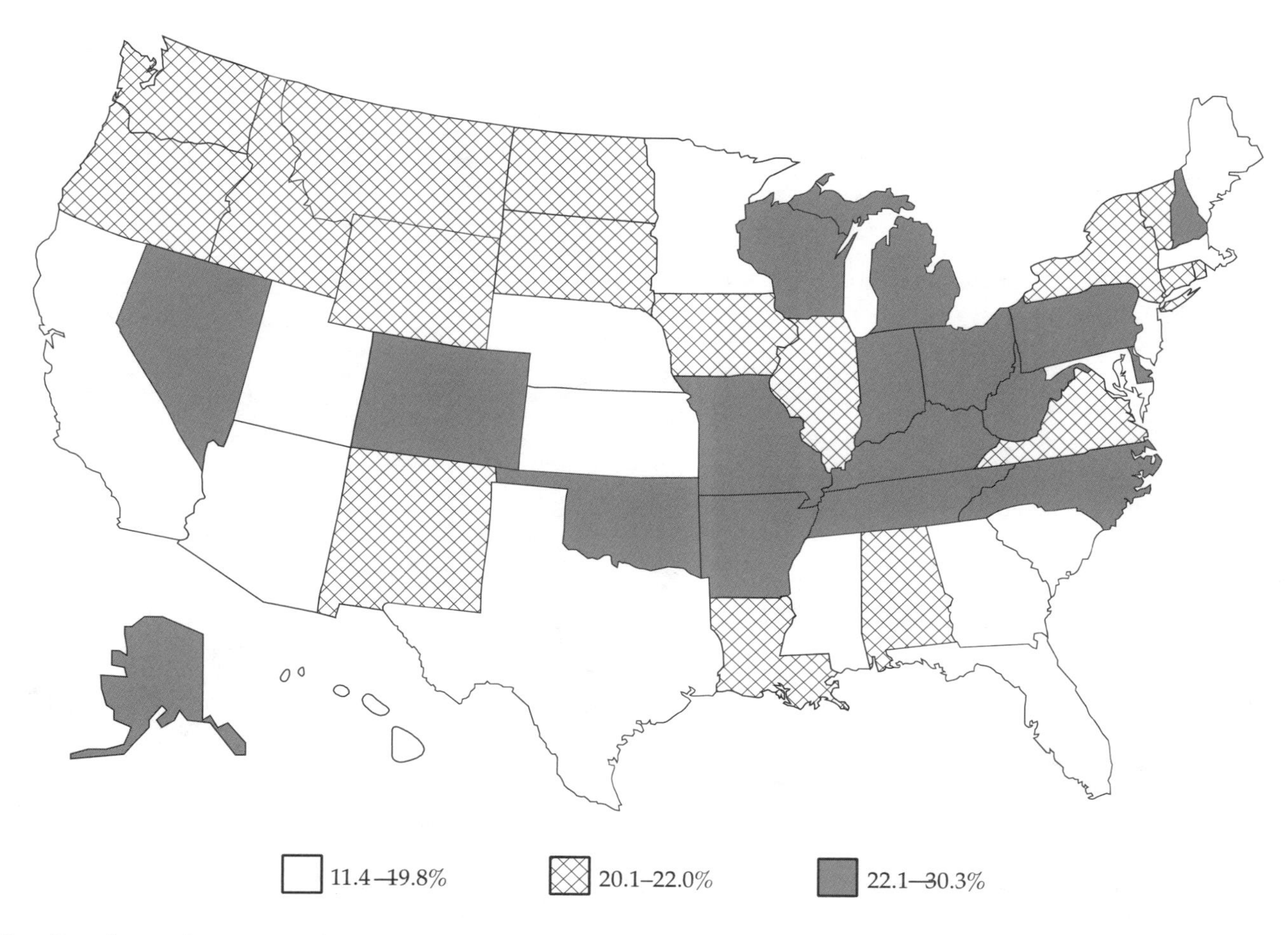


*Note:* Prevalence of current smoking is the percentage of all persons in each state who reported smoking ≥ 100 cigarettes in their lifetime and who smoked at the time of the survey. Categories were based on tertiles of smoking prevalence.
Sources: Centers for Disease Control and Prevention, Division of Adult and Community Health, public use data tape, 1999.

since 1981 may have contributed to the decline in the mean number of cigarettes smoked per day (Giovino et al. 1994).

Among female smokers aged 18 through 64 years, NHIS data showed that the proportion of heavy smokers increased during 1965–1979 and then declined (Table 2.5). Heavy smoking among women aged 65 years or older increased during 1965–1974 and then decreased, but not significantly. In 1998, the proportion of heavy smokers among women smokers aged 45 through 64 years (16.8 percent) was greater than that among younger women.

The proportion of heavy smokers among both white women and black women who smoked rose during 1965–1979, but this increase was significant only among white women (Table 2.5). Between 1979 and 1998, heavy smoking declined among white, black, and Hispanic women. Because the sample size was small for black women and Hispanic women, the results should be interpreted with caution. However, analysis of NHIS data for the combined years 1978–1980 through the combined years 1994–1995 also showed a significant decrease among Hispanic women. The prevalence of heavy smoking among

**Table 2.5. Distribution (% and 95% confidence interval) of the number of cigarettes smoked and percentage smoking 25 or more cigarettes per day, among women current smokers aged 18 years or older, by selected characteristics, National Health Interview Survey, United States, 1965–1998**

| Characteristic | 1965 | 1970 | 1974 |
|---|---|---|---|
| Women | | | |
| Number of cigarettes/day | | | |
| <15 | 44.4 (±1.2) | 38.8 (±1.2) | 38.3 (±1.6) |
| 15–24 | 41.8 (±1.2) | 43.1 (±1.1) | 43.0 (±1.5) |
| ≥ 25 | 13.8 (±0.9) | 18.1 (±0.8) | 18.7 (±1.3) |
| Percent smoking ≥ 25 cigarettes/day | 13.8 (±0.9) | 18.1 (±0.8) | 18.7 (±1.3) |
| Age (years) | | | |
| 18–24 | 8.8 (±1.7) | 12.1 (±1.4) | 13.8 (±2.2) |
| 25–44 | 16.4 (±1.3) | 21.7 (±1.3) | 22.5 (±2.3) |
| 45–64 | 13.6 (±1.7) | 17.7 (±1.2) | 16.9 (±2.0) |
| ≥ 65 | 6.4 (±3.1) | 11.3 (±2.5) | 16.2 (±4.3) |
| Race/ethnicity† | | | |
| White, non-Hispanic | 14.8 (±1.0) | 19.4 (±0.8) | 20.5 (±1.4) |
| Black, non-Hispanic | 5.7 (±1.8) | 7.2 (±1.6) | 6.6 (±2.2)* |
| Hispanic | NA‡ | NA | NA |
| Education (number of years)§ | | | |
| ≤ 8 | NA | 16.0 (±1.7) | 13.8 (±2.7) |
| 9–11 | NA | 21.2 (±1.7) | 23.6 (±3.4) |
| 12 | NA | 19.8 (±1.3) | 20.1 (±2.1) |
| 13–15 | NA | 21.1 (±2.9) | 24.5 (±4.0) |
| ≥ 16 | NA | 17.1 (±3.1) | 13.5 (±4.2) |
| Men smoking ≥ 25 cigarettes/day | 24.8 (±0.9) | 28.0 (±1.1) | 31.1 (±1.6) |

*Note:* Current smoking is the prevalence of all persons in each demographic category who reported smoking ≥ 100 cigarettes in their lifetime and who smoked at the time of the survey. Since 1992, estimates of current smoking explicitly include persons who smoked only on some days.

*Estimate should be interpreted with caution because of the small number of respondents.

American Indian or Alaska Native women and among Asian or Pacific Islander women was unchanged from 1978–1980 through 1994–1995 (USDHHS 1998). In all years, white women who smoked were more likely to be heavy smokers than were black women or Hispanic women. This finding was also reported by other investigators (Holck et al. 1982; Marcus and Crane 1985; Hahn et al. 1990; USDHHS 1990a, 1997; Resnicow et al. 1991; Winkleby et al. 1995) and is consistent with earlier surveys, such as the 1947 survey in Columbus, Ohio (Mills and Porter 1953), a 1952–1954 survey in Texas (Kirchoff and Rigdon 1956), and the 1955 Current Population Survey (Haenszel et al. 1956). Other analyses of NHIS data for 1978–1995 reported that white women who smoked were more likely to be heavy smokers than were American Indian or Alaska Native women or Asian or Pacific Islander women, but the CIs were large (USDHHS 1998).

In the 1998 NHIS, among women who smoked, white women (14.0 percent) were more likely to be heavy smokers than were black women (4.5 percent) or Hispanic women (2.1 percent) (Table 2.5). The mean number of cigarettes smoked per day was 16.1 (±0.4) for white women who smoked, 11.0 (±1.0) for black women who smoked, and 9.1 (± 0.9) for Hispanic women who smoked (NCHS, NHIS, public use data tape, 1998). In data from the Stanford Five-City Project,

| 1979 | 1985 | 1990 | 1992 | 1995 | 1998 |
|---|---|---|---|---|---|
| 34.1 (±1.6) | 36.9 (±1.4) | 40.2 (±1.5) | 43.7 (±2.0) | 46.8 (±2.5) | 48.2 (±1.8) |
| 43.9 (±1.7) | 42.5 (±1.5) | 43.2 (±1.5) | 41.0 (±1.9) | 39.1 (±2.4) | 39.7 (±1.7) |
| 22.0 (±1.3) | 20.6 (±1.3) | 16.6 (±1.2) | 15.3 (±1.4) | 14.1 (±1.7) | 12.1 (±1.2) |
| 22.0 (±1.3) | 20.6 (±1.3) | 16.6 (±1.2) | 15.3 (±1.4) | 14.1 (±1.7) | 12.1 (±1.2) |
| 15.7 (±2.7) | 11.7 (±2.3) | 6.7 (±3.0) | 8.4 (±3.0) | 9.6 (±4.9)* | 5.1 (±2.4)* |
| 24.6 (±2.1) | 23.9 (±1.9) | 17.1 (±1.6) | 15.3 (±2.1) | 12.1 (±2.4) | 11.5 (±1.7) |
| 24.8 (±2.5) | 22.7 (±2.3) | 21.8 (±2.4) | 18.7 (±2.9) | 19.0 (±3.4) | 16.8 (±2.6) |
| 12.7 (±3.8) | 13.4 (±3.7) | 11.9 (±2.7) | 15.3 (±4.5) | 16.2 (±5.3) | 10.9 (±3.6) |
| 24.4 (±1.5) | 23.2 (±1.5) | 19.0 (±1.4) | 17.4 (±1.6) | 15.9 (±2.1) | 14.0 (±1.5) |
| 9.2 (±2.6) | 7.6 (±2.0) | 4.3 (±1.7) | 5.2 (±2.0) | 5.7 (±2.9)* | 4.5 (±2.1)* |
| 11.0 (±4.2)* | 13.0 (±5.6)* | 3.4 (±2.0)* | 5.1 (±2.9)* | 9.9 (±4.8)* | 2.1 (±1.4)* |
| 20.3 (±4.5) | 18.4 (±4.8) | 22.0 (±4.7) | 19.3 (±7.1) | 22.7 (±7.7) | 15.0 (±6.0) |
| 24.0 (±3.1) | 25.1 (±3.4) | 19.9 (±3.2) | 22.3 (±4.3) | 17.4 (±5.2) | 23.6 (±6.0) |
| 24.2 (±2.5) | 23.2 (±2.2) | 19.0 (±1.9) | 16.4 (±2.2) | 15.8 (±2.7) | 13.9 (±2.2) |
| 26.3 (±3.8) | 20.5 (±3.2) | 15.9 (±2.8) | 13.6 (±3.4) | 12.1 (±3.5) | 10.8 (±2.4) |
| 19.3 (±4.6) | 21.2 (±4.2) | 11.9 (±3.1) | 11.1 (±3.6) | 8.1 (±3.9)* | 5.5 (±2.4)* |
| 32.4 (±1.5) | 32.4 (±1.6) | 28.5 (±1.6) | 27.0 (±1.8) | 25.5 (±2.3) | 22.6 (±1.7) |

†Ethnicity was not determined in 1965, 1970, or 1974. Thus, estimates for whites and for blacks during these years likely include data for some persons of Hispanic origin.
‡NA = Not available.
§For women aged ≥ 25 years. Data for the five education categories were not available for 1965.
Sources: National Center for Health Statistics, public use data tapes, 1965, 1970, 1974, 1979, 1985, 1990, 1992, 1995, 1998.

Hispanic women who smoked consumed fewer cigarettes per day than did white women who smoked, regardless of educational attainment (Winkleby et al. 1995). Among Hispanic women who smoked, the 1982–1983 HHANES showed that Mexican American women (18.8 percent) were less likely to be heavy smokers (≥ 1 pack of cigarettes per day) than were Puerto Rican American women (35.1 percent) or Cuban American women (48.6 percent) (Haynes et al. 1990). NHIS data from 1987, 1988, 1990, and 1991 (aggregate data) showed that heavy smoking among Hispanic women who smoked was highest among "other Hispanics" (17.5 percent) and Cuban Americans (10.5 percent) and lowest among Puerto Rican Americans (6.6 percent) and Mexican Americans (4.0 percent). No CIs were provided (USDHHS 1998). The proportion of heavy smokers (≥ 25 cigarettes per day) among American Indian or Alaska Native women was not significantly different in the combined years 1978–1980 (12.7 percent) than in the combined years 1994–1995 (12.0 percent) (USDHHS 1998). BRFSS data for 1988–1992 showed that the proportion of heavy smokers among American Indian or Alaska Native women who smoked varied from 6.9 percent among women living in the northern plains to 1.2 percent among women living in the Southwest; these differences were not statistically significant (USDHHS 1998).

Novotny and coworkers (1988) concluded that differences by race in the number of cigarettes smoked per day persisted even after adjustment for gender and socioeconomic factors, such as occupation, employment, education, poverty level, and marital status. In the control group in a hospital-based, case-control study, differences by race in the number of cigarettes smoked per day remained significant after adjustment for degree of inhalation, length of the cigarette butt, duration of smoking, tar level, use of menthol cigarettes, time to the first cigarette after awakening, and educational level (Kabat et al. 1991). It is not clear whether racial or ethnic differences in the metabolism or elimination of nicotine (Wagenknecht et al. 1990a) or cultural factors are responsible for the differences in the number of cigarettes smoked per day (Caraballo et al. 1998; Pérez-Stable et al. 1998).

NHIS data also showed that the proportion of heavy smokers among women smokers with 12 years of education increased during 1970–1979, but no change occurred among women in other categories of educational attainment (Table 2.5). During 1979–1998, heavy smoking declined among women with 12 or more years of education. In 1998, women smokers with 9 to 11 years of education were more likely to be heavy smokers than were those with 12 or more years of education; similar patterns were reported for NHSDA data (USDHHS 1997). In NHIS during 1970–1998, a decline in heavy smoking occurred among men with 12 or more years of education (NCHS, public use data tape, 1998).

The prevalence of heavy smoking among both women and men who smoked increased during 1965–1979 and then declined during 1979–1998 (Table 2.5). NHIS data for 1965 and 1998 showed that among both women and men, the proportion of light smokers was higher in 1998. Among men, the proportion of moderate smokers was lower in 1998 than in 1965. The proportion of heavy smokers was comparable among both women and men in 1965 and in 1998. In the 1955 Current Population Survey (Haenszel et al. 1956) and for all years of NHIS, women were less likely than men to be heavy smokers. This finding was confirmed by other studies (Killen et al. 1988; Rogers and Crank 1988; Rimer et al. 1990; Rogers 1991; Giovino et al. 1994; USDHHS 1997) (Table 2.5) and was seen in NHIS data, even after adjustment for demographic factors (Novotny et al. 1988; Rogers et al. 1995). Among smokers, the 1998 NHIS data showed that 12.1 percent of women and 22.6 percent of men were heavy smokers. Among racial and ethnic groups, a significant difference by gender was observed among white non-Hispanics, black non-Hispanics, and Hispanics. Sample sizes were too small to assess gender differences among Asians and Pacific Islanders or among American Indians and Alaska Natives (NCHS, public use data tape, 1998). However, in NHIS data for the combined years 1978–1980 through the combined years 1992–1993, American Indian and Alaska Native women consistently smoked fewer cigarettes than did men (USDHHS 1998).

## Cigarette Brand Preference Among Women

In 1933, the three brands preferred by women were Chesterfield (31 percent), Lucky Strike (31 percent), and Camel (23 percent). In 1935, women smoked Chesterfield (30 percent), Camel (22 percent), Lucky Strike (16 percent), Philip Morris (9 percent), and Kool (8 percent) (Link 1935).

Recent national data on preferences for cigarette brands among women are lacking, and data are even more limited for assessing brand preferences by race or ethnicity. The 1978, 1979, 1980, and 1987 NHIS; the 1986 AUTS; and the 1999 NHSDA asked respondents about their preferences for cigarette brand. As reported in these surveys, women's preferences varied significantly by race and ethnicity and by age. Data from the combined 1978–1980 NHIS indicated that the 3 most popular brands among white women were Marlboro (14.4 percent), Winston (10.8 percent), and Salem (10.3 percent), and that the 3 most popular brands among black women were Kool (24.4 percent), Salem (19.4 percent), and Winston (10.3 percent); 27.5 percent of white women but only 15.6 percent of black women smoked brands other than the 12 most commonly used brands (USDHHS 1998).

Data from the 1986 AUTS also showed that Marlboro (23.7 percent), Salem (10.4 percent), and Winston (8.8 percent) were the most popular brands among white women and that Newport (20.5 percent), Kool (20.3 percent), and Salem (19.7 percent) were the most popular among black women (USDHHS 1998). The 1987 NHIS data showed similar results (USDHHS 1998). A 1993 study of smoking patterns among black women in Ohio found that four cigarette brands (Newport, Kool, Salem, and Benson & Hedges) accounted for 78 percent of the brands smoked and that 90 percent of black women who smoked used mentholated cigarettes (Ahijevych and Wewers 1993).

Published data from the 1999 NHSDA on brand used most often during the past month is available for women current smokers by age, but not by other demographic characteristics (SAMHSA 2000). In 1999, the brand used most often by women aged 26 years or older was Marlboro (29.1 percent). Each of the other specific brands was used by less than 8 percent of women.

National data on the preferences of Hispanic women for cigarette brand are limited. In the 1982–1984 HHANES, 30.4 percent of Mexican American women who smoked used Marlboro cigarettes, 15.7 percent Salem, 13.6 percent Winston, and 9.9 percent Benson & Hedges (Haynes et al. 1990). Among Puerto Rican American women who smoked, 22.0 percent used Newport cigarettes, 20.5 percent Marlboro, 17.6 percent Winston, and 8.5 percent Kool. Among Cuban American women who smoked, 18.7 percent used Benson & Hedges cigarettes, 16.2 percent Winston, 15.6 percent Salem, and 15.4 percent Marlboro. Cuban American women (25.7 percent) were more likely than Mexican American women (19.0 percent) or Puerto Rican American women (9.8 percent) to choose a brand other than one of the top seven brands (Haynes et al. 1990).

Brand preference appears to vary with age. At older ages, women were increasingly likely to purchase brands other than Marlboro. In the 1986 AUTS, Marlboro was the preference for more than 50 percent of women aged 18 through 24 years, 24 percent of women aged 25 through 44 years, and about 6 percent of women aged 45 years or older (USDHEW, public use data tape, 1986). Similarly, in a 1990 California survey, Marlboro was purchased by 69.4 percent of women aged 18 through 24 years, 49.5 percent of women aged 25 through 29 years, 33.0 percent of women aged 30 through 44 years, and 12.7 percent of women aged 45 years or older (Pierce et al. 1991a). Published data from the 1999 NHSDA noted that 56.6 percent of women smokers aged 18 through 25 years reported that the brand that they used most often in the past month was Marlboro. Newport was used by 16.5 percent of these women, and Camel by 9.2 percent. No other brand was used by more than 2.5 percent, and 10.4 percent chose a brand in the category "all other brands." For women smokers 26 years of age or older, however, only 29.1 percent reported that Marlboro was the brand used most frequently in the past month. Basic was used by 7.3 percent, Virginia Slims and Doral each by 6.7 percent, Newport by 6.6 percent, and Winston by 4.9 percent; 35.4 percent chose a brand in the category "all other brands" (SAMHSA 2000).

In the 1986 AUTS data, women most often reported smoking Marlboro (21.3 percent), Salem (11.4 percent), and Winston (8.4 percent); men most often chose Marlboro (30.2 percent), Winston (12.7 percent), and Salem (7.2 percent) (USDHEW, public use data tape, 1986). In a 1990 California study, comparable proportions of women (59.0 ± 4.8 percent) and men (66.8 ± 5.0 percent) aged 18 through 29 years purchased Marlboro cigarettes, but women older than age 29 years were less likely than men this age to purchase Marlboro (Pierce et al. 1991a). With increasing age, both women and men chose brands other than the top-selling ones, but women aged 45 years or older were considerably more likely than men in this age group to choose brands other than Marlboro. In published data from the 1999 NHSDA, Marlboro was used by 29.1 percent of women smokers and 41.0 percent of men smokers aged 26 years or older (SAMHSA 2000).

Market share of generic cigarettes increased dramatically from 1990 through 1993. A California study conducted in 1992 found that women were more likely than men to smoke generic brands, even after adjustment for household income (Cavin and Pierce 1996). Women were also more likely than men to smoke generic brands in a 1993 study of the 18 communities in the Community Intervention Trial for Smoking Cessation (COMMIT) (Cummings et al. 1997). Women smokers aged 45 years or older were more likely than younger women to smoke generic brands, and generic was the option most frequently selected by women smokers aged 45 years or older (15.7 percent).

In the United States, production of filter-tipped cigarettes increased from 0.6 percent of all cigarettes produced in 1950 to 97.5 percent in 1992 (Creek et al. 1994). The proportion was 98 percent for 1998 (Federal Trade Commission 2000). National surveys reveal that the use of filter-tipped cigarettes among women increased from 76.6 percent in 1964 to 90.6 percent in 1975. Early national data showed that women were more likely than men to smoke filter-tipped cigarettes (90.6 vs. 79.3 percent in 1975) (Schuman 1977), and results in other studies confirm this finding (Hammond and Garfinkel 1961; Wynder et al. 1984). In a 1984–1985 study of current smokers in New Mexico, however, Coultas and coworkers (1993) suggested that the gender gap had narrowed considerably: 92.9 percent of white women and 94.6 percent of Hispanic women smoked filter-tipped cigarettes, and 90.0 percent of white men and 87.0 percent of Hispanic men.

Since their introduction in the 1970s, consumption of cigarettes with low tar content, as measured by machine smoking, has increased dramatically in the United States (USDHHS 1981). About 13 percent of cigarettes consumed in 2000 had tar levels of 0 to 6 mg, and 52 percent had tar levels of 7 to 15 mg (Maxwell

2000). Hahn and colleagues (1990) found that 37 percent of white women reported trying cigarettes that were low in tar and nicotine, but only 27 percent of black women reported trying these products. Other data also suggested that white women are more likely than black women to choose low-tar or low-nicotine cigarettes (Wagenknecht et al. 1990a). In CPS-II, women were considerably more likely than men to choose cigarettes with tar yields less than 12.0 mg (51.6 vs. 34.8 percent) and were less likely to choose cigarettes with tar yields of 20.2 mg or more (3.6 vs. 8.8 percent) (Stellman and Garfinkel 1986). Other studies consistently showed that women are more likely than men to choose low-tar cigarettes (Hammond and Garfinkel 1961; USDHHS 1983; Wynder et al. 1984; Hahn et al. 1990; Coultas et al. 1993; Giovino et al. 1995) and are more likely to switch from high-nicotine to low-nicotine cigarettes (Grunberg et al. 1991).

The 1987 NHIS included a question on beliefs about the safety of low-tar and low-nicotine cigarettes. Among smokers, 30 percent of women and 34 percent of men believed that people who smoke low-tar and low-nicotine cigarettes are less likely to get cancer than are people who smoke high-tar and high-nicotine cigarettes (NCHS 1989). Thus, the differences in choice of cigarettes by women and men do not appear to be based on differences in the perceived safety of these types of cigarettes.

### Summary

Cigarette smoking became prevalent among women after it did among men. The prevalence of current smoking for women aged 18 years or older increased from probably less than 6 percent in 1924 to 33.9 percent in 1965 and then declined to 22.0 percent in 1998. In 1998, the prevalence of smoking was higher for women of reproductive age (25.3 percent) than for women overall (22.0 percent). Prevalence of current smoking peaked among women born in 1925–1944. Current smoking has been lower among women than among men across all surveys, but the decline in smoking prevalence was greater for men than for women from 1965 through 1985, and thus the gap narrowed over time. Since 1985, the pattern of change in prevalence has been comparable among women and men.

In 1997–1998, the prevalence of current smoking was highest among American Indian and Alaska Native women (34.5 percent), intermediate among white women (23.5 percent) and black women (21.9 percent), and lowest among Hispanic women (13.8 percent) and Asian or Pacific Islander women (11.2 percent). Prevalence was also higher among women with 9 to 11 years of education than among women with fewer or more years of education. During 1970–1998, smoking prevalence declined among women at all levels of educational attainment. During the same period, however, no decline was observed in prevalence among women of reproductive age with 12 years of education.

The prevalence of heavy smoking (≥ 25 cigarettes per day) among women who smoked increased from 13.8 percent in 1965 to 22.0 percent in 1979 and then decreased to 12.1 percent in 1998. Among women who smoked in 1998, white women (14.0 percent) were more likely to be heavy smokers than were black women (4.5 percent) or Hispanic women (2.1 percent). Among smokers, women (12.1 percent) were less likely than men (22.6 percent) to be heavy smokers.

## Cigarette Smoking Among Young Women

Initiation of tobacco use is largely complete by age 25 years (USDHHS 1994). Although 82 percent of smokers first try a cigarette before age 18 years, another 16 percent first try a cigarette between the ages of 18 and 24 years. As programs and policies increasingly focus on reducing tobacco use among minors, it will be even more important to monitor smoking among young adults, both to determine whether trends in adolescent smoking persist into adulthood and to monitor the potential increased initiation of tobacco use by young adults. In the analysis of data on cigarette smoking among young women (aged 18 through 24 years), because of small sample sizes in individual years, data from some survey years were combined to yield more stable estimates. Combined data were used for the following years: 1965–1966, 1978–1980, 1983 and 1985 (1983/1985), 1990–1991, 1992–1993, 1994–1995, and 1997–1998.

| 1983/1985 | 1990–1991 | 1992–1993 | 1994–1995 | 1997–1998 |
|---|---|---|---|---|
| 43.1 (±1.7) | 31.2 (±1.6) | 30.4 (±2.1) | 31.7 (±2.3) | 32.9 (±2.0) |
| | | | | |
| 47.6 (±2.0) | 38.5 (±2.0) | 37.6 (±2.7) | 39.3 (±3.0) | 41.1 (±2.8) |
| 32.6 (±3.9) | 15.1 (±2.3) | 11.1 (±3.1) | 12.3 (±3.4) | 12.4 (±2.8) |
| 26.0 (±4.3) | 16.8 (±3.2) | 17.8 (±4.4) | 21.6 (±4.7) | 19.1 (±3.6) |
| | | | | |
| 57.5 (±9.6) | 36.6 (±9.7) | 36.7 (±13.3)§ | 33.4 (±15.0)§ | 32.9 (±11.2) |
| 70.6 (±4.8) | 55.2 (±5.7) | 54.7 (±7.4) | 40.9 (±7.6) | 47.3 (±6.4) |
| 52.2 (±2.9) | 39.0 (±2.7) | 37.3 (±4.0) | 42.5 (±4.9) | 40.3 (±3.8) |
| 29.7 (±2.6) | 22.2 (±2.2) | 23.2 (±3.0) | 27.8 (±3.5) | 28.3 (±2.9) |
| 40.0 (±2.0) | 33.6 (±1.8) | 35.1 (±2.5) | 36.8 (±2.8) | 39.1 (±2.0) |

†NA = Not available.
‡For women aged 20–24 years. Data for four education categories not available for 1965.
§Estimate should be interpreted with caution because of the small number of respondents.
Sources: National Center for Health Statistics, public use data tapes, 1965–1966, 1970, 1974, 1978–1980, 1983, 1985, 1990–1995, 1997–1998.

for the 1997–1998 NHSDA (combined data) (data not shown) (SAMHSA, public use data tapes, 1997, 1998; Gfroerer et al. 1997b). In two self-administered mail surveys based on convenience samples of lesbians, prevalence of current smoking was 45 percent among women aged 17 through 24 years in 1984–1985 (Bradford et al. 1994) and 45 percent among women aged 18 through 25 years in the late 1980s (Skinner and Otis 1996).

The prevalence of current smoking from NHIS data was lower among young women (25.1 percent) than among young men (31.5 percent) (Table 2.7), a pattern also found in the 1997–1998 NHSDA. Within racial and ethnic subgroups, the prevalence of smoking was generally lower among young women than among young men. These findings were statistically significant in NHIS and NHSDA, except among whites in NHIS (data not shown) (NCHS, public use data tapes, 1997, 1998; SAMHSA, public use data tapes, 1997, 1998). A survey of more than 14,000 college students (60 percent of those to whom questionnaires were sent) who were attending 119 nationally representative four-year colleges found the prevalence of cigarette use within the past 30 days was nearly identical among women (28.5 percent) and men (28.4 percent) (Rigotti et al. 2000).

## Summary

Smoking among young women (aged 18 through 24 years) declined from 37.3 percent in 1965–1966 to 25.1 percent in 1997–1998. Most of this decline occurred from 1965–1966 through 1970 and from 1983/1985 (combined data) through 1990–1991, and smoking prevalence remained unchanged through 1997–1998. The decline in prevalence of smoking between 1965–1966 and 1983/1985 was greater among young men than among young women, but a decline between 1983/1985 and 1997–1998 only occurred among young women. Young black women had a dramatic decrease in smoking prevalence between 1983/1985 (27.8 percent) and 1997–1998 (9.6 percent). A substantial decline in smoking prevalence occurred among young Hispanic women between 1978–1980 (29.6 percent) and 1997–1998 (12.0 percent). The decline among young white women between 1965 and 1998 was small (6 percentage points). Since 1992–1993, smoking prevalence has been lower among young women than among young men.

**Table 2.7. Prevalence (% and 95% confidence interval) of current smoking among young women aged 18–24 years, by selected characteristics, National Health Interview Survey, United States, 1965–1998**

| Characteristic | 1965–1966 | 1970 | 1974 | 1978–1980 |
|---|---|---|---|---|
| Young women | 37.3 (±1.3) | 32.7 (±1.4) | 34.1 (±2.0) | 32.7 (±1.7) |
| Race/ethnicity* | | | | |
| White, non-Hispanic | 37.9 (±1.3) | 33.0 (±1.6) | 34.0 (±2.2) | 33.6 (±1.8) |
| Black, non-Hispanic | 34.7 (±3.7) | 32.2 (±3.7) | 35.6 (±5.3) | 30.4 (±4.4) |
| Hispanic | NA[†] | NA | NA | 29.6 (±5.0) |
| Education (number of years)[‡] | | | | |
| ≤ 8 | NA | 43.3 (±7.2) | 35.4 (±12.0)[§] | 36.9 (±8.5) |
| 9–11 | NA | 48.4 (±3.6) | 55.3 (±6.6) | 59.2 (±5.3) |
| 12 | NA | 37.0 (±2.6) | 35.8 (±3.2) | 35.0 (±2.6) |
| ≥ 13 | NA | 26.8 (±2.1) | 26.4 (±3.6) | 21.2 (±2.5) |
| Young men | 54.1 (±1.5) | 44.3 (±1.6) | 42.1 (±2.2) | 35.5 (±1.8) |

*Note:* Prevalence of current smoking is the percentage of all persons in each demographic category who reported smoking ≥ 100 cigarettes in their lifetime and who smoked at the time of the survey. Since 1992, estimates explicitly include persons who smoked only on some days.

*Ethnicity was not determined in 1965, 1966, 1970, or 1974. Thus, estimates for whites and for blacks during these years likely include data for some persons of Hispanic origin.

# Cigarette Smoking Among Girls

Smoking among adolescents is critically important because most tobacco use begins before age 18 years. Adolescents who use tobacco often become addicted and experience withdrawal symptoms similar to those reported by adults. Smoking during adolescence also produces significant health problems among young persons, including cough, phlegm production, increased number and severity of respiratory illnesses, decreased physical fitness, and reduced lung function (USDHHS 1994).

## Methodologic Issues and Definitions in Measurement of Smoking Among Girls

Methodologic issues exist regarding the measurement of smoking behavior among children and adolescents. In addition, the definitions used to assess smoking status among children and adolescents are different from those used for adults.

Several surveys (see Appendix 1) have assessed smoking behavior among girls (aged 12 through 17 or 18 years). Data from NTTS (girls aged 12 through 18 years) and NYTS (grades 6 through 12) were not analyzed independently for this report, but published estimates are presented here. For this report, primary data were analyzed from NHSDA (girls aged 12 through 17 years), MTF Surveys (8th-, 10th-, and 12th-grade girls), YRBSS (high school girls <18 years of age), the 1989 TAPS I (girls aged 12 through 18 years), and the 1993 TAPS II (girls aged 10 through 22 years). Published data for all five surveys are also cited in this report. NHSDA is a household survey, MTF Survey and YRBSS are self-administered surveys conducted in schools, and the 1989 TAPS I and 1993 TAPS II were telephone surveys that included household interviews of persons who could not be contacted by telephone. The data from these surveys are not directly comparable because of age differences of the populations and differences in survey methods, response rates, sampling error, and the settings of interviews (Gfroerer et al. 1997a). (See Appendix 1 and Appendix 3.)

| 1983/1985 | 1990–1991 | 1992–1993 | 1994–1995 | 1997–1998 |
|---|---|---|---|---|
| 33.0 (±1.6) | 22.4 (±1.4) | 24.3 (±2.0) | 23.5 (±2.1) | 25.1 (±1.7) |
| | | | | |
| 36.2 (±1.9) | 27.8 (±1.8) | 30.3 (±2.6) | 29.5 (±2.8) | 31.6 (±2.4) |
| 27.8 (±3.7) | 11.0 (±2.1) | 9.3 (±2.9) | 9.8 (±3.0) | 9.6 (±2.5) |
| 18.1 (±3.7) | 11.8 (±3.1) | 13.1 (±4.0) | 14.9 (±4.0) | 12.0 (±2.3) |
| | | | | |
| 48.5 (±9.6) | 28.4 (±8.8) | 34.1 (±13.1)§ | 29.7 (±14.7)§ | 27.0 (±11.4)§ |
| 57.8 (±5.2) | 46.3 (±5.7) | 50.4 (±7.4) | 34.6 (±7.8) | 42.8 (±6.5) |
| 40.5 (±2.9) | 28.0 (±2.4) | 28.6 (±3.8) | 30.5 (±4.4) | 30.8 (±3.7) |
| 20.0 (±2.2) | 14.2 (±1.7) | 17.6 (±2.7) | 19.3 (±3.1) | 19.8 (±2.3) |
| 30.5 (±1.8) | 25.1 (±1.7) | 28.3 (±2.3) | 28.8 (±2.6) | 31.5 (±2.0) |

†NA = Not available.
‡For women aged 20–24 years. Data for four education categories not available for 1965.
§Estimate should be interpreted with caution because of the small number of respondents.
Sources: National Center for Health Statistics, public use data tapes, 1965–1966, 1970, 1974, 1978–1980, 1983, 1985, 1990–1995, 1997–1998.

Self-administered school surveys generally offer greater confidentiality and anonymity than household surveys. Thus, underreporting of smoking is generally a greater issue for household surveys. Williams and colleagues (1979) found that adolescents accurately reported smoking status if confidentiality was stressed. For girls aged 12 through 17 years, NHSDA estimates are used because they allow assessment of time trends since 1975 (see also Appendix 1). However, the potential for underreporting exists, as described below. For high school seniors, MTF Survey estimates are used because they provide data on trends since 1975 and because there is less underreporting in school-based surveys. The 1993 TAPS II was primarily a follow-up survey of the 1989 respondents; it cannot be used for estimates of the prevalence of tobacco use because of differential loss to follow-up among smokers and nonsmokers (see Appendix 1). The survey is used, however, to provide estimates of use of cigarette brands by current smokers.

NHSDA is a household survey conducted periodically to measure the prevalence of use of illicit drugs, alcohol, and tobacco. Before 1994, NHSDA interviewers questioned respondents aloud, which tended to diminish privacy and confidentiality if other persons in the household were present. In the absence of a special effort to ensure privacy of responses, household surveys have been found to underreport the prevalence of tobacco use, particularly among younger adolescents (USDHHS 1994). Consequently, starting in 1994, information on sensitive topics, such as tobacco use and illicit drug use, was collected through a self-administered, written questionnaire to increase the privacy of responses. In 1994, both the old and new methods were used in a split-sample design. The 1994-A data were obtained through personal interviews, and the 1994-B data were obtained by respondents recording their own answers, which the interviewers did not see. Because respondents recorded their own answers, skip patterns used in the personal interviews could not be used (see definition for "skip pattern" in Appendix 2). In the 1994-B and subsequent surveys, responses were edited to make the initial answers on smoking status consistent with later answers. This increased editing and the change in methods significantly increased the estimate of current smoking (Brittingham et al. 1998). Estimates in the 1994-B NHSDA were two times higher than those in the 1994-A survey overall and three times higher for 12- and 13-year-olds (SAMHSA 1995b). The 1994-B estimates are more comparable to those from self-administered school surveys.

Children who participated in NHSDA during 1974–1977 were categorized as ever having smoked if they reported that they had ever smoked a cigarette. In the 1979–1994-A NHSDA, ever smoked was defined as the converse of never having smoked a cigarette. In the 1994-B and subsequent NHSDA surveys, persons who had ever smoked were respondents who reported ever having smoked a cigarette, even one or two puffs. In the YRBS, ever trying smoking was defined as ever having tried a cigarette, even one or two puffs. For all surveys, current smoking was defined as any cigarette smoking during the 30 days before the survey.

## Trends in Ever Trying Smoking or Ever Smoking Among Girls

Trend data for 1968–1979 on the prevalence of adolescent girls ever trying smoking are available from NTTS (USDHEW 1979b). However, comparing these data with the more recent trend data from NHSDA is difficult because in NTTS, data were combined for persons who had never smoked (never tried a cigarette, not even a few puffs) and "experimenters" (persons who had at least a few puffs but had not smoked 100 cigarettes). The NHSDA data include experimenters with persons who had ever smoked. Thus, NTTS data provide lower estimates of the prevalence of ever smoking than do NHSDA data.

The NTTS data showed that the prevalence of ever trying smoking (i.e., former and current smoking combined) increased among females aged 12 through 18 years between 1968 and 1974; it then decreased between 1974 and 1979. NTTS data also indicated that never smoking or only experimenting with cigarettes decreased somewhat with age, whereas current smoking increased with age (USDHEW 1979b).

In the 1974–1994-A NHSDA, the prevalence of ever smoking among girls aged 12 through 17 years declined, on average, 0.86 percentage points per year (Figure 2.6). Comparing these trends to patterns after 1994 is difficult because of the 1994 changes in survey methods. Among girls, however, the new methods increased the estimate of ever smoking by 2 percentage points. The prevalence of ever smoking among girls was essentially unchanged in NHSDA between 1994-B and 1998.

Among adolescents aged 12 through 18 years in NTTS, girls were less likely than boys to have ever tried smoking, but the gap narrowed over time. The prevalence of ever trying smoking was 13.1 percent in 1968, 18.3 percent in 1972, and 18.9 percent in 1979 among girls, and 22.9 percent in 1968, 26.0 percent in 1972, and 19.2 percent in 1979 among boys (USDHEW 1979b). NHSDA data showed no significant gender-specific differences in ever smoking from 1976 through 1985 (Figure 2.6). In 1988–1992, however, the prevalence of ever smoking was significantly lower among girls than among boys. The 1989 TAPS I and the 1992 MTF Survey also found slightly lower estimates among girls than among boys for this period (Bachman et al. 1993b). For example, in the 1989 TAPS I, the prevalence of ever trying smoking was 44.4 percent among girls and 48.2 percent among boys (Moss et al. 1992). However, Kann and colleagues (1993) found no significant gender differences in YRBS. In the 1993–1998 NHSDA, gender-specific differences were generally not significant, a pattern also noted in the 1993, 1995, 1997, and 1999 YRBS and the 1993–1998 MTF Surveys (University of Michigan, Institute for Social Research, public use data tapes, 1993–1998; Kann et al. 1995, 1996, 1998, 2000).

## Ever Trying Smoking and Ever Smoking Among Girls by Demographic Characteristics

The prevalence of ever trying smoking or ever smoking varies by age or grade; differences by race or by gender are less consistent. The 1998 NHSDA and the 1999 YRBS were used to estimate the prevalence of ever trying smoking or ever smoking among adolescent girls (Table 2.8). The proportion who had ever tried smoking or who had ever smoked varied dramatically across surveys, ranging from 35.5 percent in NHSDA to 69.1 percent in YRBS. Published 1999 NHSDA data for lifetime smoking among girls aged 12 through 17 years was 36.3 percent (SAMHSA 2000). In the 1999 NYTS, 63.0 (±3.5) percent of high school girls had ever used cigarettes (CDC 2000b). The higher estimates for all demographic categories of YRBS are consistent with the older age of participants in the high school YRBS (generally aged 14 through 17 years); NHSDA assessed adolescents aged 12 through 17 years. The lower NHSDA estimates are also consistent with the underestimation generally found in household surveys. NHSDA estimates were essentially unchanged after adjustment for demographic factors (USDHHS 1997).

In both NHSDA and YRBS, the percentage of girls who had ever tried smoking or who had ever smoked a cigarette increased with age: girls aged 15 through 17 years were more likely than those aged 12 through 14 years to have tried a cigarette or to have ever smoked (Table 2.8). Among girls in the 1998 MTF

**Figure 2.6. Prevalence (%) of ever trying smoking and current smoking among adolescents aged 12–17 years, by gender, National Household Survey on Drug Abuse, United States, 1974–1998**

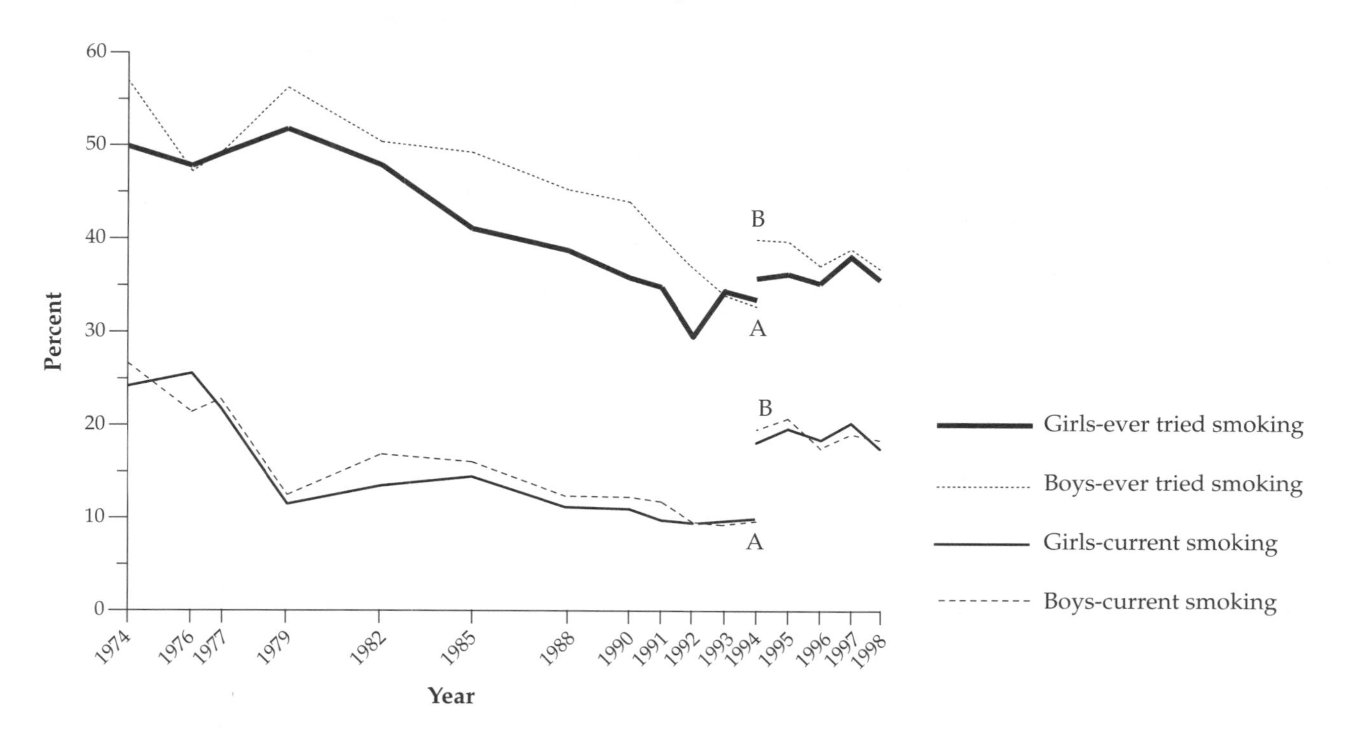


*Note:* The data changed abruptly in 1994 because of a change in survey methodology, questions, and editing procedures. The 1994 survey used a split-sample design; 1994-A used the same method of personal interview as in previous years; 1994-B used a more private self-administered answer sheet and different editing procedures that were also used in subsequent years. In 1974–1977, ever tried smoking is the percentage of all persons in each demographic category who reported ever having smoked. In 1979–1994-A, smoking status was determined by response to the question, "About how old were you when you first tried a cigarette?" If any age was given, the person was considered to have ever tried smoking. For 1994-B–1998, respondents who ever tried smoking were those who had ever smoked a cigarette, even one or two puffs. Prevalence of current smoking is the percentage of all persons in each demographic category who smoked during the 30 days before the survey.

Sources: Alcohol, Drug Abuse, and Mental Health Administration, public use data tapes, 1974, 1976, 1977, 1979, 1982, 1985, 1988, 1990–1992; Substance Abuse and Mental Health Services Administration, public use data tapes, 1993–1998.

Survey, the prevalence of ever trying smoking increased with grade in school: 45.0 percent for 8th graders, 58.7 percent for 10th graders, and 63.4 percent for 12th graders (University of Michigan, Institute for Social Research, public use data tape, 1998). These findings are consistent with those from other studies in which ever trying smoking or ever smoking increased with increasing age or grade in school (CDC 1989, 1991a, 1992; Moss et al. 1992; USDHHS 1994). In published data for the 1999 YRBS, the prevalence of ever trying cigarettes increased from grade 9 through grade 10, then remained unchanged through grade 12 (Kann et al. 2000). In 1999 NYTS data, the prevalence of ever smoking cigarettes was 27.7 (±3.7) percent for middle school girls and 63.0 (±3.5) percent for girls in high school (CDC 2000b).

Although the 1999 YRBS data showed no racial or ethnic differences, in the 1998 NHSDA, white girls were more likely than black girls or Hispanic girls to have ever tried smoking (Table 2.8). Data from the 1989 TAPS I and the 1996–1998 MTF Surveys also indicated that the prevalence of ever trying smoking was higher among white girls than among black girls (Moss et al. 1992; University of Michigan, Institute for Social Research, public use data tapes, 1996–1998). Data from the 1989 TAPS I and the 1994 MTF Survey

**Table 2.8. Prevalence (% and 95% confidence interval) of ever trying smoking or ever smoking and current smoking among girls less than 18 years of age, by selected characteristics, National Household Survey on Drug Abuse (NHSDA) and Youth Risk Behavior Survey (YRBS), United States, 1998–1999**

| | Ever trying smoking or ever smoking* | | Current smoking† | |
|---|---|---|---|---|
| Characteristic | 1998 NHSDA (ages 12–17) | 1999 YRBS (grades 9–12) | 1998 NHSDA (ages 12–17) | 1999 YRBS (grades 9–12) |
| Girls | 35.5 (±2.5) | 69.1 (±3.1) | 17.7 (±2.0) | 33.7 (±2.6) |
| Age (years) | | | | |
| 12–14 | 21.8 (±3.1) | 58.5 (±8.3) | 10.7 (±2.3) | 22.9 (±5.9) |
| 15–17 | 49.0 (±3.6) | 70.4 (±2.7) | 24.7 (±3.1) | 35.0 (±2.9) |
| Race/ethnicity | | | | |
| White, non-Hispanic | 40.9 (±3.4) | 69.4 (±4.0) | 21.0 (±2.8) | 37.9 (±4.0) |
| Black, non-Hispanic | 22.6 (±3.9) | 69.0 (±6.6) | 10.6 (±2.8) | 17.7 (±4.1) |
| Hispanic | 30.7 (±3.9) | 70.4 (±4.2) | 14.7 (±3.2) | 31.1 (±4.7) |
| Boys | 36.1 (±2.4) | 68.9 (±4.6) | 18.7 (±1.9) | 32.5 (±3.0) |

*Note:* NHSDA is a household survey that includes adolescents 12–17 years of age; 67.0% were 14–17 years of age. YRBS is a school-based survey that includes high school students in grades 9–12; these analyses were restricted to those less than 18 years of age; of these, 99.8% were 14–17 years of age. Data are not comparable across surveys due to differences in ages surveyed and survey methods.

*For NHSDA, prevalence of ever smoking is the percentage of all persons in each demographic category who reported having smoked at least one or two puffs from a cigarette. For YRBS, prevalence of ever trying smoking is the percentage of all persons in each demographic category who reported ever trying cigarette smoking, even one or two puffs.

†For NHSDA, prevalence of current smoking is the percentage of all persons in each demographic category who reported any cigarette smoking during the 30 days before the survey. For YRBS, current smoking status is based on response to the question, "How often have you smoked cigarettes during the past 30 days?" Those reporting any cigarette smoking during the 30 days before the survey were classified as current smokers.

Sources: **NHSDA:** Substance Abuse and Mental Health Services Administration, public use data tape, 1998. **YRBS:** Centers for Disease Control and Prevention, Division of Adolescent and School Health, public use data tape, 1999.

indicated that the prevalence of ever trying smoking was higher among white girls than among Hispanic girls (USDHHS 1994). The 1997 YRBS for all high school students who attended schools funded by the Bureau of Indian Affairs found that the percentage who had ever tried a cigarette was substantially higher among these girls (93.5 percent) than that among high school girls overall (69.3 percent) (Bureau of Indian Affairs 1997; CDC 1998a; Kann et al. 1998).

Both NHSDA and YRBS data showed no significant gender-specific differences in the prevalence of ever trying or ever smoking (Table 2.8), a finding also noted in the 1999 NYTS (CDC 2000b). Data from several other sources indicated that gender-specific differences in the prevalence of ever smoking are small (USDHHS 1994).

## Trends in Current Smoking Among Girls

NHSDA data indicated that the prevalence of current smoking among girls aged 12 through 17 years decreased, on average, 0.71 percentage points per year from 1974 through 1994 (Figure 2.6). Most of the decline occurred from 1974 through 1979; the prevalence changed little from 1982 through 1994. The prevalence of current smoking also declined among boys aged 12 through 17 years from 1974 through 1994; the average rate of decline was 0.85 percentage points per year. Comparing these trends with patterns after 1994 is difficult because the changes in NHSDA methods increased the estimate of current smoking by 8 percentage points among girls and 10 percentage points among boys. From 1994 through 1998, current smoking was

**Figure 2.7. Prevalence (%) of current smoking among girls, by grade in school, Monitoring the Future Survey, United States, 1975–2000**

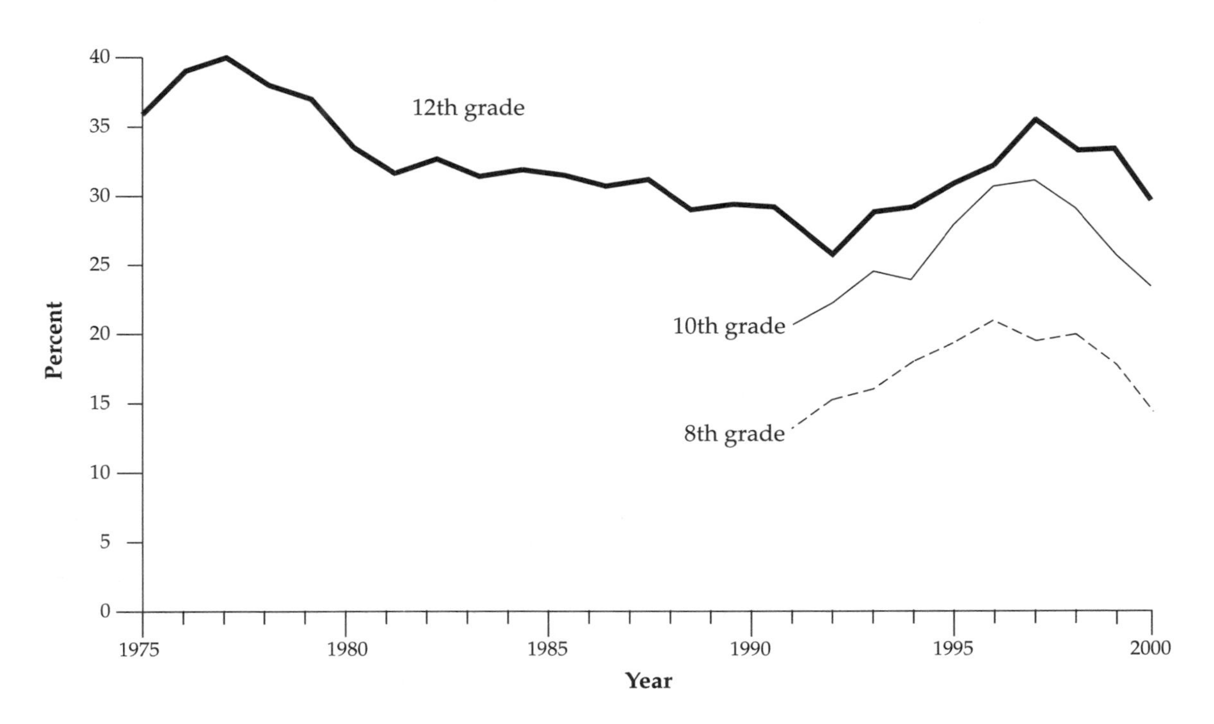


*Note:* Prevalence of current smoking is the percentage of all persons in each demographic category who reported smoking ≥ 1 cigarette during the previous 30 days.
Sources: University of Michigan, Institute for Social Research, public use data tapes, 1975–1998; University of Michigan 1999b, 2000.

unchanged among girls and boys. No gender-specific differences in prevalence for 1974–1998 were noted.

Beginning in 1991, MTF Surveys assessed current smoking among 8th- and 10th-grade girls (Figure 2.7). During 1991–1996, the prevalence of current smoking increased from 13.1 to 21.1 percent among 8th-grade girls; prevalence then decreased to 14.7 percent in 2000. Among 10th-grade girls, the prevalence of current smoking increased from 20.7 percent in 1991 to 31.1 percent in 1997; prevalence then decreased to 23.6 percent in 2000 (University of Michigan 2000).

In reporting smoking prevalence by race, two-year rolling averages (see Appendix 2) were used to generate more stable estimates. NHSDA data showed that the prevalence of current smoking decreased between 1974–1976 (combined data) and 1993–1994-A (combined data) among both white girls and black girls (Figure 2.8). The decline was significantly greater among black girls (average, 1.23 percentage points per year) than among white girls (average, 0.73 percentage points per year), but most of the decline among both white girls and black girls occurred from 1976–1977 through 1985–1988. Comparing these trends with patterns after 1994 is difficult because of changes in NHSDA methods. These changes increased the prevalence estimates by 7 percentage points among white girls and 12 percentage points among black girls. Between 1994 and 1998, current smoking among white girls and black girls was unchanged.

## Current Smoking Among Girls by Demographic Characteristics

The association between various demographic characteristics and current smoking was assessed using 1998 NHSDA and the 1999 YRBS data. Estimates of the prevalence of current smoking in 1998–1999 varied markedly by survey, ranging from 17.7 percent (NHSDA) to 33.7 percent (YRBS) (Table 2.8); the lower NHSDA estimate probably reflects the younger age of

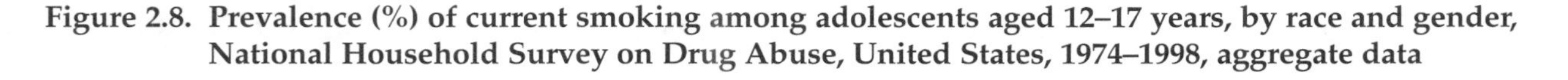
**Figure 2.8. Prevalence (%) of current smoking among adolescents aged 12–17 years, by race and gender, National Household Survey on Drug Abuse, United States, 1974–1998, aggregate data**

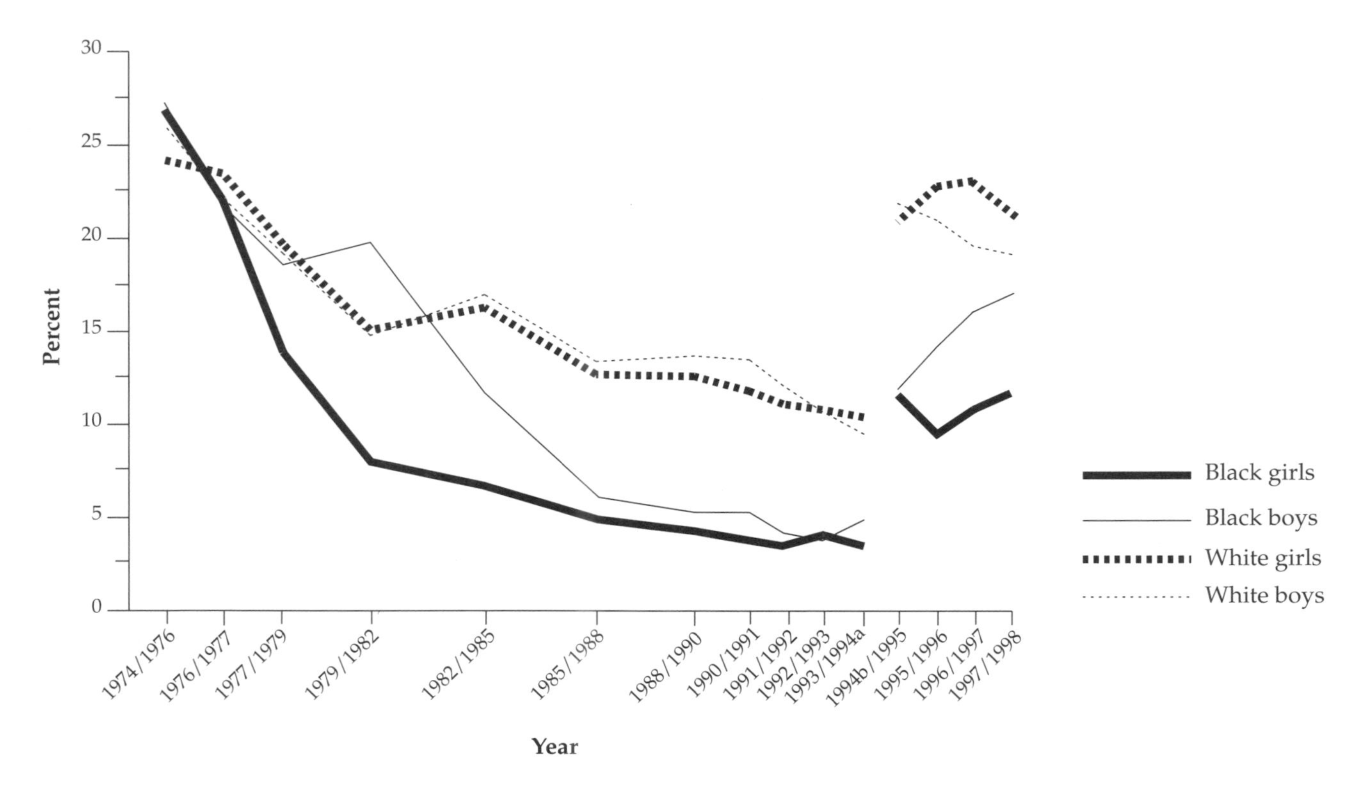


*Note:* Prevalence was calculated by using averages for combined years. Prevalence of current smoking is the percentage of all persons in each demographic category who reported any cigarette smoking during the 30 days preceding the survey. Except for 1985, data include respondents of Hispanic origin. There is an abrupt change in the data points in 1994 because the 1994 survey used a split-sample design: 1994-A used the same method of personal interview as in previous years; 1994-B used a more private self-administered answer sheet and different editing procedures that were also used in subsequent years.
Sources: Alcohol, Drug Abuse, and Mental Health Administration, public use data tapes, 1974, 1976, 1977, 1979, 1982, 1985, 1988, 1990–1992; Substance Abuse and Mental Health Services Administration, public use data tapes, 1993, 1994-A, 1994-B, 1995–1998.

respondents as well as the underreporting generally found in household surveys, where privacy may be compromised. Published data from the 1999 NHSDA showed a similar prevalence of current smoking among girls 12 through 17 years of age (15.0 percent) (SAMHSA 2000). In the 1999 NYTS, 28.2 (±3.3) percent of high school girls had smoked cigarettes in the previous month (CDC 2000b).

In both surveys, girls aged 15 through 17 years were significantly more likely to smoke cigarettes than were girls aged 12 through 14 years. For example, the 1998 NHSDA data showed 10.7 percent of girls aged 12 through 14 years and 24.7 percent of girls aged 15 through 17 years were current smokers. The 2000 MTF Survey data indicated that the prevalence of current smoking among girls was directly associated with grade in school: 14.7 percent for 8th graders, 23.6 percent for 10th graders, and 29.7 percent for 12th graders (Figure 2.7) (University of Michigan 2000). A similar pattern was noted in published data for all high school girls in the 1999 YRBS; the prevalence of current smoking was 40.5 percent for 12th-grade girls but only 29.2 percent for 9th-grade girls (Kann et al. 2000). In the 1999 NYTS, the prevalence of current smoking was 28.2 (±3.3) percent for high school girls but 8.9 (±1.7) percent for middle school girls (CDC 2000b).

Both NHSDA and YRBS data showed that white girls were more likely than black girls to be current smokers (Table 2.8). The NHSDA data also indicated that white girls were more likely than Hispanic girls to be current smokers. Similar patterns were noted among all high school girls in the 1999 YRBS (Kann et al. 2000). Data on current smoking among girls of other racial and ethnic groups are limited, but a representative 1991 survey of Navajo girls aged 12 through 19 years found a smoking prevalence of 9 percent (Freedman et al. 1997). In contrast, the 1993 YRBS of American Indians who lived on or near Montana reservations reported that the prevalence of cigarette smoking among girls in grades 9 through 12 was 57 percent (Nelson et al. 1997), and the 1997 YRBS data from schools funded by the Bureau of Indian Affairs reported that the prevalence of smoking among all high school girls was 65.1 percent (Bureau of Indian Affairs 1997).

Although sexual orientation is not broken down by category or by gender, state YRBS data represent some of the strongest data available on smoking among gay, lesbian, and bisexual youth in that YRBS uses a probability-based, representative sample instead of a random sample in restricted geographic areas or a convenience sample. Research suggests that the prevalence of current smoking is higher among lesbian, gay, and bisexual youth than among youth in general. The 1993 and 1995 Massachusetts YRBS included a question on sexual orientation. Current smoking among lesbian, gay, and bisexual (data not broken down by category) students was 38.2 ± 12.3 percent in 1993 and 59.3 percent ($p < 0.00001$ compared with youth who were not lesbian, gay, or bisexual) in 1995 (Faulkner and Cranston 1998; Garofalo et al. 1998). This prevalence was greater than current smoking prevalence among students overall in the Massachusetts YRBS (30.2 percent in 1993 and 35.7 percent in 1995) (Kann et al. 1995, 1996).

NHSDA and YRBS data demonstrated that current smoking was equally prevalent among girls and boys (Table 2.8) (CDC 1998a). Similarly, in an examination of adolescent smoking trends, in which MTF Survey, NHSDA, and NHIS data were used, Nelson and coworkers (1995) and others (USDHHS 1994) found that, as of 1991, the prevalence of current smoking was similar among adolescent girls and boys. No gender-specific differences in smoking prevalence were noted in the 1999 NYTS (CDC 2000b).

## Trends in Ever Smoking Among High School Senior Girls

Some of the earliest estimates of ever smoking among adolescents are from a study conducted by ACS in 1958 among 21,980 high school students in the area of Portland, Oregon. In this study, the prevalence of ever smoking among high school senior girls was 68.3 percent and was lower than the 81.0 percent for senior boys (Horn et al. 1959).

MTF Survey data indicated that the prevalence of ever smoking among high school senior girls was 74.8 percent in 1976; it declined to 59.9 percent in 1992 (average annual decline, 0.93 percentage points), but was 63.4 percent in 1998 (average annual increase, 0.58 percentage points) (Table 2.9). The decline in ever smoking from 1976 through 1998 was greater among black high school senior girls (33.0 ± 7.2 percentage points) than among white high school senior girls (6.0 ± 3.7 percentage points). Except for 1981–1982, when the prevalence of ever smoking was higher among senior girls than among senior boys, and 1992, when the prevalence of ever smoking was lower among girls than among boys, no gender-specific differences in ever smoking were noted for MTF Surveys for 1976–1997. In 1998, the prevalence of ever smoking was lower among girls than among boys—this finding was of borderline statistical significance. The average rate of decline in smoking prevalence in 1976–1998 was comparable among girls and boys.

## Trends in Current and Daily Smoking Among High School Senior Girls

In 1958, the prevalence of current smoking among high school senior girls was 16.5 percent in the area of Portland, Oregon (Horn et al. 1959). In the NTTS telephone survey of girls 17 through 18 years of age, the prevalence increased from 21.0 percent in 1968 to 27.0 percent in 1979 (USDHEW 1979b). Estimates of current smoking in the late 1970s from NTTS data were lower than those from MTF Survey data, a finding consistent with the methodologic difference between household and school-based surveys. In MTF Surveys, the prevalence of current smoking among high school senior girls declined from 39.9 percent in 1977 to 25.8 percent in 1992, then increased to 35.3 percent in 1997 (Table 2.9 and Figure 2.7). Prevalence decreased to 29.7 percent in 2000 (Figure 2.7) (University of Michigan 2000). Smoking prevalence in 2000 was the same as in 1988. NHSDA data also indicated a peak prevalence of current smoking among 17- to 18-year-old girls in the late 1970s (SAMHSA, public use data tapes, 1976, 1977).

MTF Survey data on senior high school students showed that prevalence of current smoking was higher among girls than among boys in the late 1970s and early 1980s, but the decline in smoking prevalence in 1976–1992 was more rapid among girls than among

**Table 2.9. Prevalence (% and 95% confidence interval) of ever smoking and current smoking among high school seniors, by gender, Monitoring the Future Survey, United States, 1976–1998**

| Year | Ever smoking* | | Current smoking† | |
|---|---|---|---|---|
| | Girls | Boys | Girls | Boys |
| 1976 | 74.8 (±1.9) | 75.8 (±1.5) | 39.0 (±2.2) | 37.8 (±1.7) |
| 1977 | 74.9 (±1.8) | 76.4 (±1.5) | 39.9 (±2.1) | 36.6 (±1.7) |
| 1978 | 75.6 (±1.7) | 74.4 (±1.4) | 38.0 (±1.9) | 34.6 (±1.5) |
| 1979 | 74.9 (±1.8) | 72.6 (±1.5) | 37.0 (±2.0) | 31.1 (±1.6) |
| 1980 | 71.7 (±1.9) | 70.0 (±1.6) | 33.5 (±2.0) | 26.6 (±1.5) |
| 1981 | 73.3 (±1.8) | 68.5 (±1.5) | 31.6 (±1.9) | 26.5 (±1.4) |
| 1982 | 72.1 (±1.8) | 68.0 (±1.5) | 32.7 (±1.9) | 26.6 (±1.4) |
| 1983 | 71.4 (±1.9) | 69.0 (±1.5) | 31.4 (±1.9) | 28.0 (±1.5) |
| 1984 | 71.4 (±1.9) | 67.0 (±1.6) | 31.9 (±2.0) | 26.0 (±1.5) |
| 1985 | 69.9 (±1.9) | 67.1 (±1.6) | 31.5 (±1.9) | 28.0 (±1.5) |
| 1986 | 68.8 (±2.0) | 66.0 (±1.7) | 30.7 (±2.0) | 27.9 (±1.6) |
| 1987 | 68.7 (±1.9) | 65.4 (±1.6) | 31.2 (±1.9) | 27.2 (±1.5) |
| 1988 | 67.3 (±1.9) | 65.3 (±1.6) | 29.0 (±1.9) | 28.0 (±1.5) |
| 1989 | 66.6 (±1.9) | 64.2 (±1.6) | 29.4 (±1.9) | 27.6 (±1.5) |
| 1990 | 64.4 (±2.1) | 64.2 (±1.6) | 29.2 (±2.0) | 29.1 (±1.5) |
| 1991 | 62.4 (±2.1) | 63.6 (±1.7) | 27.3 (±2.0) | 28.8 (±1.6) |
| 1992 | 59.9 (±2.0) | 63.7 (±1.7) | 25.8 (±1.8) | 29.3 (±1.6) |
| 1993 | 60.2 (±2.0) | 63.4 (±1.7) | 28.6 (±1.9) | 30.6 (±1.6) |
| 1994 | 60.9 (±2.0) | 63.2 (±1.7) | 29.4 (±2.0) | 33.0 (±1.6) |
| 1995 | 63.6 (±2.0) | 64.6 (±1.7) | 31.8 (±2.0) | 34.7 (±1.7) |
| 1996 | 62.1 (±2.1) | 64.4 (±1.7) | 32.4 (±2.1) | 35.0 (±1.7) |
| 1997 | 64.4 (±2.0) | 65.9 (±1.7) | 35.3 (±2.0) | 37.4 (±1.7) |
| 1998 | 63.4 (±2.1) | 67.1 (±1.6) | 33.4 (±2.0) | 36.2 (±1.7) |

*Note:* Confidence intervals are asymmetric; the number presented here reflects the largest value for each confidence interval to provide the most conservative estimates.
*Based on response to the question, "Have you ever smoked cigarettes?" Prevalence of ever smoking is the percentage of all persons in each demographic category who reported ever having smoked a cigarette, even once or twice.
†Based on response to the question, "How frequently have you smoked cigarettes during the past 30 days?" Prevalence of current smoking is the percentage of all persons in each demographic category who reported smoking ≥ 1 cigarette during the previous 30 days.
Sources: University of Michigan, Institute for Social Research, public use data tapes, 1976–1998.

boys (average, 0.83 vs. 0.53 percentage points per year); the increase during 1992–1998 averaged 1.27 percentage points per year for girls and 1.15 percentage points per year for boys (Table 2.9). As a result, prevalence has been comparable among girls and boys since the mid-1980s. In 1998, the prevalence of current smoking was not significantly different among girls (33.4 percent) and boys (36.2 percent). From MTF Surveys, much of the decline in the prevalence of current smoking among high school senior girls occurred from 1976 through 1981. Among girls, the prevalence decreased, on average, 1.48 percentage points per year from 1976 through 1981 and 0.53 percentage points per year from 1981 through 1992. Among boys, the prevalence decreased, on average, 2.26 percentage points per year from 1976 through 1981 and 0.25 percentage points per year from 1981 through 1992. Similar patterns were seen among 17- and 18-year-olds in NHSDA: current smoking among girls declined, on average, 3.04 percentage points per year from 1976 through 1985 but only 1.2 percentage points per year from 1988 through 1994; it remained unchanged from 1994 through 1998 (SAMHSA, public use data tapes, 1976–1998).

For reporting smoking prevalence by race, two-year rolling averages were used to generate more stable estimates. MTF Survey data showed a decline in the prevalence of current smoking among both white and black high school senior girls between 1976–1977 (combined data) and 1991–1992 (combined data). The decline was dramatic among black girls: from 37.5 ± 3.7 percent in 1976–1977 to 7.0 ± 3.5 percent in 1991–1992 (average, 1.9 percentage points per year). The corresponding decrease among white girls was from 39.9 ± 1.9 to 31.2 ± 1.9 percent (average, 0.54 percentage points per year). Most of the decline among white girls occurred from 1976–1977 through 1981–1982. From 1991–1992 through 1997–1998, prevalence increased among both white and black high school senior girls (from 31.2 ± 1.9 to 41.3 ± 2.1 percent and from 7.0 ± 3.5 to 12.1 ± 2.4 percent, respectively); this increase was statistically significant only among white girls. NHSDA data also showed a decline in current smoking from 1976–1977 through 1993–1994 that was 1.9 times greater among black females than among white females aged 17 or 18 years. No significant change in prevalence was noted among either white girls or black girls from 1994–1995 through 1997–1998 (SAMHSA, public use data tapes, 1976–1998). MTF Survey data for 1976–1979 showed that smoking prevalence among high school senior girls was 55.3 percent among American Indians or Alaska Natives, 39.1 percent among whites, 33.6 percent among blacks, 31.4 percent among Hispanics, and 24.4 percent among Asians or Pacific Islanders (USDHHS 1998). In 1990–1994, smoking prevalence among high school senior girls was highest among American Indians or Alaska Natives (39.4 percent) and whites (33.1 percent), intermediate among Hispanics (19.2 percent) and Asians or Pacific Islanders (13.8 percent), and lowest among blacks (8.6 percent). However, no CIs were provided (USDHHS 1998). In an analysis of combined data from the 1985–1989 MTF Surveys, Bachman and colleagues (1991b) found that the prevalence of current smoking was 24.7 percent among Puerto Rican American and Latin American girls and 18.7 percent among Mexican American girls.

To assess racial differences in smoking before 1976, published data from Burns and colleagues (1997) on smoking among birth cohorts of women over time were used to derive estimates of smoking prevalence among 18-year-old girls and boys. Data for 1976–1998 were obtained directly from MTF Surveys of high school seniors (Figure 2.9). These analyses showed that in the first half of the century, smoking prevalence was high among both white and black 18-year-old boys and low, but increasing, among both white and black 18-year-old girls. After 1950, smoking prevalence decreased among white boys and black boys and continued to increase among white girls and black girls. As a result of these patterns, the prevalence of smoking was comparable among all four racial and gender groups in the mid-to-late 1970s. Subsequently, prevalence decreased among black girls and boys but remained higher among white girls and boys.

MTF Survey data were also used to assess the prevalence of daily smoking among high school senior girls. Temporal patterns similar to those described for current smoking were found (Figure 2.10). In 1976, 28.8 percent of girls were daily smokers. The prevalence of daily smoking declined among high school senior girls between 1977 and 1981 (from 30.3 to 21.7 percent), but remained essentially stable from 1981 (21.7 percent) through 1987 (20.4 percent). It then decreased to 16.5 percent in 1992, increased to 21.6 percent in 1998, and then decreased to 19.7 percent in 2000 (University of Michigan, Institute for Social Research, public use data tapes, 1976–1998; University of Michigan, unpublished data, 2000). The prevalence of daily smoking was higher among girls than among boys during 1979–1987, but during 1988–1998, there was no gender-specific difference in smoking prevalence (Husten et al. 1996; University of Michigan, Institute for Social Research, public use data tape, 1998). Gender differences remained small in 1999 and 2000 (University of Michigan, unpublished data, 1999, 2000). The 1989 TAPS I data had consistent findings: daily smoking was similar by gender among adolescents aged 16 through 18 years (46.1 percent among girls and 48.7 percent among boys) (CDC, Office on Smoking and Health, public use data tape, 1989).

MTF Survey data on daily smoking were analyzed by race by using two-year rolling averages. Among white high school senior girls, daily smoking declined substantially between 1976–1977 and 1980–1981 (from 30.4 ± 1.8 to 24.0 ± 1.6 percent) but then decreased at a slower rate between 1980–1981 and 1991–1992 (to 20.6 ± 1.6 percent). Daily smoking prevalence increased significantly to 28.3 ± 1.9 percent in 1997–1998 (University of Michigan, Institute for Social Research, public use data tapes, 1976–1998). Among black high school senior girls, daily smoking continued to decline dramatically between 1976–1977 and 1992–1993 (from 24.7 ± 3.3 to 2.4 ± 1.2 percent) (Husten et al. 1996), but increased between 1992–1993 and 1997–1998 (5.4 ± 1.7 percent). For all years, prevalence of daily smoking was higher among white high school senior girls than among black high school senior girls (University of Michigan, Institute for Social Research, public use data tapes, 1976–1998; Patrick O'Malley, unpublished data). Estimates of daily smoking by race in the 1989 TAPS I also showed daily smoking to be higher among white girls than among black girls (Moss et al. 1992). Between 1976 and 1989, the prevalence of daily smoking decreased among Mexican American, Puerto Rican American,

**Figure 2.9. Prevalence (%) of current smoking among young adults aged 18 years, for 1904–1969, National Health Interview Survey (NHIS), and high school seniors, for 1976–1998, Monitoring the Future (MTF) Survey, by gender and race, United States**

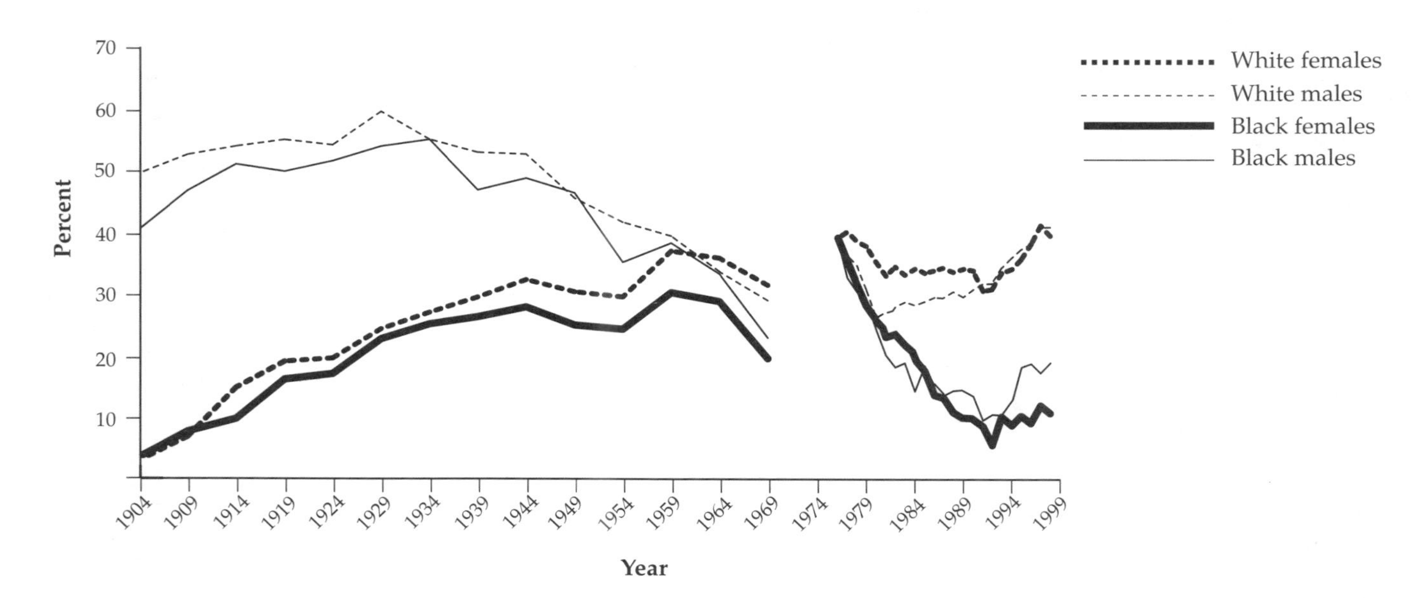


*Note:* Estimates of prevalence for 1904–1969 were derived from an analysis of NHIS data on recalled age of initiation and recalled age of cessation done by Burns et al. 1997. Data reflect estimated prevalence among persons at age 18 years. Estimates for 1976–1998 were obtained directly from MTF Surveys and are the percentage of all high school seniors who reported smoking ≥ 1 cigarette in the previous 30 days.
Sources: **NHIS:** Burns et al. 1997. **MTF Survey:** University of Michigan, Institute of Social Research, public use data tapes, 1976–1998.

and Latina high school senior girls (Bachman et al. 1991b).

## Smoking Intensity Among Girls

Heavy smoking among girls and boys is defined here as smoking about one-half pack of cigarettes (6 to 15 cigarettes) or more per day (USDHHS 1994). In the 1998 NHSDA, 5.0 percent of all adolescent girls aged 12 through 17 years were heavy smokers; among adolescent girls who smoked, 29.9 percent were heavy smokers. Among smokers, black girls (9.7 percent) and Hispanic girls (15.8 percent) were less likely than white girls (34.2 percent) to be heavy smokers (Table 2.10). Comparable estimates were obtained from the 1999 YRBS of high school students less than 18 years of age. In the 1999 NYTS, 12.3 (±3.3) percent of girls in middle school and 25.2 (±3.7) percent of girls in high school reported that they smoked 6 or more cigarettes on the days they smoked. Although girls were somewhat less likely than boys to smoke heavily, the difference was not statistically significant (CDC 2000b). Using combined data from MTF Surveys for 1985–1989, Bachman and coworkers (1991b) reported the following prevalence of heavy smoking (one-half pack or more per day) among current smokers: 23.4 percent among Native American girls, 13.3 percent among white girls, 4.5 percent among Asian girls, 4.2 percent among Puerto Rican American and Latin American girls, 2.5 percent among Mexican American girls, and 2.2 percent among black girls.

Another measure of smoking intensity is frequent smoking, which is defined here as having smoked on 20 or more of the past 30 days (USDHHS 1994). Among girls aged 12 through 17 years who smoked, 44.8 percent were frequent smokers in the 1998 NHSDA (Table 2.10). Comparable estimates were obtained by analyzing data from the 1999 YRBS data for high school students less than 18 years of age. In the 1998 NHSDA data, white girls who smoked

**Figure 2.10. Prevalence (%) of daily smoking among high school seniors, by gender, Monitoring the Future Survey, United States, 1976–2000**

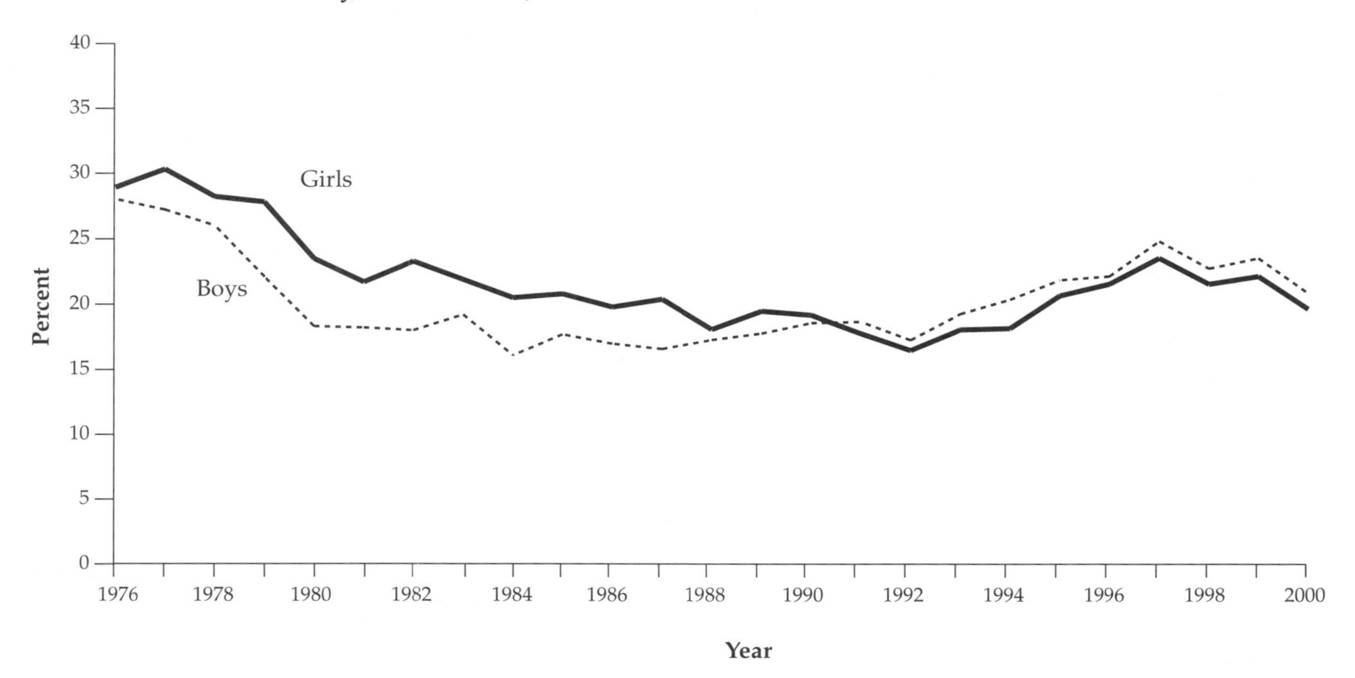


*Note:* Estimates for daily smoking are based on responses to the question, "How frequently have you smoked cigarettes in the past 30 days?" Persons reporting smoking ≥ 1 cigarette/day during the previous 30 days were classified as daily smokers.
Sources: University of Michigan, Institute for Social Research, public use data tapes, 1976–1998; University of Michigan 2000.

were more likely than Hispanic girls who smoked to be frequent smokers; the percentage for non-Hispanic black girls was intermediate to the percentages for white girls and Hispanic girls. Among current smokers in the 1997 YRBS, 47.5 percent of the girls in grades 9 through 12 and less than 18 years of age in schools funded by the Bureau of Indian Affairs smoked at least 20 of the last 30 days (CDC, Division of Adolescent and School Health, public use data tape, 1997).

In both NHSDA and YRBS data, the prevalence of heavy or frequent smoking was generally somewhat lower among girls aged 12 through 14 years than among girls aged 15 through 17 years, but these differences were not statistically significant (Table 2.10). Other data have shown that the prevalence of frequent smoking increased as grade in school increased (Johnston et al. 2000a; Kann et al. 1998, 2000).

No significant gender-specific differences were found in the prevalence of heavy or frequent smoking in either survey (Table 2.10). In the 1989 TAPS I, among adolescents aged 12 through 18 years who smoked, 23.5 percent of girls and 27.6 percent of boys smoked 10 to 19 cigarettes per day, and 12.1 percent of girls and 19.2 percent of boys smoked 20 or more cigarettes per day. However, smoking on 10 to 29 days of the past month was equally common among girls (26.2 percent) and boys (26.6 percent), as was daily smoking (40.6 vs. 41.0 percent) (Moss et al. 1992).

## Relationship of Smoking to Socioeconomic and Other Factors

Socioeconomic status and social bonding in school and with peers are strongly associated with initiation of cigarette smoking among adolescents (Conrad et al. 1992; USDHHS 1994; Distefan et al. 1998; Flay et al. 1998; Harrell et al. 1998). MTF Surveys elicited data on several of the sociodemographic risk factors for ever smoking and current smoking among high school senior girls; data for 1994–1998 were combined to provide stable estimates (Table 2.11).

Students' household structure was related to both ever smoking and current smoking. MTF Survey data showed that high school senior girls who lived with both parents or with only their mother had the lowest

**Table 2.10. Percentage (and 95% confidence interval) of girls less than 18 years of age who were current smokers who reported frequent or heavy use of cigarettes, by selected characteristics, National Household Survey on Drug Abuse (NHSDA) and Youth Risk Behavior Survey (YRBS), United States, 1998–1999**

| | Heavy use* | | Frequent use† | |
|---|---|---|---|---|
| Characteristic | 1998 NHSDA (ages 12–17) | 1999 YRBS (grades 9–12) | 1998 NHSDA (ages 12–17) | 1999 YRBS (grades 9–12) |
| Girls | 29.9 (±6.1) | 24.5 (±3.6) | 44.8 (±7.0) | 44.1 (±5.5) |
| Age (years) | | | | |
| 12–14 | 18.8 (±10.9)‡ | 27.8 (±9.5)‡ | 33.3 (±13.9) | 36.7 (±11.3) |
| 15–17 | 34.0 (±7.3) | 24.3 (±3.9) | 48.7 (±8.1) | 44.7 (±5.8) |
| Race/ethnicity | | | | |
| White, non-Hispanic | 34.2 (±7.4) | 27.5 (±5.2) | 48.5 (±8.3) | 49.3 (±7.1) |
| Black, non-Hispanic | 9.7 (±7.5)‡ | 11.5 (±7.6)‡ | 35.5 (±17.0)‡ | 30.8 (±20.1) |
| Hispanic | 15.8 (±8.8)‡ | 12.7 (±5.7) | 23.7 (±11.5)‡ | 25.1 (±7.4) |
| Boys | 32.1 (±5.8) | 30.2 (±3.9) | 43.9 (±6.4) | 48.5 (±5.3) |

*Note:* NHSDA is a household survey that includes adolescents 12–17 years of age; 67.0% were 14–17 years of age. YRBS is a school-based survey that includes high school students in grades 9–12; these analyses were restricted to those less than 18 years of age; of these, 99.8% were 14–17 years of age. Data are not comparable across surveys due to differences in ages surveyed and survey methods.

*For NHSDA, prevalence of heavy use of cigarettes is based on response to the question, "When you smoked cigarettes during the past 30 days, how many did you usually smoke each day?" For YRBS, prevalence of heavy use is based on response to the question, "During the past 30 days, on the days you smoked, how many cigarettes did you smoke per day?" In both surveys, prevalence of heavy use is the percentage of all persons in each demographic category who reported smoking about one half pack/day or more on the days they smoked during the past 30 days. In NHSDA, responses were coded as 6–15 cigarettes/day or more, and a comparable code was used in YRBS.

†Based on response to the question, "During the past 30 days, on how many days did you smoke cigarettes?" Prevalence of frequent use is the percentage of all persons in each demographic category who reported smoking on ≥ 20 of the past 30 days.

‡Estimate should be interpreted with caution because of the small number of respondents.

Sources: **NHSDA:** Substance Abuse and Mental Health Services Administration, public use data tape, 1998. **YRBS:** Centers for Disease Control and Prevention, Division of Adolescent and School Health, public use data tape, 1999.

prevalence of ever smoking and current smoking (Table 2.11). In published data from the 1994-B–1995 NHSDA (combined data), girls and boys aged 12 through 17 years who lived in a family structure other than a two-biological-parent family were more likely to have smoked in the past year than were those who lived with both biological parents (USDHHS 1997). For girls aged 12 through 17 years, the 1989 TAPS I data showed that 14.5 (± 3.4) percent of girls who spent 10 or more hours a week at home without a parent or another adult present, and 8.2 (±1.6) percent of girls who were never home alone, were current smokers (NCHS, public use data tape, 1989).

In MTF Surveys, level of parental education, defined as the highest grade either parent had completed, was generally not related to smoking status among high school senior girls (Table 2.11). In the 1992 YRBS, after adjustment for age, gender, race and ethnicity, and school enrollment, the likelihood that adolescents aged 12 through 17 years smoked cigarettes was inversely related to the number of years of education completed by the responsible adult or to the 1986–1990 family income (Lowry et al. 1996). Conversely, a representative national sample of students enrolled in four-year colleges in the United States in 1993 found that female students with at least one parent who graduated from college were 1.19 (95 percent CI, 1.06 to 1.33) times as likely to have smoked in the past 30 days as students whose parents did not graduate from college (Emmons et al. 1998). Emmons and associates also controlled for other demographic factors, lifestyle choices, and risk behaviors. Prospective studies that examined the influence of parental education on smoking initiation have also yielded conflicting results. Some studies

**Table 2.11. Prevalence (% and 95% confidence interval) of ever smoking and current smoking among high school seniors, by gender and sociodemographic risk factors, Monitoring the Future Survey, United States, 1994–1998, aggregate data**

| | Ever smoking* | | Current smoking† | |
|---|---|---|---|---|
| **Sociodemographic risk factor** | **Girls** | **Boys** | **Girls** | **Boys** |
| Household structure | | | | |
| Lives with both parents | 61.9 (±1.3) | 64.3 (±1.0) | 32.0 (±1.3) | 34.5 (±1.0) |
| Lives with mother only | 62.7 (±2.4) | 65.2 (±2.1) | 30.8 (±2.3) | 34.6 (±2.1) |
| Lives with father only | 71.7 (±5.6) | 69.9 (±3.6) | 41.4 (±6.1) | 39.1 (±3.9) |
| Lives alone | 70.0 (±17.9) | 69.3 (±9.6) | 47.2 (±19.5) | 48.1 (±10.3) |
| Other | 68.7 (±4.1) | 69.4 (±3.2) | 36.6 (±4.3) | 41.2 (±3.4) |
| Parental education level | | | | |
| Some high school or less | 61.2 (±3.9) | 65.7 (±3.4) | 28.8 (±3.6) | 32.5 (±3.3) |
| Completion of high school | 64.8 (±2.3) | 66.1 (±1.8) | 34.0 (±2.3) | 35.9 (±1.8) |
| Some college | 63.5 (±2.4) | 65.3 (±1.9) | 31.8 (±2.3) | 35.2 (±1.9) |
| Completion of college | 62.3 (±2.1) | 64.7 (±1.6) | 32.6 (±2.0) | 35.4 (±1.6) |
| Graduate/professional | 62.5 (±2.6) | 64.8 (±1.9) | 33.4 (±2.5) | 35.5 (±1.9) |
| Population density of locale where respondent grew up | | | | |
| Farm | 63.0 (±5.3) | 67.8 (±3.3) | 32.9 (±5.2) | 38.5 (±3.5) |
| Country | 63.5 (±3.1) | 67.7 (±2.3) | 33.9 (±3.1) | 37.4 (±2.4) |
| Small city | 64.3 (±2.1) | 66.7 (±1.6) | 34.5 (±2.0) | 37.5 (±1.6) |
| Medium-sized city or suburb | 63.4 (±2.5) | 65.5 (±2.0) | 32.5 (±2.4) | 34.7 (±2.0) |
| Large city or suburb | 61.7 (±2.7) | 62.2 (±2.1) | 30.2 (±2.6) | 32.3 (±2.0) |
| Very large city or suburb | 59.7 (±3.4) | 61.8 (±2.4) | 29.3 (±3.2) | 31.5 (±2.3) |
| Self-reported overall academic performance | | | | |
| Above average | 54.7 (±1.9) | 58.7 (±1.4) | 25.7 (±1.7) | 29.0 (±1.3) |
| Slightly above average | 63.8 (±2.3) | 64.9 (±1.8) | 32.2 (±2.2) | 34.4 (±1.8) |
| Average | 68.5 (±1.8) | 69.4 (±1.4) | 37.2 (±1.8) | 39.7 (±1.5) |
| Below average | 73.9 (±4.3) | 74.8 (±2.7) | 43.2 (±4.8) | 47.3 (±3.1) |
| Plans to complete 4 years of college | | | | |
| Definitely or probably will | 60.7 (±1.3) | 61.7 (±1.0) | 30.0 (±1.2) | 31.1 (±1.0) |
| Definitely or probably will not | 72.3 (±2.4) | 73.9 (±1.6) | 41.8 (±2.6) | 46.2 (±1.8) |
| Importance of religion | | | | |
| Very important | 50.2 (±2.0) | 56.4 (±1.8) | 20.2 (±1.6) | 25.4 (±1.6) |
| Important | 66.2 (±2.1) | 67.6 (±1.6) | 34.8 (±2.1) | 37.0 (±1.7) |
| Not or somewhat important | 72.4 (±1.8) | 68.9 (±1.3) | 42.1 (±1.9) | 40.7 (±1.3) |
| Weekly personal income | | | | |
| ≤ $10 | 49.7 (±3.0) | 51.3 (±2.5) | 20.5 (±2.4) | 22.1 (±2.0) |
| $11–50 | 60.0 (±2.1) | 61.5 (±1.7) | 28.6 (±1.9) | 30.4 (±1.6) |
| ≥ $51 | 68.1 (±1.5) | 69.0 (±1.1) | 37.5 (±1.5) | 39.8 (±1.1) |

*Prevalence of ever smoking is the percentage of all persons in each demographic category who reported ever having smoked cigarettes at least once or twice.

†Prevalence of current smoking is the percentage of all persons in each demographic category who reported having smoked ≥ 1 cigarette in the 30 days before the survey.

Sources: University of Michigan, Institute for Social Research, public use data tapes, 1994–1998.

showed that less parental education predicted smoking initiation, but other studies found no relationship (Conrad et al. 1992; Harrell et al. 1998).

MTF Survey data for high school senior girls showed an inverse relationship between academic performance and prevalence of ever smoking and current smoking (Table 2.11). This relationship was also observed among girls aged 12 through 17 years in the 1989 TAPS I (NCHS, public use data tape, 1989). The prevalence of ever smoking was 23.9 (±2.1) percent among girls with above-average performance, 36.2 (±2.6) percent among girls with average performance, and 63.1 (± 9.2) percent among girls with below-average performance. The prevalence of current smoking was 8.9 (±1.3) among girls with above-average performance, 15.6 (±2.1) percent among girls with average performance, and 43.4 (±10.0) percent among girls with below-average performance. Using longitudinal data from TAPS (1989–1993), Distefan and colleagues (1998) observed that youth with average or below-average school performance at baseline were 1.34 (95 percent CI, 1.11 to 1.63) times as likely to have tried a cigarette at follow-up as those with above-average performance.

Plans for education after graduation also were strongly associated with smoking status. In MTF Surveys, high school senior girls who did not plan to complete four years of college were more likely than those who planned to complete college to ever smoke (72.3 vs. 60.7 percent) or to smoke currently (41.8 vs. 30.0 percent) (Table 2.11). TAPS I data also were analyzed by "dropout" status: 17 percent of girls who were high school students or graduates, but 33 percent of girls who dropped out of high school, had smoked in the past week (USDHHS 1994). In the 1998 NHSDA data, among adolescent girls aged 12 through 17 years, 61.2 (±17.0) percent of those who dropped out of high school, but 17.2 (±2.2) percent of girls who remained in school, had smoked in the past month (SAMHSA, public use data tape, 1998). Among the college-age population (aged 17 through 22 years) in the 1998 NHSDA, 54.9 (±8.5) percent of girls who dropped out of high school, 45.4 (±6.2) percent of high school graduates who were not attending college, and 37.3 (± 9.3) percent of those attending college, had smoked in the past month (SAMHSA, public use data tape, 1998). The follow-up surveys of the high school graduating classes of 1976–1994 (modal ages, 19 through 22 years) showed that girls who did not go to college were more likely to smoke one-half pack of cigarettes or more each day than were girls attending college (Bachman et al. 1997). Academic values and expectations were also consistent predictors of smoking initiation in several prospective studies of adolescents (Conrad et al. 1992; Flay et al. 1998).

The prevalence of both ever smoking and current smoking among high school senior girls was inversely related to the self-reported importance of religion. MTF Survey data showed that girls for whom religion was not important or was only somewhat important had the highest prevalence of ever smoking (72.4 percent) and current smoking (42.1 percent) (Table 2.11). Similarly, in the 1989 TAPS I, 18.5 (±3.3) percent of girls aged 12 through 17 years who never attended religious services, but 7.7 (±1.4) percent of girls this age who often attended religious services, were current smokers (NCHS, public use data tape, 1989). In the 1993 national survey of students in four-year colleges, Emmons and colleagues (1998) observed that female students who viewed religion as not important were 1.71 (95 percent CI, 1.41 to 2.07) times as likely to have smoked in the past 30 days as those who viewed religion as important.

Weekly personal income among high school senior girls was directly related to the prevalence of both ever smoking and current smoking. Data from the MTF Survey indicated that as personal income increased from $10 or less to $51 or more, the prevalence of ever smoking increased from 49.7 to 68.1 percent and the prevalence of current smoking increased from 20.5 to 37.5 percent (Table 2.11). This finding may reflect the fact that adolescents with the highest academic performance are less likely to have jobs (Johnston et al. 1982; University of Michigan, Institute for Social Research, public use data tapes, 1994–1998). In both TAPS I and TAPS II, the prevalence of ever smoking was lower among adolescent girls whose weekly discretionary income was $1 to $20 than among adolescents who had no discretionary income or whose income was more than $20. The difference was statistically significant only in comparison to girls who had more than $20 of discretionary income (CDC, Office on Smoking and Health, public use data tapes, 1989, 1993). A similar relationship was found for current smoking. The relationship between smoking initiation and religiousness or availability of spending money generally has not been examined in prospective studies (Conrad et al. 1992).

MTF Surveys found few gender-specific differences in the sociodemographic factors related to ever smoking and current smoking (Table 2.11). Among high school seniors who considered religion to be very important, those with above-average academic performance, and those who lived with both parents, girls were less likely than boys to be ever smokers or current smokers.

An analysis of the association of these same demographic factors with experimental smoking showed that only the self-reported importance of religion and weekly personal income were associated with experimental smoking. (Experimental smoking is defined here as having ever smoked, but never regularly). Girls who reported that religion was very important were less likely to have experimented with smoking than were girls who reported that religion was important. Girls who had a weekly personal income of $10 or less were less likely to have experimented with smoking than were girls with a weekly personal income of $11 or more. Among boys, similar relationships with the importance of religion and personal income were observed, but boys who reported no plans to attend college also demonstrated a lower prevalence of experimental smoking (University of Michigan, Institute for Social Research, public use data tapes, 1994–1998). In contrast, Distefan and colleagues (1998) used longitudinal data from TAPS (1989–1993) and observed that youth with average or below-average school performance at baseline were 1.34 (95 percent CI, 1.11 to 1.63) times as likely to have experimented with smoking but not yet smoked 100 cigarettes at follow-up and were 1.68 (95 percent CI, 1.14 to 2.48) times as likely to have progressed from experimentation to established smoking as those with above-average performance.

## Attitudes About Smoking Among Girls

MTF Survey data for 1998 indicated that 64.8 percent of high school senior girls reported preferring to date people who do not smoke and that 42.4 percent reported strongly disliking being near people who are smoking (Table 2.12). Only 39.2 percent reported that they did not mind being around people who are smoking. Most girls (66.9 percent) disapproved of adults who smoke one or more packs of cigarettes per day, thought that becoming a smoker reflects poor judgment (54.1 percent), thought that their close friends would disapprove of them smoking one or more packs of cigarettes per day (72.7 percent), and believed that smoking is a dirty habit (72.4 percent). Young adolescents and young adults may be even more likely than high school seniors to have negative perceptions about smoking (Johnston et al. 2000a,b). In the 1989 TAPS I, 86.0 (±1.1) percent of girls aged 12 through 17 years reported that they would rather date people who do not smoke, and in the 1993 TAPS II, 68.2 (±1.6) percent of girls aged 10 through 17 years reported that they strongly dislike being around people who are smoking (NCHS, public use data tapes, 1989, 1993). In the 1993 MTF Survey of college students and young adults, 76.0 percent of those aged 19 through 22 years, 77.4 percent of those aged 23 through 26 years, and 86.8 percent of those 27 through 30 years reported that their friends would disapprove of their smoking one pack of cigarettes a day (Johnston et al. 1994b).

Perceptions about smoking are related to the smoking status of respondents (USDHHS 1994; Otero-Sabogal et al. 1995). For example, in the 1989 MTF Survey, 80 percent of nonsmokers and only 50 percent of smokers classified smoking as a dirty habit (USDHHS 1994). More than 85 percent of nonsmokers, but only about one-third of smokers, reported that they preferred to date nonsmokers (USDHHS 1994). In the 1999 NYTS, of girls in middle school, 93.8 (±1.5) percent of never smokers and 92.3 (±3.1) percent of current smokers thought persons can get addicted to cigarettes; for girls in high school, the percentages were 94.1 (±3.1) and 94.6 (±2.2), respectively. Among girls in middle school, 95.4 (±0.9) percent of never smokers and 76.2 (±6.4) percent of current smokers did not think it was safe to smoke 1 to 2 years and then quit; for girls in high school, the percentages were 97.2 (±1.0) and 84.8 (±2.9), respectively. Among girls in middle school, 91.8 (± 1.9) percent of never smokers and 88.4 (±3.8) percent of current smokers thought that smoking one or more packs per day was a health risk; among girls in high school, the percentages were 93.7 (±3.4) and 95.3 (±1.5), respectively (CDC 2000b). In a TAPS cohort analysis, female Hispanics aged 12 through 18 years who did not dislike being around smokers were twice as likely as those who disliked being around smokers to have initiated smoking by the time they were resurveyed at ages 15 through 22 (Cowdery et al. 1997).

MTF Surveys showed that the social desirability of smoking was unchanged from 1981 through 1998 among high school senior girls, except for attitudes about dating smokers and adult smoking (Table 2.12). The percentage of girls who preferred to date nonsmokers increased from 1981 through 1991, then decreased nonsignificantly through 1998. Significantly fewer high school senior girls disapproved of adult smoking in 1998 than in 1986. The overall pattern from 1981 through 1998 among high school senior girls largely reflects trends among whites, the majority of the population.

In the 1960s and 1970s, high school students reported that peers and friends were more likely to disapprove of smoking by girls than to disapprove of smoking by boys (Zagona 1967; Johnston et al. 1980a,b). In a more recent study of seventh-grade

**Table 2.12. Trends (% and 95% confidence interval) in the beliefs and attitudes of high school seniors about smoking and smokers, by gender, Monitoring the Future Survey, United States, 1981–1998**

| Beliefs and attitudes | 1981 Girls | 1981 Boys | 1986 Girls | 1986 Boys | 1991 Girls | 1991 Boys | 1996 Girls | 1996 Boys | 1998 Girls | 1998 Boys |
|---|---|---|---|---|---|---|---|---|---|---|
| I prefer to date people who don't smoke.* | 62.2 (±4.6) | 71.3 (±3.5) | 69.0 (±4.6) | 73.5 (±3.8) | 74.4 (±4.8) | 74.0 (±3.9) | 67.6 (±5.2) | 65.0 (±4.6) | 64.8 (±5.3) | 67.7 (±4.4) |
| I strongly dislike being near people who are smoking.* | NA[†] | NA | 46.1 (±5.0) | 44.5 (±4.3) | 50.4 (±5.6) | 48.2 (±4.5) | 45.9 (±5.5) | 39.1 (±4.7) | 42.4 (±5.5) | 39.9 (±4.6) |
| I personally don't mind being around people who are smoking.* | 42.7 (±4.7) | 33.5 (±3.6) | 39.2 (±4.9) | 34.6 (±4.1) | 36.6 (±5.4) | 29.2 (±4.1) | 39.7 (±5.4) | 38.6 (±4.7) | 39.2 (±5.5) | 37.4 (±4.6) |
| Do you disapprove of people (age ≥ 18 years) who smoke one or more packs of cigarettes per day?[‡] | 69.4 (±4.1) | 71.2 (±3.3) | 76.4 (±4.0) | 74.0 (±3.4) | 73.9 (±4.7) | 68.8 (±3.8) | 65.6 (±2.6) | 59.1 (±2.3) | 66.9 (±2.6) | 58.4 (±2.3) |
| I think that becoming a smoker reflects poor judgement.* | 53.9 (±4.7) | 60.8 (±3.8) | 57.5 (±4.9) | 62.0 (±4.2) | 60.0 (±5.4) | 62.6 (±4.4) | 55.3 (±5.5) | 55.0 (±4.8) | 54.1 (±5.6) | 55.4 (±4.7) |
| How do you think your close friends feel (or would feel) about your smoking one or more packs of cigarettes per day?[‡§] | 73.9 (±4.1) | 74.0 (±3.4) | 77.1 (±4.2) | 74.9 (±3.7) | 76.9 (±4.7) | 72.1 (±4.1) | 73.4 (±5.2) | 65.0 (±4.6) | 72.7 (±5.1) | 65.8 (±4.6) |
| Smoking is a dirty habit.* | 66.7 (±4.5) | 64.7 (±3.7) | 69.6 (±4.6) | 67.3 (±4.0) | 73.1 (±4.9) | 70.2 (±4.1) | 72.2 (±5.0) | 63.7 (±4.6) | 72.4 (±5.0) | 68.6 (±4.4) |

*Percentage who agree.
[†]NA = Not available.
[‡]Percentage who disapprove.
[§]Possible responses included "not disapprove," "disapprove," and "strongly disapprove." Percentages include those who "disapprove" or "strongly disapprove."
Sources: University of Michigan, Institute for Social Research, public use data tapes, 1981, 1986, 1991, 1996, 1998.

students, girls were less likely than boys to believe that their friends approved of smoking (Flay et al. 1994). In the 1998 MTF Survey, girls were more likely than boys to disapprove of adults smoking one or more packs of cigarettes per day (Table 2.12).

When asked in the 1998 MTF Survey how smoking makes a "girl" their age look, a substantial majority responded that it did not make her look "conforming," "independent and liberated," "mature, sophisticated," or "cool, calm, in control" (Table 2.13). They viewed smoking by a "guy" their age in a similar way. These perceptions changed little between 1981 and 1998. The 1998 MTF Survey found no gender-specific differences in how girls and boys who smoked were perceived except that boys were more likely than girls to report that smoking by a "guy" made him look "mature, sophisticated." Only 7.5 percent of boys, however, agreed with this assessment. In the 1999 NYTS, among girls in middle school, 10.8 (±1.9) percent of never smokers and 37.5 (±5.6) percent of current smokers thought smokers have more friends; among girls in high school, the percentages were 12.2 (±2.5) and 20.0 (±3.5), respectively. Among girls in middle school, 4.8 (±1.0) of never smokers and 25.3 (±5.7) percent of current smokers thought smokers looked cool; among girls in high school, the percentages were 5.1 (±1.6) and 12.4 (±2.3), respectively (CDC 2000b). (See "Factors Influencing Initiation of

**Table 2.13. Trends (% and 95% confidence interval) in the opinions* of high school seniors about smokers, by gender, Monitoring the Future Survey, United States, 1981, 1990, 1998**

| Opinions | 1981 | | 1990 | | 1998 | |
|---|---|---|---|---|---|---|
| | Girls | Boys | Girls | Boys | Girls | Boys |
| In my opinion, when a girl my age is smoking a cigarette, it makes her look... | | | | | | |
| ...like she's trying to appear mature and sophisticated | 64.8 (±4.6) | 65.0 (±3.7) | 62.2 (±5.5) | 66.6 (±4.2) | 56.2 (±5.5) | 49.8 (±4.7) |
| ...insecure | 45.9 (±4.7) | 49.4 (±3.9) | 50.0 (±5.6) | 52.3 (±4.4) | 42.2 (±5.5) | 40.0 (±4.6) |
| ...conforming | 25.5 (±4.2) | 28.2 (±3.5) | 19.5 (±4.5) | 19.7 (±3.6) | 18.8 (±4.4) | 19.3 (±3.8) |
| ...independent and liberated | 10.9 (±3.0) | 12.0 (±2.5) | 9.7 (±3.3) | 9.8 (±2.7) | 8.5 (±3.1) | 9.0 (±2.7) |
| ...mature, sophisticated | 6.8 (±2.4) | 7.4 (±2.1) | 4.1 (±2.2) | 5.1 (±2.0) | 4.5 (±2.3) | 5.6 (±2.2) |
| ...cool, calm, in control | 5.7 (±2.2) | 5.5 (±1.8) | 4.1 (±2.2) | 4.2 (±1.8) | 5.9 (±2.6) | 4.7 (±2.0) |
| In my opinion, when a guy my age is smoking a cigarette, it makes him look... | | | | | | |
| ...like he's trying to appear mature and sophisticated | 61.6 (±4.6) | 61.9 (±3.7) | 60.4 (±5.5) | 62.3 (±4.3) | 55.6 (±5.5) | 48.4 (±4.7) |
| ...insecure | 38.9 (±4.6) | 45.2 (±3.8) | 46.6 (±5.6) | 44.6 (±4.4) | 35.8 (±5.3) | 34.7 (±4.5) |
| ...conforming | 24.9 (±4.1) | 26.4 (±3.4) | 17.6 (±4.3) | 17.1 (±3.3) | 17.9 (±4.3) | 21.2 (±3.9) |
| ...rugged, tough, independent | 9.1 (±2.7) | 8.6 (±2.2) | 11.7 (±3.6) | 8.5 (±2.4) | 10.0 (±3.3) | 11.8 (±3.0) |
| ...mature, sophisticated | 4.9 (±2.1) | 6.1 (±1.8) | 2.2 (±1.7) | 3.9 (±1.7) | 3.0 (±1.9) | 7.5 (±2.5) |
| ...cool, calm, in control | 6.5 (±2.3) | 6.4 (±1.9) | 5.1 (±2.5) | 5.5 (±2.0) | 6.6 (±2.7) | 9.1 (±2.7) |

*Percentage who agree.
Sources: University of Michigan, Institute for Social Research, public use data tapes, 1981, 1990, 1998.

Smoking" in Chapter 4 and "Gender-Specific Similarities and Differences in Motives and Barriers to Stop Smoking" in Chapter 5 for further information about sociodemographic and behavioral factors associated with smoking.)

## Cigarette Brand Preference Among Girls

A 1990 study of preference for cigarette brand among smokers aged 12 through 17 years in California found that the market share of both Marlboro and Camel cigarettes increased from 1986 through 1990 among girls (Pierce et al. 1991a). In the 1993 TAPS II, 90 percent of girls aged 10 through 17 years who smoked purchased Marlboro (63.1 percent), Newport (16.9 percent), or Camel cigarettes (10.0 percent) (Table 2.14)—the three most heavily advertised brands in 1993 (Maxwell 1994). In published data from the 1999 NHSDA, the most frequent brands used in the past month by girls aged 12 through 17 years were Marlboro (55.6 percent), Newport (22.6 percent), and Camel (8.3 percent) (SAMHSA 2000). Similar proportions were noted in the 1998 MTF Survey for grades 8, 10, and 12 combined (Marlboro, 61.9 percent; Newport, 18.6 percent; Camel, 5.8 percent) (University of Michigan 1999a). In the 1999 NYTS, 39.8 percent of girls in middle school identified Marlboro as the usual brand of cigarette smoked in the 30 days preceding the survey; 26.2 percent smoked Newport, 5.7 percent smoked Camel, 13.1 percent smoked "another" brand, and 15.1 percent reported that they had no usual brand. Among girls in high school, 56.8 percent

**Table 2.14. Prevalence (% and 95% confidence interval) of use of cigarette brands among current smokers aged 10–17 years, by gender and race, Teenage Attitudes and Practices Survey II, United States, 1993**

| Gender and race | Marlboro | Newport | Camel |
|---|---|---|---|
| Girls | 63.1 (±7.2) | 16.9 (±5.6) | 10.0 (±4.2)* |
| White, non-Hispanic | 68.9 (±7.6) | 10.2 (±5.0)* | 11.1 (±4.8)* |
| Black, non-Hispanic | 20.6 (±26.1)* | 64.1 (±28.3)* | 0.0* |
| Hispanic | 36.4 (±28.7)* | 49.6 (±29.8)* | 5.8 (±11.2)* |
| Boys | 54.8 (±7.4) | 12.6 (±4.3) | 16.6 (±6.1) |
| White, non-Hispanic | 62.2 (±8.3) | 4.1 (±2.8)* | 19.2 (±7.2) |
| Black, non-Hispanic | 0.0* | 72.6 (±20.5)* | 0.0* |
| Hispanic | 30.9 (±20.3)* | 32.9 (±22.2)* | 14.1 (±15.2)* |

*Note:* Cigarette brand is based on response to the question, "What brand do you usually buy?" Current smoking is defined as any cigarette smoking during the 30 days before the survey.
*Results, particularly by race and ethnicity, should be interpreted with caution because of the small sample sizes.
Sources: Centers for Disease Control and Prevention, Office on Smoking and Health, public use data tape, 1993.

smoked Marlboro, 18.4 percent smoked Newport, 7.0 percent smoked Camel, 10.0 percent smoked "other," and 7.8 percent reported no usual brand (CDC 2000b). This concentration of brand use has been noted by others (Cummings et al. 1997).

No gender-specific differences in brand preference were noted in the 1993 TAPS II (Table 2.14). However, a 1993 California study reported that girls were less likely than boys to choose Camel cigarettes (Cavin and Pierce 1996)—a finding also noted in the 18 communities that were part of COMMIT (Cummings et al. 1997), in published data from the 1999 NHSDA (SAMHSA 2000), and in data from the 1998 MTF Survey (University of Michigan 1999a). Both COMMIT and the 1999 NHSDA also found that adolescent girls had little interest in generic cigarettes.

Data from the 1993 TAPS II showed that cigarette brand preference differed by race and ethnicity. Newport cigarettes were the most commonly purchased brand among black girls (64.1 percent) and Hispanic girls (49.6 percent); white girls preferred Marlboro cigarettes (68.9 percent). Results from the 1989 TAPS I and the 1998 MTF Survey also indicated a race-specific difference for brand preference: white adolescents preferred the Marlboro brand, and black adolescents preferred the Newport brand (Allen et al. 1993; University of Michigan 1999a).

In the 1993 TAPS II, 52.7 percent of girls smoked regular cigarettes, and 47.3 percent smoked light or ultralight cigarettes. Girls were almost twice as likely as boys to smoke light or ultralight cigarettes (47.3 vs. 25.3 percent) (NCHS, public use data tape, 1993; Giovino et al. 1996).

## Summary

Household surveys provide lower estimates than school-based surveys, but the patterns of tobacco use were similar regardless of the source of data. The prevalence of current smoking among girls 12 through 17 years of age declined between 1974 and 1998, but most of the decline occurred between 1974 and the early 1980s. The decline in prevalence was greater among black girls than among white girls. Smoking prevalence increased among 8th-, 10th-, and 12th-grade girls between 1991–1992 and 1996–1997. In 1999, the prevalence of current smoking was 17.7 percent among 8th-grade girls, 25.8 percent among 10th-grade girls, and 33.5 percent among high school senior girls; the prevalence of daily smoking among high school senior girls was 22.2 percent. Thus, much of the progress in reducing smoking prevalence among girls in the 1970s and 1980s was lost with the increased prevalence in the 1990s; current smoking among high school senior girls in 2000 was the same as in 1988. Among high school seniors, smoking prevalence was higher among girls than among boys in the 1970s and early 1980s, but comparable since the mid-1980s.

In 1998–1999, prevalence of ever smoking, current smoking, heavy smoking, and frequent smoking was directly associated with age or grade; the prevalences of current, heavy, and frequent smoking were lower among black girls than among white girls. The patterns among Hispanic girls were less clear for ever and current smoking, but for heavy or frequent smoking, the prevalence among Hispanic girls in 1998 was lower than that among white girls. In 1993, 90 percent of girls aged 10 through 17 years who smoked cigarettes purchased the three most heavily advertised brands.

Socioeconomic and other factors related to smoking patterns among adolescent girls include household structure, school performance and educational plans, religiousness, and level of discretionary income. Measures of the social desirability of smoking, as viewed by high school senior girls, showed little change from 1981 through 1998, except for disapproval of adult smoking, which was lower in 1998 than in 1986. Nevertheless, most high school senior girls disapprove of adults smoking and associate smoking with negative qualities. These girls also have a negative view of peers who smoke.

## Cigarette Smoking Among Pregnant Women and Girls

Cigarette smoking during pregnancy increases the risk of intrauterine growth retardation, low birth weight, and other unfavorable pregnancy outcomes (USDHHS 1989) (see "Reproductive Outcomes" and "Birth Outcomes" in Chapter 3). Historical data are available from the National Natality Survey, which provides data for samples of married women whose infants were born alive in 1967 or 1980. Among married mothers younger than age 20 years, smoking prevalence during pregnancy remained about the same between the two survey years: about 39 percent among white women and 27 percent among black women. Smoking prevalence among mothers aged 20 years or older declined from 40 to 25 percent among white women and from 33 to 23 percent among black women (Kleinman and Kopstein 1987).

The National Survey of Family Growth collected data in 1982, 1988, and 1995 on the smoking behavior of girls and women aged 15 through 44 years during their most recent pregnancy. The prevalence of smoking during pregnancy declined from 31 percent in 1982 to 27.5 percent in 1988. The prevalences for the two survey years, respectively, were 32.8 and 30.5 percent among white mothers, 29.2 and 23.4 percent among black mothers, and 17.2 and 13.7 percent among Hispanic mothers (Pamuk and Mosher 1988; Chandra 1995). Data from the 1995 National Survey of Family Growth indicated that 17.8 percent of pregnant and postpartum women smoked (NCHS 1997); data were not reported by race.

In the 1985 and 1990 NHIS, questions related to smoking were asked of women aged 18 through 44 years who had given birth within the past five years. In 1985, 31.8 percent of women reported that they smoked during the 12 months before giving birth, and 25.1 percent reported that they smoked after learning they were pregnant. In 1990, the prevalences were 23.7 and 18.3 percent, respectively. These prevalences were consistently higher among white mothers (33.2 and 26.0 percent in 1985, and 25.3 and 19.7 percent in 1990) than among black mothers (27.5 and 22.6 percent in 1985, and 19.0 and 14.1 percent in 1990) or among Hispanic mothers (16.8 and 10.3 percent in 1985, and 12.1 and 8.0 percent in 1990) (Floyd et al. 1993).

Data from the 1988 National Maternal and Infant Health Survey are available for white, black, and American Indian women. These data indicated that the proportion of women who smoked cigarettes in the 12 months before giving birth was similar among American Indian women (35 percent) and white women (32 percent) but slightly lower among black women (27 percent) (Sugarman et al. 1994).

The National Pregnancy and Health Survey, which was conducted from October 1992 through August 1993, provided nationally representative data on the prevalence of prenatal use of drugs among women aged 15 through 44 years. In these data, 20.4 percent of women reported smoking cigarettes during pregnancy. Statistically significant differences were noted by race and ethnicity: 24.4 percent of white women, 19.8 percent of black women, and 5.8 percent of Hispanic women reported smoking during pregnancy (USDHHS 1996b).

Since 1989, data on smoking during pregnancy have been available from information collected on the revised U.S. Standard Certificate of Live Birth. These data are currently available from birth certificates in 46 states, New York City, and the District of Columbia and are included as part of the final natality statistics compiled each year (see "Natality Statistics" in Appendix 1). At the time of birth, mothers in these states and localities are asked whether they used tobacco "during pregnancy" and the average number of cigarettes smoked per day (NCHS 1992, 1994a; Ventura et al. 1995, 1997, 1999, 2000; Matthews 1998). The proportion of women and girls who had live births who reported being smokers during pregnancy declined from 19.5 percent in 1989 to 12.9 percent in 1998 (Table 2.15). Analysis of BRFSS data suggested that the decline was primarily due to a decrease in smoking initiation among women of childbearing age rather than an increase in smoking cessation during

**Table 2.15. Trends (%) in live births in which mothers reported smoking during pregnancy, by selected characteristics, United States, 1989–1998**

| Characteristic | 1989 | 1991 | 1993 | 1995 | 1997 | 1998 |
|---|---|---|---|---|---|---|
| Overall* | 19.5 | 17.8 | 15.8 | 13.9 | 13.2 | 12.9 |
| Age (years)* | | | | | | |
| <18 | 18.3 | 16.0 | 14.4 | 14.2 | 15.1 | 15.1 |
| 18–24 | 23.6 | 21.2 | 19.2 | 17.4 | 17.2 | 17.1 |
| 25–49 | 17.2 | 15.8 | 13.9 | 12.1 | 11.0 | 10.5 |
| Race/ethnicity† | | | | | | |
| White, non-Hispanic | 21.7 | 20.5 | 18.6 | 17.1 | 16.5 | 16.2 |
| Black, non-Hispanic | 17.2 | 14.6 | 12.7 | 10.6 | 9.8 | 9.6 |
| Hispanic | 8.0 | 6.3 | 5.0 | 4.3 | 4.1 | 4.0 |
| American Indian or Alaska Native | 23.0 | 22.6 | 21.6 | 20.9 | 20.8 | 20.2 |
| Asian or Pacific Islander | 5.7 | 5.2 | 4.3 | 3.4 | 3.2 | 3.1 |
| Education (number of years)‡ | | | | | | |
| ≤ 8 | 20.8 | 18.3 | 15.2 | 12.6 | 12.1 | 11.7 |
| 9–11 | 35.0 | 31.9 | 29.0 | 26.2 | 25.7 | 25.5 |
| 12 | 22.2 | 20.6 | 19.3 | 17.7 | 17.1 | 16.8 |
| 13–15 | 13.6 | 12.4 | 11.3 | 10.5 | 9.9 | 9.6 |
| ≥ 16 | 5.0 | 4.2 | 3.1 | 2.7 | 2.4 | 2.2 |
| Number of cigarettes/day | | | | | | |
| ≤ 10 | 57.8 | 60.4 | 62.7 | 65.4 | 67.9 | 68.6 |
| 11–20 | 35.6 | 33.8 | 32.1 | 30.1 | 28.1 | 27.6 |
| ≥ 21 | 6.6 | 5.8 | 5.2 | 4.6 | 4.0 | 3.8 |

*Note:* Percentage excludes live births for mothers with unknown smoking status.

*Includes data for 43 states and the District of Columbia (DC) in 1989; 46 states and DC in 1991–1993; and 46 states, DC, and New York City in 1995–1998. Excludes data for California, Indiana, New York State, and South Dakota for all years; Louisiana, Nebraska, and Oklahoma in 1989; and New York City in 1989–1993, which did not require the reporting of mother's tobacco use during pregnancy on the birth certificate.

†For American Indians or Alaska Natives and Asians or Pacific Islanders, includes data for 43 states and DC in 1989; 46 states and DC in 1991–1993; and 46 states, DC, and New York City in 1995–1998. Excludes data for California, Indiana, New York State, and South Dakota for all years; Louisiana, Nebraska, and Oklahoma in 1989; and New York City in 1989–1993, which did not require the reporting of mother's tobacco use during pregnancy on the birth certificate. For white non-Hispanics, black non-Hispanics, and Hispanics, includes data for 42 states and DC in 1989; 45 states and DC in 1991; 46 states and DC in 1993; and 46 states, DC, and New York City in 1995–1998. Excludes data for California, Indiana, New York State, and South Dakota for all years; Louisiana, Nebraska, and Oklahoma in 1989; New Hampshire in 1989–1991; and New York City in 1989–1993, which did not require the reporting of mother's tobacco use during pregnancy or mother's Hispanic origin on the birth certificate.

‡Includes data for 42 states and DC in 1989; 45 states and DC in 1991; 46 states and DC in 1993; and 46 states, DC, and New York City in 1995–1998. Excludes data for California, Indiana, New York State, and South Dakota for all years; Louisiana, Nebraska, and Oklahoma in 1989; Washington in 1989–1991; and New York City in 1989–1993, which did not require the reporting of mother's tobacco use during pregnancy or mother's education on the birth certificate.

Sources: National Center for Health Statistics 1992, 1994a; Ventura et al. 1995, 1997, 1999, 2000; Mathews 1998.

pregnancy (Ebrahim et al. 2000). Because most mothers who stop smoking during pregnancy relapse to smoking after delivery (Fingerhut et al. 1990; Mullen et al. 1997), the percentage of women who report smoking during pregnancy is substantially lower than the prevalence of smoking among all women of reproductive age (18 through 44 years). Researchers found that some pregnant women and girls conceal their smoking from the clinician (Windsor et al. 1993; Kendrick et al. 1995; Ford et al. 1997). Such concealment would result in underreporting of smoking prevalence during pregnancy on birth certificates. Underreporting also occurs if information on smoking from the hospital medical record is not transferred onto the birth certificate (Dietz et al. 1998). Point prevalence data on smoking among pregnant women from the 1996 BRFSS was 12 percent (Ebrahim et al. 2000). A report of the combined 1994-B–1995 NHSDA data estimated that 21.5 percent of pregnant girls and women aged 12 through 44 years smoked in the past month (USDHHS 1997). Data from the Pregnancy Risk Assessment Monitoring System in 13 states for 1997 showed that the reported prevalence of smoking during the last three months of pregnancy ranged from 11 to 24 percent (Gilbert et al. 1999).

Smoking prevalence during pregnancy differs by age and by race and ethnicity. Although the prevalence declined in all age groups and in all racial and ethnic groups between 1989 and 1998, it was consistently highest among women aged 18 through 24 years, lower among girls, and generally lowest among women aged 25 through 49 years (Table 2.15). The greatest decline occurred among black mothers (from 17.2 percent in 1989 to 9.6 percent in 1998) and white mothers (from 21.7 to 16.2 percent). The prevalence decreased from 5.7 to 3.1 percent among Asian or Pacific Islander mothers and from 8.0 to 4.0 percent among Hispanic mothers. Tobacco use during pregnancy by American Indian or Alaska Native mothers was higher than that in any other group, but the prevalence decreased from 23.0 percent in 1989 to 20.2 percent in 1998. Published data from the natality statistics reported that among Asian or Pacific Islander women, prevalence was highest among pregnant Hawaiian and part-Hawaiian women and lower among pregnant Chinese, Filipinos, Japanese, and other Asians or Pacific Islanders (Ventura et al. 1999). For pregnant Hispanic women, prevalence was highest among Puerto Rican, other Hispanic, and women of unknown Hispanic status. Prevalence was lower among pregnant Cuban, Mexican American, and Central and South American women.

Smoking during pregnancy is particularly uncommon among Mexican women and Asian or Pacific Islander women born outside the United States (Ventura et al. 1995). In 1993, for example, the prevalence of smoking during pregnancy was 6 percent among Mexican mothers born in the United States, and only 2 percent among Mexican mothers born elsewhere. Similarly, 12 percent of Asian or Pacific Islander mothers born in the United States were smokers, but only 3 percent of those born elsewhere were smokers.

The prevalence of maternal smoking also differs by educational attainment (Table 2.15). In 1998, the prevalence of smoking during pregnancy was only 2.2 percent among mothers with 16 or more years of education, 9.6 percent for 13 to 15 years of education, 16.8 percent for 12 years of education, 25.5 percent for 9 to 11 years of education, and 11.7 percent for 8 or fewer years of education. From 1989 through 1998, the prevalence declined among mothers at all levels of education, but the decline was much greater among women with fewer than 12 years of education (NCHS 1992, 1994a; Ventura et al. 1995, 1997, 1999, 2000; Matthews 1998).

The proportion of pregnant smokers who smoke more than 10 cigarettes per day also has declined steadily (Table 2.15). The proportion of mothers who smoked 21 or more cigarettes per day during pregnancy decreased from 6.6 percent in 1989 to 3.8 percent in 1998, and the proportion who smoked 11 to 20 cigarettes per day decreased from 35.6 to 27.6 percent. The proportion who smoked 10 or fewer cigarettes per day increased from 57.8 to 68.6 percent (NCHS 1992, 1994a; Ventura et al. 1995, 1997, 1999, 2000; Matthews 1998).

## Summary

Birth certificate data indicate that tobacco use during pregnancy declined from 19.5 percent in 1989 to 12.9 percent in 1998. The number of cigarettes smoked per day by pregnant women and girls who smoke also decreased. However, pregnant women and girls may conceal their smoking from clinicians, and this concealment could result in an underestimation of smoking prevalence from data on birth certificates. Survey data suggest that up to 22 percent of pregnant women and girls smoke.

# Smoking Initiation

Age at initiation of smoking is an important indicator of smoking behavior. Persons who start smoking when they are young are more likely to smoke heavily and to become dependent on nicotine than are those who start smoking later in life. They are also at increased risk for smoking-related illnesses or death (Schuman 1977; USDHHS 1989; Breslau and Peterson 1996; Chassin et al. 1996; Chen and Millar 1998).

Several studies suggested that persons who began smoking at ages 14 through 16 years are more likely to become nicotine dependent than are persons who started smoking at an older age (Breslau 1993; Breslau et al. 1993a,b). However, initiation of smoking before age 14 years was not associated with a further increase in nicotine dependence, presumably because such initiation was associated with a slower progression to daily smoking than was initiation at ages 14 through 16 years. However, Everett and coworkers (1999b) found that among high school students aged 16 years or older, early age of initiation was directly related to current, frequent, and daily smoking.

In NHIS data by birth cohorts, a direct relationship was found between age at smoking initiation and the number of cigarettes smoked per day (USDHHS 1986b). This relationship was shown for women and for men. In 1955 Current Population Survey data for women aged 35 through 44 years, 19.7 percent of those who started smoking before age 18 years but only 8.8 percent of those who started smoking after age 22 years smoked more than one pack of cigarettes per day (Haenszel et al. 1956). In a study of almost 12,000 women, the age at smoking initiation was related to the intensity of smoking: 26.9 percent of women who started smoking at or before age 16 years and 15.4 percent of those who started at age 20 years or older smoked 31 or more cigarettes per day in adulthood (Taioli and Wynder 1991).

NHIS data also showed that persons who became smokers at earlier ages were more likely to continue smoking—a finding that was consistent across birth cohorts. For example, nearly 70 percent of women born in 1920–1929 who started to smoke before age 14 years, but 62 percent of women in the same birth cohort who began to smoke at age 18 or 19 years, were still smoking in 1980 (USDHHS 1986b). Similar conclusions were reported from CPS-I (Hammond and Garfinkel 1968), the 1975 AUTS (USDHEW 1976), and the U.S. Nurses' Health Study (Myers et al. 1987). In NHANES data, however, smoking initiation at an older age was not a predictor of successful cessation (McWhorter et al. 1990).

Three main measures are used to present data on smoking initiation patterns: the median or mean age at initiation, the percentage of smokers who started to smoke by a certain age, and the smoking initiation rate. To determine the median or mean age at smoking initiation or the estimated percentage of persons who had ever smoked by a certain age, researchers use the reconstructed prevalence of ever smoking by birth cohorts or the recalled age at initiation reported by persons at various ages over multiple survey years. The smoking initiation rate is calculated as the number of persons who started to smoke in a particular year, divided by the number who had not started smoking before that year. Trends in these measures of age at initiation and in initiation rates, as well as the methods used to derive them, are discussed here.

## Median Age at Smoking Initiation

### Women Born in 1885–1944

The median age at smoking initiation among women born between 1885 and 1944 was determined by reconstructing the prevalence of ever smoking for birth cohorts with use of NHIS data for 1970, 1978, 1979, 1980, 1987, and 1988 (Burns et al. 1997). Using the age at which respondents reported beginning to smoke, Burns and colleagues determined the percentage who had ever smoked in each birth cohort by age, race, and gender. For this analysis, the median age at smoking initiation was the age at which one-half of the persons who had ever smoked in each cohort were smoking, that is, the age at which one-half of the maximum prevalence of ever smoking was attained for that cohort. For example, the maximum prevalence of ever smoking among white women born in 1900–1904 was 26.4 percent, and the age by which one-half of these women (13.2 percent) were smoking was 26.2 years. The median age at smoking initiation decreased dramatically among women born in 1885–1914; the median age at initiation occurred 20 years earlier among women born in 1910–1914 than among women born in 1885–1889.

Among white women, the median age at smoking initiation declined from age 39.5 to 17.5 years in successive cohorts born in 1885–1944; most of the

**Figure 2.11. Median age at smoking initiation among adults aged 18 years or older, by race, gender, and birth cohort, United States, 1885–1944**

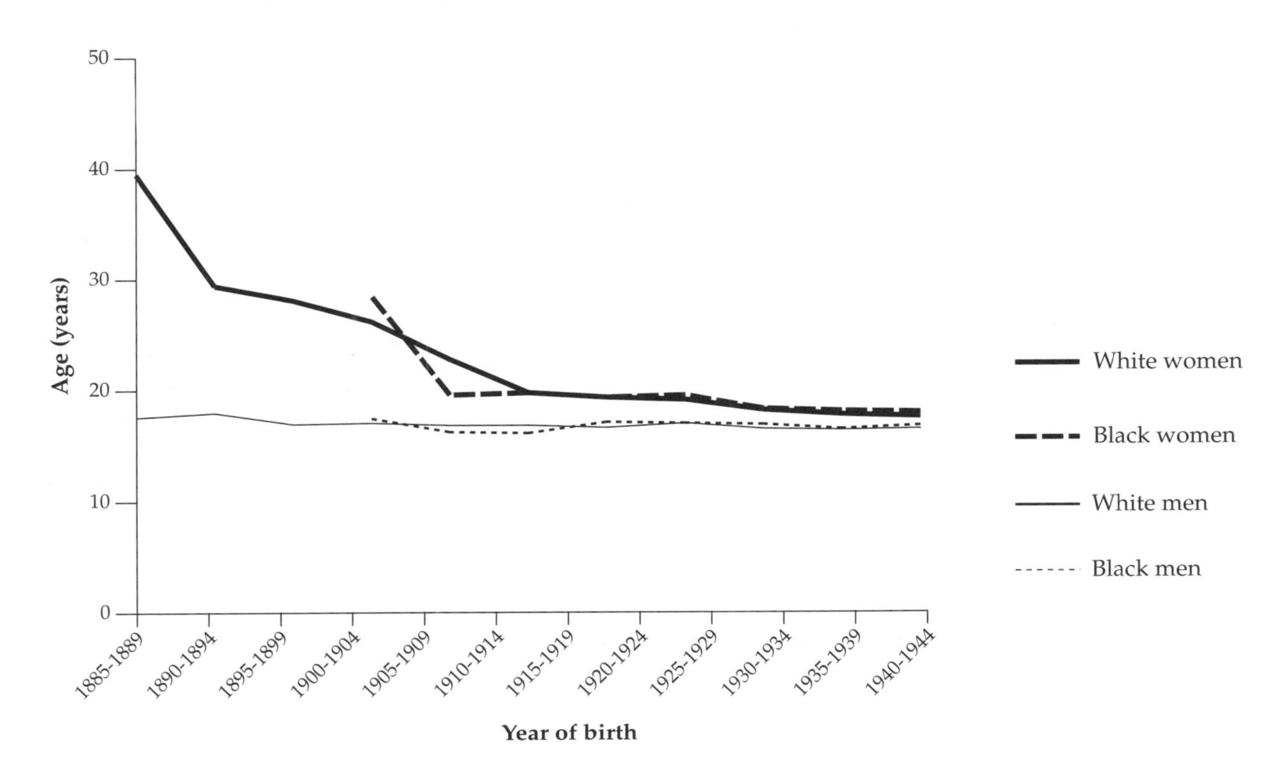


*Note:* Estimates for smoking initiation are based on responses to the question, "How old were you when you began to smoke cigarettes fairly regularly?" Age at which respondents reported beginning to smoke was used to determine the percentage who ever smoked, by birth cohort. Median age at smoking initiation was age at which one-half of persons who ever smoked in each cohort were smoking.
Source: Burns et al. 1997. Estimates derived from analyses of National Health Interview Survey data for 1970–1988.

decrease (from 39.5 to 19.8 years) occurred in the cohorts born in 1885–1914 (Figure 2.11). Among black women, the median age at smoking initiation declined from 28.5 to 17.9 years among cohorts born in 1900–1944. There were no consistent differences in the median age at initiation among black women and white women.

Among all cohorts, the median age at smoking initiation was later among women than among men. Among white women born before 1930, the median age at initiation was older than 18 years; among those born in 1930 through 1944, it was younger than 18 years. Among black women, the median age at initiation was younger than 18 years for the 1940–1944 cohort only. In contrast, the median age at initiation was younger than 18 years among almost all cohorts of men (Shopland 1995; Burns et al. 1997). In other cohort analyses of NHIS data for women, the trends for mean ages at smoking initiation (USDHHS 1980; Harris 1983) and the patterns by gender (USDHHS 1980; Harris 1983; CDC 1991b) were similar to those reported here.

Findings in the 1955 Current Population Survey were also consistent with results in these cohort analyses. The median age at smoking initiation among women declined from 35.3 years among women born in 1891–1900 to 21.3 years among women born in 1911–1920 (Burbank 1972). Although the median age at smoking initiation decreased dramatically among women born in 1890–1910, the rate of decline slowed (decrease of only two years) among women born in 1910–1940 (Haenszel et al. 1956). Further evidence consistent with these findings comes from birth cohort analyses of self-reported age at smoking initiation in CPS-I and CPS-II (Stellman and Garfinkel 1986; Garfinkel and Silverberg 1990). The trend from the 1890–1894 cohort through the 1930–1934 cohort is comparable to estimates reconstructed from NHIS data. Both analyses showed a 12-year decrease in the age at initiation among white women, but the estimates of age from CPS-I and CPS-II are consistently two to four years older than those obtained from NHIS data. This discrepancy is probably because CPS-I and CPS-II data are for volunteers who were predominantly middle class, white, well educated, and older than women in the general U.S. population (Stellman et al. 1988).

## Mean Age at Smoking Initiation

### Women Born in 1931–1962

Because smoking initiation must be completed before a median age at initiation can be determined, the median age cannot be determined for recent cohorts of smokers. However, the mean age at smoking initiation can be assessed in surveys of persons aged 30 through 39 years. By restricting analyses to this age group, researchers can assume that smoking initiation is nearly complete and that differential mortality is not yet an issue, but data may be skewed by recall bias. Because the age of survey participants is restricted and is similar over time, however, recall bias probably does not affect trends. The mean age at smoking initiation may be higher than the reconstructed median age because of outlier values, which represent persons who started smoking at an unusually late age.

In the 1959 CPS-I, the mean age at smoking initiation was 20.2 years among women aged 30 through 39 years at the time of the survey (born in 1920–1929) (Hammond and Garfinkel 1961). In 1970, 1978–1980 (combined data), 1988, and 1992, NHIS included questions about smoking initiation. Thus, the mean age at smoking initiation for persons aged 30 through 39 years can be determined among persons born in 1931–1962. Mean age was based on the question "How old were you when you started smoking cigarettes fairly regularly?" The mean age at initiation of regular smoking decreased from 19.3 years among women born in 1931–1940 to 17.7 years among women born in 1953–1962 (Table 2.16)—a decrease of about 1.5 years. The only racial or ethnic difference in the mean age at initiation of regular smoking was older mean age among black women than among white women for the 1931–1940 and 1949–1958 birth cohorts. Among all four cohorts (1931–1940, 1940–1949, 1949–1958, and 1953–1962) and the three racial and ethnic groups (whites, blacks, and Hispanics) examined, the mean age at initiation was older among women than among men.

### Women Born in 1961–1979

Mean age at smoking initiation can also be determined from surveys of young adults or adolescents. These data are more current than information obtained by the other methods, and they minimize recall bias. However, smoking initiation may not be complete among these respondents, particularly adolescents, and the estimates derived from such surveys tend to be lower than those obtained by the other methods. Because initiation largely occurs before age 18 years, surveys of young adults but not surveys of adolescents were used to estimate age at smoking initiation for this report.

**Table 2.16. Mean age (years and 95% confidence interval) at smoking initiation of regular smoking for selected birth cohorts, by gender and race or ethnicity, United States, 1931–1962**

| Birth cohort | All women | White, non-Hispanic women | Black, non-Hispanic women | Hispanic women | All men |
|---|---|---|---|---|---|
| 1931–1940 | 19.3 (±0.2) | 19.2 (±0.2) | 20.0 (±0.5) | NA* | 17.6 (±0.1) |
| 1940–1949 | 18.5 (±0.3) | 18.4 (±0.3) | 19.0 (±0.7) | 18.8 (±1.4) | 17.2 (±0.2) |
| 1949–1958 | 18.1 (±0.2) | 17.9 (±0.2) | 18.8 (±0.5) | 18.9 (±0.8) | 17.3 (±0.2) |
| 1953–1962 | 17.7 (±0.3) | 17.5 (±0.3) | 18.6 (±1.1) | 18.4 (±1.4) | 16.9 (±0.4) |

*Note:* Smoking initiation is based on response to the question, "How old were you when you first started smoking cigarettes fairly regularly?" Respondents were women aged 30–39 years in National Health Interview Surveys in 1970–1992 (e.g., women born in 1931–1962). Some birth cohorts overlap slightly, reflecting years that data were available.

*NA = Not available. Ethnicity was not determined in 1970, so for women born 1931–1940, estimates for whites and for blacks likely include data for some persons of Hispanic origin.

Sources: National Center for Health Statistics, public use data tapes, 1970, 1979, 1988, 1992.

Data from the 1982, 1985, 1988, 1991, 1994, and 1997 NHSDA were used to determine trends in mean recalled age at smoking initiation among women 18 through 21 years old (i.e., women born in 1961–1979) who had ever smoked (Table 2.17). NHSDA data on the age at first trying a cigarette are available for 1982–1997, and NHSDA data on the age at starting to smoke daily are available for 1985–1997. The mean recalled age at first use of a cigarette was older (14.3 years) among young women born in 1976–1979 than among young women born in 1964–1973. The mean recalled age at initiation of daily smoking was older (16.0 years) among young women born in 1967–1970 than among young women born in 1964–1967. The mean recalled age at initiation of daily smoking was 15.8 years among young women born in 1976–1979. For both measures, the mean ages did not differ by gender.

Rogers and Crank (1988) used data for persons aged 17 through 24 years, but they used earlier NHIS data (1979–1980) to determine the average age at smoking initiation. The average age was 19.6 years among women and 17.2 years among men. The mean age at smoking initiation was highest (20.5 years) among Mexican American women, intermediate among black women (19.9 years), and lowest among white women (19.6 years). The mean age at smoking initiation was significantly higher among women than among men in all three racial and ethnic groups.

## Percentage of Women Who Smoked by a Certain Age

### Birth Cohort Analyses

Estimates can also be constructed for prevalence of ever smoking by a certain age (e.g., 18 or 20 years). This method of reconstructing prevalence provides estimates of smoking initiation for years before 1965, when ongoing surveillance of smoking behavior began. However, reconstructed estimates are subject to biases from the differential mortality of smokers (Tolley et al. 1991; Burns et al. 1997). Smokers who began smoking at a young age are more likely than other smokers to die prematurely and not be available to participate in a survey. This bias increases the estimated average age at smoking initiation for early cohorts, but some investigators, such as Burns and coworkers (1997), adjusted for this differential mortality. Biases can also be introduced if older persons are less likely than younger persons to accurately recall their age at smoking initiation. Although Harris (1983) suggested that the accuracy of recall for age at smoking initiation and cessation decreased as age increased, Gilpin and colleagues (1994) found that the distribution of reported age at smoking initiation among birth cohorts was consistent across survey years.

**Table 2.17. Mean recalled age (years and 95% confidence interval) at smoking initiation among persons who ever smoked, by gender, United States, 1961–1979**

| | Mean age at first use of a cigarette* | | Mean age at start of daily smoking† | |
|---|---|---|---|---|
| Birth cohort | Women | Men | Women | Men |
| 1961–1964 | 13.0 (±1.2) | 12.9 (±1.4) | NA‡ | NA‡ |
| 1964–1967 | 12.2 (±0.6) | 12.9 (±0.9) | 14.9 (±0.6) | 15.7 (±0.7) |
| 1967–1970 | 13.4 (±0.4) | 12.7 (±0.7) | 16.0 (±0.4) | 15.4 (±0.8) |
| 1970–1973 | 13.3 (±0.4) | 13.2 (±0.4) | 15.7 (±0.4) | 15.9 (±0.3) |
| 1973–1976 | 13.9 (±0.4) | 13.3 (±0.5) | 15.6 (±0.4) | 15.7 (±0.4) |
| 1976–1979 | 14.3 (±0.4) | 13.7 (±0.4) | 15.8 (±0.3) | 15.8 (±0.3) |

*Note:* Respondents were aged 18–21 years in the National Household Surveys on Drug Abuse in 1982–1997 (e.g., born in 1961–1979). For 1991 and preceding years, ever smoking is defined as having smoked ≥ 100 cigarettes (about 5 packs) in their lifetime. For 1994-B and subsequent years, ever smoking is defined as having smoked ≥ 100 days in their lifetime.

*For 1991 and preceding years, respondents were asked, "About how old were you when you first tried a cigarette?" For 1994-B and subsequent years, respondents were asked, "How old were you the first time you smoked a cigarette, even one or two puffs?"

†Respondents were asked, "About how old were you when you first started smoking daily?"

‡NA = Not available.

Sources: Alcohol, Drug Abuse, and Mental Health Administration, public use data tapes, 1982, 1985, 1988, 1991; Substance Abuse and Mental Health Services Administration, public use data tapes, 1994-B, 1997.

NHIS data suggested that of the women who had ever smoked, 42 percent started smoking before age 20 years in the 1910–1919 birth cohort, 49 percent in the 1920–1929 birth cohort, and 84 percent in the 1950–1959 birth cohort (USDHHS 1986b). Cohort analysis of NHSDA data suggested that among women who had ever smoked, 51 percent started smoking before age 21 years in the 1919–1929 birth cohort, 70 percent in the 1956–1960 cohort, and 68 percent in the 1966–1970 birth cohort (Johnson and Gerstein 1998). Other analyses of NHIS data have also shown that, over time, proportionally more women began to smoke before age 18 or 20 years (USDHHS 1986b, 1989).

Pierce and colleagues (1991b) used NHIS data for 1978, 1979, 1980, and 1987 to reconstruct the prevalence of smoking among birth cohorts of women and men from 1920–1924 through 1955–1959 and then determined the proportion among persons who had ever smoked who became regular smokers before age 25 years. The proportion was 75.8 percent among the 1920–1924 birth cohort of women and 96.7 percent among the 1950–1954 cohort. The researchers concluded that smoking initiation generally occurs before age 25 years, particularly among recent birth cohorts of women.

In the U.S. Nurses' Health Study, the percentage of women who started to smoke before age 20 years increased for each successive birth cohort, from 23.8 percent among women born in 1921–1926 to 37.5 percent among women born in 1942–1946 (Myers et al. 1987). The greatest percent increase in the prevalence of smoking occurred at ages 20 through 25 years for the two older cohorts (born in 1921–1931) and at ages 15 through 20 years for the three younger cohorts (born in 1932–1946).

Burns and coworkers (1997) analyzed NHIS data by birth cohort. The analysis revealed that, among women who had ever smoked, the percentage who started smoking fairly regularly before age 18 years increased with each successive cohort from 1900–1904 through 1940–1944 (Figure 2.12). The increase in smoking initiation before age 18 years was greater among white women (29 percentage points) than among black women (24 percentage points). The percentage of women who had ever smoked and who started smoking by age 15 years increased 8 percentage points among white women and 5 percentage points among black women between the 1900–1904 cohort and the 1950–1954 cohort. Among those who had ever smoked, for all cohorts examined, a greater percentage of men than women had started smoking by age 15 or 18 years. However, the proportion of men who had ever smoked and started smoking by age 15 years was greater among the 1900–1904 cohort than among the 1950–1954 cohort, and the increase in the proportion of men from those cohorts who started smoking by age 18 years was less than the increase in the proportion for women.

An analysis of the 1991–1993 NHSDA found that among the cohort of women born in 1919–1929, 51 percent reported any cigarette use by age 21 years. This percentage increased to 67 percent by the 1941–1945 birth cohort and remained at about 67 percent through the 1971–1975 birth cohort. The percentage of women who reported regular use of cigarettes by age 21 years increased from 19 percent among the 1919–1929 birth cohort to 35 percent among the 1941–1945 birth cohort, then remained fairly constant (around 35 percent) through the 1971–1975 birth cohort. The ratio of females to males who started using cigarettes daily before age 21 years was about 0.65 among the 1919–1929 birth cohort, 0.80 among the 1941–1945 birth cohort, 0.90 among the 1956–1960 cohort, and nearly 1.00 among the 1971–1975 birth cohort (Johnson and Gerstein 1998).

All these results are consistent with those for other analyses of NHIS data (USDHHS 1986b, 1989, 1994). Over time, a greater proportion of women started to smoke cigarettes before age 18 years, and this increase was more striking among women than among men. However, data for all birth cohorts consistently showed that a lower percentage of women than men began smoking fairly regularly before age 18 years. This pattern reflects the findings that men born in earlier cohorts started smoking before age 18 years but that smoking was started before age 18 years only among more recent birth cohorts of women (USDHHS 1986b).

#### Women Aged 30 Through 39 Years

The percentage of women who smoked by a certain age can also be calculated by surveys that assess the recalled age at initiation for women aged 30 through 39 years. By restricting analyses to this age group, researchers can assume that initiation is nearly complete and that differential mortality is not yet an issue. However, these analyses are limited in that they cannot provide information on initiation behavior among cohorts born after 1968.

Data from the 1998 NHSDA provided the age at which women aged 30 through 39 years recalled having first tried a cigarette or recalled smoking cigarettes daily (Table 2.18). Of all women in the survey, 8.0 percent first tried a cigarette before age 12 years, and 55.6 percent did so before age 18 years; 22.9 percent

**Figure 2.12. Percentage of persons aged 18 years or older who ever smoked who started smoking fairly regularly by age 15 or 18 years, by race, gender, and birth cohort, United States, 1900–1954**

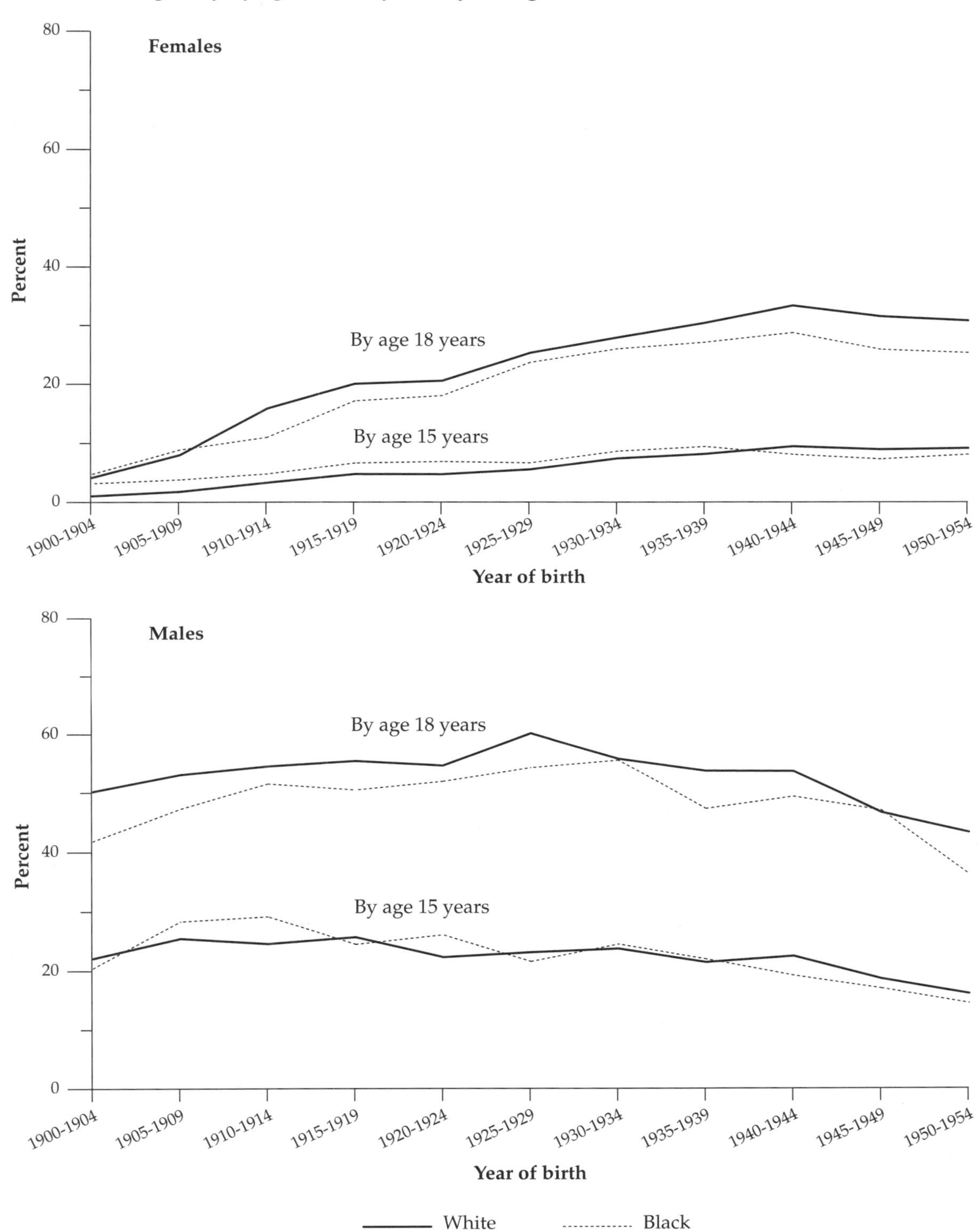


*Note:* Persons who ever smoked are those who reported smoking ≥ 100 cigarettes in their lifetime. Age of initiation was determined by responses to the question, "How old were you when you began to smoke cigarettes fairly regularly?"
Source: Burns et al. 1997. Estimates derived from analysis of National Health Interview Survey data for 1970–1988.

**Table 2.18. Cumulative percentage (and 95% confidence interval) of recalled age at which respondents aged 30–39 years first tried a cigarette or began to smoke daily, by gender, National Household Survey on Drug Abuse, United States, 1998**

| Age (years) | All persons | | | | Persons who ever smoked daily | | | |
|---|---|---|---|---|---|---|---|---|
| | First tried a cigarette* | | Began smoking daily† | | First tried a cigarette* | | Began smoking daily† | |
| | Women | Men | Women | Men | Women | Men | Women | Men |
| <12 | 8.0 (±1.8) | 12.8 (±2.4) | 1.1 (±0.8)‡ | 1.3 (±0.8)‡ | 10.3 (±2.9) | 13.1 (±4.2) | 2.7 (±1.8) | 3.4 (±2.1) |
| <14 | 23.4 (±2.7) | 26.8 (±3.1) | 4.6 (±1.4) | 3.8 (±1.4) | 34.5 (±4.8) | 31.4 (±5.4) | 11.4 (±3.4) | 10.2 (±3.5) |
| <16 | 41.6 (±3.1) | 46.0 (±3.5) | 12.0 (±2.0) | 8.5 (±1.8) | 62.6 (±5.0) | 57.9 (±5.9) | 29.7 (±4.6) | 22.8 (±4.7) |
| <18 | 55.6 (±3.1) | 60.0 (±3.5) | 22.9 (±2.7) | 18.3 (±2.7) | 80.6 (±4.2) | 80.8 (±4.6) | 56.7 (±5.1) | 49.2 (±5.9) |
| <19 | 61.5 (±3.0) | 65.8 (±3.4) | 28.0 (±2.9) | 23.5 (±3.0) | 89.5 (±3.0) | 88.3 (±3.7) | 69.4 (±4.7) | 63.1 (±5.8) |
| <20 | 63.5 (±3.0) | 68.8 (±3.3) | 29.6 (±2.9) | 26.5 (±3.2) | 91.8 (±2.7) | 90.8 (±3.4) | 73.3 (±4.5) | 71.2 (±5.4) |
| <25 | 69.3 (±2.8) | 74.4 (±3.1) | 36.9 (±3.1) | 34.8 (±3.4) | 97.7 (±1.2) | 97.8 (±2.4) | 91.6 (±2.6) | 93.5 (±3.1) |
| <30 | 70.8 (±2.8) | 76.0 (±3.0) | 39.1 (±3.1) | 36.8 (±3.5) | 99.7 (±0.3) | 100.0 (±0.0) | 97.0 (±1.6) | 98.9 (±1.1) |
| ≤ 39 | 71.6 (±2.7) | 76.2 (±3.0) | 40.3 (±3.1) | 37.2 (±3.5) | 100.0 (±0.0) | 100.0 (±0.0) | 100.0 (±0.0) | 100.0 (±0.0) |

*Respondents were asked, "How old were you the first time you smoked a cigarette, even one or two puffs?"
†Respondents were asked, "How old were you when you first started smoking cigarettes every day?"
‡Estimate should be interpreted with caution because of the small number of respondents.
Source: Substance Abuse and Mental Health Services Administration, public use data tape, 1998.

smoked daily before age 18 years. Published data from the 1994–1995 NHSDA showed that white women (7.8 percent) were more likely than black women (4.6 percent) or Hispanic women (3.5 percent) to first try a cigarette before age 12 years and more likely to try a cigarette before age 18 years (67.5, 43.9, and 33.9 percent, respectively) (USDHHS 1998).

Of women who had ever smoked, 10.9 percent first tried a cigarette before age 12 years and 80.4 percent before age 18 years (SAMHSA, public use data tape, 1998). Because the recalled age is about the same among women who had ever smoked and among those who had ever smoked daily, detailed data are presented only for women who had ever smoked daily (Table 2.18). Of these women, 10.3 percent first tried a cigarette before age 12 years and 80.6 percent before age 18 years, whereas 2.7 percent smoked daily before age 12 years and 56.7 percent smoked daily before age 18 years. Published analyses reported that among women who had ever smoked daily, 8.9 percent of whites, 6.9 percent of Hispanics, and 5.9 percent of blacks first tried a cigarette before age 12 years and 85.9 percent of whites, 68.6 percent of Hispanics, and 66.8 percent of blacks first tried a cigarette before age 18 years (USDHHS 1998). Among women who had ever smoked daily, 1.6 percent of whites, 1.6 percent of blacks, and 0.7 percent of Hispanics smoked daily before age 12 years. Among women who had ever smoked daily, 58.3 percent of whites, 41.8 percent of blacks, and 35.4 percent of Hispanics began smoking daily before age 18 years. No CIs were provided.

Girls experimented with cigarettes at older ages than did boys: fewer women than men first tried a cigarette before age 12 years (8.0 vs. 12.8 percent) (Table 2.18). However, girls and boys were equally likely to have tried a cigarette and to have smoked daily before age 18 years.

### Young Women

The percentage of women who smoked by a certain age can be calculated by using surveys that assess the recalled age at initiation among young women or adolescents. Although these data reflect current patterns of initiation and minimize recall bias, smoking initiation may not be complete among these respondents, particularly adolescents. Thus, estimates derived from such surveys tend to be lower than those obtained by other methods. Because initiation largely occurs before age 18 years, surveys of young adults were used to estimate recent patterns of smoking initiation for this report.

Data from the Current Population Survey showed that the percentage of women aged 18 through 24 years who had started smoking by age 15 years was 2.1 percent in 1955 and 8.4 percent in 1966. The proportion of young women who had started to smoke by age 18 years was 15.9 percent in 1955 and 29.9 percent in 1966 (NCHS 1970; Schuman 1977).

**Table 2.19. Cumulative percentage (and 95% confidence interval) of recalled age at which respondents aged 18–21 years first tried a cigarette or began to smoke daily, by gender, National Household Survey on Drug Abuse, United States, 1998**

| | All persons | | | | Persons who ever smoked daily | | | |
|---|---|---|---|---|---|---|---|---|
| | First tried a cigarette* | | Began smoking daily† | | First tried a cigarette | | Began smoking daily | |
| Age (years) | Young women | Young men | Young women | Young men | Young women | Young men | Young women | Young men |
| <12 | 6.3 (±1.8) | 8.8 (±2.2) | 1.0 (±0.6)‡ | 1.1 (±0.7)‡ | 14.1 (±4.9) | 14.1 (±4.6) | 3.1 (±1.9) | 3.2 (±1.9) |
| <14 | 17.1 (±2.7) | 23.5 (±3.2) | 3.3 (±1.4) | 4.2 (±1.4) | 36.9 (±6.6) | 36.7 (±6.4) | 10.4 (±4.3) | 12.0 (±4.0) |
| <16 | 35.2 (±3.5) | 42.3 (±3.7) | 9.9 (±2.3) | 11.7 (±2.4) | 67.8 (±6.7) | 62.8 (±6.5) | 31.5 (±6.4) | 33.2 (±6.1) |
| <18 | 55.1 (±3.5) | 63.5 (±3.5) | 23.5 (±3.2) | 26.0 (±3.4) | 95.5 (±3.1) | 95.4 (±2.1) | 74.8 (±6.4) | 74.3 (±5.9) |
| Mean age | NA§ | NA | NA | NA | 14.1 (±0.3) | 14.2 (±0.3) | 16.1 (±0.3) | 16.1 (±0.3) |

*Respondents were asked, "How old were you the first time you smoked a cigarette, even one or two puffs?"
†Respondents were asked, "How old were you when you first started smoking cigarettes every day?"
‡Estimate should be interpreted with caution because of the small number of respondents.
§NA = Not applicable.
Source: Substance Abuse and Mental Health Services Administration, public use data tape, 1998.

The 1998 NHSDA data were used to determine the cumulative percentages of young women aged 18 through 21 years who first smoked a cigarette by a given age and the age at which they first started smoking daily (Table 2.19). Among these young women, 6.3 percent had tried a cigarette before age 12 years and 55.1 percent before age 18 years; 23.5 percent began smoking daily before age 18 years. Among those who were ever daily smokers, 14.1 percent tried a cigarette before age 12 years and 95.5 percent before age 18 years; 74.8 percent were daily smokers before age 18 years. Fewer young women than young men first tried a cigarette by age 18 years, but the age at first smoking daily did not differ by gender. Similarly, the data from the 1992 YRBS, a household survey, found that among young women aged 18 through 21 years who had ever smoked, 7.9 percent smoked their first whole cigarette at or before age 10 years and 37.1 percent did so at 11 through 14 years of age (Adams et al. 1995).

## Initiation Rate

Another method used to assess smoking initiation is the smoking initiation rate: the proportion of persons at risk for initiation of smoking who begin to smoke by a certain age or date. The rate is generally calculated as the number of persons who started to smoke in a particular year, divided by the number of persons who had not started smoking before that year. Lee and colleagues (1993) used data on recalled age at smoking initiation that were collected by NHIS for selected years between 1970 and 1988 for women aged 20 through 50 years. The analysis was restricted to women participants in this age group to avoid bias due to differential mortality. They calculated initiation rates by age for female participants aged 12 through 24 years in 1950, 1965, or 1980. In 1950, the highest yearly increase in smoking initiation occurred among those 18 years of age, and the second-highest increase occurred among those 20 years of age. By 1980, the greatest increases were among girls aged 16 or 18 years.

Another analysis, by Pierce and Gilpin (1995), used the 1955 Current Population Survey as well as the 1970, 1978, 1980, 1987, and 1988 NHIS. The investigators restricted the analysis to women 20 years of age or older at the time of the survey and made no adjustment for differential mortality. Initiation rates were calculated for females aged 10 through 25 years for the years 1910–1977. During 1910–1925, initiation rates among girls aged 10 through 13 years remained low. For those aged 14 through 21 years, the rates increased slightly and for women aged 22 through 25 years, the rates were stable. During 1926–1939, initiation rates among girls aged 10 through 13 years remained stable, but rates increased among female participants aged 14 through 25 years. During 1940–1967, initiation rates increased among female participants aged 10 through 21 years, but they did not change among women aged 22 through 25 years. For the period 1968–1977, the initiation rates increased slightly among girls aged 10 through 13 years, whereas they increased significantly among girls aged 14 through 17 years and decreased among women aged 18 through 25 years.

NHIS data for 1970, 1978, 1980, 1987, and 1988 were used to calculate initiation rates, on the basis of recalled age at smoking initiation, for all respondents 20 years of age or older (Burns et al. 1995, 1997). Estimates of rates were adjusted for differential mortality. Rates decreased among white women born during 1940–1954. The rate among the 1955–1959 cohort was higher than that among the 1950–1954 cohort, but the rate among the 1960–1964 cohort was comparable to that among the 1950–1954 cohort. In contrast, among young men, smoking initiation rates estimated from recalled age at initiation were consistently lower for these birth cohorts. NHIS data for women aged 20 through 50 years were also used to construct age-specific rates of smoking initiation among women aged 10 through 24 years during 1944–1985 (Gilpin et al. 1994; Pierce et al. 1994b). Smoking initiation rates among young women began to decline in the 1950s and early 1960s. However, among girls, smoking initiation rates increased from 1944 until the mid-1970s and then declined. The increase from the late 1960s to mid-1970s was particularly pronounced among girls 12 through 17 years of age; this increase was 1.7 times greater among girls who did not go on to college than among those who did go on to college.

The 1992–1993 Current Population Survey was used to estimate initiation rates among adolescents (aged 14 through 17 years) or young adults (aged 18 through 21 years) during 1980–1989. Among adolescents, the initiation rate decreased slightly during 1980–1984, then increased during 1984–1989; the largest annual increase occurred in 1988. Among young adults, initiation rates decreased during 1980–1989. No gender-specific differences in initiation rates were noted for either age group (CDC 1995c). Data from the 1990 YRBS of high school students showed that the smoking initiation rate among girls was greatest for girls at ages 13 and 14 years. Initiation rates were similar among girls and boys, except boys were more likely than girls to start smoking before age 9 years (Escobedo et al. 1993).

### Summary

Historically, women started to smoke at a later age than men. Beginning with the 1960 cohort, however, the mean age at smoking initiation has not differed by gender. The median age at smoking initiation decreased dramatically among women born in 1885–1914; the median age at initiation occurred 20 years earlier among women born in 1910–1914 than among women born in 1885–1889. Among cohorts of women born in 1931–1962, the mean age at smoking initiation declined about 1.5 years, but the mean age at first use of a cigarette (14.3 years) among young women born in 1976–1979 was not significantly different than among women born in 1961–1976. Because smoking initiation is not complete by age 21 years, this estimate is somewhat lower than it eventually may be.

## Nicotine Dependence Among Women and Girls

Symptoms associated with nicotine withdrawal include nausea, headache, constipation, diarrhea, increased appetite, drowsiness, fatigue, insomnia, inability to concentrate, irritability, hostility, anxiety, and craving for tobacco (Shiffman 1979; Hatsukami et al. 1985). In its *Diagnostic and Statistical Manual of Mental Disorders*, fourth edition (*DSM-IV*), the American Psychiatric Association (APA) recognized nicotine dependence as a mental disorder due to psychoactive substance abuse (APA 1994).

Data suggest that heavy smokers and smokers who are dependent on nicotine are less likely to quit smoking than those who are not dependent on nicotine (USDHHS 1988b; Killen et al. 1992; Breslau and Peterson 1996) (see "Trends in Quantity of Cigarettes Smoked" earlier in this chapter). Among persons aged 21 through 30 years who had ever smoked, 84 percent of those who ever met the criteria of the *Diagnostic and Statistical Manual of Mental Disorders*, third edition, revised (*DSM-III-R*) for nicotine dependence had smoked in the previous year, compared with 64 percent of those who never met the criteria (Breslau et al. 1993b). In a study of 622 students in grades 6 through 12, however, smoking cessation was not related to negative symptoms associated with withdrawal, such as feeling sick, dizzy, or shaky; having a stomachache or headache; gaining weight; or experiencing increased appetite (Ershler et al. 1989).

Estimates of the prevalence of several measures of nicotine dependence among girls and women who smoke are discussed here. These measures include time to the first cigarette after awakening, reasons for smoking, withdrawal symptoms, and other indicators of nicotine dependence. (See "Nicotine Pharmacology and Addiction" in Chapter 3 for further discussion of nicotine dependence, and "Smoking Cessation and Nicotine Addiction Treatment Methods" in Chapter 5 for further information on the relationship of heavy smoking with smoking cessation and relapse.)

## Time to First Cigarette After Awakening

Smoking within 30 minutes of awakening is a component in the Fagerström nicotine addiction scale (Fagerström 1978), and time to the first cigarette of the day has been associated with successful smoking cessation (Kabat and Wynder 1987; Hymowitz et al. 1997). For this report, time to the first cigarette was evaluated by using the 1993 TAPS II data for girls aged 10 through 17 years and young women aged 18 through 22 years. The 1987 NHIS data were used for young women 18 through 24 years and women aged 25 years or older.

### Women

In the 1987 NHIS data, 36.8 percent of women smokers aged 18 years or older smoked their first cigarette within 10 minutes of awakening, and 60.5 percent did so within 30 minutes of awakening (Table 2.20). These percentages were comparable across all age groups of women, even after stratification by the number of cigarettes smoked per day. In a survey of members of the American Association of Retired Persons (AARP), 66 percent of smokers aged 50 through 102 years smoked within 30 minutes of awakening (Rimer et al. 1990).

In the 1987 NHIS data, white women (38.0 percent) and black women (34.9 percent) who smoked were equally likely to smoke the first cigarette within 10 minutes of awakening, but white women (63.2 percent) were more likely than black women (52.1 percent) to smoke within 30 minutes of awakening (Table 2.20). White women also smoke more cigarettes per day than do black women (see "Trends in Quantity of Cigarettes Smoked" earlier in this chapter). However, when the data were stratified by smoking intensity (quantity of cigarettes smoked), black women who smoked fewer than 25 cigarettes per day were significantly more likely than their white counterparts to smoke within 10 minutes of awakening. Of those who smoked fewer than 15 cigarettes per day, black women were significantly more likely than white women to smoke within 30 minutes of awakening. In baseline data from COMMIT, a community-based smoking intervention trial conducted in 1988–1993 in 22 communities in the United States and Canada, black women who smoked were more likely than white women who smoked to smoke the first cigarette within 10 minutes of awakening (Royce et al. 1993). Black women may be more sensitive than white women to the dependence-producing properties of nicotine; serum cotinine levels have been found to be higher among black women than among white women, even though black women smoked fewer cigarettes per day (Caraballo et al. 1998). Wagenknecht and associates (1990a) hypothesized that black women may smoke cigarettes with a higher nicotine content or inhale more deeply than do white women.

Gender-specific differences regarding time to the first cigarette appear to exist. Among persons who smoked 25 or more cigarettes per day, women were more likely than men to smoke within 10 minutes of awakening (69.0 vs. 58.6 percent), but this difference was largely a result of significant gender-specific differences for women aged 18 through 24 years (NCHS, public use data tape, 1987). As age increased, the difference by gender became nonsignificant. COMMIT, which did not report data by age groups, found that women who were light smokers (≤ 15 cigarettes per day) or moderate smokers (≤ 24 cigarettes per day) were more likely than their male counterparts to report smoking within 10 minutes of awakening (Royce et al. 1997).

### Girls and Young Women

In 1992, 33 percent of adolescent current smokers aged 12 through 17 years reported smoking within 30 minutes of arising; 64 percent of heavy smokers reported smoking within 30 minutes of arising (George H. Gallup International Institute 1992). (For this analysis, heavy smoking was defined as smoking ≥ 5 cigarettes daily on ≥ 10 days in the preceding month.) In the 1993 TAPS II data, 42.0 (±8.4) percent of girls aged 10 through 17 years who were current regular smokers smoked a cigarette within 30 minutes of awakening (data not shown). (For this analysis, current regular smokers were defined as smokers who had smoked ≥ 2 cigarettes daily on ≥ 3 days in the past week.) The percentage who smoked within 30 minutes of awakening increased as the number of

**Table 2.20. Percentage (and 95% confidence interval) of current women smokers aged 18 years or older who reported that they smoked their first cigarette within 10 or 30 minutes of awakening, by selected characteristics, National Health Interview Survey, United States, 1987**

| Characteristic | Smoke within 10 minutes of awakening | Smoke within 30 minutes of awakening |
|---|---|---|
| Women | 36.8 (±2.1) | 60.5 (±2.1) |
| <15 cigarettes/day* | 15.6 (±2.7) | 32.5 (±3.2) |
| 15–24 cigarettes/day | 38.7 (±3.1) | 68.3 (±3.1) |
| ≥ 25 cigarettes/day | 69.0 (±4.2) | 91.6 (±2.5) |
| Race/ethnicity | | |
| White, non-Hispanic | 38.0 (±2.4) | 63.2 (±2.3) |
| <15 cigarettes/day* | 12.8 (±3.1) | 30.5 (±4.0) |
| 15–24 cigarettes/day | 37.6 (±3.3) | 68.5 (±3.4) |
| ≥ 25 cigarettes/day | 69.1 (±4.3) | 91.4 (±2.6) |
| Black, non-Hispanic | 34.9 (±5.3) | 52.1 (±5.5) |
| <15 cigarettes/day* | 24.9 (±5.8) | 41.3 (±6.2) |
| 15–24 cigarettes/day | 52.8 (±10.2) | 71.9 (±9.9) |
| ≥ 25 cigarettes/day | 78.2 (±16.4)† | 97.7 (±3.3)† |
| Men | 37.8 (±2.1) | 64.4 (±2.1) |
| <15 cigarettes/day* | 11.9 (±2.8) | 26.3 (±3.8) |
| 15–24 cigarettes/day | 36.8 (±3.5) | 69.5 (±3.5) |
| ≥ 25 cigarettes/day | 58.6 (±3.7) | 88.0 (±2.3) |

*Note:* Current smokers were persons who reported smoking ≥ 100 cigarettes in their lifetime and who smoked at the time of the survey.
*Includes persons who did not smoke daily.
†Estimate should be interpreted with caution because of the small number of respondents.
Source: National Center for Health Statistics, public use data tape, 1987.

cigarettes smoked per day increased (Figure 2.13). Although some sample sizes were small, the test for trend was highly significant ($p < 0.001$). Girls and boys who smoked regularly were equally likely to smoke within 30 minutes of awakening. However, because some adolescents may have to wait until they leave home before they can smoke the first cigarette of the day, smoking within 30 minutes of awakening may be a less valid measure for adolescents than for adults.

TAPS II reported that, among young women aged 18 through 22 years who smoked regularly, 21.6 (±4.6) percent smoked within 10 minutes of awakening and 40.6 (±5.2) percent smoked within 30 minutes of awakening (data not shown). The proportion who smoked within 30 minutes of awakening increased directly with the number of cigarettes smoked per day (Figure 2.13), and the test for trend was highly significant ($p < 0.0001$). Young women (21.6 ± 4.6 percent) and young men (21.8 ± 3.7 percent) who smoked regularly were equally likely to smoke within 10 minutes of awakening, but young women (40.6 ± 5.2 percent) were less likely than young men (50.4 ± 4.6 percent) to smoke within 30 minutes of awakening (data not shown). These findings had borderline statistical significance.

In the 1987 NHIS data, among young women aged 18 through 24 years who smoked, 30.7 (±4.9) percent smoked within 10 minutes of awakening and 49.0 (±6.0) percent did so within 30 minutes of awakening (NCHS, public use data tape, 1987). The percentage who smoked within 10 or 30 minutes of awakening increased directly with the number of cigarettes smoked per day, and the test for trend was highly significant ($p < 0.0001$). Even among young women who smoked fewer than 15 cigarettes per day, more than one-fourth smoked within 30 minutes of awakening. On the basis of time to the first cigarette after awakening, young women who smoke appear to

**Figure 2.13. Percentage of young female current smokers aged 10–22 years who smoked their first cigarette within 30 minutes of awakening, by age and quantity of cigarettes smoked, Teenage Attitudes and Practices Survey II, United States, 1993**

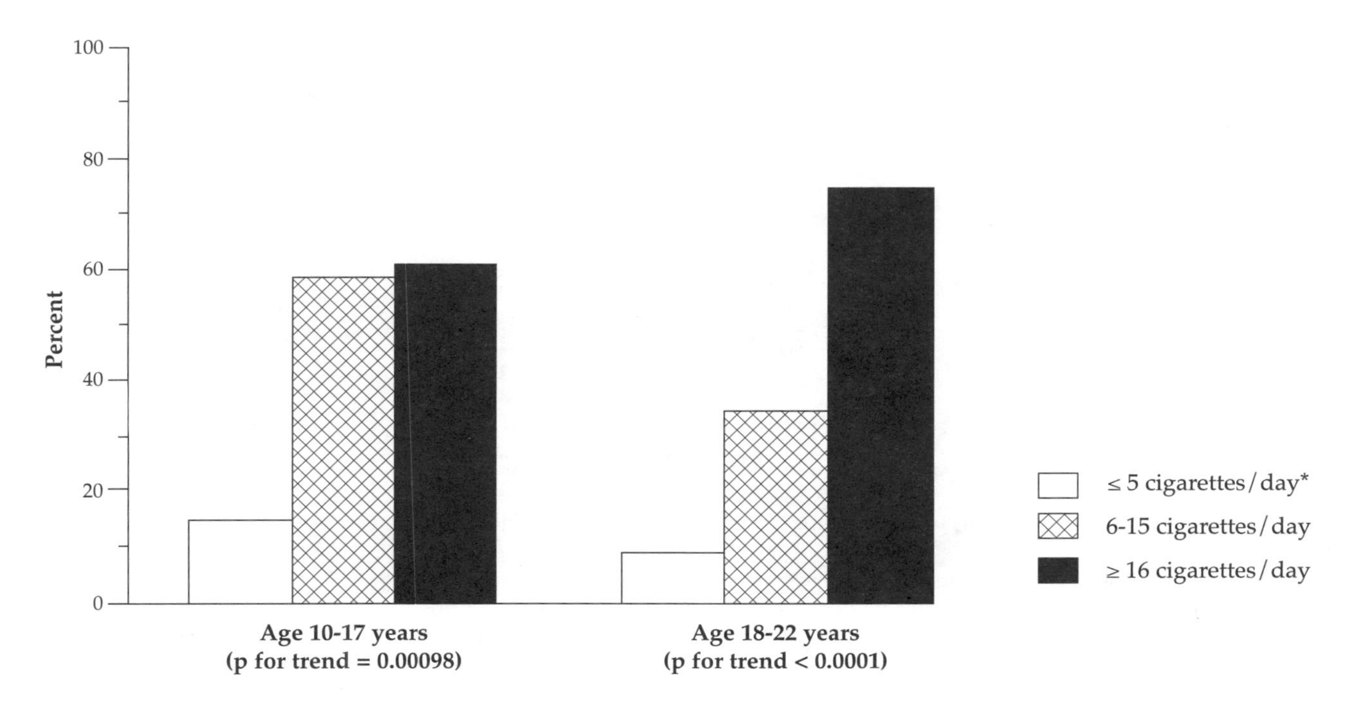


*Note:* Question was only asked of persons who smoked ≥ 2 cigarettes on ≥ 3 days in the week before the survey.
*Includes persons who did not smoke daily.
Source: Centers for Disease Control and Prevention, Office on Smoking and Health, public use data tape, 1993.

be as dependent as older women on nicotine. In a study of smoking cessation among 45 women, O'Hara and Portser (1994) found that women aged 20 through 49 years and women aged 50 through 75 years were equally likely to be classified as highly dependent smokers.

## Reasons for Cigarette Use by Girls and Young Women

In the 1993 TAPS II data, among current smokers who had smoked in the previous 30 days, 67.9 percent of girls aged 10 through 17 years and 75.5 percent of young women aged 18 through 22 years said they smoked because smoking relaxed or calmed them (Table 2.21). Even among girls who smoked five or fewer cigarettes per day, 60.7 percent reported that smoking relaxed or calmed them. The percentage of female smokers (girls and young women) who gave this response increased as the number of cigarettes smoked per day increased, and the test for trend was highly significant ($p < 0.003$). Charlton (1984) also found that 55 percent of girls aged 11 through 13 years and 76 percent of girls aged 14 through 16 years who smoked one or more cigarettes per week did so to calm nerves. McNeill and colleagues (1987) reported that the most common subjective effect reported by children who smoked was feeling calmer (64 percent among daily smokers and 38 percent among nondaily smokers). The researchers noted that reports of feeling calmer, which may be a surrogate for nicotine dependence, were directly associated with reports of having withdrawal symptoms among persons attempting to quit smoking: 82 percent of respondents who reported feeling calmer by smoking, and 40 percent of respondents who did not report feeling calmer by smoking, had at least one withdrawal symptom. This relationship was found even for children and adolescents who had been smoking for less than one year.

**Table 2.21. Prevalence (% and 95% confidence interval) of selected reasons of current smokers for using cigarettes, among girls aged 10–17 years and young women aged 18–22 years, by selected characteristics, Teenage Attitudes and Practices Survey II, United States, 1993**

| Characteristic | "It relaxes or calms me" | "It's really hard to quit" |
|---|---|---|
| Female smokers | | |
| Aged 10–17 years | 67.9 (±6.0) | 56.0 (±6.3) |
| ≤ 5 cigarettes/day* | 60.7 (±8.1) | 38.3 (±8.7) |
| 6–15 cigarettes/day | 72.9 (±10.4) | 78.1 (±9.3) |
| ≥ 16 cigarettes/day | 88.0 (±11.4)† | 80.3 (±15.4)† |
| Aged 18–22 years | 75.5 (±3.6) | 61.6 (±4.2) |
| ≤ 5 cigarettes/day* | 67.8 (±6.6) | 33.9 (±7.6) |
| 6–15 cigarettes/day | 79.1 (±5.2) | 70.4 (±6.0) |
| ≥ 16 cigarettes/day | 80.8 (±7.4) | 87.4 (±5.5) |
| Male smokers | | |
| Aged 10–17 years | 58.7 (±6.6) | 57.7 (±7.2) |
| Aged 18–22 years | 63.3 (±4.0) | 63.1 (±4.2) |

*Note:* Current smokers were persons in each demographic category who reported that they smoked cigarettes during the past 30 days.
*Includes persons who did not smoke daily.
†Estimate should be interpreted with caution because of the small number of respondents.
Source: Centers for Disease Control and Prevention, Office on Smoking and Health, public use data tape, 1993.

Girls and young women who had smoked in the previous 30 days were equally likely to report that they did so because it was "really hard" to quit smoking (Table 2.21). Even among girls who smoked five or fewer cigarettes per day, 38.3 percent reported that it was really hard to quit smoking. The percentage who gave this response increased as the number of cigarettes smoked per day increased, and the test for trend was highly significant ($p < 0.0001$). Among young women, 33.9 percent of those who smoked 5 or fewer cigarettes per day and 87.4 percent of those who smoked 16 or more cigarettes per day said it was really hard to quit smoking. When results were stratified by the number of cigarettes smoked per day, there were no significant differences between data for girls and young women.

Although no significant gender-specific differences were found among children, among young adults who smoked 16 or more cigarettes per day, women (80.8 ± 7.4 percent) were more likely than men (64.8 ± 6.8 percent) to report that they smoked because smoking relaxed or calmed them or that it was really hard to quit (87.4 ± 5.5 vs. 75.4 ± 5.7 percent) (CDC, Office on Smoking and Health, public use data tape, 1993).

## Indicators of Nicotine Dependence

### Women

The 1992–1994-A NHSDA (combined data) was used to assess self-reported indicators of nicotine dependence among women: "felt [they needed] or were dependent on cigarettes," "needed larger amounts [more cigarettes] to get the same effect," "felt unable to cut down on [their] use, even though [they] tried," and "had withdrawal symptoms, that is, felt sick because [they] stopped or cut down on cigarette use" (Table 2.22). Of the women who were current smokers, 77.5 percent reported one or more indicators of nicotine dependence, and 71.0 percent reported feeling dependent on cigarettes. Among women who had tried to cut back on their smoking, 79.2 percent reported being unable to do so, and 33.4 percent reported feeling sick when they tried to do so. On the basis of self-reports of three or more measures from *DSM-III-R*, Anthony and associates (1994) estimated that one of three tobacco smokers aged 15 through 54 years is nicotine dependent. However, in a small, local survey of 46 persons in Burlington, Vermont, about 75 percent of women who were current smokers met *DSM-III-R* criteria for nicotine dependence and 71 percent of women had withdrawal symptoms when

**Table 2.22. Percentage (and 95% confidence interval) of current women smokers aged 18 years or older who reported selected indicators of nicotine dependence, by race or ethnicity and quantity of cigarettes smoked, National Household Survey on Drug Abuse, United States, 1992–1994, aggregate data**

| | Indicators of nicotine dependence | | | | |
|---|---|---|---|---|---|
| Characteristic | Felt dependent on cigarettes | Needed more cigarettes for same effect | Unable to | Felt sick when cut down on smoking* | Any dependence indicator[†] |
| Women overall | 71.0 (±3.1) | 14.8 (±2.4) | 79.2 (±3.1) | 33.4 (±3.8) | 77.5 (±2.8) |
| ≤ 15 cigarettes/day[‡] | 61.7 (±4.9) | 10.5 (±2.2) | 70.2 (±4.9) | 27.8 (±4.8) | 68.9 (±4.7) |
| 16–25 cigarettes/day | 80.2 (±3.6) | 13.8 (±3.3) | 85.5 (±4.0) | 35.3 (±5.2) | 85.4 (±3.1) |
| ≥ 26 cigarettes/day | 78.6 (±9.2) | 29.0 (±9.0) | 90.8 (±7.7) | 44.8 (±11.1) | 86.1 (±5.7) |
| Race/ethnicity | | | | | |
| White | 74.2 (±3.6) | 14.6 (±2.8) | 79.6 (±3.6) | 33.8 (±4.4) | 79.8 (±3.3) |
| ≤ 15 cigarettes/day[‡] | 65.0 (±6.5) | 9.6 (±2.7) | 68.3 (±6.4) | 27.4 (±5.9) | 71.0 (±6.2) |
| 16–25 cigarettes/day | 82.4 (±3.6) | 12.9 (±3.3) | 86.3 (±4.3) | 35.8 (±5.6) | 86.6 (±3.3) |
| ≥ 26 cigarettes/day | 78.9 (±9.9) | 29.4 (±9.5) | 91.2 (±7.9) | 44.0 (±11.6) | 86.6 (±6.0) |
| Black | 56.1 (±5.4) | 15.3 (±5.1) | 76.7 (±6.6) | 29.8 (±6.5) | 67.7 (±5.2) |
| ≤ 15 cigarettes/day[‡] | 55.7 (±6.0) | 13.4 (±4.2) | 75.4 (±7.8) | 28.2 (±8.4) | 65.8 (±6.5) |
| 16–25 cigarettes/day | 53.0 (±14.0) | 20.1 (±17.6) | 80.5 (±16.1) | 28.6 (±10.3) | 71.5 (±9.9) |
| ≥ 26 cigarettes/day | 70.8 (±13.8) | 19.4 (±15.1)[§] | 79.0 (±24.5) | 54.6 (±24.1)[§] | 75.4 (±12.9) |
| Hispanic | 56.8 (±5.7) | 15.6 (±4.6) | 78.8 (±6.9) | 33.9 (±6.8) | 65.8 (±5.5) |
| ≤ 15 cigarettes/day[‡] | 46.5 (±6.2) | 12.8 (±4.8) | 78.6 (±6.9) | 30.8 (±8.7) | 57.7 (±6.2) |
| 16–25 cigarettes/day | 82.8 (±7.7) | 21.0 (±12.7) | 75.8 (±18.1) | 33.9 (±15.3) | 85.5 (±7.2) |
| ≥ 26 cigarettes/day | 86.6 (±12.3) | 31.5 (±29.5)[§] | 93.0 (±9.1) | 66.6 (±24.7)[§] | 91.8 (±6.6) |
| Men overall | 66.2 (±3.1) | 13.2 (±2.3) | 75.6 (±3.6) | 35.7 (±5.2) | 72.1 (±2.9) |
| ≤ 15 cigarettes/day[‡] | 51.2 (±4.0) | 11.2 (±3.4) | 62.1 (±5.4) | 28.4 (±5.7) | 60.0 (±4.1) |
| 16–25 cigarettes/day | 72.6 (±5.2) | 13.3 (±3.9) | 80.3 (±5.7) | 33.3 (±6.8) | 78.7 (±4.7) |
| ≥ 26 cigarettes/day | 78.8 (±6.6) | 16.1 (±5.8) | 88.6 (±5.3) | 50.6 (±11.8) | 80.4 (±6.6) |

*Note:* Current smokers were persons who reported smoking ≥ 100 cigarettes (about 5 packs) during their lifetime and who smoked at the time of the survey. Indicators of nicotine dependence were (1) "felt [they needed] or were dependent on cigarettes," (2) "needed larger amounts [more cigarettes] to get the same effect," (3) "felt unable to cut down on [their] use, even though [they] tried," and (4) "had withdrawal symptoms, that is, felt sick because [they] stopped or cut down on cigarette use."

*Analysis of "unable to cut down" and "felt sick" was restricted to persons who reported trying to reduce their use of cigarettes during the preceding 12 months. In addition, for indicator "unable to cut down," because of the question design, respondents who reported not trying to reduce any drug use during the preceding 12 months were excluded from this analysis.

[†]Current smokers who reported ≥ 1 of the 4 indicators of nicotine dependence.

[‡]Includes smokers who did not smoke daily.

[§]Estimate should be interpreted with caution because of the small number of respondents.

Sources: Alcohol, Drug Abuse, and Mental Health Administration, public use data tape, 1992; Substance Abuse and Mental Health Services Administration, public use data tapes, 1993, 1994-A.

they tried to reduce or stop smoking (Hale et al. 1993). Beginning with the 1994-B NHSDA, only two measures of nicotine dependence were used: smoking cigarettes more than intended in the past 12 months, and tolerance to cigarettes built up in the past 12 months. In the 1997–1998 NHSDA (combined data), one-half of the women who smoked reported at least one of these measures of nicotine dependence (data not shown) (SAMHSA, public use data tapes, 1997–1998).

In the 1992–1994-A NHSDA data, the percentage of women who reported indicators of nicotine dependence increased as the number of cigarettes smoked per day increased, particularly as daily smoking increased from 15 or fewer cigarettes per day to 16 to 25 cigarettes per day (Table 2.22). Similar patterns were noted for the indicators of nicotine dependence in the 1997–1998 NHSDA (combined data), although for these indicators the most dramatic increase occurred as daily smoking increased from 16 to 25 cigarettes per day to 26 or more cigarettes per day (data not shown). Other studies confirm that smokers who are dependent on nicotine consume more cigarettes per day than do nondependent smokers (Killen et al. 1988; Breslau et al. 1993b).

The 1992–1994-A NHSDA data indicated that black women (67.7 percent) and Hispanic women (65.8 percent) who smoked were less likely than white women who smoked (79.8 percent) to report one or more indicators of nicotine dependence (Kandel et al. 1997a) (Table 2.22). White women were more likely to report feeling dependent on cigarettes than were black women or Hispanic women. These findings may reflect differences in numbers of cigarettes smoked per day across racial and ethnic groups. Despite the higher likelihood that white women will report nicotine dependence, black women have been reported to have higher blood levels of cotinine (a nicotine metabolite) than do white women for comparable quantities of cigarettes smoked (Ahijevych et al. 1996; Caraballo et al. 1998).

The 1992–1994-A and 1997–1998 NHSDA data showed that women and men were equally likely to report one or more indicators of nicotine dependence, and no significant gender-specific differences were noted for individual indicators. In other studies, researchers have reported that women are more likely than men to describe themselves as "hooked on" or addicted to cigarettes (Eiser and Van Der Pligt 1986). This difference may reflect cultural rather than physiologic factors: in NHSDA data, no gender-specific differences were found for reporting withdrawal symptoms or feeling unable to cut down on smoking among adults who had tried to reduce smoking. Investigators in still other studies reported no gender-specific differences in prevalence of withdrawal symptoms determined either objectively or subjectively (Gunn 1986; Svikis et al. 1986; Pirie et al. 1991). Thus, several researchers have concluded that the prevalence of nicotine dependence is about the same among women and men (Svikis et al. 1986; Breslau et al. 1993a; Breslau 1995). However, some study findings suggested that women report more symptoms of nicotine dependence, more severe withdrawal symptoms, or longer duration of withdrawal symptoms than do men (Guilford 1967; Shiffman 1979; Pomerleau and Pomerleau 1994; Kandel et al. 1997a; Kandel and Chen 2000). Any gender-specific differences in withdrawal symptoms could be due to differences in attention to or reporting of symptoms, rather than to a biological difference (Waldron 1983).

Study results also differ on whether nicotine affects women and men differently (Pomerleau 1996). Some investigators reported few gender-specific differences in the subjective, behavioral, or physiologic effects of nicotine (Perkins 1995). Depending on the nicotine effect examined (e.g., dose-related withdrawal response or weight gain), others reported that women exhibit either less or greater sensitivity to nicotine than do men. Silverstein and coworkers (1980) suggested that, because women are more likely to report feeling sick after smoking their very first cigarette, they may be more sensitive than men to nicotine. Some researchers have attributed this increased sensitivity to women's smaller size, higher percentage of body fat, and slower clearance of nicotine from the body (Gorrod and Jenner 1975; Benowitz and Jacob 1984; Grunberg et al. 1991). Others have concluded that any gender-specific differences in the physiologic response to nicotine have a minor influence on differences in smoking behavior of women and men (Waldron 1991), or they have attributed a difference in the effect of nicotine to gender-specific differences in smoking patterns (Schievelbein et al. 1978).

### Girls and Young Women

The 1993 TAPS II was used to assess symptoms of nicotine withdrawal among girls aged 10 through 17 years and among young women aged 18 through 22 years who had smoked in the previous seven days and had attempted to quit smoking in the past. The items used to assess symptoms of withdrawal were having a strong need or urge to smoke; feeling more irritable; finding it hard to concentrate; feeling restless; feeling hungry more often; and feeling sad, blue, or depressed.

Of respondents who smoked in the previous seven days, 86.8 (±5.7) percent of girls and 90.0 (±3.1) percent of young women reported one or more symptoms of nicotine withdrawal during previous attempts to quit smoking. More than one-half of each group reported feeling a strong need or urge to smoke, feeling more irritable, feeling restless, and feeling hungry more often (NCHS, public use data tape, 1993).

In TAPS II data, the percentage of girls or young women who reported withdrawal symptoms during previous attempts to quit smoking increased with the number of cigarettes smoked per day (Figure 2.14). This finding is consistent with Stanton's (1995) study of 18-year-olds in which the number of cigarettes smoked per day was associated with dependence on tobacco. In TAPS II data, no significant differences were found between girls and young women in the reporting of symptoms of nicotine withdrawal. These findings have also been noted in other studies (CDC 1995a).

Ershler and coworkers (1989) found that 53.7 percent of adolescent smokers reported feeling worse when they stopped smoking. Adverse symptoms were reported by a greater proportion of heavy smokers (>10 cigarettes per day) (66.0 percent) than daily smokers (≤ 10 cigarettes per day) (55.1 percent) and by a much lower proportion of occasional smokers (sporadic, "bingey," or less than daily smoking) (15.4 percent). In a study of 24 high schools in California and Illinois in 1988–1992 by Sussman and colleagues (1998), 68 percent of high school girls reported that it bothered them to go a whole day without smoking, and 61 percent reported that they did not feel right if they went too long without a cigarette. McNeill and colleagues (1986) found that among British girls aged 11 through 17 years, 74 percent of daily smokers and 47 percent of occasional smokers who had ever tried to stop smoking permanently reported withdrawal symptoms: 13 percent of all girls who smoked reported being unable to concentrate, 33 percent being hungry, 22 percent having increased irritability, 38 percent having a strong need to smoke, and 16 percent being restless. It may be that the prevalences reported by McNeill and colleagues were lower than the prevalences from TAPS II because the mean number of cigarettes smoked per day by respondents in the study by McNeill and colleagues was lower (6.8 cigarettes per day) than that in TAPS II (7.8 cigarettes per day). Girls were as likely as young women to report withdrawal symptoms, even after adjustment for the number of cigarettes smoked per day. In a New Zealand study of 18-year-olds who had smoked every day for at least one month in the past year, Stanton (1995) found that 61 percent reported craving cigarettes, 43 percent being irritable, 46 percent being restless, 25 percent having difficulty concentrating, 45 percent having increased appetite or weight gain, and 20 percent feeling depressed when they had tried to quit smoking.

In the 1992–1994-A NHSDA (combined data), the prevalence of self-reported indicators of nicotine dependence was assessed for girls aged 12 through 17 years and young women aged 18 through 24 years who had smoked within the past 30 days (Table 2.23). These indicators included "felt [they needed] or were dependent on cigarettes," "needed larger amounts [more cigarettes] to get the same effect," "felt unable to cut down on [their] use, even though [they] tried," and "had withdrawal symptoms, that is, felt sick because [they] stopped or cut down on cigarette use." Among girls who smoked, 63.1 percent reported one or more indicators and 51.6 percent reported feeling dependent on cigarettes. Among those who had tried to cut down on their smoking, 70.0 percent felt unable to do so and 28.2 percent had withdrawal symptoms when they did so. The percentage of girls who smoked who reported one or more indicators of nicotine dependence increased as the number of cigarettes smoked per day increased: 58.3 (±11.5) percent of girls who smoked 5 or fewer cigarettes per day and 96.9 (±3.5) percent of those who smoked 16 or more cigarettes per day reported one or more indicators of nicotine dependence (Figure 2.15) (Alcohol, Drug Abuse, and Mental Health Administration, public use data tape, 1992; SAMHSA, public use data tapes, 1993, 1994-A).

In the 1997–1998 NHSDA (combined data), nearly one-half of the girls aged 12 through 17 years reported either having used cigarettes more than intended in the past 12 months or having built up tolerance to cigarettes in the past 12 months. The prevalence of these indicators increased as the intensity of smoking increased (data not shown) (SAMHSA, public use data tapes, 1997–1998).

In the 1992–1994-A NHSDA data, 81.2 percent of the young women aged 18 through 24 years who smoked reported one or more of these indicators (Table 2.23); 74.6 percent reported feeling dependent on cigarettes. Among those who had tried to cut down on their smoking, 79.0 percent reported being unable to do so and 32.3 percent reported withdrawal symptoms. The prevalence of indicators of nicotine dependence generally increased as the intensity of smoking increased (Figure 2.15). Similarly, in the 1997–1998 NHSDA data, more than one-half of young

**Figure 2.14. Percentage of girls aged 10–17 years and young women aged 18–22 years who smoked during the past week who reported selected symptoms of nicotine withdrawal during previous attempts to stop smoking, by quantity of cigarettes smoked, Teenage Attitudes and Practices Survey II, United States, 1993**

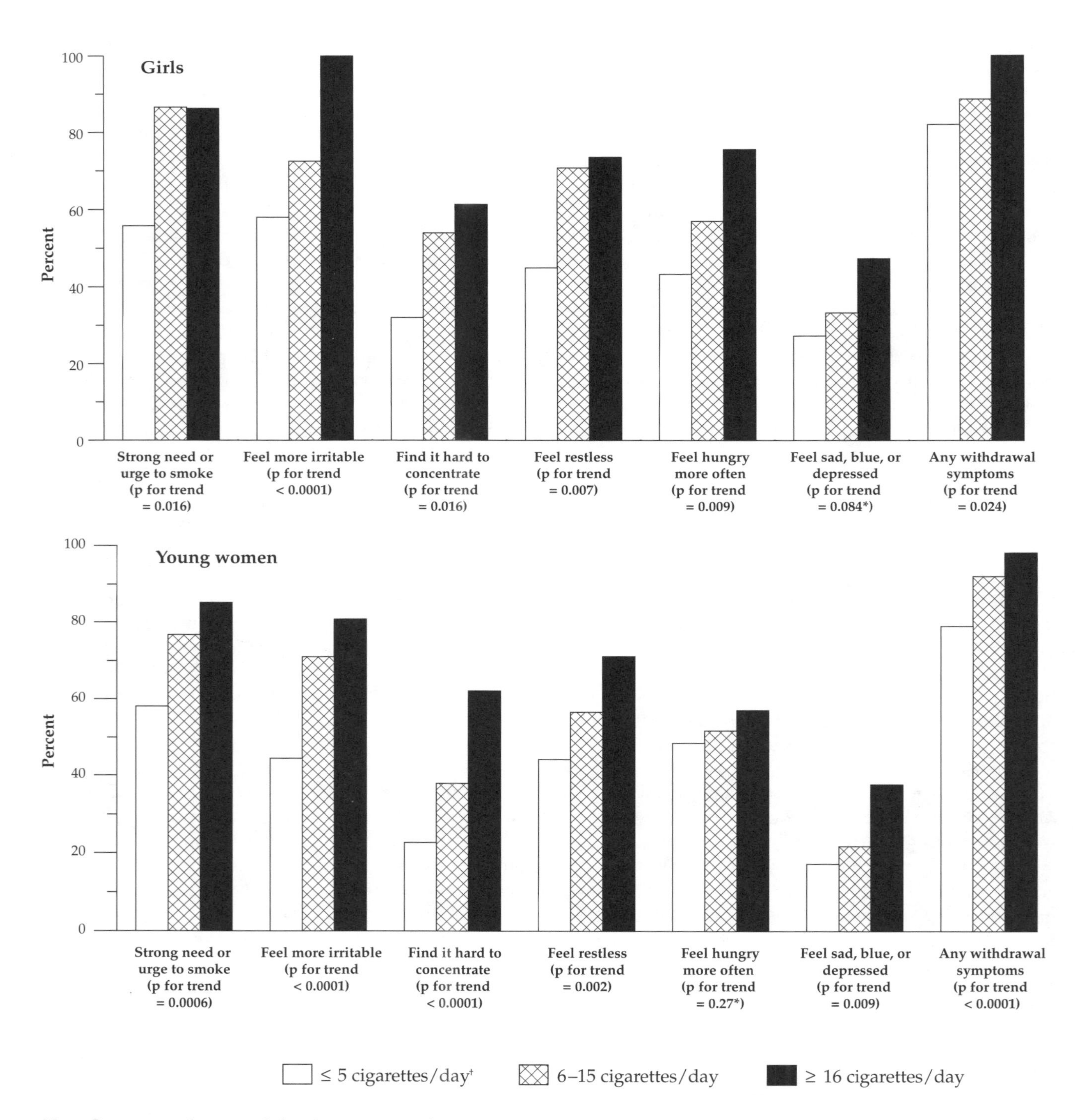


*Note:* Current smokers are defined as persons who reported smoking during the 7 days before the survey.
*Not significant.
†Includes persons who did not smoke daily.
Source: Centers for Disease Control and Prevention, Office on Smoking and Health, public use data tape, 1993.

**Table 2.23. Percentage (and 95% confidence interval) of adolescents aged 12–17 years and young adults aged 18–24 years who were current smokers who reported selected indicators of nicotine dependence, by gender and age, National Household Survey on Drug Abuse, United States, 1992–1994, aggregate data**

| | Indicators of nicotine dependence | | | | |
|---|---|---|---|---|---|
| **Characteristic** | **Felt dependent on cigarettes** | **Needed more cigarettes for same effect** | **Unable to** | **Felt sick when cut down on smoking*** | **Any dependence indicator†** |
| Female smokers | | | | | |
| Aged 12–17 years | 51.6 (±7.2) | 22.4 (±5.9) | 70.0 (±8.4) | 28.2 (±8.5) | 63.1 (±6.1) |
| Aged 18–24 years | 74.6 (±4.0) | 18.2 (±3.3) | 79.0 (±4.5) | 32.3 (±4.5) | 81.2 (±3.6) |
| Male smokers | | | | | |
| Aged 12–17 years | 50.6 (±7.1) | 22.7 (±6.3) | 68.6 (±10.1) | 31.9 (±9.7) | 61.7 (±7.3) |
| Aged 18–24 years | 60.5 (±3.6) | 18.5 (±3.1) | 68.0 (±4.9) | 29.1 (±4.9) | 70.6 (±3.5) |

*Note:* For adolescents aged 12–17 years, current smokers were persons who reported smoking cigarettes during the preceding 30 days. For young adults aged 18–24 years, current smokers were persons who reported that they had smoked ≥ 100 cigarettes (about 5 packs) in their lifetime and smoked during the preceding 30 days. Current smokers may include nondaily smokers. Indicators of nicotine dependence were (1) "felt [they needed] or were dependent on cigarettes," (2) "needed larger amounts [more cigarettes] to get the same effect," (3) "felt unable to cut down on [their] use, even though [they] tried," and (4) "had withdrawal symptoms, that is, felt sick because [they] stopped or cut down on cigarette use."

*The analysis of "unable to cut down" and "felt sick" was restricted to persons who reported trying to reduce their use of cigarettes during the preceding 12 months. In addition, for indicator "unable to cut down," because of the question design, respondents who reported not trying to reduce any drug use during the preceding 12 months were excluded from this analysis.

†Current smokers who reported ≥ 1 of the 4 indicators of nicotine dependence.

Sources: Alcohol, Drug Abuse, and Mental Health Administration, public use data tape, 1992; Substance Abuse and Mental Health Services Administration, public use data tapes, 1993, 1994-A.

women aged 18 through 24 years reported having one or both of the measures of nicotine dependence, and the prevalence of these measures increased as the intensity of smoking increased (data not shown) (SAMHSA, public use data tapes, 1997–1998).

In the 1992–1994-A NHSDA data, young women who smoked were more likely than girls to report one or more indicators of nicotine dependence (Table 2.23), but no age-specific difference was found when results were stratified by intensity of smoking (data not shown). This finding is consistent with studies showing that girls inhale cigarette smoke, even at very early stages of smoking (McNeill et al. 1989). In the 1997–1998 NHSDA, young women were more likely than girls to report one or more of these indicators of nicotine dependence, but differences for each measure alone were not statistically significant and no differences by age were noted after stratification by number of cigarettes smoked per day (data not shown) (SAMHSA, public use data tapes, 1997–1998).

For both TAPS and NHSDA data on nicotine dependence, the prevalence of reported indicators was similar among girls and boys (CDC, Office on Smoking and Health, public use data tape, 1993; Kandel et al. 1997a). In a study of 24 high schools, Sussman and colleagues (1998) found that girls were more likely than boys to report three measures of nicotine dependence. In the 1992–1994-A NHSDA data, among young adults who smoke, women were more likely than men to report one or more indicators of nicotine dependence. They were also more likely than young men to report feeling dependent on cigarettes and being unable to cut down on their smoking (Table 2.23). Although the differences were not always statistically significant, these patterns were also found when results were stratified by intensity of smoking (data not shown). For the 1997–1998 NHSDA data, however, no gender-specific differences were noted in the reporting of indicators of nicotine dependence (data not shown) (SAMHSA, public use data tapes, 1997–1998).

**Figure 2.15. Percentage of girls aged 12–17 years and young women aged 18–24 years who were current smokers who reported selected indicators of nicotine dependence, by age and quantity of cigarettes smoked, National Household Survey on Drug Abuse, United States, 1992–1994, aggregate data**

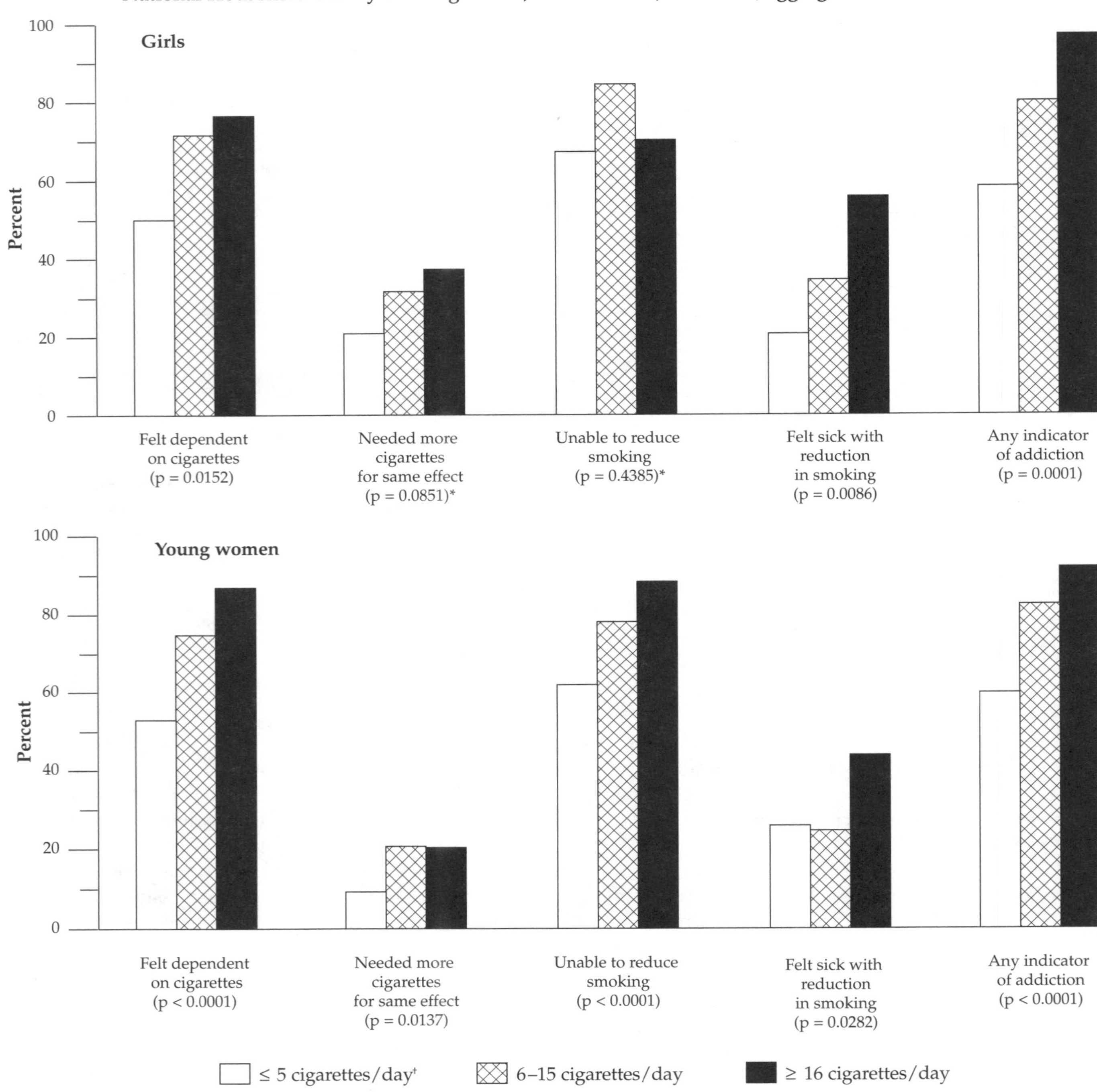


*Note:* For girls aged 12–17 years, current smokers were persons who reported smoking cigarettes during the preceding 30 days. For young women aged 18–24 years, current smokers were persons who reported that they had smoked ≥ 100 cigarettes (about 5 packs) in their lifetime and smoked during the preceding 30 days.

*NS = Not significant.

†Includes persons who did not smoke daily.

Sources: Alcohol, Drug Abuse, and Mental Health Administration, public use data tape, 1992; Substance Abuse and Mental Health Services Administration, public use data tapes, 1993, 1994-A.

### Nicotine Withdrawal Symptoms and Smoking Cessation

In the 1993 TAPS II data, girls aged 10 through 17 years who had tried to quit smoking and failed (i.e., had smoked in the past 30 days) were significantly more likely than those who had successfully quit smoking to report having had one or more symptoms of nicotine withdrawal during previous attempts to quit smoking (82.0 ± 6.1 vs. 48.6 ± 8.9 percent) (NCHS, public use data tape, 1993). This pattern was also found for each withdrawal symptom. These symptoms were feeling sad, blue, or depressed; a strong need or urge to smoke; irritability; difficulty concentrating; restlessness; and hunger. Similar results were found for young women aged 18 through 22 years: current smokers (86.8 ± 3.5 percent) were significantly more likely than former smokers (50.2 ± 7.3 percent) to report any of the symptoms of nicotine withdrawal during previous attempts to quit smoking. Other researchers have reported that smokers who tried unsuccessfully to quit smoking were more likely to be nicotine dependent than were those who successfully quit smoking (Pirie et al. 1991; Breslau et al. 1993b). TAPS II data showed no gender-specific differences among current smokers or former smokers in the reporting of nicotine withdrawal symptoms during previous attempts at smoking cessation (NCHS, public use data tape, 1993).

### Summary

The quantity of cigarettes smoked per day is strongly associated with the level of nicotine dependence. When results are stratified by number of cigarettes smoked per day, girls and women who smoke appear to be equally dependent on nicotine, as measured by time to the first cigarette after awakening, smoking for a calming or relaxing effect, or reporting of withdrawal symptoms or other indicators of nicotine dependence. After stratification of the number of cigarettes smoked per day, black women appear to be more likely than white women to smoke within 30 minutes of awakening. Few gender-specific differences were found in indicators of nicotine dependence among adolescents, young adults, or adults overall. The gender-specific differences that were found in indicators of nicotine dependence occurred primarily among young adults: young women were more likely than young men to report that they smoked because it calmed or relaxed them, that they felt dependent on cigarettes, and that they were unable to cut down on their use of cigarettes.

## Smoking Cessation

Although decreasing smoking initiation is critical to reducing tobacco use long term, reducing morbidity and mortality in the short term can only occur by increasing smoking cessation among current smokers. Smoking cessation has major and immediate health benefits for women of all ages (USDHHS 1990d).

National survey data are used here to estimate the percentage of women aged 18 years or older, young women aged 18 through 24 years, girls less than 18 years of age, and pregnant women and girls who have quit smoking. Besides these estimates, self-reported interest in quitting smoking, reasons for quitting, and reasons for relapse to smoking are also described. This section discusses the smoking continuum, which describes the current smoking status of women who had ever smoked, ranging from those who had never tried to quit smoking to those who had been abstinent for 10 or more years. Other topics addressed are the number of attempts to quit smoking, physicians' advice about smoking, and methods used to quit smoking.

### Interest in Quitting Smoking and Attempts to Quit

#### Women

Most smokers want to stop. The 1995 NHIS was used to examine interest in and attempts to quit smoking (see Appendix 2 for definitions) among women who were daily smokers. Of the women queried, 75.2 percent reported wanting to quit smoking completely, and 46.6 percent reported having tried to quit in the previous year (Table 2.24). Other studies also reported that most women want to quit smoking (USDHEW 1977; CDC 1993; Sandoval and Larsen 1995).

**Table 2.24. Percentage (and 95% confidence interval) of current women smokers aged 18 years or older who reported an interest in quitting smoking or who recently attempted to stop smoking, by selected characteristics, National Health Interview Survey, United States, 1995**

| Characteristic | Wants to quit smoking* | Attempt to stop smoking in the past year† |
|---|---|---|
| Women | 75.2 (±2.2) | 46.6 (±2.7) |
| Age (years) | | |
| 18–24 | 76.4 (±7.0) | 65.2 (±8.7) |
| 25–44 | 78.7 (±2.9) | 48.1 (±3.8) |
| 45–64 | 73.9 (±4.1) | 40.5 (±4.8) |
| ≥ 65 | 58.0 (±6.9) | 35.8 (±7.4) |
| Race/ethnicity | | |
| White, non-Hispanic | 75.6 (±2.5) | 46.4 (±3.1) |
| Black, non-Hispanic | 74.8 (±5.8) | 50.0 (±7.3) |
| Hispanic | 72.9 (±6.5) | 42.9 (±9.3) |
| Education (number of years)‡ | | |
| ≤ 8 | 72.6 (±7.6) | 33.5 (±9.6) |
| 9–11 | 78.3 (±5.9) | 44.4 (±7.2) |
| 12 | 74.4 (±3.5) | 42.0 (±4.0) |
| 13–15 | 75.1 (±4.9) | 47.5 (±6.4) |
| ≥ 16 | 74.2 (±7.0) | 55.2 (±8.3) |
| Men | 72.8 (±2.5) | 45.1 (±2.8) |

*Based on the question, "Would you like to completely quit smoking cigarettes?" Measured for current smokers. Current smokers were persons who reported smoking ≥ 100 cigarettes in their lifetime and who smoked every day or some days at the time of the survey.

†Based on the question, "During the past 12 months, have you stopped smoking for 1 day or longer?" Measured for current daily smokers. Current daily smokers were persons who reported smoking ≥ 100 cigarettes in their lifetime and smoked daily at the time of the survey.

‡For women aged ≥ 25 years.

Source: National Center for Health Statistics, public use data tape, 1995.

In NHIS data (Table 2.24), smokers 65 years or older were less interested in quitting smoking than were younger smokers, a finding also reported by others (Rimer et al. 1990; CDC 1993; Fortmann and Killen 1994). NHIS data showed that only 35.8 percent of women aged 65 years or older had tried to stop smoking in the previous year, which is significantly less than the 65.2 percent of women aged 18 through 24 years and the 48.1 percent of women aged 25 through 44 years who had tried to stop smoking in the previous year. Other data support these findings (Hatziandreu et al. 1990; Rimer et al. 1990; Derby et al. 1994). According to NHIS data, the percentage of women who wanted to or had tried to quit smoking did not differ by racial or ethnic group (Table 2.24). Desire to quit smoking did not differ significantly by level of education, but women with 16 or more years of education were more likely to have attempted to quit smoking in the past year than were women with 8 years or fewer or with 12 years of education.

In the early 1980s, men were more likely than women to state that they wanted to quit smoking (Sorensen and Pechacek 1987; Blake et al. 1989). More recent data on gender-specific differences are more equivocal. In the 1993 NHIS (CDC 1994c) and in a study of heavy smokers (Fortmann and Killen 1994), women were more likely than men to want to completely quit smoking. In the 1995 NHIS data for daily smokers, however, no gender-specific differences were found in the proportion of persons who wanted to quit smoking (Table 2.24). This finding is consistent with other data (Royce et al. 1997). In 1998, 42.3 (±2.0) percent of women reported that they had stopped smoking for more than one day in the previous 12 months because they were trying to quit smoking. No gender-specific differences were noted (NCHS, public use data tape, 1998).

Although earlier data suggested that women are less likely than men to be successful in their attempts to stop smoking (Pierce et al. 1989b), more recent data showed that women are equally or more likely to have attempted to stop smoking in the previous year and equally likely to have maintained abstinence (USDHHS 1980; CDC 1993; Derby et al. 1994; Rose et al. 1996; Whitlock et al. 1997). In the 1995 NHIS data, women and men were equally likely to report that they wanted to quit smoking or had tried to stop in the previous year. Only 17.0 (±2.2) percent of women and 19.6 (±2.3) percent of men reported that they had neither wanted to nor tried to quit smoking in the previous year (NCHS, public use data tape, 1995).

### Girls

Data for high school senior girls in MTF Surveys were combined over several years, so that sample sizes were adequate for making estimates and evaluating trends (University of Michigan, Institute for Social Research, public use data tapes, 1976–1998). Current smokers were defined as having smoked cigarettes in the past 30 days. Daily smokers were defined as averaging one or more cigarettes per day in the past 30 days. In 1996–1998 (combined data), 42.0 (±6.3) percent of high school senior girls who were current smokers and 43.5 (±7.0) percent of those who were daily smokers wanted to quit smoking (University of Michigan, Institute for Social Research, public use data tapes, 1996–1998); comparable estimates have been reported by others (Sussman et al. 1998). In the 1999 NYTS, 54.7 (±9.8) percent of girls in middle school and 57.9 (±4.0) percent of girls in high school reported that they wanted to completely stop smoking cigarettes (CDC 2000b). For current smokers, the percentage who reported interest in quitting smoking was lower in 1996–1998 (combined data) (42.0 ± 6.3 percent) than in 1976–1979 (combined data) (53.9 ± 3.9 percent); for daily smokers, the percentage was similar for the years 1976–1979 (combined data) (46.7 ± 4.6 percent) and 1996–1998 (combined data) (43.5 ± 7.0 percent). In MTF Survey data and in other data (Pirie et al. 1991; Burt and Peterson 1998; Sussman et al. 1998; CDC 2000b), interest in quitting did not differ by gender (University of Michigan, Institute for Social Research, public use data tapes, 1976–1998).

Data from a 1975 ACS survey of 267 girls aged 13 through 17 years found that 58 percent of those who smoked expressed some eagerness to quit (USDHEW 1977). Data from the 1989 TAPS I (Moss et al. 1992; Allen et al. 1993) also suggested that most girls who smoked wanted to quit: 52.7 percent of girls aged 12 through 18 years who were current smokers did not expect to be smoking one year later. In a cohort with an eight-year follow-up period, Pirie and coworkers (1991) reported that 72.4 percent of young women (average age, 19.2 years) who were current smokers wanted to quit smoking.

In combined data from MTF Surveys for the years 1996–1998, 32.6 (±5.2) percent of high school senior girls who were current smokers and 45.3 (±6.8) percent of girls who were daily smokers had tried to stop smoking at some point but could not stop (University of Michigan, Institute for Social Research, public use data tapes, 1996–1998). Among both current and daily smokers, the percentage was the same in 1976–1979 (combined data) and 1996–1998 (combined data) (University of Michigan, Institute for Social Research, public use data tapes, 1976–1998). In the 1999 NYTS, 59.2 (± 5.0) percent of girls in middle school and 57.9 (± 3.3) percent of girls in high school who were current smokers reported that they had seriously tried to quit in the previous 12 months (CDC 2000b). In data from MTF Surveys and in other data (Pirie et al. 1991; Burt et al. 1998), the percentages of current smokers who tried to stop smoking but were unable to do so did not differ by gender. In a study by Sussman and colleagues (1998), however, high school boys were more likely than girls to report that they had ever really tried to quit smoking.

In the 1989 TAPS I data, 76.8 percent of girls aged 12 through 18 years who had ever smoked regularly and who were current smokers had made at least one serious attempt to quit smoking; 58.6 percent had attempted to quit in the previous six months (Moss et al. 1992). The proportion who had tried to quit smoking in the past six months varied inversely with age, from 75.2 percent among girls aged 12 through 13 years to 53.3 percent among girls aged 16 through 18 years. In the 1993 TAPS II data, 89 percent of girls aged 12 through 17 years who had ever smoked regularly and who were current smokers had ever tried to quit smoking. Among girls who had ever tried to quit, 81 percent had tried in the previous six months (NCHS, public use data tape, 1993); again, attempts to quit smoking decreased with age. The 1992 YRBS (a household survey) reported that 57.1 percent of girls and young women aged 12 through 21 years who smoked had tried to quit smoking in the previous six months. Again, the proportion decreased as age increased, from 69.1 percent for girls aged 12 through 13 years to 61.5 percent for girls aged 14 through 17 years and 52.3 percent for young women aged 18 through 21 years (Adams et al. 1995).

These and other data (McNeill et al. 1986, 1987; Ershler et al. 1989; Pirie et al. 1991; Stanton et al. 1996a) suggest that more than one-half of adolescents and young adults who smoke try to quit smoking each year. Smoking cessation does not appear to be any easier for children, adolescents, or young adults than for older adults. Children and adolescents make frequent and unsuccessful attempts to quit smoking, and they report the same problems reported by adults. Study findings suggest that the patterns of relapse to smoking are similar for adolescents and adults. Hansen (1983) studied high school students who were current smokers but had tried to quit smoking; 65 percent had relapsed within one month of cessation and 82 percent within six months. These percentages are comparable to those for young adults (Moss 1979). Ershler and colleagues (1989) found that, of almost 100 girls and boys in grades 6 through 12 who had tried to quit smoking, 28.6 percent relapsed within one week and 53.1 percent relapsed within the first month; only 22.4 percent successfully abstained for six months. Study results suggest that reasons for relapse (withdrawal symptoms and social pressure) are similar for young persons and adults (Skinner et al. 1985; McNeill et al. 1986; Ershler et al. 1989; Flay et al. 1992).

### Number of Cessation Attempts

Most smokers attempt to quit smoking multiple times before being successful (Hazelden Foundation 1998). The 1992 NHIS was used to assess, among current smokers, the mean number of attempts to quit smoking in the past 12 months and the mean number of attempts in a lifetime (Table 2.25). (In this survey, an attempt to quit smoking was defined as having stopped smoking for ≥ 1 day.) Respondents often remember only the most recent attempts to quit smoking; they frequently forget short-term attempts that took place more than a few months before the interview (Gilpin and Pierce 1994). Thus, these data probably underestimate the actual number of attempts to quit smoking.

In 1992, women had made, on average, 2.7 attempts to quit smoking in the previous 12 months (Table 2.25). No differences were noted by age, race, education, or gender in the mean number of attempts.

Women who were current smokers reported an average of 6.3 lifetime attempts to quit smoking. The number of attempts tended to increase with age until age 64 years and then to decrease, but the differences were not statistically significant (Table 2.25). In a study of AARP members, 70.0 percent of smokers aged 50 through 102 years had made one or more attempts to quit smoking; most had tried to quit one to three times (Rimer et al. 1990). In the 1986 AUTS, little difference was found in history of smoking cessation by age, and the 1992 NHIS data showed no difference among racial and ethnic groups in the mean number of lifetime attempts to quit smoking (Table 2.25). In a population-based study of 2,626 persons in Minneapolis, Minnesota, the mean number of attempts to quit smoking was 3.0 among black women and 6.0 among white women (Hahn et al. 1990). (In this study, an attempt to quit smoking was defined as having quit smoking for ≥ 1 week.) In NHIS data, women with 9 to 11 years of education had made the fewest lifetime attempts to quit smoking (3.3), and women with 16 or more years of education had made the most attempts (9.3) (Table 2.25).

The number of lifetime attempts to quit smoking was greater among men (8.8) than among women (6.3) (Table 2.25). However, when the data were examined by age, the gender-specific difference was significant only among smokers aged 25 through 44 years (Table 2.25). Other reports noted that current smokers of both genders have made about the same number of attempts. For example, in national data from 1964, 1966, and 1970, no gender-specific differences were found in the proportion of smokers who had tried to quit smoking two or more times (Schuman 1977). In 1984 data from 10 worksites, the percentage of current smokers who had made at least one attempt to quit smoking and the mean number of attempts in the past year were about the same among women and men (Sorensen and Pechacek 1986).

Data from current smokers may underestimate the number of attempts to stop smoking. Although the mean number of lifetime attempts reported by current smokers in NHIS averages 7.6, the Hazelden Foundation (1998) found that, on average, former smokers took 18.6 years to quit smoking and tried an average of 10.8 times.

## Cessation Methods

A variety of methods, both effective and ineffective, are used by smokers in their attempts to quit smoking (Fiore et al. 1996, 2000). Methods used by women (both current and former smokers) in the most recent attempt were examined by analyzing the 1992 NHIS data. Respondents could select more than one method. Because of the small sample size, the

Table 2.25. Mean number (and 95% confidence interval) of attempts to quit smoking among current smokers aged 18 years or older, by gender and selected characteristics, National Health Interview Survey, United States, 1992

| Characteristic | Mean number of attempts to quit smoking in past 12 months* | | Mean number of attempts to quit smoking in lifetime* | |
|---|---|---|---|---|
| | Women | Men | Women | Men |
| Overall | 2.7 (±0.3) | 3.2 (±0.6) | 6.3 (±1.0) | 8.8 (±1.4) |
| Age (years) | | | | |
| 18–24 | 2.9 (±0.8) | 3.7 (±1.5) | 4.7 (±1.0) | 8.5 (±4.3) |
| 25–44 | 2.6 (±0.4) | 3.5 (±1.0) | 5.9 (±1.0) | 8.9 (±1.9) |
| 45–64 | 2.8 (±0.6) | 2.6 (±0.5) | 8.1 (±3.2) | 8.7 (±2.0) |
| ≥ 65 | 2.8 (±1.0) | 2.0 (±0.5) | 4.9 (±1.8) | 8.9 (±6.9) |
| Race/ethnicity | | | | |
| White, non-Hispanic | 2.5 (±0.3) | 3.0 (±0.8) | 6.1 (±1.2) | 7.3 (±1.2) |
| Black, non-Hispanic | 3.3 (±0.6) | 3.7 (±0.8) | 8.1 (±3.0) | 16.1 (±6.3) |
| Hispanic | 4.1 (±2.5) | 3.0 (±0.8) | 6.8 (±2.6) | 8.5 (±3.2) |
| Education (number of years)† | | | | |
| ≤ 8 | 2.6 (±1.1) | 1.4 (±0.3) | 4.5 (±2.0) | 7.9 (±8.2) |
| 9–11 | 2.4 (±0.6) | 2.9 (±1.3) | 3.3 (±0.8) | 5.1 (±1.2) |
| 12 | 2.7 (±0.5) | 3.2 (±1.2) | 6.4 (±1.2) | 8.9 (±2.2) |
| 13–15 | 2.2 (±0.3) | 2.2 (±0.5) | 8.1 (±4.4) | 8.0 (±2.0) |
| ≥ 16 | 3.6 (±1.5) | 4.7 (±1.7) | 9.3 (±3.8) | 15.4 (±6.3) |

*Note:* Current smokers were persons who reported smoking ≥ 100 cigarettes in their lifetime and who smoked at the time of the survey.
*Any attempt to quit smoking for ≥ 1 day.
†For women aged ≥ 25 years.
Source: National Center for Health Statistics, Cancer Control Supplement, public use data tape, 1992.

results were not stratified by the number of cigarettes smoked per day. Because female smokers consume fewer cigarettes per day than do male smokers, any gender-specific differences might reflect differences in the amount smoked. Also, if heavy smokers are more likely to reduce the number of cigarettes smoked and light smokers are more likely to quit smoking abruptly, these differences could affect the apparent success of one method compared with the success of another.

In the 1992 NHIS data, of the women who had quit smoking, 88.1 percent stopped "cold turkey" (stopping all at once, without cutting down), 25.4 percent decreased the number of cigarettes smoked, 17.7 percent switched to a low-tar or low-nicotine cigarette, and 10.5 percent quit smoking along with friends (method not specified) (Table 2.26). (Results total >100 percent because respondents could select more than one method.) These were also the most common methods noted in the 1986 AUTS (Fiore et al. 1990) and the 1987 NHIS. A 1998 study commissioned by the American Lung Association reported that 49 percent of women quit smoking cold turkey and 13 percent slowly reduced the number of cigarettes smoked (Yankelovich Partners 1998). Reports suggest that methods used to stop smoking do not differ by race or ethnicity: Winkleby and coworkers (1995) found that Hispanic women and white women were equally likely to have quit smoking on their own, and Hahn and colleagues (1990) found that white women and black women were equally likely to consider decreasing the number of cigarettes they smoked as part of a strategy to stop smoking.

In the 1970s and 1980s, more than 90 percent of smokers who had quit smoking reportedly did so without using formal interventions for smoking cessation (USDHEW 1979b; Fiore et al. 1990). The 1992 NHIS data showed that only 3.4 percent of women former smokers used a formal smoking cessation program to

**Table 2.26. Percentage (and 95% confidence interval) of women aged 18 years or older who used selected methods to quit smoking during most recent attempt, by smoking status, National Health Interview Survey, United States, 1987 and 1992**

| Methods used for most recent attempt to quit smoking | 1987 Former smokers | 1987 Current smokers | 1992 Former smokers | 1992 Current smokers* |
|---|---|---|---|---|
| "Stop cold turkey"† | 87.4 (±1.4) | 73.0 (±2.2) | 88.1 (±2.2) | 87.2 (±2.6) |
| Gradually decrease number of cigarettes smoked in a day | 9.5 (±1.3) | 17.9 (±1.8) | 25.4 (±2.9) | 53.0 (±3.5) |
| Switch to lower-tar or lower-nicotine cigarettes | 4.1 (±0.9) | 6.6 (±1.2) | 17.7 (±2.6) | 47.2 (±3.6) |
| Stop smoking along with friends or relatives | 4.1 (±0.9) | 5.8 (±1.1) | 10.5 (±2.0) | 15.1 (±3.0) |
| Follow instructions in book or pamphlet | 1.0 (±0.4)‡ | 4.0 (±0.9) | 3.9 (±1.5) | 6.5 (±2.0) |
| Use a stop-smoking clinic or program | NA§ | NA | 3.4 (±1.3) | 5.4 (±1.7) |
| Use Nicorette gum△ | 2.0 (±0.7) | 4.6 (±1.0) | 2.4 (±1.2)‡ | 5.8 (±1.9) |
| Use special filters¶ | 2.2 (±0.7) | 2.7 (±0.9) | NA | NA |
| Participate in Great American Smoke-Out | 1.3 (±0.5)‡ | 2.7 (±0.7) | NA | NA |
| Use some other method | 6.1 (±1.1) | 7.1 (±1.4) | 9.0 (±1.9) | 9.1 (±2.3) |

*Note:* Results total >100% because multiple responses were possible. Current smokers were persons who reported smoking ≥ 100 cigarettes in their lifetime and who smoked at the time of the survey. Former smokers had smoked ≥ 100 cigarettes in their lifetime and were not smoking at the time of the survey.

*Current smokers who had attempted to quit smoking for reasons other than sickness.

†Defined as "stopping all at once without cutting down."

‡Estimate should be interpreted with caution because of the small number of respondents.

§NA = Not available.

△A prescription nicotine chewing gum.

¶To regulate amount of smoke inhaled.

Sources: National Center for Health Statistics, Cancer Control Supplements, public use data tapes, 1987, 1992.

help them in the most recent attempt to quit smoking (Table 2.26). In another survey, only 3 percent of smokers who recently quit smoking had participated in a cessation program during the year in which they stopped (Hahn et al. 1990). In a 1996 study in California, however, 22 percent of women used assistance in attempting to quit smoking (self-help materials, counseling advice, or nicotine replacement therapy) (Zhu et al. 2000). A 1998 study commissioned by the American Lung Association found that 24 percent of women used nicotine replacement therapy on their last attempt to quit smoking and that 3 percent used another prescription medication; only 1 percent used counseling (Yankelovich Partners 1998).

Women unsuccessful in their efforts to quit smoking were significantly more likely than successful women to report having switched to a low-tar cigarette. This finding is consistent with the conclusion of the Drug Abuse Advisory Committee of the U.S. Food and Drug Administration (1994) that the amount of nicotine delivered by all currently marketed cigarettes is likely to lead to addiction in the typical smoker. Women unsuccessful in their efforts to quit smoking were also significantly more likely than those who were successful to report having decreased the number of cigarettes smoked as part of the attempt to quit smoking (Table 2.26) (Guilford 1967; Smith 1981; Fiore et al. 1990).

In the 1986 AUTS data, smokers who tried unsuccessfully to quit smoking were more likely than those who were successful to have used nicotine gum during the most recent attempt to quit smoking (Fiore et al. 1990). A similar pattern was found in the 1992 NHIS data, but the sample sizes were small, so the findings should be interpreted with caution (Table 2.26). More recent data, however, have shown that use of tobacco use treatments, (e.g., self-help materials, counseling advice, or nicotine replacement therapy) doubled cessation rates. This finding occurred even though heavy smokers were more likely than light smokers to use assistance. Women were more likely than men to use assistance, and the use of assistance increased with age. Whites were more likely than other racial and ethnic groups to use nicotine replacement therapy (Zhu et al. 2000).

Compared with the data from the 1986 AUTS and the 1987 NHIS, the 1992 NHIS data included many more women who had attempted to quit smoking by switching to low-tar or low-nicotine cigarettes and by decreasing the number of cigarettes smoked (Table 2.26). Significantly more women attempted to quit smoking along with friends in 1992 than in 1987. The proportion of women unsuccessful at smoking cessation who attempted to quit smoking cold turkey also increased between 1987 and 1992, but the proportion who used nicotine gum (Nicorette) was not significantly different. A small percentage of women who attempted to quit smoking in 1987 tried special cigarette filters, but those filters were no longer available in 1992. Otherwise, the percentage who used other methods remained the same or increased between 1987 and 1992. These patterns appear to be due to an increase in the number of methods of smoking cessation used by women who attempted to stop smoking. The mean number of methods used among women successful at smoking cessation increased from 1.1 (95 percent CI, 1.1–1.2) in 1987 to 1.6 (95 percent CI, 1.5–1.6) in 1992 (NCHS, public use data tapes, 1987, 1992). The mean number of methods used among women unsuccessful at smoking cessation increased from 1.2 (95 percent CI, 1.2–1.3) to 2.1 (95 percent CI, 2.0–2.1). In 1992, however, women who successfully quit smoking cold turkey still used fewer methods (average, 1.6 ± 0.1 methods) than did women who quit by gradually decreasing the number of cigarettes smoked (2.6 ± 0.1 methods) or by switching to low-tar or low-nicotine cigarettes (2.9 ± 0.2 methods).

In the 1992 NHIS data, women (88.1 ± 2.2 percent) were significantly less likely than men (92.3 ± 1.7 percent) to have quit smoking cold turkey (NCHS, public use data tape, 1992), a finding consistent with the results of Blake and associates (1989). However, the percentage of persons who tried to quit smoking (successfully or unsuccessfully) by reducing the number of cigarettes smoked did not differ by gender. In contrast to that finding, Blake and colleagues (1989) reported that, in their survey of six Midwest communities in the Minnesota Heart Health Program, women were more likely than men to reduce the number of cigarettes smoked, rather than stop smoking completely. Both Blake and colleagues (1989) and Sorensen and Pechacek (1987) also found that, among persons planning to quit smoking, women were more likely than men to plan to reduce the number of cigarettes smoked, whereas men were more likely to plan to completely stop smoking. In the 1992 NHIS, women (10.5 ± 2.0 percent) were more likely than men (7.9 ± 1.6 percent) to quit smoking along with relatives and friends (NCHS, public use data tape, 1992); this finding is consistent with earlier data (Schoenborn and Boyd 1989). However, women and men were equally unlikely to have attended a smoking cessation clinic or program during a successful attempt to quit smoking (NCHS, public use data tape, 1992). In the 1998 study commissioned by the American Lung Association, women were more likely than men to have used nicotine replacement therapy on their last attempt to quit smoking (24 percent vs. 17 percent) and somewhat more likely to have used another prescription medication (3 percent vs. 1 percent). Women (1 percent) and men (0 percent) were equally unlikely to have used counseling during their last attempt to quit smoking (Yankelovich Partners 1998). No CIs were given. Although some smaller studies have suggested that women use a greater number and variety of cessation strategies, in the 1992 NHIS data, no gender-specific differences were found for the mean number of methods used or the combinations of cessation strategies used by persons who used more than one cessation strategy in the last attempt at cessation (successful or unsuccessful) (NCHS, public use data tape, 1992).

## Smoking Cessation Among Women

### Trends in Smoking Cessation

Smoking cessation is associated with major and immediate health benefits for women of all ages. Monitoring of smoking cessation is a critical element of tobacco surveillance. The 1955 Current Population Survey provided the first nationally representative data on smoking cessation among women; ongoing surveillance began in 1965. In 1955, 4 percent of women in the United States were former smokers (Haenszel et al. 1956; NCHS 1970). The 1959 CPS-I showed that 5.6 percent of predominantly white, middle-class women aged 30 years or older were former smokers (Hammond and Garfinkel 1961; Garfinkel and Silverberg 1990). In NHIS, 7 to 8 percent of women were former smokers in 1966 (NCHS 1970; Giovino et al. 1994), 18 percent in 1985 (NCHS 1985; Giovino et al. 1994), and 18.8 percent in 1998 (NCHS, public use data tape, 1998).

A more commonly used measure of smoking cessation is the percentage of persons who had ever smoked who have quit smoking (formerly known as the "quit ratio") (see "Percentage of Smokers Who Quit Smoking" in Appendix 2). Several data sources showed an increase over time in the percentage of women smokers who have quit smoking. In the 1955 Current Population Survey, the percentage of women smokers who had quit was 11 percent (Haenszel et al. 1956); in the 1966 Current Population Survey, it was 16 percent (NCHS 1970). Similarly, the percentage of women smokers who had quit smoking was estimated at 19 percent in the 1964 AUTS and 22 percent in the 1966 AUTS (USDHEW 1969). The U.S. Nurses' Health Study (Myers et al. 1987) found that the percentage of smokers who had quit smoking increased threefold from the 1921–1926 through the 1942–1946 birth cohorts of women.

In NHIS data, the percentage of women smokers overall who had quit smoking increased steadily from 19.1 percent in 1965 to 46.0 percent in 1990 (Table 2.27). During 1990–1992, a decrease was observed in the reported percentage of women smokers who had quit smoking, probably because of the change in definition of current smokers to explicitly include intermittent smokers (see "Current Smoker" in Appendix 2). This change in definition resulted in more women who had ever smoked being classified as current smokers. The decrease in cessation was greatest among young women, blacks, Hispanics, and persons with a college education—the groups most likely to be intermittent smokers (Husten et al. 1998). The percentage of women smokers who had quit smoking then increased during 1992–1998 (Table 2.27). In all years, the percentage of women smokers who had quit smoking increased with increasing age, a finding noted by others (Resnicow et al. 1991). This pattern also was evident in earlier data (Hammond and Garfinkel 1961). The association with age held, even after adjustment for other demographic factors (Freund et al. 1992). The increase with age in the percentage of smokers who have quit smoking occurs because, as smokers age, a greater percentage have quit smoking (Kirscht et al. 1987; Pierce et al. 1989b; Hatziandreu et al. 1990; McWhorter et al. 1990; CDC 1993) and because continuing smokers are more likely than former smokers to die (differential mortality) (Pierce et al. 1989b; USDHHS 1990c).

NHIS data showed that the percentage of women smokers who quit smoking increased during 1965–1998 among all age groups (Table 2.27). The rate of increase was lowest among women aged 18 through 24 years and greatest among women aged 65 years or older, a pattern reported by others (Novotny et al. 1990). Among women of reproductive age (18 through 44 years), 34.5 percent of smokers had quit smoking in 1998, whereas 46.1 percent of women of all ages had (Table 2.27) (NCHS, public use data tape, 1998). During 1985–1998, the percentage of smokers who had quit smoking did not increase among women aged 18 through 44 years, but the percentage did increase significantly among women aged 45 years or older.

In NHIS data, the percentage of smokers who had quit smoking increased significantly among white women (from 19.6 percent in 1965 to 47.4 percent in 1998) and among black women (from 14.5 to 34.7 percent) (Table 2.27). The percentage of smokers who had quit smoking was higher among white women than among black women for all years. The rate of increase during 1965–1998 was also higher among white women (27.8 ± 1.8 percentage points) than among black women (20.2 ± 4.5 percentage points). The percentage of smokers who had quit smoking increased among Hispanic women (from 36.8 in 1979 to 48.1 in 1998). Other analyses also found a significant increase when data were combined for 1978–1980 and 1994–1995 (USDHHS 1998). Similar racial and ethnic patterns were noted for women of reproductive age (data not shown). Among American Indian or Alaska Native women, the percentage of smokers who had quit smoking was unchanged between 1978–1980 (36.5 percent) and 1994–1995 (37.2 percent). Among Asian or Pacific Islander women, the percentage of ever smokers who had quit smoking increased between 1978–1980 (36.9 percent) and 1994–1995 (62.2 percent); this increase was of borderline statistical significance, probably because of small sample size (USDHHS 1998).

Among women overall, the percentage of smokers who had quit smoking increased over time for all levels of education (Pierce et al. 1989a; Giovino et al. 1994) (Table 2.27). However, among women of reproductive age, the percentage was unchanged from 1970 through 1998 for women with 12 or fewer years of education (data not shown) (NCHS, NHIS, public use data tapes, 1970–1998). Among women overall (Table 2.27) and among women of reproductive age (NCHS, public use data tapes, 1970–1998), the greatest increase in smoking cessation occurred among those with 16 or more years of education (Schuman 1977; Pierce et al. 1989a; Freund et al. 1992).

NHIS data showed that during 1985–1998, among women living below the poverty level, the percentage of smokers who had quit smoking changed little (from 27.3 to 28.9 percent), but among women living at or above the poverty level, it increased significantly (from 41.3 to 48.2 percent) (Table 2.27). In the 1955 Current Population Survey, employment status was associated with smoking cessation: housewives (13.0 percent) were more likely to have quit smoking than were employed women (8.2 percent) or unemployed women who were looking for work (6.6 percent) (Haenszel et al. 1956). In 1978–1990, the percentage of smokers who had quit smoking was highest among women who were not employed and not looking for work, and it was higher among employed women than among unemployed women who were looking for work. Being either employed or not employed and not looking for work was positively associated with smoking cessation, even after adjustment for demographic variables (Novotny et al. 1988; Waldron and Lye 1989).

### Smoking Cessation by Demographic Characteristics

Smoking cessation among women varies by age, race and ethnicity, level of education, and income. Estimates of the percentage of women who had ever smoked who have quit smoking, by various demographic characteristics, were obtained from the 1997–1998 NHIS and the 1997–1998 NHSDA (combined data) (Table 2.28). In the 1997–1998 NHIS, the estimate was 46.2 percent; estimates were somewhat lower for NHSDA (42.4 percent). The percentage of women smokers who had quit smoking increased directly with age for both surveys, a finding reported by others (Giovino et al. 1995). Studies suggest that this pattern holds, even after adjustment for the number of cigarettes smoked per day and for other demographic variables (McWhorter et al. 1990; Hibbard 1993). Older persons may be more motivated than younger persons to maintain abstinence when they try to quit smoking (Kirscht et al. 1987; Pierce et al. 1989b; Hatziandreu et al. 1990; McWhorter et al. 1990; CDC 1993). This motivation may result from smoking-related diseases that occur primarily after age 40 years (Hatziandreu et al. 1990; McWhorter et al. 1990; Resnicow et al. 1991). Garvey and colleagues (1983) found that, among healthy men, age did not significantly predict smoking cessation.

The data for both surveys showed that the percentage of smokers who had quit smoking was greater among white women than among black women (Table 2.28). Other studies found that, even after adjustment for the number of cigarettes smoked per day and demographic and socioeconomic factors, blacks were significantly less likely than whites to have quit smoking (Novotny et al. 1988; Fiore et al. 1990; Hatziandreu et al. 1990; McWhorter et al. 1990). In the 1997–1998 NHIS, the percentage of smokers who had quit smoking was lowest among black non-Hispanic women (34.3 percent) and highest among white non-Hispanic women (47.7 percent) and Hispanic women (45.9 percent), a finding noted by others (USDHHS 1998). Among American Indian or Alaska Native women, the percentage of smokers who had quit smoking varied by region: it was highest among women in the Southwest (50.3 percent), Pacific Northwest (48.5 percent), and Oklahoma (47.1 percent) and lowest among women in the northern plains (30.3 percent) (USDHHS 1998). However, these differences were not statistically significant.

In both surveys (Table 2.28), the percentage of smokers who had quit smoking was lowest among women with 9 to 11 years of education, although this finding was statistically significant only for NHIS. The 1985 NHIS data showed that education had the strongest association with smoking cessation, even after adjustment for several demographic variables, including gender (Novotny et al. 1988). In a cohort study of women enrolled in a health maintenance organization, a case-control study conducted in six cities, and a study in 90 worksites, education was significantly associated with smoking cessation (Gritz et al. 1998), even after adjustment for the number of cigarettes smoked per day (Kabat and Wynder 1987; Hibbard 1993).

The 1997–1998 NHIS showed that the percentage of smokers who had quit smoking was higher among women living at or above the poverty level (48.1 percent) than among those living below the poverty level

**Table 2.27. Percentage (and 95% confidence interval) of women smokers aged 18 years or older who have quit smoking, by selected characteristics, National Health Interview Survey, United States, 1965–1998**

| Characteristic | 1965 | 1970 | 1974 | 1979 |
|---|---|---|---|---|
| Women | 19.1 (±0.8) | 26.9 (±0.9) | 28.3 (±1.1) | 33.4 (±1.5) |
| Age (years) | | | | |
| 18–24 | 14.0 (±2.0) | 19.7 (±1.8) | 18.6 (±2.4) | 22.8 (±2.5) |
| 25–44 | 18.2 (±1.3) | 27.4 (±1.2) | 26.5 (±1.5) | 31.2 (±2.1) |
| 45–64 | 21.1 (±1.6) | 27.0 (±1.3) | 30.8 (±2.6) | 36.5 (±2.6) |
| ≥ 65 | 32.2 (±4.7) | 41.0 (±3.1) | 46.9 (±4.1) | 51.3 (±4.2) |
| Race/ethnicity* | | | | |
| White, non-Hispanic | 19.6 (±0.8) | 27.8 (±0.9) | 29.6 (±1.3) | 34.3 (±1.7) |
| Black, non-Hispanic | 14.5 (±2.6) | 18.4 (±2.1) | 17.4 (±3.0) | 24.4 (±3.7) |
| Hispanic | NA[†] | NA | NA | 36.8 (±6.5) |
| Education (number of years)[‡] | | | | |
| ≤ 8 | NA | 26.3 (±1.9) | 29.5 (±3.3) | 35.8 (±3.6) |
| 9–11 | NA | 22.6 (±1.6) | 21.3 (±2.5) | 26.9 (±3.0) |
| 12 | NA | 28.7 (±1.4) | 29.5 (±1.9) | 34.2 (±2.4) |
| 13–15 | NA | 30.9 (±3.1) | 36.4 (±3.9) | 38.4 (±3.2) |
| ≥ 16 | NA | 42.8 (±3.6) | 44.7 (±5.0) | 49.0 (±3.6) |
| Socioeconomic status[§] | | | | |
| Below poverty level | NA | NA | NA | NA |
| At or above poverty level | NA | NA | NA | NA |
| Unknown | NA | NA | NA | NA |
| Men | 27.6 (±0.7) | 37.4 (±1.0) | 39.2 (±1.1) | 43.1 (±1.3) |

*Note:* Percentage of smokers who have quit smoking is the percentage of all persons in each demographic category who reported smoking ≥ 100 cigarettes in their lifetime who are former smokers.
*Ethnicity not determined in 1965, 1970, or 1974. Thus, estimates for whites and for blacks during these years likely include data for some persons of Hispanic origin.

(30.1 percent) (Table 2.28). McWhorter and colleagues (1990) reported that household income was a significant predictor of smoking cessation, even after adjustment for other demographic factors and the number of cigarettes smoked per day. Similarly, Novotny and coworkers (1988) found that living above the poverty level was significantly associated with smoking cessation, even after adjustment for sociodemographic factors.

Other studies have reported that, among employed women, the percentage of smokers who had quit smoking was highest among professional women and among women in management, intermediate among clerical and sales workers, and very low among women in blue-collar jobs (Sorensen and Pechacek 1986; Covey et al. 1992; Gritz et al. 1998). Even after adjustment for the number of cigarettes smoked per day and for education, women in professional or managerial positions were more likely to quit smoking than were women who were in service positions or who performed manual labor (Hibbard 1993).

### Gender-Specific Differences in Smoking Cessation

In 1955, the percentage of persons who had ever smoked who had quit smoking was 10.8 percent among women and 11.4 percent among men (Haenszel et al. 1956). In 1965, 19.1 percent of women who had ever smoked and 27.6 percent of men who had ever smoked had quit smoking. Thus, the gender-specific difference widened over the 10-year period (Waldron

| 1985 | 1990 | 1992 | 1995 | 1998 |
|---|---|---|---|---|
| 39.4 (±1.3) | 46.0 (±1.1) | 43.0 (±1.6) | 46.2 (±1.9) | 46.1 (±1.4) |
| | | | | |
| 24.0 (±3.2) | 30.6 (±3.5) | 17.7 (±3.7) | 28.7 (±6.5) | 25.2 (±4.5) |
| 36.1 (±1.7) | 40.2 (±1.6) | 36.7 (±2.2) | 38.7 (±2.8) | 36.7 (±2.0) |
| 41.7 (±2.2) | 49.7 (±2.1) | 48.0 (±2.8) | 49.4 (±3.2) | 51.3 (±2.3) |
| 61.1 (±2.8) | 67.0 (±2.4) | 65.9 (±3.4) | 69.9 (±3.4) | 70.7 (±2.7) |
| | | | | |
| 41.0 (±1.3) | 46.9 (±1.2) | 44.4 (±1.8) | 47.6 (±2.1) | 47.4 (±1.5) |
| 27.9 (±3.3) | 38.4 (±3.5) | 31.9 (±4.0) | 36.4 (±5.3) | 34.7 (±3.7) |
| 37.8 (±6.2) | 46.4 (±5.1) | 38.5 (±5.3) | 43.4 (±5.5) | 48.1 (±4.2) |
| | | | | |
| 41.6 (±3.5) | 48.5 (±4.2) | 44.1 (±5.6) | 48.0 (±5.8) | 49.3 (±5.4) |
| 31.8 (±3.0) | 36.0 (±3.0) | 39.0 (±4.2) | 38.0 (±4.9) | 36.0 (±3.5) |
| 38.1 (±1.8) | 43.9 (±1.8) | 40.9 (±2.3) | 45.0 (±2.9) | 44.1 (±2.3) |
| 45.4 (±2.8) | 51.8 (±2.4) | 48.9 (±3.5) | 51.0 (±3.7) | 50.1 (±2.6) |
| 60.1 (±3.2) | 64.5 (±2.9) | 59.7 (±3.8) | 59.7 (±4.3) | 64.3 (±3.3) |
| | | | | |
| 27.3 (±2.9) | 27.5 (±2.8) | 26.7 (±4.0) | 30.1 (±4.1) | 28.9 (±3.1) |
| 41.3 (±1.4) | 48.8 (±1.2) | 45.2 (±1.8) | 48.9 (±2.0) | 48.2 (±1.7) |
| 39.4 (±3.0) | 42.8 (±3.9) | 43.7 (±4.7) | 40.1 (±6.9) | 48.1 (±3.1) |
| | | | | |
| 48.7 (±1.3) | 51.5 (±1.2) | 50.1 (±1.5) | 50.5 (±2.0) | 50.9 (±1.3) |

†NA = Not available.
‡For women aged ≥ 25 years. Data for five education categories were not available for 1965.
§Definition of poverty status changed in 1997. (See Appendix 2 for definitions.)
Sources: National Center for Health Statistics, public use data tapes, 1965, 1970, 1974, 1979, 1985, 1990, 1992, 1995, 1998.

1991). Data for 1956–1978 from the Framingham study also showed this pattern (Sorlie and Kannel 1990).

In NHIS data for 1965–1998, the percentage of smokers who had quit smoking was lower among women aged 18 years or older than among men of comparable age (Schuman 1977; USDHHS 1989, 1990d; Resnicow et al. 1991; Covey et al. 1992) (Table 2.27 and Figure 2.16); in 1998, 46.1 percent of women and 50.9 percent of men who had ever smoked had quit. Other studies showed that this gender-specific difference persisted even after adjustment for race, employment status, occupation, education, marital status, and poverty level (Novotny et al. 1988; Rogers et al. 1995). However, between 1965 and 1998, the increase in the percentage of smokers who had quit smoking was slightly greater among women (27.0 ± 1.6 percentage points) than among men (23.3 ± 1.6 percentage points) (Table 2.27 and Figure 2.16) (Fiore et al. 1989; USDHHS 1989, 1990d; Fiore 1992; Giovino et al. 1994). Also, the gender gap narrowed from 8.5 ± 1.2 percentage points in 1965 to 4.8 ± 1.9 percentage points in 1998, a finding also reported by others (Ockene 1993). Moreover, the increase in the percentage of smokers who had quit smoking slowed during 1990–1998 for both women and men (Table 2.27 and Figure 2.16).

The gender-specific difference in the percentage of smokers who have quit smoking is due to several factors. Smoking prevalence peaked in the 1950s

**Table 2.28. Percentage (and 95% confidence interval) of smokers aged 18 years or older who have quit smoking, by gender and selected characteristics, National Health Interview Survey (NHIS) and National Household Survey on Drug Abuse (NHSDA), United States, 1997–1998**

| | NHIS, 1997–1998 | | NHSDA, 1997–1998 | |
|---|---|---|---|---|
| Characteristic | Women | Men | Women | Men |
| Overall | 46.2 (±0.9) | 50.1 (±0.9) | 42.4 (±2.0) | 47.5 (±2.0) |
| Age (years) | | | | |
| 18–24 | 23.8 (±2.9) | 19.3 (±2.7) | 15.4 (±2.5) | 9.8 (±1.9) |
| 25–44 | 36.9 (±1.4) | 35.3 (±1.4) | 33.2 (±2.6) | 32.4 (±3.0) |
| 45–64 | 52.7 (±1.6) | 57.4 (±1.5) | 49.4 (±3.9) | 57.9 (±3.6) |
| ≥ 65 | 70.0 (±1.9) | 83.2 (±1.3) | 64.3 (±5.1) | 77.8 (±4.3) |
| Race/ethnicity | | | | |
| White, non-Hispanic | 47.7 (±1.1) | 52.7 (±1.1) | 43.8 (±2.3) | 50.0 (±2.4) |
| Black, non-Hispanic | 34.3 (±2.5) | 35.8 (±2.6) | 34.9 (±3.7) | 34.5 (±4.0) |
| Hispanic | 45.9 (±2.9) | 42.8 (±2.5) | 35.4 (±4.8) | 41.0 (±3.9) |
| American Indian or Alaska Native | 38.4 (±10.2) | 33.3 (±11.3) | 25.4 (±16.5)* | 43.7 (±28.2)* |
| Asian or Pacific Islander | 40.0 (±8.9) | 51.2 (±6.3) | 53.3 (±19.5) | 40.1 (±13.4) |
| Education (number of years)[†] | | | | |
| ≤ 8 | 49.2 (±3.8) | 56.3 (±2.9) | 44.8 (±8.7) | 55.8 (+6.7) |
| 9-11 | 39.1 (±2.4) | 43.6 (±2.4) | 33.6 (±5.2) | 36.5 (±5.7) |
| 12 | 43.2 (±1.6) | 48.1 (±1.7) | 40.3 (±3.5) | 46.9 (±3.8) |
| 13-15 | 49.6 (±1.8) | 52.6 (±1.8) | 46.1 (±4.1) | 53.4 (±4.5) |
| ≥ 16 | 66.2 (±2.2) | 69.8 (±1.9) | 63.0 (±4.9) | 64.9 (±4.8) |
| Socioeconomic status[‡] | | | | |
| Below poverty level | 30.1 (±2.1) | 31.6 (±2.6) | NA[§] | NA |
| At or above poverty level | 48.1 (±1.1) | 51.5 (±1.1) | NA | NA |
| Unknown | 49.0 (±2.2) | 53.0 (±2.2) | NA | NA |

*Note:* Percentage of smokers who have quit smoking in NHIS is the percentage of all persons in each demographic category who reported smoking ≥ 100 cigarettes in their lifetime who are former smokers. Prevalence for NHSDA is the percentage of all persons in each demographic category who reported smoking ≥ 100 days in their lifetime who are former smokers.

*Estimate should be interpreted with caution because of the small number of respondents.

[†]For women aged ≥ 25 years.

[‡]See Appendix 2 for definitions.

[§]NA = Not available.

Sources: **NHIS:** National Center for Health Statistics, public use data tapes, 1997, 1998. **NHSDA:** Substance Abuse and Mental Health Services Administration, public use data tapes, 1997, 1998.

among men but not until 1965 among women (Burns et al. 1997), and men preceded women in smoking cessation. The percentage of smokers who have quit smoking is cumulative over time; thus, the percentage is higher among men because they began to quit smoking earlier in this century than did women (Pierce et al. 1989b).

In two large prospective studies (the Framingham study and CPS-I), the percentage of smokers who quit smoking was substantially higher among men than among women in the late 1950s and 1960s (Hammond and Garfinkel 1968; Gordon et al. 1975). The 1971–1975 NHANES I data and the 1982–1984 follow-up data showed that, even after adjustment for demographic

**Figure 2.16. Percentage of smokers who have quit smoking among adults aged 18 years or older and young adults aged 18–24 years, by gender, National Health Interview Survey, United States, 1965–1998**

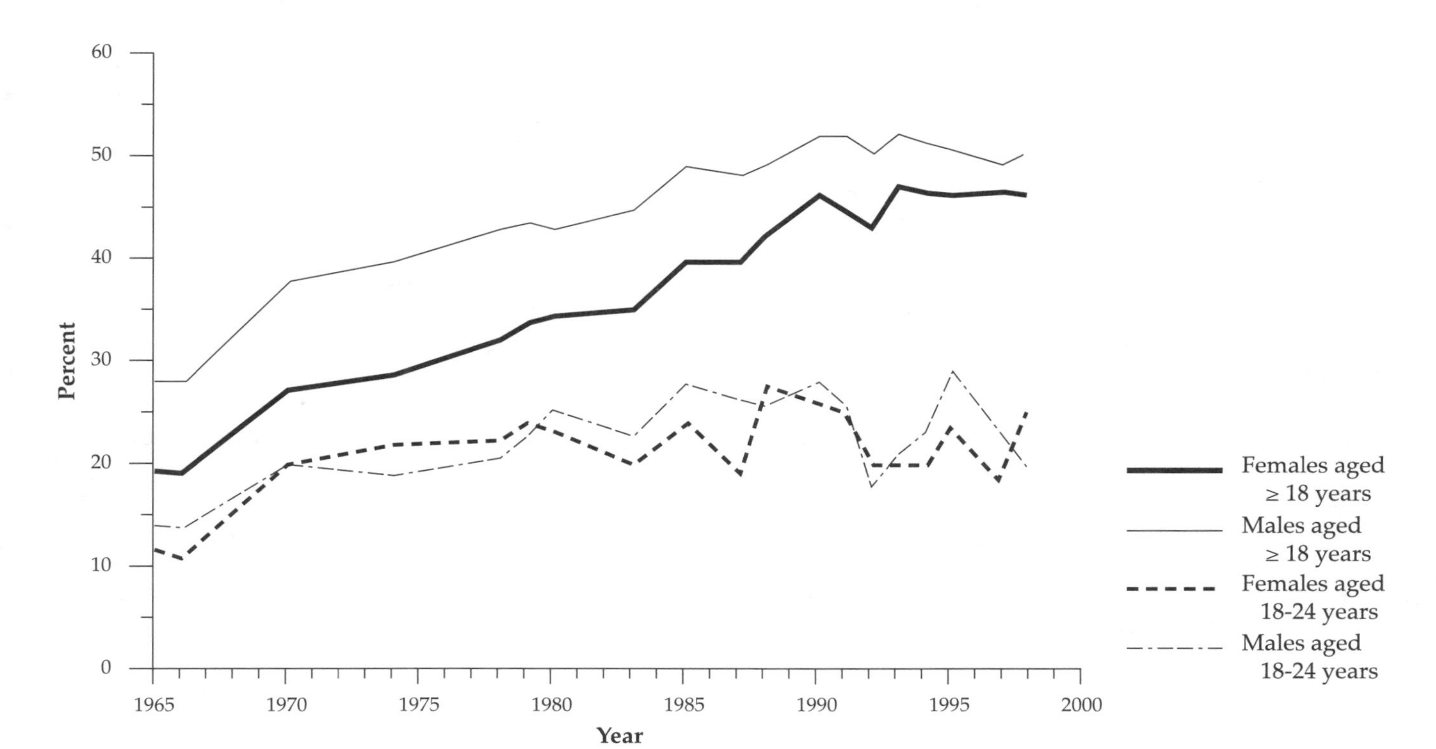


*Note:* Percentage of smokers who have quit smoking is the percentage of persons who reported smoking ≥ 100 cigarettes in their lifetime who are former smokers.
Sources: National Center for Health Statistics, public use data tapes, 1965–1998.

variables, women who had tried to quit smoking were more likely than men to relapse (McWhorter et al. 1990). Findings from several studies, however, suggested that, by the late 1970s or early 1980s, the probability of attempting to stop smoking and the probability of succeeding were equally high among women and men (USDHHS 1980; Kirscht et al. 1987; Orlandi 1987; Cohen et al. 1989; Fiore et al. 1989; Pierce et al. 1989b; Hellman et al. 1991; Coambs et al. 1992; Fiore 1992; Wagenknecht et al. 1993a; Derby et al. 1994; Whitlock et al. 1997; Gritz et al. 1998), even after adjustment for the number of cigarettes smoked per day and for demographic factors (Hatziandreu et al. 1990; Fiore 1992; CDC 1993). In birth cohort data for persons aged 30 years or older, the cessation rate began to accelerate by 1960 among men but not until 1970 among women (Harris 1983). In NHIS data for birth cohorts, the cessation rate was lower among white women than among white men in cohorts born before 1950; in later cohorts, the cessation rate was comparable for these two groups (Burns et al. 1997). However, not all studies have found an equally high rate of smoking cessation among women and men (Hubert et al. 1987; Bjornson et al. 1995; Hymowitz et al. 1997; Royce et al. 1997; Ward et al. 1997).

Another reason for findings of gender-specific differences in the percentage of smokers who have quit smoking is that this measure does not take into account other tobacco use. Men who quit smoking are more likely than women to switch to or to continue to use other tobacco products (pipes, cigars, or chewing tobacco). If users of other tobacco products are *not* counted as having quit, the gender gap narrows dramatically or disappears (Jarvis 1984; Jarvis and Jackson 1988; Schoenborn and Boyd 1989; USDHHS 1990d; Freund et al. 1992; Giovino et al. 1993; Ockene

1993). The percentage of smokers who have quit smoking is also affected by the duration of smoking, age at smoking initiation, socioeconomic status, and other parameters that have changed differently by gender over time (Gritz 1980).

In NHIS data for 1965–1998, the percentage of smokers who had quit smoking was lower among white women than among white men (NCHS, public use data tapes, 1965–1998). Rogers (1991) used NHIS data for 1985 and found that this gender-specific difference persisted after adjustment for demographic factors. Among Hispanics, the percentage of smokers who had quit smoking was comparable among women and men in 1979–1998 (NCHS, public use data tapes, 1979–1998). In another study, gender parity among Mexican Americans persisted even after adjustment for age, gender, and ethnicity (Rogers 1991). In 1965–1985, the percentage of black smokers who had quit smoking was lower among women than among men, but not significantly so (NCHS, public use data tapes, 1965–1985). Estimates for the mid-1980s that were adjusted for demographic factors also showed that black men were more likely than black women to be former smokers (Rogers 1991), but the unadjusted estimates for the percentage of smokers who have quit smoking were comparable among black women and black men in NHIS data for the 1990s (NCHS, public use data tapes, 1990, 1995, 1998).

Although the percentage of smokers who had quit smoking in 1998 was lower among women than among men (Table 2.28), patterns varied by age. The percentage was generally higher among women than among men aged 18 through 24 years, comparable among women and men aged 25 through 44 years, and generally lower among women than among men aged 45 years or older. Similar patterns were noted in other data (King et al. 1990). The gender- and age-specific differences in the percentage of persons who had ever smoked who have quit smoking probably reflect birth cohort differences.

**Reported Reasons for Smoking Cessation**

In the 1964 and 1966 AUTS (USDHEW 1969), the reasons most commonly given by female current smokers for trying to quit smoking were as follows: "wish to improve general physical condition," "have had some symptoms that might be caused by smoking cigarettes," "feel smoking may cause serious illness," and "too expensive to smoke." Prospective population studies and studies of women who entered smoking cessation programs reported similar reasons for wanting to quit smoking: concern about health, someone important to them wanting them to quit, the belief that smoking is a dirty habit, and a desire for the benefits of a more active lifestyle (O'Hara and Portser 1994; Rose et al. 1996).

In the 1964 and 1966 AUTS, women former smokers were asked why they had quit smoking (USDHEW 1969). The most common reasons given in 1964 were as follows: "don't really enjoy cigarettes" (35 percent), "wish to improve general physical condition" (34 percent), "have [had] some symptoms that might be caused by smoking cigarettes" (12 percent), "feel [felt] smoking may cause serious illness" (12 percent), "people who care about me [spouse] asked me to cut down" (11 percent), and "too expensive to smoke" (11 percent). In 1966, the reasons given for smoking cessation were as follows: "wish to improve physical condition" (31 percent), "don't really enjoy cigarettes" (29 percent), "have [had] some symptoms that might be caused by smoking cigarettes" (28 percent), "too expensive to smoke" (15 percent), and doctor or physician "advised me to quit or cut down" (11 percent).

In the 1992 NHIS data, reasons for smoking cessation were obtained from women former smokers. The reason most commonly given was concern about health. In 1992, 55.9 (± 3.5) percent of women who were former smokers had stopped smoking because of concerns about future health, and 22.9 (±2.9) percent stopped because of concerns about current health. The next most common reason given for smoking cessation was pressure from family or friends (18.3 ± 2.6 percent). Other reasons given by more than 10 percent of respondents were pregnancy (11.2 ± 2.1 percent) and cost (11.1 ± 2.2 percent) (NCHS, public use data tape, 1992). Reports from the 1986 AUTS and the 1987 NHIS showed a similar ranking of concerns (NCHS, public use data tape, 1987; Gilpin et al. 1992; Orleans et al. 1994).

In the 1992 NHIS data, women and men both cited concern for health as the main reason for smoking cessation; no significant gender-specific differences were found in the reasons for cessation, except for pregnancy (NCHS, public use data tape, 1992). However, two studies (Pirie et al. 1991; Royce et al. 1997) reported that women were more likely than men to report feeling social pressure to stop smoking.

Few studies have been done on reasons for wanting to stop smoking among girls. In a study of 24 high schools in California and Illinois, Sussman and colleagues (1998) reported that requests to quit smoking by a boyfriend, health-related reasons (someone close died because of smoking and "to live longer"), a physician's advice to quit, and cost were the primary reasons cited by girls for wanting to stop smoking. No gender-specific differences were noted in the reasons for wanting to quit.

### Reported Reasons for Relapse to Smoking

In the 1964 AUTS data, women who had made a serious but unsuccessful attempt to stop smoking were asked why they had relapsed to smoking. The reasons most commonly given were as follows: smoking is relaxing (23 percent), lack of willpower (20 percent), find smoking enjoyable (10 percent), and weight control (7 percent). Results from the 1966 AUTS data were similar (USDHEW 1969). In the 1986 AUTS data, the most frequent reasons given for relapse were irritability, weight gain, fear of weight gain, friction with family members, and inability to concentrate (USDHHS 1990a; Orleans et al. 1994).

Data from the 1987 NHIS were used to determine the reasons for relapse that were given by women current smokers who had made at least one attempt to quit smoking (see Appendix 2). Multiple reasons could be given by each respondent. The reason most frequently given by women for relapse was being nervous or tense (36.2 ± 2.4 percent). The next most common reasons were habit or being in a situation in which they used to smoke regularly, addiction or craving, a stressful life event, and the pleasure of smoking (each about 11 to 12 ± 1.6–1.7 percent). Reasons reported by less than 10 percent of respondents were "others smoking around me" (9.6 ± 1.5 percent) and actual weight gain (7.7 ± 1.4 percent). Less than 5 percent of women reported "didn't try hard enough" (4.6 ± 1.1 percent), "bored, blue, or depressed" (4.2 ± 0.9 percent), "fear of gaining weight" (3.6 ± 0.9 percent) and "not ready to stop smoking" (3.6 ± 1.0 percent) as reasons for relapse (NCHS, public use data tape, 1987).

The most frequent reasons given for relapse were generally similar for women and men. Women and men were equally likely to report addiction to or craving for cigarettes and the pleasure of smoking as the reason for relapse. Women were more likely than men to report fear of weight gain or actual weight gain as reasons for relapse, but the proportion of women citing fear of gaining weight (3.6 ± 1.0 percent) or actual weight gain (7.7 ± 1.4 percent) was small. Men (15.9 ± 2.1 percent) were more likely than women (12.0 ± 1.7 percent) to cite habit or being in a situation in which they used to smoke regularly as a reason for relapse, and women (36.2 ± 2.4 percent) were more likely than men (27.4 ± 2.5 percent) to cite being nervous or tense. Although other data suggested that having personal problems is a reason for relapse given by women more often than men (Guilford 1972), the 1987 NHIS data suggested that women and men were equally likely to report a stressful life event as a reason for relapse (NCHS, public use data tape, 1987).

### Trends in Smoking Continuum for Ever Smoking

A smoking continuum is used to more completely describe the dynamic process of smoking cessation (see "Smoking Cessation and Nicotine Addiction Treatment Methods" in Chapter 5). The continuum describes the timing and duration of attempts to stop smoking among all persons who had ever smoked cigarettes (Pierce et al. 1989b; USDHHS 1989, 1990d). Data from the 1979 and 1990 NHIS were used to construct a smoking continuum for women who had ever smoked cigarettes. The continuum included the proportions of female current smokers who had ever tried to stop smoking and of those who had tried to stop in the past year, as well as the duration of smoking cessation among female former smokers. Smoking continuums using the 1986 AUTS data have also been published (Pierce et al. 1989b; USDHHS 1989).

Women are moving through the smoking continuum over time. Among women who had ever smoked, the proportion who were current smokers who had never tried to stop smoking decreased from 29.5 percent in 1979 to 20.4 percent in 1990 (Figure 2.17). In both 1979 and 1990, a similar proportion of women who had ever smoked were current smokers who had tried to stop, but not in the past year. In 1979, however, 17.5 percent of women who had ever smoked were current smokers who had tried to stop smoking in the past year, whereas 13.0 percent in 1990 did so, and in 1990, a greater percentage (2.2 vs. 1.5 percent in 1979) who had ever smoked had quit smoking in the three months before the survey. In 1979, 6.5 percent of women who had ever smoked had quit for 5 to 9 years before the survey compared with 8.5 percent in 1990. The proportion who had quit smoking for 10 or more years before the survey doubled between 1979 and 1990 (from 10.7 to 20.9 percent). This finding is further evidence that women are moving through the continuum over time. Although NHIS data were not stratified by race, other studies showed that the mean number of years since quitting smoking was the same among white women and black women (Hahn et al. 1990) and among white women and Hispanic women (Winkleby et al. 1995).

NHIS data for 1979 showed that 30.1 (±1.4) percent of all women who smoked in the year before the survey had tried to stop smoking during that year; in 1990, 30.7 (±1.3) percent had tried to stop. The percentage

**Figure 2.17. Smoking continuum among women aged 18 years or older who ever smoked, National Health Interview Survey, United States, 1979 and 1990**

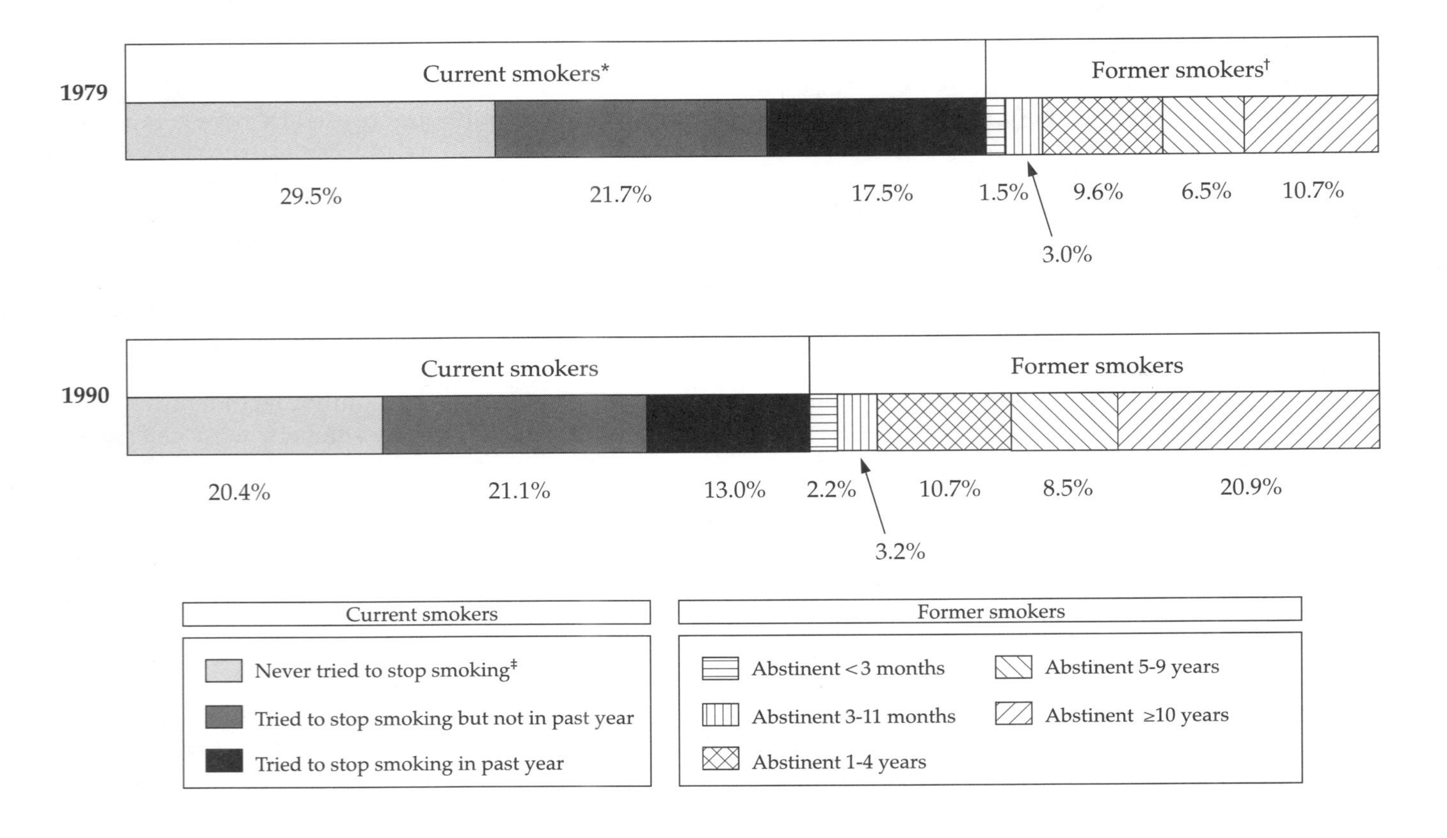


*Current smokers are persons who reported smoking ≥ 100 cigarettes in their lifetime and who smoked at the time of the survey.
†Former smokers are persons who reported smoking ≥ 100 cigarettes in their lifetime and who were not smoking at the time of the survey.
‡Based on the question, "Have you ever made a SERIOUS attempt to stop smoking cigarettes?"
Source: National Center for Health Statistics, public use data tapes, 1979, 1990.

still abstinent was significantly higher in 1990 (9.0 ± 0.8 percent) than in 1979 (6.2 ± 0.7 percent) (NCHS, public use data tapes, 1979, 1990).

Among persons who had ever smoked in 1979, women were significantly more likely than men to be current smokers who had never tried to stop smoking, but no gender-specific differences were noted in 1990 (NCHS, NHIS, public use data tapes, 1979, 1990). In this NHIS analysis and in a study by Pierce and colleagues (1989b), the major difference by gender related to long-term former smokers. In 1990, although women and men who had ever smoked were equally likely to be former smokers who had quit smoking for 1 through 9 years before the survey, women who had ever smoked (20.9 ± 1.0 percent) were less likely than men (27.6 ± 1.1 percent) to be former smokers who had quit for 10 or more years (NCHS, public use data tape, 1990). Pierce and associates (1989b), using 1986 AUTS data, found that women were as likely as men to have quit smoking for 1 to 5 years before the survey but less likely than men to have quit smoking for 5 or more years before the survey. In 1986, these gender-specific differences began at 5 years of smoking cessation, but in 1990 they were only evident for 10 or more years of cessation. These findings are not surprising because the decline in smoking prevalence began later among women than among men (Hammond and Garfinkel 1961).

**Table 2.29. Stages of smoking cessation (% and 95% confidence interval) among women smokers aged 18 years or older, by selected characteristics, National Health Interview Survey, United States, 1992**

| Characteristic | Ever quit smoking for ≥ 1 day* | Quit smoking for ≥ 1 day in past 12 months* | Seriously considering stopping smoking within next 6 months† | Planning to stop smoking within 30 days† |
|---|---|---|---|---|
| Women | 80.8 (±2.7) | 37.1 (±3.2) | 45.4 (±3.3) | 13.7 (±2.2) |
| Age (years) | | | | |
| 18–24 | 77.2 (±8.9) | 48.9 (±9.6) | 43.8 (±9.6) | 12.9 (±6.0)‡ |
| 25–44 | 82.9 (±3.2) | 36.8 (±4.1) | 46.3 (±4.5) | 13.7 (±3.2) |
| 45–64 | 83.3 (±4.6) | 36.4 (±5.9) | 49.6 (±6.3) | 15.2 (±4.3) |
| ≥ 65 | 66.7 (±10.8) | 23.5 (±8.2) | 30.2 (±9.1) | 10.2 (±6.3)‡ |
| Race/ethnicity | | | | |
| White, non-Hispanic | 80.5 (±3.0) | 35.1 (±3.5) | 44.5 (±3.6) | 12.9 (±2.3) |
| Black, non-Hispanic | 82.2 (±6.2) | 50.6 (±8.8) | 52.5 (±9.2) | 17.7 (±7.7) |
| Hispanic | 87.4 (±6.5) | 42.8 (±12.6) | 54.0 (±13.3) | 18.3 (±11.9)‡ |
| Education (number of years)§ | | | | |
| ≤ 8 | 74.8 (±11.8) | 26.6 (±10.4)‡ | 24.9 (±10.0)‡ | 10.4 (±7.1)‡ |
| 9–11 | 74.5 (±6.5) | 27.0 (±6.3) | 40.4 (±7.3) | 8.4 (±4.0)‡ |
| 12 | 82.3 (±3.7) | 37.2 (±4.7) | 46.6 (±5.2) | 15.7 (±3.7) |
| 13–15 | 82.6 (±5.8) | 37.0 (±7.0) | 48.3 (±8.0) | 13.6 (±5.0)‡ |
| ≥ 16 | 91.3 (±5.3) | 44.0 (±10.2) | 63.5 (±10.5) | 17.1 (±8.4)‡ |
| Men | 82.4 (±2.6) | 37.3 (±3.1) | 43.2 (±3.2) | 12.8 (±2.3) |

*Measured for daily smokers. Current smokers were persons who reported smoking ≥ 100 cigarettes in their lifetime and who smoked at the time of the survey. Daily smokers were current smokers who responded "every day" to the question, "Do you smoke every day, some days, or not at all?"

†Measured for current smokers. Current smokers were persons who reported smoking ≥ 100 cigarettes in their lifetime and who smoked at the time of the survey. Current smokers responded "every day" or "some days" to the question, "Do you smoke every day, some days, or not at all?"

‡Estimate should be interpreted with caution because of the small number of respondents.

§For women aged ≥ 25 years.

Source: National Center for Health Statistics, 1992 Cancer Control Supplement, public use data tape, 1992.

In the 1990 NHIS data, women who smoked in the past year (30.7 ± 1.3 percent) were as likely as men who smoked in the past year (28.5 ± 1.4 percent) to have tried to stop smoking and to still be abstinent at the time of the survey (both 9.0 percent) (NCHS, public use data tape, 1990). These findings were also true among women and men in the 1991 survey (CDC 1993).

### Stages of Cessation Among Current Smokers

Readiness to quit smoking is commonly measured by using a stages-of-change model (precontemplation, contemplation, action, and maintenance) (DiClemente et al. 1991). Survey measures have been developed to measure these stages of change (Crittenden et al. 1994). The 1992 NHIS was used to assess the stages of cessation among women who were current daily smokers (Table 2.29). Current daily smokers were asked if they had ever stopped smoking for 1 day or longer and if they had stopped smoking in the past 12 months for 1 day or longer; current smokers were asked whether they were seriously considering stopping smoking within the next 6 months, and whether they were planning to stop within the next 30 days. Of the women who were current daily smokers, 19.2 percent had never tried to stop smoking (precontemplation stage), 80.8 percent had quit smoking for at least 1 day in the past, and 37.1 percent had tried to stop smoking in the 12 months before the survey. In 1992, 45.4 percent of the women current smokers reported seriously considering stopping smoking in the next

6 months (contemplation stage), and 13.7 percent reported planning to stop smoking in the next 30 days.

Women aged 65 years or older were significantly less likely than women aged 25 through 64 years to have ever tried to quit smoking, less likely than women aged 18 through 44 years to have tried to quit smoking in the previous 12 months, and less likely than women aged 25 through 64 years to be seriously thinking about stopping smoking in the next 6 months. White women (35.1 percent) were less likely than black women (50.6 percent) to have tried to stop smoking in the past 12 months. No racial or ethnic differences were found among women planning to stop smoking, a finding consistent with other data (Kviz et al. 1994). Women with 16 or more years of education (44.0 percent) were more likely than women with less than 12 years of education (about 27 percent) to have stopped smoking for at least 1 day in the previous year (Table 2.29), a finding noted by others (Hatziandreu et al. 1990). Women with 16 or more years of education were more likely than women with 12 or fewer years of education to be considering smoking cessation in the next 6 months.

Among adult current daily smokers, no gender-specific differences were found for persons who ever attempted to quit smoking for at least 1 day, quit for at least 1 day in the previous year, seriously considered stopping in the next six months, or planned to stop within 30 days (Table 2.29). Other studies have also shown that women are as likely as men to have ever tried to quit smoking (Sorensen and Pechacek 1986, 1987; Blake et al. 1989; Derby et al. 1994) or to have recently attempted to quit smoking (Sorensen and Pechacek 1986; Blake et al. 1989; Pierce et al. 1989b; Hatziandreu et al. 1990; Fortmann and Killen 1994). Some studies found no differences in the percentages of women and men who planned to change their smoking behavior in the next year (Sorensen and Pechacek 1986; Blake et al. 1989), although one study reported that women were less likely than men to plan to stop smoking within the next three months (Kviz et al. 1994). In the 1992 NHIS data, the association between education and planning to stop smoking in the next six months was stronger for women than for men (data not shown). Among women with 16 or more years of education, 63.5 percent were planning to stop smoking in the next six months; only 24.9 percent of women with 8 or fewer years of education were planning to do so (Table 2.29). The comparable estimates for men were 48.4 (±10.1) and 31.7 (±12.5) percent, respectively (NCHS, public use data tape, 1992).

## Smoking Cessation Among Young Women

Smoking cessation efforts historically have focused on middle-aged smokers because they are at greater risk for smoking-related diseases. However, other investigators have suggested that cessation efforts need to focus on young adults (Wechsler 1998; Everett et al. 1999a). Smoking cessation before age 35 years eliminates nearly all of the excess mortality attributed to smoking (Doll et al. 1994). The NHIS data for 1965–1966 through 1997–1998 were used to determine trends in the percentage of young women smokers aged 18 through 24 years who quit smoking (Table 2.30 and Figure 2.16). The percentage of young women who had ever smoked who had quit smoking increased 10.0 (±3.0) percentage points, from 13.8 percent in 1965–1966 to 23.8 percent in 1997–1998 (Table 2.30) (Giovino et al. 1994). The increase was significant from 1965–1966 (combined data) through 1970 and again from 1983/1985 (combined data) through 1990–1991 (combined data); from then through 1992–1993 (combined data) it declined significantly (possibly a result of the change in the question used to assess smoking status) and remained unchanged through 1997–1998. Patterns of cessation among black women and among Hispanic women must be interpreted with caution because of small sample sizes. However, the percentage of smokers who had quit smoking appears to be lower among young black women than among young white women from 1965–1966 through 1983/1985 and then comparable in the 1990s. The percentage of smokers who had quit smoking was generally higher among young women with more than 12 years of education than among those with fewer than 12 years of education. Young women who smoked were equally likely as young men who smoked to have quit smoking. These findings are consistent with other data (Breslau and Peterson 1996).

Smoking cessation among young women varies by demographic characteristics (Table 2.30). NHIS data showed that in 1997–1998, 23.8 percent of young adult women smokers had quit smoking. The estimates from the 1997–1998 NHSDA (combined data) were somewhat lower (data not shown). The percentage of smokers who had quit smoking was higher among young Hispanic women than among young non-Hispanic white women and young non-Hispanic black women, but this finding was not significant for young non-Hispanic black women. Similar patterns were noted for the 1997–1998 NHSDA, but the differences were not statistically significant (data not shown). The percentage of young female smokers who had quit smoking was higher among those with more than 12 years of education than among those with fewer than 12 years of education. In the 1997–1998 NHSDA, the percentage of young female smokers who had quit smoking was higher among those with more than 12 years of education than among those with 12 or fewer years of education. The difference was statistically significant only among young women with 12 years of education, but not for young women with less than 12 years of education (data not shown). The percentage of smokers who had quit smoking was higher among young women than among young men in the 1997–1998 NHSDA and NHIS surveys, although the difference was not significant in NHIS (Table 2.30) (SAMHSA, public use data tapes, 1997, 1998).

## Smoking Cessation Among Girls

Only 14 percent of high school girls who were ever daily smokers who had ever tried to quit smoking were former smokers at the time of survey (CDC 1998b). Similar findings have been reported by others (Johnston et al. 1995b). In MTF Surveys of 1976–1986, 44 percent of daily smokers believed that they would not be smoking in five years, but 73 percent remained daily smokers five to six years later (USDHHS 1994).

The percentage of high school senior girls who had smoked regularly at some time but had not smoked in the past 30 days was considered to be the percentage of smokers who had quit smoking. This percentage was assessed by using the 1976–1998 MTF Survey data (University of Michigan, Institute for Social Research, public use data tapes, 1976–1998). The percentage of smokers who had quit smoking increased from 16.3 (±2.8) percent in 1976 to 20.9 (± 3.2) percent in 1981, then decreased to 13.0 (±2.9) percent in 1998.

Gender-specific differences in smoking cessation have been small and inconsistent among adolescents. Generally, girls and boys were equally likely to be unsuccessful in their attempts to stop smoking (Ershler et al. 1989; Waldron et al. 1991). MTF Survey data confirm this finding. In 1976, the percentage of smokers who had quit smoking was 17.1 (±2.4) percent among boys and 16.3 (±2.8) percent among girls. In 1998, the percentage was 15.6 (±2.5) percent among boys and 13.0 (±2.9) percent among girls (University of Michigan, Institute for Social Research, public use data tapes, 1976–1998). An analysis based on 633 adolescent smokers in TAPS I (1989) who were followed up in TAPS II (1993) found no significant difference in quit rates by gender (16.1 percent for females and 15.0 percent for males) (Zhu et al. 1999).

## Smoking Cessation Among Pregnant Women and Girls

Smoking cessation is particularly important during pregnancy. In the 1986 Linked Telephone Survey, white women aged 20 through 44 years who were respondents to the 1985 NHIS were interviewed again (Fingerhut et al. 1990). Of those who smoked before pregnancy, 39 percent stopped smoking while they were pregnant (27 percent on learning they were pregnant and 12 percent later during pregnancy). Smoking cessation increased as the level of education increased (Fingerhut et al. 1990).

In the 1991 NHIS, questions related to smoking cessation after learning of pregnancy were asked of women aged 18 through 44 years who had given birth within the past five years. In 1991, 30.8 (±2.3) percent of women who were smoking when they became pregnant reported having quit smoking after learning of the pregnancy (NCHS, public use data tape, 1991). The percentage was 30.9 (±2.6) among white women and 31.8 (±5.8) among black women. As the level of education increased, the likelihood of quitting smoking also increased. In 1991, 21.1 (± 3.9) percent of women with fewer than 12 years of education, but 45.4 (±10.5) percent of women with 16 or more years of education, quit smoking during pregnancy. This finding is consistent with previously published studies (O'Campo et al. 1992; Floyd et al. 1993).

In an analysis of data from the 1988 National Maternal and Infant Health Survey, Sugarman and colleagues (1994) reported that the percentage of smokers who reported having quit smoking for at least one week during the pregnancy was higher among American Indian mothers (64 percent) than among white mothers (57 percent) or black mothers (49 percent).

Pregnant women generally stopped smoking because of concerns about potential adverse outcomes during pregnancy or negative effects on infant health (O'Campo et al. 1992). Many pregnant women, however, consider smoking cessation during pregnancy to be a temporary abstinence. Although considerable efforts have been made to promote smoking cessation during pregnancy, pregnant women who stop smoking are typically abstinent for five to seven months and enter the postpartum period as likely to relapse to smoking as nonpregnant smokers who have just stopped smoking. Within one year of delivery, 70 percent of women who had quit smoking during pregnancy had relapsed. The majority of mothers resume smoking within six months after delivery (Fingerhut et al. 1990; Mullen et al. 1990; McBride et al. 1992;

**Table 2.30. Percentage (and 95% confidence interval) of young women smokers aged 18–24 years who have quit smoking, by selected characteristics, National Health Interview Survey, United States, 1965–1998**

| Characteristic | 1965–1966 | 1970 | 1974 | 1978–1980 |
|---|---|---|---|---|
| Young women | 13.8 (±1.4) | 19.7 (±1.8) | 18.6 (±2.4) | 22.6 (±2.1) |
| Race/ethnicity* | | | | |
| White, non-Hispanic | 14.6 (±1.4) | 20.7 (±1.9) | 19.5 (±2.6) | 23.9 (±2.3) |
| Black, non-Hispanic | 5.9 (±3.1) | 10.5 (±3.3) | 8.8 (±5.4)† | 13.1 (±5.6)† |
| Hispanic | NA‡ | NA | NA | 26.0 (±7.9) |
| Education (number of years)§ | | | | |
| <12 | NA | 15.1 (±3.4) | 11.3 (±4.8)† | 14.5 (±4.2) |
| 12 | NA | 19.1 (±2.8) | 23.0 (±4.3) | 26.5 (±3.7) |
| >12 | NA | 31.0 (±4.7) | 19.5 (±4.6) | 29.5 (±5.1) |
| Young men | 11.4 (±1.1) | 19.5 (±1.6) | 21.6 (±3.0) | 23.0 (±2.0) |

*Note:* Percentage of smokers who have quit smoking is the percentage of persons who reported smoking ≥ 100 cigarettes in their lifetime who are former smokers.

*Ethnicity not determined in 1965, 1966, 1970, or 1974. Thus, estimates for whites and for blacks during these years likely include data for some persons of Hispanic origin.

†Estimate should be interpreted with caution because of the small number of respondents.

Floyd et al. 1993; Stotts et al. 1996). Age, race, marital status, and education have not been significantly associated with postpartum relapse to smoking (Fingerhut et al. 1990; O'Campo et al. 1992). (See "Postpartum Smoking" in Chapter 5.)

## Physicians' Advice About Smoking

### Advice to Women

According to the 1991 NHIS data, 79 percent of women who smoked saw a physician in the year before the survey (NCHS, public use data tape, 1991); the percentage was comparable in the 1992 NHIS (NCHS, public use data tape, 1992). In a study using the 1988 NHIS data, 70 percent of female smokers who considered themselves to be in excellent health reported seeing a physician each year (Ockene 1993). Physicians, therefore, have many opportunities to advise women to quit smoking, and study findings showed that physicians' advice to quit smoking increases cessation rates (Fiore et al. 1996, 2000).

In the 1964 AUTS data, only 16.6 percent of women who smoked reported ever having received advice to quit smoking from a physician (USDHEW 1969; USDHHS 1990d). The percentage of smokers who had ever received such advice increased steadily over time. Still, in the 1975 AUTS data (USDHEW 1976), only 38 percent of women who smoked reported that a physician had advised them to do something about their smoking. A 1975 ACS household survey of 559 young women aged 18 through 35 years reported that only 27 percent of the women had been cautioned by their health care provider about the dangers of smoking (USDHEW 1977). In a 1980–1983 survey of 1,652 adults in Michigan (Anda et al. 1987), 46 percent of women who smoked reported ever having been told by a physician to quit smoking. According to the 1987 NHIS data, 54 percent of women who smoked reported ever having received advice from a physician to quit smoking (Schoenborn and Boyd 1989; USDHHS 1990d). In the 1991 NHIS, 62.4 percent of women who smoked reported ever having received advice to quit smoking from a physician or other health professional. In the 1992 NHIS data, 69.4 percent of women smokers reported ever having received such advice from a physician or dentist (NCHS, public use data tapes, 1991, 1992).

The 1964 AUTS data reported that women (16.6 percent) and men (15.0 percent) who currently smoked were equally likely to report ever having received a physician's advice to quit smoking (USDHEW 1969; USDHHS 1990a). Over time, however, a gender-specific difference developed; women who smoked became more likely than men to report having received such advice. In 1980–1983 (combined data), women were slightly, but not significantly,

| 1983/1985 | 1990–1991 | 1992–1993 | 1994–1995 | 1997–1998 |
|---|---|---|---|---|
| 23.2 (±2.0) | 27.9 (±2.4) | 19.9 (±3.0) | 25.7 (±3.9) | 23.8 (±2.9) |
| | | | | |
| 23.8 (±2.3) | 27.8 (±2.5) | 19.3 (±3.3) | 25.0 (±4.2) | 23.1 (±3.3) |
| 14.5 (±5.4) | 26.5 (±7.8) | 16.4 (±9.9)† | 21.0 (±13.3)† | 22.6 (±9.9)† |
| 30.4 (±9.8) | 29.5 (±9.7) | 26.7 (±12.8)† | 30.0 (±10.5)† | 37.2 (±9.5) |
| | | | | |
| 17.7 (±4.5) | 17.0 (±5.1) | 7.7 (±4.2)† | 14.1 (±7.9)† | 17.0 (±6.8) |
| 22.3 (±3.4) | 28.1 (±4.0) | 23.2 (±5.2) | 28.0 (±7.2) | 23.0 (±5.7) |
| 32.3 (±4.5) | 36.1 (±4.7) | 23.7 (±5.9) | 30.3 (±6.6) | 30.0 (±5.1) |
| 23.4 (±2.2) | 25.5 (±3.1) | 19.6 (±3.6) | 21.5 (±3.7) | 19.3 (±2.7) |

‡NA = Not available.
§For women aged 20–24 years. Data for these education categories were not available for 1965.
Sources: National Center for Health Statistics, public use data tapes, 1965–1966, 1970, 1974, 1978–1980, 1983, 1985, 1990–1995, 1997–1998.

more likely to report having received such advice (46 vs. 42 percent) (Anda et al. 1987; Ockene et al. 1987). The questions used to assess whether a person received a physician's advice to quit smoking were slightly different in the 1991 and 1992 NHIS, but in both years, women who smoked were significantly more likely than men to report having received such advice (69.4 vs. 60.7 percent in 1992) (NCHS, public use data tapes, 1991, 1992).

Data from the 1991 NHIS were used to assess the percentage of female smokers who, within the past year, had seen a physician and reported receiving advice to quit smoking from a physician or another health care professional (Table 2.31). The data indicated that 38.9 percent of these women reported that they had received such advice. A population-based study in Rhode Island from 1990 reported that 48 percent of women who had visited a health care setting in the previous year reported receiving advice to quit smoking (Goldstein et al. 1997). In the 1991 NHIS, physicians' advice to quit smoking was most common (44.5 percent) among women aged 45 through 64 years (Table 2.31). Of women aged 65 years or older, 34.9 percent reported having received advice to quit smoking within the previous year. Similarly, in a survey of AARP members, 39 percent of persons aged 50 through 102 years reported having been advised by their physician in the previous year to stop smoking (Rimer et al. 1990).

In the 1991 NHIS data, black women (38.1 percent) were as likely as white women (39.8 percent) to report having received a physician's advice to quit smoking in the previous year (Table 2.31). An earlier study using aggregated data from 1980 and 1983 in Michigan had reported that black women were less likely than white women to have received such advice (Anda et al. 1987). In NHIS, Hispanic women who smoked were less likely than white women to report having received advice to quit smoking (Table 2.31). This difference occurred despite a comparable number of visits to a physician by Hispanic women and white women (NCHS, public use data tape, 1991). In another study, 27 percent of Hispanic women and 67.7 percent of white women with fewer than 12 years of education reported ever having received a physician's advice to quit smoking (Winkleby et al. 1995). The difference by race and ethnicity was not explained by a difference in language barriers or by a difference in access to care, and the number of visits to physicians was comparable. Because of the fairly low prevalence of smoking among Hispanic women, clinicians may not have assessed smoking in this population. No difference by race or ethnicity was seen for women with 12 or more years of education.

Among all women, no significant difference was observed by education in reported physicians' advice to quit smoking in the previous year. The prevalence of reporting such advice increased as the number of

**Table 2.31. Percentage (and 95% confidence interval) of persons aged 18 years or older who had smoked in the previous 12 months who reported receiving advice to quit smoking from a physician or other health care professional in the preceding 12 months, by gender and selected characteristics, National Health Interview Survey, United States, 1991**

| Characteristic | Women | Men |
|---|---|---|
| Overall | 38.9 (±1.6) | 35.2 (±1.8) |
| Age (years) | | |
| 18–24 | 35.9 (±4.5) | 16.9 (±4.2) |
| 25–44 | 37.6 (±2.3) | 33.4 (±2.5) |
| 45–64 | 44.5 (±3.0) | 43.1 (±3.7) |
| ≥ 65 | 34.9 (±4.4) | 43.3 (±5.7) |
| Race/ethnicity | | |
| White, non-Hispanic | 39.8 (±1.8) | 36.3 (±2.1) |
| Black, non-Hispanic | 38.1 (±4.0) | 30.5 (±4.8) |
| Hispanic | 30.6 (±6.7) | 30.5 (±7.7) |
| Education (number of years)* | | |
| ≤ 8 | 37.8 (±6.5) | 41.8 (±6.5) |
| 9–11 | 44.0 (±4.4) | 34.3 (±5.1) |
| 12 | 39.4 (±2.6) | 37.8 (±3.0) |
| 13–15 | 38.1 (±3.6) | 38.4 (±4.3) |
| ≥ 16 | 36.8 (±4.5) | 35.4 (±4.8) |
| Number of visits | | |
| 1 | 29.2 (±2.9) | 27.2 (±2.7) |
| 2–3 | 36.6 (±2.7) | 35.8 (±3.4) |
| ≥ 4 | 46.4 (±2.5) | 43.9 (±3.4) |
| Number of cigarettes/day | | |
| <15 | 36.0 (±2.7) | 30.0 (±3.3) |
| 15–24 | 43.3 (±2.7) | 38.8 (±3.2) |
| ≥ 25 | 50.2 (±4.2) | 43.7 (±3.8) |

*Note:* 79.0 (±1.2)% of women smokers and 62.0 (±1.5)% of men smokers had visited a physician in the past year. Mean number of visits: 5.2 for women, 3.2 for men. Smokers receiving advice to quit smoking were among persons who had seen a physician or other health care professional in the past year.
*For women aged ≥ 25 years.
Source: National Center for Health Statistics, public use data tape, 1991.

visits to a physician increased (Table 2.31); this finding has also been reported by other investigators (Anda et al. 1987). In NHIS data, advice from a physician to quit smoking also increased as the number of cigarettes smoked per day increased (Table 2.31).

In the 1991 NHIS data, among smokers who had visited a physician in the past year, women (38.9 percent) were slightly more likely than men (35.2 percent) to report having received advice to quit smoking in the past year (Table 2.31), a pattern also reported in the population-based study in Rhode Island (Goldstein et al. 1997). In the 1992 NHIS, which had a much smaller sample size and which asked about advice from a medical doctor, the gender-specific difference for those receiving advice from a medical doctor was much greater (53.4 percent for women vs. 49.7 percent for men) but was not statistically significant (NCHS, public use data tape, 1992; Tomar et al. 1996). Further analysis of the 1991 NHIS data for smokers showed that, in the previous year, women made more visits to physicians (5.2) than did men (3.2) (NCHS, public use data tape, 1991). No gender-specific difference was noted when having received advice was stratified by the number of visits. The finding of no difference by gender is consistent with other data (Royce et al. 1997).

In the 1991 NHIS data, young women aged 18 through 24 years who smoked were much more likely (35.9 percent) than their male counterparts (16.9 percent) to report having received advice from a physician to quit smoking (Table 2.31). This pattern was also true in combined data from 1980 and 1983 (Anda et al. 1987). The 1991 NHIS data showed that young women made a greater number of visits to a physician (6.5) than did young men (2.0), but when the data were stratified by the number of visits young women were still more likely to report having received a physician's advice to quit smoking (NCHS, public use data tape, 1991). This advice may have been given because of the types of visits made by young women (i.e., for contraceptive counseling or pregnancy). Anda and colleagues (1987) found, however, that women who used oral contraceptives were no more likely than those who did not use them to be advised to quit smoking.

### Advice to Girls

In 1991, about 83 percent of girls had visited a physician within the previous year and 93 percent within the previous two years. Multiple visits were common—about four contacts with a physician per year (Adams and Benson 1992). Thus, physicians had multiple opportunities to advise girls on smoking prevention and cessation. A 1975 ACS survey of girls aged 13 through 17 years found, however, that only 30 percent reported having been cautioned by a health care provider about the dangers of smoking (USDHEW 1977). Similarly, in 1993, only 26.5 percent of girls and young women aged 10 through 22 years remembered that a health care provider had ever talked to them about smoking. White females (27.9 percent) were more likely than black (22.5 percent), Hispanic (23.5 percent), or Alaska Native and American Indian (15.7 percent) females to have been counseled by a health care provider on cigarette smoking. Sample sizes were too small to assess physicians' advice to Asians or Pacific Islander females (CDC 1995d). In the 1999 NYTS, among girls in middle school, 30.6 (±3.1) percent of never smokers and 31.7 (±5.9) percent of current smokers had talked to a doctor about the danger of tobacco use; among girls in high school, the percentages were 26.4 (±3.5) and 31.2 (±3.9), respectively (CDC 2000b). No gender-specific differences were noted.

## Summary

In 1997–1998, the percentage of persons who had ever smoked who had quit smoking was lower among women (46.2 percent) than among men (50.1 percent), probably because men began to quit smoking earlier in this century than did women and because these data do not take into account that men are more likely than women to switch to or to continue to use other tobacco products when they stop smoking cigarettes. Since the late 1970s or early 1980s, the probability of attempting to quit smoking and succeeding has been equally high among women and men.

In 1998, only 13.0 percent of high school senior girls who had ever smoked regularly had quit smoking. In 1997–1998, 23.8 percent of young women who had ever smoked had quit smoking. In 1998, 34.5 percent of women smokers of reproductive age (18 through 44 years) and 46.1 percent of women overall had quit smoking. The percentage of smokers who have quit smoking increases with age because of increases in the number of smokers who have quit and because of differential mortality between continuing smokers and those who have quit smoking.

In 1996–1998, 43.5 percent of high school senior girls who smoked daily wanted to quit smoking; 45.3 percent had tried at some point and could not quit. In 1995, 75.2 percent of women who were daily smokers wanted to quit smoking completely, and 46.6 percent had tried to quit smoking in the previous year. Women cited concern for health as the primary reason they wanted to quit smoking. The reason most frequently given by women for relapse to smoking was being nervous or tense.

Women are progressing through the smoking continuum over time. The proportion of women who had ever smoked who had quit smoking for 10 or more years doubled between 1979 (10.7 percent) and 1990 (20.9 percent). In 1992, among adult current daily smokers, no gender-specific differences were observed in ever attempting to quit smoking, attempts to quit in the previous 12 months, serious consideration of stopping within the next 6 months, or plans to stop within the next 30 days. Women smokers had made, on average, 6.3 lifetime attempts to quit smoking and 2.7 attempts in the previous 12 months.

In 1991, only 38.9 percent of women smokers who had seen a physician or other health care professional in the previous year reported having received advice to quit smoking. In 1993, only 26.5 percent of girls and young women aged 10 through 22 years remembered a health care provider ever having talked to them about smoking. Although women were slightly more likely than men to report having received such advice during the previous year, when the results were stratified by the number of visits to a physician, no gender-specific difference was found. Hispanic women were less likely than white women to have received advice to quit smoking, even though the number of physicians' visits was comparable.

In 1992, most women smokers who had successfully quit smoking (88.1 percent) cited abrupt cessation (cold turkey) as one of the methods used. Only 3.4 percent of women former smokers used a formal cessation program in their last attempt to quit smoking. However, new therapies, particularly pharmacotherapies, have been introduced in recent years, and recent studies suggested that a substantial minority of smokers are using these therapies. From 1987 through 1992, the average number of methods women used during their last attempt to quit smoking increased. Women who quit smoking cold turkey used fewer methods than did women who quit by gradually decreasing the number of cigarettes smoked or by switching to low-tar cigarettes.

# Other Tobacco Use

Smokeless tobacco is causally associated with oral leukoplakia and oral cancer and may increase the risk for cancer at other anatomic sites (USDHHS 1986a). Study findings suggest that it also increases the risk of tooth loss, periodontitis, and gingival recession (Novotny and Giovino 1998). In studies limited to men, some evidence suggests that the use of smokeless tobacco may also increase the risk of cardiovascular disease (Benowitz 1992; Bolinder et al. 1994). Results of other studies indicate that the use of a pipe or cigar increases the risk for laryngeal, oral, esophageal, and lung cancers (USDHHS 1982), although again, analyses are limited to men. More recent reviews have concluded that cigar smoking causes cancer of the lung, oral cavity, larynx, esophagus, and probably the pancreas. Persons who smoke cigars heavily and those who inhale cigar smoke deeply are at increased risk for coronary heart disease, aortic aneurysm, and chronic obstructive pulmonary disease (Shanks and Burns 1998). Recent evidence suggests that teens use cigars as "blunts" (i.e., replacing all or part of the tobacco with marijuana) (USDHHS 1999b).

Other tobacco products, such as bidis and kreteks, are being smoked in the United States. Bidis are small, brown, hand-rolled cigarettes from India and other Southeast Asian countries consisting of tobacco wrapped in a tendu or temburni leaf and tied at one end with a string. Bidis are available in different flavors (e.g., cherry, chocolate, mango). When tested on a standard smoking machine, bidis produce higher levels of carbon monoxide, nicotine, and tar than do cigarettes. Because of the low combustability of the wrapper, bidi smokers inhale more often and more deeply than do cigarette smokers (CDC 1999a). Studies suggest that bidi users are at increased risk for coronary heart disease and several cancers (oral cavity, lung, pharynx, larynx, esophagus, stomach, and liver). Kreteks are clove cigarettes made in Indonesia that contain clove extract and tobacco.

## Cigars

### Women

National data from the 1964 and 1966 AUTS indicated that 0.2 to 0.4 percent of women smoked cigars (USDHEW 1969). Data from the 1970, 1987, 1991, 1992, and 1998 NHIS data indicated that ever smoking and current smoking of cigars by women remained low, but increased during 1970–1998 (ever smoking, from 0.44 percent in 1970 to 5.9 percent in 1998; current smoking, from 0.19 percent in 1970 to 0.7 percent in 1998) (Table 2.32). Results from the 1986 AUTS are comparable (AUTS, public use data tape, 1986). In the 1998 NHIS, cigar use among women was inversely associated with age (Table 2.32). From 1992 through 1998, the percentage of women who had ever smoked a cigar increased; this increase occurred primarily among women 18 through 44 years of age but not among older women. Other data also suggested that cigar smoking is increasing in popularity among women (Martin and Elkin 1995; Somasundaram 1996). Surveys of tobacco use that were conducted among adults in California in both 1990 and 1996 included questions about current use of cigars. The prevalence of current cigar use among women increased fivefold between 1990 (0.2 ±

**Table 2.32. Prevalence (% and 95% confidence interval) of ever and current cigar smoking among women aged 18 years or older, by selected characteristics, National Health Interview Survey, United States, 1970–1998**

| Characteristic | 1970 | 1987 | 1991 | 1992 | 1998 |
|---|---|---|---|---|---|
| Ever smoking | | | | | |
| Women | 0.44 (±0.08) | 3.6 (±0.4) | 3.1 (±0.3) | 3.7 (±0.5) | 5.9 (±0.4) |
| Aged 18–24 years | 0.43 (±0.16)* | 4.5 (±1.3) | 2.7 (±0.7) | 5.0 (±1.7) | 9.6 (±1.7) |
| Aged 25–44 years | 0.51 (±0.14) | 4.3 (±0.6) | 3.6 (±0.4) | 4.0 (±0.8) | 7.2 (±0.7) |
| Aged 45–64 years | 0.42 (±0.14) | 3.3 (±0.7) | 3.4 (±0.5) | 3.7 (±1.0) | 5.0 (±0.7) |
| Aged ≥ 65 years | 0.35 (±0.18)* | 1.6 (±0.6) | 1.7 (±0.4) | 2.2 (±0.9)* | 1.7 (±0.5) |
| Men | 32.16 (±0.95) | 36.3 (±1.3) | 35.5 (±1.0) | 40.2 (±1.7) | 35.1 (±1.0) |
| Current smoking | | | | | |
| Women | 0.19 (±0.05) | 0.06 (±0.03)* | 0.05 (±0.03)* | 0.02 (±0.05)* | 0.7 (±0.1) |
| Men | 16.22 (±0.56) | 5.3 (±0.4) | 3.5 (±0.3) | 3.3 (±0.5) | 8.4 (±0.5) |

*Note:* Prevalence of ever cigar smoking is the percentage of all persons in each demographic category who reported that they ever smoked cigars. For 1970, prevalence of current cigar smoking is the percentage of all persons in each demographic category who smoked at the time of the survey. For 1987, 1991, and 1992, prevalence of current cigar smoking is the percentage of all persons in each demographic category who reported smoking ≥ 50 cigars in their lifetime and who smoked at the time of the survey. For 1998, prevalence of current cigar smoking is the percentage of all persons in each demographic category who reported that they ever smoked cigars and smoked cigars at the time of the survey.
*Estimate should be interpreted with caution because of the small number of respondents.
Sources: National Center for Health Statistics, public use data tapes, 1970, 1987, 1991, 1992, 1998.

0.1 percent) and 1996 (1.1 ± 0.3 percent). Although prevalence of cigar smoking among men increased at a slower rate, it nearly doubled during this period and remained significantly higher (8.9 ± 0.7 percent in 1996) than prevalence among women (Gerlach et al. 1998).

In all years, women were considerably less likely than men to have ever smoked a cigar or to be a current cigar smoker. Although overall use of cigars among women has traditionally been low, it has been higher among some demographic groups of women. Aggregate data from the 1987 and 1991 NHIS showed that cigar use was somewhat higher among American Indian and Alaska Native women (0.2 percent) than among women of other racial and ethnic groups (0.1 percent) (USDHHS 1998). Data from the 1995–1996 Current Population Survey also showed a somewhat higher prevalence of cigar use among American Indian and Alaska Native women (0.5 percent) (Gerlach et al. 1998).

The 1998 NHSDA data reported cigar use over a lifetime and in the past month, by age and gender. Lifetime cigar use ranged from 24.5 (±2.2) percent among women aged 18 through 25 years to 14.5 (±1.5) percent among women aged 35 years or older. Current cigar use (in the past month) decreased from 4.6 (±1.0) percent among women aged 18 through 25 years to 1.5 (± 0.5) percent among women aged 35 years or older (SAMHSA, public use data tape, 1998). This finding is in contrast to the results of the 1995–1996 Current Population Survey, which found no age pattern (Gerlach et al. 1998). In the 1998 NHSDA data, lifetime cigar use among women aged 18 through 25 years was 46 percent of that among men in the same age group, and among women aged 35 years or older it was only 24 percent of that among men of comparable age. Current cigar use among women aged 18 through 25 years was one-fourth that among men in the same age group, and among women aged 35 years or older it was one-seventh that among men of comparable age (SAMHSA, public use data tape, 1998).

### Girls

The prevalence of cigar use appears to be higher among adolescent girls than among women. The 1998 NHSDA data showed that 14.8 (±1.9) percent of girls aged 12 through 17 years had ever smoked a cigar. This prevalence of ever smoking was about two-thirds that among boys. In the 1999 NYTS, 10.9 (±2.0) percent of middle school girls and 31.9 (±2.8) percent

**Table 2.33. Prevalence (% and 95% confidence interval) of current cigar smoking among adolescents less than 18 years of age, by gender and selected characteristics, National Household Survey on Drug Abuse (NHSDA) and Youth Risk Behavior Survey (YRBS), United States, 1998–1999**

| Characteristic | 1998 NHSDA* (ages 12–17) Girls | 1998 NHSDA* (ages 12–17) Boys | 1999 YRBS† (grades 9–12) Girls | 1999 YRBS† (grades 9–12) Boys |
|---|---|---|---|---|
| Overall | 3.7 (±1.0) | 7.5 (±1.3) | 9.8 (±2.4) | 24.3 (±2.2) |
| Age (years) | | | | |
| 12–14 | 2.1 (±1.0) | 2.0 (±0.9) | 8.6 (±3.3) | 15.8 (±5.8) |
| 15–17 | 5.4 (±1.6) | 13.4 (±2.5) | 9.9 (±2.7) | 25.4 (±2.2) |
| Race/ethnicity | | | | |
| White, non-Hispanic | 4.2 (±1.4) | 8.5 (±1.8) | 8.8 (±2.9) | 27.3 (±3.3) |
| Black, non-Hispanic | 2.3 (±1.3)‡ | 4.7 (±2.1)‡ | 12.3 (±4.3) | 14.5 (±3.3) |
| Hispanic | 3.9 (±1.7) | 6.6 (±2.3) | 10.7 (±2.7) | 22.4 (±3.8) |

*Note:* NHSDA is a household survey that includes adolescents 12–17 years of age; 67.0% were 14–17 years of age. YRBS is a school-based survey that includes high school students in grades 9–12; these analyses were restricted to those less than 18 years of age; of these, 99.8% were 14–17 years of age. Data are not comparable across surveys due to differences in ages surveyed and survey methods.

*For NHSDA, prevalence of current cigar smoking is the percentage of all persons in each demographic category who reported smoking cigars in the 30 days preceding the survey.

†For YRBS, prevalence of current cigar smoking is the percentage of all persons in each demographic category who reported smoking cigars on one or more days in the 30 days preceding the survey.

‡Estimate should be interpreted with caution because of the small number of respondents.

Sources: **NHSDA:** Substance Abuse and Mental Health Services Administration, public use data tape, 1998. **YRBS:** Centers for Disease Control and Prevention, Division of Adolescent and School Health, public use data tape, 1999.

of high school girls had ever smoked cigars, compared with 20.1 (±2.2) percent of middle school boys and 51.1 (±3.1) percent of high school boys (CDC 2000b).

In the 1999 YRBS data, 9.8 percent of high school girls less than 18 years of age and 9.9 percent of all high school girls had smoked a cigar in the month preceding the survey (Table 2.33) (Kann et al. 2000). Estimates were somewhat lower for NHSDA; the 1998 NHSDA data showed that 3.7 (±1.0) percent of girls aged 12 through 17 years had smoked a cigar in the past month. No racial or ethnic differences in prevalence were found. Prevalence of cigar smoking did not vary by age for girls in YRBS, although higher prevalence at age 15 years was noted in NHSDA. In contrast, prevalence increased with age for boys in both surveys. Girls were significantly less likely than boys to be current cigar users (Table 2.33) (Kann et al. 2000). A 1996 national survey conducted by The Robert Wood Johnson Foundation estimated that 16.0 percent (1.7 million) of adolescent girls aged 14 through 19 years had smoked a cigar in the past year; the prevalence among boys was 37.0 percent (CDC 1997a). Among girls, the prevalence of cigar smoking in the past month was about one-half that among boys (SAMHSA, public use data tape, 1998). In the 1999 NYTS, 4.4 (±1.3) percent of girls in middle school and 10.2 (±1.6) percent of girls in high school reported smoking cigars in the previous month. Girls were about half as likely as boys to be current cigar users (CDC 2000b).

## Pipes

### Women

National data from the 1964 and 1966 AUTS indicated that 0.3 percent of women smoked a pipe (USDHEW 1969). In the 1986 AUTS and the 1970, 1987, 1991, and 1992 NHIS, pipe smoking among women was low (0.0 to 0.1 percent) (NCHS, public use data tapes, 1970, 1987, 1991, 1992; USDHHS, public use data tape, 1986; Giovino et al. 1993; Nelson et al. 1996). Aggregate data from the 1987 and 1991 NHIS showed that pipe use was low among white women

(0.1 percent) and among women of other racial and ethnic groups (0.0 percent) (USDHHS 1998). In all years, women were much less likely than men to smoke a pipe (NCHS, public use data tapes, 1970, 1987, 1991, 1992; USDHHS, public use data tape, 1986).

### Girls

In the 1999 NYTS, 1.4 (±0.6) percent of girls in middle school and 1.4 (±0.5) percent of girls in high school reported that they had smoked a pipe in the preceding month. Current pipe use among girls was 33 to 40 percent that of boys (CDC 2000b).

## Smokeless Tobacco

### Women

Data from the 1964 and 1966 AUTS indicated that about 2.0 percent of women used snuff and about 0.4 percent used chewing tobacco (USDHEW 1969). In the 1985 NHSDA data, 3 percent of women aged 21 years or older reported ever using smokeless tobacco, whereas 1 percent reported use in the past year. Among women who reported ever using smokeless tobacco, 26 percent reported use almost every day in the past year (Rouse 1989).

In NHIS data, current use of smokeless tobacco is defined as reported use of snuff or chewing tobacco at least 20 times and at the time of the survey. Because of the small sample size, multiple years of data were combined to derive some estimates. Use of smokeless tobacco by women decreased significantly from 1970 through 1991–1992 and 1994 (1991/1992/1994, combined data), and the decline was significant among women in almost all demographic groups (Table 2.34). Further declines occurred through 1998 among women 65 years of age or older. Declines that were borderline statistically significant were found among women overall, black non-Hispanic women, and women who reside in the South. In 1998 data, use of smokeless tobacco was more prevalent among older women than among younger women. Other surveys have also found a higher prevalence of smokeless tobacco use among older women (Bauman et al. 1989; Giovino et al. 1995).

In NHIS data for 1998, black women (1.0 percent) were more likely than white women (0.2 percent) to use smokeless tobacco (Table 2.34). This finding holds for all regions of the country (NCHS, public use data tape, 1998) and is consistent with the results of other surveys (Bauman et al. 1989; Marcus et al. 1989; Giovino et al. 1995). In the 1970 NHIS data, 24.5 percent of black women aged 65 years or older currently used smokeless tobacco (NCHS, public use data tape, 1970). The 1985 NHSDA data found a high prevalence of use among black women aged 55 years or older: 19 percent had used smokeless tobacco in their lifetime, and 12 percent were current daily users (Rouse 1989). A 1985 study of current use of smokeless tobacco in 10 areas of the Southeast also reported prevalence to be particularly high among black women aged 70 years or older (18.6 percent) (Bauman et al. 1989). This prevalence was higher than that for any other age, race (black or white), or gender group.

Aggregated data from the 1987 and 1991 NHIS showed that use of smokeless tobacco was reported by 2.9 percent of black women, 1.2 percent of American Indian or Alaska Native women, 0.3 percent of white women, 0.1 percent of Hispanic women, and 0 percent of Asian or Pacific Islander women (Giovino et al. 1994; USDHHS 1998). Two studies have examined use of smokeless tobacco among American Indian women in the Lumbee tribe in southeastern North Carolina and in the Cherokee tribe in western North Carolina (CDC 1995b; Spangler et al. 1997a,b). They found that a significant percentage of the women reported current use of smokeless tobacco (23 and 8 percent, respectively). In both studies, use was higher among older women, women with fewer than 12 years of education, and women with a low income level. The study of Lumbee women found that 28 percent of the women who had ever used smokeless tobacco started using it by the age of 6 years (CDC 1995b). In other studies, smokeless tobacco use was low (2 percent) among American Indian women in Montana (Nelson et al. 1997) but relatively high among Navajo women (10 percent) (Strauss et al. 1997). Alaska Native women have a higher prevalence of smokeless tobacco use (11 percent) than do American Indian women in the continental United States (1 percent) (Kaplan et al. 1997). Although Glover and Glover (1992) reported that gender is not a predictor of smokeless tobacco use among American Indian or Alaska Natives, national data suggested that among American Indian or Alaska Natives, women were less likely than men to use smokeless tobacco (USDHHS 1998).

In NHIS data, women with 12 or more years of education were less likely than women with less than 12 years of education to use smokeless tobacco (Table 2.34). Less than 1 percent of women with 12 or more years of education were users of smokeless tobacco. For all women except for those with 9 to 11 years of education, the use of smokeless tobacco decreased during 1970–1998. Use of smokeless tobacco among women was more likely in rural areas than in urban areas and more likely in the South than in other

**Table 2.34. Prevalence (% and 95% confidence interval) of current use of smokeless tobacco among adults aged 18 years or older, by gender and selected characteristics, National Health Interview Survey, United States, 1970 and 1991, 1992, 1994 (aggregate data) and 1998**

| | 1970 | | 1991/1992/1994 | | 1998 | |
|---|---|---|---|---|---|---|
| Characteristic | Women | Men | Women | Men | Women | Men |
| Overall | 1.8 (±0.3) | 5.2 (±0.6) | 0.5 (±0.1) | 5.6 (±0.4) | 0.3 (±0.1) | 5.1 (±0.5) |
| Age (years) | | | | | | |
| 18–44 | 0.6 (±0.2) | 2.9 (±0.4) | 0.1 (±0.1) | 6.3 (±0.6) | 0.1 (±0.1)* | 6.4 (±0.7) |
| 45–64 | 2.3 (±0.5) | 5.8 (±0.8) | 0.5 (±0.2) | 4.3 (±0.6) | 0.4 (±0.3)* | 3.2 (±0.6) |
| ≥ 65 | 4.8 (±0.9) | 12.7 (±1.6) | 1.5 (±0.3) | 4.9 (±0.9) | 0.6 (±0.3) | 3.5 (±0.9) |
| Race/ethnicity† | | | | | | |
| White, non-Hispanic | 1.2 (±0.3) | 5.0 (±0.6) | 0.3 (±0.1) | 6.6 (±0.5) | 0.2 (±0.1)* | 6.3 (±0.6) |
| Black, non-Hispanic | 7.5 (±2.0) | 7.4 (±1.4) | 2.2 (±0.8) | 2.9 (±0.7) | 1.0 (±0.4) | 0.8 (±0.4)‡ |
| Education (number of years)‡ | | | | | | |
| ≤ 8 | 6.5 (±1.2) | 12.9 (±1.1) | 3.7 (±0.8) | 8.9 (±1.4) | 2.6 (±1.2) | 6.1 (±1.9) |
| 9–11 | 1.2 (±0.3) | 4.5 (±0.7) | 0.8 (±0.4) | 7.1 (±1.4) | 1.2 (±0.6)* | 7.7 (±1.8) |
| ≥ 12 | 0.3 (±0.1) | 2.4 (±0.4) | 0.1 (±0.0) | 4.6 (±0.4) | 0.1 (±0.0)* | 4.4 (±0.5) |
| Region | | | | | | |
| South | 5.0 (±1.0) | 9.2 (±1.5) | 1.2 (±0.3) | 8.8 (±1.0) | 0.7 (±0.2) | 7.0 (±0.9) |
| Other | 0.4 (±0.1) | 3.4 (±0.5) | 0.1 (±0.0) | 4.1 (±0.4) | 0.1 (±0.0)* | 4.0 (±0.5) |
| Residence | | | | | | |
| Rural | 3.7 (±0.8) | 9.8 (±0.9) | 1.2 (±0.4) | 11.3 (±1.4) | 0.7 (±0.3)* | 9.9 (±1.3) |
| Urban | 0.8 (±0.3) | 2.7 (±0.4) | 0.3 (±0.1) | 4.0 (±0.4) | 0.2 (±0.1) | 3.7 (±0.5) |

*Note:* In 1970, prevalence of current use of smokeless tobacco was the percentage of all persons in each demographic category who reported that they used snuff or chewing tobacco at the time of the survey. In 1991/1992/1994 and 1998, prevalence of current use of smokeless tobacco was the percentage of all persons in each demographic category who reported that they used snuff or chewing tobacco ≥ 20 times during their lifetime and who used snuff or chewing tobacco at the time of the survey.

*Estimate should be interpreted with caution because of the small number of respondents.

†Ethnicity was not determined in 1970. Thus, estimates for whites and for blacks for that year likely include data for some persons of Hispanic origin.

‡For women aged ≥ 25 years.

Sources: National Center for Health Statistics, public use data tapes, 1970, 1991, 1992, 1994, 1998.

regions (Table 2.34). In the 1995–1996 Current Population Survey, smokeless tobacco use among women was low overall and did not exceed 2.1 percent in any state. A clear pattern of higher use, however, was observed in the Southeast (data not shown) (U.S. Bureau of the Census, public use data tape, 1995–1996).

A 1995 survey of the U.S. Department of Defense reported that 0.7 percent of military women used smokeless tobacco (Bray et al. 1996). Use was highest among women in the U.S. Marine Corps (1.6 ± 0.8 percent) and lowest among women in the U.S. Navy (0.3 ± 0.3 percent).

Gender-specific differences in smokeless tobacco use are long-standing. In AUTS data for 1964, the same proportion of men as women (2 percent) used snuff, but in the 1966 AUTS data, 3.1 percent of men and 2.1 percent of women used snuff. In both survey years, the proportion of women who used chewing tobacco was considerably lower than that for men (0.5 vs. 5.1 percent in 1964, and 0.4 vs. 7.1 percent in 1966) (USDHEW 1969). Data from the 1985 NHSDA showed that 3 percent of women had ever used smokeless tobacco and 1 percent had used it in the past year, whereas 20 percent of men had ever used smokeless tobacco and 12 percent had used it in the past year. However, women who had ever used smokeless tobacco were as likely as men to have used it almost daily in the past year (Rouse 1989). In the 1991/1992/1994 NHIS data, women were significantly less likely than men to use smokeless tobacco (0.5 vs. 5.6 percent) (Table 2.34).

NHIS data showed a decline in use of smokeless tobacco between 1970 and 1991/1992/1994 among women, but the prevalence of use of all types of smokeless tobacco (chewing tobacco and snuff combined) among men did not change during this period (Table 2.34). From 1970 through 1991/1992/1994, women and men aged 45 years or older showed declines in smokeless tobacco use. During this period, use declined among women aged 18 through 44 years and increased significantly among men in the same age group. Smokeless tobacco use by women was higher for women aged 65 years or older than for women of younger ages. Use by men was higher among those 65 years or older in 1978, but higher for those aged 18 through 44 years in the 1990s. In addition, although smokeless tobacco use was more prevalent among black women than among white women in all years, the reverse was true among men in the 1990s. Among all racial and ethnic groups except blacks, women were much less likely than men to use smokeless tobacco (USDHHS 1998).

### Girls

Findings in a study using cohort data from the 1989 TAPS I and the 1993 TAPS II suggested that about 1.7 percent of females aged 11 through 19 years experiment with smokeless tobacco use each year but that few of them become regular users (Tomar and Giovino 1998). However, results of more recent school-based surveys (MTF Survey) suggested that the prevalence of smokeless tobacco use among girls may be increasing (Johnston et al. 1995b). In the 1999 NYTS, 3.3 (±0.8) percent of middle school girls and 7.6 (±1.5) percent of high school girls reported ever using smokeless tobacco (CDC 2000b).

In the 1998 MTF Survey, 1.5 percent of 8th-grade girls, 1.8 percent of 10th-grade girls, and 1.5 percent of 12th-grade girls reported using smokeless tobacco in the preceding month (University of Michigan, Institute for Social Research, public use data tape, 1998). In an analysis of 1999 YRBS data for high school students less than 18 years of age, 1.4 (±0.6) percent of girls had used smokeless tobacco in the past month (CDC, Division of Adolescent and School Health, public use data tape, 1999). Similarly, in the NYTS, 1.3 (±0.5) percent of girls in middle school and 1.5 (±0.6) percent of girls in high school had used smokeless tobacco in the previous month (CDC 2000b). Published data from the 1999 YRBS found that 1.4 (±0.6) percent of all girls in grades 9 through 12 used smokeless tobacco in the past month; white girls were more likely than black girls to have used smokeless tobacco (Kann et al. 2000).

Although the prevalence of smokeless tobacco use is low for girls overall, it is higher for girls in specific geographic regions (e.g., the Southeast and rural Alaska) (CDC 1987a) and in certain racial and ethnic groups (American Indian or Alaska Native). For example, a 1987 study found that 15.3 percent of adolescent girls in the Southeast had tried smokeless tobacco. The rate of trying smokeless tobacco was highest among American Indian girls (20.2 percent) and lowest among black girls (10.8 percent) (Riley et al. 1990). A 1987–1988 study of use of smokeless tobacco among sixth-grade students reported that 28.7 percent of girls at three Indian Health Service sites currently used smokeless tobacco (Backinger et al. 1993). Similarly, 30 percent of American Indian girls who lived on or near reservations in Montana used smokeless tobacco (Nelson et al. 1997). However, a representative 1991 household survey of Navajo females aged 12 through 19 years reported a prevalence of smokeless tobacco use of only 3 percent (Freedman et al. 1997), and the 1997 YRBS survey of high schools that are funded by the Bureau of Indian Affairs found a 16-percent prevalence of smokeless tobacco use (Bureau of Indian Affairs 1997).

Use of smokeless tobacco is much lower among girls than among boys (USDHHS 1994; CDC 2000b). In the 1998 MTF Survey, 1.5 percent of high school senior girls, but 15.7 percent of high school senior boys, used smokeless tobacco in the past month (University of Michigan, Institute for Social Research, public use data tape, 1998). The 1999 YRBS found that 1.3 (±0.5) percent of high school girls less than 18 years of age but 14.2 (±3.8) percent of their male counterparts used smokeless tobacco in the past month (CDC, Division of Adolescent and School Health, public use data tape, 1999). Similar patterns were noted among all high school students (Kann et al. 2000).

## Other Tobacco Products

### Bidis

In the 1999 NYTS, 4.1 (±1.1) percent of girls in middle school and 11.5 (±2.5) percent of girls in high school had ever smoked bidis (CDC 2000b). No gender differences were noted for middle school students, but high school girls (11.5 ± 2.5 percent) were less likely than high school boys (16.6 ± 2.5 percent) to have ever smoked bidis. In the 1999 NYTS, 1.8 (±0.6) percent of girls in middle school and 3.8 (±1.0) percent of girls in high school reported smoking bidis in the preceding month; use may be higher in some urban areas (CDC 1999a). Girls were less likely than boys to have smoked bidis in the past month.

### Kreteks

In the 1999 NYTS, 1.7 (±0.7) percent of girls in middle school and 5.3 (±1.5) percent of girls in high school reported smoking kreteks in the previous month (CDC 2000b). No gender-specific differences in kretek use were noted.

## Summary

Although cigar use is lower among women than among men, the fivefold increase in current use among women in California from 1990 through 1996 and the high prevalence of use among girls in other surveys suggested that cigar smoking is becoming more prevalent among women and girls. Pipe smoking among women is low, and women are much less likely than men to smoke a pipe.

The prevalence of use of smokeless tobacco among girls and women is low and remains considerably lower than that among boys and men. Use of smokeless tobacco is higher among black women and American Indian or Alaska Native women, women with fewer than 12 years of education, and women who live either in rural areas or in the South. Among girls, use may be highest among American Indian or Alaska Native girls. For "other" tobacco use among high school girls, cigar use is the most common, bidi use and kretek use are intermediate, and pipe use and smokeless tobacco use are the least common.

# Exposure to Environmental Tobacco Smoke

Exposure to environmental tobacco smoke (ETS) has emerged as a public health problem. In 1992, the U.S. Environmental Protection Agency (EPA) released a report concluding that ETS is a group A (known human) carcinogen responsible for about 3,000 lung cancer deaths per year in nonsmokers (EPA 1992). Although this finding was set aside by a judicial verdict, other organizations have concluded that ETS is a human carcinogen (National Cancer Institute 1999). Other studies suggest that ETS increases the risk of cardiovascular disease as well as adverse reproductive outcomes. (See "Environmental Tobacco Smoke" in Chapter 3 for a review of effects of ETS exposure on health.) A national study (Pirkle et al. 1996) found that 88 percent of non-tobacco users 4 years of age or older had detectable cotinine levels, a finding that indicated widespread exposure of the U.S. population to ETS.

Respondents to the 1966 AUTS were asked whether it was annoying to be near a person who is smoking (USDHEW 1969); 55.0 percent of women said yes. Women who had never smoked (71.3 percent) were more likely to agree with this statement than were women current smokers (27.2 percent) or former smokers (56.9 percent). Women (55 percent) were more likely than men (41 percent) to report being annoyed by being near a person who is smoking. Two decades later, the 1987 NHIS determined whether respondents believed that smoke from someone else's cigarette was harmful to them; 82.9 percent of women and 79.7 percent of men believed so (Schoenborn and Boyd 1989).

## Home

In a 1963 household survey in Maryland, 64.2 percent of women who were nonsmokers reported being exposed to ETS in the home (Sandler et al. 1989). Exposure decreased with increasing age and educational attainment. Married women were more likely than unmarried women to be exposed to ETS at home, and women living in households having more than one adult were also more likely to be exposed to ETS at home. Women (64.2 percent) were considerably more likely than men (30.0 percent) to report exposure to ETS, a finding that most likely reflects the higher prevalence of smoking among men than among women in the early 1960s.

Among Hispanic nonsmoking girls and women who participated in the 1982–1983 HHANES, the proportion who reported ETS exposure at home ranged from 31 percent (among Puerto Rican American women aged 40 through 49 years) to 62 percent (among Mexican American girls and young women aged 12 through 19 years) (Pletsch 1994). Among both

Mexican Americans and Puerto Rican Americans, adolescents had significantly higher levels of exposure in the home than did older groups.

A study of cardiovascular risk factors among urban young adults assessed exposure to ETS (Wagenknecht et al. 1993b). In 1985–1986, 28.7 percent of nonsmoking white women and 34.6 percent of nonsmoking black women with a high school education or less had a detectable cotinine level, indicating exposure to ETS. Among white women and black women with more than a high school education, the percentages were 21.3 percent and 27.5 percent, respectively.

A 1986 study of exposure to ETS in the home and workplace among adults attending a screening clinic found that 75.1 percent of nonsmoking women were exposed to ETS in the home sometime in their adult lifetime; 66 percent of these women reported ETS exposure from their spouse (Cummings et al. 1989). Thus, most of the women who reported a history of ETS exposure in the home as an adult were exposed to ETS by their husbands. Nonsmoking women in older age groups reported higher lifetime exposure to ETS in the home. This finding probably reflects the higher prevalence of smoking among older cohorts of men. Women (75.1 percent) were more likely than men (51.1 percent) to report lifetime exposure to ETS in the home.

In NHANES data for 1988–1991, 18.3 percent of nonsmoking females 17 years of age or older lived in homes where a member of the household smoked in the home (Pirkle et al. 1996). Exposure was greatest among females aged 17 through 19 years (31.9 percent). However, this same study reported that although only 37 percent of all nonsmokers reported home or work exposure to ETS, 88 percent of nonsmokers in the sample had detectable levels of cotinine, a fact that indicated widespread exposure to ETS.

In NHIS data for 1994, 13.2 (± 0.9) percent of women who were currently nonsmokers reported that someone living in the home smoked inside the home; exposure to ETS was highest among women nonsmokers aged 18 through 24 years (19.3 ± 3.7 percent) and lowest among those aged 65 years or older (7.6 ± 1.4 percent) (NCHS, public use data tape, 1994). Consistent with other data (Matanoski et al. 1995), ETS exposure decreased with increasing level of education; only 7.1 (±1.5) percent of women nonsmokers with 16 or more years of education reported exposure to ETS. Black women reported the highest exposure to ETS (16.2 ± 3.1 percent), and Hispanic women reported the lowest exposure (10.2 ± 2.5 percent). Aggregate NHIS data for 1991–1993 found that the percentage of women nonsmokers exposed to ETS in the home on three or more days per week was highest among American Indians or Alaska Natives (17.8 percent), intermediate among Asians or Pacific Islanders (15.5 percent) and blacks (15.1 percent), and lowest among whites (13.1 percent) and Hispanics (13.0 percent), but these differences were not statistically significant (USDHHS 1998). No gender-specific differences were noted overall, but among persons 65 years of age or older, women (7.6 ± 1.4 percent) were less likely than men (12.1 ± 2.1 percent) to report exposure by someone living in the home (NCHS, public use data tape, 1994).

In the 1994 NHIS, among women nonsmokers who reported ETS exposure in the home, 86.2 (±1.3) percent reported that smoking, either by someone living in the home or by visitors, occurred frequently (≥ 4 days per week) (NCHS, public use data tape, 1994). Women aged 65 years or older were less likely to report frequent smoking in the home than were women aged 25 through 64 years. Women with 16 or more years of education were less likely than women with 9 to 12 years of education to report frequent exposure to ETS in the home. Hispanic women were less likely than white women to report frequent exposure to ETS at home. Men nonsmokers were as likely as women nonsmokers to report that smoking frequently occurred in the home.

In a 1993 California survey, 52 percent of the women reported a complete ban on smoking in their homes, and 21 percent reported a partial ban (Pierce et al. 1994a). Hispanic women and Asian or Pacific Islander women were more likely than white women or black women to have a total ban on smoking in the home. Women with 16 or more years of education were also more likely to report a total ban than were women with less education.

## Workplace

The National Institute for Occupational Safety and Health (NIOSH) has concluded that the risk for lung cancer and possibly heart disease is increased among workers who are occupationally exposed to ETS, and NIOSH has recommended that ETS be classified as a potential occupational carcinogen (NIOSH 1991). A 1997 study among nurses suggested that regular exposure to ETS at work increases the risk of heart disease among women (Kawachi et al. 1997) (see "Environmental Tobacco Smoke and Coronary Heart Disease" in Chapter 3). Many state and local governments have passed legislation to limit exposure to ETS in the workplace. Many businesses have also established their own policies to promote smoke-free indoor air. In the 1992–1993 Current Population Survey, 51 percent of women reported a smoke-free policy in the workplace, 19 percent had a smoke-free policy in work areas only, and 30 percent either had a workplace that allowed smoking anywhere or had no policy on smoking in the workplace (Gerlach et al. 1997).

A 1986 survey of persons who had never smoked found that 75.0 percent of working women reported current exposure to the tobacco smoke of others in the workplace (Cummings et al. 1989). Women younger than 40 years of age were more likely than those aged 40 through 79 years to report such exposure. Younger women also reported significantly more hours of exposure at work per week than did the older women. However, women (75.0 percent) were less likely than men (93.0 percent) to report ETS exposure at work.

In NHANES data for 1988–1991, 19.7 percent of females aged 17 years or older reported work exposure to ETS (Pirkle et al. 1996). Exposure was greatest for women aged 20 through 29 years (31.1 percent). However, this same study reported that although only 37 percent of all nonsmokers 17 years of age or older reported home or work exposure to ETS, 88 percent of nonsmokers in the sample had detectable levels of cotinine, indicating widespread exposure to ETS.

The 1992 NHIS asked whether smoking had occurred in the immediate work area in the two weeks before the survey; workers who reported exposure were then asked if they were bothered by smoking in the immediate work area in those two weeks. In 1992, 16.6 percent of nonsmoking women reported that smoking had occurred in the immediate work area (Table 2.35). This finding is consistent with a 1993 statewide survey from California, which found that 17.2 percent of women nonsmokers were exposed to ETS in indoor workplaces (Pierce et al. 1994a). In NHIS data, women aged 18 through 44 years were somewhat more likely than older women to be exposed, but this finding was not statistically significant (Table 2.35). No differences were found by race, but women with 12 or fewer years of education and workers in service or blue-collar positions were more likely to report recent ETS exposure in the immediate work area. Women were less likely than men to report ETS exposure in the immediate work area.

**Table 2.35. Percentage (and 95% confidence interval) of nonsmoking women aged 18 years or older who reported that anyone smoked in their immediate work area and the proportion of those exposed who reported being bothered by cigarette smoke in their immediate work area, by selected characteristics, National Health Interview Survey, United States, 1992**

| Characteristic | Exposed to smoking in immediate work area* | Bothered by cigarette smoke in immediate work area† |
|---|---|---|
| Women | 16.6 (±1.8) | 60.0 (±5.6) |
| Age (years) | | |
| 18–44 | 18.0 (±2.2) | 60.7 (±6.7) |
| ≥45 | 13.4 (±3.0) | 57.5 (±12.1) |
| Race/ethnicity | | |
| White, non-Hispanic | 16.6 (±2.2) | 59.5 (±6.8) |
| Black, non-Hispanic | 21.3 (±5.8) | 55.8 (±13.0) |
| Education (number of years)‡ | | |
| ≤12 | 21.6 (±3.4) | 54.4 (±8.5) |
| >12 | 10.4 (±1.8) | 64.0 (±9.8) |
| Occupational category | | |
| White collar | 14.1 (±1.9) | 61.9 (±6.9) |
| Service or blue collar | 28.4 (±5.1) | 56.3 (±10.5) |
| Men | 26.1 (±3.1) | 46.9 (±6.3) |

*Based on the question, "During the past 2 weeks, has anyone smoked in your immediate work area?"
†Based on the question, "During the past 2 weeks, have you ever been bothered by cigarette smoke in your immediate work area?" Analysis was restricted to those who reported that someone had smoked in their immediate work area.
‡For women aged ≥25 years.
Source: National Center for Health Statistics, Cancer Control Supplement, public use data tape, 1992.

A 1993 statewide survey from California found that ETS exposure was reported by 8.1 percent of female nonsmokers whose workplaces prohibited smoking in all areas, 28.8 percent whose workplaces banned smoking in work areas but allowed it in common areas, and 79.1 percent whose workplaces allowed smoking in some or all work areas (Pierce et al. 1994a). Female nonsmokers whose workplaces prohibited smoking either in all areas or in work areas were less likely to report exposure than were male nonsmokers working under similar policies. However, female nonsmokers whose workplaces had few or no restrictions were more likely to report exposure than were male nonsmokers whose workplaces had few or no restrictions.

In the 1992 NHIS, among women nonsmokers who reported exposure to ETS at work in the previous two weeks, 60.0 percent reported being bothered by exposure to smoke (Table 2.35). No differences were noted by age, education, race, or occupational category, but CIs were large. Nonsmoking women were more likely than nonsmoking men to report being bothered by smoke in the immediate work area. In particular, nonsmoking women with 12 or fewer years of education (54.4 ± 8.5 percent) were more likely than nonsmoking men with comparable educational attainment (36.3 ± 4.3 percent) to report being bothered by ETS in the immediate work area (NCHS, public use data tape, 1992) (data not shown). Hispanic nonsmoking women (85.5 ± 13.0 percent) were more likely than Hispanic nonsmoking men (40.6 ± 19.2 percent) to report being bothered by ETS exposure. White nonsmoking women (59.5 ± 6.8 percent) were more likely than white nonsmoking men (46.7 ± 7.0 percent) to report being bothered, but the differences were not statistically significant. No significant gender-specific differences were noted by age or occupational category (NCHS, NHIS, public use data tape, 1992).

### Summary

In 1994, 13.2 percent of women who did not smoke reported that someone living in the home smoked inside the home. Among nonsmoking women who were exposed to ETS in the home, 86.2 percent reported frequent exposure (≥ 4 days per week). In 1992, 16.6 percent of women who did not smoke reported that smoking had occurred in the immediate work area in the two weeks before the survey.

## Other Issues

Other issues related to women and smoking include body weight, other drug use, and mental health. The focus here is on prevalence data from large-scale, nationally representative surveys. Other chapters discuss some of these topics in depth (see "Body Weight and Fat Distribution" and "Depression and Other Psychiatric Disorders" in Chapter 3 and "Weight Control" and "Depression" in Chapter 5).

### Smoking and Body Weight

Several studies of adolescents and adults found relationships between smoking and body image, body weight, and dieting behavior (USDHHS 1988b; Fisher et al. 1991; Gritz and Crane 1991; Klesges et al. 1991; Croft et al. 1992; Klesges and Klesges 1993; Page et al. 1993; French et al. 1994; Welch and Fairburn 1998). Women's concerns about weight may encourage smoking initiation, may be a barrier to smoking cessation, and may increase relapse rates among women who stop smoking (Sorensen and Pechacek 1987; Klesges and Klesges 1988; Gritz et al. 1989; Klesges et al. 1989, 1997; USDHHS 1990a; Pirie et al. 1991; French et al. 1992, 1994; Gritz and St. Jeor 1992; Weekley et al. 1992; Camp et al. 1993; French and Jeffery 1995; Welch and Fairburn 1998). However, two prospective studies in working populations found that weight concerns did not predict cessation (French et al. 1995; Jeffery et al. 1997). Although smokers weigh less than nonsmokers and gain weight after they quit smoking, changes in body weight with changes in smoking status are generally small, and the health benefits of smoking cessation greatly outweigh any risks associated with weight gain (Williamson et al. 1991; Colditz et al. 1992; Audrain et al. 1995; Flegal et al. 1995).

#### Smoking and Attempted Weight Loss Among Girls

Data from the 1999 school-based YRBS indicated that most girls (66.4 percent) in grades 9 through 12 (and <18 years of age) who currently smoked were

**Table 2.36. Percentage (and 95% confidence interval) of adolescents in grades 9–12 and less than 18 years of age who were attempting to lose weight, by gender and smoking status, Youth Risk Behavior Survey, United States, 1999**

| Characteristic | Girls | Boys |
|---|---|---|
| Overall | | |
| Current smokers* | 66.4 (±3.6) | 25.5 (±4.0) |
| Noncurrent smokers† | 59.4 (±3.6) | 30.2 (±4.4) |
| Never smoked‡ | 52.4 (±4.3) | 25.5 (±4.0) |
| White, non-Hispanic | | |
| Current smokers | 66.2 (±4.8) | 25.0 (±5.6) |
| Noncurrent smokers | 62.4 (±6.8) | 28.9 (±6.4) |
| Never smoked | 56.6 (±6.4) | 24.6 (±4.0) |
| Black, non-Hispanic | | |
| Current smokers | 59.8 (±10.7) | 23.8 (±5.2) |
| Noncurrent smokers | 44.7 (±7.1) | 26.7 (±12.3) |
| Never smoked | 47.9 (±7.9) | 16.4 (±5.0) |
| Hispanic | | |
| Current smokers | 76.6 (±6.3) | 39.0 (±8.6) |
| Noncurrent smokers | 65.6 (±6.4) | 42.2 (±8.5) |
| Never smoked | 51.1 (±7.5) | 34.3 (±10.3) |

*Note:* Estimates of the percentage of those attempting to lose weight are based on response to the question, "Which of the following are you trying to do about your weight?" Those answering "lose weight" were included.
*Current smokers are persons who reported smoking in the past 30 days.
†Noncurrent smokers are persons who reported trying cigarette smoking, even one or two puffs, but did not smoke in the past 30 days.
‡Never smokers are persons who never smoked a cigarette, not even one or two puffs.
Source: Centers for Disease Control and Prevention, Division of Adolescent and School Health, public use data tape, 1999.

attempting to lose weight (Table 2.36). This percentage is significantly higher than that for girls who never smoked (52.4 percent); the percentage of girls who had smoked previously who were attempting weight loss (59.4 percent) is intermediate. The differences between the percentages of girls who currently smoked and girls who had never smoked and between the percentages of girls who had previously smoked and girls who had never smoked were statistically significant among Hispanic girls. Among current smokers, Hispanic girls were more likely than black girls to be trying to lose weight; this finding was of borderline statistical significance. In contrast, no relationship between smoking and attempted weight loss was found among boys. Regardless of smoking status or racial or ethnic group, adolescent girls were much more likely than adolescent boys to be trying to lose weight. In the 1989 TAPS I data, both girls and boys who smoked were more likely than nonsmokers to believe that smoking helps to keep weight down (Moss et al. 1992). Several local school-based studies reported similar relationships between smoking and weight (see "Concerns About Weight Control" in Chapter 4).

### Smoking and Perception of Body Weight Among Women

The relationship between perceived weight and smoking status among women was examined in the 1991 NHIS data. Women who were overweight (for women aged <20 years, a body mass index [BMI] ≥ 25.7; for women aged ≥ 20 years, a BMI ≥ 27.3) on the basis of self-reported weight and height (USDHHS 1995) were excluded from the analysis. Among normal weight and underweight women, former smokers were the most likely to perceive themselves as overweight, and current smokers were more likely than women who had never smoked to perceive themselves as overweight (Table 2.37). However, the relationship between smoking status and perceived

**Table 2.37. Perception of overweight (% and 95% confidence interval) among normal and underweight women aged 18 years or older, by smoking status and selected characteristics, National Health Interview Survey, United States, 1991**

| Characteristic | Current smokers* | Former smokers† | Never smoked‡ |
|---|---|---|---|
| Women | 37.9 (±1.5) | 42.8 (±1.8) | 33.2 (±1.0) |
| Age (years) | | | |
| 18–24 | 35.9 (±4.6) | 31.2 (±7.7) | 27.0 (±2.7) |
| 25–44 | 40.4 (±2.2) | 41.9 (±2.9) | 36.4 (±1.6) |
| 45–64 | 40.3 (±3.0) | 51.4 (±3.5) | 40.4 (±2.4) |
| ≥ 65 | 21.9 (±3.9) | 36.2 (±3.7) | 24.6 (±1.9) |
| Race/ethnicity | | | |
| White, non-Hispanic | 38.5 (±1.7) | 43.2 (±1.9) | 34.7 (±1.2) |
| Black, non-Hispanic | 29.7 (±4.5) | 33.7 (±7.3) | 28.3 (±3.1) |
| Hispanic | 45.0 (±7.6) | 43.6 (±8.8) | 33.2 (±3.6) |
| Men | 18.9 (±1.4) | 27.8 (±1.7) | 17.8 (±1.1) |

*Note:* Perception of overweight is determined by the question, "Do you consider yourself overweight, underweight, or just about right?" This analysis excludes those who were actually overweight (body mass index ≥ 25.7 for women <20 years of age; body mass index ≥ 27.3 for women ≥ 20 years of age) based on self-reported weight and height.
*Current smokers reported smoking ≥ 100 cigarettes in their lifetime and smoked at the time of the survey.
†Former smokers reported smoking ≥ 100 cigarettes in their lifetime but did not smoke at the time of the survey.
‡Never smokers did not smoke ≥ 100 cigarettes in their lifetime.
Source: National Center for Health Statistics, public use data tape, 1991.

weight varied substantially by age. Among young women aged 18 through 24 years, current smokers were more likely than those who had never smoked to perceive themselves as overweight. Among women aged 25 through 44 years, both former smokers and current smokers were more likely than those who had never smoked to perceive themselves as overweight. For the older age groups (45 through 64 years and 65 years or older), former smokers were more likely than those who had never smoked and current smokers to view themselves as overweight. In contrast, for all age groups, self-reported body weight adjusted for height was similar among former smokers and those who had never smoked and lowest among current smokers (NCHS, public use data tape, 1991).

When examined by race and ethnicity, the overall relationship between smoking status and perceived weight was found among white women only (Table 2.37). No statistically significant difference in perceived weight by smoking status was observed among black women, and regardless of smoking status, black women were the least likely to perceive themselves as overweight. Among Hispanic women, current smokers were more likely than those who had never smoked to view themselves as overweight.

In the 1991 NHIS, women were much more likely than men, regardless of smoking status, to perceive themselves as overweight (Table 2.37). In contrast to women, similar percentages of men current smokers and men who had never smoked perceived themselves as overweight, and men former smokers were the most likely to perceive themselves as overweight. This pattern was true for all racial and ethnic groups. However, no differences in perception of being overweight were found among men aged 18 through 24 years, regardless of smoking status. Among men aged 45 through 64 years, current smokers were less likely than those who had never smoked to perceive themselves as overweight (NCHS, public use data tape, 1991).

When overweight women were included in the analysis of the 1991 NHIS data, perception of weight among smokers was not associated with attempts to quit smoking: 39.7 (±2.1) percent of women who perceived themselves as overweight and 37.6 (±2.5) percent of those who perceived their weight as "just about right" had quit smoking for at least one day in the previous year (NCHS, public use data tape, 1991). In addition, no difference by self-perceived weight was found in the number of attempts to quit smoking in the past year (average, 2.8 ± 0.2 attempts) (NCHS, public use data tape, 1991). No gender-specific differences in these relationships were observed. NHIS did not assess concern about postcessation weight gain, but such concern has been associated with decreased smoking cessation in some studies (Sorensen and Pechacek 1987; Gritz et al. 1989; Weekley et al. 1992; French and Jeffery 1995) but not others (French et al. 1995; Jeffery et al. 1997).

### Smoking and Actual Body Mass Index Among Women

Despite self-perceptions of body weight, data from NHANES III (1988–1996) showed that BMI among women was significantly less among current smokers than among former smokers or among those who had never smoked; BMI was calculated from weight and height at examination (Table 2.38). (This table includes data on overweight women.) Among women aged 45 years or older and among all three racial and ethnic groups, significant differences in BMI were found by smoking status. However, among white women and Mexican American women, differences in BMI between current smokers and those who had never smoked were not statistically significant.

The relationship between smoking status and body weight was similar for women and men, although the difference among former smokers and those who had never smoked was statistically significant among men (Table 2.38). Similar patterns were found for all ages and racial and ethnic groups among men, except that among men aged 25 through 44 years, current smokers had significantly lower BMIs than did former smokers or those who had never smoked and that among men aged 45 through 64 years and among whites, differences between former smokers and those who had never smoked were statistically significant (NCHS, public use data tapes, 1988–1996).

A study of all U.S. Air Force Basic Military Training recruits also observed no relationship between current smoking and body weight among young women (Klesges et al. 1998). Using data from NHANES III, phase I (1988–1991), Flegal and colleagues (1995) found that current smokers, both women and men, had the lowest age-adjusted prevalence of overweight and the lowest mean BMI. In addition, persons who had quit smoking within the previous 10 years had gained, over the 10 years, significantly more weight than did current smokers or those who had never smoked. However, no difference in mean BMI or in the prevalence of overweight was observed between former smokers who had quit smoking more than 10 years earlier and those who had never smoked. This finding suggested that weight gain occurs shortly after smoking cessation and that former smokers do not continue to gain weight at a higher rate than those who had never smoked.

**Table 2.38. Average body mass index (and 95% confidence interval) among women aged 18 years or older, by smoking status and selected characteristics, National Health and Nutrition Examination Survey III, United States, 1988–1994**

| Characteristic | Current smokers* | Former smokers† | Never smoked‡ |
|---|---|---|---|
| Women | 25.5 (±0.4) | 27.1 (±0.6) | 26.5 (±0.4) |
| Age (years) | | | |
| 18–24 | 24.1 (±1.0) | 24.4 (±1.9) | 23.8 (±0.6) |
| 25–44 | 25.5 (±0.5) | 26.5 (±1.2) | 26.2 (±0.5) |
| 45–64 | 26.8 (±0.8) | 28.7 (±0.8) | 28.3 (±0.5) |
| ≥65 | 24.7 (±0.9) | 27.1 (±0.6) | 26.7 (±0.4) |
| Race/ethnicity | | | |
| White, non-Hispanic | 25.2 (±0.5) | 26.9 (±0.6) | 26.0 (±0.5) |
| Black, non-Hispanic | 27.2 (±0.7) | 29.7 (±0.8) | 29.0 (±0.5) |
| Mexican American | 27.5 (±0.8) | 29.2 (±0.7) | 27.7 (±0.4) |
| Men | 25.7 (±0.3) | 27.5 (±0.3) | 26.5 (±0.3) |

*Note:* Body mass index (weight in kilograms divided by height in meters squared) is based on height and weight measured during physical examination. Table includes data on all women, including overweight women.

*Current smokers reported smoking ≥ 100 cigarettes in their lifetime and smoked at the time of the survey.

†Former smokers reported smoking ≥ 100 cigarettes in their lifetime but did not smoke at the time of the survey.

‡Never smokers did not smoke ≥ 100 cigarettes in their lifetime.

Sources: National Center for Health Statistics, public use data tapes, 1988–1994.

## Smoking and Other Drug Use Among Girls and Young Women

The consumption patterns for the combined use of cigarettes and alcohol, marijuana, or cocaine among girls and women have been examined in several studies using different methods (USDHHS 1988b, 1994; Willard and Schoenborn 1995; Everett et al. 1998). Local and national surveys have consistently shown that girls and women who smoke are more likely than those who do not smoke to use alcohol, marijuana, or cocaine (Kandel et al. 1992; Schorling et al. 1994; Willard and Schoenborn 1995; Escobedo et al. 1997; Emmons et al. 1998; Everett et al. 1998). National data indicate that, for most young women who have ever smoked, cigarette smoking occurs before use of these other drugs (Johnston et al. 1994b). The prevalence of alcohol and drug use has remained lower among girls than among boys during the past 20 years (Johnston et al. 2000a).

Data from the 1998 NHSDA among adolescents aged 12 through 17 years and the 1999 YRBS among high school students less than 18 years of age indicated that adolescent girls who smoke are much more likely than girls who do not smoke to use alcohol or marijuana or to engage in binge drinking (Table 2.39). Differences in the prevalence of drug use between the surveys are most likely due to YRBS surveying older

**Table 2.39. Prevalence (% and 95% confidence interval) of other drug use among girls and boys less than 18 years of age, by gender and smoking status, National Household Survey on Drug Abuse (NHSDA) and Youth Risk Behavior Survey (YRBS), United States, 1998–1999**

| | NHSDA 1998 (ages 12–17) | | YRBS 1999 (grades 9–12) | |
|---|---|---|---|---|
| **Substance used/smoking status** | **Girls** | **Boys** | **Girls** | **Boys** |
| Alcohol use* | | | | |
| Current smokers† | 65.1 (±8.6) | 71.6 (±7.2) | 77.7 (±4.8) | 82.3 (±5.7) |
| Noncurrent smokers‡ | 19.3 (±14.0)§ | 53.7 (±18.3)§ | 40.6 (±4.5) | 47.8 (±5.0) |
| Never smoked∆ | 13.8 (±1.9) | 13.4 (±1.8) | 18.3 (±2.9) | 19.9 (±3.0) |
| Binge drinking¶ | | | | |
| Current smokers | 39.3 (±9.3) | 45.4 (±8.5) | 56.8 (±5.0) | 63.9 (±5.6) |
| Noncurrent smokers | 3.9 (±4.8)§ | 19.4 (±15.3)§ | 16.8 (±3.3) | 26.8 (±5.2) |
| Never smoked | 3.4 (±0.9) | 4.9 (±1.1) | 6.0 (±1.9) | 7.4 (±1.6) |
| Marijuana use** | | | | |
| Current smokers | 44.3 (±9.0) | 45.8 (±8.3) | 49.6 (±5.3) | 59.7 (±6.1) |
| Noncurrent smokers | 13.2 (±12.4)§ | 18.4 (±15.6)§ | 12.2 (±2.7) | 23.7 (±5.6) |
| Never smoked | 3.9 (±0.9) | 4.6 (±1.0) | 3.0 (±1.6) | 4.8 (±2.0) |

*Note:* NHSDA is a household survey that includes adolescents 12–17 years of age; 67.0% were 14–17 years of age. YRBS is a school-based survey that includes high school students in grades 9–12; analyses were restricted to those less than 18 years of age—among this group, 99.8% were 14–17 years of age. Data are not comparable across surveys due to differences in ages and survey methods.

*Prevalence of alcohol use is the percentage of all persons in each demographic category who reported any use of alcohol during the past month.

†Current smokers are persons who reported that they smoked in the past 30 days.

‡Noncurrent smokers are persons who reported that they smoked previously, but not in the past 30 days.

§Estimate should be interpreted with caution because of the small number of respondents.

∆Never smokers are persons who reported that they never smoked a cigarette.

¶Prevalence of binge drinking is percentage of all persons in each demographic category who reported that they drank ≥ 5 drinks in a row on ≥ 1 day in the past month.

**Prevalence of marijuana use is the percentage of all persons in each demographic category who reported any use of marijuana during the past month.

Sources: **NHSDA:** Substance Abuse and Mental Health Services Administration, public use data tape, 1998. **YRBS:** Centers for Disease Control and Prevention, Division of Adolescent and School Health, public use data tape, 1999.

adolescents and to different survey methods. YRBS, a school-based survey, provides more privacy than NHSDA, a household survey (Gfroerer et al. 1997a).

The 1999 YRBS showed that high school girls less than 18 years of age who were current smokers were more than four times as likely than girls who had never smoked to have used alcohol during the past month (Table 2.39). Most girls (77.7 percent) who smoked in the past month had used alcohol, and one-half (56.8 percent) had engaged in binge drinking or had used marijuana during the past month (49.6 percent). In comparison, 18.3 percent of girls who had never smoked had used alcohol, 6.0 percent had engaged in binge drinking, and 3.0 percent had used marijuana. In addition, 7.7 (±2.4) percent of girls who smoked had used cocaine (CDC, Division of Adolescent and School Health, public use data tape, 1999). Because of small sample size, estimates of cocaine use among girls who had never smoked could not be calculated. Using data from the 1995 YRBS for all high school girls, Everett and colleagues (1998) observed a significant dose-response relationship between smoking and the odds of binge drinking or current alcohol, marijuana, or cocaine use.

In both the 1998 NHSDA and the 1999 YRBS data, girls who were noncurrent smokers were also more likely than girls who had never smoked to have used alcohol, participated in binge drinking, and used marijuana in the past month; these differences were statistically significant for YRBS (Table 2.39). In NHSDA, the prevalence of alcohol use, binge drinking, and marijuana use was lower among current smokers, noncurrent smokers, and girls who had never smoked, but the data are consistent with YRBS data in that girls who smoked were most likely, noncurrent smokers were intermediate, and nonsmokers were the least likely to have used alcohol or marijuana. Similar relationships between smoking status and use of alcohol, marijuana, and cocaine were observed among boys.

Data from the 1998 MTF Survey showed similar patterns of substance use among high school senior girls. Current smokers were much more likely than noncurrent smokers and girls who had never smoked to have used marijuana or alcohol in the past month or to have participated in binge drinking in the past two weeks (Figure 2.18). Use of cocaine and inhalants was also higher among current smokers than among noncurrent smokers and girls who had never smoked (University of Michigan, Institute for Social Research, public use data tape, 1998). Among high school seniors, the relationship between smoking status and use of alcohol and other drugs was similar among girls and boys.

Patterns similar to those among girls were found among young women aged 18 through 24 years and among women aged 25 years or older in the 1997–1998 NHSDA (Table 2.40). Among both age groups, current smokers were more likely than former smokers or women who had never smoked to use alcohol, to engage in binge drinking, or to use marijuana. Among both age groups, former smokers were more likely than women who had never smoked to engage in alcohol use, but former smokers and women who never smoked were equally likely to engage in binge drinking and marijuana use. Except for alcohol use among former smokers and women who had never smoked, regardless of smoking status, the maximum prevalence of use of substances other than tobacco occurred among women aged 18 through 24 years.

In NHSDA data, the relationship between smoking status and other substance use was generally similar among women and men. However, the difference in the prevalence of alcohol use between former smokers and persons who had never smoked was statistically significant among women but not among men (Table 2.40). Regardless of smoking status or age, however, women were less likely than men to engage in these behaviors except that among former smokers, the prevalence of alcohol use was similar among young women and young men.

Data from the 1997–1998 NHSDA were used to examine the relationship between the initiation of cigarette smoking and the start of other drug use among adults aged 18 through 24 years (Table 2.41). Among most young women, smoking initiation preceded or was concurrent with the start of other drug use. The proportion of women for whom smoking preceded drug use ranged from 47.9 percent among those who had also tried alcohol to 90.3 percent among those who had also tried cocaine. Smoking initiation was concurrent with the start of alcohol use among 23.8 percent of the women, marijuana use among 18.4 percent, and cocaine use among 6.1 percent. In contrast, the proportion of women for whom drug use preceded smoking ranged from 3.6 percent for cocaine use to 28.4 percent for alcohol use. Young women were slightly less likely than young men to have tried alcohol before trying cigarettes.

These patterns are reflected in the mean age at which young adults began to use cigarettes, alcohol, and other drugs, as shown in data from the 1997–1998 NHSDA (Table 2.42). Among young women who had both smoked and used alcohol, the mean age at smoking initiation (14.3 years) was significantly lower than the mean age at first use of alcohol (15.3 years). Among

**Figure 2.18. Prevalence (%) of alcohol and marijuana use among high school senior girls, by smoking status, Monitoring the Future Survey, United States, 1998**

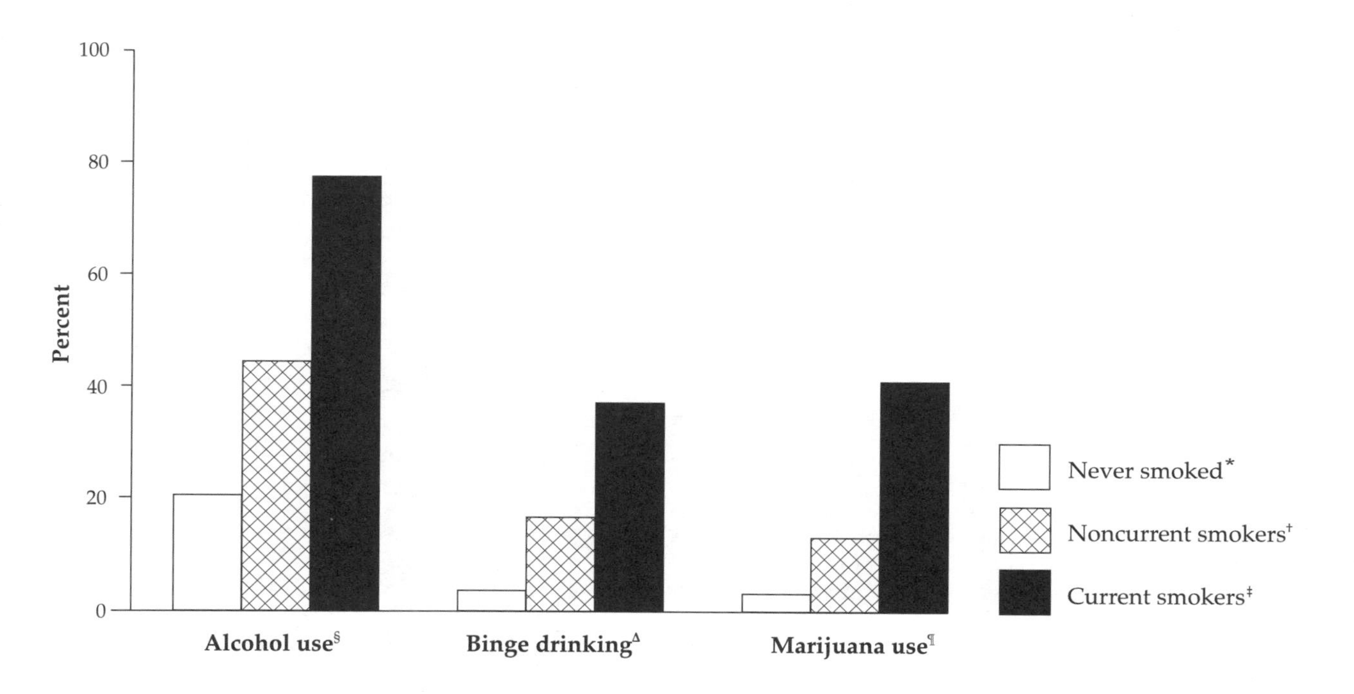


*Never smokers are persons who never smoked a cigarette.
†Noncurrent smokers are persons who smoked previously, but not in the past 30 days.
‡Current smokers are persons who smoked in the past 30 days.
§Prevalence of alcohol use is the percentage of all persons who reported any use of alcohol in the past month.
∆Prevalence of binge drinking is the percentage of all persons who reported that they drank ≥ 5 alcoholic drinks at one time in the past 2 weeks.
¶Prevalence of marijuana use is the percentage of all persons who reported any use of marijuana in the past month.
Source: University of Michigan, Institute for Social Research, public use data tape, 1998.

young women who had used both, the mean age at first use of cigarettes was also lower than the mean age at first use of marijuana or cocaine. On average, women reported using cigarettes 1.0 years before using alcohol, 2.0 years before using marijuana, and 4.3 years before using cocaine. The average age at smoking initiation was 13.3 years for women who had both smoked cigarettes and used cocaine and 15.6 years for women who had used cigarettes only. These and other data (Kandel et al. 1992; USDHHS 1994; Willard and Schoenborn 1995) demonstrate that cigarette smoking generally occurs at an earlier age than other drug use. Among young men who had smoked and used alcohol, marijuana, or cocaine, the mean age at smoking initiation was also younger than the mean age at first use of those substances.

## Smoking and Mental Health Among Women and Girls

The prevalence of cigarette smoking tends to be higher among persons with psychiatric disorders such as schizophrenia, mania, personality disorders (Hughes et al. 1986), depression (Anda et al. 1990; Glassman et al. 1990; Pérez-Stable et al. 1990b; Breslau et al. 1991; Kendler et al. 1993), and panic disorders (Breslau et al. 1991; Pohl et al. 1992). The causal direction of these associations is unclear. Depressed smokers are also less likely to quit smoking (Anda et al. 1990; Glassman et al. 1990), and smokers with a history of depression have a greater risk of relapse to smoking after a cessation attempt (Fiore et al. 1996). Covey and associates (1990) reported that smoking

**Table 2.40. Prevalence (% and 95% confidence interval) of alcohol and marijuana use among adults aged 18 years or older, by gender, smoking status, and age, National Household Survey on Drug Abuse, United States, 1997–1998**

| | Aged 18–24 years | | Aged ≥ 25 years | |
|---|---|---|---|---|
| **Substance used/smoking status** | **Women** | **Men** | **Women** | **Men** |
| Alcohol use* | | | | |
| Current smokers† | 72.6 (±3.6) | 85.3 (±2.5) | 58.8 (±2.7) | 70.8 (±2.7) |
| Former smokers‡ | 53.8 (±8.6) | 64.4 (±9.6) | 52.2 (±3.3) | 60.1 (±3.1) |
| Never smoked§ | 41.9 (±2.3) | 54.5 (±2.7) | 40.8 (±1.8) | 59.1 (±2.3) |
| Binge drinking^Δ^ | | | | |
| Current smokers | 35.5 (±3.9) | 59.0 (±3.6) | 16.8 (±2.0) | 35.4 (±2.9) |
| Former smokers | 12.9 (±5.6) | 35.0 (±9.6) | 5.3 (±1.6) | 16.8 (±2.4) |
| Never smoked | 12.2 (±1.7) | 30.3 (±2.6) | 3.7 (±0.6) | 17.9 (±1.8) |
| Marijuana use¶ | | | | |
| Current smokers | 22.9 (±3.4) | 33.9 (±3.5) | 6.3 (±1.3) | 10.7 (±1.9) |
| Former smokers | 3.5 (±2.4)** | 15.3 (±6.8) | 0.8 (±0.5) | 2.5 (±1.1) |
| Never smoked | 4.9 (±1.0) | 8.3 (±1.4) | 0.7 (±0.2) | 2.4 (±0.6) |

*Prevalence of alcohol use is the percentage of all persons in each demographic category who reported that they drank ≥ 1 alcoholic drink in the 30 days before the survey.
†Current smokers were persons who reported that they had smoked for ≥ 100 days in their lifetime and smoked at the time of the survey.
‡Former smokers were persons who reported that they had smoked for ≥ 100 days in their lifetime but did not smoke at the time of the survey.
§Never smokers were persons who reported that they had never smoked for 100 days.
ΔPrevalence of binge drinking is the percentage of all persons in each demographic category who reported that they drank ≥ 5 alcoholic drinks in a row on ≥ 1 day in the 30 days before the survey.
¶Prevalence of marijuana use is the percentage of all persons in each demographic category who reported that they used marijuana in the 30 days before the survey.
**Estimate should be interpreted with caution because of the small number of respondents.
Sources: Substance Abuse and Mental Health Services Administration, public use data tapes, 1997, 1998.

**Table 2.41. Patterns of initiation of smoking and use of other substances (% and 95% confidence interval) among young adults aged 18–24 years who ever used cigarettes and another substance, by gender, National Household Survey on Drug Abuse, United States, 1997–1998**

| | Young women | | | Young men | | |
|---|---|---|---|---|---|---|
| **Substance used** | **Initiation of cigarette use preceded substance use** | **Initiation of cigarette use concurrent with substance use** | **Initiation of substance use preceded cigarette use** | **Initiation of cigarette use preceded substance use** | **Initiation of cigarette use concurrent with substance use** | **Initiation of substance use preceded cigarette use** |
| Alcohol* | 47.9 (±2.6) | 23.8 (±2.2) | 28.4 (±2.4) | 44.3 (±2.6) | 21.7 (±2.2) | 33.9 (±2.5) |
| Marijuana† | 69.9 (±3.1) | 18.4 (±2.6) | 11.7 (±2.2) | 66.2 (±3.0) | 20.2 (±2.5) | 13.6 (±2.1) |
| Cocaine‡ | 90.3 (±5.0) | 6.1 (±4.4) | 3.6 (±2.7)§ | 92.8 (±3.2) | 5.0 (±2.9) | 2.1 (±1.5)§ |

*Note:* Initiation of smoking is based on response to the question, "About how old were you when you first tried a cigarette?"
*Respondents were asked, "About how old were you the first time you had a glass of beer or wine or a drink of liquor, such as whiskey, gin, scotch, etc.? Do not include childhood sips that you might have had from an older person's drink."
†Respondents were asked, "About how old were you the first time you actually used marijuana or hash, even once?"
‡Respondents were asked, "About how old were you the first time you actually used cocaine, in any form, even once?"
§Estimate should be interpreted with caution because of the small number of respondents.
Sources: Substance Abuse and Mental Health Services Administration, public use data tapes, 1997, 1998.

**Table 2.42. Mean age (years and 95% confidence interval) at first use of cigarettes and other substances among young adults aged 18–24 years who had ever smoked cigarettes, by gender, National Household Survey on Drug Abuse, United States, 1997–1998**

| | Young women | | Young men | |
|---|---|---|---|---|
| Other substance used | Age first used cigarettes* | Age first used other substance | Age first used cigarettes | Age first used other substance |
| None | 15.6 (±1.1) | — | 14.9 (±1.0) | — |
| Alcohol[†] | 14.3 (±0.2) | 15.3 (±0.2) | 14.3 (±0.2) | 14.9 (±0.2) |
| Marijuana[‡] | 14.1 (±0.2) | 16.1 (±0.2) | 14.1 (±0.2) | 15.9 (±0.2) |
| Cocaine[§] | 13.3 (±0.5) | 17.6 (±0.3) | 13.1 (±0.4) | 17.9 (±0.3) |

*Note:* Persons who ever smoked cigarettes were those who smoked ≥ 100 days in their lifetime.
*Respondents were asked, "About how old were you when you first tried a cigarette?"
[†]Respondents were asked, "About how old were you the first time you had a glass of beer or wine or a drink of liquor, such as whisky, gin, scotch, etc.? Do not include childhood sips that you might have had from an older person's drink."
[‡]Respondents were asked, "About how old were you the first time you actually used marijuana or hash, even once?"
[§]Respondents were asked, "About how old were you the first time you actually used cocaine, in any form, even once?"
Sources: Substance Abuse and Mental Health Services Administration, public use data tapes, 1997, 1998.

cessation caused more intense depressed mood among smokers with a history of depression and that these symptoms were related to lower success rates for cessation. The prevalence of depression among women is twice that among men (Weissman et al. 1991; APA 1994), indicating that these associations may be particularly important among women. Similar patterns have been noted among adolescents. In a longitudinal study, Kandel and Davies (1986) reported that depressed adolescents were more likely than nondepressed adolescents to report daily smoking nine years later. Other data have shown an association between heavy smoking and depression among adolescents (Covey and Tam 1990) (see "Depression and Other Psychiatric Disorders" in Chapter 3).

The 1991 NHIS included questions on the emotional and mental health of respondents. Questions were specifically related to experiences of boredom, restlessness, depression, loneliness, and upset in the two weeks preceding the survey. Substantial proportions of women reported the following feelings: 11.4 percent depression, 11.2 percent boredom, 10.3 percent restlessness, 5.8 percent loneliness, and 4.5 percent upset (Schoenborn and Horm 1993). Current smokers were more likely than those who had never smoked to report feelings of boredom (17.1 vs. 9.5 percent), restlessness (15.4 vs. 8.7 percent), depression (15.9 vs. 9.6 percent), loneliness (8.7 vs. 4.8 percent), and upset (2.9 vs. 1.4 percent) (Table 2.43). Overall, women who were former smokers were similar to those who had never smoked in their reporting of all categories of negative moods. However, the prevalences of feelings of boredom and restlessness were significantly higher among women who were abstinent (self-reported) fewer than 12 months than among women who were abstinent for 12 or more months. Women abstinent fewer than 12 months reported feelings similar to those of current smokers, whereas women abstinent 12 or more months reported feelings similar to those of women who had never smoked. Across all smoking categories, women were more likely than men to report feelings of boredom, depression, and loneliness but equally likely to report feeling restless; data were less clear for feeling upset.

Schoenborn and Horm (1993) analyzed the same data and controlled for age, race, education, income, marital status, and health status. They reported that the relative risk (RR) for smoking was higher among women who reported feelings of depression (RR, 1.5; 95 percent CI, 1.4 to 1.7), loneliness (RR, 1.6; 95 percent CI, 1.4 to 1.9), restlessness (RR, 1.7; 95 percent CI, 1.5 to 1.9), or boredom (RR, 1.7; 95 percent CI, 1.5 to 1.9) than among those who did not report negative moods.

Analyses of data from the 1989 TAPS I resulted in similar findings among girls aged 12 through 17 years (NCHS, public use data tape, 1989). Respondents were asked if they had experienced certain negative emotions—specifically, feelings of depression, nervousness, or hopelessness—in the year preceding the survey. Current smokers were more likely than those who had never smoked to report that they often had feelings of unhappiness, sadness, or depression (32.9 ± 4.7 vs. 13.7 ± 1.5 percent), nervousness or tension

**Table 2.43. Prevalence (% and 95% confidence interval) of selected feelings* during the 2 weeks before the survey among adults aged 18 years or older, by gender and smoking status, National Health Interview Survey, United States, 1991**

| | Felt bored | | Felt restless[†] | | Felt depressed or very low | | Felt very lonely or abandoned | | Felt upset | |
|---|---|---|---|---|---|---|---|---|---|---|
| **Smoking status** | **Women** | **Men** | **Women** | **Men** | **Women** | **Men** | **Women** | **Men** | **Women** | **Men** |
| Current smokers[‡] | 17.1 (±1.2) | 14.1 (±1.1) | 15.4 (±1.1) | 15.0 (±1.2) | 15.9 (±1.1) | 10.4 (±0.9) | 8.7 (±0.8) | 5.3 (±0.6) | 2.9 (±0.5) | 1.4 (±0.3) |
| Former smokers[§] | 9.1 (±1.0) | 7.6 (±0.8) | 9.0 (±0.9) | 9.3 (±0.9) | 11.2 (±1.0) | 6.0 (±0.7) | 5.2 (±0.7) | 3.1 (±0.5) | 1.4 (±0.4) | 1.0 (±0.3) |
| Abstinent <12 months | 15.8 (±4.2) | 14.7 (±4.6) | 16.0 (±4.1) | 13.4 (±4.3) | 13.0 (±3.6) | 8.0 (±3.4)[Δ] | 5.8 (±2.3)[Δ] | 3.2 (±1.8)[Δ] | 1.5 (±1.1)[Δ] | 2.4 (±1.7)[Δ] |
| Abstinent ≥ 12 months | 8.5 (±1.1) | 7.2 (±0.8) | 8.4 (±1.0) | 9.0 (±1.0) | 11.1 (±1.0) | 6.0 (±0.8) | 5.1 (±0.7) | 3.2 (±0.6) | 1.5 (±0.5) | 0.8 (±0.3) |
| Never smoked[¶] | 9.5 (±0.7) | 7.5 (±0.7) | 8.7 (±0.6) | 9.4 (±0.8) | 9.6 (±0.6) | 5.7 (±0.6) | 4.8 (±0.4) | 2.2 (±0.3) | 1.4 (±0.2) | 0.7 (±0.2) |

*Possible responses included "never," "rarely," "sometimes," "often," "very often"; percentages include those who responded "often" or "very often."
[†]Defined as "so restless that you could hardly sit still."
[‡]Current smokers were persons who reported that they smoked ≥100 cigarettes in their lifetime and smoked at the time of the survey.
[§]Former smokers were persons who reported that they smoked ≥100 cigarettes in their lifetime but did not smoke at the time of the survey.
[Δ]Estimate should be interpreted with caution because of the small number of respondents.
[¶]Never smokers were persons who reported that they never smoked 100 cigarettes.
Source: National Center for Health Statistics, public use data tape, 1991.

(33.8 ± 4.5 vs. 16.2 ± 1.5 percent), or hopelessness (18.2 ± 3.8 vs. 6.3 ± 1.0 percent). Among current or former smokers, girls were more likely than boys to report feelings of unhappiness, hopelessness, or nervousness. A longitudinal analysis using the 1989 TAPS I and the 1993 TAPS II found that smoking status at baseline was the most significant predictor of depressive symptoms among girls (Choi et al. 1997). Girls who were current smokers at baseline were twice as likely as girls who had never smoked to develop depressive symptoms. However, a study of substance use and psychiatric disorders among 1,285 adolescents aged 9 through 18 years in three states and Puerto Rico did not find a significant increase in anxiety or mood disorders among females who were daily smokers (Kandel et al. 1997b).

In data from the 1996 NHSDA among girls aged 12 through 17 years, 37.4 percent of those with high scores for psychosocial problems, but 14.0 percent of those with low scores, were smokers (SAMHSA 1998a). Similarly, 30.3 percent of girls with high scores for emotional problems were smokers, whereas 16.9 percent of girls with low scores were smokers. Among girls with high scores for behavioral problems, 42.0 percent were smokers, but only 12.7 percent of those with low scores were smokers. Among girls and boys with high scores in any of the three problem areas, girls were more likely to be smokers, although CIs were not provided. Among girls and boys with low scores in any of the three problem areas, no gender-specific differences were noted in smoking prevalence.

## Summary

Women who are current smokers weigh less than women who had never smoked. However, among normal weight and underweight women, current smokers are more likely than those who had never smoked to perceive themselves as overweight. Adolescent girls who are current smokers are also more likely than those who had never smoked to be trying to lose weight. These findings suggest that body weight, body image, and concerns about weight are related to smoking among women. Girls and women who smoke are more likely than those who do not smoke to use alcohol or other drugs, and the initiation of cigarette smoking generally occurs before the start of other substance use. Cigarette smoking may, therefore, be considered a "gateway" drug in the sequence of drug use among women because it frequently precedes, and is associated with, the use of other drugs.

Adult current smokers were more likely than those who had never smoked and former smokers who have been abstinent 12 months or more to report negative moods or emotions, including boredom, restlessness, depression, or loneliness. The association between cigarette smoking and these moods was found across age groups. Further research is needed to explore these relationships, the direction of causality, and implications for smoking initiation and cessation. (See "Depression and Other Psychiatric Disorders" in Chapter 3 for a review of evidence of an association between depression and smoking cessation.)

## International Patterns of Smoking Prevalence Among Women

Because of increased concern about the hazards of tobacco use, many countries and international organizations have attempted to collect data on smoking prevalence. In most developed and some developing countries, smoking behavior is measured through sample surveys of the population, and occasionally, questions on smoking are included on census questionnaires, but the frequency and coverage of such surveys is far from systematic. Depending on how a smoker is defined (e.g., by the number of cigarettes smoked per day, frequency of smoking, or cumulative lifetime consumption of cigarettes), the percentage of the population classified as regular smokers can vary significantly. Differences in sampling procedures (e.g., survey of specific population groups only) or in interview methods can seriously affect the degree to which the results of smoking prevalence surveys are representative and comparable. Therefore, reported differences in smoking prevalence among countries may not, in fact, indicate real differences in prevalence. In countries where smoking among women is socially unacceptable, prevalence estimates for women that are based on direct interviews may substantially underestimate true smoking behavior because of misrepresentation of smoking status. Thus, international comparisons of smoking prevalence must be made with caution.

The smoking epidemic may be a cohort phenomenon. Typically, initiation of smoking has increased first among young men and boys, followed several decades later by an increase among young women and girls. Social norms and customs have acted to discourage smoking among women and girls, and prevalence only begins to rise when these taboos are weakened. This weakening usually occurs first among younger, more educated women (Borras et al. 2000) because they are more likely to question traditional social values. Subsequently, smoking spreads to other socioeconomic groups and, with the aging of cohorts, to older age groups. In general, better educated persons are more responsive to health education messages about smoking hazards; hence, this group is more likely to have higher rates of smoking cessation than less educated persons. Populations in which smoking prevalence is common at all ages and in both genders and in which smoking cessation is also relatively widespread might be considered to be populations with a "mature" smoking epidemic.

Overall smoking prevalence at any point in time reflects the balance between increased smoking initiation and smoking cessation in different age groups. Assessing the current phase of the tobacco epidemic in a population requires data on age-specific trends in both initiation and cessation of smoking. Unfortunately, detailed, reliable, and comparable data on these trends are not available for most countries.

The different smoking histories of women and men reflect different sociocultural constraints, which have acted—at different times in different countries—to discourage tobacco use among women. However, these constraints have weakened in many countries, and smoking prevalence among women has risen, often accelerated by aggressive advertising campaigns targeted directly to women. In some countries, the prevalence of smoking among women is still increasing. This pattern, which was seen in many industrialized countries throughout the twentieth century, seems likely to be repeated in developing countries during this century unless effective tobacco control measures are implemented. Thwarting an increase in tobacco use among women in developing countries represents one of the greatest opportunities for disease prevention in the world today (World Bank 1999; WHO 1999).

## Current Prevalence

About one-third of all regular smokers in developed countries are women, but in the developing world, only one in eight women is a regular smoker. (All of Europe [including the newly independent states of the former USSR] and North America, as well as Australia, Japan, and New Zealand, are considered developed regions and countries; all other regions are classified as developing.) Globally, an estimated 12 percent of women smoke. Overall, smoking prevalence among women is 24 percent in developed countries and 7 percent in developing countries (WHO 1997). Although in some areas of the world women have traditionally practiced some forms of tobacco use, cultural norms have served as a powerful deterrent to women's smoking in most developing countries. By World Bank region, the prevalence of cigarette smoking among females aged 15 years or older in 1995 was estimated to be 1 percent in south Asia, 4 percent in east Asia and the Pacific, 5 percent in the Middle East and North Africa, 10 percent in sub-Saharan Africa, 21 percent in the Caribbean and Latin America, and 26 percent in central Asia and Eastern Europe. In addition, approximately 3 percent of women in south Asia smoked bidis, a traditional hand-rolled tobacco product (World Bank 1999). An estimated 200 million women worldwide were smokers in 1995, 100 million in developed countries and 100 million in developing countries (*WHO Tobacco Alert* 1996). By the year 2025, if current patterns continue, approximately 500 million women worldwide will be smokers (Judith Mackay, e-mail to Leslie Norman, September 22, 2000).

Even within regions, the prevalence of smoking among women often varies substantially across countries (Table 2.44). For example, within Europe, prevalence is high in Denmark (37.0 percent), Norway (35.5 percent), and the Czech Republic (31.0 percent) but relatively low in Portugal (15.0 percent). Although smoking prevalence is generally high in industrialized countries, it is relatively low among women in Japan (14.8 percent) and Singapore (2.7 percent) (WHO 1997).

These overall estimates may conceal important differences within subgroups. In New Zealand, 57 percent of Maori women and two-thirds of pregnant Maori women smoked in 1991 (New Zealand Public Health Commission 1994). In 1991, 57 percent of native Canadian Indian women smoked (Health Canada 1994). Although overall smoking prevalence among South African women in 1995 was 17 percent, marked differences were noted among subgroups. For example, 59 percent of "colored" women smoked (Reddy et al. 1996). Overall estimates of smoking prevalence may also conceal important differences by age group. For example, the WHO MONICA survey in Catalonia, Spain, indicated that 48 percent of the women aged 25 through 34 years, but 4 percent of the women aged 55 through 64 years, were regular smokers (Molarius et al. 2001).

The pattern by which smoking first becomes most prevalent among young women is reflected in data for European countries bordering the Mediterranean Sea. In 1994, the prevalence of smoking by age for women in France, Greece, and Italy was similar to that in Spain. The prevalence of smoking was much lower among older women than among younger women, which indicates that the tobacco epidemic is still maturing. Thus, in the European countries around the Mediterranean Sea, where the epidemic is in mid-development, smoking among women is confined primarily to young and middle-aged women.

In some nonindustrialized countries, patterns of smoking by age differ from those in industrialized countries. These patterns may reflect differences in the acceptability of tobacco use, including traditional tobacco products, by women in different age groups. Overall, smoking prevalence among women is low in most developing countries. For example, among the black population of the Cape Peninsula in South Africa, overall smoking prevalence among women was 8.4 percent. However, prevalence was much higher among women aged 55 through 64 years (12.2 percent) than among women aged 20 through 24 years (6.6 percent) (Steyn et al. 1994). Similarly, this distinct pattern is seen in some Asian countries where tobacco use by older women has traditionally been tolerated. For example, in China, Korea, and Thailand, the overall prevalence of smoking among women is about 4 to 8 percent; prevalence is 10 to 20 times higher among women aged 50 years or older than among younger women. This unique pattern does not detract from the pattern of broader diffusion outlined earlier, whereby as the modern tobacco epidemic takes root, smoking is initially more common among younger women than among older women (Liu et al. 1998).

The pattern of smoking in Japan illustrates how East Asian countries could soon progress to the pattern of Mediterranean European countries. In the late 1960s, smoking prevalence among Japanese women aged 60 years or older was about 20 percent, which was twice that among women aged 20 through 29 years. By 1999, the prevalence for all age groups was 13.4 percent, but by then it was over threefold higher among women aged 20 through 29 years (23.2

**Table 2.44. Estimated smoking prevalence among females and males aged 15 years or older, by country and gender, latest available year (ranked in order of female smoking prevalence)**

| Rank | Country (year of survey) | Females | Males | Rank | Country (year of survey) | Females | Males |
|---|---|---|---|---|---|---|---|
| 1 | Denmark (1993) | 37.0 | 37.0 | 45 | Bulgaria (1989) | 17.0 | 49.0 |
| 2 | Norway (1994) | 35.5 | 36.4 | 45 | South Africa (1995) | 17.0 | 52.0 |
| 3 | Czech Republic (1994) | 31.0 | 43.0 | 47 | Bangladesh (1990) | 15.0 | 60.0 |
| 4 | Fiji (1988) | 30.6 | 59.3 | 47 | Portugal (1994) | 15.0 | 38.0 |
| 5 | Israel (1989) | 30.0 | 45.0 | 49 | Japan (1994) | 14.8 | 59.0 |
| 5 | Russian Federation (1993) | 30.0 | 67.0 | 50 | Mexico (1990) | 14.4 | 38.3 |
| 7 | Canada (1991) | 29.0 | 31.0 | 51 | Tonga (1991) | 14.0 | 65.0 |
| 7 | The Netherlands (1994) | 29.0 | 36.0 | 52 | Dominican Republic (1990) | 13.6 | 66.3 |
| 7 | Poland (1993) | 29.0 | 51.0 | 53 | Jamaica (1990) | 13.0 | 43.0 |
| 10 | Greece (1994) | 28.0 | 46.0 | 53 | Peru (1989) | 13.0 | 41.0 |
| 10 | Iceland (1994) | 28.0 | 31.0 | 55 | El Salvador (1988) | 12.0 | 38.0 |
| 10 | Ireland (1993) | 28.0 | 29.0 | 55 | Kuwait (1991) | 12.0 | 52.0 |
| 10 | Papua New Guinea (1990) | 28.0 | 46.0 | 55 | Latvia (1993) | 12.0 | 67.0 |
| 14 | Austria (1992) | 27.0 | 42.0 | 58 | Honduras (1988) | 11.0 | 36.0 |
| 14 | France (1993) | 27.0 | 40.0 | 59 | Seychelles (1989) | 10.3 | 50.9 |
| 14 | Hungary (1989) | 27.0 | 40.0 | 60 | Algeria (1980) | 10.0 | 53.0 |
| 17 | Uruguay (1990) | 26.6 | 40.9 | 60 | Lithuania (1992) | 10.0 | 52.0 |
| 18 | Cook Islands (1988) | 26.0 | 44.0 | 62 | Morocco (1990) | 9.1 | 39.6 |
| 18 | Italy (1994) | 26.0 | 38.0 | 63 | Philippines (1987) | 8.0 | 43.0 |
| 18 | Luxembourg (1993) | 26.0 | 32.0 | 63 | Swaziland (1989) | 8.0 | 33.0 |
| 18 | Slovakia (1992) | 26.0 | 43.0 | 65 | Albania (1990) | 7.9 | 49.8 |
| 18 | Switzerland (1992) | 26.0 | 36.0 | 66 | Cyprus (1990) | 7.2 | 42.5 |
| 18 | United Kingdom (1994) | 26.0 | 28.0 | 67 | China (1984) | 7.0 | 61.0 |
| 24 | Brazil (1989) | 25.4 | 39.9 | 67 | Mongolia (1990) | 7.0 | 40.0 |
| 25 | Chile (1990) | 25.1 | 37.9 | 69 | Republic of Korea (1989) | 6.7 | 68.2 |
| 26 | Spain (1993) | 25.0 | 48.0 | 69 | Nigeria (1990) | 6.7 | 24.4 |
| 27 | Cuba (1990) | 24.5 | 49.3 | 71 | Bahrain (1991) | 6.0 | 24.0 |
| 28 | Estonia (1994) | 24.0 | 52.0 | 72 | Paraguay (1990) | 5.5 | 24.1 |
| 28 | Sweden (1994) | 24.0 | 22.0 | 73 | Iraq (1990) | 5.0 | 40.0 |
| 28 | Turkey (1988) | 24.0 | 63.0 | 74 | Pakistan (1980) | 4.4 | 27.4 |
| 31 | Argentina (1992) | 23.0 | 40.0 | 75 | Indonesia (1986) | 4.0 | 53.0 |
| 31 | Slovenia (1994) | 23.0 | 35.0 | 75 | Malaysia (1986) | 4.0 | 41.0 |
| 33 | United States of America (1993) | 22.5 | 27.7 | 75 | Thailand (1995) | 4.0 | 49.0 |
| 34 | New Zealand (1992) | 22.0 | 24.0 | 78 | Bahamas (1989) | 3.8 | 19.3 |
| 35 | Germany (1992) | 21.5 | 36.8 | 79 | Mauritius (1992) | 3.7 | 47.2 |
| 36 | Bolivia (1992) | 21.4 | 50.0 | 80 | India (1980s) | 3.0 | 40.0 |
| 37 | Australia (1993) | 21.0 | 29.0 | 81 | Singapore (1995) | 2.7 | 31.9 |
| 38 | Costa Rica (1988) | 20.0 | 35.0 | 82 | Egypt (1986) | 1.0 | 39.8 |
| 39 | Colombia (1992) | 19.1 | 35.1 | 82 | Lesotho (1989) | 1.0 | 38.3 |
| 40 | Belgium (1993) | 19.0 | 31.0 | 82 | Uzbekistan (1989) | 1.0 | 40.0 |
| 40 | Finland (1994) | 19.0 | 27.0 | 85 | Sri Lanka (1988) | 0.8 | 54.8 |
| 42 | Samoa (1994) | 18.6 | 53.0 | 86 | Turkmenistan (1992) | 0.5 | 26.6 |
| 43 | Malta (1992) | 18.0 | 40.0 | 87 | Saudi Arabia (1990) | NA* | 52.7 |
| 44 | Guatemala (1989) | 17.7 | 37.8 | | | | |

*NA = Not available.
Source: World Health Organization 1997.

percent) than among women aged 60 through 69 years (7.2 percent) (Ministry of Health and Welfare 2000).

## Trends

Large numbers of women first began to smoke in Great Britain and the United States during the 1920s and 1930s. In other industrialized countries, widespread smoking by women occurred some years later. By the 1960s, smoking prevalence had reached 25 to 35 percent in most industrialized countries, although in a few such countries (e.g., Japan and Portugal), overall smoking prevalence among women still does not exceed about 15 percent. Smoking among women never attained the prevalence of 60 percent or greater seen among men in Great Britain immediately after World War II and more recently in China, Japan, and Korea.

In many industrialized countries, smoking prevalence among women remained at about 30 to 40 percent until the 1970s to early 1980s, when a gradual decline began in some countries (Table 2.45). From the early 1970s to the early 1990s, prevalence declined by about 10 percentage points in Ireland, the Netherlands, New Zealand, Sweden, and the United Kingdom and by smaller amounts in Australia, Canada, and the United States. Prevalence remained relatively unchanged in Denmark, Finland, and Japan and, until more recently, in France. Conversely, prevalence rose among women in Greece, Portugal, and Spain. WHO sponsored community-based surveys over a 10-year period in 36 populations, primarily European; the initial surveys generally occurred in the mid-1980s and the final surveys in the mid-1990s (Molarius et al. 2001). Among women, overall smoking prevalence increased over time by more than 5 percentage points in 6 (17 percent) of the 36 populations and decreased in 9 (25 percent) of the 36. In many of the populations, prevalence increased among the younger age groups. Populations of women with low baseline prevalence tended to experience increases in smoking prevalence over time (e.g., in Poland, Russia, and Spain), whereas populations with higher baseline prevalence, especially among the younger age group(s), experienced decreases (e.g., in Australia, the United Kingdom, and the United States).

Because it is generally younger women who begin smoking first in a population, the ratio of prevalence among young women to that among older women is a good indicator of the "maturity" of the smoking epidemic in a population. Smoking among younger women is also an indicator of the probable extent of smoking attributable deaths in the future and of the effectiveness of strategies for preventing smoking initiation. Trends in smoking among young women have varied from country to country. In Norway, smoking prevalence among girls and women aged 16 through 24 years was about 40 percent in the mid-1970s; it steadily decreased to about 25 percent in 1994. In Great Britain, the prevalence among girls and women aged 16 through 24 years peaked at just over 50 percent in 1970 and declined to about 30 percent by 1992 (Thomas et al. 1994). Similarly, in Ireland, the prevalence of smoking among girls and women aged 16 through 24 years declined from 42 percent in 1972 to 27 percent in 1993 (Shelley et al. 1996). In Spain, almost 40 percent of women aged 18 through 24 years smoked in 1993; in Greece, the prevalence among women and girls aged 15 through 24 years was 41 percent in 1994. Only about 15 percent of young Portuguese women smoked in 1977, whereas 31 percent smoked in 1988, although more recent surveys suggested that the prevalence may have fallen slightly. In China, according to a 1996 survey, 4.2 percent of women aged 15 years or older smoked, but in the age group 15 through 19 years, 10 percent of women were smokers (Tomlinson 1998). For many countries, particularly developing countries, population-based data on smoking prevalence are sparse or nonexistent. For example, relatively little is known about recent trends in smoking prevalence among young women in Asian countries, where cigarette marketing targeted to women has increased markedly (Mackay 1989).

## Other Tobacco Use

In most industrialized countries, women have smoked manufactured cigarettes; very few have smoked pipes, cigars, or roll-your-own cigarettes, nor have they been consumers of other forms of tobacco such as snuff or chewing tobacco. However, in Denmark, about 10 percent of women smoked cigars, cigarillos, or pipes in 1970, although the prevalence by the early 1990s was only about 2 percent. In 1989–1990, the overall prevalence of snuff use among Swedish women and girls aged 16 years or older was 2 percent, ranging from 0 percent among women aged 55 years or older to 5 percent among those aged 16 through 24 years.

In central, south, and Southeast Asia, smokeless tobacco use includes nass, naswar, khaini, mishri, gudakhu, and betelquid. The prevalence of smokeless tobacco is relatively high among women in some developing countries, where its use is considered more socially acceptable than smoking for women. Surveys suggested that, in certain areas of India, about 57 percent of women use smokeless tobacco, which is similar to the pattern of use among men (55.6 percent) (Gupta et al. 1992; Gupta 1996). Data from other countries in south Asia suggested that many women in the region regularly chew tobacco. These patterns correlate with the incidence of oropharyngeal cancer, which is found among women of this region to be the highest in the world (Coleman et al. 1993).

The use of smokeless tobacco in South Africa is common not only among Indian women but also among black women of the Cape Peninsula area. Among black women in South Africa aged 45 through 54 years, the prevalence of snuff use has been reported to be as high as 67.5 percent and the prevalence of chewing tobacco use is 12.0 percent. Snuff use accounts for 23.3 percent of tobacco use among black women and only 0.4 percent among black men (Steyn et al. 1994). In Sudan, toombak, a form of oral snuff, is also widely used. The reported prevalence of toombak use is much lower among women than among men (1.7 vs. 23.0 percent) and is more common among older women than among younger women (Idris et al. 1998).

## Summary

The prevalence of smoking and trends in smoking among women over time vary markedly across countries, even across industrialized countries for which the most reliable data exist. With notable exceptions, smoking prevalence among females has generally been highest in developed countries and lowest in less developed countries. Prevalence appears to have peaked and to have begun to decline in many industrialized countries, while increases are occurring in several industrialized countries and many less developed areas of the world. Thwarting an increase in tobacco use among women, especially in countries where prevalence is still relatively low, represents one of the greatest disease prevention opportunities in the world today.

**Table 2.45. Smoking prevalence (%) among women in selected countries, 1970–1994**

| | Australia | Canada | Denmark | Finland | France | Greece | Ireland | Japan |
|---|---|---|---|---|---|---|---|---|
| 1970 | | 35 | 36 | | | | | 16 |
| 1971 | | | | | | | 42 | |
| 1972 | 29 | 35 | | | | | | |
| 1973 | 29 | | | | | | | |
| 1974 | 30 | 34 | | | | | 36 | 17 |
| 1975 | 29 | 34 | 38 | | | 10 | | 15 |
| 1976 | 29 | | | 17 | | | | |
| 1977 | 29 | 34 | | | 29 | | 33 | |
| 1978 | 29 | | | | | | | |
| 1979 | | 33 | | 18 | | | | |
| 1980 | 26 | | 38 | 17 | | | 32 | 14 |
| 1981 | | 32 | 38 | 19 | | | | |
| 1982 | | | 38 | 16 | | | | |
| 1983 | 25 | 31 | 38 | 19 | 29 | | | |
| 1984 | | | 39 | 17 | 33 | | | 14 |
| 1985 | | | 37 | 14 | | | | |
| 1986 | | 28 | | 18 | 30 | | | |
| 1987 | | | | 21 | | 25 | | |
| 1988 | | | | 20 | | 24 | | |
| 1989 | | 31 | | 19 | 33 | 27 | | |
| 1990 | | | | 20 | | 26 | 29 | 14 |
| 1991 | 21 | 29 | 39 | 22 | 35 | 26 | 27 | |
| 1992 | | | | 20 | 33 | 24 | 26 | 13 |
| 1993 | 21 | | 37 | 19 | 27 | | 28 | |
| 1994 | | 29 | | 19 | | 28 | | 15 |

Sources: Nicolaides-Bouman et al. 1993; Joossens et al. 1994; World Health Organization database 1996, unpublished data; World Health Organization 1997.

| The Netherlands | New Zealand | Norway | Portugal | Spain | Sweden | United Kingdom | United States |
|---|---|---|---|---|---|---|---|
| 42 | | 37 | | | | 44 | 31 |
| | | 35 | | | | 42 | |
| 40 | | 38 | | | | 41 | |
| | | 38 | | | | 43 | |
| | 31 | 37 | | | | 41 | 31 |
| 36 | | 39 | | | | 43 | 29 |
| | 32 | 38 | | | 34 | 38 | 33 |
| | | 40 | 3 | | | 41 | 31 |
| | | 40 | | 17 | | 37 | 30 |
| 38 | | 39 | | | | 39 | 29 |
| | | 39 | 1 | | 29 | 37 | 30 |
| | 29 | 38 | | | | 36 | |
| | | 39 | | 20 | | 33 | |
| 37 | | 41 | 9 | | | 35 | 29 |
| | | 40 | 10 | | 28 | 32 | |
| | 30 | 39 | 9 | | | 34 | 28 |
| | | | | | | | |
| | | | 5 | 23 | | | |
| | | | 12 | | | | |
| | | | | 21 | | | |
| 31 | 27 | 33 | | | 26 | 29 | 23 |
| 30 | 25 | | | | | | 24 |
| 31 | 22 | 31 | | | | 28 | 24 |
| | | 33 | | 25 | | | 23 |
| 29 | | 26 | 15 | | 24 | 26 | |

# Conclusions

1. Cigarette smoking became prevalent among women after it did among men, and smoking prevalence has always been lower among women than among men. The gender-specific difference in smoking prevalence narrowed between 1965 and 1985. Since 1985, the decline in prevalence has been comparable among women and men.
2. The prevalence of current smoking among women increased from less than 6 percent in 1924 to 34 percent in 1965, then declined to 22 to 23 percent in the late 1990s. In 1997–1998, smoking prevalence was highest among American Indian or Alaska Native women (34.5 percent), intermediate among white women (23.5 percent) and black women (21.9 percent), and lowest among Hispanic women (13.8 percent) and Asian or Pacific Islander women (11.2 percent). By educational level, smoking prevalence is nearly three times higher among women with 9 to 11 years of education (30.9 percent) than among women with 16 or more years of education (10.6 percent).
3. Much of the progress in reducing smoking prevalence among girls in the 1970s and 1980s was lost with the increase in prevalence in the 1990s: current smoking among high school senior girls was the same in 2000 as in 1988. Although smoking prevalence was higher among high school senior girls than among high school senior boys in the 1970s and early 1980s, prevalence has been comparable since the mid-1980s.
4. Smoking declined substantially among black girls from the mid-1970s through the early 1990s; the decline among white girls for this same period was small. As adolescents age into young adulthood, these patterns are now being reflected in the racial and ethnic differences in smoking among young women. Data are not available on long-term trends in smoking prevalence among high school seniors of other racial and ethnic groups.
5. Smoking during pregnancy appears to have decreased from 1989 through 1998. Despite increased knowledge of the adverse health effects of smoking during pregnancy, estimates of women smoking during pregnancy range from 12 percent based on birth certificate data to as high as 22 percent based on survey data.
6. Historically, women started to smoke at a later age than did men, but beginning with the 1960 cohort, the mean age at smoking initiation has not differed by gender.
7. Nicotine dependence is strongly associated with the number of cigarettes smoked per day. Girls and women who smoke appear to be equally dependent on nicotine when results are stratified by number of cigarettes smoked per day. Few gender-specific differences have been found in indicators of nicotine dependence among adolescents, young adults, or adults overall.
8. The percentage of persons who have ever smoked and who have quit smoking is somewhat lower among women (46.2 percent) than among men (50.1 percent). This finding is probably because men began to stop smoking earlier in this century than did women and because these data do not take into account that men are more likely than women to switch to or to continue to use other tobacco products when they stop smoking cigarettes. Since the late 1970s or early 1980s, the probability of attempting to quit smoking and to succeed has been equally high among women and men.
9. Prevalence of the use of cigars, pipes, and smokeless tobacco among women is generally low, but recent data suggested that cigar smoking among women and girls is increasing.
10. Smoking prevalence among women varies markedly across countries; the percentages range from an estimated 7 percent in developing countries to 24 percent in developed countries. Thwarting further increases in tobacco use among women is one of the greatest disease prevention opportunities in the world today.

# Appendix 1: Sources of Data

Data in Chapter 2 were obtained primarily from national surveys (Table 2.1). For primary data analyses, when sample sizes for a single year were too small for estimating the prevalence of smoking in a particular subgroup, data for several years were combined. This approach increased the reliability and stability of the prevalence estimates (Frazier et al. 1992).

## Adult Use of Tobacco Survey

The Adult Use of Tobacco Survey (AUTS) was conducted in 1964, 1966, 1970, 1975, and 1986 by the Office on Smoking and Health, formerly the National Clearinghouse for Smoking and Health (U.S. Department of Health, Education, and Welfare [USDHEW] 1969, 1973, 1976; U.S. Department of Health and Human Services [USDHHS] 1990a). The 1966 and 1970 surveys included interviews of respondents to previous surveys. The 1964 and 1966 surveys were conducted through in-person household interviews. Beginning in 1970, the surveys were conducted by telephone. Respondents were drawn from the U.S. civilian, noninstitutionalized, adult population and were asked about their knowledge, attitudes, and practices regarding tobacco use. Data were collected from a national probability sample of adults aged 21 years or older in 1964, 1966, 1970, and 1975 and adults aged 17 years or older in 1986. A two-stage, cluster-sampling procedure was used, and data were weighted to provide national estimates.

## Behavioral Risk Factor Surveillance System

Since 1981, the National Center for Chronic Disease Prevention and Health Promotion, Centers for Disease Control and Prevention (CDC), has coordinated state surveillance of behavioral risk factors through the Behavioral Risk Factor Surveillance System (BRFSS) (Gentry et al. 1985; Remington et al. 1985, 1988; Frazier et al. 1992; Powell-Griner et al. 1997; Nelson et al. 1998). Each state that participates in BRFSS provides estimates of risk behaviors for its population aged 18 years or older. A multistage cluster design is used to select households from which an adult is selected for a telephone interview. Fifty states, the District of Columbia, and Puerto Rico participated in 1999. Data were weighted to provide state-specific estimates.

## Current Population Survey

The U.S. Bureau of the Census has conducted the Current Population Survey for more than 50 years to assess employment in the United States (U.S. Bureau of the Census 1995, 1996a,b). Households are selected on the basis of area of residence to represent the nation as a whole and individual states. The sample is drawn from the U.S. civilian, noninstitutionalized, population aged 15 years or older. Data are collected monthly through household interviews by using a stratified cluster design. Questions on tobacco use were added as a special National Cancer Institute Tobacco Use Supplement to the monthly Current Population Survey for three months in 1995 and 1996 (September 1995, January 1996, and May 1996) (U.S. Bureau of the Census 1995, 1996a,b). For this report, these data were combined and used to produce state and national estimates for the period. The estimates include both self-reported and proxy-reported data.

## Monitoring the Future Survey

Supported by grants from the National Institute on Drug Abuse (NIDA), the University of Michigan's Institute for Social Research has surveyed nationally representative samples of high school seniors in the spring of each year since 1975 as part of the Monitoring the Future (MTF) Survey (Bachman et al. 1980a,b, 1981, 1984, 1985, 1987, 1991a, 1993a,b; Johnston et al. 1980a,b, 1982, 1984, 1986, 1991, 1992, 1993, 1994a, 1995a,b, 1996, 1997, 1999, 2000a). Beginning in 1991, surveys were also conducted among 8th- and 10th-grade students. Multistage sampling designs were used to randomly select students in public and private schools within the 48 contiguous states. Self-administered questionnaires were distributed to students in classrooms by trained personnel, and standardized procedures were followed. Between 123 and 146 high schools were selected each year; 51 to 72 percent of selected schools participated, and 79 to 87 percent of sampled students participated (Johnston et al. 1997, 2000a; Patrick O'Malley, e-mail to Linda Pederson, December 14, 2000). (Nonparticipation was primarily due to absenteeism.) This report uses MTF Survey data from public use data tapes for 1976–1998 and from published reports for 1999 and 2000. The data were weighted to provide national estimates, and confidence intervals were calculated by using formulas provided by the Institute for Social Research (Johnston et al. 2000a). Confidence intervals for MTF Survey data are asymmetric; the numbers presented in this chapter reflect the larger value for each confidence interval to provide the most conservative estimates. Trends in current smoking prevalence by race are calculated by using two-year rolling averages to generate more stable estimates.

Since 1980, NIDA has also surveyed a nationally representative sample of college students who were part of the previous MTF surveys. College students are defined as full-time students, one to four years after high school, enrolled in a two- or four-year college in March during the year of the survey. This definition generally encompasses more than 70 percent of all undergraduate college students enrolled full time. The survey does not use a cluster-sample design, because the heterogeneity in the student populations is greater in postsecondary institutions than in high schools (Johnston et al. 2000b).

## Natality Statistics

In this report, the data on smoking among women who gave birth are from birth certificates for 1989, 1991, 1993, 1995, 1997, and 1998. These data are provided to the National Center for Health Statistics (NCHS) through the Vital Statistics Cooperative Program. Although the birth data are not subject to sampling error, they may be affected by random variation in the number of births. The 1989 revision of the U.S. Standard Certificate of Live Birth included several new items on medical and lifestyle risk factors of pregnancy and birth, including tobacco use and the number of cigarettes smoked per day by the mother. Data on tobacco use during pregnancy were available for 43 states and the District of Columbia in 1989 and for 46 states and the District of Columbia in 1991–1994. In 1995–1998, 46 states, the District of Columbia, and New York City were included; the reporting area excluded California, Indiana, the rest of New York, and South Dakota and accounted for 81.0 percent of U.S. births. All information was provided as a check mark on the certificate and certified by an attendant (Tolson et al. 1991; NCHS 1992, 1994a; Ventura et al. 1995, 1997, 1999, 2000; Matthews 1998).

## National Health and Nutrition Examination Survey

NCHS conducted the third National Health and Nutrition Examination Survey (NHANES III) (NCHS 1994b) in 1988–1994. A stratified, multistage probability design was used to obtain a sample that was representative of the total noninstitutionalized U.S. civilian population aged two months or older. Persons aged two months to 5 years, persons aged 60 years or older, blacks, and Mexican Americans were oversampled (i.e., sampled in greater numbers than their proportion in the population, to obtain adequate sample size). The survey was conducted in two phases; each phase comprised a national probability sample. Data were weighted to provide national estimates, and confidence intervals were calculated by using standard errors generated by the software Survey Data Analysis (SUDAAN) (Shah et al. 1997).

Between 1982 and 1983, NCHS also conducted the Hispanic Health and Nutrition Examination Survey (HHANES), which was a probability-based survey of Mexican Americans residing in the Southwest; Cuban Americans residing in Dade County (Miami), Florida; and Puerto Ricans residing in the greater New York City area. This survey was conducted in either English or Spanish and included civilian, noninstitutionalized persons aged six months to 74 years (Haynes et al. 1990).

## National Health Interview Survey

NCHS has been collecting health data on tobacco from a probability sample of the U.S. civilian, noninstitutionalized, adult population since 1965 (NCHS 1975; Kovar and Poe 1985; Schoenborn 1988; Schoenborn and Marano 1988; Massey et al. 1989; USDHHS 1999a). To determine cigarette smoking trends among adults (aged ≥ 18 years), data were used from the National Health Interview Survey (NHIS) for 1965, 1966, 1970, 1974, 1978, 1979, 1980, 1983, 1985, 1987, 1988, 1990, 1991, 1992, 1993, 1994, 1995, 1997, and 1998. Proxy responses were allowed in the 1965, 1966, and 1970 surveys. The sample design was changed in 1985 to oversample blacks and thereby produce more precise estimates. Most interviews were conducted in the home; telephone interviews were conducted when respondents could not be interviewed in person. The sample was weighted to provide national estimates. For 1965, confidence intervals were calculated by using variance curves (NCHS 1978). For later years, confidence intervals were calculated by using standard errors generated by SUDAAN (Shah et al. 1997).

## National Household Survey on Drug Abuse

Since 1974, first NIDA (Alcohol, Drug Abuse, and Mental Health Administration) then the Substance Abuse and Mental Health Services Administration (SAMHSA) has conducted the National Household

Survey on Drug Abuse (NHSDA), a periodic household survey of the civilian, noninstitutionalized population aged 12 years or older, to measure the prevalence of use of illicit drugs, alcohol, and tobacco (Abelson and Atkinson 1975; Abelson and Fishburne 1976; Abelson et al. 1977; Miller et al. 1983; USDHHS 1988a, 1990b, 1991; SAMHSA 1993, 1995a,b, 1996, 1997, 1998a,b, 2000). Data from 1974, 1976, 1977, 1979, 1982, 1985, 1988, 1990, 1991, 1992, 1993, 1994, 1995, 1996, 1997, and 1998 were used in this report. A multistage sampling design was used to randomly sample household units. The 48 contiguous states were included through 1990; since 1991, the survey has also included Alaska and Hawaii. Respondents were interviewed in person in their homes by trained interviewers. The response rate averaged 80 percent across survey years (J. Gfroerer, e-mail to Alyssa Easton, December 9, 1999), and the data were weighted to provide national estimates. Starting in 1994, information on sensitive topics, such as tobacco use and illicit drug use, was collected through a personal interview with a self-administered answer sheet to increase the privacy of responses. This change in method also resulted in the elimination of skip patterns (see definition for "skip pattern" in Appendix 2), and the initial response was edited to be consistent with later answers (Brittingham et al. 1998). In 1994, both the old and new methods were used in a split-sample design. The 1994-A data were obtained through personal interviews, and the 1994-B data were obtained by using a self-administered answer sheet. Since 1995, only the self-administered format was used. These data were also weighted to provide national estimates, and confidence intervals were calculated by using SUDAAN (Shah et al. 1997).

## National Teenage Tobacco Survey

USDHEW conducted the National Teenage Tobacco Survey (NTTS) (USDHEW 1972, 1979b) in 1968, 1970, 1972, 1974, and 1979 to obtain information on the prevalence of smoking and related factors among adolescents. A three-stage, stratified, random probability sample was used to obtain a representative sample of persons aged 12 through 18 years. The 1968 survey was conducted by telephone interview or by in-person interview in households not having a telephone. Surveys in subsequent years were conducted by telephone interview only. Results were not weighted.

## National Youth Tobacco Survey

The American Legacy Foundation conducted the National Youth Tobacco Survey (NYTS) (CDC 2000b) in 1999 to obtain information on the prevalence of tobacco use and related factors and to provide data to support the design, implementation, and evaluation of comprehensive tobacco control interventions. Similar state Youth Tobacco Surveys, conducted by CDC, began in 1998. Published data from the National Youth Tobacco Survey are used in this report. A three-stage cluster sample design produced a nationally representative sample of students in grades 6 through 12 in public and private schools in the United States. This self-administered school questionnaire was distributed in the classroom by trained data collectors. The data were weighted to provide national estimates, and confidence intervals were calculated by using standard errors generated by SUDAAN (Shah et al. 1997).

## Teenage Attitudes and Practices Survey

In 1989 and 1993, the U.S. Public Health Service (Office on Smoking and Health and NCHS) used the Teenage Attitudes and Practices Survey (TAPS) to collect self-reported data on tobacco use by adolescents (Allen et al. 1991, 1993; Moss et al. 1992; NCHS, public use data tape, 1993; CDC 1994a,d). The 1989 TAPS I collected information from a national household sample of young persons aged 12 through 18 years. Adolescents were selected from households that had been sampled in the 1988–1989 NHIS. TAPS I was conducted by computer-assisted telephone interview; a questionnaire was mailed to persons who could not be reached by telephone. The 1993 TAPS II was also a telephone survey, but it included household interviews of persons who could not be contacted by telephone. The TAPS II sample had two components: a longitudinal component consisting only of the respondents to the 1989 TAPS I telephone interview (aged 15 through 22 years in 1993), and a new probability sample of persons aged 10 through 15 years, obtained from the last half of the 1991 NHIS and the first three months of the 1992 NHIS sample frames. The 1989 and 1993 data were weighted to provide national population estimates. Confidence intervals were calculated by using standard errors generated by SUDAAN (Shah et al. 1997). Because part of the 1993 survey was a follow-up survey of respondents from 1989, the 1993 survey cannot be used for tobacco prevalence estimates (smokers were more likely to be lost to follow-up).

## Youth Risk Behavior Surveillance System

CDC developed the Youth Risk Behavior Surveillance System (YRBSS) in 1990 to measure six categories of priority health risk behaviors, including tobacco use among adolescents. Data were collected through national, state, and local school-based surveys of high school students that were conducted during the spring of 1991, 1993, 1995, 1997, and 1999 and through a national household-based survey of youth aged 12 through 21 years conducted during 1992 (Kolbe 1990; CDC 1992; Kann et al. 1993, 1995, 1996, 1998, 2000; Kolbe et al. 1993). Data from the 1999 national school-based survey are used in this report.

The 1999 Youth Risk Behavior Survey (YRBS) used a three-stage, cluster-sample design to draw a nationally representative sample of 9th- through 12th-grade students in public and private schools in all 50 states and the District of Columbia. Schools having a substantial proportion of black students and Hispanic students were oversampled. The questionnaire was administered in the classroom by trained data collectors. The data were weighted to provide national estimates, and confidence intervals were calculated by using standard errors generated by SUDAAN (Shah et al. 1997).

Analyses done for this report restricted the YRBS sample to students less than 18 years of age (see Tables 2.8, 2.10, and 2.39). Of the students in this group, 99.8 percent were between 14 and 17 years of age. However, published YRBS data, including publications cited in this report, include information on students 18 years of age or older. Because of the age restrictions used in data analyses for this report, the estimates in this report may be different from the published estimates.

# Appendix 2: Definitions

Measures of cigarette smoking differ among surveys and between surveys of children and adults. Five surveys (MTF Survey, NHSDA, NYTS, TAPS, and YRBS) provide information about smoking among children and adolescents, and four surveys (BRFSS, NHIS, NHSDA, and the Current Population Survey) provide information about smoking among adults. For each smoking measure, the definitions used in the various surveys are summarized here.

## Attempts to Quit Smoking

An attempt to quit smoking is defined as having quit smoking for one or more days. Depending on the year of the survey, NHIS asked about attempts to quit in the past year or in a lifetime. Examples of questions are, "During the past 12 months, have you quit smoking for one day or longer?" and "Have you EVER stopped smoking for one day or longer?" In the 1998 NHIS, the question was revised to, "During the past 12 months, have you stopped smoking for more than one day because you were trying to quit smoking?"

## Bidis

Bidis are small, brown, hand-rolled cigarettes from India and other southeast Asian countries. They consist of tobacco wrapped in a tendu or temburni leaf and are tied at one end with a string. In NYTS, ever use of bidis was defined as having ever tried bidis, even one or two puffs. In NYTS, current use of bidis was defined as use on 1 or more of the 30 days preceding the survey.

## Body Weight

Body mass index (BMI) (weight in kilograms divided by height in meters squared) is used as the measure of body weight. In NHANES III, weight (in kilograms to two decimal places) and height (to the nearest millimeter) were measured at examination. For persons aged 20 years or older, overweight was defined as BMI equal to or greater than 27.3 for women and 27.8 for men. These values are based on the gender-specific 85th percentile of BMI from NHANES II for persons aged 20 through 29 years. For persons aged 18 or 19 years, overweight was defined as BMI of at least 25.7 for women and 25.8 for men, on the basis of the gender-specific 85th percentile of BMI from NHANES II for persons aged 18 or 19 years.

The classification of weight perception varies by survey. In NHIS, adults responded to the question, "Do you consider yourself overweight, underweight, or just about right?" NHIS analyses on weight perception in this report excluded persons who were overweight according to BMI on the basis of self-reported weight and height.

## Cigar Use

### Adults

Among adult respondents in NHIS, ever smoking a cigar was determined by persons self-reporting that they had ever smoked cigars. For the 1970 NHIS, prevalence was based on persons who reported smoking cigars at the time of the survey. Current cigar smokers in NHIS for 1987, 1991, and 1992 included respondents who smoked at least 50 cigars in their entire lifetime and who smoked at the time of the survey. For the 1998 NHIS, current cigar smokers were respondents who reported that they ever smoked cigars and smoked cigars at the time of survey.

### Children and Adolescents

In the 1999 NYTS, ever use of cigars was defined as ever trying cigars, cigarillos, or little cigars, even one or two puffs. In the 1999 NYTS, the 1998 NHSDA, and the 1999 YRBS, current cigar smoking among adolescents was defined as having smoked cigars on at least 1 of the 30 days preceding the survey.

## Current Smoker

### Adults

NHIS for 1965–1991 defined current smokers as respondents who have smoked at least 100 cigarettes and who answered yes to the question, "Do you smoke cigarettes now?" Beginning in 1992, NHIS assessed whether respondents smoked every day, some days, or not at all. Persons who smoked every day or some days were classified as current smokers. The 1995–1996 Current Population Survey also included information on lifetime cigarette smoking ($\geq$ 100 cigarettes) and distinguished between current smokers who consumed cigarettes every day or only some days. Estimates of prevalence of current smoking included persons who smoked either every day or only some days. For the 1974–1994-A NHSDA data used in this report, a current smoker was defined as a person who has smoked 100 or more cigarettes (about 5 packs) in his or her entire lifetime and who smoked in the 30 days before the survey. For the NHSDA data since the 1994-B survey, a current smoker was defined as a person who has smoked for 100 or more days and who smoked in the 30 days before the survey.

#### Children and Adolescents

In the surveys of children and adolescents, current cigarette smoking among adolescents was defined as having smoked on at least 1 of the 30 days preceding the survey.

### Ever Smoked

#### Adults

In NHIS, BRFSS, and the Current Population Survey, adults who had ever smoked were respondents who had smoked at least 100 cigarettes in their entire lifetime. In NHSDA for 1974–1994-A, adults who had ever smoked were respondents who had smoked at least 100 cigarettes (about 5 packs) in their entire lifetime; since the 1994-B survey, persons who had ever smoked were respondents who had smoked at least 100 days in their entire lifetime.

#### Children and Adolescents

In the 1974–1977 NHSDA, children and adolescents who had ever smoked were those who reported that they had ever smoked a cigarette. In the 1979–1994-A NHSDA, ever smoked was defined as the inverse of never having smoked a cigarette. In the 1994-B survey and in subsequent years, persons who had ever smoked were respondents who reported ever having smoked a cigarette, even one or two puffs. In the MTF Survey, those who reported that they had ever smoked cigarettes, even once or twice, were classified as having ever smoked.

### Ever Tried Smoking

#### Children and Adolescents

In NYTS, TAPS, and YRBS, persons who had ever tried smoking are those respondents who had tried a cigarette, even one or two puffs. In the 1979–1994-A NHSDA, smoking status was determined by response to the question, "About how old were you when you first tried a cigarette?" If any age was given, the person was considered to have ever tried smoking.

### Former Smoker

#### Adults

In NHIS, BRFSS, and the Current Population Survey, former smokers were respondents who had smoked at least 100 cigarettes in their lifetime but did not smoke at the time of the survey. No time frame for not smoking was specified, but some analyses specify former smokers who have not smoked in one year or in the past 12 months. In NHSDA for 1974–1994-A, former smokers had smoked at least 100 cigarettes but had not smoked in the past 30 days; since the 1994-B survey, former smokers had smoked at least 100 days but had not smoked in the past 30 days.

#### Children and Adolescents

In TAPS II, respondents who reported having smoked cigarettes regularly in the past, but not in the past 30 days, and who stated that they had quit smoking were classified as former smokers. In the MTF Survey, persons who had ever used cigarettes regularly but had not smoked in the past 30 days were classified as former smokers.

### Initiation

For this report, smoking initiation was defined as the age at which a person first tried a cigarette (NHSDA), first smoked a whole cigarette (TAPS and YRBS), or first became a daily smoker (NHSDA and YRBS). The MTF Survey measured the school grade in which respondents first smoked a cigarette and first smoked daily. NHIS measured the recalled age at which adult respondents first started smoking fairly regularly (self-defined); this response was used to estimate the percentage of adults who became regular smokers during their adolescent years. Results from the different measures were not combined and are clearly identified in the tables and text.

### Kreteks

Kreteks are clove cigarettes made in Indonesia that contain clove extract and tobacco. In NYTS, current use of kreteks was defined as use on 1 or more of the 30 days preceding the survey.

## Never Smoked

### Adults

In NHIS, BRFSS, and the Current Population Survey, persons who had never smoked were those who had not smoked 100 cigarettes in their entire lifetime. In NHSDA for 1974–1994-A, persons who had never smoked were those who had not smoked 100 cigarettes (about 5 packs) in their entire lifetime. In NHSDA since the 1994-B survey, persons who had never smoked had not smoked for 100 days in their entire lifetime.

### Children and Adolescents

In TAPS and YRBS, persons who had never smoked were those who had never tried a cigarette, not even a puff. In the MTF Survey, persons who had never smoked were defined as persons who had never smoked, not even once or twice. In NHSDA, persons who had never smoked were those who had never tried cigarettes.

## Noncurrent Smoker

In YRBS, MTF Survey, and NHSDA data, noncurrent smoker was used to describe adolescents who had ever tried a cigarette, even one or two puffs or only once or twice (ever smoked), but who had not smoked in the 30 days before the survey.

## Percentage of Smokers Who Quit Smoking

The percentage of smokers who quit smoking was calculated for adults as the percentage of former smokers who had ever smoked at least 100 cigarettes. For children and adolescents, the percentage of smokers who quit smoking was defined as the proportion of children or adolescents who had ever smoked regularly (self-defined) who quit smoking.

## Pipe Use

### Adults

Current pipe smokers in NHIS were categorized as having smoked a pipe at least 50 times during their lifetime and by use at the time of the interview. Current pipe smoking in AUTS was determined by self-reporting of ever smoking a pipe and smoking a pipe at the time of the survey.

### Children and Adolescents

In NYTS, current pipe smokers had smoked a pipe on 1 or more of the 30 days preceding the survey.

## Quantity of Cigarettes Smoked

### Adults

For this report, heavy smoking among adults was defined as smoking 25 or more cigarettes per day. NHIS was used to assess the number of cigarettes smoked per day among adults. Until 1992, NHIS asked all current smokers, "On the average, how many cigarettes do you now smoke a day?" Since 1992, this same question was asked of daily smokers, but persons who smoked only on some days were asked the number of cigarettes smoked on the days they smoked. To combine these responses into a comparable measure per day, responses from persons who smoked only on some days were multiplied by the fraction of days of smoking per month. Data from NHIS are also recoded as 25 or more cigarettes per day. The data used here for pregnant women were published data from NHIS, which defined heavy smoking as smoking 21 or more cigarettes per day.

NHSDA asked, "How many cigarettes have you smoked per day, on the average, during the past 30 days?" Responses were coded as 25 or fewer cigarettes and 26 or more cigarettes. This coding resulted in a definition of heavy smoking that is slightly inconsistent between NHSDA and NHIS.

### Children and Adolescents

To measure the quantity of cigarettes smoked, NHSDA, YRBS, and TAPS assessed the number of cigarettes smoked per day. NHSDA asked, "When you smoked cigarettes during the past 30 days, how many did you usually smoke each day?" Categories were coded as 5 or fewer, 6 to 15, and 16 or more cigarettes per day. NYTS and YRBS asked, "During the past 30 days, on the days you smoked, how many cigarettes did you smoke per day?" Categories were coded as less than 1 per day, 1 per day, 2 to 5 per day, 6 to 10 per day, 11 to 20 per day, and more than 20 per day. TAPS asked, "I'm going to ask you to think about your cigarette smoking on each of the last seven days. Let's start with yesterday, which was [day]. Please think back carefully and tell me how many cigarettes you smoked [day]? Now, how many cigarettes did you smoke the day before that, which was [day]?" The actual number was recorded. For the present report, heavy smoking among young persons was defined as smoking about one-half pack of cigarettes per day, but due to NHSDA coding categories, this resulted in the category being 6 to 15 or more cigarettes per day.

## Rolling Averages

When sample sizes were small, yearly trend data were based on two-year rolling averages to increase subgroup sample sizes and generate more stable and reliable estimates. (Percentages were calculated by averaging the data for the specified year and the previous year.) The two-year periods reported have overlap (e.g., 1976–1977, 1977–1978, 1978–1979).

## Skip Pattern

A skip pattern directs the respondent to the next relevant question on the basis of his or her specific response to a previous question.

## Smokeless Tobacco Use

### Adults

Smokeless tobacco use includes use of chewing tobacco and snuff. For NHIS, current smokeless tobacco use identifies persons who have used snuff or chewing tobacco at least 20 times during their lifetime and who used it at the time of the interview.

### Children and Adolescents

In NYTS, ever use of smokeless tobacco was determined by asking, "Have you ever used chewing tobacco, snuff, or dip, such as Redman, Levi Garrett, Beechnut, Skoal, Skoal Bandits, or Copenhagen?"

In MTF Surveys, current smokeless tobacco use among adolescents was defined as having used smokeless tobacco on at least 1 of the 30 days preceding the survey. In NYTS and YRBS, smokeless tobacco use was defined as having used chewing tobacco or snuff on at least 1 of the 30 days preceding the survey.

## Socioeconomic Status

In this report, socioeconomic status is defined by income level: below the poverty level, at or above the poverty level, or unknown. In 1965–1995, poverty status was based on income earned in the year before the survey and on definitions developed by the Social Security Administration in 1964, modified by federal interagency committees in 1969 and 1980, and prescribed by the Office of Management and Budget as the standard to be used by federal agencies for statistical purposes. In 1997 and 1998, the 1996 poverty thresholds from the Bureau of the Census were used.

Educational attainment is the most commonly used single indicator of social class; it is considered a reliable but limited indicator of socioeconomic status (Liberatos et al. 1988; Montgomery and Carter-Pokras 1993). Educational attainment has been associated with certain health risk factors, including cigarette smoking, even after income and occupation are controlled for (Winkleby et al. 1990). For most analyses, educational attainment was categorized as 8 or fewer years, 9 to 11 years, 12 years, 13 to 15 years, or 16 or more years. Persons with fewer than 12 years of education were not grouped together (unless small sample sizes necessitated broader categories) because both historical data (Green and Nemzer 1973; USDHEW 1976; Schuman 1977) and recent data (CDC 1994c; Zhu et al. 1996) suggest that the prevalence of smoking is much lower among persons with 8 or fewer years of education than among those with 9 to 11 years of education (Andersen et al. 1979).

# Appendix 3: Validity of Self-Reported Data

Some researchers express concern that self-reported current smoking status may be increasingly underreported because of the increased social disapproval of smoking, and a study by Warner (1978) supports this view. However, Warner compared data from early years (derived from in-person interviews) with data from recent years (derived from telephone interviews). Estimates from telephone interviews are generally lower than those from in-person interviews because of nonresponse from population subgroups at higher risk from smoking and because of sampling bias from population subgroups without telephone service (Andersen et al. 1979), so the apparent decline in reporting over time may result from use of different interview methods (USDHHS 1989).

Other research suggests that underreporting of cigarette use has not increased over time. Hatziandreu and colleagues (1989) compared total self-reported cigarette consumption (based on 1974–1985 data from NHIS and NHSDA) with adjusted consumption data (based on cigarette excise taxes) from the U.S. Department of Agriculture for the same period. The researchers found no increase in the underreporting of cigarette smoking and concluded that cross-sectional surveys of self-reported smoking status are reliable. They also found no change when they compared their data with results from comparable surveys conducted in the 1960s.

Biochemical validation studies also suggested that data on self-reported cigarette consumption are valid, except in certain situations, such as in conjunction with intense smoking cessation programs, and with certain populations, such as pregnant women or adolescents (USDHHS 1990d, 1994; Kendrick et al. 1995; Velicer et al. 1992). A meta-analysis of 26 validation studies found that self-reported smoking status is generally accurate (Patrick et al. 1994), particularly when interviewer-administered questionnaires are used.

Underreporting may vary by race and ethnicity (Brownson et al. 1999), but not all studies found racial or ethnic differences in underreporting (Wills and Cleary 1997). A study by Bauman and Ennett (1994) found that blacks were more likely than whites to underreport tobacco use. Wagenknecht and coworkers (1992) found that misclassification was low among adults aged 18 through 30 years overall but relatively high among blacks and among respondents with a high school education or less. For some subgroups, the misclassification rate could be as high as 4 percent. In HHANES, 6.3 percent of Mexican Americans who self-reported that they were nonsmokers were classified as smokers on the basis of serum cotinine levels (Pérez-Stable et al. 1992). In another study, self-reported prevalence was 4 percentage points lower than the cotinine-validated prevalence among Hispanic women in New Mexico (Coultas et al. 1988). Wewers and colleagues (1995) found that smoking was significantly underreported among Southeast Asian immigrant women, particularly Cambodian and Laotian women. Misclassification may also be more common among occasional smokers; Wells and colleagues (1998) reported that misclassification rates (female smokers misclassified as females who had never smoked) was 0.8 percent among majority (white) regular smokers, 6.0 percent among majority occasional smokers, 2.8 percent among minority (black, Latino) regular smokers, and 15.3 percent among minority occasional smokers.

Even if estimates of smoking prevalence are reliable, smokers may misreport the number of cigarettes smoked per day because of digit preference (preference for multiples of 10). In the 1976–1980 NHANES II, persons who had smoked more heavily, whites, and those with less education were more likely to show digit preference (Klesges et al. 1995). Smokers may also underreport the number of cigarettes smoked per day (Warner and Murt 1982). In HHANES data, 3 percent of Mexican American women who reported smoking 20 or more cigarettes per day and 25 percent of Mexican American women who reported smoking 1 to 9 cigarettes per day had cotinine levels indicating higher consumption (Pérez-Stable et al. 1990a). Explanations for these findings may include racial and ethnic differences in underreporting, cotinine metabolism, depth of inhalation, and the quantity of cigarettes smoked.

Underreporting of cigarette smoking status may be more of a problem among children and adolescents than among adults. Williams and associates (1979) found, however, that adolescents reported their smoking status accurately when confidentiality was stressed. Dolcini and colleagues (1996), in their review of 28 studies, concluded that assuring adolescents of confidentiality, and if possible, anonymity, should increase reporting accuracy. Traditionally, self-administered school surveys provide more confidentiality and anonymity than household surveys, and self-reports of current smoking from school surveys appear to be valid (Bauman et al. 1982). Traditional household surveys that use face-to-face interviews tend to underreport prevalence of tobacco use, particularly among young adolescents (Rootman and Smart 1985; USDHHS 1994; Hedges and Jarvis 1998). Telephone surveys of adolescents and young adults may also underestimate smoking prevalence (Luepker et al. 1989). However, in a comparison of responses from self-administered, school-based and household-based questionnaires among white, middle-class high school students, Zanes and Matsoukas (1979) did not find any statistically significant differences in the reported use of legal or illegal drugs. A study of telephone versus in-person interviews among Latino girls also found no difference in the reporting of smoking-related behaviors (Kaplan and Tanjasiri 1996). Dolcini and colleagues (1996) noted that adolescent self-report is generally accurate, but that accuracy may be improved if adolescents expect external confirmation of their smoking status.

The 1974–1993 NHSDA surveys were standard household surveys in which respondents were interviewed aloud by trained interviewers, which would tend to lessen the confidentiality of responses if others in the household were present. Beginning with the 1994 NHSDA, survey methods were changed from an interview format to a self-completed written questionnaire to increase confidentiality of responses. This change in method also resulted in the elimination of skip patterns (see definition for "skip pattern" in Appendix 2), and the initial response was edited to be consistent with later answers (Brittingham 1998). A split sample was used in 1994 to assess the effect of the change. The new method resulted in prevalence estimates of smoking that were two times higher overall and three times higher among adolescents aged 12 through 13 years (SAMHSA 1995b). These prevalence estimates from the new methodology are more comparable to those from self-administered school surveys.

Measures using recall about smoking initiation or past attempts to quit smoking may be less accurate than data about current smoking behavior; however, Gilpin and colleagues (1994) found that the distribution of reported age at smoking initiation among birth cohorts was consistent across survey years. Gilpin and Pierce (1994) also found that smokers did not recall unsuccessful cessation attempts that occurred far in the past or were of short duration, a finding also reported by Stanton and colleagues (1996b).

# References


Abelson HI, Atkinson RB. *Public Experience with Psychoactive Substances: a Nationwide Study among Adults and Youth.* Princeton (NJ): Response Analysis Corporation, 1975.

Abelson HI, Fishburne PM. *Nonmedical Use of Psychoactive Substances: 1975/6 Nationwide Study Among Youth and Adults. Part I: main findings.* Princeton (NJ): Response Analysis Corporation, 1976.

Abelson HI, Fishburne PM, Cisin I. *National Survey on Drug Abuse: 1977: A Nationwide Study—Youth, Young Adults, and Older People. Volume 1: Main Findings.* Rockville (MD): U.S. Department of Health, Education and Welfare, Public Health Service, Alcohol, Drug Abuse, and Mental Health Administration, National Institute on Drug Abuse, Division of Research, 1977. DHEW Publication No. (ADM) 78-618.

Adams PF, Benson V. Current estimates from the National Health Interview Survey, 1991. *Vital and Health Statistics.* Series 10, No. 184. Hyattsville (MD): U.S. Department of Health and Human Services, Public Health Service, Centers for Disease Control, National Center for Health Statistics, 1992. DHHS Publication No. (PHS) 93-1512.

Adams PF, Schoenborn CA, Moss AJ, Warren CW, Kann L. Health risk behaviors among our nation's youth: United States, 1992. *Vital and Health Statistics.* Series 10, No. 192. Hyattsville (MD): U.S. Department of Health and Human Services, Public Health Service, Centers for Disease Control and Prevention, National Center for Health Statistics, 1995. DHHS Publication No. (PHS) 95-1520.

Ahijevych K, Gillespie J, Demirci M, Jagadeesh J. Menthol and nonmenthol cigarettes and smoke exposure in black and white women. *Pharmacology, Biochemistry and Behavior* 1996;53(2):355–60.

Ahijevych K, Wewers ME. Factors associated with nicotine dependence among African American women cigarette smokers. *Research in Nursing and Health* 1993;16(4):283–92.

Allen K, Simpson G, Winn D, Giovino G. Response rates and characteristics of adolescents in the 1989 Teenage Attitudes and Practices Survey. In: *American Statistical Association: 1991 Proceedings of the Section on Survey Research Methods.* Paper presented at the Annual Meeting of the American Statistical Association, Atlanta, GA, Aug 18–22, 1991, under the sponsorship of the Section on Survey Research methods. Alexandria (VA): American Statistical Association, 1991:575–80.

Allen KF, Moss AJ, Giovino GA, Shopland DR, Pierce JP. Teenage tobacco use: data estimates from the Teenage Attitudes and Practices Survey, United States, 1989. *Advance Data.* No. 224. Hyattsville (MD): U.S. Department of Health and Human Services, Public Health Service, Centers for Disease Control and Prevention, National Center for Health Statistics, 1993. DHHS Publication No. (PHS) 93-1250.

American Psychiatric Association. *Diagnostic and Statistical Manual of Mental Disorders: DSM-IV.* 4th ed. Washington: American Psychiatric Association, 1994.

Anda RF, Remington PL, Sienko DG, Davis RM. Are physicians advising smokers to quit? The patient's perspective. *Journal of the American Medical Association* 1987;257(14):1916–9.

Anda RF, Williamson DF, Escobedo LG, Mast EE, Giovino GA, Remington PL. Depression and the dynamics of smoking: a national perspective. *Journal of the American Medical Association* 1990;264(12):1541–5.

Andersen R, Kasper J, Frankel MR. *Total Survey Error: Applications to Improve Health Surveys.* San Francisco: Jossey-Bass Publishers, 1979.

Anthony JC, Warner LA, Kessler RC. Comparative epidemiology of dependence on tobacco, alcohol, controlled substances, and inhalants: basic findings from the National Comorbidity Survey. *Experimental and Clinical Psychopharmacology* 1994;2(3):244–68.

Arday DR, Tomar SL, Nelson DE, Merritt RK, Schooley MW, Mowery P. State smoking prevalence estimates: a comparison of the behavioral risk factor surveillance system and current population surveys. *American Journal of Public Health* 1997;87(10):1665–9.

Audrain JE, Klesges RC, Klesges LM. Relationship between obesity and the metabolic effects of smoking in women. *Health Psychology* 1995;14(2):116–23.

Bachman JG, Johnston LD, O'Malley PM. *Monitoring the Future: Questionnaire Responses from the Nation's High School Seniors 1976.* Ann Arbor (MI):

University of Michigan, Institute for Social Research, Survey Research Center, 1980a.

Bachman JG, Johnston LD, O'Malley PM. *Monitoring the Future: Questionnaire Responses from the Nation's High School Seniors, 1978.* Ann Arbor (MI): University of Michigan, Institute for Social Research, Survey Research Center, 1980b.

Bachman JG, Johnston LD, O'Malley PM. *Monitoring the Future: Questionnaire Responses from the Nation's High School Seniors, 1980.* Ann Arbor (MI): University of Michigan, Institute for Social Research, Survey Research Center, 1981.

Bachman JG, Johnston LD, O'Malley PM. *Monitoring the Future: Questionnaire Responses from the Nation's High School Seniors, 1982.* Ann Arbor (MI): University of Michigan, Institute for Social Research, Survey Research Center, 1984.

Bachman JG, Johnston LD, O'Malley PM. *Monitoring the Future: Questionnaire Responses from the Nation's High School Seniors, 1984.* Ann Arbor (MI): University of Michigan, Institute for Social Research, Survey Research Center, 1985.

Bachman JG, Johnston LD, O'Malley PM. *Monitoring the Future: Questionnaire Responses from the Nation's High School Seniors, 1986.* Ann Arbor (MI): University of Michigan, Institute for Social Research, Survey Research Center, 1987.

Bachman JG, Johnston LD, O'Malley PM. *Monitoring the Future: Questionnaire Responses from the Nation's High School Seniors, 1988.* Ann Arbor (MI): University of Michigan, Institute for Social Research, Survey Research Center, 1991a.

Bachman JG, Johnston LD, O'Malley PM. *Monitoring the Future: Questionnaire Responses from the Nation's High School Seniors, 1990.* Ann Arbor (MI): University of Michigan, Institute for Social Research, Survey Research Center, 1993a.

Bachman JG, Johnston LD, O'Malley PM. *Monitoring the Future: Questionnaire Responses from the Nation's High School Seniors, 1992.* Ann Arbor (MI): University of Michigan, Institute for Social Research, Survey Research Center, 1993b.

Bachman JG, Wadsworth KN, O'Malley PM, Johnston LD, Schulenberg JE, editors. *Smoking, Drinking, and Drug Use in Young Adulthood: the Impacts of New Freedoms and New Responsibilities.* Mahwah (NJ): Lawrence Erlbaum Associates, 1997.

Bachman JG, Wallace JM Jr, O'Malley PM, Johnston LD, Kurth CL, Neighbors HW. Racial/ethnic differences in smoking, drinking, and illicit drug use among American high school seniors, 1976–89. *American Journal of Public Health* 1991b;81(3):372–7.

Backinger CL, Bruerd B, Kinney MB, Szpunar SM. Knowledge, intent to use, and use of smokeless tobacco among sixth grade schoolchildren in six selected U.S. sites. *Public Health Reports* 1993; 108(5):637–42.

Bauman KE, Ennett SE. Tobacco use by black and white adolescents: the validity of self-reports. *American Journal of Public Health* 1994;84(3):394–8.

Bauman KE, Koch GG, Bryan ES. Validity of self-reports of adolescent cigarette smoking. *International Journal of the Addictions* 1982;17(7):1131–6.

Bauman KE, Koch GG, Fisher LA, Bryan ES. Use of smokeless tobacco by age, race, and gender in ten standard metropolitan statistical areas of the Southeast United States. In: *Smokeless Tobacco Use in the United States.* National Cancer Institute Monograph. Bethesda (MD): U.S. Department of Health and Human Services, Public Health Service, National Institutes of Health, National Cancer Institute, 1989:35–7.

Benowitz NL. Pharmacology of smokeless tobacco use: nicotine addiction and nicotine-related health consequences. In: *Smokeless Tobacco or Health: an International Perspective*. Smoking and Tobacco Control Monograph 2. U.S. Department of Health and Human Services, Public Health Service, National Institutes of Health, 1992. NIH Publication No. 92-3461.

Benowitz NL, Jacob P III. Daily intake of nicotine during cigarette smoking. *Clinical Pharmacology and Therapeutics* 1984;35(4):499–504.

Berman BA, Gritz ER. Women and smoking: current trends and issues for the 1990s. *Journal of Substance Abuse* 1991;3(2):221–38.

Bjornson W, Rand C, Connett JE, Lindgren P, Nides M, Pope F, Buist AS, Hoppe-Ryan C, O'Hara P. Gender differences in smoking cessation after 3 years in the Lung Health Study. *American Journal of Public Health* 1995;85(2):223–30.

Blake SM, Klepp K-I, Pechacek TF, Folsom AR, Luepker RV, Jacobs DR, Mittelmark MB. Differences in smoking cessation strategies between men and women. *Addictive Behaviors* 1989;14(4):409–18.

Bolinder G, Alfredsson L, Englund A, de Faire U. Smokeless tobacco use and increased cardiovascular mortality among Swedish construction workers. *American Journal of Public Health* 1994;84(3): 399–404.

Borras JM, Fernandez E, Schiaffino A, Borrell C, La Vecchia C. Pattern of smoking initiation in Catalonia, Spain, from 1948 to 1992. *American Journal of Public Health* 2000;90(9):1459–62.

Brackbill R, Frazier T, Shilling S. Smoking characteristics of U.S. workers, 1978–1980. *American Journal of Industrial Medicine* 1988;13(1):5–41.

Bradford J, Ryan C, Rothblum ED. National Lesbian Health Care Survey: implications for mental health care. *Journal of Counseling and Clinical Psychology* 1994;62(2):228–42.

Bray RM, Kroutil LA, Wheeless SC, Marsden ME, Fairbank JA, Harford TC. *Highlights 1995 Department of Defense Survey of Health Related Behaviors Among Military Personnel.* Research Triangle Park (NC): Research Triangle Institute, 1996. RTI/6019/06-FR.

Bray RM, Sanchez RP, Ornstein ML, Lentine D, Vincus AA, Baird TU, Walker JA, Wheeless SC, Guess LL, Kroutil LA, Iannacchione VG. *1998 Department of Defense Survey of Health Related Behaviors Among Military Personnel.* Research Triangle Park (NC): Research Triangle Institute, 1999. RTI/7034/006-FR.

Breslau N. Daily cigarette consumption in early adulthood: age of smoking initiation and duration of smoking. *Drug and Alcohol Dependence* 1993;33(3):287–91.

Breslau N. Psychiatric comorbidity of smoking and nicotine dependence. *Behavior Genetics* 1995;25(2):95–101.

Breslau N, Fenn N, Peterson EL. Early smoking initiation and nicotine dependence in a cohort of young adults. *Drug and Alcohol Dependence* 1993a;33(2):129–37.

Breslau N, Kilbey M, Andreski P. Nicotine dependence, major depression, and anxiety in young adults. *Archives of General Psychiatry* 1991;48(12):1069–74.

Breslau N, Kilbey MM, Andreski P. Vulnerability to psychopathology in nicotine-dependent smokers: an epidemiologic study of young adults. *American Journal of Psychiatry* 1993b;150(6):941–6.

Breslau N, Peterson EL. Smoking cessation in young adults: age at initiation of cigarette smoking and other suspected influences. *American Journal of Public Health* 1996;86(2):214–20.

Brittingham A, Tourangeau R, Kay W. Reports of Smoking in a National Survey: data from screening and detailed interviews, and from self- and interviewer-administered questions. *Annals of Epidemiology* 1998;8:393–401.

Brooks JE. *The Mighty Leaf: Tobacco Through the Centuries.* Boston: Little, Brown, and Company, 1952.

Brownson RC, Eyler AA, King AC, Shyu Y-L, Brown DR, Homan SM. Reliability of information on physical activity and other chronic disease risk factors among US women aged 40 years or older. *American Journal of Epidemiology* 1999;149(4):379–91.

Burbank F. U.S. lung cancer death rates begin to rise proportionately more rapidly for females than for males: a dose-response effect? *Journal of Chronic Diseases* 1972;25(8):473–9.

Bureau of Indian Affairs. *Youth Risk Behavior Survey of High School Students Attending Bureau Funded Schools.* U.S. Department of the Interior, Bureau of Indian Affairs, Office of Indian Education Programs, 1997.

Burns D, Pierce JP. *Tobacco use in California, 1990–1991.* Sacramento (CA): California Department of Health Services, 1992.

Burns DM, Lee L, Shen LZ, Gilpin E, Tolley HD, Vaughn J, Shanks TG. Cigarette smoking behavior in the United States. In: Shopland R, Burns DM, Garfinkel L, Samet JM, editors. *Changes in Cigarette-Related Disease Risks and Their Implication for Prevention and Control.* Smoking and Tobacco Control Monograph 8. U.S. Department of Health and Human Services, Public Health Service, National Institutes of Health, National Cancer Institute, 1997: 13–42. NIH Publication No. 97-4213.

Burns DM, Lee L, Vaughn JW, Chiu YK, Shopland DR. Rates of smoking initiation among adolescents and young adults, 1907–81. *Tobacco Control* 1995; 4(Suppl 1):S2–S8.

Burt RD, Peterson AV. Smoking cessation among high school seniors. *Preventive Medicine* 1998;27(3):319–27.

Camp DE, Klesges RC, Relyea G. The relationship between body weight concerns and adolescent smoking. *Health Psychology* 1993;12(1):24–32.

Caraballo RS, Giovino GA, Pechacek TF, Mowery PD, Richter PA, Strauss WJ, Sharp DJ, Eriksen MP, Pirkle JL, Maurer KR. Racial and ethnic differences in serum cotinine levels of cigarette smokers. Third National Health and Nutrition Examination Survey, 1988–1991. *Journal of the American Medical Association* 1998;280(2):135–9.

Cavin SW, Pierce JP. Low-cost cigarettes and smoking behavior in California, 1990–1993. *American Journal of Preventive Medicine* 1996;12(1):17–21.

Centers for Disease Control. Smokeless tobacco use in rural Alaska. *Morbidity and Mortality Weekly Report* 1987a;36(10):140–3.

Centers for Disease Control. Cigarette smoking in the United States, 1986. *Morbidity and Mortality Weekly Report* 1987b;36(35):581–5.

Centers for Disease Control. Results from the National Adolescent Student Health Survey. *Morbidity and Mortality Weekly Report* 1989;38(9):147–50.

Centers for Disease Control. Tobacco use among high school students—United States, 1990. *Morbidity and Mortality Weekly Report* 1991a;40(36):617–9.

Centers for Disease Control. Differences in the age of smoking initiation between blacks and whites—United States. *Morbidity and Mortality Weekly Report* 1991b;40(44):754–7.

Centers for Disease Control. Tobacco, alcohol, and other drug use among high school students—United States, 1991. *Morbidity and Mortality Weekly Report* 1992;41(37):698–703.

Centers for Disease Control and Prevention. Smoking cessation during previous year among adults—United States, 1990 and 1991. *Morbidity and Mortality Weekly Report* 1993;42(26):504–7.

Centers for Disease Control and Prevention. Changes in the cigarette brand preferences of adolescent smokers—United States 1989–1993. *Morbidity and Mortality Weekly Report* 1994a;43(32):577–81.

Centers for Disease Control and Prevention. Cigarette smoking among adults—United States, 1992, and changes in the definition of current cigarette smoking. *Morbidity and Mortality Weekly Report* 1994b;43(19):342–6.

Centers for Disease Control and Prevention. Cigarette smoking among adults—United States, 1993. *Morbidity and Mortality Weekly Report* 1994c;43(50): 925–29.

Centers for Disease Control and Prevention. Reasons for tobacco use and symptoms of nicotine withdrawal among adolescent and young adult tobacco users—United States, 1993. *Morbidity and Mortality Weekly Report* 1994d;43(41):745–50.

Centers for Disease Control and Prevention. Indicators of nicotine addiction among women—United States, 1991–1992. *Morbidity and Mortality Weekly Report* 1995a;44(6):102–5.

Centers for Disease Control and Prevention. Smokeless tobacco use among American Indian Women—Southeastern North Carolina, 1991. *Morbidity and Mortality Weekly Report* 1995b;44(6): 113–7.

Centers for Disease Control and Prevention. Trends in smoking initiation among adolescents and young adults—United States, 1980–1989. *Morbidity and Mortality Weekly Report* 1995c;44(28):521–5.

Centers for Disease Control and Prevention. Healthcare provider advice on tobacco use to persons aged 10–22 years—United States, 1993. *Morbidity and Mortality Weekly Report* 1995d;44(44):826–30.

Centers for Disease Control and Prevention. Cigarette smoking among adults—United States, 1994. *Morbidity and Mortality Weekly Report* 1996;45(27): 588–90.

Centers for Disease Control and Prevention. Cigar smoking among teenagers—United States, Massachusetts, and New York, 1996. *Morbidity and Mortality Weekly Report* 1997a;46(20):433–40.

Centers for Disease Control and Prevention. State-specific prevalence of cigarette smoking among adults, and children's and adolescents' exposure to environmental tobacco smoke—United States, 1996. *Morbidity and Mortality Weekly Report* 1997b; 46(44):1038–43.

Centers for Disease Control and Prevention. Cigarette smoking among adults—United States, 1995. *Morbidity and Mortality Weekly Report* 1997c;46(51): 1217–20.

Centers for Disease Control and Prevention. Tobacco use among high school students—United States, 1997. *Morbidity and Mortality Weekly Report* 1998a; 47(12):229–33.

Centers for Disease Control and Prevention. Selected cigarette smoking initiation and quitting behaviors among high school students—United States, 1997. *Morbidity and Mortality Weekly Report* 1998b; 47(19):386–9.

Centers for Disease Control and Prevention. Bidi use among urban youth—Massachusetts, March–April 1999. *Morbidity and Mortality Weekly Report* 1999a; 48(36):796–99.

Centers for Disease Control and Prevention. Cigarette smoking among adults—United States, 1997. *Morbidity and Mortality Weekly Report* 1999b;48(43): 994–6.

Centers for Disease Control and Prevention. Cigarette smoking among adults—United States, 1998. *Morbidity and Mortality Weekly Report* 2000a;49(39): 881–4.

Centers for Disease Control and Prevention. Youth tobacco surveillance—United States, 1998–1999. *Morbidity and Mortality Weekly Report* 2000b;49(SS-10):1–94.

Chandra A. Health aspects of pregnancy and childbirth: United States, 1982–1988. *Vital and Health Statistics.* Series 23, No. 18. Hyattsville (MD): U.S. Department of Health and Human Services, Public Health Service, Centers for Disease Control and Prevention, National Center for Health Statistics, 1995. DHHS Publication No. (PHS) 95-1994.

Charlton A. Children's opinions about smoking. *Journal of the Royal College of General Practitioners* 1984; 34(266):483–7.

Chassin L, Presson CC, Rose JS, Sherman SJ. The natural history of cigarette smoking from adolescence to adulthood: demographic predictors of continuity and change. *Health Psychology* 1996;15(6): 478–84.

Chen J, Millar WJ. Age of smoking initiation: implications for quitting. *Health Reports* 1998;9(4):39–46.

Choi WS, Patten CA, Gillin JC, Kaplan RM, Pierce JP. Cigarette smoking predicts development of depressive symptoms among U.S. adolescents. *Annals of Behavioral Medicine* 1997;19(1):42–50.

Coambs RB, Li S, Kozlowski LT. Age interacts with heaviness of smoking in predicting success in cessation of smoking. *American Journal of Epidemiology* 1992;135(3):240–6.

Cohen S, Lichtenstein E, Prochaska JO, Rossi JS, Gritz ER, Carr CR, Orleans CT, Schoenbach VJ, Biener L, Abrams D, DiClemente C, Curry S, Marlatt GA, Cummings KM, Emont SL, Giovino G, Ossip-Klein D. Debunking myths about self-quitting: evidence from 10 prospective studies of persons who attempt to quit smoking by themselves. *American Psychologist* 1989;44(11):1355–65.

Colditz GA, Segal MR, Myers AH, Stampfer MJ, Willett W, Speizer RE. Weight change in relation to smoking cessation among women. *Journal of Smoking-Related Disorders* 1992;3(2):145–53.

Coleman MP, Esteve J, Damiecki P, Arsla A, Renard H. *Trends in Cancer Incidence and Mortality*. IARC Scientific Publication No. 121. Lyon (France): International Agency for Research on Cancer, 1993.

Conover AG. Discussion of Elmo Jackson's paper. *Journal of Farm Economics* 1950;32 (4 Pt 2):923–4.

Conrad KM, Flay BR, Hill D. Why children start smoking cigarettes: predictors of onset. *British Journal of Addiction* 1992;87(12):1711–24.

Coriell M, Adler NE. Socioeconomic status and women's health: how do we measure SES among women? *Women's Health: Research on Gender, Behavior, and Policy* 1996;2(3):141–56.

Coultas DB, Howard CA, Peake GT, Skipper BJ, Samet JM. Discrepancies between self-reported and validated cigarette smoking in a community survey of New Mexico Hispanics. *American Review of Respiratory Disease* 1988;137(4):810–4.

Coultas DB, Stidley CA, Samet JM. Cigarette yields of tar and nicotine and markers of exposure to tobacco smoke. *American Review of Respiratory Disease* 1993;148(2):435–40.

Covey LS, Glassman AH, Stetner F. Depression and depressive symptoms in smoking cessation. *Comprehensive Psychiatry* 1990;31(4):350–4.

Covey LS, Tam D. Depressive mood, the single-parent home, and adolescent cigarette smoking. *American Journal of Public Health* 1990;80(11):1330–3.

Covey LS, Zang EA, Wynder EL. Cigarette smoking and occupational status: 1977 to 1990. *American Journal of Public Health* 1992;82(9):1230–4.

Cowdery JE, Fitzhugh EC, Wang MQ. Sociobehavioral influences on smoking initiation of Hispanic adolescents. *Journal of Adolescent Health* 1997;20(1): 46–50.

Creek L, Capehart T, Grise V. *U.S. Tobacco Statistics, 1935–1992.* Statistical Bulletin No. 869. Washington: U.S. Department of Agriculture, Economic Research Service, Commodity Economics Division, 1994.

Crittenden KS, Manfredi C, Lacey L, Warnecke R, Parsons J. Measuring readiness and motivation to quit smoking among women in public health clinics. *Addictive Behaviors* 1994;19(5):497–507.

Croft JB, Strogatz DS, James SA, Keenan NL, Ammerman AS, Malarcher AM, Haines PS. Socioeconomic and behavioral correlates of body mass index in Black adults: the Pitt County Study. *American Journal of Public Health* 1992;82(6):821–6.

Cummings KM, Hyland A, Pechacek TF, Orlandi M, Lynn WR. Comparison of recent trends in adolescent and adult cigarette smoking behaviour and brand preferences. *Tobacco Control* 1997;6(Suppl 2): S31–S37.

Cummings KM, Markello SJ, Mahoney MC, Marshall JR. Measurement of lifetime exposure to passive smoke. *American Journal of Epidemiology* 1989; 130(1):122–32.

Denny CH, Holtzman D. *Health Behaviors of American Indians and Alaska Natives: Findings from the Behavioral Risk Factor Surveillance System, 1993–1996.* Atlanta: Centers for Disease Control and Prevention, 1999.

Denny CH, Taylor TL. American Indian and Alaska Native health behavior: findings from the Behavioral Risk Factor Surveillance System, 1992–1995. *Ethnicity and Disease* 1999;9(3):403–9.

Derby CA, Lasater TM, Vass K, Gonzalez S, Carleton RA. Characteristics of smokers who attempt to quit and of those who recently succeeded. *American Journal of Preventive Medicine* 1994;10(6):327–34.

DiClemente CC, Prochaska JO, Fairhurst SK, Velicer WF, Valasquez MM, Rossi JS. The process of smoking cessation: an analysis of precontemplation, contemplation, and preparation stages of change. *Journal of Consulting and Clinical Psychology* 1991; 59(2):295–304.

Dietz PM, Adams MM, Kendrick JS, Mathis MP, the PRAMS Working Group. Completeness of ascertainment of prenatal smoking using birth certificates and confidential questionnaires. *American Journal of Epidemiology* 1998;148(11):1048–54.

Distefan JM, Gilpin EA, Choi WS, Pierce JP. Parental influences predict adolescent smoking in the United States, 1989–1993. *Journal of Adolescent Health* 1998;22(6):466–74.

Dolcini MM, Adler NE, Ginsberg D. Factors influencing agreement between self-reports and biological measures of smoking among adolescents. *Journal of Research on Adolescence* 1996;6(4):515–42.

Doll R, Peto R, Wheatley K, Gray R, Sutherland I. Mortality in relation to smoking: 40 years' observations on male British doctors. *British Medical Journal* 1994;309(6959):901–11.

Ebi-Kryston KL, Higgins MW, Keller JB. Health and other characteristics of employed women and homemakers in Tecumseh, 1959–1978: I. Demographic characteristics, smoking habits, alcohol consumption, and pregnancy outcomes and conditions. *Women and Health* 1990;16(2):5–21.

Ebrahim SH, Floyd RL, Merritt RK Jr, Decoufle P, Holtzman D. Trends in pregnancy-related smoking rates in the United States, 1987–1996. *Journal of the American Medical Association* 2000;283(3):361–6.

Eiser JR, Van Der Pligt J. "Sick" or "hooked": smokers' perceptions of their addiction. *Addictive Behaviors* 1986;11(1):11–5.

Emmons KM, Wechsler H, Dowdall G, Abraham M. Predictors of smoking among US college students. *American Journal of Public Health* 1998;88(1):104–7.

Environmental Protection Agency. *Respiratory Health Effects of Passive Smoking: Lung Cancer and Other Disorders*. Washington: U.S. Environmental Protection Agency, Office of Research and Development, Office of Air Radiation, 1992. Report No. EPA/600/6-90/0006F.

Ernster VL. Mixed messages for women. A social history of cigarette smoking and advertising. *New York State Journal of Medicine* 1985;85(7):335–40.

Ershler J, Leventhal H, Fleming R, Glynn K. The quitting experience for smokers in sixth through twelfth grades. *Addictive Behaviors* 1989;14(4):365–78.

Escobedo LG, Marcus SE, Holtzman D, Giovino GA. Sports participation, age at smoking initiation, and the risk of smoking among U.S. high school students. *Journal of the American Medical Association* 1993;269(11):1391–5.

Escobedo LG, Peddicord JP. Smoking prevalence in US birth cohorts: the influence of gender and education. *American Journal of Public Health* 1996;86(2):231–6.

Escobedo LG, Reddy M, DuRant RH. Relationship between cigarette smoking and health risk and problem behaviors among US adolescents. *Archives of Pediatrics and Adolescent Medicine* 1997;151(1):66–71.

Escobedo LG, Remington PL. Birth cohort analysis of prevalence of cigarette smoking among Hispanics in the United States. *Journal of the American Medical Association* 1989;261(1):66–9.

Escobedo LG, Remington PL, Anda RF. Long-term age-specific prevalence of cigarette smoking among Hispanics in the United States. *Journal of Psychoactive Drugs* 1989;21(3):307–18.

Everett SA, Giovino GA, Warren CW, Crossett L, Kann L. Other substance use among high school students who use tobacco. *Journal of Adolescent Health* 1998;23(5):289–96.

Everett SA, Husten CG, Kann L, Warren CW, Sharp D, Crossett L. Smoking initiation and smoking patterns among US college students. *Journal of American College Health* 1999a;48(2):55–60.

Everett SA, Warren CW, Sharp D, Kann L, Husten CG, Crossett LS. Initiation of cigarette smoking and subsequent smoking behavior among U.S. high school students. *Preventive Medicine* 1999b;29(5):327–33.

Fagerström K-O. Measuring degree of physical dependence to tobacco smoking with reference to individualization of treatment. *Addictive Behaviors* 1978;3(3–4):235–41.

Faulkner AH, Cranston K. Correlates of same-sex sexual behavior in a random sample of Massachusetts high school students. *American Journal of Public Health* 1998;88(2):262–6.

Federal Trade Commission. *Report to Congress for 1998: Pursuant to the Federal Cigarette Labeling and Advertising Act*. Washington: Federal Trade Commission, 2000.

Fingerhut LA, Kleinman JC, Kendrick JS. Smoking before, during, and after pregnancy. *American Journal of Public Health* 1990;80(5):541–4.

Fiore MC. Trends in cigarette smoking in the United States: the epidemiology of tobacco use. *Medical Clinics of North America* 1992;76(2):289–303.

Fiore MC, Bailey WC, Cohen SJ, Dorfman SF, Goldstein MG, Gritz ER, Heyman RB, Holbrook J, Jaen CR, Kottke TE, Lando HA, Mecklenburg R,

Mullen PD, Nett LM, Robinson K, Stitzer ML, Tommasello AC, Villejo L, Wewers ME. *Smoking Cessation.* Clinical Practice Guideline No. 18. Rockville (MD): U.S. Department of Health and Human Services, Public Health Service, Agency for Health Care Policy and Research, 1996. AHCPR Publication No. 96-0692.

Fiore MC, Bailey WC, Cohen SJ, Dorfman SF, Goldstein MG, Gritz ER, Heyman RB, Jaén CR, Kottke TE, Lando HA, Mecklenburg R, Mullen PD, Nett LM, Robinson K, Stitzer ML, Tommasello AC, Villejo L, Wewers ME. *Treating Tobacco Use and Dependence.* Clinical Practice Guideline. Rockville (MD): U.S. Department of Health and Human Services, Public Health Service, 2000.

Fiore MC, Novotny TE, Pierce JP, Giovino GA, Hatziandreu EJ, Newcomb PA, Surawicz TS, Davis RM. Methods used to quit smoking in the United States: do cessation programs help? *Journal of the American Medical Association* 1990;263(20): 2760–5.

Fiore MC, Novotny TE, Pierce JP, Hatziandreu EJ, Patel KM, Davis RM. Trends in cigarette smoking in the United States: the changing influence of gender and race. *Journal of the American Medical Association* 1989;261(1):49–55.

Fisher M, Schneider M, Pegler C, Napolitano B. Eating attitudes, health-risk behaviors, self-esteem, and anxiety among adolescent females in a suburban high school. *Journal of Adolescent Health* 1991; 12(5):377–84.

Flay BR, Hu FB, Richardson J. Psychosocial predictors of different stages of cigarette smoking among high school students. *Preventive Medicine* 1998; 27(5 Pt 3):A9–A18.

Flay BR, Hu FB, Siddiqui O, Day LE, Hedeker D, Petraitis J, Richardson J, Sussman S. Differential influence of parental smoking and friends' smoking on adolescent initiation and escalation of smoking. *Journal of Health and Social Behavior* 1994; 35(3):248–65.

Flay BR, Ockene JK, Tager IB. Smoking: epidemiology, cessation, and prevention. *Chest* 1992;102(3 Suppl): 277S–301S.

Flegal KM, Troiano RP, Pamuk ER, Kuczmarski RJ, Campbell SM. The influence of smoking cessation on the prevalence of overweight in the United States. *New England Journal of Medicine* 1995; 333(18):1165–70.

Floyd RL, Rimer BK, Giovino GA, Mullen PD, Sullivan SE. A review of smoking in pregnancy: effects on pregnancy outcomes and cessation efforts. In: Omenn GS, Fielding JE, Lave LB, editors. *Annual Review of Public Health* 1993;14:379–411.

Ford RPK, Tappin DM, Schluter PJ, Wild CJ. Smoking during pregnancy: how reliable are maternal self reports in New Zealand? *Journal of Epidemiology and Community Health* 1997;51(3):246–51.

Fortmann SP, Killen JD. Who shall quit? Comparison of volunteer and population-based recruitment in two minimal-contact smoking cessation studies. *American Journal of Epidemiology* 1994;140(1):39–51.

*Fortune Magazine*. The Fortune survey III. Cigarettes. *Fortune Magazine* 1935;12(1):68, 111–6.

Frazier EL, Franks AL, Sanderson LM. Behavioral risk factor data. In: *Using Chronic Disease Data: A Handbook for Public Health Practitioners.* Atlanta: U.S. Department of Health and Human Services, Public Health Service, Centers for Disease Control, National Center for Chronic Disease Prevention and Health Promotion, Office of Surveillance and Analysis, 1992;4-1–4-17.

Freedman DS, Serdula MK, Percy CA, Ballew C, White L. Obesity, levels of lipids and glucose, and smoking among Navajo adolescents. *Journal of Nutrition* 1997;127:2120S–2127S.

French SA, Jeffery RW. Weight concerns and smoking: a literature review. *Annals of Behavioral Medicine* 1995;17(3):234–44.

French SA, Jeffery RW, Pirie PL, McBride CM. Do weight concerns hinder smoking cessation efforts? *Addictive Behaviors* 1992;17(3):219–26.

French SA, Perry CL, Leon GR, Fulkerson JA. Weight concerns, dieting behavior, and smoking initiation among adolescents: a prospective study. *American Journal of Public Health* 1994;84(11):1818–20.

French SA, Story M, Downes B, Resnick MD, Blum RW. Frequent dieting among adolescents: psychosocial and health behavior correlates. *American Journal of Public Health* 1995;85(5):695–701.

Freund KM, D'Agostino RB, Belanger AJ, Kannel WB, Stokes J III. Predictors of smoking cessation: the Framingham Study. *American Journal of Epidemiology* 1992;135(9):957–64.

Gallup GH. *The Gallup Poll: Public Opinion 1935–1971. Volume One: 1935–1948.* New York: Random House, 1972a.

Gallup GH. *The Gallup Poll: Public Opinion 1935–1971. Volume Two: 1949–1958.* New York: Random House, 1972b.

Garfinkel L, Silverberg E. Lung cancer and smoking trends in the United States over the past 25 years. *Annals of the New York Academy of Science* 1990;609: 146–54.

Garofalo R, Wolf RC, Kessel S, Palfrey J, DuRant RH. The association between health risk behaviors and sexual orientation among a school-based sample of adolescents. *Pediatrics* 1998;101(5):895–902.

Garvey AJ, Bosse R, Glynn RJ, Rosner B. Smoking cessation in a prospective study of healthy adult males: effects of age, time period, and amount smoked. *American Journal of Public Health* 1983; 73(4):446–50.

Gentry EM, Kalsbeek WD, Hogelin GC, Jones JT, Gaines KL, Forman MR, Marks JS, Trowbridge FL. The Behavioral Risk Factor Surveys: II. Design, methods, and estimates from combined state data. *American Journal of Preventive Medicine* 1985;1(6): 9–14.

George H. Gallup International Institute. *Teen-Age Attitudes and Behavior Concerning Tobacco: Report of the Findings*. Princeton (NJ): George H. Gallup International Institute, 1992.

Gerlach KK, Cummings KM, Hyland A, Gilpin EA, Johnson M, Pierce JP. Trends in cigar consumption and smoking prevalence. In: *Cigars: Health Effects and Trends*. Smoking and Tobacco Control Monograph 9. U.S. Department of Health and Human Services, Public Health Service, National Institutes of Health, 1998:21–53. NIH Publication No. 98–4302.

Gerlach KK, Shopland DR, Hartman AM, Gibson JT, Pechacek TF. Workplace smoking policies in the United States: results from a national survey of more than 100,000 workers. *Tobacco Control* 1997; 6(3):199–206.

Gfroerer J, Wright D, Kopstein A. Prevalence of youth substance use: the impact of methodological differences between two national surveys. *Drug and Alcohol Dependence* 1997a;47(1):19–30.

Gfroerer JC, Greenblatt JC, Wright DA. Substance use in the US college-age population: differences according to educational status and living arrangement. *American Journal of Public Health* 1997b; 87(1):62–5.

Gilbert BJC, Johnson CH, Morrow B, Gaffield ME, Ahluwalia I, PRAMS Working Group. Prevalence of selected maternal and infant characteristics, Pregnancy Risk Assessment Monitoring System (PRAMS), 1997. *Morbidity and Mortality Weekly Report* 1999;48(SS-5):1–37.

Gilpin E, Pierce JP. Measuring smoking cessation: problems with recall in the 1990 California Tobacco Survey. *Cancer Epidemiology, Biomarkers and Prevention* 1994;3(7):613–7.

Gilpin E, Pierce JP, Goodman J, Burns D, Shopland D. Reasons smokers give for stopping smoking: do they relate to success in stopping? *Tobacco Control* 1992;1(4):256–63.

Gilpin EA, Lee L, Evans N, Pierce JP. Smoking initiation rates in adults and minors: United States, 1944–1988. *American Journal of Epidemiology* 1994; 140(6):535–43.

Giovino GA, Henningfield JE, Tomar SL, Escobedo LG, Slade J. Epidemiology of tobacco use and dependence. *Epidemiologic Reviews* 1995;17(1):48–65.

Giovino GA, Schooley MW, Zhu B-P, Chrismon JH, Tomar SL, Peddicord JP, Merritt RK, Husten CG, Eriksen MP. Surveillance for selected tobacco-use behaviors—United States, 1900–1994. *Morbidity and Mortality Weekly Report* 1994;43(SS-3):1–43.

Giovino GA, Shelton DM, Schooley MW. Trends in cigarette smoking cessation in the United States. *Tobacco Control* 1993;2(Suppl):S3–S16.

Giovino GA, Tomar SL, Reddy MN, Peddicord JP, Zhu B-P, Escobedo LG, Eriksen MP. Attitudes, knowledge, and beliefs about low-yield cigarettes among adolescent and adults. In: *The FTC Cigarette Test Method for Determining Tar, Nicotine, and Carbon Monoxide Yields of U.S. Cigarettes: Report of the NCI Expert Committee.* Smoking and Tobacco Control Monograph 7. Rockville (MD): U.S. Department of Health and Human Services, Public Health Service, National Institutes of Health, National Cancer Institute, 1996;39–57. NIH Publication No. 96-4028.

Giuliano A, Papenfuss M, De Zapien JG, Tilousi S, Nuvayestewa L. Prevalence of chronic disease risk and protective behaviors among American Indian women living on the Hopi reservation. *Annals of Epidemiology* 1998;8(3):160–7.

Glassman AH, Helzer JE, Covey LS, Cottler LB, Stetner F, Tipp JE, Johnson J. Smoking, smoking cessation, and major depression. *Journal of the American Medical Association* 1990;264(12):1546–9.

Glover ED, Glover PN. The smokeless tobacco problem: risk groups in North America. In: *Smokeless Tobacco or Health: an International Perspective.* Smoking and Tobacco Control Monograph 2. U.S. Department of Health and Human Services, Public Health Service, National Institutes of Health, 1992. NIH Publication No. 92-3461.

Goldstein MG, Niaura R, Wiley-Lessne C, DePue J, Eaton C, Rakowski W, Dubé C. Physicians counseling smokers. A population-based survey of patients' perceptions of health care provider-delivered smoking cessation interventions. *Archives of Internal Medicine* 1997;157(12):1313–19.

Gordon T, Kannel WB, Dawber TR, McGee D. Changes associated with quitting cigarette smoking: the Framingham Study. *American Heart Journal* 1975;90(3):322–8.

Gorrod JW, Jenner P. The metabolism of tobacco alkaloids. In: Hayes WJ Jr, editor. *Essays in Toxicology.* Vol. 6. New York: Academic Press, 1975:35–78.

Gottsegen JJ. *Tobacco: A Study of Its Consumption in the United States*. New York: Pitman Publishing, 1940.

Green DE, Nemzer DE. Changes in cigarette smoking by women—an analysis, 1966 and 1970. *Health Services Reports* 1973;88(7):631–6.

Gritz ER. Problems related to the use of tobacco by women. In: Kalant OJ, editor. *Alcohol and Drug Problems in Women. Research Advances in Alcohol and Drug Abuse,* Vol. 5. New York: Plenum Press, 1980.

Gritz ER, Crane LA. Use of diet pills and amphetamines to lose weight among smoking and nonsmoking high school seniors. *Health Psychology* 1991;10(5):330–5.

Gritz ER, Klesges RC, Meyers AW. The smoking and body weight relationship: implications for intervention and postcessation weight control. *Annals of Behavioral Medicine* 1989;11(4):144–53.

Gritz ER, St. Jeor ST. Task Force 3: implications with respect to intervention and prevention. *Health Psychology* 1992;11(Suppl):17–25.

Gritz ER, Thompson B, Emmons K, Ockene JK, McLerran DF, Nielsen IR, for the Working Well Research Group. Gender differences among smokers and quitters in the Working Well Trial. *Preventive Medicine* 1998;27(4):553–61.

Grunberg NE, Winders SE, Wewers ME. Gender differences in tobacco use. *Health Psychology* 1991; 10(2):143–53.

Guilford JS. Sex differences between successful and unsuccessful abstainers from smoking. In: Zagona SV, editor. *Studies and Issues in Smoking Behavior.* Tucson (AZ): University of Arizona Press, 1967: 95–102.

Guilford JS. Group treatment versus individual initiative in the cessation of smoking. *Journal of Applied Psychology* 1972;56(2):162–7.

Gunn RC. Reactions to withdrawal symptoms and success in smoking cessation clinics. *Addictive Behaviors* 1986;11(1):49–53.

Gupta PC. Survey of sociodemographic characteristics of tobacco use among 99,598 individuals in Bombay, India using handheld computers. *Tobacco Control* 1996;5(2):114–20.

Gupta PC, Hamner JE, Murti PR, editors. *Control of Tobacco-Related Cancers and Other Diseases.* Proceedings of an International Symposium; 1990 Jan 15–19; Bombay. Bombay: Oxford University Press, 1992.

Haenszel W, Shimkin MB, Miller HP. *Tobacco Smoking Patterns in the United States.* Public Health Monograph 45. Washington: U.S. Department of Health, Education, and Welfare, Public Health Service, 1956. Publication No. (PHS) 463.

Hahn LP, Folsom AR, Sprafka JM, Norsted SW. Cigarette smoking and cessation behaviors among urban blacks and whites. *Public Health Reports* 1990;105(3):290–5.

Hale KL, Hughes JR, Oliveto AH, Helzer JE, Higgins ST, Bickel WK, Cottler LB. Nicotine dependence in a population-based sample. In: Harris L, editor. *Problems of Drug Dependence, 1992: Proceedings of the 54th Annual Scientific Meeting, the College on Problems of Drug Dependence.* NIDA Research Monograph 132. Rockville (MD): U.S. Department of Health and Human Services, Public Health Service, National Institutes of Health, National Institute on Drug Abuse, 1993. NIH Publication No. 93-3505.

Hammond EC, Garfinkel L. Smoking habits of men and women. *Journal of the National Cancer Institute* 1961;27(2):419–42.

Hammond EC, Garfinkel L. Changes in cigarette smoking. *Journal of the National Cancer Institute* 1964;33(1):49–64.

Hammond EC, Garfinkel L. Changes in cigarette smoking, 1959–1965. *American Journal of Public Health* 1968;58(1):30–45.

Hansen WB. Behavioral predictors of abstinence: early indicators of a dependence on tobacco among adolescents. *International Journal of the Addictions* 1983;18(7):913–20.

Harrell JS, Bangdiwala SI, Deng S, Webb JP, Bradley C. Smoking initiation in youth. The roles of gender, race, socioeconomics, and developmental status. *Journal of Adolescent Health* 1998;23(5):271–9.

Harris JE. Cigarette smoking among successive birth cohorts of men and women in the United States during 1900–80. *Journal of the National Cancer Institute* 1983;71(3):473–9.

Hatsukami D, Hughes JR, Pickens R. Characterization of tobacco withdrawal: physiological and subjective effects. In: Grabowski J, Hall SM, editors.

*Pharmacological Adjuncts in Smoking Cessation*. National Institute on Drug Abuse Monograph 53. U.S. Department of Health and Human Services, Public Health Service, Alcohol, Drug Abuse, and Mental Health Administration, 1985:56–67. DHHS Publication No. (ADM) 85-1333.

Hatziandreu EJ, Pierce JP, Fiore MC, Grise V, Novotny TE, Davis RM. The reliability of self-reported cigarette consumption in the United States. *American Journal of Public Health* 1989;79(8):1020–3.

Hatziandreu EJ, Pierce JP, Lefkopoulou M, Fiore MC, Mills SL, Novotny TE, Giovino GA, Davis RM. Quitting smoking in the United States in 1986. *Journal of the National Cancer Institute* 1990;82(17):1402–6.

Haynes SG, Harvey C, Montes H, Nickens H, Cohen BH. VIII. Patterns of cigarette smoking among Hispanics in the United States: results from HHANES 1982–84. *American Journal of Public Health* 1990;80(Suppl):47–54.

Hazelden Foundation. National survey shows it takes smokers an average 11 attempts before they quit for good [press release]. Center City (MN): Hazelden Foundation, 1998 Nov. 12.

Health Canada. *Smoking Among Aboriginal People in Canada, 1991*. Ottawa: Minister of Supply and Services Canada, 1994.

Hedges B, Jarvis M. Cigarette smoking. In: Prescott-Clarke P, Primatesta P, editors. *Health Survey for England: The Health of Young People '95–97*. London: The Stationery Office, 1998:191–221.

Heimann RK. *Tobacco and Americans*. New York: McGraw-Hill, 1960.

Hellman R, Cummings KM, Haughey BP, Zielezny MA, O'Shea RM. Predictors of attempting and succeeding at smoking cessation. *Health Education Research* 1991;6(1):77–86.

Hibbard JH. Social roles as predictors of cessation in a cohort of women smokers. *Women and Health* 1993; 20(4):71–80.

Holck SE, Warren CW, Rochat RW, Smith JC. Lung cancer mortality and smoking habits: Mexican-American women. *American Journal of Public Health* 1982;72(1):38–42.

Hoover IH. Hail to the Chief. *Saturday Evening Post* 1934 May 5:14–15, 42, 44, 45.

Horn D, Courts FA, Taylor RM, Solomon ES. Cigarette smoking among high school students. *American Journal of Public Health* 1959;49(11):1497–511.

Howe H. An historical review of women, smoking and advertising. *Health Education* 1984;15(3):3–9.

Hubert HB, Eaker ED, Garrison RJ, Castelli WP. Lifestyle correlates of risk factor change in young adults: an eight-year study of coronary heart disease risk factors in the Framingham offspring. *American Journal of Epidemiology* 1987;125(5):812–31.

Hughes JR, Hatsukami DK, Mitchell JE, Dahlgren LA. Prevalence of smoking among psychiatric outpatients. *American Journal of Psychiatry* 1986;143(8):993–7.

Husten CG, Chrismon JH, Reddy MN. Trends and effects of cigarette smoking among girls and women in the United States, 1965–1993. *Journal of the American Medical Women's Association* 1996; 51(1-2):11–8.

Husten CG, McCarty MC, Giovino GA, Chrismon JH, Zhu BP. Intermittent smokers: a descriptive analysis of persons who have never smoked daily. *American Journal of Public Health* 1998;88(1):86–9.

Hymowitz N, Cummings KM, Hyland A, Lynn WR, Pechacek TF, Hartwell TD. Predictors of smoking cessation in a cohort of adult smokers followed for five years. *Tobacco Control* 1997;6(Suppl 2):S57–S62.

Idris M, Ibrahim YE, Warnakulasuriya KA, Cooper DJ, Johnson NW, Nilsen R. Toombak use and cigarette smoking in the Sudan: estimates of prevalence in the Nile state. *Preventive Medicine* 1998; 27(4):597–603.

Jarvis M. Gender and smoking: do women really find it harder to give up? *British Journal of Addiction* 1984;79(4):383–7.

Jarvis M, Jackson P. Cigar and pipe smoking in Britain: implications for smoking prevalence and cessation. *British Journal of Addiction* 1988;83(3):323–30.

Jeffery RW, Boles SM, Strycker LA, Glasgow RE. Smoking-specific weight gain concerns and smoking cessation in a working population. *Health Psychology* 1997;16(5):487–9.

Johnson RA, Gerstein DR. Initiation of use of alcohol, cigarettes, marijuana, cocaine, and other substances in U.S. birth cohorts since 1919. *American Journal of Public Health* 1998;88(1):27–33.

Johnston LD, Bachman JG, O'Malley PM. *Monitoring the Future: Questionnaire Responses from the Nation's High School Seniors 1977*. Ann Arbor (MI): University of Michigan, Institute for Social Research, Survey Research Center, 1980a.

Johnston LD, Bachman JG, O'Malley PM. *Monitoring the Future: Questionnaire Responses from the Nation's High School Seniors, 1979*. Ann Arbor (MI): University of Michigan, Institute for Social Research, Survey Research Center, 1980b.

Johnston LD, Bachman JG, O'Malley PM. *Monitoring the Future: Questionnaire Responses from the Nation's High School Seniors, 1981*. Ann Arbor (MI): University of Michigan, Institute for Social Research, Survey Research Center, 1982.

Johnston LD, Bachman JG, O'Malley PM. *Monitoring the Future: Questionnaire Responses from the Nation's High School Seniors, 1983*. Ann Arbor (MI): University of Michigan, Institute for Social Research, Survey Research Center, 1984.

Johnston LD, Bachman JG, O'Malley PM. *Monitoring the Future: Questionnaire Responses from the Nation's High School Seniors, 1985*. Ann Arbor (MI): University of Michigan, Institute for Social Research, Survey Research Center, 1986.

Johnston LD, Bachman JG, O'Malley PM. *Monitoring the Future: Questionnaire Responses from the Nation's High School Seniors, 1987*. Ann Arbor (MI): University of Michigan, Institute for Social Research, Survey Research Center, 1991.

Johnston LD, Bachman JG, O'Malley PM. *Monitoring the Future: Questionnaire Responses from the Nation's High School Seniors, 1989*. Ann Arbor (MI): University of Michigan, Institute for Social Research, Survey Research Center, 1992.

Johnston LD, Bachman JG, O'Malley PM. *Monitoring the Future: Questionnaire Responses from the Nation's High School Seniors, 1991*. Ann Arbor (MI): University of Michigan, Institute for Social Research, Survey Research Center, 1993.

Johnston LD, Bachman JG, O'Malley PM. *Monitoring the Future: Questionnaire Responses from the Nation's High School Seniors, 1993*. Ann Arbor (MI): University of Michigan, Institute for Social Research, Survey Research Center, 1995a.

Johnston LD, Bachman JG, O'Malley PM. *Monitoring the Future: Questionnaire Responses from the Nation's High School Seniors, 1995*. Ann Arbor (MI): University of Michigan, Institute for Social Research, Survey Research Center, 1997.

Johnston LD, O'Malley PM, Bachman JG. *National Survey Results on Drug Use from the Monitoring the Future Study, 1975–1993. Volume I: Secondary School Students*. Rockville (MD): U.S. Department of Health and Human Services, Public Health Service, National Institutes of Health, National Institute on Drug Abuse, 1994a.

Johnston LD, O'Malley PM, Bachman JG. *National Survey Results on Drug Use from the Monitoring the Future Study, 1975–1993. Volume II: College Students and Young Adults*. Rockville (MD): U.S. Department of Health and Human Services, Public Health Service, National Institutes of Health, National Institute on Drug Abuse, 1994b.

Johnston LD, O'Malley PM, Bachman JG. *National Survey Results on Drug Use from the Monitoring the Future Study, 1975–1994. Volume I: Secondary School Students*. Rockville (MD): U.S. Department of Health and Human Services, Public Health Service, National Institutes of Health, National Institute on Drug Abuse, 1995b. NIH Publication No. 95-4026.

Johnston LD, O'Malley PM, Bachman JG. *National Survey Results on Drug Use from the Monitoring the Future Study, 1975–1995. Volume I: Secondary School Students*. Rockville (MD): U.S. Department of Health and Human Services, Public Health Service, National Institutes of Health, National Institute on Drug Abuse, 1996.

Johnston LD, O'Malley PM, Bachman JG. *National Survey Results on Drug Use from the Monitoring the Future Study, 1975–1998. Volume I: Secondary School Students*. Bethesda (MD): U.S. Department of Health and Human Services, Public Health Service, National Institutes of Health, National Institute on Drug Abuse, 1999.

Johnston LD, O'Malley PM, Bachman JG. *National Survey Results on Drug Use from the Monitoring the Future Study, 1975–1999. Volume I: Secondary School Students*. Bethesda (MD): U.S. Department of Health and Human Services, National Institutes of Health, National Institute on Drug Abuse, 2000a.

Johnston LD, O'Malley PM, Bachman JG. *National Survey Results on Drug Use from the Monitoring the Future Study, 1975–1999. Volume II: College Students and Adults Ages 19–40*. Bethesda (MD): U.S. Department of Health and Human Services, National Institute on Drug Abuse, 2000b.

Joossens L, Naett C, Howie C, Muldoon A. *Tobacco and Health in the European Union: An Overview*. Brussels: European Bureau for Action on Smoking Prevention, 1994.

Kabat GC, Morabia A, Wynder EL. Comparison of smoking habits of blacks and whites in a case-control study. *American Journal of Public Health* 1991;81(11):1483–6.

Kabat GC, Wynder EL. Determinants of quitting smoking. *American Journal of Public Health* 1987; 77(10):1301–5.

Kandel D, Chen K, Warner LA, Kessler RC, Grant B. Prevalence and demographic correlates of symptoms of last year dependence on alcohol, nicotine, marijuana and cocaine in the U.S. population. *Drug and Alcohol Dependence* 1997a;44(1):11–29.

Kandel DB, Chen K. Extent of smoking and nicotine dependence in the United States: 1991–1993. *Nicotine and Tobacco Research* 2000;2(3):263–74.

Kandel DB, Davies M. Adult sequelae of adolescent depressive symptoms. *Archives of General Psychiatry* 1986;43(3):255–62.

Kandel DB, Johnson JG, Bird HR, Canino G, Goodman SH, Lahey BB, Regier DA, Schwab-Stone M. Psychiatric disorders associated with substance use among children and adolescents: findings from the Methods for the Epidemiology of Child and Adolescent Mental Disorders (MECA) Study. *Journal of Abnormal Child Psychology* 1997b;25(2): 121–32.

Kandel DB, Yamaguchi K, Chen K. Stages of progression in drug involvement from adolescence to adulthood: further evidence for the gateway theory. *Journal of Studies on Alcohol* 1992;53(5):447–57.

Kann L, Kinchen SA, Williams BI, Ross JG, Lowry R, Grunbaum JA, Kolbe LJ. Youth risk behavior surveillance—United States, 1999. *Morbidity and Mortality Weekly Report* 2000;49(SS-5):1–96.

Kann L, Kinchen SA, Williams BI, Ross JG, Lowry R, Hill CV, Grunbaum JA, Blumson PS, Collins JL, Kolbe LJ. Youth risk behavior surveillance—United States, 1997. *Morbidity and Mortality Weekly Report* 1998;47(SS-3):1–91.

Kann L, Warren CW, Collins JL, Ross J, Collins B, Kolbe LJ. Results from the national school-based 1991 Youth Risk Behavior Survey and progress toward achieving related health objectives for the nation. *Public Health Reports* 1993;108(Suppl 1): 47–55.

Kann L, Warren CW, Harris WA, Collins JL, Douglas KA, Collins ME, Williams BI, Ross JG, Kolbe LJ. Youth risk behavior surveillance—United States, 1993. *Morbidity and Mortality Weekly Report* 1995; 44(SS-1):1–56.

Kann L, Warren CW, Harris WA, Collins JL, Williams BI, Ross JG, Kolbe LJ. Youth Risk Behavior Surveillance—United States, 1995. *Morbidity and Mortality Weekly Report* 1996;45(SS-4):1–84.

Kaplan CP, Tanjasiri SP. The effects of interview mode on smoking attitudes and behavior: self-report among female Latino adolescents. *Substance Use and Misuse* 1996;31(8):947–63.

Kaplan SD, Lanier AP, Merritt RK, Siegel PZ. Prevalence of tobacco use among Alaska Natives: a review. *Preventive Medicine* 1997;26(4):460–5.

Kawachi I, Colditz GA, Speizer FE, Manson JE, Stampfer MJ, Willett WC, Hennekens CH. A prospective study of passive smoking and coronary heart disease. *Circulation* 1997;95(10):2374–9.

Kendler KS, Neale MC, MacLean CJ, Heath AC, Eaves LJ, Kessler RC. Smoking and major depression: a causal analysis. *Archives of General Psychiatry* 1993; 50(1):36–43.

Kendrick JS, Zahniser SC, Miller N, Salas N, Stine J, Gargiullo PM, Floyd RL, Spierto FW, Sexton M, Metzger RW, Stockbauer JW, Hannon WH, Dalmat ME. Integrating smoking cessation into routine public prenatal care: the Smoking Cessation in Pregnancy Project. *American Journal of Public Health* 1995;85(2):217–22.

Killen JD, Fortmann SP, Kraemer HC, Varady A, Newman B. Who will relapse? Symptoms of nicotine dependence predict long-term relapse after smoking cessation. *Journal of Consulting and Clinical Psychology* 1992;60(5):797–801.

Killen JD, Fortmann SP, Telch MJ, Newman B. Are heavy smokers different from light smokers? A comparison after 48 hours without cigarettes. *Journal of the American Medical Association* 1988;260(11): 1581–5.

King AC, Taylor CB, Haskell WL. Smoking in older women: is being female a "risk factor" for continued cigarette use? *Archives of Internal Medicine* 1990;150(9):1841–6.

Kirchoff H, Rigdon RH. Smoking habits of 21,612 individuals in Texas. *Journal of the National Cancer Institute* 1956;16(5):1287–304.

Kirscht JP, Brock BM, Hawthorne VM. Cigarette smoking and changes in smoking among a cohort of Michigan adults, 1980–82. *American Journal of Public Health* 1987;77(4):501–2.

Klatsky AL, Armstrong MA. Cardiovascular risk factors among Asian Americans living in northern California. *American Journal of Public Health* 1991; 81(11):1423–8.

Kleinman JC, Kopstein A. Smoking during pregnancy, 1967–1980. *American Journal of Public Health* 1987; 77(7):823–5.

Klesges RC, Debon M, Ray JW. Are self-reports of smoking rate biased? Evidence from the Second National Health and Nutrition Examination Survey. *Journal of Clinical Epidemiology* 1995;48(10): 1225–33.

Klesges RC, Elliott VE, Robinson LA. Chronic dieting and the belief that smoking controls body weight in a biracial, population-based adolescent sample. *Tobacco Control* 1997;6(2):89–94.

Klesges RC, Klesges LM. Cigarette smoking as a dieting strategy in a university population. *International Journal of Eating Disorders* 1988;7(3):413–9.

Klesges RC, Klesges LM. The relationship between body mass and cigarette smoking using a biochemical index of smoking exposure. *International Journal of Obesity* 1993;17(10):585–91.

Klesges RC, Klesges LM, Meyers AW. Relationship of smoking status, energy balance, and body weight: analysis of the Second National Health and Nutrition Examination Survey. *Journal of Consulting and Clinical Psychology* 1991;59(6):899–905.

Klesges RC, Meyers AW, Klesges LM, LaVasque ME. Smoking, body weight, and their effects on smoking behavior: a comprehensive review of the literature. *Psychological Bulletin* 1989;106(2):204–30.

Klesges RC, Zbikowski SM, Lando HA, Haddock CK, Talcott GW, Robinson LA. The relationship between smoking and body weight in a population of young military personnel. *Health Psychology* 1998;17(5):454–8.

Klevens RM, Giovino GA, Peddicord JP, Nelson DE, Mowery P, Grummer-Strawn L. The association between veteran status and cigarette-smoking behaviors. *American Journal of Preventive Medicine* 1995;11(4):245–50.

Kolbe LJ. An epidemiological surveillance system to monitor the prevalence of youth behaviors that most affect health. *Health Education* 1990;21(6):44–8.

Kolbe LJ, Kann L, Collins JL. Overview of the Youth Risk Behavior Surveillance System. *Public Health Reports* 1993;108(Suppl 1):2–10.

Kovar MG, Poe GS. The National Health Interview Survey design, 1973–84, and procedures, 1975–83. *Vital and Health Statistics*. Series 1, No. 18. Hyattsville (MD): U.S. Department of Health and Human Services, Public Health Service, National Center for Health Statistics, 1985. DHHS Publication No. (PHS) 85-1320.

Kviz FJ, Clark MA, Crittenden KS, Freels S, Warnecke RB. Age and readiness to quit smoking. *Preventive Medicine* 1994;23(2):211–22.

Lander M. *The Tobacco Problem*. 3rd ed. Boston: De Wolfe, Fiske and Company, 1885.

Lee L, Gilpin E, Pierce JP. Changes in the patterns of initiation of cigarette smoking in the United States, 1950, 1965, and 1980. *Cancer Epidemiology, Biomarkers and Prevention* 1993;2(6):593–7.

Lefkowitz D, Underwood C. *Personal Health Practices: Findings from the Survey of American Indians and Alaskan Natives. National Medical Expenditure Survey. Research Findings 10.* Rockville (MD): U.S. Department of Health and Human Services, Public Health Service, Agency for Health Care Policy and Research, Center for General Health Services Intramural Research, 1991. AHCPR Publication No. 91-0034.

Liberatos P, Link BG, Kelsey JL. The measurement of social class in epidemiology. *Epidemiologic Reviews* 1988;10:87–121.

Link HC. Significance of change in cigarette preference. *Advertising and Selling* 1935 June 6:27, 44.

Liu B-Q, Peto R, Chen Z-M, Boreham J, Wu Y-P, Li J-Y, Campbell TC, Chen J-S. Emerging tobacco hazards in China: 1. Retrospective proportional mortality study of one million deaths. *British Medical Journal* 1998;317(7170):1411–22.

Lowry R, Kann L, Collins JL, Kolbe LJ. The effect of socioeconomic status on chronic disease risk behaviors among US adolescents. *Journal of the American Medical Association* 1996;276(10):792–7.

Luepker RV, Pallonen UE, Murray DM, Pirie PL. Validity of telephone surveys in assessing cigarette smoking in young adults. *American Journal of Public Health* 1989;79(2):202–4.

Mackay J. Battlefield for the tobacco war. *Journal of the American Medical Association* 1989;261(1):28–9.

Marcus AC, Crane LA. Smoking behavior among Hispanics: a preliminary report. *Progress in Clinical and Biological Research* 1984;156:141–51.

Marcus AC, Crane LA. Smoking behavior among U.S. Latinos: an emerging challenge for public health. *American Journal of Public Health* 1985;75(2):169–72.

Marcus AC, Crane LA, Shopland DR, Lynn WR. Use of smokeless tobacco in the United States: recent estimates from the Current Population Survey. In: *Smokeless Tobacco Use in the United States*. NCI Monograph 8. Bethesda (MD): U.S. Department of Health and Human Services, Public Health Service, National Institutes of Health, National Cancer Institute, 1989:17–23.

Markides KS, Coreil J, Ray LA. Smoking among Mexican Americans: a three-generation study. *American Journal of Public Health* 1987;77(6):708–11.

Martin G, Elkin EJ. Aficionadas: women and their cigars. *Cigar Aficionado* 1995;3(4):142–59.

Massey JT, Moore TF, Parsons VL, Tadros W. Design and estimation of the National Health Interview Survey, 1985–94. *Vital and Health Statistics*. Series 2, No. 110. Hyattsville (MD): U.S. Department of Health and Human Services, Public Health Service, Centers for Disease Control, National Center for Health Statistics, 1989. DHHS Publication No. (PHS) 89-1384.

Matanoski G, Kanchanaraksa S, Lantry D, Chang Y. Characteristics of nonsmoking women in NHANES I and NHANES I Epidemiologic

Follow-up Study with exposure to spouses who smoke. *American Journal of Epidemiology* 1995; 142(2):149–57.

Mathews TJ. Smoking during pregnancy, 1990–96. *National Vital Statistics Report* 1998;47(10):1–12.

Maxwell JC Jr. *The Maxwell Consumer Report: First-Quarter 1994 Sales Estimates for the Cigarette Industry*. Wheat First Butcher Singer, 1994.

Maxwell JC Jr. *The Maxwell Report: Fourth Quarter and Year-End 1999 Sales Estimates for the Cigarette Industry*. Richmond (VA): Davenport & Company, 2000.

McBride CM, Pirie PL, Curry SJ. Postpartum relapse to smoking: a prospective study. *Health Education Research* 1992;7(3):381–90.

McGinnis JM, Shopland D, Brown C. Tobacco and health: trends in smoking and smokeless tobacco consumption in the United States. In: Breslow L, Fielding JE, Lane LB, editors. *Annual Review of Public Health* 1987;8:441–67.

McKinney WP, McIntire DD, Carmody TJ, Joseph A. Comparing the smoking behavior of veterans and nonveterans. *Public Health Reports* 1997;112(3): 212–7.

McNeill AD, Jarvis M, West R. Subjective effects of cigarette smoking in adolescents. *Psychopharmacology* 1987;92(1):115–7.

McNeill AD, Jarvis MJ, Stapleton JA, West RJ, Bryant A. Nicotine intake in young smokers: longitudinal study of saliva cotinine concentrations. *American Journal of Public Health* 1989;79(2):172–5.

McNeill AD, West RJ, Jarvis M, Jackson P, Bryant A. Cigarette withdrawal symptoms in adolescent smokers. *Psychopharmacology* 1986;90(4):533–6.

McWhorter WP, Boyd GM, Mattson ME. Predictors of quitting smoking: the NHANES I followup experience. *Journal of Clinical Epidemiology* 1990;43(12): 1399–405.

Metropolitan Insurance Companies. Cigarette smoking among U.S. adults, 1985–1990, and smoking among selected occupational groups, 1990. *Statistical Bulletin—Metropolitan Insurance Companies* 1992;73(4):12–9.

Miller JD, Cisin IH, Gardner-Keaton H, Harrell AV, Wirtz PW, Abelson HI, Fishburne PM. *National Survey on Drug Abuse: Main Findings 1982*. Rockville (MD): U.S. Department of Health and Human Services, Public Health Service, Alcohol, Drug Abuse, and Mental Health Administration, National Institute on Drug Abuse, 1983. DHHS Publication No. (ADM) 83-1263.

Mills CA, Porter MM. Tobacco-smoking habits in an American city. *Journal of the National Cancer Institute* 1953;13:1283–97.

*Milwaukee Journal*. Consumer analysis of the greater Milwaukee market. *Milwaukee Journal* 1935–1979.

Ministry of Health and Welfare. *Report on National Survey on Smoking and Health in 1999*. Japan: Health Services Bureau, Ministry of Health and Welfare, 2000.

Molarius A, Parsons RW, Dobson AJ, Evans A, Fortmann SP, Jamrozik K, Kuulasmaa K, Moltchanov V, Sans S, Tuomilehto J, Puska P for the WHO MONICA Project. Trends in cigarette smoking in 36 populations from the early 1980s to the mid-1990s: findings from the WHO MONICA Project. *American Journal of Public Health* 2001;91(2):206–12.

Montgomery LE, Carter-Pokras O. Health status by social class and/or minority status: implications for environmental equity research. *Toxicology and Industrial Health* 1993;9(5):729–73.

Moss AJ. Changes in cigarette smoking and current smoking practices among adults. United States, 1978. *Advance Data*. No. 52. U.S. Department of Health, Education, and Welfare, Public Health Service, National Center for Health Statistics, Office of Health Research, Statistics, and Technology, 1979.

Moss AJ, Allen KF, Giovino GA, Mills SL. Recent trends in adolescent smoking, smoking-uptake correlates, and expectations about the future. *Advance Data*. No. 221. Hyattsville (MD): U.S. Department of Health and Human Services, Public Health Service, Centers for Disease Control, National Center for Health Statistics, 1992.

Mullen PD, Quinn VP, Ershoff DH. Maintenance of nonsmoking postpartum by women who stopped smoking during pregnancy. *American Journal of Public Health* 1990;80(8):992–4.

Mullen PD, Richardson MA, Quinn VP, Ershoff DH. Postpartum return to smoking: who is at risk and when. *American Journal of Health Promotion* 1997; 11(5):323–30.

Myers AH, Rosner B, Abbey H, Willet W, Stampfer MJ, Bain C, Lipnick R, Hennekens C, Speizer F. Smoking behavior among participants in the Nurses' Health Study. *American Journal of Public Health* 1987;77(5):628–30.

National Cancer Institute. *Health Effects of Exposure to Environmental Tobacco Smoke: The Report of the California Environmental Protection Agency*. Smoking and Tobacco Control Monograph 10. Bethesda (MD): U.S. Department of Health and Human Services, National Institutes of Health, National Cancer Institute, 1999. NIH Publication No. 99-4645.

National Center for Health Statistics, Ahmed PI, Gleeson GA. Changes in cigarette smoking habits between 1955 and 1966. *Vital and Health Statistics.* Series 10, No. 59. Rockville (MD): U.S. Department of Health, Education, and Welfare, Public Health Service, Health Services and Mental Health Administration, National Center for Health Statistics, 1970. Publication No. (PHS) 1000.

National Center for Health Statistics. Health interview survey procedures, 1957–1974. *Vital and Health Statistics*. Series 1, No. 11. Rockville (MD): U.S. Department of Health, Education, and Welfare, Public Health Service, Health Resources Administration, National Center for Health Statistics, 1975. DHEW Publication No. (HRA) 75-1311.

National Center for Health Statistics. Current estimates from the Health Interview Survey: United States—1977. *Vital and Health Statistics*. Series 10, No. 126. Hyattsville (MD): U.S. Department of Health, Education, and Welfare, Public Health Service, National Center for Health Statistics, 1978. DHEW Publication No. (PHS) 78-1554.

National Center for Health Statistics. Provisional data from the Health Promotion and Disease Prevention Supplement to the National Health Interview Survey: United States, January–March 1985. *Advance Data*. No. 113. Hyattsville (MD): U.S. Department of Health and Human Services, Public Health Service, National Center for Health Statistics, 1985. DHHS Publication No. (PHS) 86-1250.

National Center for Health Statistics. Smoking and other tobacco use: United States, 1987. *Vital and Health Statistics*. Series 10, No. 169. Hyattsville (MD): U.S. Department of Health and Human Services, Public Health Service, Centers for Disease Control, National Center for Health Statistics, 1989. DHHS Publication No. (PHS) 89-1597.

National Center for Health Statistics. Advance report of new data from the 1989 birth certificate. *Monthly Vital Statistics Report* 1992:40(12 Suppl).

National Center for Health Statistics. Advance report of maternal and infant health data from the birth certificate, 1991. *Monthly Vital Statistics Report* 1994a:42(11 Suppl).

National Center for Health Statistics. Plan and operation of the third National Health and Nutrition Examination Survey, 1988–94. *Vital and Health Statistics.* Series 1, No. 32. Hyattsville (MD): U.S. Department of Health and Human Services, Public Health Service, Centers for Disease Control and Prevention, National Center for Health Statistics, 1994b. DHHS Publication No. (PHS) 94-1308.

National Center for Health Statistics. Fertility, family planning, and women's health: new data from the 1995 National Survey of Family Growth. *Vital and Health Statistics*. Series 23, No. 19. Hyattsville (MD): U.S. Department of Health and Human Services, Public Health Service, Centers for Disease Control and Prevention, National Center for Health Statistics, 1997.

National Institute for Occupational Safety and Health. *Environmental Tobacco Smoke in the Workplace: Lung Cancer and Other Health Effects.* Current Intelligence Bulletin 54. U.S. Department of Health and Human Services, Public Health Service, Centers for Disease Control, and National Institute for Occupational Safety and Health, Division of Standards Development and Technology Transfer, Division of Surveillance, Hazard Evaluations, and Field Studies, 1991. DHHS (NIOSH) Publication No. 91-108.

Nelson DE, Davis RM, Chrismon JH, Giovino GA. Pipe smoking in the United States, 1965–1991: prevalence and attributable mortality. *Preventive Medicine* 1996;25(2):91–9.

Nelson DE, Emont SL, Brackbill RM, Cameron LL, Peddicord J, Fiore MC. Cigarette smoking prevalence by occupation in the United States: a comparison between 1978 to 1980 and 1987 to 1990. *Journal of Occupational Medicine* 1994;36(5):516–25.

Nelson DE, Giovino GA, Shopland DR, Mowery PD, Mills SL, Eriksen MP. Trends in cigarette smoking among U.S. adolescents, 1974 through 1991. *American Journal of Public Health* 1995;85(1):34–40.

Nelson DE, Holtzman D, Waller M, Leutzinger C, Condon K. Objectives and design of the Behavioral Risk Factor Surveillance System. Proceedings of the American Statistical Association Annual Conference, Dallas, TX, August 1998.

Nelson DE, Moon RW, Holtzman D, Smith P, Siegel PZ. Patterns of health risk behaviors for chronic disease: a comparison between adolescent and adult American Indians living on or near reservations in Montana. *Journal of Adolescent Health* 1997; 21(1):25–32.

New Zealand Public Health Commission. *Tobacco Products: The Public Health Commission's Advice to the Minister of Health, 1993–1994.* Wellington: Public Health Commission, 1994.

Nicolaides-Bouman A, Wald N, Forey B, Lee P, editors. *International Smoking Statistics*. London: Wolfson Institute of Preventive Medicine, Oxford University Press, 1993.

Novotny TE, Fiore MC, Hatziandreu EJ, Giovino GA, Mills SL, Pierce JP. Trends in smoking by age and sex, United States, 1974–1987: the implications for disease impact. *Preventive Medicine* 1990;19(5): 552–61.

Novotny TE, Giovino GA. Tobacco use. In: Brownson RC, Remington PL, Davison JR, editors. *Chronic Disease Epidemiology and Control*. 2nd ed. Washington: American Public Health Association Press, 1998:117–48.

Novotny TE, Warner KE, Kendrick JS, Remington PL. Smoking by Blacks and Whites: socioeconomic and demographic differences. *American Journal of Public Health* 1988;78(9):1187–9.

O'Campo P, Faden RR, Brown H, Gielen AC. The impact of pregnancy on women's prenatal and postpartum smoking behavior. *American Journal of Preventive Medicine* 1992;8(1):8–13.

Ockene JK. Smoking among women across the life span: prevalence, interventions, and implications for cessation research. *Annals of Behavioral Medicine* 1993;15(2–3):135–48.

Ockene JK, Hosmer DW, Williams JW, Goldberg RJ, Ockene IS, Biliouris T, Dalen JE. The relationship of patient characteristics to physician delivery of advice to stop smoking. *Journal of General Internal Medicine* 1987;2(5):337–40.

O'Hara P, Portser SA. A comparison of younger-aged and older-aged women in a behavioral self-control smoking program. *Patient Education and Counseling* 1994;23(2):91–6.

Orlandi MA. Gender differences in smoking cessation. *Women and Health* 1987;11(3–4):237–51.

Orleans TC, Jepson C, Resch N, Rimer BK. Quitting motives and barriers among older smokers. *Cancer* 1994;74(7 Suppl):2055–61.

Otero-Sabogal R, Sabogal F, Pérez-Stable EJ. Psychosocial correlates of smoking among immigrant Latina adolescents. *Journal of the National Cancer Institute Monographs* 1995;18:65–71.

Page RM, Allen O, Moore L, Hewitt C. Weight-related concerns and practices of male and female adolescent cigarette smokers and nonsmokers. *Journal of Health Education* 1993;24(6):339–46.

Pamuk ER, Mosher WD. Health aspects of pregnancy and childbirth: United States, 1982. *Vital and Health Statistics*. Series 23, No. 16. Hyattsville (MD): U.S. Department of Health and Human Services, Public Health Service, Centers for Disease Control, National Center for Health Statistics, 1988. DHHS Publication No. (PHS) 89-1992.

Patrick DL, Cheadle A, Thompson DC, Diehr P, Koepsell T, Kinne S. The validity of self-reported smoking: a review and meta-analysis. *American Journal of Public Health* 1994;84(7):1086–93.

Pérez-Stable EJ, Herrera B, Jacob P III, Benowitz NL. Nicotine metabolism and intake in black and white smokers. *Journal of the American Medical Association* 1998;280(2):152–6.

Pérez-Stable EJ, Marín BV, Marín G, Brody DJ, Benowitz NL. Apparent underreporting of cigarette consumption among Mexican American smokers. *American Journal of Public Health* 1990a; 80(9):1057–61.

Pérez-Stable EJ, Marín G, Marín BV, Benowitz NL. Misclassification of smoking status by self-reported cigarette consumption. *American Review of Respiratory Disease* 1992;145(1):53–7.

Pérez-Stable EJ, Marín G, Marín BV, Katz MH. Depressive symptoms and cigarette smoking among Latinos in San Francisco. *American Journal of Public Health* 1990b;80(12):1500–2.

Perkins KA. Individual variability in responses to nicotine. *Behavior Genetics* 1995;25(2):119–32.

Pierce JP, Evans N, Farkas AJ, Cavin SW, Berry C, Kramer M, Kealey S, Rosbrook B, Choi W, Kaplan RM. *Tobacco Use in California: An Evaluation of the Tobacco Control Program 1989–1993*. La Jolla (CA): University of California, San Diego, 1994a.

Pierce JP, Fiore MC, Novotny TE, Hatziandreu EJ, Davis RM. Trends in cigarette smoking in the United States: educational differences are increasing. *Journal of the American Medical Association* 1989a; 261(1):56–60.

Pierce JP, Gilpin E, Burns DM, Whalen E, Rosbrook B, Shopland D, Johnson M. Does tobacco advertising target young people to start smoking? Evidence from California. *Journal of the American Medical Association* 1991a;266(22):3154–8.

Pierce JP, Gilpin EA. A historical analysis of tobacco marketing and the uptake of smoking by youth in the United States: 1890–1977. *Health Psychology* 1995;14(6):500–8.

Pierce JP, Giovino G, Hatziandreu E, Shopland D. National age and sex differences in quitting smoking. *Journal of Psychoactive Drugs* 1989b;21(3): 293–8.

Pierce JP, Lee L, Gilpin EA. Smoking initiation by adolescent girls, 1944–1988: an association with targeted advertising. *Journal of the American Medical Association* 1994b;271(8):608–11.

Pierce JP, Naquin M, Gilpin E, Giovino G, Mills S, Marcus S. Smoking initiation in the United States: a role for worksite and college smoking bans. *Journal of the National Cancer Institute* 1991b;83(14): 1009–13.

Pirie PL, Murray DM, Luepker RV. Gender differences in cigarette smoking and quitting in a cohort of young adults. *American Journal of Public Health* 1991;81(3):324–7.

Pirkle JL, Flegal KM, Bernert JT, Brody DJ, Etzel RA, Maurer KR. Exposure of the U.S. population to environmental tobacco smoke: the Third National Health and Nutrition Examination Survey, 1988 to 1991. *Journal of the American Medical Association* 1996;275(16):1233–40.

Pletsch PK. Environmental tobacco smoke exposure among Hispanic women of reproductive age. *Public Health Nursing* 1994;11(4):229–35.

Pohl R, Yeragani VK, Balon R, Lycaki H, McBride R. Smoking in patients with panic disorder. *Psychiatry Research* 1992;43(3):253–62.

Pomerleau CS. Smoking and nicotine replacement treatment issues specific to women. *American Journal of Health Behavior* 1996;20(5):291–9.

Pomerleau CS, Pomerleau OF. Gender differences in frequency of smoking withdrawal symptoms. *Annals of Behavioral Medicine* 1994;16(Suppl):S118.

Powell-Griner E, Anderson JE, Murphy W. State- and sex-specific prevalence of selected characteristics—Behavioral Risk Factor Surveillance System, 1994 and 1995. *Morbidity and Mortality Weekly Report* 1997;46(SS-3):1–31.

Reddy P, Meyer-Weitz A, Yach D. Smoking status, knowledge of health effects and attitudes towards tobacco control in South Africa. *South African Medical Journal* 1996;86(11):1389–93.

Remington PL, Forman MR, Gentry EM, Marks JS, Hogelin GC, Trowbridge FL. Current smoking trends in the United States: the 1981–1983 Behavioral Risk Factor Surveys. *Journal of the American Medical Association* 1985;253(20):2975–8.

Remington PL, Smith MY, Williamson DF, Anda RF, Gentry EM, Hogelin GC. Design, characteristics, and usefulness of state-based behavioral risk factor surveillance: 1981–87. *Public Health Reports* 1988;103(4):366–75.

Resnicow K, Kabat G, Wynder E. Progress in decreasing cigarette smoking. In: DeVita VT Jr, Hellman S, Rosenberg SA, editors. *Important Advances in Oncology 1991*. Philadelphia: J.B. Lippincott, 1991: 205–13.

Rigotti NA, Lee JE, Wechsler H. US college students' use of tobacco products: results of a national survey. *Journal of the American Medical Association* 2000;284(6):699–705.

Riley WT, Barenie JT, Mabe A, Myers DR. Smokeless tobacco use in adolescent females: prevalence and psychosocial factors among racial/ethnic groups. *Journal of Behavioral Medicine* 1990;13(2):207–20.

Rimer BK, Orleans CT, Keintz MK, Cristinzio S, Fleisher L. The older smoker: status, challenges and opportunities for intervention. *Chest* 1990; 97(3):547–53.

Robert JC. *The Story of Tobacco in America*. New York: Alfred A. Knopf, 1952.

Rogers RG. Demographic characteristics of cigarette smokers in the United States. *Social Biology* 1991; 38(1–2):1–12.

Rogers RG, Crank J. Ethnic differences in smoking patterns: findings from NHIS. *Public Health Reports* 1988;103(4):387–93.

Rogers RG, Nam CB, Hummer RA. Demographic and socioeconomic links to cigarette smoking. *Social Biology* 1995;42(1–2):1–21.

Rootman I, Smart RG. A comparison of alcohol, tobacco and drug use as determined from household and school surveys. *Drug and Alcohol Dependence* 1985;16(2):89–94.

Rose JS, Chassin L, Presson CC, Sherman SJ. Prospective predictors of quit attempts and smoking cessation in young adults. *Health Psychology* 1996; 15(4):261–8.

Rouse BA. Epidemiology of smokeless tobacco use: a national study. In: *Smokeless Tobacco Use in the United States*. National Cancer Institute Monograph 8. Bethesda (MD): U.S. Department of Health and Human Services, Public Health Service, National Institutes of Health, National Cancer Institute, 1989:29–33.

Royce JM, Corbett K, Sorensen G, Ockene J. Gender, social pressure, and smoking cessations: the Community Intervention Trial for Smoking Cessation (COMMIT) at baseline. *Social Science and Medicine* 1997;44(3):359–70.

Royce JM, Hymowitz N, Corbett K, Hartwell TD, Orlandi MA. Smoking cessation factors among African Americans and Whites. *American Journal of Public Health* 1993;83(2):220–6.

Sandler DP, Helsing KJ, Comstock GW, Shore DL. Factors associated with past household exposure to tobacco smoke. *American Journal of Epidemiology* 1989;129(2):380–7.

Sandoval JSO, Larsen MD. *National Adult Smoking Study*. Rockville (MD): Gallup Organization, 1995.

Schievelbein H, Heinemann G, Loschenkohl K, Troll C, and Schlegel J. Metabolic aspects of smoking behaviour. In: Thornton RE, editor. *Smoking Behaviour: Physiological and Psychological Influences.* Edinburgh: Churchill Livingstone, 1978.

Schoenborn CA. Health promotion and disease prevention: United States, 1985. *Vital and Health Statistics.* Series 10, No. 163. Hyattsville (MD): U.S. Department of Health and Human Services, Public Health Service, Centers for Disease Control, National Center for Health Statistics, 1988. DHHS Publication No. (PHS) 88-1591.

Schoenborn CA, Boyd G. Smoking and other tobacco use: United States, 1987. *Vital and Health Statistics.* Series 10, No. 169. Hyattsville (MD): U.S. Department of Health and Human Services, Public Health Service, Centers for Disease Control, National Center for Health Statistics, 1989. DHHS Publication No. (PHS) 89-1597.

Schoenborn CA, Horm J. Negative moods as correlates of smoking and heavier drinking: implications for health promotion. *Advance Data.* No. 236. Hyattsville (MD): U.S. Department of Health and Human Services, Public Health Service, Centers for Disease Control and Prevention, National Center for Health Statistics, 1993.

Schoenborn CA, Marano M. Current estimates from the National Health Interview Survey, United States, 1987. *Vital and Health Statistics.* Series 10, No. 166. Hyattsville (MD): U.S. Department of Health and Human Services, Public Health Service, Centers for Disease Control, National Center for Health Statistics, 1988. DHHS Publication No. (PHS) 88-1594.

Schorling JB, Gutgesell M, Klas P, Smith D, Keller A. Tobacco, alcohol and other drug use among college students. *Journal of Substance Abuse* 1994;6(1): 105–15.

Schuman LM. Patterns of smoking behavior. In: Jarvik ME, Cullen JW, Gritz ER, Vogt TM, West LJ, editors. *Research on Smoking Behavior*. NIDA Research Monograph 17. U.S. Department of Health, Education, and Welfare, Public Health Service, Alcohol, Drug Abuse, and Mental Health Administration, National Institute on Drug Abuse, 1977: 36–66. DHEW Publication No. (ADM) 78-581.

Shah BV, Barnwell BG, Bieler GS. *SUDAAN User's Manual, Release 7.5.* Research Triangle Park (NC): Research Triangle Institute, 1997.

Shanks TG, Burns DM. Disease consequences of cigar smoking. In: Shopland DR, Burns DM, Hoffman D, Cummings KM, editors. *Cigars: Health Effects and Trends.* Smoking and Tobacco Control Monograph 9. U.S. Department of Health and Human Services, Public Health Service, National Institutes of Health, National Cancer Institute, 1998:105–60. NIH Publication No. 98-4302.

Shelley E, Collins C, Daly L. Trends in smoking prevalence: the Kilkenny Health Project Population Surveys 1985 to 1991. *Irish Medical Journal* 1996;89(5): 182–5.

Shiffman SM. The tobacco withdrawal syndrome. In: Krasnegor NA, editor. *Cigarette Smoking as a Dependence Process.* National Institute on Drug Abuse Research Monograph 23. U.S. Department of Health, Education, and Welfare, Public Health Service, Alcohol, Drug Abuse and Mental Health Administration, National Institute on Drug Abuse, 1979:158–84.

Shopland DR. Tobacco use and its contribution to early cancer mortality with a special emphasis on cigarette smoking. *Environmental Health Perspectives* 1995;103(Suppl 8):131–41.

Silverstein B, Feld S, Kozlowski LT. The availability of low-nicotine cigarettes as a cause of cigarette smoking among teenage females. *Journal of Health and Social Behavior* 1980;21(4):383–8.

Skinner WF, Massey JL, Krohn MD, Lauer RM. Social influences and constraints on the initiation and cessation of adolescent tobacco use. *Journal of Behavioral Medicine* 1985;8(4):353–76.

Skinner WF, Otis MD. Drug and alcohol use among lesbian and gay people in a southern U.S. sample: epidemiological, comparative, and methodological findings from the Trilogy Project. *Journal of Homosexuality* 1996;30(3):59–91.

Smith KA. Cigarette smoking. A phenomenological analysis of the experience of women in their successful versus unsuccessful attempts to quit smoking. *Dissertation Abstracts International* 1981;43(1): 297B–298B.

Sobel R. *They Satisfy. The Cigarette in American Life.* Garden City (NY): Anchor Press/Doubleday, 1978.

Somasundaram M. Cigars' rebound puffs up Culbro's profit. *Wall Street Journal* 1996 Feb 16;Sect A:4B (Col 1).

Sorensen G, Pechacek T. Occupational and sex differences in smoking and smoking cessation. *Journal of Occupational Medicine* 1986;28(5):360–4.

Sorensen G, Pechacek TF. Attitudes toward smoking cessation among men and women. *Journal of Behavioral Medicine* 1987;10(2):129–37.

Sorlie PD, Kannel WB. A description of cigarette smoking cessation and resumption in the Framingham Study. *Preventive Medicine* 1990;19(3): 335–45.

Spangler JG, Bell RA, Dignan MB, Michielutte R. Prevalence and predictors of tobacco use among Lumbee Indian women in Robeson county, North Carolina. *Journal of Community Health* 1997a;22(2): 115–126.

Spangler JG, Dignan MB, Michielutte R. Correlates of tobacco use among Native American women in western North Carolina. *American Journal of Public Health* 1997b;87(1):108–11.

Stanton WR. DSM-III-R tobacco dependence and quitting during late adolescence. *Addictive Behaviors* 1995;20(5):595–603.

Stanton WR, Lowe JB, Gillespie AM. Adolescents' experiences of smoking cessation. *Drug and Alcohol Dependence* 1996a;43(1–2):63–70.

Stanton WR, McClelland M, Elwood C, Ferry D, Silva PA. Prevalence, reliability and bias of adolescents' reports of smoking and quitting. *Addiction* 1996b; 91(11):1705–14.

Stellman SD, Boffetta P, Garfinkel L. Smoking habits of 800,000 American men and women in relation to their occupations. *American Journal of Industrial Medicine* 1988;13(1):43–58.

Stellman SD, Garfinkel L. Smoking habits and tar levels in a new American Cancer Society prospective study of 1.2 million men and women. *Journal of the National Cancer Institute* 1986;76(6):1057–63.

Stellman SD, Stellman JM. Women's occupations, smoking, and cancer and other diseases. *CA—A Cancer Journal for Clinicians* 1981;31(1):29–43.

Sterling TD, Weinkam JJ. Smoking characteristics by type of employment. *Journal of Occupational Medicine* 1976;18(11):743–54.

Sterling TD, Weinkam JJ. Smoking patterns by occupation, industry, sex and race. *Archives of Environmental Health* 1978;33(6):313–7.

Steyn K, Bourne LT, Jooste PL, Fourie JM, Lombard CJ, Yach D. Smoking in the black community of the Cape Peninsula, South Africa. *East African Medical Journal* 1994;71(12):784–9.

Stotts AL, DiClemente CC, Carbonari JP, Mullen PD. Pregnancy smoking cessation: a case of mistaken identity. *Addictive Behaviors* 1996;21(4):459–71.

Strauss KF, Mokdad A, Ballew C, Mendlein JM, Will JC, Goldberg HI, White L, Serdula MK. The health of Navajo women: findings from the Navajo Health and Nutrition Survey, 1991–1992. *Journal of Nutrition* 1997;127(10 Suppl):2128S–2133S.

Substance Abuse and Mental Health Services Administration. *National Household Survey on Drug Abuse: Main Findings 1991.* Rockville (MD): U.S. Department of Health and Human Services, Public Health Service, Substance Abuse and Mental Health Services Administration, Office of Applied Studies, 1993. DHHS Publication No. (SMA) 93-1980.

Substance Abuse and Mental Health Services Administration. *National Household Survey on Drug Abuse: Main Findings 1992.* Rockville (MD): U.S. Department of Health and Human Services, Public Health Service, Substance Abuse and Mental Health Services Administration, Office of Applied Studies, 1995a. DHHS Publication No. (SMA) 94-3012.

Substance Abuse and Mental Health Services Administration. *National Household Survey on Drug Abuse: Population Estimates 1994.* Rockville (MD): U.S. Department of Health and Human Services, Public Health Service, Substance Abuse and Mental Health Services Administration, Office of Applied Studies, 1995b. DHHS Publication No. (SMA) 95-3063.

Substance Abuse and Mental Health Services Administration. *National Household Survey on Drug Abuse: Population Estimates 1995.* Rockville (MD): U.S. Department of Health and Human Services, Public Health Service, Substance Abuse and Mental Health Services Administration, Office of Applied Studies, 1996. DHHS Publication No. (SMA) 96-3095.

Substance Abuse and Mental Health Services Administration. *National Household Survey on Drug Abuse: Population Estimates 1996.* Rockville (MD): U.S. Department of Health and Human Services, Public Health Service, Substance Abuse and Mental Health Services Administration, Office of Applied Studies, 1997. DHHS Publication No. (SMA) 97-3137.

Substance Abuse and Mental Health Services Administration. *National Household Survey on Drug Abuse: Main Findings 1996.* Rockville (MD): U.S. Department of Health and Human Services, Public Health Service, Substance Abuse and Mental Health Services Administration, Office of Applied Studies, 1998a.

Substance Abuse and Mental Health Services Administration. *National Household Survey on Drug Abuse: Population Estimates 1997.* Rockville (MD): U.S. Department of Health and Human Services, Public Health Service, Substance Abuse and Mental Health Services Administration, Office of Applied Studies, 1998b. DHHS Publication No. (SMA) 98-3250.

Substance Abuse and Mental Health Services Administration. *Summary of Findings from the 1999 National Household Survey on Drug Abuse.* Rockville (MD):

U.S. Department of Health and Human Services, Substance Abuse and Mental Health Services Administration, Office of Applied Studies, 2000.

Sugarman JR, Brenneman G, LaRoque W, Warren CW, Goldberg HI. The urban American Indian oversample in the 1988 National Maternal and Infant Health Survey. *Public Health Reports* 1994;109(2): 243–50.

Sullivan M. *Our Times. The United States 1900–1925. Volume III: Pre-War America.* New York: Charles Scribner's Sons, 1930.

Sussman S, Dent CW, Nezami E, Stacy AW, Burton D, Flay BR. Reasons for quitting and smoking temptation among adolescent smokers: gender differences. *Substance Use and Misuse* 1998;33(14): 2703–20.

Svikis DS, Hatsukami DK, Hughes JR, Carroll KM, Pickens RW. Sex differences in tobacco withdrawal syndrome. *Addictive Behaviors* 1986;11(4):459–62.

Taioli E, Wynder EL. Effect of the age at which smoking begins on frequency of smoking in adulthood. *New England Journal of Medicine* 1991;325(13):968–9.

Tennant RB. *The American Cigarette Industry: A Study in Economic Analysis and Public Policy.* New Haven (CT): Archon Books, 1971.

Thomas M, Goddard E, Hickman M, Hunter P. *General Household Survey 1992.* Series GHS, No. 23 London: Office of Population Censuses and Surveys, Social Survey Division and the Government Statistical Service, 1994.

Tolley HD, Crane L, Shipley N. Smoking prevalence and lung cancer death rates. In: Shopland DR, Burns DM, Samet JM, Gritz ER, editors. *Strategies to Control Tobacco Use in the United States: A Blueprint for Public Health Action in the 1990s.* U.S. Department of Health and Human Services, Public Health Service, National Institutes of Health, National Cancer Institute, 1991. Publication No. (NIH) 92-3316.

Tolson GC, Barnes JM, Gay GA, Kowaleski JL. The 1989 revision of the U.S. standard certificates and reports. *Vital and Health Statistics.* Series 4, No. 28. Hyattsville (MD): U.S. Department of Health and Human Services, Public Health Service, Centers for Disease Control, National Center for Health Statistics, 1991. DHHS Publication No. (PHS) 91-1465.

Tomar SL, Giovino GA. Incidence and predictors of smokeless tobacco use among U.S. youth. *American Journal of Public Health* 1998;88(1):20–6.

Tomar SL, Husten CG, Manley MW. Do dentists and physicians advise tobacco users to quit? *Journal of the American Dental Association* 1996;127(2):259–65.

Tomlinson R. China [news item]. *British Medical Journal* 1998;316:723.

University of Michigan. Cigarette brands smoked by American teens: one brand predominates, three account for nearly all teen smoking [press release]. Ann Arbor (MI): University of Michigan News and Information Services, 1999a Apr 13.

University of Michigan. Cigarette smoking among American teens continues gradual decline [press release]. Ann Arbor (MI): University of Michigan News and Information Services, 1999b Dec 17.

University of Michigan. Cigarette use and smokeless tobacco use decline substantially among teens [press release]. Ann Arbor (MI): University of Michigan News and Information Services, 2000 Dec 14.

U.S. Bureau of the Census. *Current Population Survey, September 1995: Tobacco Use Supplement, Technical Documentation (for machine-readable data).* Washington: U.S. Department of Commerce, Bureau of the Census, 1995.

U.S. Bureau of the Census. *Current Population Survey, January 1996: Tobacco Use Supplement, Technical Documentation (for machine-readable data).* Washington: U.S. Department of Commerce, Bureau of the Census, 1996a.

U.S. Bureau of the Census. *Current Population Survey, May 1996: Tobacco Use Supplement, Technical Documentation (for machine-readable data).* Washington: U.S. Department of Commerce, Bureau of the Census, 1996b.

U.S. Department of Health, Education, and Welfare. *Use of Tobacco: Practices, Attitudes, Knowledge, and Beliefs, United States—Fall 1964 and Spring 1966.* U.S. Department of Health, Education, and Welfare, Public Health Service, Health Services and Mental Health Administration, National Clearinghouse for Smoking and Health, 1969.

U.S. Department of Health, Education, and Welfare. *Teenage Smoking: National Patterns of Cigarette Smoking, Ages 12 through 18, in 1968 and 1970.* Rockville (MD): U.S. Department of Health, Education, and Welfare, Public Health Service, Health Services and Mental Health Administration, Regional Medical Programs Services, National Clearinghouse for Smoking and Health, 1972. DHEW Publication No. (HSM) 72-7508.

U.S. Department of Health, Education, and Welfare. *Adult Use of Tobacco 1970.* Atlanta: U.S. Department of Health, Education, and Welfare, Public Health Service, Center for Disease Control, National Clearinghouse for Smoking and Health, 1973.

U.S. Department of Health, Education, and Welfare. *1975 Adult Use of Tobacco*. Atlanta: U.S. Department of Health, Education, and Welfare, Public Health Service, Centers for Disease Control, Bureau of Health Education, 1976.

U.S. Department of Health, Education, and Welfare. *Cigarette Smoking Among Teen-Agers and Young Women*. U.S. Department of Health, Education, and Welfare, Public Health Service, National Institutes of Health, National Cancer Institute, 1977. DHEW Publication No. (NIH) 77-1203.

U.S. Department of Health, Education, and Welfare. *Teenage Smoking: Immediate and Long Term Patterns*. Washington: U.S. Department of Health, Education, and Welfare, National Institute of Education, Program on Educational Policy and Organization, 1979.

U.S. Department of Health and Human Services. *The Health Consequences of Smoking for Women. A Report of the Surgeon General*. Washington: U.S. Department of Health and Human Services, Public Health Service, Office of the Assistant Secretary for Health, Office on Smoking and Health, 1980.

U.S. Department of Health and Human Services. *The Health Consequences of Smoking: the Changing Cigarette. A Report of the Surgeon General*. Rockville (MD): U.S. Department of Health and Human Services, Public Health Service, Office on Smoking and Health, 1981. DHHS Publication No. (PHS) 81-50156.

U.S. Department of Health and Human Services. *The Health Consequences of Smoking: Cancer. A Report of the Surgeon General*. Rockville (MD): U.S. Department of Health and Human Services, Public Health Service, Office on Smoking and Health, 1982. DHHS Publication No. (PHS) 82-50179.

U.S. Department of Health and Human Services. *The Health Consequences of Smoking: Cardiovascular Disease. A Report of the Surgeon General*. Rockville (MD): U.S. Department of Health and Human Services, Public Health Service, Office on Smoking and Health, 1983. DHHS Publication No. (PHS) 84-50204.

U.S. Department of Health and Human Services. *The Health Consequences of Using Smokeless Tobacco. A Report of the Advisory Committee to the Surgeon General, 1986*. Bethesda (MD): U.S. Department of Health and Human Services, Public Health Service, National Institutes of Health, 1986a. NIH Publication No. 86-2874.

U.S. Department of Health and Human Services. *Smoking and Health: A National Status Report. A Report to Congress*. Rockville (MD): U.S. Department of Health and Human Services, Public Health Service, Centers for Disease Control, Center for Health Promotion and Education, Office on Smoking and Health, 1986b. DHHS/PHS/CDC Publication No. (CDC) 87-8396.

U.S. Department of Health and Human Services. *National Household Survey on Drug Abuse: Main Findings 1985*. Rockville (MD): U.S. Department of Health and Human Services, Public Health Service, Alcohol, Drug Abuse, and Mental Health Administration, National Institute on Drug Abuse, Division of Epidemiology and Statistical Analysis, 1988a. DHHS Publication No. (ADM) 88-1586.

U.S. Department of Health and Human Services. *The Health Consequences of Smoking: Nicotine Addiction. A Report of the Surgeon General*. Atlanta: U.S. Department of Health and Human Services, Public Health Service, Centers for Disease Control, National Center for Chronic Disease Prevention and Health Promotion, Office on Smoking and Health, 1988b. DHHS Publication No. (CDC) 88-8406.

U.S. Department of Health and Human Services. *Reducing the Health Consequences of Smoking: 25 Years of Progress. A Report of the Surgeon General*. Rockville (MD): U.S. Department of Health and Human Services, Public Health Service, Centers for Disease Control, National Center for Chronic Disease Prevention and Health Promotion, Office on Smoking and Health, 1989. DHHS Publication No. (CDC) 89-8411.

U.S. Department of Health and Human Services. *Tobacco Use in 1986: Methods and Basic Tabulations from Adult Use of Tobacco Survey*. Rockville (MD): U.S. Department of Health and Human Services, Public Health Service, Centers for Disease Control, Center for Chronic Disease Prevention and Health Promotion, Office on Smoking and Health, 1990a. DHHS Publication No. OM90-2004.

U.S. Department of Health and Human Services. *National Household Survey on Drug Abuse: Main Findings 1988*. Rockville (MD): U.S. Department of Health and Human Services, Public Health Service, Alcohol, Drug Abuse, and Mental Health Administration, National Institute on Drug Abuse, Division of Epidemiology and Prevention Research, 1990b. DHHS Publication No. (ADM) 90-1682.

U.S. Department of Health and Human Services. *Smoking, Tobacco, and Cancer Program: 1985–1989 Status Report*. Rockville (MD): U.S. Department of

Health and Human Services, Public Health Service, National Institutes of Health, National Cancer Institute, 1990c. NIH Publication No. 90-3107.

U.S. Department of Health and Human Services. *The Health Benefits of Smoking Cessation. A Report of the Surgeon General.* Atlanta: U.S. Department of Health and Human Services, Public Health Service, Centers for Disease Control, National Center for Chronic Disease Prevention and Health Promotion, Office on Smoking and Health, 1990d. DHHS Publication No. (CDC) 90-8416.

U.S. Department of Health and Human Services. *National Household Survey on Drug Abuse: Main Findings 1990.* Rockville (MD): U.S. Department of Health and Human Services, Public Health Service, Alcohol, Drug Abuse, and Mental Health Administration, National Institute on Drug Abuse, Division of Epidemiology and Prevention Research, 1991. DHHS Publication No. (ADM) 91-1788.

U.S. Department of Health and Human Services. *Preventing Tobacco Use Among Young People. A Report of the Surgeon General.* Atlanta: U.S. Department of Health and Human Services, Public Health Service, Centers for Disease Control and Prevention, National Center for Chronic Disease Prevention and Health Promotion, Office on Smoking and Health, 1994.

U.S. Department of Health and Human Services. *Healthy People 2000; Midcourse Review and 1995 Revisions.* Washington: U.S. Department of Health and Human Services, Public Health Service, 1995.

U.S. Department of Health and Human Services. *Health United States, 1995.* Hyattsville (MD): U.S. Department of Health and Human Services, Public Health Service, Centers for Disease Control and Prevention, National Center for Health Statistics, 1996a. DHHS Publication No. (PHS) 96-1232.

U.S. Department of Health and Human Services. *National Pregnancy and Health Survey. Drug Use Among Women Delivering Livebirths: 1992.* Rockville (MD): U.S. Department of Health and Human Services, National Institutes of Health, National Institute on Drug Abuse, 1996b. NIH Publication No. 96-3819.

U.S. Department of Health and Human Services. *Substance Use Among Women in the United States.* Rockville (MD): U.S. Department of Health and Human Services, Public Health Services, Substance Abuse and Mental Health Services Administration, Office of Applied Studies, 1997. DHHS Publication No. (SMA) 97-3162.

U.S. Department of Health and Human Services. *Tobacco Use Among U.S. Racial/Ethnic Minority Groups—African Americans, American Indians and Alaska Natives, Asian Americans and Pacific Islanders, and Hispanics: A Report of the Surgeon General.* Atlanta: U.S. Department of Health and Human Services, Centers for Disease Control and Prevention, National Center for Chronic Disease Prevention and Health Promotion, Office on Smoking and Health, 1998.

U.S. Department of Health and Human Services. *1997 National Health Interview Survey (NHIS) Provisional Public Use Data Release.* Hyattsville (MD): U.S. Department of Health and Human Services, Centers for Disease Control and Prevention, National Center for Health Statistics, Division of Health Interview Statistics, 1999a.

U.S. Department of Health and Human Services. *Youth Use of Cigars: Patterns of Use and Perceptions of Risk.* U.S. Department of Health and Human Services, Office of Inspector General, Office of Evaluation and Inspections, 1999b. Publication No. OEI-06-98-00030.

U.S. Food and Drug Administration Center for Drug Evaluation and Research. Summary Minutes for the 27th Meeting of the Drug Abuse Advisory Committee; 1994 August 1–3; Silver Spring, MD.

Valanis BG, Bowen DJ, Bassford T, Whitlock E, Charney P, Carter RA. Sexual orientation and health: comparisons in the Women's Health Initiative sample. *Archives of Family Medicine* 2000;9(9): 843–53.

Velicer WF, Prochaska JO, Rossi JS, Snow MG. Assessing outcome in smoking cessation studies. *Psychological Bulletin* 1992:111(1):23–41.

Ventura SJ, Martin JA, Curtin SC, Mathews TJ. Report of final natality statistics, 1995. *Monthly Vital Statistics Report* 1997;45(11 Suppl):1–57.

Ventura SJ, Martin JA, Curtin SC, Mathews TJ. Births: final data for 1997. *National Vital Statistics Report* 1999;47(18):1–96.

Ventura SJ, Martin JA, Curtin SC, Mathews TJ, Park MM. Births: final data for 1998. *National Vital Statistics Reports* 2000;48(3):1–100.

Ventura SJ, Martin JA, Taffel SM, Mathews TJ, Clarke SC. Advance report of final natality statistics, 1993. *Monthly Vital Statistics Report* 1995;44(3 Suppl): 1–83.

Wagenknecht LE, Burke GL, Perkins LL, Haley NJ, Friedman GD. Misclassification of smoking status in the CARDIA Study: a comparison of self-report with serum cotinine levels. *American Journal of Public Health* 1992;82(1):33–6.

Wagenknecht LE, Cutter GR, Haley NJ, Sidney S, Manolio TA, Hughes GH, Jacobs DR. Racial differences in serum cotinine levels among smokers in the Coronary Artery Risk Development in (Young) Adults Study. *American Journal of Public Health* 1990a;80(9):1053–6.

Wagenknecht LE, Manolio TA, Lewis CE, Perkins LL, Lando HA, Hulley SB. Race and education in relation to stopping smoking in the U.S.: the CARDIA Study. *Tobacco Control* 1993a;2(4):286–92.

Wagenknecht LE, Manolio TA, Sidney S, Burke GL, Haley NJ. Environmental tobacco smoke exposure as determined by cotinine in black and white young adults: the CARDIA Study. *Environmental Research* 1993b;63(1);39–46.

Wagenknecht LE, Perkins LL, Cutter GR, Sidney S, Burke GL, Manolio TA, Jacobs DR, Liu K, Friedman GD, Hughes GH, Hulley SB. Cigarette smoking behavior is strongly related to educational status: the CARDIA Study. *Preventive Medicine* 1990b; 19(2):158–69.

Wagner S. *Cigarette Country: Tobacco in American History and Politics.* New York: Praeger, 1971.

Waldron I. Employment and women's health. An analysis of causal relationships. *International Journal of Health Services* 1980;10(3):435–54.

Waldron I. Sex differences in illness incidence, prognosis and mortality: issues and evidence. *Social Science and Medicine* 1983;17(16):1107–23.

Waldron I. Patterns and causes of gender differences in smoking. *Social Science and Medicine* 1991;32(9): 989–1005.

Waldron I, Lye D. Employment, unemployment, occupation, and smoking. *American Journal of Preventive Medicine* 1989;5(3):142–9.

Waldron I, Lye D, Brandon A. Gender differences in teenage smoking. *Women and Health* 1991;17(2): 65–90.

Ward KD, Klesges RC, Zbikowski SM. Gender differences in the outcome of an unaided smoking cessation attempt. *Addictive Behaviors* 1997;22(4)521–33.

Warner KE. Possible increases in the underreporting of cigarette consumption. *Journal of the American Statistical Association* 1978;73(362):314–8.

Warner KE, Murt HA. Impact of the antismoking campaign on smoking prevalence: a cohort analysis. *Journal of Public Health Policy* 1982;3(4):374–90.

Wechsler H, Rigotti NA, Giedhill-Hoyt J, Lee H. Increased levels of cigarette use among college students: a cause for national concern. *Journal of the American Medical Association* 1998;280(19): 1673–8.

Weekley CK, Klesges RC, Relyea G. Smoking as a weight-control strategy and its relationship to smoking status. *Addictive Behaviors* 1992;17(3): 259–71.

Weissman MM, Bruce ML, Leaf PJ, Florio LP, Holzer C III. Affective disorders. In: Robins LN, Regier DA, editors. *Psychiatric Disorders in America: the Epidemiologic Catchment Area Study*. Toronto: Free Press, 1991:53–80.

Welch SL, Fairburn CG. Smoking and bulimia nervosa. *International Journal of Eating Disorders* 1998;23(4): 433–7.

Wells AJ, English PB, Posner SF, Wagenknecht LE, Pérez-Stable EJ. Misclassification rates for current smokers misclassified as nonsmokers. *American Journal of Public Health* 1998;88(10):1503–9.

Welty TK, Lee ET, Yeh J, Cowan LD, Go O, Fabsitz RR, Le N-A, Oopik AJ, Robbins DC, Howard BV. Cardiovascular disease risk factors among American Indians: the Strong Heart Study. *American Journal of Epidemiology* 1995;142(3):269–87.

Wessel CA. The first sixty billions are the hardest for cigarette industry. *Printers' Ink* 1924;126(5):3–6, 137–46.

Wewers ME, Dhatt RK, Moeschberger ML, Guthrie RM, Kuun P, Chen MS. Misclassification of smoking status among Southeast Asian adult immigrants. *American Journal of Respiratory and Critical Care Medicine* 1995;152(6 Pt 1):1917–21.

Whitlock EP, Ferry LH, Burchette RJ, Abbey D. Smoking characteristics of female veterans. *Addictive Behaviors* 1995;20(4):409–26.

Whitlock EP, Vogt TM, Hollis JF, Lichtenstein E. Does gender affect response to a brief clinic-based smoking intervention? *American Journal of Preventive Medicine* 1997;13(3):159–66.

Willard JC, Schoenborn CA. Relationship between cigarette smoking and other unhealthy behaviors among our Nation's youth: United States, 1992. *Advance Data.* No. 263. Hyattsville (MD): U.S. Department of Health and Human Services, Public Health Service, Centers for Disease Control and Prevention, National Center for Health Statistics, 1995. DHHS Publication No. (PHS) 95-1250.

Williams CL, Eng A, Botvin GJ, Hill P, Wynder EL. Validation of students' self-reported cigarette smoking status with plasma cotinine levels. *American Journal of Public Health* 1979;69(12):1272–4.

Williamson DF, Madans J, Anda RF, Kleinman JC, Giovino GA, Byers T. Smoking cessation and severity of weight gain in a national cohort. *New England Journal of Medicine* 1991;324(11):739–45.

Wills TA, Cleary SD. The validity of self-reports of smoking: analyses by race/ethnicity in a school sample of urban adolescents. *American Journal of Public Health* 1997;87(1):56–61.

Wills WD, Wills HO. Women and cigarettes. *Printers' Ink* 1932;158(7):25–7.

Windsor RA, Lowe JB, Perkins LL, Smith-Yoder D, Artz L, Crawford M, Amburgy K, Boyd NR Jr. Health education for pregnant smokers: its behavioral impact and cost benefit. *American Journal of Public Health* 1993;83(2):201–6.

Winkleby MA, Fortmann SP, Barrett DC. Social class disparities in risk factors for disease: eight-year prevalence patterns by level of education. *Preventive Medicine* 1990;19(1–2):1–12.

Winkleby MA, Schooler C, Kraemer HC, Lin J, Fortmann SP. Hispanic versus white smoking patterns by sex and level of education. *American Journal of Epidemiology* 1995;142(4):410–8.

World Bank. *Curbing the Epidemic: Governments and the Economics of Tobacco Control.* Washington: World Bank, 1999.

World Health Organization. *Tobacco or Health: A Global Status Report.* Geneva: World Health Organization, 1997.

World Health Organization. *The World Health Report 1999: Making a Difference.* Geneva: World Health Organization, 1999.

*World Health Organization Tobacco Alert*. The tobacco epidemic: a global public health emergency. *World Health Organization Tobacco Alert* 1996; special issue:1–28.

Wynder EL, Goodman MT, Hoffmann D. Demographic aspects of the low-yield cigarette: considerations in the evaluation of health risk. *Journal of the National Cancer Institute* 1984;72(4):817–22.

Yankelovich Partners. *Smoking Cessation Study.* Report prepared for Ketchum Public Relations and their client American Lung Association. Norwalk (CT): Yankelovich Partners, July 27, 1998; <http://www.lungusa.org/partner/yank/1.html>; accessed: August 15, 2000.

Zagona SV. Psycho-social correlates of smoking behavior and attitudes for a sample of Anglo-American, Mexican-American, and Indian-American high school seniors. In: Zagona SV, editor. *Studies and Issues in Smoking Behavior.* Tucson (AZ): University of Arizona Press, 1967:157–80.

Zanes A, Matsoukas E. Different settings, different results? A comparison of school and home responses. *Public Opinion Quarterly* 1979;43(4):550–7.

Zhu B-P, Giovino GA, Mowery PD, Eriksen MP. The relationship between cigarette smoking and education revisited: implications for categorizing persons' educational status. *American Journal of Public Health* 1996;86(11):1582–9.

Zhu S-H, Melcer T, Sun J, Rosbrook B, Pierce JP. Smoking cessation with and without assistance: a population-based analysis. *American Journal of Preventive Medicine* 2000;18(4):305–11.

Zhu S-H, Sun J, Billings SC, Choi WS, Malarcher A. Predictors of smoking cessation in U.S. adolescents. *American Journal of Preventive Medicine* 1999;16(3):202–7.

# Chapter 3. Health Consequences of Tobacco Use Among Women

# Introduction

This chapter reviews the evidence for a relationship between smoking, as well as exposure to environmental tobacco smoke (ETS), and a wide range of diseases and health-related conditions among women. It begins with a section on the impact of smoking on mortality from all causes combined among women who smoke compared with women who have never smoked. Most of the remainder of the chapter is devoted to the effects of active smoking on specific health outcomes among women, ranging from cancer to bone density. Lung cancer is discussed first because of the strength of its association with smoking and because smoking is responsible for lung cancer becoming the leading cause of cancer death among U.S. women by the late 1980s, a position it continues to hold. Female-specific cancers are discussed next, followed by other cancers. Because coronary heart disease constitutes the major overall cause of death among women and because of the well-established association of smoking with heart disease and stroke, a section devoted to cardiovascular disease appears next. After that, another important cause of smoking-related morbidity and mortality, chronic obstructive pulmonary disease, is discussed. A brief section on sex hormones, thyroid disorders, and diabetes follows. Next reviewed are areas of unique concern among women, namely the effects of smoking on menstrual function and menopause and on reproductive hormones. Other sections review a variety of diseases (e.g., eye disease, gastrointestinal disease) or physiologic effects (e.g., bone density, nicotine addiction) that have been examined in relation to smoking among women. The chapter concludes with sections on the effect of ETS on female lung cancer, heart disease, and reproductive outcomes. Our knowledge base regarding the effects of smoking on women's health has grown enormously since the Surgeon General's first report on women and smoking was published in 1980 (U.S. Department of Health and Human Services [USDHHS] 1980). The physiologic effects of smoking are broad ranging and, in addition to the health risks shared with men who smoke, women smokers experience unique risks such as those related to reproduction and menopause. Since 1980, approximately three million U.S. women have died prematurely as a result of a smoking-related disease. In 1997 alone, an estimated 165,000 U.S. women died prematurely of a smoking-related disease.

Because numerous experts contributed to this report, with varying preferences for use of terms to report outcome measures and statistical significance, the editors chose certain simplifying conventions in reporting research results. In particular, the term "relative risk" generally was adopted throughout this chapter for ratio measures of association—whether original study results were reported as relative risks, estimated relative risks, odds ratios, rate ratios, risk ratios, or other terms that express risk for one group of individuals (e.g., smokers) as a ratio of another (e.g., nonsmokers). Moreover, relative risks and confidence intervals were generally rounded to one decimal place, except when rounding could change a marginally statistically significant finding to an insignificant finding; thus, only when the original confidence limit was within 0.95 to 0.99 or within 1.01 to 1.04 were two decimal places retained in the reporting of results.

# Total Mortality

Women in the United States began regular cigarette smoking in large numbers decades before women in most other countries did; among women born before 1960, adolescent girls took up regular smoking at progressively earlier ages (Burns et al. 1997a) (see Chapter 2). Thus, U.S. women have been at the forefront of an emerging worldwide epidemic of deaths from smoking, and their experience underscores the need to curtail tobacco marketing worldwide. Women in the United States make up approximately 20 percent of women in the developed world. In 1990, they accounted for more than 40 percent of all deaths attributable to smoking among women in developed countries (Peto et al. 1994).

**Figure 3.1. All-cause death rates for current smokers and lifelong nonsmokers, by age and gender, Cancer Prevention Study II, 1982–1988**

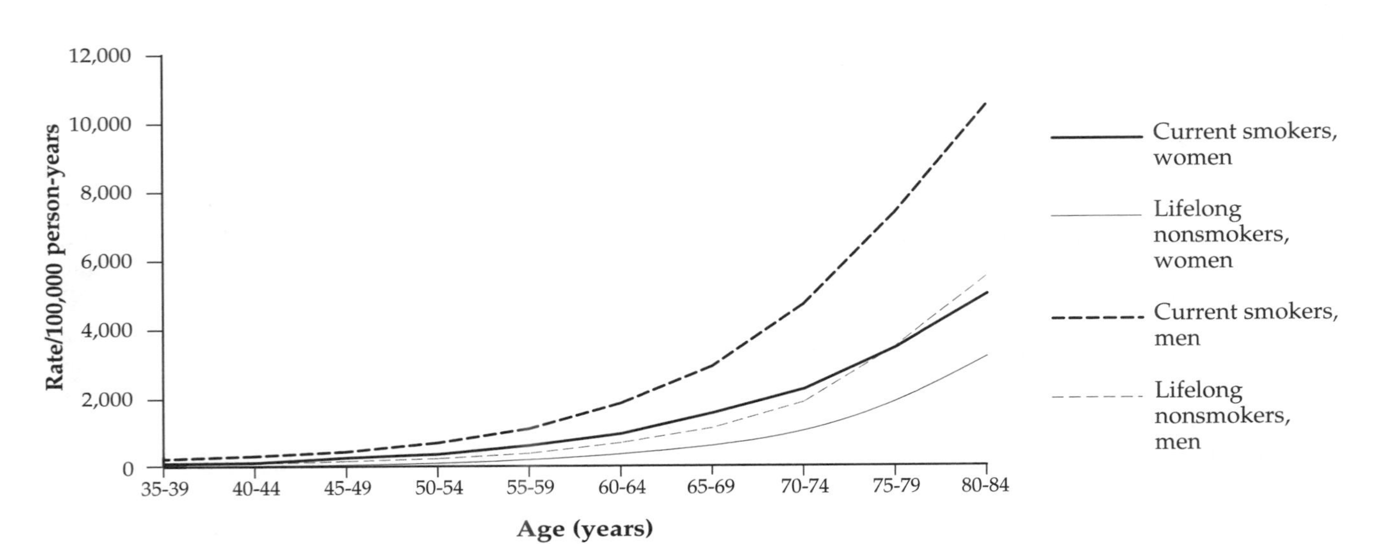


Sources: Thun et al. 1997a,c.

In this section of Chapter 3, the death rate from all causes combined among women who continue to smoke (current smokers) is compared with the rate in those who have never smoked regularly. The risk from smoking depends on the duration of smoking, the number of cigarettes smoked per day, the age of the smoker, and the epidemiologic measure used to assess risk. By all measures, however, risk increased dramatically among U.S. women from the 1950s through the late 1980s. This finding is clearly demonstrated by the results of at least eight large prospective studies from North America.

## Age-Specific and Smoking-Specific Death Rates

The largest contemporary study of smoking and mortality in the United States is the American Cancer Society (ACS) Cancer Prevention Study II (CPS-II)—a prospective, epidemiologic study of more than one million adults that was begun by ACS in 1982 (Garfinkel 1985; Stellman and Garfinkel 1986; Garfinkel and Stellman 1988; Thun et al. 1995, 1997a). Descriptions of CPS-II and of other epidemiologic studies discussed in this section are provided in the Appendix to this chapter.

As illustrated in Figure 3.1 and Table 3.1, overall death rates in CPS-II were substantially higher among women who currently smoked cigarettes when enrolled than among those who had never smoked regularly (lifelong nonsmokers). The death rate (per 100,000 person-years at risk) among women who smoked was approximately twice that among women who had never smoked in every age group from 45 through 74 years (Table 3.1). Although death rates were lower among women than among men (Figure 3.1), the relationship of smoking to all-cause death rates was similar among women and men. The large size of CPS-II allows death rates to be estimated fairly precisely by gender and smoking status and within five-year intervals of age at the time of follow-up.

CPS-II data on the relationship of smoking and the risk for death from all causes combined are shown in Table 3.1. This relationship was measured in three ways. (1) The death rate, defined as deaths per 100,000 person-years at risk, reflects the absolute probability (risk) of death per year (also see Figure 3.1). (2) Relative risk (RR), defined as the death rate among smokers divided by the rate among those who had never smoked, expresses the risk among smokers as a multiple of the annual risk among those who had never smoked. (3) Rate difference, defined as the death rate among smokers minus the rate among those who had never smoked, reflects the absolute excess risk for death per year among smokers compared with those who had never smoked. The CPS-II results illustrate that the impact of smoking on deaths

**Table 3.1. All-cause mortality among women for lifelong nonsmokers and current smokers, by age, Cancer Prevention Study II, 1982–1988**

| | Age specific | | | | | |
|---|---|---|---|---|---|---|
| | Lifelong nonsmokers | | Current smokers | | | |
| Age (years) | Number of deaths | Death rate* | Number of deaths | Death rate* | Relative risk | Rate difference* |
| 35–39 | 40 | 80.6 | 22 | 88.8 | 1.1 | 8.2 |
| 40–44 | 93 | 109.3 | 50 | 110.9 | 1.0 | 1.6 |
| 45–49 | 255 | 122.4 | 256 | 252.6 | 2.1 | 130.2 |
| 50–54 | 564 | 182.1 | 501 | 348.5 | 1.9 | 166.4 |
| 55–59 | 927 | 268.2 | 874 | 598.8 | 2.2 | 330.6 |
| 60–64 | 1,401 | 411.4 | 1,140 | 936.3 | 2.3 | 525.0 |
| 65–69 | 1,871 | 666.5 | 1,243 | 1,533.7 | 2.3 | 867.2 |
| 70–74 | 2,216 | 1,073.9 | 1,020 | 2,227.0 | 2.1 | 1,153.1 |
| 75–79 | 2,487 | 1,838.7 | 658 | 3,417.9 | 1.9 | 1,579.1 |
| 80–84 | 2,245 | 3,154.2 | 285 | 4,959.2 | 1.6 | 1,805.0 |
| Total | 12,099 | | 6,049 | | | |

| | Age standardized to age distribution in 1980 U.S. population | |
|---|---|---|
| | Lifelong nonsmokers | Current smokers |
| Death rate* | 475.0 | 913.5 |
| 95% CI[†] | 465.6–484.3 | 885.2–941.8 |
| Relative risk | 1.0 | 1.9 |
| 95% CI | NA[‡] | 1.9–2.0 |
| Rate difference* | 0 | 438.5 |
| 95% CI | NA | 408.7–468.3 |

*Note:* Analyses restricted to women aged 35–84 years to maximize stability and validity of results.
*Death rate and rate difference, for all causes, per 100,000 person-years.
[†]CI = Confidence interval.
[‡]NA = Not applicable.
Sources: Thun et al. 1997a,c.

from all causes varies at different ages for each of the three measures of risk (Thun et al. 1997c). Beginning at approximately age 45 years, the death rate from all causes was progressively higher among women who smoked than among those who had never smoked (Figure 3.1). The absolute increase in risk associated with smoking became greater with age, as measured by the increase in the rate difference from ages 45 through 84 years (Table 3.1). In contrast, the value for RR associated with any current smoking increased from approximately 1.0 among women younger than 45 years to a maximum of 2.3 at ages 60 through 69 years, then decreased to 1.6 at ages 80 through 84 years (Table 3.1).

Measured in absolute terms, smoking becomes more, rather than less, hazardous with increasing age. Older smokers incur a larger individual risk for dying prematurely from their smoking than do younger smokers, and the total number of smoking attributable deaths is greater among older smokers than among younger smokers. On the other hand, trends in RR reflect first the increase and later the decrease, with age, of the proportionate contribution of smoking to deaths among smokers. In the CPS-II data, the RR associated with smoking among women peaked at 2.3 at ages 60 through 69 years (Table 3.1). The corresponding RR among British male physicians and men in CPS-II who continued to smoke cigarettes was approximately 3.0 at approximately 40 through 60 years of age (Doll et al. 1994; Thun et al. 1997c). The proportionately smaller contribution of smoking to death among older smokers indicated that death rates from factors unrelated to smoking increase even faster at older ages than do the increasing hazards from smoking.

## Changes over Time in the Association Between Smoking and All-Cause Death Rates

Changes in women's smoking behavior, particularly the trend up to 1960 among adolescent girls to start smoking at progressively earlier ages, underlie the gradual increase in smoking-associated RR for death among women smokers in the last half-century. A unique longitudinal perspective on how smoking behavior and smoking-specific death rates changed among U.S. women from the late 1950s through the 1980s may be seen by comparing the results of CPS-II with its predecessor, the Cancer Prevention Study I (CPS-I), which was conducted by ACS in 1959–1965 (USDHHS 1989b; Thun et al. 1995, 1997a). In CPS-I, methods of recruitment and follow-up were similar to those in CPS-II (see Appendix to this chapter). In general, women in CPS-I who smoked began to smoke regularly just before, during, or after World War II, and relatively few had smoked for more than 20 years. In contrast, many women enrolled in CPS-II had smoked regularly for 30 to 40 years. Women in CPS-II started smoking in larger numbers at younger ages and, in every age group, the mean number of cigarettes smoked daily at baseline was greater (Thun et al. 1997a,c).

Two major temporal trends are evident in the comparison of age-specific and smoking-specific all-cause death rates in CPS-I and CPS-II. The first trend (Figure 3.2) is that the difference in female age-specific, all-cause death rates (rate difference) between current smokers and women who had never smoked (as reported at enrollment) was much greater in CPS-II than in CPS-I at age 45 years and older. Tables 3.1 (CPS-II) and 3.2 (CPS-I) present age-specific, all-cause death rates among women for the two studies directly standardized to the age distribution of the U.S. population in 1980. The rate difference between women who were current smokers and those who had never smoked almost doubled, from 238.4 in CPS-I (Table 3.2) to 438.5 in CPS-II (Table 3.1). Similarly, the RR associated with current

**Figure 3.2. All-cause death rates among women for current smokers and lifelong nonsmokers, by age, Cancer Prevention Study I (CPS-I), 1959–1965, and Cancer Prevention Study II (CPS-II), 1982–1988**

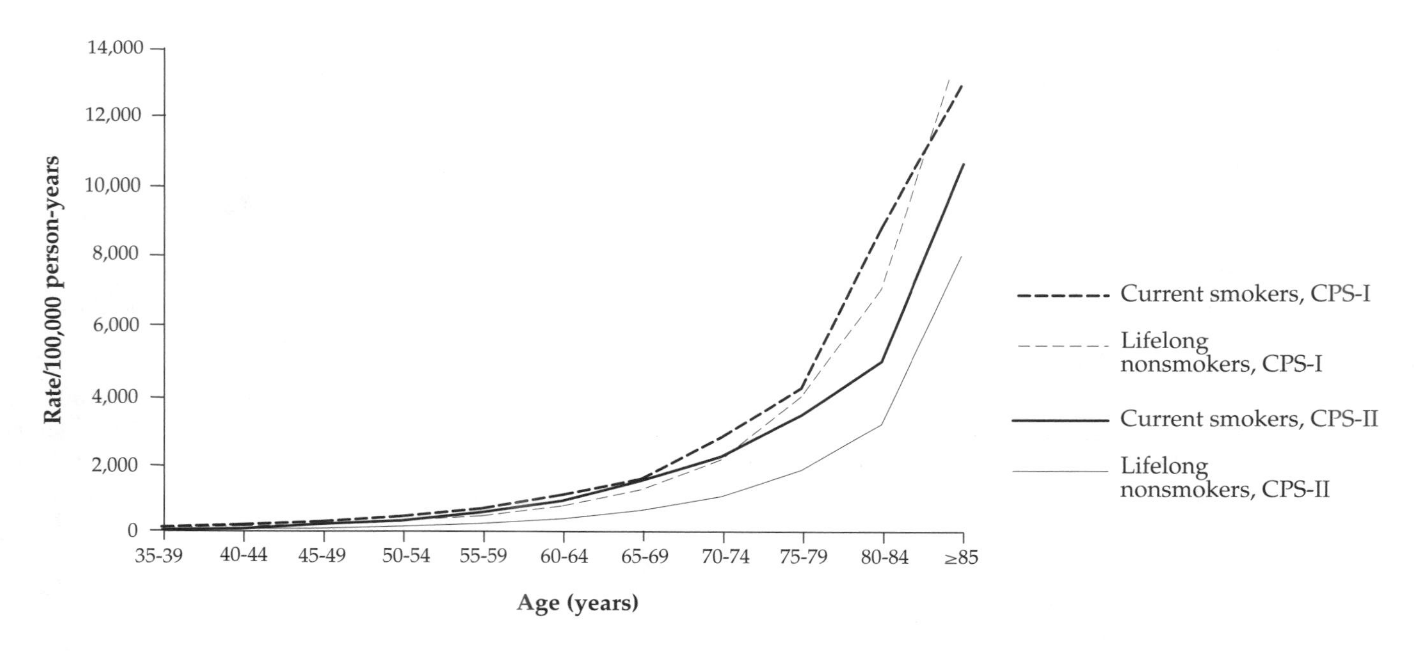


Source: Thun et al. 1997a.

smoking increased from 1.3 (Table 3.2) to 1.9 (Table 3.1). These large increases during the two decades between the two ACS studies in both the rate difference and the RR for U.S. women who smoked reflect the emergence of the full effect of smoking-related deaths among women who were long-term smokers.

The second important difference between CPS-I and CPS-II is the decline in background rates of all-cause mortality in the time period between the two studies. This mortality rate difference was largely due to the decline over the past several decades in death rates for cardiovascular diseases—the leading cause of death in the United States among women and men. Table 3.2 (CPS-I) and Table 3.1 (CPS-II) show the age-adjusted, all-cause death rates among smokers and among persons who had never smoked. The all-cause death rate among women who had never smoked was approximately 50 percent lower for those in CPS-II than for those in CPS-I, but only 22 percent lower among current smokers in CPS-II than among current smokers in CPS-I. This difference largely reflects the decline in death rates for cardiovascular disease over these two decades, and the decline in cardiovascular disease death rates between the two studies was smaller among women who smoked than among women who had never smoked.

**Table 3.2. All-cause mortality among women for lifelong nonsmokers and current smokers, by age, Cancer Prevention Study I, 1959–1965**

| | Age specific | | | | | |
|---|---|---|---|---|---|---|
| | Lifelong nonsmokers | | Current smokers | | | |
| Age (years) | Number of deaths | Death rate* | Number of deaths | Death rate* | Relative risk | Rate difference* |
| 35–39 | 73 | 100.1 | 67 | 111.4 | 1.1 | 11.3 |
| 40–44 | 230 | 150.7 | 230 | 199.2 | 1.3 | 48.5 |
| 45–49 | 638 | 211.4 | 600 | 291.6 | 1.4 | 80.2 |
| 50–54 | 1,247 | 320.9 | 932 | 442.0 | 1.4 | 121.1 |
| 55–59 | 1,696 | 454.2 | 906 | 673.1 | 1.5 | 218.9 |
| 60–64 | 2,371 | 749.5 | 756 | 1,076.6 | 1.4 | 327.1 |
| 65–69 | 3,140 | 1,234.7 | 545 | 1,545.4 | 1.3 | 310.7 |
| 70–74 | 3,700 | 2,101.1 | 425 | 2,739.9 | 1.3 | 638.8 |
| 75–79 | 3,933 | 3,925.1 | 241 | 4,162.7 | 1.1 | 237.6 |
| 80–84 | 3,406 | 7,031.6 | 147 | 8,802.4 | 1.3 | 1,770.8 |
| Total | 20,434 | | 4,849 | | | |

| | Age standardized to age distribution in 1980 U.S. population | |
|---|---|---|
| | Lifelong nonsmokers | Current smokers |
| Death rate* | 927.6 | 1,166.0 |
| 95% CI[†] | 914.2–941.0 | 1,107.9–1,224.1 |
| Relative risk | 1.0 | 1.3 |
| 95% CI | NA[‡] | 1.2–1.3 |
| Rate difference* | 0 | 238.4 |
| 95% CI | NA | 178.8–298.1 |

*Note:* Analyses restricted to women aged 35–84 years to maximize stability and validity of results.
*Death rate and rate of difference, for all causes, per 100,000 person-years.
[†]CI = Confidence interval.
[‡]NA = Not applicable.
Sources: Thun et al. 1997a,c.

## Consistency of Temporal Trends Across Studies

Beside the results of CPS-I and CPS-II, other prospective studies since the late 1940s suggested a temporal trend of increasing RR for death from all causes among female smokers and an increasing proportion of deaths attributable to smoking (Figure 3.3). None of these cohort studies (see Appendix to this chapter) was designed specifically to assess a temporal trend in risk. Collectively, however, their results suggested that the all-cause RR associated with current smoking for women was similar across studies and that the RR increased from approximately 1.2 in the 1950s and early 1960s to a range of 1.8 to 1.9 by the 1980s. In the earlier studies, including the British doctors' study (Doll et al. 1980), a large census-based study in Japan (Hirayama 1990), and CPS-I (Thun et al. 1997a), women who smoked had usually begun to smoke regularly less than 20 years before the start of the study. In the more recent studies, including the U.S. Nurses' Health Study (Kawachi et al. 1993a), the Kaiser Permanente Medical Care Program cohort study (Friedman et al. 1997), a study of three U.S.

**Figure 3.3. Age-adjusted total mortality ratios among women (and 95% confidence interval) for current smokers compared with lifelong nonsmokers, prospective studies**

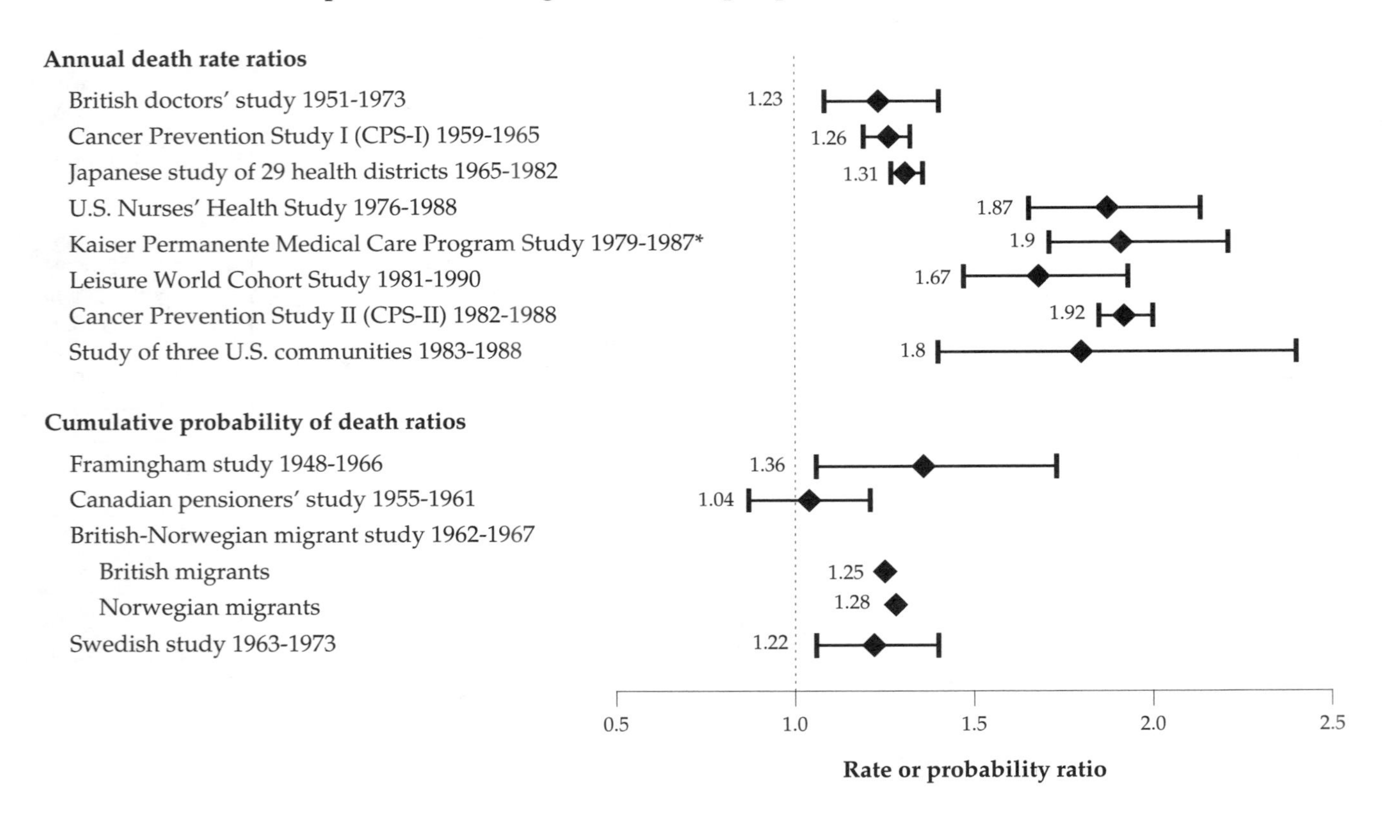


*Note:* All confidence intervals shown represent 95% except the study in Japan (90%). Age standardized to 1980 U.S. population.

*Data for white women.

†Data not available to compute 95% confidence intervals.

Sources: **British doctors' study:** Doll et al. 1980. **CPS-I and CPS-II:** Thun et al. 1995. **Japanese study of 29 health districts:** Hirayama 1990. **U.S. Nurses' Health Study:** Kawachi et al. 1993a, 1997b. **Kaiser Permanente Medical Care Program Study:** Friedman et al. 1997. **Leisure World Cohort Study:** Paganini-Hill and Hsu 1994. **Study of three U.S. communities:** LaCroix et al. 1991. **Framingham study:** Shurtleff 1974; Cupples and D'Agostino 1987; Freund et al. 1993. **Canadian pensioners' study:** Best et al. 1961; Canadian Department of National Health and Welfare 1966. **British-Norwegian migrant study:** Pearl et al. 1966; U.S. Department of Health and Human Services 1980. **Swedish study:** Cederlöf et al. 1975.

communities (LaCroix et al. 1991), and CPS-II (Thun et al. 1997a), women who reported current smoking had smoked for longer periods of time than they did in the earlier studies. In a recent cohort study, the estimated RR for death from all causes combined was slightly lower (1.7; 95 percent confidence interval [CI], 1.5 to 1.9) than in the other studies (Paganini-Hill and Hsu 1994). Participants in that study, however, were members of the Leisure World retirement community of southern California and were substantially older at the time of enrollment (median age, 73 years) than were the participants in most of the other studies.

The investigators of four studies (Canadian Department of National Health and Welfare 1966; Shurtleff 1974; Cederlöf et al. 1975; USDHHS 1980) measured the excess risk among smokers by calculating the cumulative probability of death ratio, which was defined as the probability of death among smokers divided by the probability among those who had never smoked, over a specified period (Kleinbaum et al. 1982). In studies with prolonged follow-ups and a common end point, the use of this ratio results in a slight underestimation of the RR (Rothman 1986). Thus, these studies are presented separately from the eight studies, including CPS-I and CPS-II, that reported annual death rate ratios (Figure 3.3 and Appendix to this chapter).

The findings in CPS-I, CPS-II, and the other studies generally support the observation that the risk for death from smoking among U.S. women has increased over time. Total mortality by amount smoked also has been reported based on pooled data from three prospective studies conducted in Copenhagen, with initial exams between 1964 and 1992 and follow-up until 1994 (Prescott et al. 1998a). RRs for all-cause mortality increased with amount smoked: compared with persons who had never smoked, the RR was 2.2 (95 percent CI, 2.0 to 2.5) among women who smoked less than 15 g of tobacco per day, 2.7 (95 percent CI, 2.4 to 3.1) among women who smoked 15 to 24 g per day, and 3.6 (95 percent CI, 2.9 to 4.5) among those who smoked 25 g or more per day.

### Adjustment for Risk Factors Other than Smoking

Although factors such as the duration of smoking, the number of cigarettes smoked per day, and the age of the smoker strongly influence the association between smoking and all-cause mortality, other demographic and behavioral factors associated with smoking also appear to affect the risks associated with smoking.

In most studies, risk estimates were not adjusted for potential confounders other than age. However, studies in which adjustment was made for other factors found little evidence that the estimates of risk associated with smoking were substantially different after adjustment. Data from the 12-year follow-up of the U.S. Nurses' Health Study showed no real difference between the estimates of RR for death from all causes combined that were adjusted for age alone and the estimates that were adjusted for age, hypertension, cholesterol, menopausal status, postmenopausal estrogen therapy, and other factors (Kawachi et al. 1993a, 1997b) (Table 3.3).

Among women in CPS-II, values for the RR for death from all causes combined were negligibly different among current smokers aged 30 years or older

**Table 3.3. Age-adjusted and multivariate relative risks (RRs) for all-cause mortality, by smoking status and number of cigarettes smoked per day, U.S. Nurses' Health Study, 1976–1988**

| | Lifelong nonsmokers | Former smokers | Current smokers | Number of cigarettes/day for current smokers | | | |
|---|---|---|---|---|---|---|---|
| | | | | 1–14 | 15–24 | 25–34 | ≥ 35 |
| Number of deaths | 933 | 799 | 1,115 | 234 | 480 | 215 | 153 |
| RR* | 1.0 | 1.3 | 1.9 | 1.4 | 1.99 | 2.1 | 2.6 |
| RR† | 1.0 | 1.3 | 1.9 | 1.5 | 2.0 | 2.1 | 2.6 |
| 95% CI‡ | | 1.1–1.5 | 1.7–2.1 | 1.3–1.8 | 1.7–2.4 | 1.7–2.6 | 2.1–3.3 |

*Adjusted for age only.
†Adjusted for age; follow-up period; body mass index (weight/height$^2$); history of hypertension, high cholesterol, or diabetes; parental history of myocardial infarction before age 60 years; postmenopausal estrogen therapy; menopausal status; previous use of oral contraceptives; and age at start of smoking.
‡CI = Confidence interval.
Sources: Kawachi et al. 1993a, 1997b.

after adjustment for age, dietary fat and vegetable consumption, physical activity, and aspirin use (ACS, unpublished data) (Table 3.4). Small changes in the RR after multivariate adjustment (Table 3.4) would result in even smaller change in the attributable fraction among persons exposed, assuming that the estimates of RR accurately reflect a causal relationship with smoking. Adjustment for covariates decreased the attributable fraction from 50 to 47 percent of all deaths among current smokers and increased it from 23 to 29 percent among former smokers (Table 3.4). Thus, when adjusted only for age, nearly one-half of all deaths among women who currently smoked and about one-fourth of deaths in former smokers were attributable to smoking. In comparison, the percentage of deaths that would be attributable to smoking among women current smokers in the earlier period of CPS-I was only 21 percent (Table 3.2 and Figure 3.3).

## Smoking Attributable Deaths Among U.S. Women

Two approaches have been used to estimate the number of deaths attributable to smoking among U.S. women and to assess how this burden has changed over time. Estimates for the U.S. Public Health Service are produced by the Centers for Disease Control and Prevention (CDC), Office on Smoking and Health, using a computer program—Smoking Attributable Mortality, Morbidity, and Economic Costs (SAMMEC 3.0), which incorporates an epidemiologic measure of risk known as the population attributable risk (USDHHS 1997). These estimates for women take three factors into account: (1) the prevalence of current and former smoking among U.S. women in a particular year, (2) the RR estimates among women in CPS-II during the initial four years of follow-up for selected conditions having a firmly established relationship to smoking, and (3) the total number of deaths coded to these conditions among U.S. women. The SAMMEC estimate has increased from 30,000 in 1965 to 106,000 in 1985 (USDHHS 1989b) and to 152,000 annually during 1990–1994 (CDC 1997). For 1995–1997, the annual SAMMEC estimates for U.S. women averaged 163,000 (CDC, unpublished data). On the basis of recent trends in these estimates, it can be projected that SAMMEC estimates among U.S. women during the years 1998–2000 will average about 170,000 (CDC, unpublished data). Thus, since the last report on the health consequences of smoking among women in 1980, it can be estimated that approximately 3 million deaths among U.S. women have been attributable to smoking (CDC, unpublished data).

An alternate technique was developed by Peto and associates (1994) to provide estimates of deaths from smoking in developed countries, even where reliable data on smoking prevalence are not available. By using the national death rate for lung cancer to index past smoking habits, Peto and associates estimated that smoking caused approximately 14,100 deaths among U.S. women in 1965 and 131,000 in 1985. Although not expected to be exact, the estimates of smoking attributable mortality generated for different countries by use of this method showed that women in the United States and the United Kingdom who have smoked longer than women in other countries are at the forefront of the emerging global epidemic of deaths from tobacco smoking (Peto et al. 1994).

## Years of Potential Life Lost

Another measure of the impact of smoking on survival is years of potential life lost (YPLL). Although less commonly used, YPLL takes into account the age at which people die, as well as the total number of deaths. Using the SAMMEC software program

**Table 3.4. Relative risks among women for death from all causes, and smoking attributable fraction of deaths among smokers ($AF_{exp}$), with adjustment for age and multiple potential risk factors, Cancer Prevention Study II, 1982–1988**

| | | Current smokers (n = 6,416) | | Former smokers (n = 4,812) | |
|---|---|---|---|---|---|
| Adjustment for: | Lifelong nonsmokers (n = 15,929) | Relative risk (95% CI)* | $AF_{exp}$ (%) | Relative risk (95% CI) | $AF_{exp}$ (%) |
| Age | 1.0 | 2.0 (2.0–2.1) | 50 | 1.3 (1.3–1.4) | 23 |
| Multiple risk factors† | 1.0 | 1.9 (1.9–2.0) | 47 | 1.4 (1.3–1.4) | 29 |

*CI = Confidence interval.
†Age, dietary fat and vegetable consumption, physical activity, and aspirin use.
Source: American Cancer Society, unpublished data.

(USDHHS 1997), CDC's Office on Smoking and Health estimated YPLL from smoking among U.S. women each year during 1990–1994 on the basis of disease-specific RRs among women smokers from CPS-II for 1982–1986, mortality data among U.S. women for 1990, and prevalence of current and former women smokers in the United States in 1990–1994 (CDC 1997). Based on survival to life expectancy, the average annual YPLL due to smoking-related deaths from neoplastic, cardiovascular, respiratory, and pediatric diseases was 2,148,000, or about 14 years for each smoking attributable death (CDC, unpublished data). This estimate did not include YPLL due to exposure to ETS. Other investigators estimated that U.S. white women who were current smokers had a life expectancy in 1986 that was three to seven years less than that of women the same age who had never smoked (Rogers and Powell-Griner 1991). A multisite, population-based, prospective study of persons aged 65 years or older found that even when level of physical activity was controlled for, women who had ever smoked lived an average of four to five years less than women who had never smoked (Ferrucci et al. 1999). On the basis of these YPLL estimates and the estimated number of deaths among U.S. women attributable to smoking, it can be estimated that since the last report on the health consequences of smoking among women in 1980, from 9 to 41 million years of potential life have been lost by U.S. women because of smoking (CDC, unpublished data).

## Effects of Smoking Cessation

Several studies examined the reduction in all-cause death rates among women that is related to smoking cessation (USDHHS 1990). In the U.S. Nurses' Health Study, to better estimate the effect of cessation, women with nonfatal coronary heart disease, stroke, or cancer (except nonmelanoma skin cancer) were excluded at baseline and at the beginning of each 2-year follow-up period. The RR for death from all causes combined during the 12-year follow-up was 1.15 (95 percent CI, 1.01 to 1.29) among women who had stopped smoking (Kawachi et al. 1993a, 1997b). This RR was substantially lower than that of 2.04 (95 percent CI, 1.85 to 2.27) among women who continued to smoke (Kawachi et al. 1993a, 1997b). The RR among former smokers decreased progressively with time since smoking cessation; 10 through 14 years after smoking cessation, the RR approached the risk among those who had never smoked (Figure 3.4).

An alternate method of expressing the benefits of smoking cessation is to present the absolute risk for death at various ages during follow-up by grouping

**Figure 3.4. Relative risks of death from all causes (and 95% confidence interval) for current smokers compared with lifelong nonsmokers, by years since smoking cessation, U.S. Nurses' Health Study, 1976–1988**

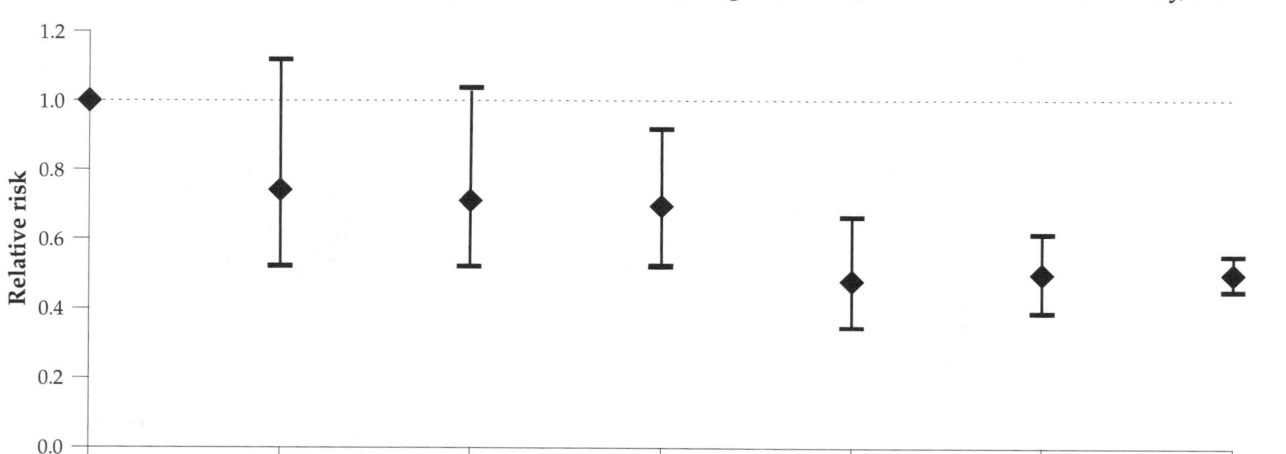


*Note:* Multivariate relative risks were adjusted for age, follow-up period, body mass index, history of hypertension, diabetes, high cholesterol level, postmenopausal estrogen therapy, menopausal status, previous use of oral contraceptives, parental history of myocardial infarction before age 60 years, and daily number of cigarettes smoked during the period prior to smoking cessation. Persons with nonfatal coronary heart disease, stroke, and cancer (except nonmelanoma skin cancer) were excluded at baseline and at the beginning of each two-year follow-up period.
Source: Kawachi et al. 1997b.

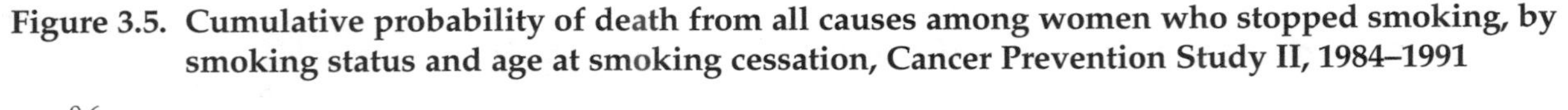

**Figure 3.5. Cumulative probability of death from all causes among women who stopped smoking, by smoking status and age at smoking cessation, Cancer Prevention Study II, 1984–1991**

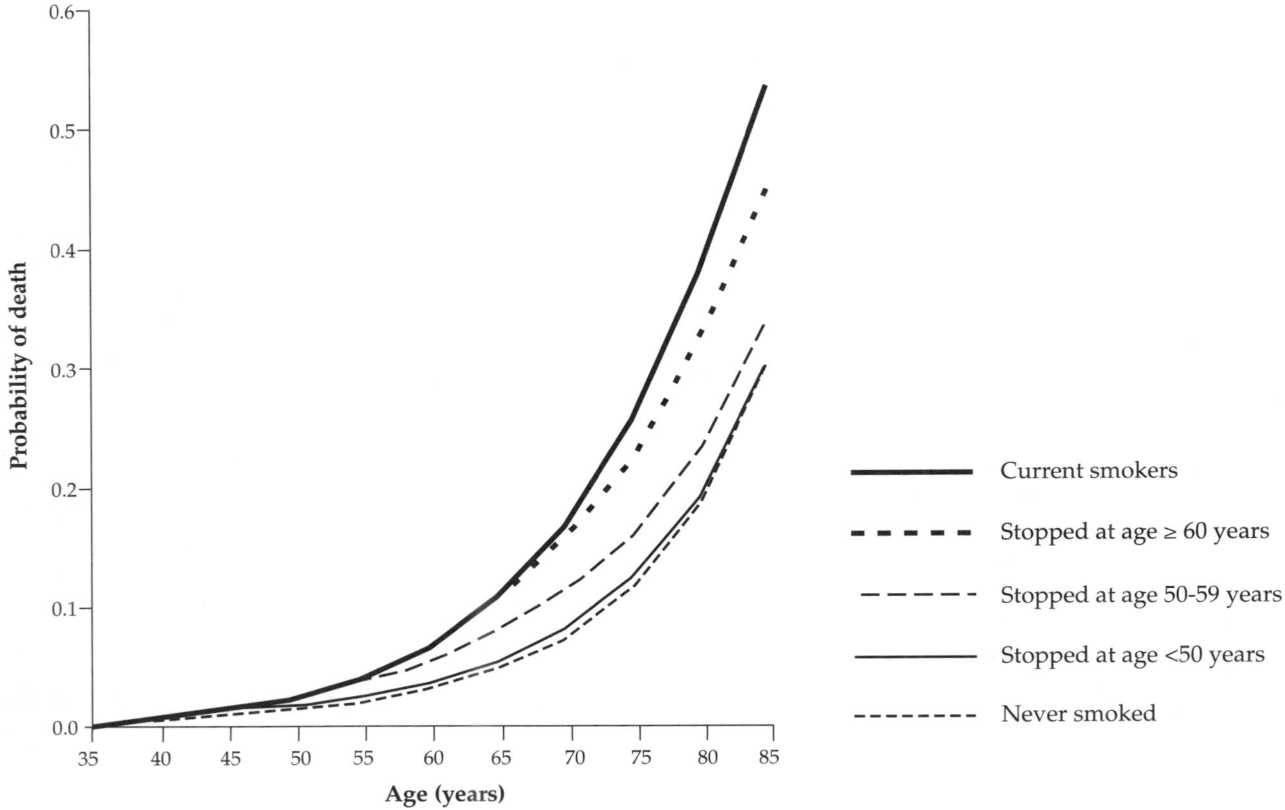


*Note:* Study excludes data from first 2 years of follow-up; persons with a history of cancer, heart disease, or stroke at enrollment; and those who stopped smoking <2 years before entering study.
Source: American Cancer Society, unpublished data.

women according to age at cessation of smoking. Figure 3.5 shows the cumulative probability that a woman in CPS-II would die during follow-up in 1984–1991 according to smoking status at study entry and, for former smokers, according to age at the time of smoking cessation (ACS, unpublished data). To minimize bias from smoking cessation due to illness, this analysis excluded data from the first two years of follow-up; persons with a history of cancer, heart disease, or stroke at study entry; and persons who had stopped smoking less than two years before enrollment. During the seven-year period, women who were current smokers at baseline had the highest cumulative probability of death during follow-up; those who had stopped smoking, particularly at younger ages, had intermediate risk; and those who had never smoked had the lowest risk. The risk among women who had stopped smoking before age 50 years was only slightly higher than that among women who had never smoked and, over time, the risk became indistinguishable from that among those who had never smoked. However, it should be stressed that the probabilities shown in Figure 3.5 are underestimates of the true cumulative risk for death at any age in the general population because the calculations are based on data from a cohort that included only women who survived and could therefore enter the study and excluded women with cancer, heart disease, or stroke at the time of enrollment, thereby making the study population healthier than the general U.S. population. Nevertheless, Figure 3.5 illustrates the substantial benefits of smoking cessation, the additional benefit for women who stop smoking at a younger age, and the optimal situation of never having started to smoke.

## Conclusions

1. Cigarette smoking plays a major role in the mortality of U.S. women.
2. The excess risk for death from all causes among current smokers compared with persons who have never smoked increases with both the number of years of smoking and the number of cigarettes smoked per day.
3. Among women who smoke, the percentage of deaths attributable to smoking has increased over the past several decades, largely because of increases in the quantity of cigarettes smoked and the duration of smoking.
4. Cohort studies with follow-up data analyzed in the 1980s show that the annual risk for death from all causes is 80 to 90 percent greater among women who smoke cigarettes than among women who have never smoked. A woman's annual risk for death more than doubles among continuing smokers compared with persons who have never smoked in every age group from 45 through 74 years.
5. In 1997, approximately 165,000 U.S. women died prematurely from a smoking-related disease. Since 1980, approximately three million U.S. women have died prematurely from a smoking-related disease.
6. U.S. females lost an estimated 2.1 million years of life each year during the 1990s as a result of smoking-related deaths due to neoplastic, cardiovascular, respiratory, and pediatric diseases as well as from burns caused by cigarettes. For every smoking attributable death, an average of 14 years of life was lost.
7. Women who stop smoking greatly reduce their risk for dying prematurely. The relative benefits of smoking cessation are greater when women stop smoking at younger ages, but smoking cessation is beneficial at all ages.

# Cancer

## Lung Cancer

When the report to the Surgeon General on smoking and health was published in 1964 (U.S. Department of Health, Education, and Welfare [USDHEW] 1964), lung cancer mortality among women was low (approximately 7 deaths per 100,000 women). The 1964 report concluded that evidence suggested a causal association between smoking and lung cancer among women but did not conclude that smoking was a cause of lung cancer among women. Subsequent reports of the Surgeon General reviewed data published after 1964, including both cohort and case-control studies of lung cancer among women, and strongly affirmed a causal relationship (USDHHS 1980, 1982, 1989b, 1990) between smoking and lung cancer among women.

Women started smoking in the 1930s and 1940s, about 20 to 30 years later than men. Thus, the sharp rise in lung cancer mortality that was so apparent among men before 1964 (from 5 deaths per 100,000 in 1930 to 45 deaths per 100,000 in 1964) did not occur until the 1970s among women (USDHHS 1989b). By 1980, when the first Surgeon General's report on women and smoking was released, lung cancer had become the second-leading cause of cancer deaths among women (USDHHS 1980). The lung cancer death rate among white women rose by over 600 percent from 1950 through 1997. This rise was equivalent to an average annual increase of 5.3 percent (Ries et al. 2000). During the 1973–1997 period, the lung cancer death rate among women increased 149 percent, but only 6.5 percent among men (Ries et al. 2000). In 1987, lung cancer surpassed breast cancer as the leading cause of cancer death among women (Figure 3.6), and in 2000, lung cancer accounted for an estimated 1 of every 4 cancer deaths and nearly 1 of every 8 newly diagnosed cancers among women (Greenlee et al. 2000). The estimates for 2000 also indicated that about 74,600 new cases of lung cancer would be diagnosed and that 67,600 deaths from the disease would occur among women (Greenlee et al. 2000).

Lung cancer incidence among women increased by 127 percent from 1973, when ongoing collection of population-based cancer incidence data by the National Cancer Institute (NCI) began, through 1997, when the annual age-adjusted incidence was 43.1 cases

**Figure 3.6. Age-adjusted death rates for lung cancer and breast cancer among women, United States, 1930–1997**

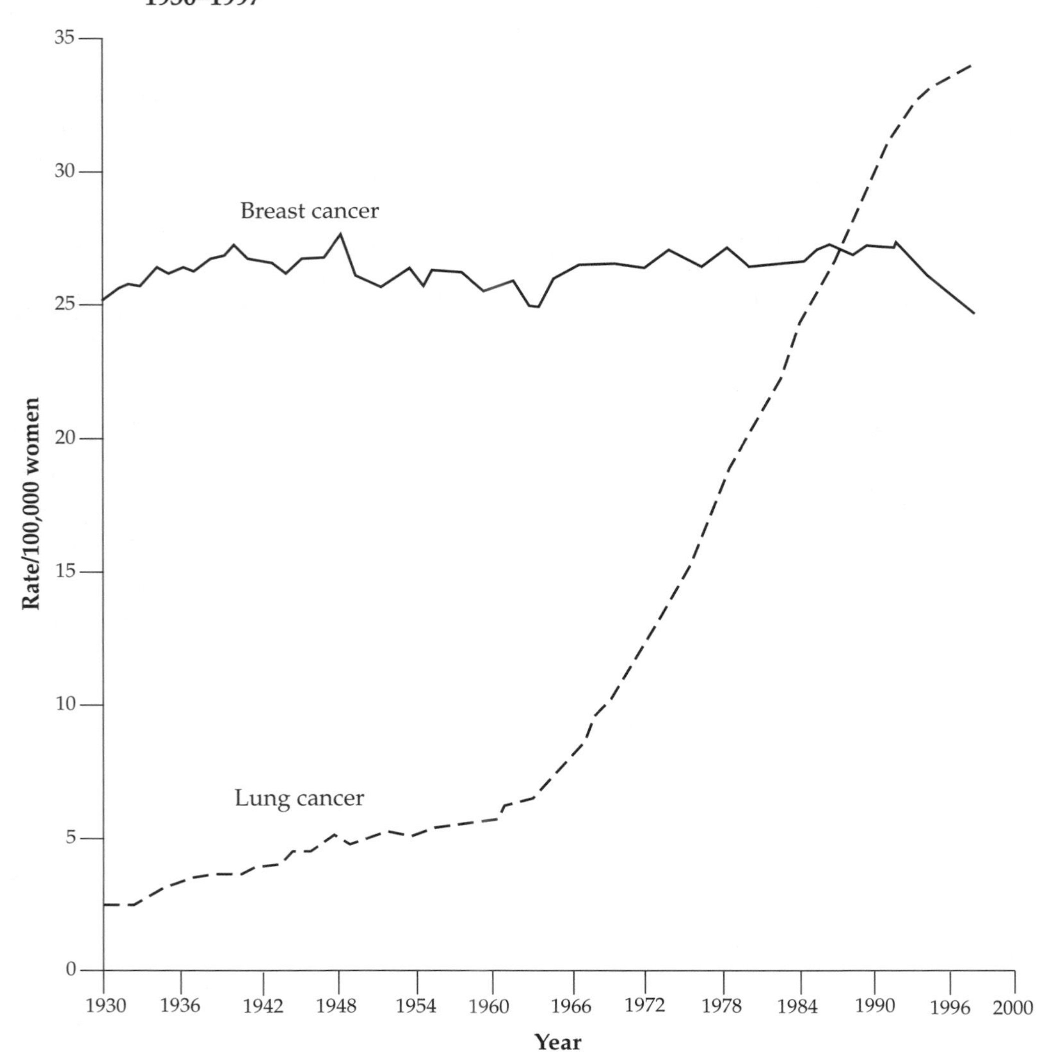


*Note:* Death rates are age-adjusted to the 1970 population.
Sources: Parker et al. 1996; National Center for Health Statistics 1999; Ries et al. 2000; American Cancer Society, unpublished data.

per 100,000 women (Ries et al. 2000). In recent years, the rate of increase has slowed—from 9.1 percent per year for 1973–1976 to 0.0 percent per year for 1991–1997. Incidence rates among women may have peaked in the 1990s (Wingo et al. 1999; Ries et al. 2000). Rates among women aged 40 through 49 years and among women aged 50 through 59 years reached a peak in the mid-1970s and late 1980s, respectively, whereas rates remained stable among women aged 60 through 69 years (Wingo et al. 1999). The overall age-adjusted incidence among men has declined steadily since 1987 (Ries et al. 2000). By 1997, the male-to-female ratio for incidence of lung cancer was 1.6:1, a change from 3:1 in 1980. In 1995–1997, the lifetime risk for developing lung cancer was 1 in 17.3 among women.

The overall incidence of lung cancer among black women resembles that among white women. In 1997, the age-adjusted incidence per 100,000 women was 42.6 among blacks and 45.0 among whites (Ries et al. 2000). In contrast, the incidence among black men was more than 50 percent higher than that among white men. In 1996–1997, lung cancer incidence rates

**Figure 3.7. Lung cancer incidence rates among white women and black women, Surveillance, Epidemiology, and End Results (SEER) Program, 1996–1997**

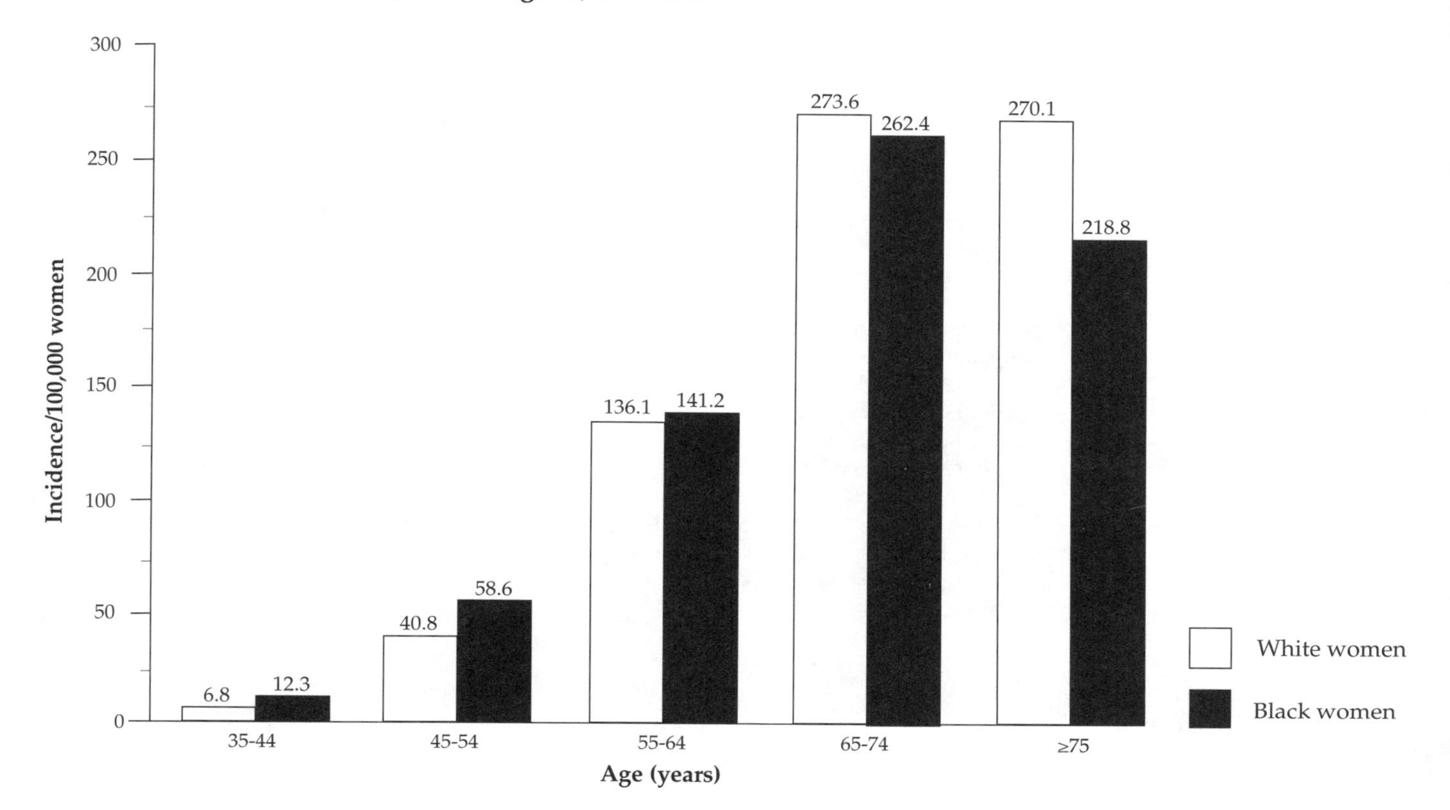


Source: Ries et al. 2000.

among women younger than age 65 years were higher among blacks than among whites (Figure 3.7). This finding suggested that differences between incidence among black women and white women may increase in the future.

In the United States, the incidence rate for 1990–1997 among Hispanic white women (20.3 per 100,000 women) was one-half that among non-Hispanic white women (45.9) (Ries et al. 2000). The rate among Asian or Pacific Islander women (22.5 per 100,000 women) was also lower than that among white women. Variation exists among subgroups of Asian women. Based on data for 1988–1992, rates were lowest among Japanese women and highest among Vietnamese women: 15.2 per 100,000 among Japanese, 16.0 among Korean, 17.5 among Filipino, 25.3 among Chinese, and 31.2 among Vietnamese women (NCI 1996b). Hawaiian women, however, developed lung cancer at approximately the same rate as did white women (43.1) (NCI 1996b). Incidence rates from California for 1991–1995 were comparable among non-Hispanic black women (48.2) and non-Hispanic white women (50.4), whereas rates among Hispanic women (19.7) and Asian women (21.7) were about 50 percent lower (Perkins et al. 1998). These differences in the incidence rate of lung cancer are likely the result of lower rates of cigarette smoking among Hispanic women and Asian women.

Because of the poor survival associated with lung cancer, mortality parallels incidence for all age and ethnic groups. The 5-year relative survival rates among black women and white women diagnosed with lung cancer in 1989–1996 were 13.5 and 16.6 percent, respectively (Ries et al. 2000). Survival was higher among women with localized disease (52.5 percent), but only 16 percent of cases among women were diagnosed at this early stage. Survival rates declined with age at diagnosis and advanced stage of disease but were higher among women than among men at all ages and stages and for all cell types. Survival rates have changed little in the past 20 years (Ries et al. 2000).

**Table 3.5. Relative risks of death from lung cancer for women and men, by quantity smoked, major prospective studies**

| Study | Women: Smoking status | Women: Relative risk | Men: Smoking status | Men: Relative risk |
|---|---|---|---|---|
| British doctors' study 1951–1973 | Nonsmokers | 1.0 | Nonsmokers | 1.0 |
| | Current smokers | 5.0 | Current smokers | 14.0 |
| | 1–14 cigarettes/day | 1.3 | 1–14 cigarettes/day | 7.8 |
| | 15–24 cigarettes/day | 6.4 | 15–24 cigarettes/day | 12.7 |
| | ≥ 25 cigarettes/day | 29.7 | ≥ 25 cigarettes/day | 25.1 |
| Cancer Prevention Study I (CPS-I) 1959–1972 | Never smoked | 1.0 | Never smoked | 1.0 |
| | Current smokers | 3.6 | Current smokers | 8.5 |
| | 1–9 cigarettes/day | 1.3 | 1–9 cigarettes/day | 4.6 |
| | 10–19 cigarettes/day | 2.4 | 10–19 cigarettes/day | 8.6 |
| | 20–39 cigarettes/day | 4.9 | 20–39 cigarettes/day | 14.7 |
| | ≥ 40 cigarettes/day | 7.5 | ≥ 40 cigarettes/day | 18.7 |
| Swedish study 1963–1979 | Nonsmokers | 1.0 | Nonsmokers | 1.0 |
| | Current smokers | 4.5 | Current smokers | 7.0 |
| | 1–7 cigarettes/day | 1.8 | 1–7 cigarettes/day | 2.3 |
| | 8–15 cigarettes/day | 11.3 | 8–15 cigarettes/day | 8.8 |
| | | | ≥ 16 cigarettes/day | 13.7 |
| Japanese study of 29 health districts 1966–1982 | Nonsmokers | 1.0 | Nonsmokers | 1.0 |
| | Current smokers | 2.0 | Current smokers | 3.8 |
| | <20 cigarettes/day | 1.9 | <20 cigarettes/day | 3.5 |
| | 20–29 cigarettes/day | 4.2 | 20–39 cigarettes/day | 5.7 |
| | | | ≥ 40 cigarettes/day | 6.5 |
| Kaiser Permanente Medical Care Program Study 1979–1987 | Nonsmokers | 1.0 | Nonsmokers | 1.0 |
| | Current smokers | 15.1 | Current smokers | 8.1 |
| | 1–19 cigarettes/day | 8.5 | 1–19 cigarettes/day | 4.7 |
| | ≥ 20 cigarettes/day | 21.7 | ≥ 20 cigarettes/day | 10.4 |
| Cancer Prevention Study II (CPS-II) 1982–1988 | Never smoked | 1.0 | Never smoked | 1.0 |
| | Former smokers | 4.7 | Former smokers | 9.4 |
| | Current smokers | 11.9 | Current smokers | 20.3 |
| | 1–9 cigarettes/day | 3.9 | 1–9 cigarettes/day | 12.2 |
| | 10–19 cigarettes/day | 8.3 | 10–19 cigarettes/day | 14.6 |
| | 20 cigarettes/day | 14.2 | 20 cigarettes/day | 21.7 |
| | 21–39 cigarettes/day | 21.4 | 21–39 cigarettes/day | 22.8 |
| | 40 cigarettes/day | 19.3 | 40 cigarettes/day | 24.2 |
| | ≥ 41 cigarettes/day | 18.2 | ≥ 41 cigarettes/day | 45.7 |

Sources: U.S. Department of Health and Human Services 1982 for British doctors' study, CPS-I, Swedish study, and Japanese study of 29 health districts; Friedman et al. 1997 for Kaiser Permanente Medical Care Program Study; Thun et al. 1997a for CPS-II.

### Smoking-Associated Risks

#### *Evidence from Cohort Studies*

Six prospective studies, which included more than one million women from four countries, provided data on smoking and risk for lung cancer among women. Many of the results from these studies were described previously (USDHHS 1982, 1989b). All showed significantly higher lung cancer mortality among smokers than among nonsmokers (Table 3.5). Together with case-control studies, these studies demonstrated that lung cancer mortality among

**Table 3.6. Age-adjusted death rates, relative risks, and rate differences for lung cancer, among women and men who were current smokers and never smokers, Cancer Prevention Study I (CPS-I), 1959–1965, and Cancer Prevention Study II (CPS-II), 1982–1988**

| | CPS–I | | CPS-II | |
|---|---|---|---|---|
| | Women | Men | Women | Men |
| Death rate* | | | | |
| Never smoked | 9.6 | 15.7 | 12.0 | 14.7 |
| Current smokers | 26.1 | 187.1 | 154.6 | 341.3 |
| Relative risk (95% CI)[†] | 2.7 (2.1–3.5) | 11.9 (9.5–14.9) | 12.8 (11.3–14.7) | 23.2 (19.3–27.9) |
| Rate difference (95% CI) | 16.5 (11–22) | 171.4 (157–186) | 142.6 (132–153) | 326.6 (309–344) |

*Per 100,000 person-years.
[†]CI = Confidence interval.
Source: Thun et al. 1997a.

women increases with increasing exposure to cigarette smoking, as measured by the number of cigarettes smoked daily, duration of smoking, depth of inhalation, age at smoking initiation, and tar content of the cigarettes smoked (USDHHS 1980, 1982, 1989b). The lower RRs observed among women than among men reflect differences in smoking habits across birth cohorts. Historically, women adopted the smoking habit at a later age than did men, smoked fewer cigarettes per day for fewer years, were less likely to inhale deeply, and were more likely to smoke filter-tipped or low-tar cigarettes (USDHHS 1980).

CPS-I, which was begun in 1959, and CPS-II, which was begun in 1982, enabled examination of changes over time in smoking-associated risk for death from lung cancer. Data from CPS-I and CPS-II confirmed that the epidemic of lung cancer among women was confined largely to smokers. The age-adjusted lung cancer death rate among women who had never smoked was about the same during the two study periods, but among current smokers, it increased nearly sixfold (Table 3.6). In CPS-I, lung cancer mortality was 2 to 3 times higher among women smokers than among women who had never smoked; 20 years later, in CPS-II, mortality was more than 12 times higher. (During this same period, the rate among men increased by a factor of 2.) Women in CPS-II began smoking earlier in life, smoked for more years, and reported inhaling moderately or deeply more often than did women in CPS-I. These findings probably largely explain the higher RR among smokers in CPS-II than in CPS-I, the corresponding greater differences in absolute risk among women smokers and nonsmokers, and the narrowing of the gender gap for these measures over time (Thun et al. 1997a) (Table 3.6).

The risk for lung cancer mortality increases with the number of cigarettes smoked (USDHHS 1989b) (Table 3.5). In CPS-II, the RR for lung cancer death increased from 3.9 among women who smoked 1 to 9 cigarettes per day to 21.4 among women who smoked one to two packs of cigarettes (21 to 39 cigarettes) per day (Thun et al. 1997a). Analyses from a cohort study of subscribers of a large health maintenance organization (HMO) (Kaiser Permanente Medical Health Care Program Study) also showed a RR of 21.7 among women who smoked 20 or more cigarettes per day (Table 3.5). The risk increased 12.0 times among women who smoked for 20 to 39 years and 27.5 times for women who smoked 40 or more years (data not shown) (Friedman et al. 1997).

The age-adjusted RR among current smokers and among persons who had never smoked varies with race and ethnicity. The RR was lower among Asian women (3.2) than among black women (23.5) or white women (18.6) in an HMO cohort study (Friedman et al. 1997). These differences may reflect racial or ethnic differences in dose, duration, and intensity of smoking (Shopland 1995). Cohort studies have not included enough minority women to allow comparison of the dose-response effect of smoking and lung cancer among racial and ethnic groups.

In CPS-II, RRs decreased after cessation of cigarette smoking. The RR for death from lung cancer among women former smokers was about 50 percent lower than that among women current smokers, but it was still higher than that among women who had never smoked (Table 3.5). The RR for lung cancer in both the HMO study and CPS-II decreased with increased duration of smoking cessation (Table 3.7). CPS-II data showed marked reductions in RR within 3 to 5 years after smoking cessation, especially among lighter smokers. However, lung cancer mortality remained higher among women former smokers than among those who had never smoked, even after more than 15 years of smoking cessation (USDHHS 1990).

*Evidence from Case-Control Studies*

More than 20 case-control studies of smoking and lung cancer that included women have been reviewed (USDHEW 1971, 1979; USDHHS 1982). Table 3.8 presents estimated RRs from 11 studies reported during 1985–1993 from the United States, Canada, and northern Europe. Each of these studies included approximately 100 or more cases of lung cancer among women. Consistent with findings in cohort studies and temporal trends in women's smoking, results of case-control investigations showed an increase in smoking-associated risk for lung cancer during the 1950s through 1970s (USDHHS 1982). A steep upward gradient in risk with the number of cigarettes smoked per day was reported from almost all case-control studies of smoking and lung cancer among women conducted during the 1980s (USDHHS 1989b). The estimated risk for lung cancer among women who smoked 20 or more cigarettes per day relative to nonsmokers (10- to 20-fold excess risk) was remarkably consistent in both hospital- and population-based studies in Europe and North America.

Lung cancer risk increased with the number of years of smoking, and this increase was independent of the number of cigarettes smoked per day (Schoenberg et al. 1989; Osann 1991). The RRs were 2 to 3 among women who smoked for shorter durations (<20 years [Osann 1991], <20 pack-years [pack-years is the number of packs of cigarettes smoked per day multiplied by the number of years of cigarette smoking] [Sellers et al. 1991], or <35 years and <20 cigarettes per day [Schoenberg et al. 1989]) and 8 to 24 among those who smoked for longer durations. The risk for lung cancer was two to four times higher among women who inhaled tobacco smoke frequently and deeply than among those who did not inhale (Potter et al. 1985; Osann 1991) (data not shown).

Age at initiation of smoking is closely associated with the number of years of smoking. Because women who smoked for the longest duration usually began to smoke at younger ages, it is difficult to separate the independent effect of each factor related to lung cancer risk (Thun et al. 1997c). Although a

**Table 3.7. Age-adjusted relative risks for lung cancer associated with smoking status and smoking cessation among women, cohort studies**

| Study | Smoking status | Number of years of cessation | Relative risk | |
|---|---|---|---|---|
| Kaiser Permanente Medical Care Program Study 1979–1987 | Never smoked | NA* | 1.0 | |
| | Former smokers | 2–10 | 8.4 | |
| | | 11–20 | 3.8 | |
| | | >20 | 4.4 | |
| Cancer Prevention Study II 1982–1988 | Never smoked | NA | 1.0 | |
| | | | Number of cigarettes/day | |
| | | | 1–19 | ≥ 20 |
| | Former smokers | <1 | 7.9 | 34.3 |
| | | 1–2 | 9.1 | 19.5 |
| | | 3–5 | 2.9 | 14.6 |
| | | 6–10 | 1.0 | 9.1 |
| | | 11–15 | 1.5 | 5.9 |
| | | ≥ 16 | 1.4 | 2.6 |

*NA = Not applicable.
Sources: U.S. Department of Health and Human Services 1990; Friedman et al. 1997.

**Table 3.8. Relative risks for lung cancer among women smokers compared with nonsmokers, by smoking status and quantity smoked, case-control studies**

| Study | Number of cases/controls | Source | Relative risk (95% confidence interval) by smoking status | | | Relative risk (95% confidence interval) by quantity/duration of smoking | | |
|---|---|---|---|---|---|---|---|---|
| | | | Ever smoked | Current smokers | Former smokers | | | |
| Humble et al. 1985 | 173/272 | Registry | —[*] | — | 6.5 (2.8–15.4) | <20 cigarettes/day | 19.2 | (6.5–60.8) |
| | | | | | | ≥ 20 cigarettes/day | 16.0 | (6.7–36.3) |
| Benhamou et al. 1987 | 96[†]/192 | Hospital | 6.6 (3.0–14.4) | — | — | <10 cigarettes/day | 1.2[‡] | |
| | | | | | | 10–19 cigarettes/day | 2.9 | (1.2–7.2) |
| | | | | | | ≥ 20 cigarettes/day | 20.0 | (6.0–66.9) |
| Schoenberg et al. 1989 | 994/995 | Population | 8.5 (6.7–10.8) | — | — | <20 cigarettes/day | | |
| | | | | | | <35 years | 3.2 | (2.3–4.4) |
| | | | | | | ≥ 35 years | 8.4 | (6.2–11.2) |
| | | | | | | ≥ 20 cigarettes/day | | |
| | | | | | | <35 years | 6.5 | (4.5–9.4) |
| | | | | | | ≥ 35 years | 16.0 | (11.9–21.7) |
| Svensson et al. 1989 | 210/209 | Population | 6.4 (4.0–10.5) | — | 2.6 (1.4–5.1) | <10 cigarettes/day | 4.6 | (2.5–9.3) |
| | | | | | | 11–20 cigarettes/day | 12.6 | (6.5–25.2) |
| | | | | | | ≥ 20 cigarettes/day | 59.0 | (7.6–)[§] |
| Katsouyanni et al. 1991 | 101/89 | Hospital | — | 3.4 (1.8–6.6) | — | ≥ 30 cigarettes/day | 7.5 | (2.4–23.2) |
| Osann 1991 | 217/217 | Registry | 6.7 (3.7–12.0) | 9.1 (4.8–17.3) | 2.5 (1.1–5.9) | <20 cigarettes/day | 2.5 | (1.2–5.2) |
| | | | | | | ≥ 20 cigarettes/day | 12.6 | (6.2–25.6) |
| | | | | | | ≤ 20 years | 1.6 | (0.7–3.5) |
| | | | | | | >20 years | 11.6 | (5.8–23.3) |
| Sellers et al. 1991 | 152/1,900 | Registry | — | 18.3 (11.1–30.3) | 5.3 (3.7–11.2) | 0–19 pack-years | 3.4 | (1.7–6.8) |
| | | | | | | 20-39 pack-years | 12.7 | (7.3–21.9) |
| | | | | | | ≥ 40 pack-years | 23.9 | (14.1–40.1) |
| Brownson et al. 1992b | 5,212/ >10,000[Δ] | Registry | 12.7 (11.5–13.9) | 13.6 (12.3–15.1) | 11.6 (10.4–13.0) | <20 cigarettes/day | 8.4 | (7.2–9.7) |
| | | | | | | ≥ 20 cigarettes/day | 17.1 | (15.3–19.1) |
| Hegmann et al. 1993 | 100/1,087 | Registry | — | — | — | Age at smoking initiation | | |
| | | | | | | ≤ 25 years | 26.8 | (15.4–46.8) |
| | | | | | | >25 years | 4.8 | (1.0–22.1) |
| Osann et al. 1993 | 833/1,656 | Registry | 15.0 (11.8–19.1) | 19.6 (15.2–25.2) | 8.1 (6.0–11.0) | <40 cigarettes/day | 14.4 | (11.0–18.9) |
| | | | | | | ≥ 40 cigarettes/day | 40.9 | (29.3–57.1) |
| Risch et al. 1993 | 442/410 | Registry | 9.2 (5.95–15.1) | 16.8 (9.9–30.6) | 8.0[¶] (4.3–15.9) | <30 pack-years | 7.3 | (4.1–13.0) |
| | | | | | | 30–59 pack-years | 26.7 | (14.0–50.6) |
| | | | | | | ≥ 60 pack-years | 81.9 | (25.2–267) |

*Dash = Data not available.
†Kreyberg I cases (squamous cell, small cell, and large cell carcinoma).
‡Not statistically significant.
§Upper confidence limit is not provided because of the small numbers in this category.
ΔThe exact number of controls is not specified, but authors state that the ratio of controls to cases was approximately 2.5.
¶Former smokers who had stopped smoking 2–10 years previously.

significant increase in risk with early age at smoking initiation was noted in one study of women (Hegmann et al. 1993), other studies showed no such increase after adjustment for duration of smoking (Svensson et al. 1989; Benhamou and Benhamou 1994). A differential effect for age at initiation, independent of the quantity of cigarettes smoked and the duration of smoking, would imply that the lung is more susceptible to the carcinogenic effects of cigarette smoke at a younger age.

Data from case-control studies generally support the association between tar level of cigarettes and lung cancer risk observed in some cohort studies (Stellman and Garfinkel 1986; Garfinkel and Stellman 1988; Sidney et al. 1993; Stellman et al. 1997). Women who smoked nonfiltered cigarettes had higher risk than did women who smoked filter-tipped brands (Pathak et al. 1986; Wynder and Kabat 1988; Lubin et al. 1984; Stellman et al. 1997). Several researchers attempted to account for variation in tar yield over time and by brand of cigarettes. Kaufman and colleagues (1989) examined dose-response relationships by using the average tar content of cigarettes smoked over a specified period. Zang and Wynder (1992) constructed an index of cumulative tar exposure. Both methods showed an increase in lung cancer risk among women with increased exposure to tar. Limitations of studies of tar exposure include use of surrogate measures for tar in some studies (e.g., presence or absence of a filter), use of a machine-derived tar yield of specific brands at a certain time or during a short interval, and failure to account for compensatory changes in smoking habits (e.g., increased depth of inhalation or number of puffs). Underestimation of actual exposure to tar levels in human-based or machine-derived results of Federal Trade Commission (FTC) testing methods to date has long been a concern (National Cancer Institute 1996a; Djordjevic et al. 2000).

Few case-control studies reported data on variation in smoking-associated risk by race or ethnicity. In a hospital-based study, the odds for lung cancer were higher among black women than among white women at each level of tar exposure (Harris et al. 1993). Although RRs were generally higher among black women across all histologic types of lung cancer, the differences were greater for the types most strongly associated with smoking. Humble and coworkers (1985) found no significant differences between non-Hispanic white women and Hispanic women in dose-response relationships. A case-control study examined risk for lung cancer by race and ethnicity among women in Hawaii who had ever smoked (Le Marchand et al. 1992). Relative to Japanese women, RRs were higher among Hawaiian (1.7), Caucasian (2.7), and Filipino (3.7) women and lower among Chinese women (0.4), after adjustment for pack-years of smoking and age. However, these results were not statistically significant. Differences across ethnic groups in the reporting of smoking habits or the intensity of smoking may be responsible for some of the observed differences in lung cancer risk.

Case-control studies of lung cancer risk among women former smokers were described previously (USDHHS 1990). Retrospective investigations reported since 1985 all showed lower risk among former smokers than among current smokers (Table 3.8). Risk declined within 5 years of smoking cessation, varied with the level of previous exposure, but remained higher than the risk among those who had never smoked, even after 20 years of abstinence. The rate of decline in risk with years of abstinence is not well characterized because of the small number of former smokers, particularly long-term former smokers, in most case-control studies.

*Differences by Gender*

Although the RR for death from lung cancer among women current smokers increased over time (Thun et al. 1997a), all but one of the six major cohort studies (Table 3.5) showed lower RRs among women than among men (Kaiser Permanente Medical Care Program Study). The difference is believed to result from the time lag in smoking initiation among women and thus the lower cumulative exposure to smoking among birth cohorts of women (Burns et al. 1997b). In CPS-I, the RRs among women smokers were approximately one-fifth as high as those among men (Thun et al. 1997a). Among women smokers in CPS-II, death rates and RRs were about one-half those among men smokers in CPS-II and were equal to those among men 20 years earlier in CPS-I (Thun et al. 1997a). Differences in RR may be due to differences between women and men in duration and intensity of smoking within each age- and quantity-specific stratum or to residual confounding within these large strata (Thun et al. 1997c). Cohort studies generally have not been large enough to allow comparison of RR for subgroups of women and men of exactly comparable age and smoking exposure. However, within categories defined by age, number of cigarettes smoked, and duration of smoking in years that were examined using CPS-II data, men generally had higher lung cancer death rates than did women (Thun et al. 1997a) and the rate ratios associated with smoking were generally higher among men than among women (Thun et al. 1997b). A pooled analysis of data from three prospective population-based studies conducted in the area of Copenhagen, Denmark (13,444 women and 17,430 men), examined risk for lung cancer by pack-years of smoking and gender. After adjustment for pack-years of smoking, the ratio of female to male smokers' RRs for developing lung cancer was 0.8 (95 percent CI, 0.3 to 2.1) (Prescott et al. 1998b). On the other hand, results from the HMO study found that risk was higher among female heavy smokers than among male heavy smokers in every age group (Friedman et al. 1997).

Some case-control studies have found RRs among women that were nearly equal to (Schoenberg et al. 1989; Osann et al. 1993) or higher than those among men (Brownson et al. 1992b; Risch et al. 1993; Zang and Wynder 1996). A lower baseline risk for lung cancer or higher cigarette consumption among women smokers could explain the higher RR associated with ever smoking cigarettes among women (Hoover 1994; Wilcox 1994). In cohort studies, however, the death rates for lung cancer have been similar among women and men who had never smoked (Burns et al. 1997a; Thun et al. 1997a), and U.S. national survey data showed that the proportion of heavy smokers has consistently been higher over the years among men, not women (see Chapter 2). Several possible reasons may explain the higher smoking-associated RRs for lung cancer among women than among men reported from some case-control studies. The smoking patterns of women and men may differ in ways that have not been entirely accounted for in the study design and analysis. Women may underreport daily consumption of cigarettes and may, therefore, appear to have a higher risk than men for a given quantity smoked. Because smoking prevalence has always been higher among men than women (even though the gender gap has narrowed over time), women who smoke may also be more likely than men to be exposed to spousal smoking, which is itself associated with an increased risk for lung cancer (see "Environmental Tobacco Smoke" later in this chapter). Even when women smoke the same number of cigarettes as men do, exposure to cigarette smoke may be greater among women than among men because of differences in puff volume, puff frequency, or depth of inhalation. Alternately, women may be more biologically susceptible to the effects of cigarette smoke (Risch et al. 1993). McDuffie and colleagues (1991) observed that women with lung cancer developed disease at a younger age than did men and had a similar level of pulmonary dysfunction, but after less exposure to cigarette smoking. It is also likely that some of the observed gender differences represent chance findings. Thus, no conclusion regarding differential gender susceptibility to smoking-related lung cancer can be made at present.

Differences by gender in the proportion of lung cancer deaths directly attributable to current smoking are small. In CPS-II, the proportion of lung cancer deaths attributable to current smoking was 92 percent among women and 95 percent among men (Thun et al. 1997c). Smoking attributable fractions of deaths among women current smokers decreased with age, from 95 percent among women aged 45 through 49 years to 86 percent among women aged 80 years or older. This decrease among older women smokers likely is a result of differences in the smoking histories of older women, including later ages of initiation and lower cumulative exposures to smoking (Burns et al. 1997b). Nearly the same proportion of lung cancer deaths among women and men could be prevented by eliminating cigarette smoking.

*Histologic Types*

Lung cancers are classified into four main categories: squamous cell carcinoma, small cell carcinoma, adenocarcinoma, and large cell carcinoma (Churg 1994). Differences in histologic type have been observed between smokers and nonsmokers, and among smokers, gender-specific differences may be seen in the distribution of lung cancers by histologic type (Muscat and Wynder 1995b) (Table 3.9). In 1962, Kreyberg hypothesized that smoking causes squamous cell, small cell, and large cell carcinomas (Kreyberg type I), but that other factors cause adenocarcinoma and bronchioloalveolar carcinoma (Kreyberg type II) (Kreyberg 1962). Squamous cell carcinoma has long been the predominant type of lung cancer found among men, and adenocarcinoma has been predominant among women. Kreyberg (1962) based his hypothesis on this difference and on differences in the smoking habits of women and men at the time.

Although some early studies suggested that smoking might not be responsible for some histologic types of lung cancer, the association between smoking and all the major histologic types has been recognized since the 1980 Surgeon General's report (USDHHS 1980). Studies conducted since that report have confirmed that smoking strongly increases the risk for the four major types of lung cancer among women (Table 3.10). The risk was significantly higher among smokers than among women who had never smoked and, in

**Table 3.9. Percent distribution of lung cancer cases, by gender, histologic type, and smoking status**

| | Women (n = 2,098) | | | Men (n = 3,756) | | |
|---|---|---|---|---|---|---|
| Histologic type | Current smokers | Former smokers | Never smoked | Current smokers | Former smokers | Never smoked |
| Adenocarcinoma | 42 | 44 | 59 | 32 | 34 | 58 |
| Squamous cell carcinoma | 20 | 20 | 12 | 35 | 37 | 19 |
| Small cell carcinoma | 19 | 12 | 3 | 15 | 11 | 0 |
| Other | 19 | 24 | 26 | 18 | 18 | 23 |

Source: Compiled from Muscat and Wynder 1995b.

general, increased as the quantity of cigarettes smoked increased (Lubin and Blot 1984; Wu et al. 1985; Schoenberg et al. 1989; Svensson et al. 1989; Katsouyanni et al. 1991; Morabia and Wynder 1991; Osann 1991; Brownson et al. 1992b; Osann et al. 1993; Zang and Wynder 1996) (Table 3.10). Risk also increased with duration of smoking (Schoenberg et al. 1989; Osann 1991; Risch et al. 1993) and depth of inhalation (Osann 1991) (data not shown). In one study, after adjustment for duration, risk did not increase with early age at smoking initiation for any histologic type of lung cancer (Svensson et al. 1989) (data not shown). Risk was generally lower among former smokers than among current smokers for each type of lung cancer (Wu et al. 1985; Svensson et al. 1989; Morabia and Wynder 1991; Osann 1991; Brownson et al. 1992b; Osann et al. 1993) (Table 3.10). Risk also decreased with duration of smoking cessation (Svensson et al. 1989; Morabia and Wynder 1991; Risch et al. 1993) (data not shown).

Among women, the RRs among smokers compared with those who had never smoked were consistently highest for small cell carcinoma (range, 37.6 to 86.0), followed by squamous cell carcinoma (range, 10.6 to 26.4), and then adenocarcinoma (range, 3.5 to 9.5) (Potter et al. 1985; Schoenberg et al. 1989; Brownson et al. 1992b; Osann et al. 1993; Risch et al. 1993) (Table 3.11). At each dose level of smoking, the RR was higher for small cell carcinoma than for squamous cell carcinoma and lowest for adenocarcinoma (Schoenberg et al. 1989; Brownson et al. 1992b; Osann et al. 1993; Zang and Wynder 1996) (data not shown). With the exception of the study by Risch and associates (1993), several investigators found that the risk among men was equally high for small cell and squamous cell carcinoma but lower for adenocarcinoma (Table 3.11). The RR among women and men who had ever smoked differed by less than a factor of 2 for adenocarcinoma (generally higher among men) and squamous cell carcinoma (higher among women in one-half of the studies), but the RR for small cell carcinoma among women consistently exceeded that among men by at least two to three times. In one study, dose-response RRs associated with specific levels of cumulative exposure to cigarette smoke (in kilograms of tar) were significantly higher by 1.5 to 1.7 times among women than among men for all three major histologic types (Zang and Wynder 1996).

Comparisons among histologic types and between women and men are subject to limitations because of diagnostic uncertainties, unstable estimates, and difficulties in assessment of cumulative exposure. Accurate classification of lung cancers into the four main histologic categories is compromised by interobserver variability and intrinsic tumor heterogeneity (Churg 1994). Comparisons of smoking-associated RR among histologic types and between genders are also limited by the small numbers of study participants who had never smoked. This limitation results in unstable risk estimates with wide, overlapping CIs. The lower smoking-associated risk for adenocarcinoma could be explained by a higher baseline risk for adenocarcinoma among women who had never smoked—a risk that is possibly due to exposure to ETS or other factors. Consistent with this explanation, adenocarcinoma does constitute a greater proportion of lung cancers among nonsmokers than among current or former smokers (Brownson et al. 1995; Muscat and Wynder 1995b). The subjective assessment of exposure to cigarette smoke may also differ between women and men.

*Temporal Trends*

Over time, the smoking habits of women have changed to more closely resemble those of men (Burns et al. 1997a). Differences between women and men in histologic patterns of lung cancer have lessened but have not disappeared (Wynder and Hoffman 1994).

The incidence of each of the main histologic types of lung cancer has increased among women since 1973, but adenocarcinoma had the greatest percent increase (206 percent during 1973–1992) (Surveillance, Epidemiology, and End Results Program, unpublished data) (Figure 3.8). Among men, the overall lung cancer rate has begun to decline, but adenocarcinoma increased by 84 percent during 1973–1992. The increasing incidence of adenocarcinoma among both women and men may reflect the increase over time in the use of filter-tipped and low-tar cigarettes, which may result in greater deposition of smoke particles in the small airways of the lung periphery (Zheng et al. 1994). Yang and colleagues (1989) observed that smoke from filter-tipped and low-tar cigarettes contains fewer large particles and more small particles and may preferentially predispose smokers to peripheral tumors such as adenocarcinoma. Case-control results support an increased risk for adenocarcinoma among smokers of low-tar cigarettes (Stellman et al. 1997).

Analyses of gender-specific lung cancer trends by histologic type from data from the United States, Switzerland, and elsewhere showed that changes over time represent birth cohort effects reflecting gender-specific and generational changes in smoking and the types of cigarettes consumed (Levi et al. 1997; Thun et al. 1997b). For example, smoking among women was on the increase when filter-tipped and lower yield cigarettes were introduced. Such products are more likely to be inhaled than high-tar, unfiltered cigarettes because they are less irritating and because smokers compensate for the lower yield by smoking more intensely (greater number and depth of puffs). Thus, carcinogens may be more likely to travel beyond the central bronchi, where squamous cell carcinomas often occur, and to reach the bronchioloalveolar regions and smaller bronchi, where adenocarcinomas typically develop. Among women, the incidence of small cell carcinoma has increased steeply since 1973 and smaller increases have been seen in squamous cell carcinoma (Dodds et al. 1986; Wu et al. 1986; Butler et al. 1987; el-Torky et al. 1990; Devesa et al. 1991; Travis et al. 1995). An increase in bronchioloalveolar carcinoma found in hospital-based studies (Auerbach and Garfinkel 1991; Barsky et al. 1994) was not confirmed in population-based studies (Zheng et al. 1994). Analysis of more recent trends showed that rates for squamous cell carcinoma among women have remained fairly stable since the mid-1980s, rates for large cell carcinoma have decreased since the late 1980s, and rates for small cell carcinoma declined between 1991 and 1996. Incidence rates for adenocarcinoma, however, continued to increase, but the rate of increase appeared to be slowing (Wingo et al. 1999). Examination of trends by birth cohort revealed a decrease in the incidence of squamous cell carcinoma among birth cohorts of women and men born since 1935 and a reduction in the rate of increase in small cell carcinoma and adenocarcinoma among birth cohorts of women born since 1940 (Zheng et al. 1994).

Changes over time in the overall age-adjusted incidence of lung cancer can be primarily attributed to changes in smoking prevalence (Burns et al. 1997a). The steep rise in the incidence among women began in the 1960s and trailed the increase among men by about 20 years—a finding that reflects the later adoption of smoking by women. The recent decline in rates for squamous and small cell carcinomas and the slower rate of increase for adenocarcinoma among younger birth cohorts (Zheng et al. 1994) may be related to the decrease in smoking prevalence among these groups. Changes in smoking prevalence, however, may not explain all of the observed male-female differences in incidence patterns by histologic type. Additional risks related to use of low-tar, low-nicotine cigarettes and increasing exposure to tobacco-specific nitrosamines (TSNAs) may partially explain the increase in adenocarcinoma among women and men beginning in the 1970s (Wynder and Hoffman 1994).

*Tobacco-Specific Nitrosamines*

Wynder and Hoffman (1994) raised concerns about the level of TSNA carcinogens in brands of cigarettes smoked by women. The level of TSNA carcinogens in tobacco products is known to vary according to blend (Fischer et al. 1989), processing (Burton et al. 1989), and storage (Andersen et al. 1982c); this variation is a concern within the tobacco industry (Fisher 2000). As part of the validation of an analytical chemistry method to measure TSNAs in cigarette tobacco, the 10 best selling brands in the United States in 1996 were tested (Song and Ashley 1999). Two cigarettes from one pack of each brand were tested for this analysis. In this report, the 10 cigarette brands were ranked in the order of increasing *N*′-nitrosonornicotine (NNN) level, and Virginia Slims cigarettes (reported as Brand J in Table 5 in the report) (David Ashley, CDC, e-mail to Patricia Richter, CDC, August 31, 2000) were found to have the highest levels of

**Table 3.10. Relative risks for lung cancer among women, by smoking status and histologic type, case-control studies**

| | | | Relative risk (95% confidence interval) | | | |
|---|---|---|---|---|---|---|
| Study | Years | Smoking status | Squamous cell carcinoma | Kreyberg I* | Small cell carcinoma | Adeno-carcinoma |
| Lubin and Blot 1984 | 1976–1980 | Never smoked | 1.0 | | 1.0 | 1.0 |
| | | Ever smoked | | | | |
| | | 1–9 cigarettes/day | 2.8† | | 2.3† | 1.0† |
| | | 10–19 cigarettes/day | 2.4† | | 2.4† | 2.0† |
| | | 20–29 cigarettes/day | 5.3† | | 6.2† | 1.1† |
| | | ≥ 30 cigarettes/day | 4.2† | | 5.6† | 2.3† |
| Potter et al. 1985 | 1976–1980 | Nonsmokers | 1.0 | | 1.0 | 1.0 |
| | | Smokers | 8.3† | | 52.3† | 4.0† |
| Wu et al. 1985 | 1981–1982 | Nonsmokers | 1.0 | | | 1.0 |
| | | Former smokers | 7.7 (0.8–70.3) | | | 1.2 (0.6–2.3) |
| | | Current smokers | 35.3 (4.7–267.3) | | | 4.1 (2.3–7.5) |
| | | 1–20 cigarettes/day | 17.7 (2.3–138.2) | | | 2.7 (1.4–5.4) |
| | | ≥ 21 cigarettes/day | 94.4 (9.9–904.6) | | | 6.5 (3.1–13.9) |
| Benhamou et al. 1987 | 1976–1980 | Nonsmokers | | 1.0 | | 1.0 |
| | | Smokers | | 6.6 (3.0–14.4) | | 2.1 (0.7–6.4) |
| Schoenberg et al. 1989 | 1982–1983 | Nonsmokers | 1.0 | | 1.0 | 1.0 |
| | | All smokers | | | | |
| | | <20 cigarettes/day | | | | |
| | | <35 years | 2.7 (1.4–5.1) | | 19.0 (6.4–56.5) | 2.0 (1.3–3.2) |
| | | ≥ 35 years | 12.0 (7.4–19.6) | | 62.5 (22.3–176.0) | 3.9 (2.6–5.9) |
| | | ≥ 20 cigarettes/day | | | | |
| | | <35 years | 7.7 (4.1–14.3) | | 40.6 (13.5–122.0) | 3.4 (2.0–5.6) |
| | | ≥ 35 years | 21.4 (13.1–34.9) | | 140.0 (49.8–391.0) | 6.8 (4.5–10.1) |
| Svensson et al. 1989 | 1983–1986 | Never smoked | 1.0 | | 1.0 | 1.0 |
| | | Former smokers | 4.0 (1.0–16.9) | | 9.1 (1.4–69.7) | 1.8 (0.8–4.3) |
| | | Current smokers | | | | |
| | | ≤ 10 cigarettes/day | 9.7 (2.9–45.9) | | 33.7 (6.9–265.3) | 2.2 (1.0–5.8) |
| | | 11–20 cigarettes/day | 36.2 (12.0–168.9) | | 72.1 (11.9–452.6) | 5.4 (2.4–13.2) |
| | | >20 cigarettes/day | 96.0 (6.9–)‡ | | 215.8 (18.3–)‡ | 19.7 (1.7–)‡ |
| Katsouyanni et al. 1991 | 1987–1989 | Nonsmokers | | 1.0 | | 1.0 |
| | | Former smokers | | 4.7 (1.05–21.1) | | 1.8 (0.4–8.7) |
| | | Current smokers | | | | |
| | | ≤ 20 cigarettes/day | | 3.2 (1.1–8.9) | | 1.4 (0.52–3.49) |
| | | >20 cigarettes/day | | 19.5 (5.4–71.1) | | 3.0 (0.76–11.41) |

*Kreyberg I includes squamous cell, small cell, and large cell carcinoma.
†95% confidence interval was not reported.
‡Upper confidence limit is not given; estimates are imprecise because of the small number of persons in the high-exposure category.

NNN: 5.60 micrograms per gram (µg/g) of tobacco with a relative standard deviation of 1.4 percent, versus 1.89 µg/g with a relative standard deviation of 11 percent for Brand A. Of the TSNAs, NNN and *N'*-nitrosoanatabine (NAT) levels correlated more closely; however, 4-(methylnitrosamino)-1-(3-pyridyl)-1-butanone (NNK) and *N'*-nitrosoanabasine (NAB) levels did not correlate with NNN or NAT levels across

**Table 3.10. Continued**

| | | | Relative risk (95% confidence interval) | | | |
|---|---|---|---|---|---|---|
| **Study** | **Years** | **Smoking status** | **Squamous cell carcinoma** | **Kreyberg I*** | **Small cell carcinoma** | **Adeno-carcinoma** |
| Morabia and Wynder 1991 | 1985–1990 | Former smokers | | | | |
| | | <20 cigarettes/day | 0.4 (0.1–1.2) | | 0.5 (0.1–2.0) | 0.7 (0.4–1.3) |
| | | ≥ 20 cigarettes/day | 2.0 (1.0–4.3) | | 1.8 (0.7–4.9) | 0.9 (0.5–1.5) |
| | | Current smokers | | | | |
| | | 1–19 cigarettes/day[§] | 1.0 | | 1.0 | 1.0 |
| | | 20–29 cigarettes/day | 1.5 (0.7–3.3) | | 1.8 (0.7–4.9) | 1.3 (0.8–2.2) |
| | | ≥ 30 cigarettes/day | 2.7 (1.3–5.7) | | 3.2 (1.2–8.1) | 1.5 (0.9–2.6) |
| Osann 1991 | 1969–1977 | Never smoked | | 1.0 | | 1.0 |
| | | Former smokers | | 12.6 (1.4–113.0) | | 1.7 (0.5–5.3) |
| | | Current smokers | | | | |
| | | <20 cigarettes/day | | 12.1 (1.5–96.3) | | 0.9 (0.3–2.7) |
| | | ≥ 20 cigarettes/day | | 71.2 (8.3–609.0) | | 3.8 (1.6–8.8) |
| Brownson et al. 1992b | 1984–1990 | Never smoked | 1.0 | | 1.0 | 1.0 |
| | | Former smokers | 19.2 (15.2–24.2) | | 29.8 (22.0–40.3) | 7.2 (6.2–8.5) |
| | | Current smokers | 20.6 (16.6–25.6) | | 42.5 (32.1–56.6) | 7.2 (6.2–8.3) |
| | | <20 cigarettes/day | 11.7 (8.7–15.8) | | 25.6 (18.1–36.3) | 5.8 (4.7–7.1) |
| | | ≥ 20 cigarettes/day | 26.1 (20.7–32.8) | | 53.1 (39.5–71.3) | 8.6 (7.3–10.1) |
| Osann et al. 1993 | 1984–1986 | Never smoked | 1.0 | | 1.0 | 1.0 |
| | | Former smokers | 13.5 (6.8–27.0) | | 43.3 (15.1–124.0) | 5.8 (3.8–9.0) |
| | | Ever smoked | | | | |
| | | <40 cigarettes/day | 24.0 (12.7–45.5) | | 76.7 (27.5–215.0) | 8.8 (6.1–12.8) |
| | | ≥ 40 cigarettes/day | 72.3 (36.8–142.0) | | 316.1 (111.0–900.0) | 24.2 (15.8–37.2) |
| Risch et al. 1993 | 1981–1985 | Never smoked | 1.0 | | 1.0 | 1.0 |
| | | Smoked ≥ 40 pack-years | 101.0 (15.3–660.0) | | 87.3 (26.7–286.0) | 8.8 (3.7–20.8) |
| Zang and Wynder 1996 | 1981–1994 | Never smoked | 1.0 | | | 1.0 |
| | | Current smokers | | | | |
| | | 1–10 cigarettes/day | 9.3 (3.9–22.1) | | | 4.5 (2.7–7.7) |
| | | 11–20 cigarettes/day | 33.0 (16.3–66.6) | | | 14.2 (9.6–20.9) |
| | | 21–40 cigarettes/day | 74.9 (37.0–151.5) | | | 27.2 (17.8–41.6) |
| | | ≥ 41 cigarettes/day | 85.3 (29.5–247.1) | | | 34.3 (16.2–72.5) |

*Kreyberg I includes squamous cell, small cell, and large cell carcinoma.
[§]Referent group.

the 10 brands. Nevertheless, Virginia Slims had the highest levels of both NAB and NAT and the second-highest level of NNK. As alleged by a former Philip Morris chemist, internal industry testing of Virginia Slims cigarettes "found levels of nitrosamines 10 times higher than other cigarettes, including Marlboros" (Geyelin 1997). Although preliminary, these findings call for the rigorous testing of Virginia Slims and other cigarette brands popular among women who smoke.

### Family History and Genetic Susceptibility Markers

Although approximately 90 percent of lung cancers are attributed to tobacco exposure, only a fraction of smokers (<20 percent) will develop lung cancer in their lifetime. Familial aggregation of lung cancer provides indirect evidence for a role of genetic predisposition to carcinogenesis from exposure to tobacco.

**Table 3.11. Relative risks for lung cancer associated with ever smoking for women and men, by histologic type**

| | | Relative risk (95% confidence interval) | | |
|---|---|---|---|---|
| **Study** | **Gender** | **Squamous cell carcinoma** | **Small cell carcinoma** | **Adenocarcinoma** |
| Potter et al. 1985 | Women | 8.3* | 52.3* | 4.0* |
| Schoenberg et al. 1989 | Women | 10.6 (6.8–16.6) | 59.0 (21.6–161) | 3.6 (2.6–5.0) |
| | Men | 18.9 (7.0–51.3) | 22.9 (3.2–166) | 4.8 (1.9–12.0) |
| Brownson et al. 1992b | Women | 20.1 (16.4–24.8) | 37.6 (28.5–49.3) | 6.9 (6.1–7.8) |
| | Men | 11.1 (9.5–12.9) | 11.4 (9.1–14.2) | 8.2 (6.9–9.7) |
| Osann et al. 1993 | Women | 26.4 (14.5–48.1) | 86.0 (31.6–234) | 9.5 (6.8–13.8) |
| | Men | 36.1 (17.8–73.3) | 37.5 (13.9–102) | 17.9 (10.4–31.0) |
| Risch et al. 1993 | Women | 25.5 (7.9–156) | 48.0 (10.5–849) | 3.5 (1.8–7.1) |
| | Men | 18.0 (5.5–111) | 6.3 (2.2–27.0) | 8.0 (2.3–50.6) |

*95% confidence interval was not reported.

Lung cancer is prevalent in certain families (Lynch et al. 1978; Paul et al. 1987). In case-control studies, patients with lung cancer were more likely than control subjects to report having relatives with lung cancer (Lynch et al. 1986; Ooi et al. 1986; Samet et al. 1986; Sellers et al. 1987; Horwitz et al. 1988; Wu et al. 1988; Osann 1991; Shaw et al. 1991), and risk appears to increase with the number of first-degree relatives affected (Shaw et al. 1991). A study in Germany examined the effects of smoking and family history of lung cancer among case patients older than age 45 years and among those aged 55 through 69 years, and among control subjects of comparable age. After adjustment for pack-years of smoking, a first-degree family history of lung cancer was associated with a significantly increased risk for lung cancer among those in the younger age group (RR, 2.6; 95 percent CI, 1.1 to 6.0) but not the older age group (RR, 1.2; 95 percent CI, 0.9 to 1.6) (Kreuzer et al. 1998). Gender-specific results were not reported in that study, but the finding of a stronger association of family history with early onset of disease is consistent with an inherited predisposition. Another German case-control study, in which 83 percent of subjects were men, also found increased smoking-adjusted RRs associated with lung cancer in a parent or sibling, again with greater elevations in RR for cases diagnosed at younger (<51 years) relative to older ages (Bromen et al. 2000). Paternal but not maternal history of lung cancer was associated with increased risk. Elsewhere, smoking was found to interact synergistically with a family history of lung cancer and to increase lung cancer risk by 30 to 47 times the risk for nonsmokers with no family history of lung cancer (Tokuhata 1963; Horwitz et al. 1988; Osann 1991). In two studies, risk was greatest among female relatives (Ooi et al. 1986) and sisters of probands (McDuffie 1991). Findings from segregation analysis were compatible with Mendelian codominant inheritance of a rare major autosomal gene for predisposition to lung cancer. These findings also supported a model in which 62 percent of the population was susceptible and women were both more susceptible and affected at an earlier age than were men (Sellers et al. 1990).

These studies on patterns of inheritance suggested that a small proportion of lung cancer resulting from cigarette smoking is due to "lung cancer genes" that are likely to be of low frequency but high penetrance. The discovery of high-penetrance/low-frequency genes for lung cancer, however, is not likely to explain the vast majority of lung cancers. Instead, there may be low-penetrance genes of relatively high frequency that interact with smoking to increase the odds of developing lung cancer and for which attributable risks may be high. This field of investigation is burgeoning (Amos et al. 1992), but few definitive conclusions can be drawn as to which specific low-penetrance genes affect lung cancer risk or whether there are differential gender-specific effects.

**Figure 3.8. Trends in lung cancer incidence among women, by histologic type, Surveillance, Epidemiology, and End Results (SEER) Program, 1973–1992**

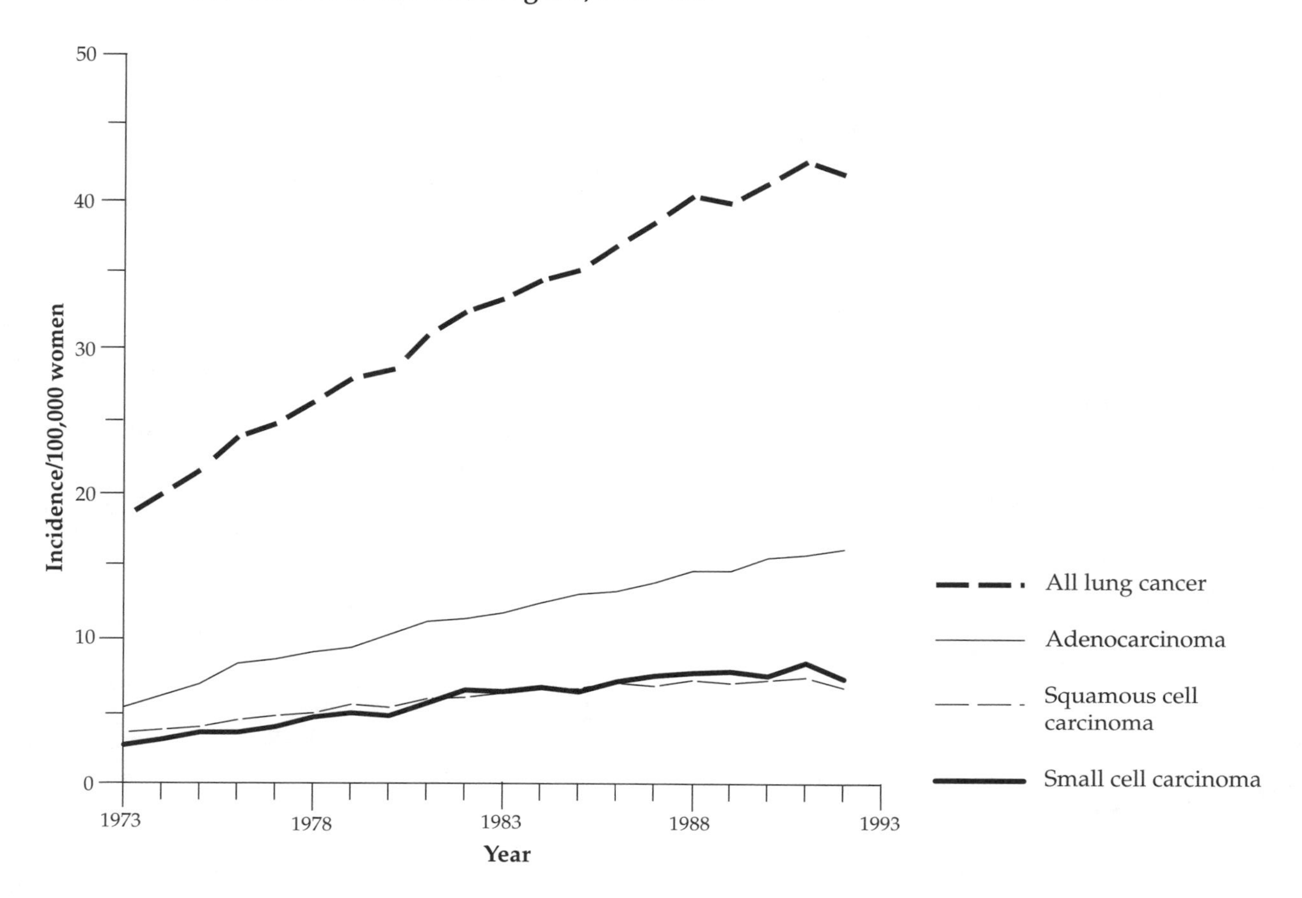


Source: SEER Program, unpublished data.

Mutations in the p53 tumor-suppressor gene are more common in lung cancers among smokers than among nonsmokers, and the p53 mutational spectra differ between smokers and nonsmokers with lung cancer (Bennett et al. 1999; Gealy et al. 1999). The frequency of mutations correlates positively with lifetime exposure to cigarette smoking, and good evidence indicated that benzo[*a*]pyrene, a chemical carcinogen in cigarettes, causes specific p53 mutations (Bennett et al. 1999).

Future research in this area may identify smokers who, by virtue of their genetic profile, are at particularly high risk and may determine whether gender-specific differences exist in the effects of genetic susceptibility markers on the risk for lung cancer associated with smoking. It is unlikely that one marker alone will be completely predictive of lung cancer risk; it is more likely that multiple susceptibility factors must be accounted for to represent the true dimensions of interactions between genes and exposure to tobacco.

### Other Risk Factors

Cigarette smoking is overwhelmingly the most important cause of lung cancer. However, other risk factors that influence susceptibility to the effects of smoking have been identified (Kabat 1993; Ernster 1994); these include exposure to carcinogens such as radon and asbestos that act synergistically with cigarette smoking to increase lung cancer risk (Reif and Heeren 1999). Selected environmental exposures and host characteristics that may alter lung cancer risk in combination with cigarette smoking are discussed here.

*Diet*

The role of diet in the etiology of lung cancer has been reviewed and is supported by a large body of experimental and epidemiologic evidence (Goodman 1984; Colditz et al. 1987; Fontham 1990; Willett 1990). Both prospective studies (Hirayama 1984b; Steinmetz et al. 1993) and retrospective studies (Fontham et al. 1988; Koo 1988; Le Marchand et al. 1989; Jain et al. 1990) of women reported a 50-percent reduction in risk for lung cancer associated with high intake of fruits and vegetables containing beta-carotene. Although three studies found a significant protective effect of these dietary factors among women nonsmokers (Koo 1988; Kalandidi et al. 1990; Mayne et al. 1994), most studies included few nonsmokers and noted a protective effect primarily among smokers. This finding suggested a possible interaction of diet with smoking (Fontham 1990). No consensus has emerged about which group of smokers may enjoy the greatest protection—current smokers (Dorgan et al. 1993), heavy smokers (Dorgan et al. 1993), light smokers (Fontham et al. 1988; Le Marchand et al. 1989), or former smokers (Samet et al. 1985; Humble et al. 1987b; Steinmetz et al. 1993). Research has shown a reduced risk for squamous and small cell carcinomas, which occur predominantly among smokers, but has not shown a reduced risk for adenocarcinoma. These findings provided additional support for a possible interaction between smoking and consumption of carotenoids (Byers et al. 1987; Fontham et al. 1988). However, other studies reported significant inverse associations between carotenoids and adenocarcinoma (Wu et al. 1985, 1988; Koo 1988), large cell carcinoma (Steinmetz et al. 1993), and lung cancers of all cell types (Dorgan et al. 1993; Wu et al. 1994).

Despite the protective effects associated with fruits and vegetables in observational studies, large-scale, randomized intervention trials showed either no benefit or a possibly harmful effect, at pharmacologic doses, of beta-carotene supplementation on lung cancer mortality, and no effect was found for alpha-tocopherol (Alpha-Tocopherol Beta-Carotene Cancer Prevention Study Group 1994; Omenn et al. 1996). Only one of the trials included women (Omenn et al. 1996).

Protective effects of preformed vitamin A (retinol) (Pastorino et al. 1987; Fontham et al. 1988; Koo 1988), vitamin C (Fontham et al. 1988; Koo 1988), vitamin E (Comstock et al. 1991; Mayne et al. 1994), and selenium (van den Brandt et al. 1993) were reported in some studies, but others reported no effect (Hinds et al. 1984; Samet et al. 1985; Wu et al. 1985, 1988; Byers et al. 1987; Humble et al. 1987b; Le Marchand et al. 1989). Epidemiologic studies of a possible increase in lung cancer risk with increased consumption of fat and cholesterol yielded conflicting results (Jain et al. 1990; Goodman et al. 1992; Alavanja et al. 1993; Wu et al. 1994). The ability to examine both independent associations and interactions of dietary factors with smoking is limited by small sample sizes and by inadequate estimation and analytic control for exposure to smoking.

*Occupation*

Few studies have examined specific occupational risks for lung cancer among women. Hazardous occupational exposures may explain 5 percent of lung cancers among women and 15 percent among men (Doll and Peto 1981). Occupational studies are often subject to limitations because of an inadequate number of women and insufficient adjustment for the effects of cigarette smoking.

Regardless of limitations of studies, investigators have identified several occupational exposures that interact synergistically with smoking to increase risk beyond that observed for smoking alone (Ives et al. 1988; Saracci and Boffetta 1994). Results of combined analysis for Japanese women and men exposed to arsenic-contaminated drinking water supported a previously observed synergistic effect for smoking and arsenic exposure (Hertz-Picciotto et al. 1992; Tsuda et al. 1995).

*Air Pollution*

Although most cohort studies conducted in the 1950s through the 1970s that considered the effects of air pollution included only men, more recent case-control studies have included women and have attempted to control for smoking and other confounders. A case-control study in New Mexico found that living in urban areas was associated with increased smoking among non-Hispanic, white female controls; however, in multivariate analyses, living in urban areas was not associated with increased risk for lung cancer (Samet et al. 1987). Researchers also noted a significant association between smoking and duration of urban residence among women in the Niagara region of Ontario (Holowaty et al. 1991). However, even after adjustment for smoking, women in Shenyang, China, had a twofold increase in risk for lung cancer that was associated with living in a smoky environment, residing near industrial factories, and using coal-burning stoves (Xu et al. 1989). In Poland, researchers found interaction between the effects of smoking and air pollution among men but not among women (Jedrychowski et al. 1990). Among women in Athens, a nonsignificant interaction between the effects of smoking duration and air pollution was reported (Katsouyanni et al. 1991). Although data are potentially consistent with a small role for air pollution in lung cancer risk, the limitations of inadequate control of confounding from smoking and occupational exposures and the difficulties in measuring cumulative exposure preclude definite conclusions.

*Radon and Ionizing Radiation*

Radon gas is released from the decay of radium in rock, soil, and water, and it accumulates in mines, caves, and buildings. Findings in studies of uranium miners indicated that radon is a cause of lung cancer and suggested a synergistic effect with cigarette smoking (Samet 1989b; Samet et al. 1989; Lubin 1994; National Research Council 1999). Because women have traditionally spent more time in the home, they have a higher risk from exposure to residential radon than do men.

Results from studies of atomic bomb survivors, who are at increased risk for lung cancer, were consistent with either a multiplicative or additive relationship among radiation, smoking, and risk (Prentice et al. 1983). Elsewhere, an excess risk for developing lung cancer 10 or more years following radiotherapy for breast cancer was observed among women smokers (Neugut et al. 1994). Compared with nonsmokers who were not exposed to radiotherapy, study participants who were exposed to radiation alone had a RR of 3, those who smoked but were not exposed to radiation had a RR of 14, and those who both smoked and were exposed to radiation had a RR of nearly 33. Because no increased risk was found for the first 10 years after radiotherapy, some doubt exists about the causal nature of the association. Current radiotherapy practices deliver substantially less radiation to the lungs than previously and reduce any potential hazard.

### Conclusions

1. Cigarette smoking is the major cause of lung cancer among women. About 90 percent of all lung cancer deaths among U.S. women smokers are attributable to smoking.
2. The risk for lung cancer increases with quantity, duration, and intensity of smoking. The risk for dying of lung cancer is 20 times higher among women who smoke two or more packs of cigarettes per day than among women who do not smoke.
3. Lung cancer mortality rates among U.S. women have increased about 600 percent since 1950. In 1987, lung cancer surpassed breast cancer to become the leading cause of cancer death among U.S. women. Overall age-adjusted incidence rates for lung cancer among women appear to have peaked in the mid-1990s.
4. In the past, men who smoked appeared to have a higher relative risk for lung cancer than did women who smoked, but recent data suggest that such differences have narrowed considerably. Earlier findings largely reflect past gender-specific differences in duration and amount of cigarette smoking.
5. Former smokers have a lower risk for lung cancer than do current smokers, and risk declines with the number of years of smoking cessation.

## International Trends in Lung Cancer Among Women

In 1990, cancers of the trachea, bronchus, and lung accounted for about 10 percent of all cancer deaths among women worldwide. The proportion of cancers varied widely among countries, which reflects the historical differences across countries in smoking initiation by women. Among women in Canada, the United Kingdom, and the United States, 20 percent or more of all cancer deaths were due to lung cancer; among women in France, Portugal, and Spain, the proportion was less than 5 percent. The estimated number of lung cancer deaths among women worldwide increased 23 percent between 1985 and 1990 (Pisani et al. 1999).

Since the early 1950s, lung cancer mortality for women in many industrialized countries has risen, on average, by more than 300 percent (Peto et al. 1994). Meanwhile, death rates among women for all other cancers combined have fallen by about 6 to 8 percent (Lopez 1995). Large prospective studies in the United Kingdom, the United States, and other industrialized countries showed that lung cancer death rates among nonsmokers have remained low, constant, and comparable among women and men (USDHHS 1989b; NCI 1997). These rates, about 5 cases per 100,000 persons (standardized to the European age structure of the World Health Organization [WHO]), are similar to the rates found for women in Southern Europe, where smoking prevalence among women has been low until recently.

Breast cancer has been the leading cause of cancer death among women in the industrialized world as a whole for about the last four decades. However, in some countries, notably Canada, Denmark, Scotland, and the United States, lung cancer now exceeds breast cancer as the principal cause of cancer death. Because lung cancer mortality is increasing among women in many countries, this crossover of death rates for the two cancer sites will probably occur in other countries as well. For women in the United States, the death rate for lung cancer also overtook the rate for colorectal cancer around 1980.

### Trends in Developed Countries

The predominant determinant of the lung cancer trends among both women and men is cigarette smoking (Peto et al. 1994). Several decades elapse between the initiation of regular smoking by a particular generation and the manifestation of smoking-related lung cancer risk in that cohort (Doll and Peto 1981; Harris 1983; Brown and Kessler 1988). In the United States, for example, cigarette consumption among women did not substantially take hold until the 1930s and 1940s (USDHHS 1980) (see "Historical Trends in Smoking" in Chapter 2), and until the early 1960s, lung cancer death rates were low.

Data from the early 1990s indicated that Denmark (35.6 per 100,000 women) and the United States (36.9 per 100,000 women) had the highest lung cancer death rates. Australia, Canada, Hungary, New Zealand, England, Wales, and Ireland had rates around 20 to 30 deaths per 100,000 women (Table 3.12). These are some of the countries in which women first began cigarette smoking and in which the prevalence of smoking among women remained at a fairly high level. Among developed countries, the lung cancer rates among women were lowest (about 10 cases or fewer per 100,000 women) in countries of Eastern and Southern Europe as well as in Finland and France.

The rate at which mortality from lung cancer has increased among women in different countries between 1985 and 1990–1993 is a public health concern (Table 3.12). Death rates rose most rapidly (about 5 percent per year) in Hungary, the Netherlands, and Switzerland; the percent increase was almost as high (3.3 to 3.7 percent per year) in several other countries, including Germany, Norway, and Sweden. Much more modest increases (about 0.5 percent per year) occurred in Bulgaria, Finland, Greece, Ireland, and Spain. In Ireland, the epidemic of lung cancer appears to have reached a plateau (Peto et al. 1994), but in Bulgaria, Finland, Greece, and Spain, low rates of increase suggested that the epidemic has yet to occur.

The range of lung cancer death rates in the early 1990s confirms that the lung cancer epidemic is heterogeneous even among women in industrialized countries (Peto et al. 1994). Countries for which data

**Table 3.12. Age-standardized average annual death rate for lung cancer among women, 1990–1993, and average annual percent increase between 1985 and 1990–1993, selected industrialized countries**

| Country | Death rate* | % increase | Country | Death rate* | % increase |
|---|---|---|---|---|---|
| United States | 36.9 | 3.3 | Austria | 13.6 | 1.8 |
| Denmark | 35.6 | 2.9 | Germany[†] | 12.8 | 3.5 |
| Canada | 31.5 | 3.1 | Japan | 12.6 | 0.9 |
| England and Wales | 30.8 | 0.8 | Switzerland | 12.0 | 5.1 |
| Ireland | 26.3 | 0.4 | Italy | 10.9 | 1.2 |
| New Zealand | 25.9 | 2.9 | Greece | 10.2 | 0.4 |
| Hungary | 23.9 | 5.2 | Finland | 10.2 | 0.6 |
| Australia | 19.2 | 2.0 | Bulgaria | 9.2 | 0.2 |
| The Netherlands | 15.5 | 4.6 | Romania | 9.0 | 0.9 |
| Norway | 15.4 | 3.4 | France | 7.7 | 2.9 |
| Sweden | 15.2 | 3.7 | Portugal | 6.8 | 3.1 |
| Poland | 14.5 | 3.1 | Spain | 5.4 | 0.6 |

*Per 100,000 women.
[†]Former Federal Republic of Germany.
Source: Calculated from unpublished data provided to the World Health Organization by respective countries.

are available can be grouped into three broad categories describing trends of about the last four decades.

- Group 1: Countries where death rates are already high (about 20 deaths or more per 100,000 women) and, in most cases, are still rising or have peaked. These countries include Australia, Canada, Denmark, Hungary, Ireland, New Zealand, the United Kingdom, and the United States.
- Group 2: Countries where death rates are still moderately low (10 to 15 deaths per 100,000 women) but are rising. These countries include Austria, Germany, Italy, Japan, the Netherlands, Norway, Poland, Sweden, and Switzerland.
- Group 3: Countries where death rates are low (about 5 to 10 deaths per 100,000 women) and roughly stable and where the lung cancer epidemic generally has not yet become apparent among women. These countries include Bulgaria, Finland, France, Greece, Portugal, Romania, and Spain.

Although the countries in each group may have similar death rates at a given time, trends in rates over time may differ. For example, unlike some countries in Group 3, which has low rates, France and Portugal have rates that are low but have been rising since about 1980. A trend of rising rates is evident in France, but it is not clear whether the increase in rates in Portugal is the beginning of an upward trend or a random fluctuation (Peto et al. 1994).

In the United Kingdom, the age-standardized lung cancer death rate among women has remained at around 31 deaths per 100,000 women since 1988. This rate, which is based on a large number of lung cancer deaths among women annually (about 12,500), suggested that the lung cancer epidemic has peaked among women in the United Kingdom. As noted earlier in this section, it also appears to have peaked in the United States (Wingo et al. 1999). The epidemic may have peaked in Australia, Ireland, and New Zealand, but because the number of lung cancer deaths in these countries is much smaller, the evidence is less conclusive.

Evidence that lung cancer rates among women in some areas may soon begin to rise was provided by trends in age-standardized death rates among women aged 35 through 54 years and among women aged 55 through 74 years. Lung cancer death rates among women aged 35 through 54 years have been declining since the late 1970s in the United Kingdom. Rates in this age group also appear to have reached their maximum level in Denmark and the United States more than a decade ago and more recently in Canada. On the other hand, rates among women aged 35 through 54 years were still rising in several countries in the early 1990s, for example in Hungary. The death rates among older women (aged 55 through 74 years) have generally continued to rise, as the cohorts most exposed to smoking have aged. However, death rates have already peaked and begun to decline among women in Ireland and the United Kingdom for this age group as well. The data for Australia and New Zealand also suggested that lung cancer mortality has peaked there among older women, but the trend is less conclusive in those two countries (Lopez 1995).

In several countries, including Austria, Germany, the Netherlands, Poland, Sweden, and Switzerland, and especially Hungary, the lung cancer death rate among women aged 35 through 54 years is relatively high compared with that among women aged 55 through 74 years. The ratios of these rates suggested that the epidemic of lung cancer is beginning among younger middle-aged women who have now been smoking long enough to incur an increased risk for developing the disease. As these cohorts of women at high risk for disease grow older, the lung cancer epidemic among women is likely to continue to develop in those countries.

If the epidemic of lung cancer among women has peaked or will soon peak in those countries where it first began, then it will have been less severe than the epidemic among men (Peto et al. 1994). In the United Kingdom, the age-standardized lung cancer death rates among men peaked at 110 deaths per 100,000 men in the early 1970s. In the United States, the peak among men was lower—about 85 deaths per 100,000 men. If the circumstances in the United Kingdom and the United States are replicated in other countries, the lung cancer death rate among women may rise to only about one-third to one-half that found among men at the height of the epidemic of lung cancer among men.

#### Trends in Developing Countries

Mortality trends for lung cancer are not known for most developing countries, because data collection systems that would yield comparable, reliable estimates of mortality over time generally have not existed. However, current available data suggest that lung cancer death rates are generally low (Pisani et al. 1999), as would be expected for populations without a long history of smoking. An exception to the general pattern is the relatively high lung cancer rate among Chinese women in Asia (Parkin et al. 1999), despite the fact that relatively few Chinese women smoke. Factors other than smoking appear to be responsible for the high lung cancer death rates among women in China, possibly factors related to indoor air pollution created by certain cooking and heating sources. Despite the low prevalence of smoking, however, case-control studies have shown that smoking is also a strong risk factor for lung cancer among Chinese women (Wu-Williams et al. 1990).

### Conclusion

1. International lung cancer death rates among women vary dramatically. This variation reflects historical differences in the adoption of cigarette smoking by women in different countries. In 1990, lung cancer accounted for about 10 percent of all cancer deaths among women worldwide and more than 20 percent of cancer deaths among women in some developed countries.

## Female Cancers

Various factors associated with smoking, such as decreased fertility, age at menopause, and low body weight, are predictors of risk for many female cancers. The recognition that smoking can affect estrogen-related diseases and events (Baron et al. 1990) provided further reason to examine the relationship between smoking and cancers influenced by endogenous hormones. Studies have also shown that smoking can influence the metabolism of exogenous hormones (Jensen et al. 1985; Cassidenti et al. 1990). These findings have prompted evaluation of combined effects of smoking and use of oral contraceptives (OCs) or menopausal estrogens, exposures that have been repeatedly examined with respect to various female cancers.

### Breast Cancer

Indirect evidence suggests the biological possibility that smoking may reduce the risk for breast cancer. It is recognized that high levels of estrogens, particularly estrone and estradiol, contribute to an increased risk for breast cancer (Bernstein and Ross 1993), and smoking is thought to have an antiestrogenic effect (see "Sex Hormones" later in this chapter). The occurrence of menopause at an earlier age among smokers than among nonsmokers is also well established, and late age at menopause has been consistently related to an increased risk for breast cancer (Alexander and Roberts 1987). Thus, smoking could reduce the risk for breast cancer. On the other hand, cigarette smoke contains numerous carcinogens that could plausibly affect the breast. Also, nicotine has been detected in the breast fluid of nonlactating women (Petrakis et al. 1978).

Multiple case-control studies and several cohort studies assessed the relationship between smoking and breast cancer risk (Palmer and Rosenberg 1993). The results of some studies, particularly hospital-based, case-control studies, must be interpreted cautiously. Smoking prevalence may be higher among hospital control subjects than among women in the general population and may result in an underestimation of the effects of smoking. Furthermore, questions have been raised about the results of some studies of women in breast cancer screening programs (Schechter et al. 1985; Meara et al. 1989) because the extent to which early detection methods are used may be correlated with smoking behaviors. Population-based studies are generally believed to provide the most valid results.

Many studies have reported no significant differences in breast cancer risk by whether participants had ever smoked (Rosenberg et al. 1984; Smith et al. 1984; Baron et al. 1986b, 1996b; Adami et al. 1988; Kato et al. 1989; London et al. 1989; Schechter et al. 1989; Ewertz 1990; Vatten and Kvinnsland 1990; Field et al. 1992; Braga et al. 1996; Engeland et al. 1996; Gammon et al. 1998; Millikan et al. 1998). (See Table 3.13 for results from case-control studies.) One study reported a lower but nonsignificant risk for breast cancer among current smokers but not among former smokers (O'Connell et al. 1987). Other studies reported a slightly to moderately higher risk among smokers (Schechter et al. 1985; Brinton et al. 1986b; Hiatt and Fireman 1986; Stockwell and Lyman 1987; Meara et al. 1989; Rohan and Baron 1989; Chu et al. 1990; Palmer et al. 1991; Bennicke et al. 1995; Morabia et al. 1996). Most elevations in RRs have been modest. Increased risk for breast cancer associated with smoking has been reported from at least two studies that used as the referent group women who were nonsmokers and who had not been exposed to ETS (Lash and Aschengrau 1999; Johnson et al. 2000).

Most studies showed that RRs were generally similar for current and former smokers (Rosenberg et al. 1984; Lund 1985; Brinton et al. 1986b; Hiatt and Fireman 1986; London et al. 1989; Rohan and Baron 1989; Chu et al. 1990; Ewertz 1990; Baron et al. 1996b; Braga et al. 1996). (See Table 3.13 for results from case-control studies.) In the few studies in which risk differed, the direction of the difference was inconsistent; some studies showed a higher risk among current smokers (Schechter et al. 1985; Stockwell and Lyman 1987; Brownson et al. 1988; Palmer et al. 1991), and other studies showed a higher risk among former smokers (Hiatt and Fireman 1986; O'Connell et al. 1987). Meara and colleagues (1989) showed a higher risk among current smokers aged 45 through 69 years in a screening program study and a decreased risk among current smokers aged 45 through 59 in a hospital-based study. One study showed an elevated risk among recent smokers that was restricted to postmenopausal women (Millikan et al. 1998). Similarly, studies that examined risk by years since smoking cessation or by age at cessation showed no substantive relationships (Chu et al. 1990; Field et al. 1992; Baron et al. 1996b).

The majority of studies have indicated no differences in risk from either long-term or high-intensity smoking. Age at initiation of smoking also seems unrelated to breast cancer risk (Brinton et al. 1986b; Adami et al. 1988; Ewertz 1990; Palmer et al. 1991; Field et al. 1992; Baron et al. 1996b; Braga et al. 1996). Furthermore, the few studies that examined risk by years since initiation of smoking showed no significant relationship (Adami et al. 1988; Braga et al. 1996). One study examined whether many years of smoking before a first-term pregnancy affected risk and found no adverse effect (Adami et al. 1988).

Some studies reported an increased risk for premenopausal breast cancer associated with ever smoking (Schechter et al. 1985), cigarette-years of smoking (Schechter et al. 1985), current but not former smoking (Brownson et al. 1988), or former smoking (Brinton et al. 1986b). Johnson and colleagues (2000) used never active smokers who had also not been exposed to ETS as the referent group and found that premenopausal women had an increased risk for breast cancer associated with active smoking and higher RRs than did postmenopausal women. In one study that focused on women whose breast cancers were detected before age 45 years, current smoking was related to reduced risk among women who began smoking before 16 years of age (Gammon et al. 1998). However, in another study, which included women with a diagnosis of breast cancer before age 36 years, smoking was not related to risk (Smith et al. 1994). Most well-conducted studies have not confirmed an association between current or former smoking and premenopausal breast cancer (Hiatt and Fireman 1986; London et al. 1989; Rohan and Baron 1989; Schechter et al. 1989; Ewertz 1990; Field et al. 1992; Baron et al. 1996b). In the large Cancer and Steroid Hormone (CASH) study in which only women younger than 55 years of age were included, Chu and associates (1990) found that smoking-associated risk for breast cancer was somewhat higher among women diagnosed before menopause; the differences by menopausal status at diagnosis were not statistically significant.

Smoking-associated risk was also examined by age at diagnosis of breast cancer, but again no definitive relationships were found. In the CASH study (Chu et al. 1990), risk was somewhat higher among women who had a diagnosis of breast cancer before age 45 years, but the interaction with age was not statistically significant. Stockwell and Lyman (1987) similarly found the highest risk when cancer was diagnosed before age 50 years, but Vatten and Kvinnsland (1990) reported no difference in the effects of smoking before and after age 51 years. In another study, women with a diagnosis of breast cancer at 65 years of age or older (Brinton et al. 1986b) had a smoking-associated RR less than 1.0. However, the data showed no trends in risk among current smokers with long duration or high intensity of smoking. Other investigators reported no substantial difference in risk for breast cancer among women by age at diagnosis (before or after age 50 years) (Palmer et al. 1991).

Although most studies did not find a significant relationship between smoking and breast cancer, the biological rationale for such a relationship has been compelling enough to motivate investigators to assess relationships within subgroups defined by hormonally related risk factors (e.g., use of exogenous hormones), hormone receptor status, and most recently, genetic polymorphisms.

Because evidence suggested that smoking might enhance the clearance of exogenous hormones, several studies evaluated whether any effects of smoking were modified by use of OCs or menopausal estrogens. In one study, cigarette smoking was strongly associated with breast cancer risk among women who had used either OCs or menopausal estrogens (Brinton et al. 1986b), but other studies failed to confirm this result (Adami et al. 1988; Chu et al. 1990; Ewertz 1990; Palmer et al. 1991; Gammon et al. 1998).

Most studies did not find the effects of smoking to be modified by additional risk factors, including parity, family history of breast cancer, body mass, alcohol consumption, dietary factors, and educational status (Rosenberg et al. 1984; Smith et al. 1984; Brinton et al. 1986b; Chu et al. 1990; Ewertz 1990; Palmer et al. 1991).

Data are conflicting on whether a different relationship might exist for smoking among estrogen

**Table 3.13. Relative risks for breast cancer for smokers compared with nonsmokers, case-control studies**

| Study | Number of cases | Number of controls | Source of controls | Relative risk (95% confidence interval) | | |
|---|---|---|---|---|---|---|
| | | | | Ever smoked | Current smokers | Former smokers |
| Rosenberg et al. 1984 | 2,160 | 717 | Other cancers | | 1.1 (0.8–1.7)* | 1.1 (0.8–1.3) |
| Smith et al. 1984 | 429 | 612 | Population | 1.2 (0.9–1.6)† | | |
| Schechter et al. 1985 | 123 | 369 | Screening program | 1.4 (0.9–2.1) | 1.9 (1.2–3.1) | 1.0 (0.6–1.7) |
| Brinton et al. 1986b | 1,547 | 1,930 | Screening program | 1.2 (1.0–1.4) | 1.2 (0.9–1.4) | 1.2 (1.0–1.5) |
| O'Connell et al. 1987 | 276 | 1,519 | Community | | 0.6 (0.3–1.1)‡ | 1.2 (0.8–1.7) |
| Stockwell and Lyman 1987 | 5,246 | 3,921 | Other cancers | | 1.3 (1.0–1.8)§ | 1.0 (0.8–1.1) |
| Adami et al. 1988 | 422 | 527 | Population | 1.0 (0.8–1.3) | 1.1 (0.7–1.8)Δ | |
| Brownson et al. 1988 | 456 | 1,693 | Screening program | 1.1 (0.9–1.4) | 1.4 (1.0–1.9) | 0.9 (0.6–1.2) |
| Kato et al. 1989 | 1,740 | 8,920 | Other cancers | 0.9 (0.7–1.0) | | |
| Meara et al. 1989 | 998 | 998 | Hospital | | | |
| | | | Ages 25–44 years | | 1.2 (0.7–1.8)¶ | 0.9 (0.6–1.5) |
| | | | Ages 45–59 years | | 0.8 (0.6–1.1)¶ | 0.9 (0.7–1.3) |
| | 118 | 118 | Screening program | | | |
| | | | Ages 45–69 years | | 2.9 (1.2–7.2)¶ | 1.0 (0.4–2.3) |
| Rohan and Baron 1989 | 451 | 451 | Population | 1.2 (0.9–1.5) | 1.4 (0.9–2.0) | 1.0 (0.7–1.5) |
| Schechter et al. 1989 | 254 | 762 | Screening program | | | |
| | | | Prevalent | 1.1 (0.9–1.5) | | |
| | | | Incident | 1.2 (0.9–1.6) | | |
| Chu et al. 1990 | 4,720 | 4,682 | Population | 1.2 (1.1–1.3) | 1.2 (1.1–1.3) | 1.1 (1.0–1.3) |

*≥25 cigarettes/day.
†Continuous smokers.
‡>20 cigarettes/day.
§>40 cigarettes/day.
Δ≥20 cigarettes/day.
¶≥5 cigarettes/day.

receptor (ER)-positive tumors and among ER-negative tumors. In one population-based, case-control study, smoking was associated with a 63-percent higher risk for ER-negative tumors, a risk that was significantly different from the null association observed for ER-positive tumors (Cooper et al. 1989). This association of smoking with ER-negative tumors was confined to women with premenopausal cancer—an effect consistent with that found in a clinical study that included only women with breast cancer (Ranocchia et al. 1991). However, a second study reported the opposite relationship—a fairly weak association with smoking for women with ER-positive tumors (London et al. 1989). A third study found that the risks for both ER-positive and ER-negative breast cancer increased with both active and passive smoking (Morabia et al. 1998). Other studies have not shown cigarette smoking to vary by the ER status of tumors (McTiernan et al. 1986; Stanford et al. 1987b; Yoo et al. 1997).

**Table 3.13. Continued**

| Study | Number of cases | Number of controls | Source of controls | Relative risk (95% confidence interval) | | |
|---|---|---|---|---|---|---|
| | | | | Ever smoked | Current smokers | Former smokers |
| Ewertz 1990 | 1,480 | 1,332 | Population | | 0.9 (0.8–1.1) | 1.0 (0.8–1.2) |
| Palmer et al. 1991 | | | | | | |
| Canada | 607 | 1,214 | Neighborhood | 1.0 (0.8–1.3) | 1.1 (0.9–1.4) | 1.0 (0.7–1.3) |
| United States | 1,955 | 805 | Other cancers | 1.2 (1.0–1.5) | 1.3 (1.1–1.6) | 1.1 (0.9–1.4) |
| Field et al. 1992 | 1,617 | 1,617 | Driver's license | 1.0 (0.9–1.2) | | |
| Smith et al. 1994 | 755 | 755 | Population | 1.0 (0.8–1.3) | | |
| Baron et al. 1996b | 6,888 | 9,529 | Driver's license and Medicare | | 1.0 (0.9–1.1) | 1.1 (1.0–1.2) |
| Braga et al. 1996 | 2,569 | 2,588 | Hospital | 0.9 (0.8–1.1) | 0.8 (0.7–1.0) | 1.1 (0.9–1.4) |
| Morabia et al. 1996 | 244 | 1,032 | Population | | 5.1 (2.1–12.6)** | |
| Gammon et al. 1998†† | 1,645 | 1,497 | Population | 0.9 (0.8–1.1) | 0.8 (0.7–1.0) | 1.0 (0.8–1.2) |
| Millikan et al. 1998 | 498 | 473 | HCFA‡‡ and state Division of Motor Vehicles | | 1.0 (0.7–1.4) | 1.3 (0.9–1.8) |
| Lash and Aschengrau 1999 | 265 | 765 | HCFA and next of kin | 2.0 (1.1–3.6)§§ | 2.3 (0.8-6.8)ΔΔ | |
| Johnson et al. 2000 | 2,317 | 2,438 | Population | Premenopausal women: 2.3 (1.2–4.5)§§<br>Postmenopausal women: 1.5 (1.0–2.3)§§ | Premenopausal women: 1.9 (0.9–3.8)§§<br>Postmenopausal women: 1.6 (1.0–2.5)§§ | Premenopausal women: 2.6 (1.3–5.3)§§<br>Postmenopausal women: 1.4 (0.9–2.1)§§ |

**≥20 cigarettes/day; reference group comprised of subjects not exposed to active or passive smoking.
††Women <45 years of age.
‡‡HCFA = Health Care Financing Administration.
§§Compared with subjects not exposed to active or passive smoking.
ΔΔPersons smoking within 5 years before diagnosis.

ACS's CPS-II prospective study reported a significant increase in breast cancer mortality among current smokers (RR, 1.3); the risk from smoking for a long duration or at high intensity was even higher (RR, 1.7 for >40 cigarettes per day) (Calle et al. 1994). The investigators hypothesized that these findings could be due to delayed diagnosis of breast cancer among smokers or to a poorer prognosis among patients with breast cancer who smoke. Consistent with a poorer prognosis are results that showed a shorter average interval to recurrence of breast cancer among smokers than among nonsmokers (Daniell 1984) and poorer survival among patients with breast cancer who smoked than among nonsmokers (Yu et al. 1997). In another study, however, diagnosis of local breast cancer, as opposed to regional or distant breast cancer, was more likely among smokers than among nonsmokers (Smith et al. 1984). Thus, additional studies are necessary to address how breast cancers are detected among smokers and how smoking affects the prognosis of the disease.

More recent studies focused on whether smoking may have unusual effects on breast cancer risk among genetically susceptible subgroups. These studies examined whether risk varied in the presence or absence of certain genetic polymorphisms involved in the activation or detoxification of carcinogens, including polymorphisms in *GSTM1*, *CYP1A1*, and *N*-acetyltransferase 2 (*NAT2*) genotypes. Although two studies did not find that the *GSTM1* genotype modified the effect of smoking on overall breast cancer risk (Ambrosone et al. 1996; Kelsey et al. 1997), one of the studies did find an increased risk for breast cancer among heavy smokers with specific polymorphisms in either the *CYP1A1* (Ambrosone et al. 1995) or *NAT2* genes (Ambrosone et al. 1996). Other studies have also identified some interaction of smoking with either the *NAT1* gene (Zheng et al. 1999), the *NAT2* gene (Morabia et al. 2000), or both genes (Millikan et al. 1998), but in the study of both genes, the effect was restricted to postmenopausal women who had smoked recently. Later data from the large prospective U.S. Nurses' Health Study did not find that the *NAT2* polymorphism increased the risk for breast cancer among smokers (Hunter et al. 1997), but did find some support for an interaction of smoking with the *CYP1A1* gene among women who began smoking early in life (Ishibe et al. 1998). Additional studies are examining potential interactions with these as well as other genetic polymorphisms. A recent study also suggested that cigarette smoking may reduce the risk for breast cancer among carriers of the highly penetrant genes *BRCA1* and *BRCA2* (Brunet et al. 1998). Studies are also beginning to assess the relationships between smoking and breast cancer within groups defined by tumor-suppressor genes; one recent investigation showed a higher risk associated with current cigarette smoking among patients with p53-positive tumors (Gammon et al. 1999). These various preliminary findings require further verification.

Correlations between the incidence of lung cancer among men and breast cancer among women in various countries and parts of the United States supported the hypothesis that ambient tobacco smoke may be related to breast cancer (Horton 1988). In a case-control study, exposure to ETS was associated with breast cancer among premenopausal women but not among postmenopausal women (Sandler et al. 1985, 1986), but the number of cases was small and the analysis was controlled only for age and level of education. In a large Japanese cohort study, Hirayama (1990) observed a significant dose-response relationship between the number of cigarettes smoked by husbands and their wives' risk for breast cancer at ages 50 through 59 years. In a case-control study of women younger than age 36 years, those exposed to ETS had an elevated risk for developing breast cancer, but the investigators noted little evidence of significant trends with increasing exposure (Smith et al. 1994).

Wells (1991, 1998) recommended further study of the effects of ETS exposure on breast cancer risk, because any risk associated with active smoking might be underestimated if the possibly confounding effect of ETS exposure is not considered. Indeed, the first study to examine this issue found a RR of 3.2 among nonsmoking women exposed to ETS compared with nonsmoking women who had not been exposed to ETS (Morabia et al. 1996). The plausibility of this finding was questionable because the RR associated with active smoking, using never active smokers as the referent group, was much higher (RR, 1.9 for smokers of >20 cigarettes per day) than that observed in other investigations. However, subsequent case-control studies that used persons who had never smoked or who had never been exposed to ETS as the referent group also found evidence of increased risk associated with ETS exposure (Lash and Aschengrau 1999; Johnson et al. 2000). In the study by Lash and Aschengrau (1999), the RRs associated with active smoking and with exposure to ETS were each 2.0, with evidence of higher risks among active smokers who smoked only before the first pregnancy and among subjects exposed to ETS before age 12 years. Similarly, in a large, population-based case-control study in Canada with adjustment for multiple potentially confounding variables, Johnson and colleagues (2000) found both ever active smoking and ETS exposure to be associated with increased risks for premenopausal and postmenopausal breast cancer after adjustment for multiple confounding variables. The referent group was women who were neither active smokers nor exposed to ETS. Millikan and associates (1998) reported positive associations between ETS exposure and breast cancer among never active smokers (RRs, 1.2 to 1.5), but the associations were weak and the findings were not statistically significant. In contrast, Wartenberg and colleagues (2000) found no association between ETS exposure and breast cancer mortality in the CPS-II cohort study. They noted that after 12 years of follow-up, the risk was similar among women who were lifelong never smokers whose spouse was a current smoker at baseline and among women whose spouse had never smoked (multivariate RR, 1.0; 95 percent CI, 0.8 to 1.2), and no dose-response relationship was found. Biologically it is implausible that ETS exposure could impart a risk that is the same as that of active smoking, but whether ETS is related to breast cancer risk remains an open question and one that is receiving attention in other investigations.

The relationship of breast cancer risk to in utero exposure to tobacco smoke is also of interest because smoking may be associated with lower estrogen levels during pregnancy (Petridou et al. 1990). Although reduced estrogen levels might be expected to lower the risk for breast cancer, Sanderson and associates (1996), in a study that evaluated effects of maternal smoking and the risk for breast cancer, reported no significant effect overall and only a slight increase in risk among women diagnosed with breast cancer at age 30 years or younger whose mothers had smoked during pregnancy. This association persisted after the investigators considered the effects of birth weight.

Thus, active smoking does not appear to appreciably affect breast cancer risk overall. However, several issues are not entirely resolved, including whether starting to smoke at an early age increases risk, whether certain subgroups defined by genetic polymorphisms are differentially affected by smoking, and whether ETS exposure affects risk.

*Benign Breast Disease*

Studies provided mixed evidence as to whether smoking affects the risk for developing various benign breast conditions (Nomura et al. 1977; Berkowitz et al. 1985; Pastides et al. 1987; Rohan et al. 1989; Parazzini et al. 1991b; Yu et al. 1992). To compare the results of these studies is difficult because they differ by the types of conditions examined (fibroadenoma, fibrocystic disease, or proliferative disorders of varying degrees of severity), by how smoking status was defined (ever, current, or former smoking), and by whether data were analyzed by menopausal status.

### Endometrial Cancer

Some researchers proposed that exposure to tobacco may reduce the risk for endometrial cancer by reducing estrogen production (MacMahon et al. 1982), a hypothesis that received some support from findings that estriol excretion is reduced among postmenopausal smokers (Key et al. 1996). Another theory is that smoking affects endometrial cancer risk by altering the metabolism, absorption, or distribution of hormones. Research has shown that smokers have higher rates of conversion of estradiol to 2-hydroxyestrones, which have low estrogenic activity (Michnovicz et al. 1986). Furthermore, antiestrogenic effects of smoking may be mediated by inducing microsomal, mixed-function oxidase systems that metabolize sex hormones (Lu et al. 1972). Both mechanisms are consistent with findings that women smokers who take oral estradiol have lower levels of unbound estradiol and higher serum hormone-binding capacity than do women nonsmokers who take estradiol (Jensen et al. 1985; Cassidenti et al. 1990). However, other mechanisms should not be dismissed. For example, several investigators believe that the effects of smoking on androgen, progestogen, or cortisol may reduce the risk for endometrial cancer among smokers (Seyler et al. 1986; Khaw et al. 1988; Baron et al. 1990; Berta et al. 1991).

Multiple case-control studies showed a reduced risk for endometrial cancer among cigarette smokers (Baron et al. 1986b; Franks et al. 1987a; Levi et al. 1987; Stockwell and Lyman 1987; Kato et al. 1989; Koumantaki et al. 1989; Dahlgren et al. 1991; Brinton et al. 1993; Parazzini et al. 1995) (Table 3.14). Several other studies found reduced risks among smokers that were not statistically significant (Smith et al. 1984; Lesko et al. 1985; Tyler et al. 1985; Lawrence et al. 1987; Weir et al. 1994). Some of these studies examined results by menopausal status and showed that the reduced risk among smokers was restricted to women with endometrial cancer diagnosed after menopause (Lesko et al. 1985; Stockwell and Lyman 1987; Koumantaki et al. 1989; Parazzini et al. 1995). Among postmenopausal women, the magnitude of the risk reduction associated with ever smoking was about 50 percent. One study found a significantly elevated risk for premenopausal endometrial cancer associated with ever smoking (Smith et al. 1984). In most studies that showed a reduced risk associated with smoking, the effect was greater among current smokers than among former smokers or was confined to current smokers.

The factors that are known to increase the risk for endometrial cancer and that are potential confounders of the association between smoking and the disease include obesity, late onset of menopause, menstrual disorders, infertility, and use of menopausal estrogens; reduced risk has been associated with use of OCs. Despite careful control for these variables, the magnitude of observed reductions in risk associated with smoking has not been substantially affected.

Beside considering confounding effects, several investigators assessed whether the presence of selected risk factors could modify the relationship between smoking and endometrial cancer risk. Three studies noted a greater reduction in smoking-associated risk

**Table 3.14. Relative risks for endometrial cancer for smokers compared with nonsmokers, case-control studies**

| Study | Number of cases | Number of controls | Source of controls | Relative risk (95% confidence interval) | | |
|---|---|---|---|---|---|---|
| | | | | Ever smoked | Current smokers | Former smokers |
| Smith et al. 1984 | 70 | 612 | Population | | 0.8 (0.4–1.5)* | |
| Lesko et al. 1985 | 510 | 727 | Other cancers | | 0.7 (0.5–1.0) | 0.9 (0.6–1.2) |
| Tyler et al. 1985 | 437† | 3,200† | Population | 0.9 (0.7–1.1) | 0.8 (0.7–1.1) | 1.0 (0.7–1.4) |
| Franks et al. 1987a | 79‡ | 416‡ | Population | 0.5 (0.3–0.8) | | |
| Lawrence et al. 1987 | 200§ | 200 | Driver's license | | 0.5Δ | 0.6Δ |
| Levi et al. 1987 | 357 | 1,122 | Hospital | | 0.4 (0.3–0.7) | 0.9 (0.5–1.5) |
| Stockwell and Lyman 1987 | 1,374 | 3,921 | Other cancers | | 0.5 (0.3–0.9)¶ | 0.6 (0.5–0.8) |
| Kato et al. 1989 | 239 | 8,920 | Other cancers | 0.4 (0.3–0.8) | | |
| Lawrence et al. 1989a | 844** | 168 | Driver's license | | 0.9Δ | 1.0Δ |
| Brinton et al. 1993 | 405 | 297 | Population | 0.8 (0.5–1.1) | 0.4 (0.2–0.7) | 1.1 (0.7–1.6) |
| Weir et al. 1994 | 73†† | 399†† | Neighbor | 0.8 (0.5–1.4) | 0.8 (0.4–1.5) | 0.8 (0.3–2.1)‡‡ |
| Parazzini et al. 1995 | 726 | 1,452 | Hospital | | 0.8 (0.7–1.1) | 0.6 (0.4–0.9) |

*Continuous smokers.
†Women 20–54 years of age.
‡Postmenopausal women >40 years of age.
§Women with early-stage tumors.
Δ>1 pack of cigarettes/day. 95% confidence interval was not reported, but the results of Lawrence et al. 1987 were reported to be statistically significant and results of Lawrence et al. 1989a were not.
¶>40 cigarettes/day.
**Women with late-stage tumors.
††Postmenopausal women.
‡‡Women who had stopped smoking ≥10 years before.

among obese women (Lawrence et al. 1987; Brinton et al. 1993; Parazzini et al. 1995). Other research indicated that obesity enhances the capacity to produce estrogens through extraovarian sources and is associated with higher levels of sex hormone-binding globulin (Siiteri 1987). Several studies reported a greater reduction in risk for smokers than nonsmokers among women taking estrogen replacement therapy (Weiss et al. 1980; Franks et al. 1987a), but not all study results supported such an effect (Brinton et al. 1993; Parazzini et al. 1995). One study found the greatest reduction in risk associated with smoking among multiparous women (Brinton et al. 1993).

Endometrial hyperplasia is generally recognized as a precursor of endometrial cancer (Kurman et al. 1985). Weir and colleagues (1994) examined the association between smoking and endometrial hyperplasia and showed a lower RR among both premenopausal and postmenopausal women smokers. The results of this study, however, were not statistically significant.

**Table 3.15. Relative risks for ovarian cancer for smokers compared with nonsmokers, case-control studies**

| Study | Number of cases | Number of controls | Source of controls | Relative risk (95% confidence interval) | | |
|---|---|---|---|---|---|---|
| | | | | Ever smoked | Current smokers | Former smokers |
| Byers et al. 1983 | 274 | 1,034 | Hospital | 0.9* | | |
| Smith et al. 1984 | 58 | 612 | Population | | 0.8 (0.4–1.6)† | |
| Tzonou et al. 1984 | 150 | 250 | Hospital | 0.8‡ | | |
| Franks et al. 1987b | 494 | 4,238 | Population | 1.0 (0.9–1.3) | 1.1 (0.9–1.4) | 0.9 (0.7–1.2) |
| Stockwell and Lyman 1987 | 889 | 3,921 | Other cancers | | 1.1 (0.6–1.9)§ | 0.9 (0.7–1.2) |
| Hartge et al. 1989 | 296 | 343 | Hospital | | 0.8 (0.6–1.3) | 1.3 (0.9–2.0) |
| Kato et al. 1989 | 417 | 8,920 | Other cancers | 0.8 (0.6–1.1) | | |
| Shu et al. 1989 | 229 | 229 | Hospital | 1.8 (0.7–4.8) | | |
| Polychronopoulou et al. 1993 | 189 | 200 | Hospital visitor | 1.0 (0.5–1.8) | | |

*Authors stated that relative risk was not statistically significant.
†Continuous smokers.
‡p = 0.08.
§Current smokers of >40 cigarettes/day.

### Ovarian Cancer

Frequency of ovulation has been hypothesized in regard to risk for epithelial ovarian cancer: the greater the number of ovulatory cycles in a lifetime, the greater the risk (Whittemore et al. 1992). If smoking interrupts ovulation, as suggested by menstrual irregularity and subfecundity among smokers (see "Menstrual Function" and "Reproductive Outcomes" later in this chapter), smoking could lower the risk for ovarian cancer. On the other hand, cigarette smoke contains carcinogens, which could increase the risk for ovarian cancer. Furthermore, enzymes in the ovaries of rodents have been shown to metabolize polycyclic aromatic hydrocarbons (PAHs) to electrophilic intermediates, and exposure to these compounds through smoking may have direct toxic effects or may stimulate ovarian atresia (imperforation or closure). Thus, the risk for ovarian cancer may be increased (Mattison and Thorgeirsson 1978). A broad range of possible biological effects of smoking on ovarian tissue or on hormones exists, but studies have not examined the relationship of smoking with risk for ovarian cancer in detail. In most studies in which the effects of smoking were evaluated, only limited information on exposure was collected, and comparisons were usually dependent on hospital-based control subjects. In fact, few studies have considered the combined influence of smoking and other risk factors for ovarian cancer. Further research is also needed on the relationship of smoking with histologic subtypes of ovarian cancer.

Most investigations of the relationship between the risk for ovarian cancer and a history of ever having smoked have found no association (Byers et al. 1983; Smith et al. 1984; Baron et al. 1986b; Franks et al. 1987b; Stockwell and Lyman 1987; Hartge et al. 1989; Kato et al. 1989; Hirayama 1990; Polychronopoulou et al. 1993; Engeland et al. 1996; Mink et al. 1996). Table 3.15 shows results of case-control studies that provided estimates of RR.

Only a few studies examined the relationship of ovarian cancer with duration or intensity of smoking. A study in Greece found a slightly reduced risk among smokers who smoked 20 or more cigarettes per day, but the relationship was not statistically significant (Tzonou et al. 1984). The CASH study reported that risk for ovarian cancer did not vary in relation to quantity of cigarettes smoked and duration of smoking, including the interval since smoking cessation, the number of pack-years of smoking, the interval since initiation of smoking, and age at initiation (Franks et al. 1987b). Furthermore, smoking effects did not vary by several other factors, including reproductive history, menopausal status, use of exogenous hormones, alcohol use, and family history of ovarian cancer. However, the CASH study included only women with a diagnosis of ovarian cancer before age 55 years, which limits the generalizability of the results. Studies that included a broader age range of women found no substantial relationship of ovarian cancer risk with current smoking or duration of smoking (Stockwell and Lyman 1987; Hartge et al. 1989).

**Cervical Cancer**

A positive correlation between the incidence of cervical cancer and other cancers known to be related to cigarette smoking across populations prompted the hypothesis that smoking may affect the risk for cervical cancer (Winkelstein 1977). Excess risk for cervical cancer among smokers was demonstrated in a number of case-control studies (Clarke et al. 1982; Marshall et al. 1983; Baron et al. 1986b; Brinton et al. 1986a; La Vecchia et al. 1986; Peters et al. 1986; Nischan et al. 1988; Licciardone et al. 1989; Bosch et al. 1992; Daling et al. 1996). (See Table 3.16 for studies that provided data on smokers and never smokers.) One cohort study also found an excess risk for cervical cancer among smokers (Greenberg et al. 1985). In these studies, the association between cervical cancer and smoking was not eliminated, even though the investigators controlled for several well-established risk factors for cervical cancer, including early age at first sexual intercourse, history of multiple sex partners, and low socioeconomic status.

Several subtypes of human papillomavirus (HPV) are recognized as the main cause of cervical cancer worldwide (Bosch et al. 1995), and the extent to which the relationship between smoking and cervical cancer reflects a causal association independent of HPV infection is not known. The association of smoking with cervical cancer may be causal, may reflect confounding or risk modification among women with HPV infection, or may even reflect an effect of smoking on risk for HPV infection. Residual confounding by sexual history may also explain observed smoking associations, and adjustment for HPV will probably address that possibility.

Most studies in which risk values were not adjusted for HPV infection reported a RR of approximately 2.0 among smokers compared with nonsmokers. Women who smoked for a long duration or at high intensity generally had the highest risk (Table 3.16). In several studies, the relationship was restricted to, or strongest among, recent or current smokers (Brinton et al. 1986a; La Vecchia et al. 1986; Licciardone et al. 1989). Two studies reported the highest risk among women who started smoking late in life (Brinton et al. 1986a; Herrero et al. 1989), but other studies reported the opposite effect, namely higher risk among women who began smoking at young ages (La Vecchia et al. 1986; Daling et al. 1996). The results from several studies showed further biological evidence to support an association between cervical cancer and smoking. The findings included an enhanced risk associated with continuous smoking (Slattery et al. 1989), use of unfiltered cigarettes (Brinton et al. 1986a), and inhaling smoke into the throat and mouth (Slattery et al. 1989). The effects of smoking appear to be restricted to squamous cell carcinoma; no relationship was observed for the rarer occurrences of adenocarcinoma or adenosquamous carcinoma (Brinton et al. 1986a).

In numerous studies, an association with smoking appears to prevail for both cervical cancer and precursor conditions, including carcinoma in situ and cervical dysplasia (also known as squamous intraepithelial neoplasia) (Harris et al. 1980; Berggren and Sjostedt 1983; Hellberg et al. 1983; Lyon et al. 1983; Trevathan et al. 1983; Clarke et al. 1985; Mayberry 1985; La Vecchia et al. 1986; Brock et al. 1989; Slattery et al. 1989; Coker et al. 1992; Gram et al. 1992; Parazzini et al. 1992a; Munoz et al. 1993; Becker et al. 1994; de Vet et al. 1994; Kjaer et al. 1996; Ylitalo et al. 1999) (Table 3.17). Most of these studies reported particularly high risk among current smokers and among those who smoked for a long time or at a high intensity, but they have been limited by the absence of information on HPV. In one study, smoking did not affect the overall risk for cervical intraepithelial neoplasia (CIN) when sexual history and HPV infection status were taken into account (Schiffman et al. 1993). However, current cigarette smoking was related to nearly a threefold increase in risk among the limited number of HPV-positive women who had a higher grade of disease (CIN II or III). Elsewhere, in a clinics-based study among HPV-infected women in which women with CIN I served as the referent group, smoking was significantly associated with CIN III (Ho et al. 1998). These findings suggested that smoking may be involved in disease progression. They were supported by results in two other studies that

**Table 3.16. Relative risks for invasive cervical cancer for smokers compared with nonsmokers and for quantity or duration of smoking, case-control studies**

| Study | Number of cases/controls | Source of controls | Relative risk (95% confidence interval) by smoking status | | | Relative risk (95% confidence interval) by quantity/duration of smoking | |
|---|---|---|---|---|---|---|---|
| | | | Ever smoked | Current smokers | Former smokers | | |
| Clarke et al. 1982 | 178/855 | Neighbor | | 2.3 (1.6–3.3) | 1.7 (1.0–2.8) | | |
| Marshall et al. 1983 | 513/490 | Hospital | | 1.6 (1.2–2.1) | 0.8 (0.5–1.4) | <½ pack/day | 1.7* |
| | | | | | | ½–1 pack/day | 1.7* |
| | | | | | | 1–2 packs/day | 1.0 |
| | | | | | | >2 packs/day | 0.4 |
| Baron et al. 1986b | 1,174/2,128 | Hospital | | | | 1–14 packs/year | 1.4* |
| | | | | | | ≥15 packs/year | 1.8* |
| Brinton et al. 1986a | 480/797 | Community | 1.5 (1.1–1.9) | 1.5 (1.2–2.0) | 1.3 (0.9–1.9) | <10 years | 1.1 |
| | | | | | | 10–19 years | 1.6* |
| | | | | | | 20–29 years | 1.3 |
| | | | | | | 30–39 years | 1.5* |
| | | | | | | ≥40 years | 2.2* |
| La Vecchia et al. 1986 | 230/230 | Hospital | | 1.7 (1.1–2.3) | 0.8 (0.4–1.7) | <15 cigarettes/day | 1.7† |
| | | | | | | ≥15 cigarettes/day | 1.8† |
| Peters et al. 1986 | 200/200 | Neighbor | | | | 2–20 years | 1.5‡ |
| | | | | | | ≥21 years | 4.0*‡ |
| Nischan et al. 1988 | 225/435 | Hospital | 1.2 (0.8–1.7) | | | <10 years | 0.7 |
| | | | | | | 10–19 years | 1.3 |
| | | | | | | 20–29 years | 1.7 |
| | | | | | | ≥30 years | 2.7* |
| Herrero et al. 1989 | 667/1,430 | Hospital/community | | 1.0 (0.7–1.2) | 1.0 (0.8–1.3) | <10 years | 1.0 |
| | | | | | | 10–19 years | 1.0 |
| | | | | | | 20–29 years | 1.1 |
| | | | | | | 30–39 years | 0.6 |
| | | | | | | ≥40 years | 1.5 |
| Licciardone et al. 1989 | 331/993 | Other cancers | | | 1.7 (1.0–2.9) | <1 pack/day | 2.2*† |
| | | | | | | ≥1 pack/day | 3.9*† |
| Bosch et al. 1992 | 436/387 | Population | 1.5 (1.0–2.2) | | | | |
| Eluf-Neto et al. 1994 | 199/225 | Hospital | 1.5 (0.99–2.3) | | | | |
| Daling et al. 1996 | 314/672 | Population | | 2.5 (1.8–3.4) | 1.5 (1.1–2.2) | <10 years | 1.0§ |
| | | | | | | 10–19 years | 2.4* |
| | | | | | | ≥20 years | 2.8* |

*Statistically significant.
†Relative risk for current smokers.
‡Relative risk for years of smoking >5 cigarettes/day. Reference group consisted of persons who smoked for ≤1 year.
§Referent group for the study by Daling et al. 1996.

**Table 3.17. Relative risks for cervical intraepithelial neoplasia for smokers compared with nonsmokers, case-control studies**

| Study | Cases | | Controls | | Relative risk (95% confidence interval) | | |
|---|---|---|---|---|---|---|---|
| | Type | Number | Source | Number | Ever smoked | Current smokers | Former smokers |
| Harris et al. 1980 | Dysplasia/ CIS‡ | 190 | Hospital | 422 | | 2.1*† | |
| Lyon et al. 1983 | CIS | 217 | Community | 243 | | 3.0 (1.9–4.8)§ | |
| Trevathan et al. 1983 | Mild, moderate dysplasia | 194 | Family-planning program | 288 | 2.4 (1.6–3.7) | 2.6 (1.7–4.1) | 1.6 (0.8–3.6) |
| | Severe dysplasia | 81 | | | 3.3 (1.9–5.8) | 3.0 (1.6–5.6) | 5.7 (2.4–13.5) |
| | CIS | 99 | | | 3.6 (2.1–6.2) | 4.2 (2.7–7.5) | 2.1 (0.8–5.6) |
| Clarke et al. 1985 | Dysplasia | 250 | Neighbor | 500 | | 3.1*† | 1.1† |
| Mayberry 1985 | CIN^Δ | 210¶ | Clinic | 317 | | 2.0 (1.3–3.0) | 1.4 (0.7–2.8) |
| La Vecchia et al. 1986 | CIN | 183 | Screening program | 183 | | 2.6 (1.3–5.2)** | 2.5 (0.9–6.7) |
| Brock et al. 1989 | CIS | 116 | Physician | 193 | | 4.5 (2.2–9.1) | 1.3 (0.6–3.0) |
| Slattery et al. 1989 | CIS | 266†† | Random digit dialing | 408 | | 3.4 (2.1–5.6) | 1.4 (0.8–2.5) |
| Coker et al. 1992 | CIN II, III | 103 | Clinic‡‡ | 268 | 1.7 (0.9–3.3) | 3.4 (1.7–7.0) | |
| Parazzini et al. 1992a | CIN I, II | 128 | Screening program | 323 | | 1.8 (1.1–2.9) | 1.1 (0.4–2.9) |
| | CIN III | 238 | | | | 2.0 (1.3–3.1) | 1.7 (0.8–3.5) |
| Munoz et al. 1993 | CIN III | 525 | Cytology | 512 | | | |
| Spain | | | | | | 1.3 (0.7–2.3) | 0.9 (0.2–3.8) |
| Colombia | | | | | | 2.0 (1.3–3.0) | 1.8 (0.9–3.5) |
| Becker et al. 1994 | CIN II, III | 201 | Colposcopy | 337 | 1.4 (1.0–2.1) | 1.8 (1.2–2.8) | 0.9 (0.5–1.5) |
| de Vet et al. 1994 | Dysplasia | 257 | Population | 705 | | 3.5 (2.1–5.9)* | 2.0 (1.1–3.4) |
| Kjaer et al. 1996 | CIS | 586 | Population | 614 | 2.3 (1.6–3.2) | 2.4 (1.7–3.4) | 1.6 (1.0–2.7) |
| Ylitalo et al. 1999 | CIS | 422 | Screening program | 422 | | 1.9 (1.3–2.8) | 1.5 (0.9–2.3) |

*≥20 cigarettes/day.
†95% confidence interval was not provided, but the results were reported as not significant.
‡CIS = Carcinoma in situ.
§90% confidence interval.
ΔCIN = Cervical intraepithelial neoplasia; CIN II and CIN III define disease progression.
¶Includes 35 women with severe dysplasia, 9 with CIS, and 10 with invasive carcinoma.
**≥15 cigarettes/day.
††Includes 36 women with invasive carcinoma.
‡‡Women with normal cervical cytologies.

were limited by the absence of data on HPV status. In those studies, smoking was a risk factor only for CIN III (Coker et al. 1992) or was a stronger risk factor for CIN III than for CIN II (Trevathan et al. 1983).

Investigators in only a few studies evaluated the interaction between smoking and other risk factors for cervical cancer. One study found no significant variation by other factors, including sexual behavior and history of sexually transmitted disease (STD) (Mayberry 1985). Two studies reported that the effects of smoking were greatest among women with a history of limited sexual activity (Nischan et al. 1988; Slattery et al. 1989). However, in another study, the effects of smoking were greatest among women who were married multiple times or who had more than one sexual partner (La Vecchia et al. 1986). Lyon and associates (1983) found the effects of smoking to be greater among Mormon women, who tend to begin to bear children at a younger age than do other women in the United States.

Because HPV infection, which is usually contracted from a sexual partner, is widely recognized as the main cause of cervical cancer, Phillips and Smith (1994) focused on ways to assess whether the association between smoking and cervical cancer is independent of HPV infection. HPV occurs frequently among women with cervical cancer but infrequently in control subjects. Thus, recent studies have examined smoking effects by status of HPV infection among subgroups of women. An early study found the effects of smoking to be most pronounced among women infected with HPV, but these results may have been limited by imprecise assays to detect HPV (Herrero et al. 1989). Several studies using reliable measures of HPV reported that smoking was not associated with risk for cervical cancer among HPV-positive women (Bosch et al. 1992; Munoz et al. 1993; Eluf-Neto et al. 1994). This finding suggested that cigarette smoking may not affect risk for cervical cancer independently of HPV infection status. However, all these studies were conducted in Latin America, where the effects of smoking on cervical cancer have been found to be weak—possibly because few women in these studies have a history of smoking for a long duration or at a high intensity (Herrero et al. 1989). Thus, it is noteworthy that two studies, one in the United States and the other in Denmark, found smoking to be a risk factor among both HPV-positive and HPV-negative women (Daling et al. 1996; Ylitalo et al. 1999).

Several research teams have attempted to define possible mechanisms by which smoking might alter the cervical epithelium. Because of the high levels of nicotine and cotinine detected in the cervical mucus of smokers, the researchers initially investigated a direct effect of smoking (Sasson et al. 1985; Schiffman et al. 1987; McCann et al. 1992). Zur Hausen (1982) also suggested that the oncogenicity of HPV may be enhanced by certain chemical compounds, including those in tobacco smoke. The results of one study supported this hypothesis (Herrero et al. 1989), but others did not find an enhanced effect of smoking among HPV-positive women (Munoz et al. 1993; Eluf-Neto et al. 1994). More recent studies reported no significant difference in smoking-related DNA damage (DNA adduct levels) in the cervical epithelium of HPV-positive and HPV-negative smokers (Simons et al. 1995). Attention also focused on whether smoking might cause local immunosuppression within the cervix as a result of a decrease in the number of Langerhans' cells (Barton et al. 1988). Some have suggested that such immunosuppression may allow the persistence of HPV. For example, one study showed that the prevalence of HPV was positively associated with the number of cigarettes smoked per day (Burger et al. 1993). Hildesheim and colleagues (1993), however, did not find smoking to be strongly associated with the risk for cervical HPV infection, when correlations with sexual behavior were taken into account. Thus, whether the relationship between smoking and cervical cancer is biological or reflects residual confounding remains unclear.

Further clues to mechanisms of the effects of smoking may be revealed by examining interaction with dietary factors. Several investigators suggested that diets low in carotenoids or vitamin C may predispose women to cervical cancer (Brock et al. 1988; La Vecchia et al. 1988; Verreault et al. 1989). The results of one study suggested that the effects of cigarette smoking were more pronounced among women with high levels of antioxidants than among those with low levels, but these findings were not statistically significant (Brock et al. 1989). Because smokers may have lower levels of plasma beta-carotene than do nonsmokers (Brock et al. 1988) and because nutrition may affect the persistence of HPV (Potischman and Brinton 1996), studies that focus on the combined effects of cigarette smoking, nutrition, and HPV persistence may prove insightful.

The effects of exposure to ETS on risk for cervical cancer began to receive attention in the 1980s. Investigators addressed these effects primarily by studying the smoking behavior of partners of women or by directly questioning women about their passive exposure to cigarette smoke. Two studies that focused on husbands found that the prevalence of smoking was higher among husbands of women with cervical cancer than among husbands of control subjects (Buckley et al. 1981; Zunzunegui et al. 1986). However, Buckley and colleagues (1981) accounted for the number of sexual partners of the husbands and found that ETS exposure did not persist as a significant predictor of risk. In a study of intraepithelial neoplasia, Coker and colleagues (1992) found no consistent association with ETS exposure. On the other hand, Slattery and associates (1989) found that women with passive exposure to cigarette smoke for three or more hours per day had nearly a threefold increase in risk. In fact, the effect was even more enhanced for women nonsmokers. Additional studies are needed to determine whether ETS exposure actually increases risk for cervical cancer or whether it appears to do so because of confounding factors that have not been adequately controlled in some of the studies to date. McCann and associates (1992) examined nicotine and cotinine levels in cervical mucus and found no real differences between nonsmoking women who did or did not report exposure to ETS.

#### Vulvar Cancer

In several studies, the risk for cancer of the vulva has been higher among smokers than among nonsmokers (Newcomb et al. 1984; Mabuchi et al. 1985; Brinton et al. 1990). In one investigation, the risk was about twice as high among current smokers than among nonsmokers or former smokers and even higher among current smokers who had smoked at a high intensity (Brinton et al. 1990). The increased risk among current smokers, which was also reported for cervical cancer, is consistent with the action of cigarette smoke as a promoter in the late stages of carcinogenesis.

Results from all studies were limited by the absence of reliable information on the status of HPV infection, which is an accepted risk factor for vulvar cancer (Andersen et al. 1991). Because the risk for vulvar cancer is higher among smokers with a history of condylomata or genital warts, which are caused by HPV infection (Brinton et al. 1990), future studies should address whether data on the effects of smoking are confounded by HPV infection status and whether risk is modified by the presence of HPV. Findings from several small clinical studies (Andersen et al. 1991; Bloss et al. 1991) supported the hypothesis that smoking may predispose women to the subset of vulvar cancers most strongly linked with HPV infection—cancers with intraepithelial-like growth patterns—rather than the well-differentiated vulvar cancers more common among older women. Zur Hausen (1982) proposed that the effect of HPV infection may be enhanced by other risk factors. Immune alterations are a plausible mechanism for this synergistic relationship. Smoking has been linked with several changes in immune function (Hughes et al. 1985; Barton et al. 1988), and HPV infection occurs more commonly among persons with immunosuppression (Sillman et al. 1984).

#### Conclusions

1. The totality of the evidence does not support an association between smoking and risk for breast cancer.
2. Several studies suggest that exposure to environmental tobacco smoke is associated with an increased risk for breast cancer, but this association remains uncertain.
3. Current smoking is associated with a reduced risk for endometrial cancer, but the effect is probably limited to postmenopausal disease. The risk for this cancer among former smokers generally appears more similar to that of women who have never smoked.
4. Smoking does not appear to be associated with risk for ovarian cancer.
5. Smoking has been consistently associated with an increased risk for cervical cancer. The extent to which this association is independent of human papillomavirus infection is uncertain.
6. Smoking may be associated with an increased risk for vulvar cancer, but the extent to which the association is independent of human papillomavirus infection is uncertain.

## Other Cancers

Smoking has been shown to increase the risk for cancer at sites outside the respiratory system, including the digestive system, the urinary tract, and the hematopoietic system. Previously, information on the effects of smoking was derived primarily from epidemiologic studies of men (USDHHS 1989b), but later data from studies of women showed generally similar patterns of risk for equivalent levels of exposure.

### Oral and Pharyngeal Cancers

Numerous cohort and case-control studies have shown that the main risk factors for cancers of the mouth and pharynx are smoking and alcohol use

(Blot et al. 1996). These associations hold for cancers of the mouth, tongue, and pharynx, almost all of which are squamous cell carcinomas, but little or no association has been shown for salivary gland tumors, which are extremely rare and are generally adenocarcinomas (Preston-Martin et al. 1988; Horn-Ross et al. 1997).

In almost all populations, oral and pharyngeal cancers occur more frequently among men than among women (Parkin et al. 1992). However, smoking increases the risk for these cancers among both genders. In CPS-II, the risk for death from oral or pharyngeal cancer was five times higher among women current smokers than among women who had never smoked (Table 3.18). In a cohort study from Sweden, women who smoked also had an increased risk for oropharyngeal cancer incidence (Nordlund et al. 1997).

In a large, population-based case-control study that included more than 350 women with cancer, the risk for oral or pharyngeal cancer rose progressively with the duration of smoking and the number of cigarettes smoked. After adjustment for alcohol intake, the risk for oral and pharyngeal cancers was 10 times greater among women who were long-term ($\geq$ 20 years), heavy ($\geq$ 2 packs per day) smokers than among women nonsmokers. Smoking cigarettes and drinking alcohol in combination greatly increased risk. The risk for these cancers was more than 10 times greater among women who had 15 or more drinks a week and smoked 20 or more cigarettes a day for 20 or more years than among women nonsmokers and nondrinkers (Blot et al. 1988). These high RRs may exceed those among men (Blot et al. 1988; Kabat et al. 1994b; Macfarlane et al. 1995; Muscat et al. 1996; Talamini et al. 1998). Among both women and men, the risk for these cancers does not appear to be elevated among persons who had stopped smoking for 10 or more years (Blot et al. 1988; Kabat et al. 1994b; Macfarlane et al. 1995). This rapid reduction in risk suggested that smoking affects a late stage in the process of oral and pharyngeal carcinogenesis and that women can substantially decrease their risk in a fairly short time if they stop smoking. About 60 percent of oral and pharyngeal cancers among women are due to the combined effects of tobacco and alcohol (Blot et al. 1988; Negri et al. 1993), but smoking-related risk for oral and pharyngeal cancer exists even among women who do not drink alcohol (Macfarlane et al. 1995; La Vecchia et al. 1999).

Use of smokeless tobacco also increases the risk for oral cancer, particularly at sites that have direct contact with the tobacco product. This finding has been reported in India and other Asian countries, where use of smokeless tobacco is common (International Agency for Research on Cancer [IARC] 1985; USDHHS 1986a; Nandakumar et al. 1990; Sankaranarayanan 1989a,b, 1990), but evidence also comes from studies of women in rural areas of the southern United States. In a study of women in North Carolina (Winn et al. 1981), the RR for cancers of the cheek and gum rose sharply with use of snuff. Among women who had used snuff for 50 or more years, the risk for oral cancer was 50 times that among women who had not used snuff. Indeed, in this population, nearly all cancers of the gum and buccal mucosa were attributable to long-term use of snuff.

**Table 3.18. Relative risks for death from selected cancers among women, by smoking status, Cancer Prevention Study II, 1982–1988**

| Cancer type | Current smokers | Former smokers |
|---|---|---|
| Oral and pharyngeal cancers | 5.1 | 2.3 |
| Laryngeal cancer | 13.0 | 5.2 |
| Esophageal | 7.7 | 2.8 |
| Stomach cancer | 1.4 | 1.4 |
| Colon cancer | 1.3 | 1.2 |
| Rectal cancer | 1.4 | 1.2 |
| Liver cancer | 1.6 | 2.1 |
| Biliary tract cancer | 0.7 | 0.5* |
| Pancreatic cancer | 2.2 | 1.5 |
| Bladder cancer | 2.2 | 1.9 |
| Kidney cancer | 1.3 | 1.0 |
| Myeloid leukemia | 1.2 | 1.3 |
| Lymphoid leukemia | 1.4* | 1.4 |
| Multiple myeloma | 1.2 | 1.1 |
| Non-Hodgkin's lymphoma | 1.3 | 0.8 |
| Hodgkin's lymphoma | 5.1* | 2.6* |

*Note:* Risk relative to women who never smoked.
*Based on <10 deaths.
Source: American Cancer Society, unpublished data.

**Laryngeal Cancer**

Laryngeal cancer is a relatively rare disease among women; the male-to-female incidence ratio is 5:1. Survival is relatively good; about 70 percent of patients live 5 or more years after diagnosis (Austin and Reynolds 1996). This cancer is caused largely by heavy smoking and heavy drinking of alcohol

(Tavani et al. 1994a; Austin and Reynolds 1996). Data are limited on the relationship between cigarette smoking and laryngeal cancer among women, but these data also showed a much higher risk among smokers than among persons who had never smoked. In CPS-II, the risk for death from laryngeal cancer among women current smokers was 13 times that among women who had never smoked (Table 3.18). Similarly, in a multisite case-control study, Williams and Horm (1977) reported a risk ratio of 17.7 for laryngeal cancer among women who had smoked more than 40 pack-years compared with women nonsmokers. In another case-control study, Wynder and Stellman (1977) found a RR of 9.0 among women who were long-term smokers (>40 years). Case-control studies from Italy and China reported even higher RRs (Zheng et al. 1992; Tavani et al. 1994a). Although the reported RR estimates were based on small numbers of subjects and consequently were not precise, they are compatible with a 10-fold higher risk among current smokers than among nonsmokers. Studies conducted largely among men indicated that smoking cessation decreases the smoking-related risks (Tuyns et al. 1988; Falk et al. 1989).

### Esophageal Cancer

Esophageal cancer is also a malignant disease that occurs among men much more often than among women (Parkin et al. 1992). The high male-to-female incidence ratio applies to both squamous cell carcinoma, the most common histologic type of esophageal cancer in most populations, and adenocarcinoma, a cell type rapidly rising in incidence in the United States and parts of Europe (Blot et al. 1991). Smoking, combined with drinking alcohol, has consistently been shown to be a strong risk factor for squamous cell esophageal cancer and appears to increase the risk for adenocarcinoma (Blot 1994; Brown et al. 1994b; Vaughan et al. 1995; Gammon et al. 1997).

Only limited data are available on the effect of smoking on the risk for esophageal cancer among women, but no evidence suggests that these effects differ among women and men. In an investigation of esophageal cancer among women in northern Italy, smoking was the main risk factor and risk increased with the amount smoked; women who smoked one or more packs of cigarettes per day had five times the risk of nonsmokers (Negri et al. 1992; Tavani et al. 1993). Among women in CPS-II, the risk for death from esophageal cancer among current smokers was almost eight times higher than that among women who had never smoked (Table 3.18). Studies of smoking cessation, largely among men, have consistently found excess risk to be reduced, but not eliminated, after cessation (IARC 1986; USDHHS 1989b; Tavani et al. 1993).

### Stomach Cancer

Smoking may increase the risk for stomach cancer (McLaughlin et al. 1990; Kneller et al. 1991; Hansson et al. 1994; Nomura 1996; Trédaniel et al. 1997), but some investigators have shown no association (Buiatti et al. 1989; Trédaniel et al. 1997). The excess risks reported have been smaller than those found for oral or esophageal cancer, and dose-response trends have been absent or relatively weak. Nonetheless, differences in diet between smokers and nonsmokers do not appear to totally explain the difference in risk (Hansson et al. 1994).

Among women participating in CPS-II, the risk for mortality from stomach cancer was 40 percent higher among current smokers and former smokers than among never smokers (Table 3.18). These findings are consistent with the evidence among men (McLaughlin et al. 1995a). In several case-control studies, differences by gender in smoking-related risks were small (Haenszel et al. 1972; Kono et al. 1988; Kato et al. 1990; Tominaga et al. 1991; Burns and Swanson 1995; Chow et al. 1999), but several investigators found indications of a weaker effect among women (Trédaniel et al. 1997; Inoue et al. 1999). In both cohort studies (USDHHS 1989b; McLaughlin et al. 1995b) and case-control studies (Hansson et al. 1994), risk for stomach cancer among former smokers was not significantly elevated compared with persons who had never smoked. Subjects in these studies were mostly men.

### Colorectal Cancer

Smoking has been associated with a twofold to threefold excess risk for colorectal adenomas, benign precursors of most colorectal cancers (Kikendall et al. 1989; Lee et al. 1993; Neugut et al. 1993; Olsen and Kronborg 1993; Giovannucci et al. 1994a; Newcomb et al. 1995), but its association with colorectal cancer has been more controversial (Kune et al. 1992; Terry and Neugut 1998). Several cohort and case-control studies of women found no excess risk for colon or rectal cancer among smokers (Sandler et al. 1988; Akiba and Hirayama 1990; Chute et al. 1991; Kune et al. 1992; Baron et al. 1994b; Boutron et al. 1995; D'Avanzo et al. 1995a; Engeland et al. 1996; Nordlund et al. 1997; Knekt et al. 1998). However, CPS-II found small increases in the risk for death from cancers of the colon (RR, 1.3) and rectum (RR, 1.4) among women current smokers on the basis of 6 years of follow-up (Table 3.18). A more detailed analysis after 14 years of follow-up of the CPS-II cohort found that, in general, risk for colorectal cancer death increased with the number of cigarettes smoked and with pack-years of smoking (Chao et al. 2000). Moreover, some cohort studies that had 20 years or more of follow-up showed a moderately elevated risk for colorectal cancer death among smokers, for both women (Doll et al. 1980) and men (Doll et al. 1994; Heineman et al. 1994). In a pair of related cohort studies (Giovannucci et al. 1994a,b), smoking was associated with an increased risk for developing colorectal cancer after a latent period of 35 years among both women and men. Risk for colorectal cancer also has been modestly associated with cigarette smoking in some case-control studies of women (Newcomb et al. 1995; Le Marchand et al. 1997; Slattery et al. 1997). In some analyses, excess risks for long-term smokers were not reduced substantially after smoking cessation (Chute et al. 1991; Heineman et al. 1994; Newcomb et al. 1995). Several other studies of women found smoking-related RRs to be greater for cancer of the rectum than for cancer of the colon (Doll et al. 1980; Inoue et al. 1995; Newcomb et al. 1995).

### Liver and Biliary Tract Cancers

Heavy alcohol use and chronic hepatitis B infection are recognized risk factors for hepatocellular carcinoma (IARC 1988), but the role of cigarette smoking is less clear. An early study reported an increased risk for hepatocellular carcinoma, even after adjustment for alcohol intake, among women and men smokers who did not have hepatitis B infection (Trichopoulos et al. 1980). Among the women in CPS-II, the mortality rate for liver cancer was 60 percent higher among current smokers than among those who had never smoked (Table 3.18). In the studies that presented data separately for women (Table 3.19), the RR estimates for liver cancer were generally similar to those among men and ranged from no association (Stemhagen et al. 1983) to a threefold excess risk among current smokers (Tsukuma et al. 1990). Risk for liver cancer rose with increasing number of

**Table 3.19. Relative risks for primary liver cancer among women for smokers compared with nonsmokers, case-control studies**

| Study | Number of cases/controls | Smoking status | Relative risk | 95% confidence interval |
|---|---|---|---|---|
| Stemhagen et al. 1983 | 151/284 | Ever smoked | 1.0 | 0.6–1.7 |
| Yu et al. 1988 | 73/202 | Former smokers | 1.2 | NR* |
| | | Current smokers | 2.1† | NR |
| Tsukuma et al. 1990 | 34/73 | Current smokers | 2.9 | 1.1–7.9 |
| Yu et al. 1991 | 25/58 | Former smokers | 1.4 | 0.3–6.5 |
| | | Current smokers | 2.4 | 0.8–6.9 |
| Tanaka et al. 1992 | 36/119 | Former smokers | 1.7 | 0.4–7.1 |
| | | Current smokers | 1.0 | 0.3–3.2 |
| Goodman et al. 1995 | 81/179,381‡ | Former smokers | 1.7 | 0.8–3.6 |
| | | Current smokers | 1.6 | 0.9–2.9 |
| Tanaka et al. 1995 | 117/257 | Ever smoked | | |
| | | 0.1–12.9 pack-years§ | 2.4 | 1.1–4.9 |
| | | ≥13.0 pack-years | 1.8 | 0.8–3.7 |

*NR = Value not specified in report of study.
†$p < 0.05$.
‡Number of cases and person-years.
§Pack-years = number of years smoking multiplied by the usual number of packs of cigarettes smoked per day.

cigarettes smoked per day in some studies (Yu et al. 1988, 1991) but not in others (Stemhagen et al. 1983; Tsukuma et al. 1990; Goodman et al. 1995; Tanaka et al. 1995). Smoking cessation has typically been associated with a modest reduction in the RR for liver cancer, particularly after sustained cessation (Yu et al. 1988, 1991; Tsukuma et al. 1990; Goodman et al. 1995), but among women in CPS-II, the RR for death from liver cancer among former smokers was not reduced (Tables 3.18 and 3.19). Thus, smoking may be a contributing factor in the development of liver cancer, but further clarification of the effect among women is needed.

Cancers of the biliary tract include malignant tumors that arise from the gallbladder, extrahepatic bile ducts, and ampulla of Vater (Fraumeni et al. 1996). Smoking-related excess risk for these tumors has been observed in a few case-control studies of women and men combined (Ghadirian et al. 1993; Chow et al. 1994; Moerman et al. 1994), but not in one other case-control study (Yen et al. 1987). Among women in CPS-II, risk for death from biliary tract cancers was lower among smokers than among women who had never smoked (Table 3.18). A nonsignificantly decreased risk for gallbladder cancer was observed in a Swedish follow-up study (Nordlund et al. 1997), but a Japanese cohort study reported a 30-percent excess mortality from this cancer among women who smoked (95 percent CI, 0 to 100 percent) (Akiba and Hirayama 1990). In a study of cancers of the extrahepatic bile duct and ampulla of Vater, the risk was three times higher among women who had smoked more than 50 pack-years than among women who had never smoked, but women who smoked less than 50 pack-years had no excess risk (Chow et al. 1994). Estimates from both the Swedish and Japanese studies were based on a few cases and were imprecise.

### Pancreatic Cancer

Studies have consistently demonstrated that smoking increases the risk for pancreatic cancer. Among women in CPS-II, the risk for death from pancreatic cancer was about twice as high among current smokers as among women who had never smoked (Table 3.18). A doubling of risk among women who smoked was also reported in the U.S. Nurses' Health Study (Fuchs et al. 1996) and the Iowa Women's Health Study (Harnack et al. 1997). Cohort studies from Ireland (Tulinius et al. 1997), Japan (Akiba and Hirayama 1990), Norway (Engeland et al. 1996), and Sweden (Nordlund et al. 1997) also indicated elevated risks for pancreatic cancer incidence or mortality among women who smoked. In a large case-control study of pancreatic cancer in the United States, risk was twice as high among current smokers as among women and men who had never smoked. The RRs were similar among women and men and increased with both the number of cigarettes smoked and the duration of smoking (Silverman et al. 1994). The risk was elevated more than threefold among smokers who smoked 40 or more cigarettes per day for at least 40 years. Other investigators found similar elevations in RRs among women and men (MacMahon et al. 1981; Kinlen and McPherson 1984; Wynder et al. 1986; Cuzick and Babiker 1989; Muscat et al. 1997).

Studies that have included both women and men make clear that the excess risk for pancreatic cancer associated with smoking declines after smoking cessation, regardless of the number of cigarettes smoked or the duration of smoking (Mack et al. 1986; Howe et al. 1991; Silverman et al. 1994; Ji et al. 1995; Fuchs et al. 1996). Nonetheless, former smokers who stop smoking for more than 10 years may retain a 20- to 30-percent excess risk (Howe et al. 1991; Silverman et al. 1994). The risk associated with smoking is not explained by the confounding effects of alcohol consumption—another suspected risk factor (Velema et al. 1986). Up to one-third of pancreatic cancers among women may be attributable to smoking (USDHHS 1989b; Silverman et al. 1994).

### Urinary Tract Cancers

Cancers of the urinary tract comprise only about 7 percent of all cancers, but their incidence is rising (Devesa et al. 1990, 1995). Bladder cancer accounts for about 67 percent of all urinary tract cancers, cancer of the renal parenchyma (renal cell cancer) 23 percent, cancer of the renal pelvis 5 percent, and ureteral and miscellaneous tumors 5 percent. For these cancers, male-to-female incidence ratios are 3.9 for bladder cancer, 2.3 for renal cell cancer, 2.3 for cancer of the renal pelvis, and 2.9 for cancer of the ureter.

Smoking is a significant risk factor for cancer of each part of the urinary tract (McLaughlin et al. 1996; Silverman et al. 1996). The transitional cell cancers of the lower urinary tract (renal pelvis, ureter, and bladder) are more strongly related to smoking than are the adenocarcinomas of the renal parenchyma (renal cell cancers). For cancers of the renal pelvis and ureter, risk increases markedly with the number of cigarettes smoked and the duration of smoking. Long-term smokers (>45 years) have up to a sevenfold excess risk (Ross et al. 1989; McLaughlin et al. 1992).

In CPS-II, mortality from bladder cancer among women was more than 100 percent higher among current smokers than among those who had never smoked (Table 3.18); mortality from kidney cancer was 30 percent higher. Similar excess risks from smoking were found for bladder cancer mortality or incidence among women in cohort studies from Japan (Akiba and Hirayama 1990), Norway (Engeland et al. 1996), and Sweden (Nordlund et al. 1997). In the largest studies of specific urinary tract cancers and smoking, the lowest RR among women was found for renal cell cancer (adenocarcinoma of the renal parenchyma) and the highest for cancer of the renal pelvis and ureter; the risk for bladder cancer was intermediate (McLaughlin et al. 1992, 1995b; Hartge et al. 1993) (Table 3.20). Dose-response patterns were found for each cancer site. For each of these cancers, the risk among former smokers was less than that among current smokers (Hartge et al. 1987, 1993; Ross et al. 1989; McLaughlin et al. 1992,

**Table 3.20. Relative risks for urinary tract cancer among women for smokers compared with nonsmokers, case-control studies**

| Study | Number of cases/controls | Exposure | Relative risk | 95% confidence interval |
|---|---|---|---|---|
| | | | Renal pelvis | |
| McLaughlin et al. 1992 | 115/181 | Never smoked | 1.0 | |
| | | Ever smoked | 2.0 | 1.2–3.5 |
| | | <20 cigarettes/day | 1.4 | 0.7–3.0 |
| | | 20–39 cigarettes/day | 2.7 | 1.4–5.2 |
| | | ≥40 cigarettes/day | 3.4 | 0.9–13.4 |
| | | | Ureter | |
| McLaughlin et al. 1992 | 56/181 | Never smoked | 1.0 | |
| | | Ever smoked | 3.1 | 1.4–7.0 |
| | | <20 cigarettes/day | 2.4 | 0.9–6.4 |
| | | 20–39 cigarettes/day | 4.2 | 1.6–11.3 |
| | | ≥40 cigarettes/day | 3.7 | 0.4–38.9 |
| | | | Bladder | |
| Hartge et al. 1993 | 666/1,401 | White women | 1.0 | |
| | | Never smoked | | |
| | | Former smokers | | |
| | | <20 cigarettes/day | 2.0 | 1.4–2.7 |
| | | ≥20 cigarettes/day | 1.3 | 0.9–2.0 |
| | | Current smokers | | |
| | | <20 cigarettes/day | 2.0 | 1.5–2.7 |
| | | ≥20 cigarettes/day | 3.1 | 2.4–4.2 |
| | | Black women | | |
| | | Never smoked | 1.0 | |
| | | Former smokers | | |
| | | <20 cigarettes/day | 3.6 | 1.0–13.0 |
| | | ≥20 cigarettes/day | 5.0 | 0.9–28.0 |
| | | Current smokers | | |
| | | <20 cigarettes/day | 1.7 | 0.6–4.7 |
| | | ≥20 cigarettes/day | 2.1 | 0.4–10.0 |
| | | | Renal parenchyma | |
| McLaughlin et al. 1995b | 682/880 | Never smoked | 1.0 | |
| | | Ever smoked | 1.2 | 0.9–1.5 |
| | | 1–20 cigarettes/day | 1.1 | 0.9–1.4 |
| | | >20 cigarettes/day | 2.2 | 1.1–3.2 |

1995b; Silverman et al. 1996). Other studies confirmed these findings (McCredie et al. 1982; Morrison et al. 1984; Piper et al. 1986; Jensen et al. 1988; Wynder et al. 1988; Burch et al. 1989; La Vecchia et al. 1990; Burns and Swanson 1991; McCredie and Stewart 1992; Nordlund et al. 1997; Yuan et al. 1998).

The large-scale studies described in Table 3.20 reported that, among women, the proportion of cancers due to smoking was 9 percent for renal cell cancer (McLaughlin et al. 1995b), 31 percent for cancer of the renal pelvis and 46 percent for cancer of the ureter (McLaughlin et al. 1992), and 32 percent for bladder cancer (Hartge et al. 1987, 1993). Other studies of renal cell cancer reported population attributable risks ranging from 14 to 24 percent among women (McLaughlin et al. 1984; McCredie and Stewart 1992).

**Thyroid Cancer**

Although thyroid cancer is often studied as a single entity, four principal histologic types are recognized: papillary, follicular (well differentiated), medullary, and anaplastic (poorly differentiated). Papillary thyroid cancer is the most common type (50 to 80 percent of thyroid cancers in a given series), and follicular thyroid cancer is the next most common type (10 to 40 percent). Mortality from anaplastic thyroid cancer is high, but the five-year survival rates among patients with the other histologic types approach 95 percent (Ron 1996). Because papillary and follicular thyroid carcinomas occur more frequently among women than among men, women have a higher overall risk for thyroid cancer than do men.

Exposure to ionizing radiation is a well-established risk factor for thyroid cancer. Thyroid diseases such as goiter, thyrotoxicosis, and benign nodules have also been associated with an increased risk (McTiernan et al. 1984b; Preston-Martin et al. 1987; Ron et al. 1987; D'Avanzo et al. 1995b; Galanti et al. 1995b). A high body mass index (BMI) may also be a risk factor (Ron et al. 1987; Goodman et al. 1992; Preston-Martin et al. 1993).

The higher incidence of thyroid cancer among women than among men suggests a causative role for female sex hormones. In fact, evidence indicated that estrogens probably act as late promoters of thyroid tumor growth in rodents (Mori et al. 1990). In epidemiologic studies of women, use of exogenous steroid hormones (OCs and hormone replacement therapy [HRT]) has inconsistently been associated with an increased risk for thyroid cancer (Franceschi et al. 1993), and reproductive history may be associated with risk (Preston-Martin et al. 1987, 1993; Ron et al. 1987; Franceschi et al. 1990; Kolonel et al. 1990; La Vecchia et al. 1993b; Levi et al. 1993; Galanti et al. 1995a; Paoff et al. 1995).

Investigations of smoking and risk for thyroid cancer have reported conflicting results. Studies that did not separate findings among women and men have not presented a consistent pattern (Ron et al. 1987; Sokic et al. 1994). Apparently no association exists specifically among men, but the data are scanty (Williams and Horm 1977; Kolonel et al. 1990; Hallquist et al. 1994). Among women, however, the majority of studies have found an inverse association between smoking and risk for thyroid cancer (McTiernan et al. 1984a; Kolonel et al. 1990; Hallquist et al. 1994; Galanti et al. 1996).

A Scandinavian case-control study has presented the most detailed data on smoking and thyroid cancer among women (Galanti et al. 1996). Risk was lower among premenopausal women who had ever smoked than among those who had never smoked (RR, 0.6; 95 percent CI, 0.4 to 0.96), particularly among those who started smoking before the age of 15 years (RR, 0.4; 95 percent CI, 0.3 to 0.8). Findings in this study also suggested a dose-response effect related to the number of cigarettes smoked per day and the duration of smoking. The results persisted after careful control of covariates such as reproductive history, use of exogenous hormones, and socioeconomic indicators.

One case-control study explored the association between maternal cigarette smoking during pregnancy and risk for thyroid cancer among their offspring (Paoff et al. 1995). More control mothers than case mothers smoked during pregnancy, but the investigators found no evidence of a dose-response relationship.

It is not clear why cigarette smoking would be associated with a reduced risk for thyroid cancer. Smokers have lower levels of thyroid-stimulating hormone than do nonsmokers (Bertelsen and Hegedüs 1994), and they could have a lower thyroid cancer risk because of reduced thyroid stimulation. However, this mechanism should lead to a reduced risk among both women and men. Another possible explanation for a reduced risk among women is the antiestrogenic effect of smoking (Baron et al. 1990), which could counteract the excess risk due to estrogen-related stimuli among women. Identification of thyroid cancer and particularly of papillary cancers among young women is, however, largely influenced by the intensity of medical surveillance (Ron 1996). Because nonsmoking women are more health conscious than are smokers, their excess risk for thyroid cancer may be partially explained by enhanced diagnosis of the disease. This possibility may also explain the inconsistent results among former smokers.

### Lymphoproliferative and Hematologic Cancers

Of the various hematopoietic malignant diseases, only acute myeloid leukemia has been consistently associated with smoking. RRs among smokers have ranged from 1.3 to nearly 3.0, but typically have been about 1.5 (Siegel 1983; Brownson et al. 1993; Kabat et al. 1994a). In CPS-II, women current smokers had an increased risk for mortality from myeloid and lymphoid leukemias (Table 3.18). A limited number of other studies presented gender-specific results. The excess risk for leukemia associated with smoking was similar among women and men in some of these studies (Williams and Horm 1977; Brownson et al. 1991), but in other investigations, the association was stronger among men (Garfinkel and Boffetta 1990; Friedman 1993). An upward trend in the risk for leukemia with increasing cigarette consumption was suggested in several studies (Kabat et al. 1994a), including one that reported separate data for women (Williams and Horm 1977). Limited evidence suggests that RRs may be reduced with increasing years of smoking cessation (Severson et al. 1990).

In general, multiple myeloma has not been associated with tobacco use (Garfinkel 1980; Boffetta et al. 1989; Brownson 1991; Heineman et al. 1992; Linet et al. 1992; Friedman 1993; Adami et al. 1998), although a few studies—generally those based on few participants—reported an increase in risk (Williams and Horm 1977; Mills et al. 1990). Findings specific among women are scant, but in both CPS-I and CPS-II, mortality from multiple myeloma was similar among women who smoked and among those who had never smoked (Garfinkel 1980) (Table 3.18). Two other cohort studies also found no association between multiple myeloma and cigarette smoking among women (Friedman 1993; Nordlund et al. 1997).

In some studies, investigators reported a modest excess risk for non-Hodgkin's lymphomas among smokers (Williams and Horm 1977; Franceschi et al. 1989; Brown et al. 1992; Linet et al. 1992; Zahm et al. 1997; De Stefani et al. 1998). In CPS-II, mortality from non-Hodgkin's lymphoma was slightly higher among women who smoked than among those who had never smoked (Table 3.18). However, other studies reported no substantial association (Hoar et al. 1986; Doll et al. 1994; Tavani et al. 1994b; McLaughlin et al. 1995a; Siemiatycki et al. 1995; Nelson et al. 1997; Herrinton and Friedman 1998). Some investigators proposed that smoking may confer higher risks among younger persons (Freedman et al. 1998) or among women (Zahm et al. 1997).

The association between Hodgkin's lymphoma and smoking has not been adequately examined. Some studies (Williams and Horm 1977; McLaughlin et al. 1995a; Siemiatycki et al. 1995; Mueller 1996; Nordlund et al. 1997; Pasqualetti et al. 1997) presented data regarding the relationship between smoking and the risk for Hodgkin's lymphoma, but the small number of cases prevents any conclusions. The risk for mortality from Hodgkin's disease was five times higher among women current smokers in CPS-II (Table 3.18) than among women who had never smoked, but this observation, based on only 10 deaths, lacks precision.

### Conclusions

1. Smoking is a major cause of cancers of the oropharynx and bladder among women. Evidence is also strong that women who smoke have increased risks for cancers of the pancreas and kidney. For cancers of the larynx and esophagus, evidence among women is more limited but consistent with large increases in risk.
2. Women who smoke may have increased risks for liver cancer and colorectal cancer.
3. Data on smoking and cancer of the stomach among women are inconsistent.
4. Smoking may be associated with an increased risk for acute myeloid leukemia among women but does not appear to be associated with other lymphoproliferative or hematologic cancers.
5. Women who smoke may have a decreased risk for thyroid cancer.
6. Women who use smokeless tobacco have an increased risk for oral cancer.

# Cardiovascular Disease

Cardiovascular diseases (CVDs) are disorders of the circulatory system, including diseases of the heart, cerebrovascular diseases, atherosclerosis, and other diseases of blood vessels. This group of diseases accounts for a greater proportion of deaths among women (42.3 percent) than among men (38.1 percent) (Murphy 2000). These disease processes interfere with the blood supply to important organs and can lead to serious clinical events such as myocardial infarction (MI; heart attack) and stroke. Impairment of the blood supply to the limbs can lead to pain and even a need for amputation. In this section, evidence on the relationship between smoking and the following cardiovascular conditions among women is reviewed: coronary heart disease (CHD), cerebrovascular disease, carotid atherosclerosis, peripheral vascular disease, abdominal aortic aneurysm, and hypertension.

## Coronary Heart Disease

### Smoking-Associated Risks

Each year, more than 500,000 women in the United States have an MI, and about one-half of them die from the event (Rich-Edwards et al. 1995). Despite a continuing decline since the 1960s in mortality from CHD, this condition still ranks first among the causes of death for middle-aged and older women (Eaker et al. 1993).

Epidemiologic data gathered during the past 40 years clearly point to the causative role of smoking in CHD: more than a dozen prospective studies indicated that women who smoke are at increased risk (Table 3.21). Studies in addition to those listed in Table 3.21 include the Tecumseh (Michigan) Community Health Study (Higgins et al. 1987), the Walnut Creek (California) Study (Perlman et al. 1988), and the Lipid Research Clinics Follow-up Study (Bush et al. 1987).

More than 20 years ago, smoking was recognized as a major independent cause of CHD among women—increasing their risk for CHD by a factor of about 2 (USDHHS 1980, 1983). The risk for CHD rises with the number of cigarettes smoked daily, the total number of years of smoking, the degree of inhalation, and early age at initiation of smoking. In the U.S. Nurses' Health Study, even women who smoked as few as one to four cigarettes per day had twice the risk for CHD as women who had never smoked (Willett et al. 1987; Kawachi et al. 1994); an analysis of data from that large cohort study after 14 years of follow-up found that 41 percent of coronary events in the study population were attributable to current smoking (Stampfer et al. 2000). Cigarette smoking acts together with other risk factors, particularly elevated serum cholesterol and hypertension, to greatly increase the risk for CHD. When the amount smoked and the duration of smoking are taken into account, the relative increase in death rates from CHD among smokers is similar for women and men, but the absolute increase in risk is higher among men (USDHHS 1983).

The effect of smoking on CHD risk among women seems to be relatively similar regardless of racial or ethnic group. In one study (Friedman et al. 1997) that included a substantial number of minority women, the age-adjusted RR for CHD mortality among current smokers compared with those who had never smoked was 2.3 ($p < 0.05$) for black women, 2.2 ($p > 0.05$) for Asian women, and 1.6 ($p < 0.05$) for white women. These RRs do not take into account the numbers of cigarettes smoked daily, so some differences in RRs may be due to differences in smoking patterns.

About 41 percent of deaths from CHD among U.S. women younger than 65 years of age and 12 percent among women older than 65 years have been attributed to cigarette smoking (USDHHS 1989b). Smoking has been associated with particularly high RRs among younger women (<50 years old) (Slone et al. 1978; Rosenberg et al. 1980a, 1985); consequently, the proportion of CHD cases attributable to cigarette smoking is high in this age group. According to one estimate in 1985, cigarette smoking may account for as much as two-thirds of the incidence of CHD among women younger than 50 years of age (Rosenberg et al. 1985).

More recent epidemiologic investigations have tended to report higher RRs for CHD among women who smoke than did earlier studies. For example, the 1989 Surgeon General's report on reducing the health consequences of smoking compared findings from the two ACS cohort studies conducted about 20 years apart (USDHHS 1989b). Both studies used identical sampling schemes. In the six-year follow-up of CPS-I in 1959–1965, the age-adjusted RRs for CHD among current smokers compared with those who had never smoked were 1.8 (95 percent CI, 1.7 to 2.0) among women aged 35 through 64 years and 1.2 (95 percent CI, 1.1 to 1.4) among women aged 65 years or older. In CPS-II, with follow-up during 1982–1986, the age-adjusted RRs for CHD were 3.0 (95 percent CI, 2.5 to 3.6) among women aged 35 through 64 years and 1.6 (95 percent CI, 1.4 to 1.8) among women aged 65 years or older. The latter findings were replicated in a six-year follow-up of CPS-II (Thun et al. 1997a).

Several factors could explain the higher RRs found in more recent studies of the association between smoking and CHD among women. These factors include the declines in overall cardiovascular mortality, as well as the higher number of cigarettes smoked daily and the longer duration of smoking among women in more recent years (Thun et al. 1997a). Early age at initiation of smoking is also associated with a markedly elevated risk for CHD, presumably because it is related to longer duration of smoking. In the U.S. Nurses' Health Study, early age at initiation was one of the strongest risk factors for CHD (Kawachi et al. 1994). Compared with women who had never smoked, women current smokers who started smoking before age 15 years had a RR of 9.3 (95 percent CI, 5.3 to 16.2). Even among women former smokers, the RR was 7.6 (95 percent CI, 2.5 to 22.5) for those who started smoking before age 15 years compared with those who had never smoked. The age at smoking initiation steadily declined for successive birth cohorts of U.S. women up to the 1960 birth cohort (see "Smoking Initiation" in Chapter 2). Data from the National Health Interview Survey (NHIS) indicated that the proportion of women who started to smoke before age 16 years increased from 7.2 percent among those born in 1910–1914 to 20.2 percent among those born in 1950–1954 (USDHHS 1989b). Thus, in more recent birth cohorts, duration of exposure to smoking has been longer because of early age at initiation.

The data on smoking cessation and CHD risk indicated a rapid, partial decline in risk followed by a gradual decline that eventually reaches the level of risk among persons who had never smoked (USDHHS 1990). The excess risk for CHD associated with smoking is reduced by 25 to 50 percent after 1 year of smoking abstinence; after 10 to 15 years of abstinence, the risk for CHD is similar to that of persons who had never smoked. Although most of the data were derived from white men, sufficient information is available about women to indicate that similar conclusions can be drawn for both genders (USDHHS 1990).

Studies of the effects of smoking cessation on the risk for CHD among women are summarized in Tables 3.22 and 3.23. The findings indicated a rapid decline in risk for CHD soon after smoking cessation. The case-control studies indicated a reduction of 30 to 45 percent in excess CHD risk among former smokers within one year of smoking cessation (Table 3.22). This reduction represents 35 to 70 percent of the eventual benefit (reduction in CHD risk) from permanent cessation. Similarly, two cohort studies (Omenn et al. 1990; Kawachi et al. 1994) found a 25-percent reduction in risk for CHD among former smokers within two years of cessation. This reduction represents one-third to one-half of the full potential benefit of cessation (Table 3.23).

These studies (Tables 3.22 and 3.23) also suggested that 10 years or more of smoking cessation must elapse before the risk for CHD among former smokers approaches that among persons who had never smoked. The case-control study by Dobson and colleagues (1991a) showed almost a complete reversal in risk after 3 years of cessation (RR, 1.3) among former smokers, but the other data summarized in Tables 3.22 and 3.23 indicated that virtually complete reversal of risk is achieved only after more prolonged cessation.

Data from two studies (LaCroix et al. 1991; Paganini-Hill and Hsu 1994) that included women older than 65 years of age demonstrated that the benefits of smoking cessation also apply to older women. Indeed, the Established Populations for Epidemiologic Studies of the Elderly found a complete reversal in risk for CHD within five years of cessation (RR, 1.0; 95 percent CI, 0.5 to 2.1) (LaCroix et al. 1991). Risk declined among women who had stopped smoking either before or after 65 years of age. In contrast, the Leisure World Cohort Study found a significant difference in RR by age at cessation (Paganini-Hill and Hsu 1994). The study indicated that women who had stopped smoking at ages younger than 65 years had a RR for CHD mortality of 1.2 (95 percent CI, 0.9 to 1.5) and that women who had stopped at age 65 years or older had a RR of 1.6 (95 percent CI, 1.2 to 2.0).

Although the RR for CHD among current smokers tends to be lower for older persons than for younger persons, smoking cessation among older persons has a greater absolute effect because the rate of CHD is much higher in this group (USDHHS 1990). For example, in CPS-II, the RR for CHD mortality was 7.2 among women current smokers aged 45 through 49 years compared with women in the same age group who had never smoked; the corresponding RR among women aged 75 through 79 years was 1.6 (Thun et al. 1997c). However, the absolute difference in CHD mortality among smokers and nonsmokers aged 45

**Table 3.21. Relative risks for coronary heart disease (CHD) among women for current smokers compared with nonsmokers, cohort studies**

| Study | Population | Number of years of follow-up | Outcome | Number of cases | Smoking status | Relative risk (95% confidence interval) |
|---|---|---|---|---|---|---|
| Cederlöf et al. 1975 | 28,000 women<br>Aged 18–69 years<br>Sweden | 10 | Death from CHD | 457 | Never smoked | 1.0 |
| | | | | | Current smokers | |
| | | | | | Aged 50–59 years | 2.6* |
| | | | | | Aged 60–69 years | 1.1* |
| Doll et al. 1980 | 6,194 women physicians<br>Aged ≥ 20 years<br>United Kingdom | 22 | Death from CHD | 179 | Never smoked | 1.0 |
| | | | | | Current smokers | |
| | | | | | 1–14 cigarettes/day | 1.0* |
| | | | | | 15–24 cigarettes/day | 2.2* |
| | | | | | ≥25 cigarettes/day | 2.1* |
| Barrett-Connor et al. 1987 | 2,048 women<br>Aged 50–79 years<br>United States | 10 | Death from CHD | 59 | Aged 50–64 years | |
| | | | | | Never smoked | 1.0 |
| | | | | | Current smokers | 2.7* |
| | | | | | Aged 65–79 years | |
| | | | | | Never smoked | 1.0 |
| | | | | | Current smokers | 1.0* |
| Hirayama 1990 | 142,857 women<br>Aged ≥ 40 years<br>Sampled from Japanese census | 17 | Death from ischemic heart disease | 1,378 | Nonsmokers[†] | 1.0 |
| | | | | | Current smokers | |
| | | | | | 1–9 cigarettes/day | 1.7 (1.4–2.5) |
| | | | | | 10–19 cigarettes/day | 2.3 (1.9–2.7) |
| | | | | | ≥20 cigarettes/day | 3.8 (2.9–4.9) |
| LaCroix et al. 1991 | 4,469 women<br>Aged ≥ 65 years<br>United States | 10 | Death from CHD | NR[‡] | Never smoked | 1.0 |
| | | | | | Current smokers | 1.7 (1.3–2.3) |
| Freund et al. 1993 | 2,587 women<br>Aged 45–84 years<br>United States | 34 | Angina<br>Coronary insufficiency<br>Myocardial infarction<br>Death from CHD | 303 | Aged 45–64 years | |
| | | | | | Nonsmokers[†] | 1.0 |
| | | | | | Current smokers | 1.2 (1.0–1.6) |
| | | | | | Aged 65–84 years | |
| | | | | | Nonsmokers | 1.0 |
| | | | | | Current smokers | 1.2 (0.9–1.6) |

*95% confidence interval was not reported.
[†]Women who were never smokers and women who were former smokers combined.
[‡]NR = Value not specified in report of study.

through 49 years was 23.8 deaths per 100,000 woman-years; among women aged 70 through 79 years, the difference was 316.6 deaths per 100,000 woman-years.

Some investigations have reported that persons who stop smoking tend to have smoked fewer cigarettes per day and to have started at an older age than those who continue to smoke (USDHHS 1990). In most of the studies discussed in this chapter, risk estimates were not adjusted for the number of cigarettes smoked per day before cessation or for age at smoking initiation—omissions that could lead to overestimation of the benefits of cessation (Kawachi et al. 1993a). In practice, however, such a bias does not seem to occur. In the U.S. Nurses' Health Study, the temporal pattern in reduction of CHD risk after smoking cessation was similar among women regardless of the number of cigarettes smoked per day before cessation, the age at smoking initiation, and

**Table 3.21. Continued**

| Study | Population | Number of years of follow-up | Outcome | Number of cases | Smoking status | Relative risk (95% confidence interval) |
|---|---|---|---|---|---|---|
| Kawachi et al. 1994 | 117,006 women nurses<br>Aged 30–55 years<br>United States | 12 | CHD incidence | 215 | Never smoked | 1.0 |
| | | | | | Current smokers | |
| | | | | 93 | 1–14 cigarettes/day | 2.5 (1.8–3.5) |
| | | | | 242 | 15–24 cigarettes/day | 4.8 (3.8–6.1) |
| | | | | 123 | 25–34 cigarettes/day | 5.5 (4.1–7.4) |
| | | | | 79 | ≥35 cigarettes/day | 5.5 (3.9–7.8) |
| Paganini-Hill and Hsu 1994 | 8,869 women<br>Median age, 73 years<br>United States | 10 | Death from CHD | NR | Never smoked | 1.0 |
| | | | | | Current smokers | 1.5 (1.1–1.9) |
| Njølstad et al. 1996 | 5,701 women<br>Aged 35–52 years<br>Norway | 12 | CHD incidence | 20 | Never smoked | 1.0 |
| | | | | 73 | Current smokers | 3.6 (2.2–6.0) |
| | | | | 19 | 1–9 cigarettes/day | 2.3 (1.2–4.2) |
| | | | | 40 | 10–19 cigarettes/day | 4.1 (2.4–7.1) |
| | | | | 13 | ≥20 cigarettes/day | 5.9 (2.9–11.8) |
| Burns et al. 1997b | 594,551 women<br>Aged >30 years<br>United States | 12 | Death from CHD | 7,065 | Never smoked | 1.0 |
| | | | | 1,248 | Current smokers | 1.4 (1.3–1.5) |
| Freidman et al. 1997 | 36,035 women<br>Aged ≥ 35 years<br>Enrolled in health maintenance organization | 6 | Death from CHD | 134 | Never smoked | 1.0 |
| | | | | | Current smokers | |
| | | | | 20 | ≤19 cigarettes/day | 1.4* |
| | | | | 30 | ≥20 cigarettes/day | 2.2* |
| Thun et al. 1997c | 676,527 women<br>Aged >30 years<br>United States | 6 | Death from CHD | 3,717 | Never smoked | 1.0 |
| | | | | 1,161 | Current smokers | 1.6 (1.4–1.7) |

*95% confidence interval was not reported.

other risk factors for CVD (Kawachi et al. 1994) (Table 3.23). Similarly, in a case-control study from Italy, Negri and colleagues (1994) reported that the time course of reduction in risk for acute MI after smoking cessation was similar among women and men who had smoked less than 30 years and among those who had smoked longer.

The benefits of smoking cessation seem to apply even among women with established coronary atherosclerosis. The Coronary Artery Surgery Study, which included 5,386 women evaluated by angiography (Omenn et al. 1990), showed that the time course of reduction in risk for CHD mortality after smoking cessation was similar among women with or without coronary atherosclerosis.

In summary, studies of smoking cessation among women indicated a substantial (25- to 45-percent) reduction in excess risk for CHD within 1 to 2 years of cessation. This immediate benefit is followed by an additional gradual benefit: at least 5 years and perhaps 10 to 15 years of cessation or more may be needed for the risk among former women smokers to be reduced to the risk among women who had never smoked. These benefits are, however, available to women regardless of current age, age at smoking initiation, age at cessation, number of cigarettes smoked daily before cessation, duration of smoking, and presence of established CHD.

### Smoking and Use of Oral Contraceptives

Epidemiologic investigation of the effects of oral contraceptives (OC) use on health is complicated because of changes in prescribing practices that resulted from early studies suggesting an association between OC use and CHD. Physicians may avoid prescribing OCs for women considered at increased risk for CHD, and heightened suspicion of disease in those who use OCs may have led to intensive investigation of symptoms (Stolley et al. 1989). Moreover, the composition of OC pills has changed over time. When OCs were introduced 30 years ago, they contained 150 µg of ethinyl estradiol and 10 mg of progestin, 5 and 10 times the current doses, respectively. As early as 1974, the estrogen component was as low as 20 µg in some preparations, but even in 1983 about one-half of OC prescriptions were still for formulations containing 50 µg or more of ethinyl estradiol (Mishell 1991). OCs now in widespread use in the United States contain 30 or 35 µg of estrogen (Petitti et al. 1996).

Studies conducted before the 1983 Surgeon General's report on smoking and CVD (USDHHS 1983) indicated that OC users had an increased risk for CHD (Stadel 1981; Sartwell and Stolley 1982). Overall, women who used OCs were reported to

**Table 3.22. Relative risks for coronary heart disease (CHD) among women, by time since smoking cessation, case-control studies**

| Study | Population | Type of CHD | Number of controls | Source of controls | Number of cases | Smoking status | Relative risk (95% confidence interval) |
|---|---|---|---|---|---|---|---|
| Thompson et al. 1989 | Women physicians | 275 definite, 84 possible | 718 | British women physicians | NR[*] | Never smoked | 1.0 |
| | Aged 45–69 years | myocardial infarctions | | | NR | Current smokers | 2.6[†] |
| | United Kingdom | | | | NR | Former smokers | 1.1[†] |
| | | | | | | Cessation for: | |
| | | | | | NR | 1–2 years | 1.9[†] |
| | | | | | NR | 3–5 years | 1.6[†] |
| | | | | | NR | 6–10 years | 1.2[†] |
| | | | | | NR | 11–15 years | 0.95[†] |
| | | | | | NR | >15 years | 0.7[†] |
| Dobson et al. 1991a | Women | Nonfatal myocardial infarction and fatal CHD | 1,031 | Participants in community survey of risk factor prevalence | 174 | Never smoked | 1.0 |
| | Aged 35–69 years | | | | 127 | Current smokers | 4.7 (3.4–6.6) |
| | Australia | | | | 86 | Former smokers | 1.5 (1.1–2.2) |
| | | | | | | Cessation for: | |
| | | | | | 15 | <6 months | 3.2 (1.2–9.2) |
| | | | | | 7 | 6–<12 months | 10.0 (2.1–47.1) |
| | | | | | 19 | 1–3 years | 2.9 (1.2–6.7) |
| | | | | | 9 | 4–6 years | 1.3 (0.5–3.4) |
| | | | | | 9 | 7–9 years | 1.3 (0.5–3.2) |
| | | | | | 7 | 10–12 years | 1.7 (0.6–4.9) |
| | | | | | 19 | >12 years | 0.7 (0.4–1.4) |
| Negri et al. 1994 | Women | Acute myocardial infarction | 130 | Hospital patients | 115[‡] | Never smoked | 1.0 |
| | Aged 24–74 years | | | | | Current smokers | 5.8[†] |
| | Italy | | | | | Former smokers | |
| | | | | | | Cessation for: | |
| | | | | | | 1–5 years | 2.5[†] |
| | | | | | | >5 years | 0.7[†] |

*NR = Value not specified in report of study.
†95% confidence interval was not reported.
‡There were 115 cases altogether; number was not split by type of smoker or by years of smoking cessation.

have about 4 times the MI risk of nonusers, but smokers who used OCs had a risk for MI about 10 times that of women who neither used OCs nor smoked (USDHHS 1983). In some studies, women who used OCs and smoked heavily (≥ 25 cigarettes per day) had up to a 40-fold increase in risk than did those who did not smoke or use OCs (Shapiro et al. 1979). Thus the risk from combined tobacco and OC exposure was greater than expected from the magnitude of the risk from OCs or smoking alone (Croft and Hannaford 1989).

The more recently available lower dose OC pills may be associated with a lower risk for CHD than are the higher dose preparations (Mant et al. 1987; Porter et al. 1987; Thorogood et al. 1991; Palmer et al. 1992; Sidney et al. 1998; Dunn et al. 1999). Nevertheless, studies continued to report a substantial excess risk for CHD among heavy smokers who currently use OCs (Rosenberg et al. 1985; Stampfer et al. 1988b; D'Avanzo et al. 1994; WHO Collaborative Study 1997) and indicated that the risk for MI associated with OCs may be concentrated among women who smoke (Stampfer et al. 1988b). In a case-control study of acute MI among women (Rosenberg et al. 1985), the RR was 3.1 (95 percent CI, 0.4 to 22.0) for current OC users who smoked 1 to 24 cigarettes per day compared with nonsmokers who used OCs. Among OC users who smoked 25 or more cigarettes per day, the RR was 23.0 (95 percent CI, 6.6 to 82.0). In the WHO Collaborative Study (1997), women who smoked 10 or more cigarettes per day and used OCs had a multivariate RR of 87.0 (95 percent CI, 29.8 to 254.0) compared with nonsmokers who did not use OCs. This elevation in risk is considerably greater than that which would be expected from the individual effects of smoking and OCs. The RR for MI associated with OC use among nonsmokers was 4.0 (95 percent CI, 1.5 to 10.4), and the RR for smoking 10 or more cigarettes per day among women who did not use OCs was 11.1 (95 percent CI, 5.7 to 21.8). Only exceedingly sparse data are currently available on the risk for CHD among smokers who use "third-generation" OCs—preparations containing 30 µg or less of ethinyl estradiol and either gestodene or desogestrel (Lewis et al. 1996).

The clinical recommendation has been that women who smoke, especially older women (e.g., >40 years), should be counseled against using OCs. A consensus panel reviewed the evidence on the health effects of OC use and smoking and recommended that women older than 35 years of age who smoke more than 15 cigarettes per day should not take OCs (Schiff et al. 1999). However, because cigarette smoking confers a higher risk for MI than does OC use, it may be more appropriate to advise women who use OCs to stop smoking (Hennekens and Buring 1985).

**Smoking and Hormone Replacement Therapy**

A meta-analysis of 31 case-control and cohort studies published before 1991 found a highly significant reduction in CHD risk (RR, 0.6; 95 percent CI, 0.5 to 0.6) for women who were taking HRT (Stampfer and Colditz 1991). Because smoking accelerates catabolism of oral estrogens, serum estrogen levels are lower among postmenopausal smokers who receive oral HRT than among nonsmokers who receive HRT (Jensen et al. 1985; Cassidenti et al. 1990). Consequently, the potential beneficial effects of HRT on CHD risk may be attenuated among smokers. This was indeed the case in one prospective study (Henderson et al. 1988), although the statistical significance of the finding was not addressed. In a case-control study, the protective effect of estrogen replacement therapy on fatal ischemic heart disease was similarly more marked among nonsmokers (Ross et al. 1981). In a case-control study of women aged 45 through 64 years, the protective effect of HRT on MI risk was also confined to nonsmokers (Mann et al. 1994). The RR among HRT users was 0.7 (95 percent CI, 0.5 to 1.0) for nonsmokers and 1.1 (95 percent CI, 0.7 to 1.5) for current smokers. However, smoking status was unknown for about one-half of the participants, and the data were more complete among case subjects than among control subjects.

A different interaction between HRT use and smoking status was reported from a 12-year follow-up study of 1,868 women aged 50 through 79 years who resided in a planned community (Criqui et al. 1988). Among HRT users, current smokers had a RR for CHD mortality of 0.4 (95 percent CI, 0.1 to 1.3), but former smokers had a RR of 2.3 (95 percent CI, 0.8 to 6.6); for women who had never smoked, the RR was 0.95 (95 percent CI, 0.5 to 2.0). In other studies, no substantial difference was observed in the effect of HRT between women who smoked and those who did not (Rosenberg et al. 1980b, 1993; Grodstein and Stampfer 1998; Hulley et al. 1998).

Thinking about the role of estrogens in heart disease is now tempered by the results of a randomized clinical trial of estrogen plus progestin for the secondary prevention of heart disease (Hulley et al. 1998) and by very preliminary results from the Women's Health Initiative, a large trial that is investigating whether HRT affects risk for CVD and other outcomes (Kolata 2000). Contrary to expectation, both studies

**Table 3.23. Relative risks for coronary heart disease (CHD) among women, by time since smoking cessation, cohort studies**

| Study | Population | Number of years of follow-up | Outcome | Number of cases | Smoking status | Relative risk (95% confidence interval) |
|---|---|---|---|---|---|---|
| Omenn et al. 1990 | 5,386 U.S. women Aged >35 years‡ | 10 | Death from CHD | NR*† | Never smoked | 1.0 |
| | | | | | Current smokers | 1.7 (1.3–2.3) |
| | | | | | Former smokers | |
| | | | | | Cessation for: | |
| | | | | | ≤ 1 year | 1.3 (0.96–1.9) |
| | | | | | 2–9 years | 1.3 (0.9–1.8) |
| | | | | | 10–19 years | 1.1 (0.7–1.9) |
| | | | | | ≥20 years | 0.9 (0.4–1.8) |
| LaCroix et al. 1991 | 4,469 women Aged ≥65 years 3 U.S. communities | 5 | Death from cardiovascular disease | NR§ | Never smoked | 1.0 |
| | | | | | Current smokers | 1.7 (1.3–2.4) |
| | | | | | Former smokers | |
| | | | | | Cessation for: | |
| | | | | | ≤5 years | 1.0 (0.5–2.1) |
| | | | | | 6–10 years | 1.0 (0.5–2.0) |
| | | | | | 11–20 years | 0.5 (0.2–1.1) |
| | | | | | >20 years | 0.8 (0.4–1.4) |
| Kawachi et al. 1994 | 117,006 U.S. women nurses Aged 30–55 years | 12 | Nonfatal myocardial infarction | 418 | Current smokers | 1.0 |
| | | | | 166 | Never smoked | 0.2 (0.2–0.3) |
| | | | | 138 | Former smokers | |
| | | | | | Cessation for: | |
| | | | | 36 | < 2 years | 0.8 (0.5–1.3) |
| | | | | 22 | 2–4 years | 0.4 (0.3–0.7) |
| | | | | 26 | 5–9 years | 0.4 (0.2–0.6) |
| | | | | 13 | 10–14 year | 0.3 (0.1–0.5) |
| | | | | 41 | ≥15 years | 0.3 (0.2–0.4) |
| | | | Death from CHD | 123 | Current smokers | 1.0 |
| | | | | 49 | Never smoked | 0.2 (0.2–0.4) |
| | | | | 47 | Former smokers | |
| | | | | | Cessation for: | |
| | | | | 7 | <2 years | 1.5 (0.4–5.2) |
| | | | | 9 | 2–4 years | 0.6 (0.2–1.4) |
| | | | | 14 | 5–9 years | 0.7 (0.4–1.4) |
| | | | | 4 | 10–14 years | 0.3 (0.1–0.9) |
| | | | | 13 | ≥15 years | 0.3 (0.2–0.7) |

*NR = Value not specified in report of study.
†392 deaths from CHD among all women (never smokers, current smokers, and former smokers).
‡75% had coronary artery disease.
§729 deaths from cardiovascular disease among men and women.

suggested the possibility of adverse cardiovascular effects. Thus, more evidence, including effects by smoking status, is clearly warranted. Regardless of any interaction between HRT and smoking, every woman who receives HRT should be counseled to stop smoking because HRT cannot negate the excess risk for CHD associated with cigarette smoking.

## Cerebrovascular Disease

### Smoking-Associated Risks

Stroke, the major form of cerebrovascular disease, is the third-leading cause of death among middle-aged and older U.S. women; it accounts for 87,000 deaths each year. Stroke is also the leading cause of

**Table 3.23. Continued**

| Study | Population | Number of years of follow-up | Outcome | Number of cases | Smoking status | Relative risk (95% confidence interval) |
|---|---|---|---|---|---|---|
| Kawachi et al. 1994 (continued) | | | CHD | 541 | Current smokers | 1.0 |
| | | | | 215 | Never smoked | 0.2 (0.2–0.3) |
| | | | | 185 | Former smokers | |
| | | | | | Cessation for: | |
| | | | | 43 | <2 years | 0.8 (0.5–1.2) |
| | | | | 31 | 2–4 years | 0.5 (0.3–0.7) |
| | | | | 40 | 5–9 years | 0.4 (0.3–0.7) |
| | | | | 17 | 10–14 years | 0.3 (0.1–0.5) |
| | | | | 54 | ≥15 years | 0.3 (0.2–0.4) |
| Paganini-Hill and Hsu 1994 | 8,869 women<br>Median age, 73 years<br>U.S. retirement community | 10 | Death from CHD | NR | Never smoked | 1.0 |
| | | | | | Current smokers | 1.5 (1.1–2.0) |
| | | | | | Former smokers | |
| | | | | | Cessation for: | |
| | | | | | ≤5 years | 1.3 (0.8–2.0) |
| | | | | | 6–10 years | 1.4 (0.9–2.2) |
| | | | | | 11–20 years | 1.5 (1.1–2.0) |
| | | | | | ≥21 years | 1.1 (0.8–1.4) |
| Burns et al. 1997b | 594,551 women<br>Aged >30 years<br>25 U.S. states | 12 | Death from CHD | NR | Never smoked | 1.0 |
| | | | | | Current smokers | 1.4 (1.3–1.5) |
| | | | | | Former smokers | |
| | | | | | Cessation for[Δ]: | |
| | | | | | 2–4 years | 2.2[¶] |
| | | | | | 5–9 years | 1.5[¶] |
| | | | | | 10–14 years | 1.0[¶] |
| | | | | | 15–19 years | 0.8[¶] |
| | | | | | 20–24 years | 0.9[¶] |
| | | | | | 25–29 years | 1.0[¶] |
| | | | | | 30–34 years | 0.6[¶] |
| | | | | | 35–39 years | 0.6[¶] |
| Friedman et al. 1997 | 36,035 U.S. women<br>Aged ≥ 35 years<br>Enrolled in health maintenance organization | 6 | Death from CHD | 134 | Never smoked | 1.0 |
| | | | | | Current smokers | |
| | | | | 7 | ≤19 cigarettes/day | 1.4[¶] |
| | | | | 13 | ≥20 cigarettes/day | 2.2[¶] |
| | | | | | Former smokers | |
| | | | | | Cessation for: | |
| | | | | 9 | 2–10 years | 1.4[¶] |
| | | | | 14 | 11–20 years | 1.4[¶] |
| | | | | 12 | >20 years | 1.1[¶] |

[Δ]Data are for white women only; number of black former smokers was insufficient for separate analyses.
[¶]95% confidence interval was not reported.

severe disability and costs about $15.3 billion annually in medical care, including rehabilitation (Eaker et al. 1993). Smoking has long been recognized as a major cause of stroke (USDHHS 1989b). In CPS-II, 55 percent (95 percent CI, 45 to 65 percent) of deaths from cerebrovascular disease among women younger than 65 years and 6 percent of deaths from cerebrovascular disease among women aged 65 years or older were attributable to smoking (USDHHS 1989b).

In a meta-analysis of 32 studies of smoking and stroke that were published before May 1988, the overall RR for stroke among women and men current smokers was 1.5 (95 percent CI, 1.5 to 1.6) (Shinton and Beevers 1989). A strong dose-response relationship was found between the risk for stroke and the number of cigarettes smoked per day. Increased risks were found for subarachnoid hemorrhage (RR, 2.9; 95 percent CI, 2.5 to 3.5) and cerebral infarction (RR, 1.9; 95 percent CI, 1.7 to 2.2), but no increase in risk was found for hemorrhagic stroke (mainly intracerebral hemorrhage) (RR, 1.01; 95 percent CI, 0.8 to 1.3) or for intracerebral hemorrhage alone (RR, 0.7; 95 percent CI, 0.6 to 0.98). The estimate for hemorrhagic stroke was based on pooled data from only four studies and was strongly influenced by a single study that showed a marked inverse association with smoking (RR, 0.2 among men) (Bell and Ambrose 1982). In 26 studies, the number of women was sufficient to allow stratification by gender. In these data, the pooled risk for any stroke was slightly higher among women smokers (RR, 1.7; 95 percent CI, 1.6 to 1.9) than among men smokers (RR, 1.4; 95 percent CI, 1.4 to 1.5) (Shinton and Beevers 1989).

Subsequent studies generally have found a twofold to threefold excess risk for ischemic stroke and subarachnoid hemorrhage among women who smoked compared with women who had never smoked; the risk has been generally higher among heavy smokers (Tables 3.24 and 3.25). A possible explanation for the increase in RR over time is that control of hypertension has improved in the United States during the past two decades. Thus, smoking is a more prominent risk factor for stroke than it was in the past (USDHHS 1990). An alternative explanation is that women who have recently reached the peak ages of stroke incidence tend to be heavier smokers than smokers in previous decades.

Although smoking is a clearly established risk factor for ischemic stroke and subarachnoid hemorrhage among both women and men, the relationship with primary intracerebral hemorrhage is less certain (Tables 3.24 and 3.25). One small population-based study found smoking to be a significant risk factor (Jamrozik et al. 1994). In contrast, a hospital-based, case-control study from Finland found that smoking was not an independent risk factor for intracerebral hemorrhage among either women or men (Juvela et al. 1995). In the U.S. Nurses' Health Study (Kawachi et al. 1993b), current smoking was associated with a multivariate-adjusted RR for cerebral hemorrhage of 1.4 (95 percent CI, 0.8 to 2.8) (Table 3.25). In the case-control study by Gill and colleagues (1989), current smoking was associated with an adjusted RR for cerebral hemorrhage of 1.3 (95 percent CI, 0.5 to 3.4) among women (Table 3.24) and 1.8 (95 percent CI, 0.9 to 3.7) among men. These data were based on few cases, however, because primary intracerebral hemorrhage tends to be the least common subtype of stroke among white women.

Smoking cessation has been reported to reduce the risk for both ischemic stroke and subarachnoid hemorrhage. After smoking cessation, the risk for stroke seems to return to the level of risk among those who had never smoked (USDHHS 1990). In some studies, the risk for stroke among women former smokers approached that of nonsmokers within 5 years of cessation (Wolf et al. 1988; USDHHS 1990 [CPS-II data for women in 50 states]). In other studies, 10 to 15 years of abstinence from smoking have been required (Rogot and Murray 1980; Donnan et al. 1989; USDHHS 1990 [CPS-II data for men in 50 states]).

Additional investigations since the late 1980s (Table 3.26) considered the relationship between duration of abstinence from smoking and the risk for stroke among women (Thompson et al. 1989; Kawachi et al. 1993b; Burns et al. 1997b; Friedman et al. 1997). In the U.S. Nurses' Health Study (Kawachi et al. 1993b), the risk for stroke among women former smokers approached the level of risk among women who had never smoked after 2 to 4 years of abstinence. The reduction of risk persisted after control for the number of cigarettes previously smoked daily, age at smoking initiation, and other known risk factors for stroke (data not shown). However, in a case-control study in the United Kingdom, only after 11 to 15 years of smoking cessation did stroke risk among female former smokers approximate that among women who had never smoked (Thompson et al. 1989).

In CPS-I, the risk for death from stroke among women former smokers approached that among women who had never smoked, at 15 to 19 years after smoking cessation (Burns et al. 1997b) (Table 3.26). The time it took for risk to decline differed by the number of cigarettes smoked daily before cessation (data not shown). For example, among women former smokers who had smoked fewer than 20 cigarettes per day, the risk approached that among women who had never smoked 5 to 9 years after cessation. Among former smokers who had smoked 20 or more cigarettes per day, an excess risk for stroke mortality persisted even after 20 to 24 years of cessation. A similar pattern was reported from a small study of men in the United Kingdom (Wannamethee et al. 1995).

In summary, the findings in most studies with data on women indicated that the increased stroke risk associated with smoking is reversible after smoking cessation. However, the duration of abstinence required for the excess risk to dissipate varied from 5 to 15 years.

### Smoking and Use of Oral Contraceptives

Smokers who use OCs are at a significantly increased risk for stroke, especially subarachnoid hemorrhage, and part of this risk may result from the combined effects of smoking and OC use (USDHHS 1983). Studies published in the 1970s (Collaborative Group for the Study of Stroke in Young Women 1975; Petitti and Wingerd 1978) reported a particularly high risk for stroke among women who were heavy smokers and who used OCs; RRs ranged from more than 4.0 to 22.0. The dose of estrogen in OC preparations has been substantially reduced since then, and the risk for CVD associated with OC use and smoking may have changed from that observed for the early higher dose preparations (USDHHS 1990).

Most studies published since 1990 found that currently prescribed lower dose OC preparations are not associated with a substantially increased risk for stroke (Hirvonen and Idänpään-Heikkilä 1990; Thorogood et al. 1992; Lidegaard 1993; Lindenstrøm et al. 1993; WHO Collaborative Study 1996a,b; Schwartz et al. 1998). However, some studies reported that smoking increases the risk for stroke associated with OCs (Hannaford et al. 1994; Petitti et al. 1996; WHO Collaborative Study 1996a,b). For example, a multicenter, hospital-based, case-control study reported an adjusted RR for ischemic stroke of 7.2 (95 percent CI, 3.2 to 16.1) among current smokers who used OCs compared with nonsmokers who did not use OCs (WHO Collaborative Study 1996a). On the other hand, some data suggested no such interaction (Lidegaard 1993; Schwartz et al. 1998).

### Smoking and Hormone Replacement Therapy

The data on the effects of HRT on the risk for stroke are sparse and inconsistent. Some investigators have observed a protective effect of HRT (Paganini-Hill et al. 1988; Finucane et al. 1993), others an increased risk (Wilson et al. 1985), and several no effect (Stampfer et al. 1991; Pedersen et al. 1997; Petitti et al. 1998).

A 12-year follow-up study of 7,060 women in the Copenhagen City Heart Study showed a statistically significant ($p < 0.04$) interaction between smoking status and HRT use (Lindenstrøm et al. 1993). HRT use appeared to be protective for stroke and transient ischemic attack (TIA) among current smokers but not among nonsmokers (both former smokers and women who had never smoked). Among current smokers who used HRT, the risk for stroke or TIA was about one-third the risk among women current smokers who did not use HRT. Among nonsmokers, however, HRT use was not associated with cerebrovascular events (RR, 1.0; 95 percent CI, 0.6 to 1.8). A similar pattern was observed in a population-based, case-control study of subarachnoid hemorrhage (Longstreth et al. 1994). In contrast, a more recent study found no interaction between HRT use and smoking in relation to stroke risk (Pedersen et al. 1997).

## Carotid Atherosclerosis

Smoking is a major cause of carotid atherosclerosis, a marker of risk for TIA and stroke (USDHHS 1983). In several cross-sectional studies that included women, atherosclerotic lesions were more severe and diffuse among current smokers than among nonsmokers (Tell et al. 1989, 1994; Ingall et al. 1991). Ingall and colleagues (1991) reported results from a cross-sectional study of 1,004 patients (404 women) aged 40 through 69 years who had intracranial carotid artery arteriography. After adjustment for other cerebrovascular risk factors, duration of smoking was a strong predictor of the severity of atherosclerosis among both women and men. A similar finding was reported for severe atherosclerosis of the extracranial carotid arteries (Whisnant et al. 1990). In a study of 49 male and female pairs of identical twins discordant for smoking status, the total area of atherosclerotic carotid plaques was 3.2 times larger among smokers than among nonsmokers (Haapanen et al. 1989).

The association of smoking with carotid atherosclerosis persists with age. In a cross-sectional study of 5,116 participants (2,837 women) older than 64 years of age who were evaluated by ultrasonography, the prevalence of clinically significant (≥ 50 percent) stenosis of the internal carotid artery was 4.4 percent among persons who had never smoked, 7.3 percent among former smokers, and 9.5 percent among current smokers ($p < 0.0001$) (Tell et al. 1994). This study also showed a dose-response relationship between pack-years of smoking and mean thickness of the carotid artery wall ($p < 0.0001$). The difference in wall thickening among current smokers and persons who had never smoked was greater than the difference associated with 10 years of aging. In the Framingham study, an association was observed between time-integrated measures of smoking and carotid artery stenosis

**Table 3.24. Relative risks for stroke among women for current smokers compared with nonsmokers, case-control studies**

| Study | Population | Number of cases | Number of controls | Source of controls | Type of stroke | Smoking status | Relative risk (95% confidence interval) |
|---|---|---|---|---|---|---|---|
| Donnan et al. 1989 | Women<br>Aged 25–85 years<br>Australia | 166 hospitalized for stroke | 166 | General population | Cerebral ischemia | Never smoked | 1.0 |
| | | | | | | Current smokers | 3.0 (1.3–7.1) |
| Gill et al. 1989 | Women<br>Mean age, 53.4 years<br>United Kingdom | 281 hospitalized for stroke | 303 | Participants in factory screening survey | Total | Never smoked | 1.0 |
| | | | | | | Current smokers | |
| | | | | | | 1–10 cigarettes/day | 1.8 (0.7–4.7) |
| | | | | | | 11–20 cigarettes/day | 1.6 (0.8–3.0) |
| | | | | | | >20 cigarettes/day | 2.8 (1.7–4.7) |
| | | | | | Cerebral infarction | Never smoked | 1.0 |
| | | | | | | Current smokers | 2.3 (1.2–4.2) |
| | | | | | Cerebral hemorrhage | Never smoked | 1.0 |
| | | | | | | Current smokers | 1.3 (0.5–3.4) |
| | | | | | Subarachnoid hemorrhage | Never smoked | 1.0 |
| | | | | | | Current smokers | 2.5 (1.4–4.5) |
| Thompson et al. 1989 | Women physicians<br>Aged 45–69 years<br>United Kingdom | 37 fatal stroke<br>207 nonfatal stroke | 488 | Women physicians | Total | Never smoked | 1.0 |
| | | | | | | Current smokers | 2.3* |
| Longstreth et al. 1992 | Women<br>≥ 18 years<br>United States | 103 subarachnoid hemorrhage | 206 | General population | Subarachnoid hemorrhage | Never smoked | 1.0 |
| | | | | | | Current smokers | 4.6 (2.6–8.1) |
| Morris et al. 1992 | Women admitted to Department of Neurosurgery<br>United Kingdom | 131 subarachnoid hemorrhage | 131 | Women admitted with nonvascular or spinal pathologic condition | Subarachnoid hemorrhage | Never smoked | 1.0 |
| | | | | | | Current smokers | 1.9 (1.4–2.6) |

*95% confidence interval was not reported.

greater than 25 percent on ultrasound among both women and men. Smoking at the time of the examination was associated with stenosis only among women (RR, 2.6; 95 percent CI, 1.6 to 4.3) (Wilson et al. 1997).

A few prospective studies have evaluated the relationship between smoking and progression of carotid atherosclerosis. In a two-year follow-up of 308 apparently healthy women in France aged 45 through 55 years (Bonithon-Kopp et al. 1993), current smoking was a strong predictor of the development of new carotid atheromatous plaques, as assessed by B-mode ultrasound (multivariate-adjusted RR, 3.6; 95 percent CI, 1.5 to 8.7). A two-year follow-up of Finnish men similarly showed that pack-years of smoking was one of the strongest predictors of progression of carotid atherosclerosis (Salonen and Salonen 1990). More than

**Table 3.24. Continued**

| Study | Population | Number of cases | Number of controls | Source of controls | Type of stroke | Smoking status | Relative risk (95% confidence interval) |
|---|---|---|---|---|---|---|---|
| Juvela et al. 1993 | Women Aged 15–60 years Finland | 133 hospitalized with subarachnoid hemorrhage | 150 | Hospitalized women | Subarachnoid hemorrhage | Never smoked | 1.0 |
| | | | | | | Current smokers | 2.4 (1.5–3.9) |
| | | | | | | ≤10 cigarettes/day | 1.2 (0.5–2.7) |
| | | | | | | 11–20 cigarettes/day | 3.6 (1.3–9.6) |
| | | | | | | >20 cigarettes/day | 2.0 (0.95–4.1) |
| Lidegaard 1993 | Women Aged 15–44 years | 321 hospitalized for stroke | 1,198 | General population | Ischemic stroke or transient ischemic attack | Never smoked | 1.0 |
| | | | | | | Current smokers | |
| | | | | | | <10 cigarettes/day | 1.6 (1.1–2.6) |
| | | | | | | ≥10 cigarettes/day | 1.5 (1.1–2.0) |
| Hannaford et al. 1994 | Denmark<br>Women physicians Aged 21–70 years United Kingdom | 253 incident stroke or amaurosis fugax | 759 | Nested in cohort | Incident stroke or amaurosis fugax | Never smoked | 1.0 |
| | | | | | | Current smokers | |
| | | | | | | 1–14 cigarettes/day | 2.1 (1.5–2.9) |
| | | | | | | ≥15 cigarettes/day | 2.5 (1.7–3.7) |
| Pedersen et al. 1997 | Women Aged 45–64 years Denmark | Hospitalized for cerebrovascular attack and surviving 160 subarachnoid hemorrhage 835 thrombo-embolic infarction 321 transient ischemic attack | 3,171 | General population | Subarachnoid hemorrhage | Never smoked | 1.0 |
| | | | | | | Current smokers | |
| | | | | | | 1–10 cigarettes/day | 3.7 (2.2–6.1) |
| | | | | | | 11–20 cigarettes/day | 4.4 (2.7–7.1) |
| | | | | | | >20 cigarettes/day | 3.7 (1.1–12.0) |
| | | | | | Thrombo-embolic infarction | Never smoked | 1.0 |
| | | | | | | Current smokers | |
| | | | | | | 1–10 cigarettes/day | 2.4 (1.8–3.2) |
| | | | | | | 11–20 cigarettes/day | 3.4 (2.6–4.5) |
| | | | | | | >20 cigarettes/day | 6.4 (3.7–11.0) |
| | | | | | Transient ischemic attack | Never smoked | 1.0 |
| | | | | | | Current smokers | |
| | | | | | | 1–10 cigarettes/day | 2.5 (1.7–3.7) |
| | | | | | | 11–20 cigarettes/day | 2.8 (1.9–4.1) |
| | | | | | | >20 cigarettes/day | 3.9 (1.7–9.0) |

10,000 women and men were followed for three years in the Atherosclerosis Risk in Communities Study (Howard et al. 1998). Current smoking was associated with a 50-percent increase in the progression of carotid atherosclerosis.

Cessation of smoking appears to slow the progression of carotid atherosclerosis. In a cross-sectional study of 1,692 patients (829 women) admitted for diagnostic evaluation of the carotid arteries, the plaque measured by B-mode ultrasonography was 0.35 mm thicker among former smokers than among persons who had never smoked (95 percent CI, 0.17 to 0.54 mm). The plaque thickness of current smokers was 0.63 mm greater than that of persons who had never smoked (95 percent CI, 0.45 to 0.81 mm; $p < 0.001$ by multivariate analysis of variance). This finding suggested that the rate of progression of carotid atherosclerosis may be slower among persons who stop smoking than among continuing smokers (Tell et al. 1989).

**Table 3.25. Relative risks for stroke among women for current smokers compared with nonsmokers, cohort studies**

| Study | Population | Number of years of follow-up | Outcome | Smoking status | Relative risk (95% confidence interval) |
|---|---|---|---|---|---|
| Hirayama 1990 | 142,857 women<br>Aged ≥40 years<br>Sampled from census<br>Japan | 17 | Death from cerebrovascular disease | Nonsmokers | 1.0 |
| | | | | Current smokers | |
| | | | | 1–9 cigarettes/day | 1.2 (1.1–1.3)* |
| | | | | 10–19 cigarettes/day | 1.1 (0.99–1.2)* |
| | | | | ≥20 cigarettes/day | 1.3 (1.1–1.6)* |
| | | | Death from subarachnoid hemorrhage | Nonsmokers | 1.0 |
| | | | | Current smokers | |
| | | | | 1–9 cigarettes/day | 1.5 (1.2–2.5) |
| | | | | 10–19 cigarettes/day | 1.4 (0.9–2.2) |
| | | | | ≥20 cigarettes/day | 2.1 (0.9–4.6) |
| Kiyohara et al. 1990 | 904 women<br>Aged >40 years<br>Japan | 23 | Nonembolic cerebral infarction | Never smoked | 1.0 |
| | | | | Current smokers | 0.8 (0.4–1.4) |
| Knekt et al. 1991 | Population samples<br>Aged 20–69 years<br>Finland | 12 | Subarachnoid hemorrhage | Nonsmokers | 1.0 |
| | | | | Current smokers | 2.4 (1.4–4.0) |
| Kawachi et al. 1993b | 117,006 women nurses<br>Aged 30–55 years<br>United States | 12 | Total stroke | Never smoked | 1.0 |
| | | | | Current smokers | |
| | | | | 1–14 cigarettes/day | 2.0 (1.3–3.1) |
| | | | | 15–24 cigarettes/day | 3.3 (2.4–4.7) |
| | | | | 25–34 cigarettes/day | 3.1 (1.9–4.9) |
| | | | | ≥35 cigarettes/day | 4.5 (2.8–7.2) |
| | | | Subarachnoid hemorrhage | Never smoked | 1.0 |
| | | | | Current smokers | 4.9 (2.9–8.1) |

*90% confidence interval.

Rogers and colleagues (1983) found significantly lower cerebral perfusion among long-term smokers than among nonsmokers; the reduction in cerebral blood flow was directly related to the number of cigarettes smoked daily. In a cross-sectional study, these investigators showed that smoking cessation was associated with a substantial improvement in cerebral perfusion within one year of cessation (Rogers et al. 1985).

## Peripheral Vascular Disease

Peripheral vascular disease is associated with both functional limitations and increased risk for mortality. For example, in a 10-year follow-up study of 309 women and 256 men (average age, 66 years) with large-vessel peripheral arterial disease, the total mortality rate was 2.7 times higher (95 percent CI, 1.2 to 6.0) among women with large-vessel disease than among women free of disease. The corresponding RR for death from CVD was 5.7 (95 percent CI, 1.4 to 23.2) (Criqui et al. 1992).

Smoking is a strong, independent risk factor for arteriosclerotic peripheral vascular disease among women, and smoking cessation improves the prognosis of the disorder and has a favorable effect on vascular potency after reconstructive surgery (USDHHS 1980; Fowkes 1989). In general, the risk for intermittent claudication, a major clinical manifestation of peripheral vascular disease, has been reported to be lower among former smokers than among current smokers (USDHHS 1990). Among patients with established peripheral artery disease,

**Table 3.25. Continued**

| Study | Population | Number of years of follow-up | Outcome | Smoking status | Relative risk (95% confidence interval) |
|---|---|---|---|---|---|
| Kawachi et al. 1993b (continued) | | | Ischemic stroke | Never smoked<br>Current smokers | 1.0<br>2.5 (1.9–3.4) |
| | | | Cerebral hemorrhage | Never smoked<br>Current smokers | 1.0<br>1.4 (0.8–2.8) |
| Lindenstrøm et al. 1993 | 7,060 women<br>Aged >35 years<br>Denmark | 12 | Total stroke or transient ischemic attack | Never smoked<br>Current smokers | 1.0<br>1.4 (1.02–1.9) |
| Burns et al. 1997b | 594,551 women<br>Aged >30 years<br>25 U.S. states | 12 | Death from stroke | Never smoked<br>Current smokers<br>Aged 35–49 years<br>Aged 50–64 years<br>Aged 65–79 years<br>Aged ≥ 80 years | 1.0<br><br>2.5[†]<br>2.2[†]<br>1.3[†]<br>0.8[†] |
| Friedman et al. 1997 (see Table 3.23) | 36,035 women<br>Aged ≥35 years<br>United States | 6 | Death from stroke | Never smoked<br>Current smokers<br>1–19 cigarettes/day<br>≥ 20 cigarettes/day | 1.0<br><br>0.9[†]<br>1.9[†] |
| Thun et al. 1997c | 676,527 women<br>Aged >30 years<br>50 U.S. states | 6 | Death from stroke | Never smoked<br>Current smokers | 1.0<br>1.5 (1.2–1.7) |

[†]95% confidence interval was not reported.

smoking cessation has also been associated with improved performance (greater maximum treadmill walking distance and reduction of pain at rest), better prognosis (longer duration between initial and subsequent operations, lower amputation rate, and greater potency of vascular grafts), and longer overall survival (USDHHS 1990).

Studies published since 1990 continued to confirm a higher risk for peripheral vascular disease among smokers than among nonsmokers. Most studies were cross-sectional rather than prospective. However, in the 34-year follow-up of participants in the Framingham study (Freund et al. 1993), current smoking was a powerful predictor of intermittent claudication; RR was 2.3 (95 percent CI, 1.4 to 3.5) for current smokers compared with nonsmokers among women 45 through 64 years old. Among women aged 65 through 84 years, the RR was 2.2 (95 percent CI, 1.3 to 3.7).

The Edinburgh Artery Study (Fowkes et al. 1994) examined the ankle brachial pressure index (ABPI) in a random population sample of 783 women and 809 men aged 55 through 74 years. (The ABPI is a validated index inversely related to the degree of peripheral atherosclerosis.) In that study, lifetime history of cigarette smoking was correlated with lower ABPI among both women and men ($r = -0.27$; $p < 0.001$). Smoking was a stronger predictor of the prevalence of peripheral vascular disease than of CHD (Fowkes et al. 1992).

Epidemiologic studies are generally concerned with establishing the association of risk factors with clinical events, such as MI, stroke, or symptomatic peripheral vascular disease. The development of clinical disease is, however, the end point of a progression of pathophysiologic changes (Kuller et al. 1994). In the past, evaluation of the extent of atherosclerosis

**Table 3.26. Relative risks of stroke for women former smokers versus women who never smoked, by time since smoking cessation, case-control and cohort studies**

| Study | Type of study | Outcome | Smoking status | Relative risk (95% confidence interval) |
|---|---|---|---|---|
| Thompson et al. 1989 (see Table 3.24) | Case-control | Total stroke | Never smoked | 1.0 |
| | | | Former smokers | |
| | | | Cessation for: | |
| | | | 1–2 years | 1.9* |
| | | | 3–5 years | 1.6* |
| | | | 6–10 years | 1.7* |
| | | | 11–15 years | 1.0* |
| | | | ≥15 years | 0.8* |
| Kawachi et al. 1993b (see Table 3.25) | Cohort | Total stroke | Current smokers | 1.0 |
| | | | Never smoked | 0.4 (0.3–0.5) |
| | | | Former smokers | |
| | | | Cessation for: | |
| | | | <2 years | 0.8 (0.5–1.5) |
| | | | 2–4 years | 0.4 (0.2–0.9) |
| | | | 5–9 years | 0.4 (0.2–0.8) |
| | | | 10–14 years | 0.8 (0.4–1.5) |
| | | | ≥15 years | 0.4 (0.2–0.7) |
| | | Ischemic stroke | Current smokers | 1.0 |
| | | | Never smoked | 0.4 (0.3–0.5) |
| | | | Former smokers | |
| | | | Cessation for: | |
| | | | <2 years | 0.6 (0.3–1.5) |
| | | | 2–4 years | 0.2 (0.04–0.96) |
| | | | 5–9 years | 0.5 (0.2–1.2) |
| | | | 10–14 years | 0.9 (0.5–1.9) |
| | | | ≥15 years | 0.4 (0.2–0.8) |
| | | Subarachnoid hemorrhage | Current smokers | 1.0 |
| | | | Never smoked | 0.2 (0.1–0.3) |
| | | | Former smokers | |
| | | | Cessation for: | |
| | | | <2 years | 1.3 (0.5–3.6) |
| | | | 2–4 years | 0.7 (0.2–2.8) |
| | | | 5–14 years | 0.5 (0.1–1.5) |
| | | | ≥15 years | 0.4 (0.1–0.97) |
| Burns et al. 1997b (see Table 3.23) | Cohort | Death from stroke | Never smoked | 1.0 |
| | | | Former smokers | |
| | | | Cessation for: | |
| | | | 2–4 years | 2.3* |
| | | | 5–9 years | 1.2* |
| | | | 10–14 years | 1.3* |
| | | | 15–19 years | 1.01* |
| | | | 20–24 years | 1.1* |
| | | | 25–29 years | 0.8* |
| | | | 30–34 years | 0.6* |
| | | | 35–39 years | 0.9* |
| Friedman et al. 1997 (see Table 3.23) | Cohort | Death from stroke | Never smoked | 1.0 |
| | | | Former smokers | |
| | | | Cessation for: | |
| | | | 1–10 years | 0.3* |
| | | | 11–20 years | 1.2* |
| | | | ≥21 years | 0.9* |

*95% confidence interval was not reported.

was limited to postmortem studies or to studies that used invasive techniques such as angiography. The advent of noninvasive diagnostic methods has made it feasible to study the extent of subclinical atherosclerosis in asymptomatic persons. Kuller and colleagues (1994) examined the relationship of smoking with subclinical atherosclerosis among 5,201 Medicare enrollees (2,955 women and 2,246 men) aged 65 years or older. Subclinical disease was defined as major electrocardiographic abnormalities, low ejection fraction or ventricular wall motion abnormality on echocardiogram, more than 25 percent stenosis or more than a 25-percent increase in wall thickness of the carotid artery or the internal carotid artery, decreased ABPI (≤ 0.9 mm Hg), and angina or intermittent claudication, as determined by a research questionnaire. In this cross-sectional study, current smoking was associated with increased risk for subclinical disease among women (RR for current smokers compared with nonsmokers, 2.0; 95 percent CI, 1.5 to 2.7) and among men (RR, 2.4; 95 percent CI, 1.6 to 3.6). In summary, current smoking among women is associated with increased risk for both clinical and subclinical peripheral vascular atherosclerosis. Smoking cessation is associated with improvement in symptoms, prognosis, and survival.

## Abdominal Aortic Aneurysm

Smoking aggravates or accelerates aortic atherosclerosis, and the death rate for ruptured aortic aneurysm is higher among smokers than among nonsmokers (USDHHS 1983; Blanchard 1999). Excess risk for aortic aneurysm remains substantial even after 20 years' cessation of cigarette smoking (USDHHS 1983). Data for women are sparse; a previous Surgeon General's report summarized data from five prospective studies that examined the risk for death from aortic aneurysm; only two of these studies included data for women (Doll et al. 1980; USDHHS 1990, p. 242 [CPS-I tabulations]). Both studies found a higher risk for mortality from aortic aneurysm among women who smoked than among women who did not smoke.

In CPS-I (Burns et al. 1997b), the RR for death from abdominal aortic aneurysm was 3.9 among women current smokers compared with women who had never smoked. Risk increased with the number of cigarettes smoked; RRs were 3.5, 4.6, or 4.8 among women who smoked 1 to 19, 20, or 21 or more cigarettes per day, respectively. In a census-based cohort study in Japan that included 142,857 women aged 40 years or older, the RR for death from aortic aneurysm was 4.4 (90 percent CI, 2.7 to 7.3) among women current smokers compared with women who had never smoked (Hirayama 1990).

In a prospective study of 43 patients (10 women) who had small abdominal aortic aneurysms (diameter <5 cm), a median growth rate of 0.13 cm/year was recorded by serial ultrasound during follow-up (mean, three years) (MacSweeney et al. 1994). The growth rate was not associated with the initial diameter of the aneurysm, systolic or diastolic blood pressure, or serum cholesterol level. However, 30 of the 43 patients were current smokers, and smoking was associated with growth of the aneurysm. The median annual growth rate of aneurysms was 0.16 cm among smokers and 0.09 cm among nonsmokers ($p = 0.03$).

In a population-based cohort study, 758 women aged 45 through 64 years were examined by radiography for the development or progression of atherosclerotic plaques in the abdominal aorta, as indicated by calcified deposits (Witteman et al. 1993). After 9 years of follow-up, the investigators reported a dose-response association between atherosclerotic change and the number of cigarettes smoked per day. In a comparison with women who had never smoked, the multivariate-adjusted RR for development or progression of aortic atherosclerosis was 1.4 (95 percent CI, 1.0 to 2.0) among women who smoked 1 to 9 cigarettes per day, 2.0 (95 percent CI, 1.6 to 2.5) among women who smoked 10 to 19 cigarettes per day, and 2.3 (95 percent CI, 1.8 to 3.0) among women who smoked 20 or more cigarettes per day. Inhaling (compared with not inhaling) and duration of smoking were also statistically significant predictors of risk, after adjustment for intensity of smoking. The RR for aortic atherosclerosis declined after smoking cessation, but a residual excess risk among women former smokers compared with women who had never smoked was still apparent 5 to 10 years after smoking cessation (RR, 1.6; 95 percent CI, 1.1 to 2.2). These data are compatible with the reported slow reversibility of smoking-induced atherosclerotic damage in the abdominal aorta (USDHHS 1983).

## Hypertension

Severe or malignant hypertension has been reported to be more common among women who smoke than among those who do not smoke (USDHHS 1980), yet epidemiologic and laboratory studies have produced conflicting results on the association between smoking and blood pressure. Several epidemiologic studies have shown that when blood pressure is measured in a physician's office, the readings among smokers are similar to or lower than those among nonsmokers, even after the lower BMI of smokers is taken into account (Greene et al. 1977; Gofin et al. 1982; Green et al. 1986). In contrast, laboratory studies have shown that cigarette smoking acutely raises blood pressure even among long-term smokers; the peak rise in blood pressure ranges from 3 to 12 mm Hg systolic pressure and 5 to 10 mm Hg diastolic pressure for a 20- to 30-minute duration of effect (Freestone and Ramsay 1982; Mann et al. 1989; Berlin et al. 1990; Groppelli et al. 1992).

Ambulatory measurement of blood pressure may clarify these results. Mann and colleagues (1991) compared blood pressure measurements taken in a physician's office with the 24-hour ambulatory blood pressure measurements for 77 women and 100 men with hypertension (diastolic blood pressure $\geq$ 90 mm Hg) who were not receiving medication. Participants in this study were 26 women and 33 men who currently smoked at least one pack of cigarettes per day and 51 women and 67 men nonsmokers. Blood pressure readings taken in a physician's office were similar among smokers and nonsmokers (means, 141/93 vs. 142/93 mm Hg). However, the mean ambulatory systolic blood pressure was much higher among smokers than among nonsmokers (145 vs. 140 mm Hg; $p < 0.05$). Findings were similar among women and men. The lack of difference in physician's office readings for smokers and nonsmokers was attributed to abstinence from smoking during the minutes or hours preceding the blood pressure measurement. This explanation may also account for the lack of association between smoking and blood pressure measurements in epidemiologic studies, in which blood pressure is often assessed without consideration of time since the last cigarette. Similar findings on ambulatory blood pressure emerged from later studies of women and men (De Cesaris et al. 1992; Narkiewicz et al. 1995; Poulsen et al. 1998), but contrary data have also been reported (Mikkelsen et al. 1997). A study of salivary cotinine levels reported data consistent with higher blood pressure among smokers: higher pressures among women and men with higher salivary cotinine levels (Istvan et al. 1999). These findings also suggested that the effects of smoking on blood pressure are transient.

## Conclusions

1. Smoking is a major cause of coronary heart disease among women. For women younger than 50 years, the majority of coronary heart disease is attributable to smoking. Risk increases with the number of cigarettes smoked and the duration of smoking.
2. The risk for coronary heart disease among women is substantially reduced within 1 or 2 years of smoking cessation. This immediate benefit is followed by a continuing but more gradual reduction in risk to that among nonsmokers by 10 to 15 or more years after cessation.
3. Women who use oral contraceptives have a particularly elevated risk of coronary heart disease if they smoke. Currently evidence is conflicting as to whether the effect of hormone replacement therapy on coronary heart disease risk differs between smokers and nonsmokers.
4. Women who smoke have an increased risk for ischemic stroke and subarachnoid hemorrhage. Evidence is inconsistent concerning the association between smoking and primary intracerebral hemorrhage.
5. In most studies that include women, the increased risk for stroke associated with smoking is reversible after smoking cessation; after 5 to 15 years of abstinence, the risk approaches that of women who have never smoked.
6. Conflicting evidence exists regarding the level of the risk for stroke among women who both smoke and use either the oral contraceptives commonly prescribed in the United States today or hormone replacement therapy.
7. Smoking is a strong predictor of the progression and severity of carotid atherosclerosis among women. Smoking cessation appears to slow the rate of progression of carotid atherosclerosis.
8. Women who are current smokers have an increased risk for peripheral vascular atherosclerosis. Smoking cessation is associated with improvements in symptoms, prognosis, and survival.
9. Women who smoke have an increased risk for death from ruptured abdominal aortic aneurysm.

# Chronic Obstructive Pulmonary Disease and Lung Function

Chronic obstructive pulmonary disease (COPD) is a term defined differently by clinicians, pathologists, and epidemiologists, and each discipline uses different criteria based on physiologic impairment, pathologic abnormalities, and symptoms (Samet 1989a). The hallmark of COPD is airflow obstruction, as measured by spirometric testing, with persistently low forced expiratory volume in one second ($FEV_1$) and low ratio of $FEV_1$ to forced vital capacity (FVC) ($FEV_1$/FVC), despite treatment.

COPD may include chronic bronchitis characterized by a chronic cough productive of sputum with airflow obstruction, and emphysema accompanied by airflow obstruction. Emphysema is defined as "a condition of the lung characterized by abnormal permanent enlargement of the airspaces distal to the terminal bronchiole, accompanied by destruction of their walls, and without obvious fibrosis" (American Thoracic Society 1987, p. 225). However, like bronchitis, emphysema is not consistently associated with airflow obstruction. Chronic bronchitis and emphysema with airflow obstruction are both included in the clinical diagnosis of COPD, but other lung diseases associated with airflow obstruction are specifically excluded from the clinical definition of COPD; these include asthma, bronchiectasis, and cystic fibrosis.

In epidemiologic studies, the diagnosis of COPD may be derived from surveys or databases. Questionnaire responses that may be used to diagnose COPD include reports of symptoms (e.g., dyspnea, cough, and phlegm), reports of physician diagnoses (e.g., emphysema, chronic bronchitis, or COPD), or both. Spirometry is often performed in epidemiologic studies to provide objective evidence of airflow obstruction among subjects with or without symptoms. Sources of data for descriptive or analytic studies of COPD include databases containing hospital discharge information or vital statistics (e.g., from death certificates). The standard terms used for COPD in these databases include terms from the *International Classification of Diseases,* ninth revision (*ICD-9*) (USDHHS 1989a)—"chronic bronchitis" (*ICD-9,* item 491); "emphysema" (*ICD-9,* item 492); and "chronic airways disease not otherwise classified" (*ICD-9,* item 496). The quality of these data sources may vary greatly.

Gender-specific differences have been observed in the likelihood of having a diagnosis of COPD, and it is unclear whether these differences result from diagnostic bias or reflect true gender-related differences in susceptibility. For example, in the Tucson (Arizona) Epidemiologic Study of Obstructive Lung Diseases, Dodge and colleagues (1986) found that, among subjects aged 40 years or older with a new diagnosis of asthma, emphysema, or chronic bronchitis based on self-report, women were more likely than men to receive a physician diagnosis of asthma or chronic bronchitis, and men were more likely to receive a diagnosis of emphysema. In the same population, Camilli and colleagues (1991) reported that a diagnosis of obstructive airways disease was stated on the death certificates of only 37 percent of 157 patients who had this diagnosis before death and that the proportion was lower among women (28 percent) than among men (42 percent).

Spirometric testing provides the most objective basis for diagnosing COPD. Among persons with a diagnosis of mild disease based on spirometric testing, reporting of obstructive airways disease on the death certificates was slightly higher among women (45 percent) than among men (34 percent), whereas for those with moderate-to-severe disease, reporting was higher among men (81 percent) than among women (57 percent). (For mild disease, the criteria were $FEV_1/FVC < 65$ percent and predicted $FEV_1$ 50 to 70 percent of that in the normal reference population. For moderate-to-severe disease, the criteria were $FEV_1/FVC < 65$ percent and predicted $FEV_1 < 50$ percent of that in the normal reference population.)

Evidence suggested that changes in the structure and function of small airways (bronchioles) are fundamental for the development of smoking-induced COPD (Wright 1992; Thurlbeck 1994). An inflammatory process of the small airways (respiratory bronchiolitis) develops in all cigarette smokers; but in susceptible smokers, this process progresses and causes narrowing of these airways (Bosken et al. 1990; USDHHS 1990; Aguayo 1994). The inflammatory process may extend into the peribronchiolar alveoli and destroy the alveolar walls, which is the hallmark of emphysema. The rate of expiratory airflow depends on elastic recoil forces from the alveoli and on the diameter of the small airways. Complex interactions between changes in the structure and function of small airways and lung parenchyma result in the physiologic finding of chronic airflow limitation.

Cigarette smoking as a cause of COPD was extensively reviewed in earlier reports of the Surgeon General (USDHHS 1980, 1984, 1989b, 1990). (In the 1980 and 1984 Surgeon General's reports, COPD was referred to as chronic obstructive lung disease [COLD].) In the 1980 Surgeon General's report on the health consequences of smoking for women (USDHHS 1980), the major conclusions relevant to COPD were as follows: (1) The death rate for COPD among women was rising, and the data available demonstrated an excess risk for death among women who smoked compared with nonsmokers, with a much greater risk for heavy smokers than for light smokers. (2) Women's overall risk for COPD appeared to be somewhat lower than men's, a difference possibly due to differences in previous smoking habits. (3) The prevalence of chronic bronchitis increased with the number of cigarettes smoked per day. (4) Evidence on differences in the prevalence of chronic bronchitis among women and men who smoked was inconsistent. (5) The presence of emphysema at autopsy exhibited a dose-response relationship with cigarette smoking during life. (6) A close relationship existed between cigarette smoking and chronic cough or chronic sputum production among women, which increased with total pack-years of smoking. (7) Women current smokers had poorer pulmonary function, by spirometric testing, than did women former smokers or nonsmokers, and the relationship was related to the number of cigarettes smoked.

In the 1984 Surgeon General's report on smoking and COPD (USDHHS 1984), the major additional conclusions relevant to morbidity and mortality from COPD among women were as follows: (1) Cigarette smoking was the major cause of COPD mortality among both women and men in the United States. (2) Both male and female smokers were found to develop abnormalities in the small airways, but the data were not sufficient to define possible gender-related differences in this response. (3) The risk for COPD mortality among former smokers did not decline to that among persons who had never smoked, even 20 years after smoking cessation.

In the 1990 Surgeon General's report on the health benefits of smoking cessation (USDHHS 1990), the major conclusions relevant to COPD were as follows: (1) Compared with continued smoking, cessation reduces rates of respiratory symptoms (e.g., cough, sputum production, and wheezing) and of respiratory infections (e.g., bronchitis and pneumonia). (2) Among persons with overt COPD, smoking cessation improves pulmonary function about 5 percent within a few months after cessation. (3) Cigarette smoking accelerates the age-related decline in lung function that occurs among persons who have never smoked, but with sustained abstinence from smoking, the rate of decline in pulmonary function among former smokers returns to that among persons who have never smoked. (4) With sustained abstinence, the COPD mortality rates among former smokers decline compared with those among continuing smokers.

Much of the more recent research on the relationship between COPD and cigarette smoking has focused on determining predictors of susceptibility (e.g., childhood respiratory illness and degree of airway hyperactivity) and on early detection (Samet 1989a; USDHHS 1994). The following discussion summarizes the research that has developed since previous Surgeon General's reports on smoking and provides more recent information on the epidemiology of COPD among women.

## Smoking and Natural History of Development, Growth, and Decline of Lung Function

Although longitudinal data on the effects of cigarette smoking and development of COPD are not available for childhood through adulthood, study findings suggested that the development of COPD among adults may result from impaired lung development and growth, premature onset of decline of lung function, accelerated decline of lung function, or any combination of these conditions (USDHHS 1990). Airway development in utero and alveolar proliferation through age 12 years are critical to the mechanical functioning of the lungs, and impaired lung growth in utero from exposure to maternal smoking may enhance susceptibility to later development of COPD. Exposure to ETS in infancy and childhood and active smoking during childhood and adolescence may further contribute to impairment of lung growth and the risk for developing COPD (Fletcher et al. 1976; Samet et al. 1983; USDHHS 1984; Tager et al. 1988; Sherrill et al. 1991; Helms 1994; Samet and Lange 1996).

### Lung Development in Utero

In utero exposure to maternal smoking is associated with wheezing and affects lung function during infancy (U.S. Environmental Protection Agency [EPA] 1992), but only limited information exists on gender-specific effects. Young and colleagues (1991) measured pulmonary function and airway hyperresponsiveness to histamine among 63 healthy infants from a prenatal clinic in Perth, Australia. The infants were categorized into four groups on the basis of family history of asthma and parental cigarette smoking during pregnancy, but prenatal and postnatal exposures to cigarette smoke could not be separated. At a mean age of 4.5 weeks, rates of forced expiratory flow did not differ among the four groups. However, airway responsiveness was greater among infants whose parents smoked during pregnancy.

Hanrahan and colleagues (1992) measured forced expiratory flow rates among 80 healthy infants (average age, four weeks) from the East Boston Neighborhood Health Center, Massachusetts. These infants included 47 born to mothers who did not smoke during pregnancy, 21 to mothers who smoked throughout pregnancy, and 12 to mothers who reported varying smoking status or who had urine cotinine levels that were inconsistent with not smoking. After adjustment for infant size, age, gender, and ETS exposure after birth, expiratory flow rates were shown to be lower among infants whose mothers smoked during pregnancy than among infants whose mothers did not smoke. To determine the longitudinal effects of maternal smoking during pregnancy, Tager and colleagues (1995) studied 159 infants from the East Boston Neighborhood Health Center and obtained follow-up pulmonary function tests at 4 through 6, 9 through 12, and 15 through 18 months of age. On average, maternal smoking during pregnancy was associated with a 16-percent reduction in the expiratory flow rate at functional residual capacity among infant girls and a 5-percent reduction among infant boys. In contrast, exposure to ETS after birth was not associated with a significant decrement in longitudinal change in pulmonary function during infancy. A consequence of reduction in expiratory airflow and airway hyperresponsiveness may be an increased risk for lower respiratory tract illnesses, including wheezing. In a sample of 97 infants from the East Boston Neighborhood Health Center, Tager and colleagues (1993) found maternal smoking during pregnancy to be associated with an elevated risk for lower respiratory tract illnesses (RR, 1.5; 95 percent CI, 1.1 to 2.0). The finding was identical among infant girls and infant boys.

The decrement in pulmonary function associated with in utero exposure to smoke that is evident at birth and throughout infancy may persist into childhood and into adulthood. In a cross-sectional survey, Cunningham and colleagues (1994) measured pulmonary function among 8,863 children, aged 8 through 12 years, from 22 North American communities. In multivariate analyses, the children whose mothers reported smoking during pregnancy had significantly lower forced expiratory flows and reduction in forced expiratory volume in three-fourths of a second ($FEV_{0.75}$) and $FEV_1/FVC$ than did the children of mothers who did not smoke during pregnancy, but absolute differences tended to be greater among boys than among girls. After adjustment for maternal smoking during pregnancy, current maternal smoking was not associated with significant decrement of lung function. Cunningham and colleagues (1995) also examined the relationship between maternal smoking during pregnancy and level of lung function among 876 Philadelphia schoolchildren aged 9 through 11 years. Overall, maternal smoking during pregnancy was associated with significant deficits in forced expiratory flow between 25 and 75 percent of FVC ($FEF_{25-75}$) (-8.1 percent; 95 percent CI, -12.9 to -3.1 percent) and $FEV_1/FVC$ (-2.0 percent; 95 percent CI, -3.0 to -0.9 percent) among the children. This association remained after adjustment for the children's height, weight, age, gender, area of residence, race, socioeconomic status, and current exposure to ETS at home. The largest effects of maternal smoking on lung function were observed among boys and among black children; the deficit among girls was not significant: $FEF_{25-75}$ was -3.1 percent (95 percent CI, -9.9 to 4.2 percent), and $FEV_1/FVC$ was -1.1 percent (95 percent CI, -2.5 to 0.4 percent).

Sherrill and colleagues (1992) in New Zealand examined the effects of maternal smoking during pregnancy among 634 children who were enrolled at age 3 years in a longitudinal study and had spirometric tests at ages 9, 11, 13, and 15 years. Gender-specific findings were not discussed, but compared with children of mothers who did not smoke, no significant changes in pulmonary function were found among children whose mothers smoked during pregnancy, within three months after childbirth, or at both times. However, details of the analysis were not presented, and power to detect differences may have been limited because most mothers who smoked during pregnancy also smoked during the three months after pregnancy (n = 219); few mothers smoked only during pregnancy (n = 10) or only after pregnancy (n = 18).

### Growth of Lung Function in Infancy and Childhood

Beside the effects of in utero exposure to maternal smoking on lung function during infancy and childhood, substantial evidence suggested that ETS is an important determinant of impaired lung function during childhood (National Research Council [NRC] 1986; USDHHS 1986b; EPA 1992). The 1992 EPA report concluded "that there is a causal relationship between ETS exposure and reductions in airflow parameters of lung function… in children" (EPA 1992, p. 7-63). However, few studies gave separate consideration to prenatal, infant, and childhood exposures to tobacco smoke, which may all be highly correlated, and few longitudinal studies on the effects of such exposure were performed. Wang and colleagues (1994b) analyzed longitudinal data on pulmonary function among 8,706 white children (4,290 girls and 4,416 boys) who did not smoke. The children entered the study at about 6 years of age and were followed up through 18 years of age to determine the association between parental cigarette smoking and growth of lung function among the children. Maternal smoking during the first five years of life and at the time of pulmonary testing was a significant predictor of lung function level among both girls and boys. In multiple regression models, current maternal smoking was the only significant predictor of growth of pulmonary function. Among children aged 6 through 10 years, rates for growth of lung function per each pack of cigarettes smoked daily by the mother were significantly lower for FVC (-2.8 mL/year), $FEV_1$ (-3.8 mL/year), and $FEF_{25-75}$ (-14.3 mL/second per year). Among children aged 11 through 18 years, current maternal smoking was significantly associated with slower growth rates only for $FEF_{25-75}$ (-7.9 mL/second per year).

In a longitudinal study in New Zealand, Sherrill and colleagues (1992) analyzed spirometric data collected bienially from 634 children ages 9 through 15 years. The $FEV_1$/FVC ratio was significantly lower among boys (-1.57 percent) but not among girls whose parents both smoked when the children were ages 7, 9, and 11, compared with those whose parents did not smoke. Among children who had wheezing or asthma by age 15 years, those whose parents smoked had lower mean $FEV_1$/FVC ratios than those whose parents did not smoke (a reduction of 2.3 percent for girls and 3.9 percent for boys). The effect of ETS on pulmonary function may have been underestimated because of misclassification of ETS exposure. A child was categorized as exposed only if parental smoking was reported consecutively during three surveys when the child was 7, 9, and 11 years old. Children were considered to be unexposed if their parents reported smoking at two or fewer of these surveys.

The association between ETS exposure in childhood and pneumonia (USDHHS 1986b; EPA 1992) provides additional evidence that may indirectly link ETS exposure and COPD in adulthood. Study findings indicated that ETS exposure increases the occurrence of lower respiratory tract illnesses, which are associated with small airway and alveolar inflammation, and that the inflammation provides a pathogenic basis for linking ETS exposure, lower respiratory tract illnesses, and development of COPD.

Beside the adverse effects on pulmonary function of in utero exposure to maternal smoking and postnatal exposure to parental smoking, active cigarette smoking in childhood and adolescence impairs growth of lung function, thus increasing the risk for COPD in adulthood (USDHHS 1994).

### Decline of Lung Function

The effects of cigarette smoking on growth and decline of lung function were examined in longitudinal studies in East Boston, Massachusetts (Tager et al. 1988), and Tucson, Arizona (Sherrill et al. 1991). In the East Boston study, estimates of the age range when lung function begins to decline were wide but tended to be at earlier ages among current smokers (19 through 29 years) than among asymptomatic nonsmokers (18 through 42 years) or symptomatic nonsmokers (21 through 35 years). On average, the decline of lung function was more rapid among current smokers (-20 mL/year) than among asymptomatic nonsmokers (-10 mL/year) and symptomatic nonsmokers (-5 mL/year). Results were not presented separately by gender, but overall, the results from this study suggested that cigarette smokers experience premature onset of the decline of lung function and a more rapid decline than do nonsmokers. These findings were consistent with those of a longitudinal analysis of lung function from the Tucson Epidemiologic Study of Obstructive Lung Diseases (Sherrill et al. 1991).

Cross-sectional and longitudinal studies of ventilatory function showed, on average, higher rates of decline of $FEV_1$ among current smokers than among former smokers and nonsmokers (Table 3.27). As the amount of cigarette smoking increased, the rate of decline of $FEV_1$ also increased (Xu et al. 1992, 1994; Vestbo et al. 1996).

Identification of the minority of smokers who will have an accelerated decline of $FEV_1$ has been the focus of an increasing number of investigations, but generally data have not been presented for women and men separately. Predictors of a rapid decline of $FEV_1$ among smokers include respiratory symptoms (Jedrychowski et al. 1988; Sherman et al. 1992; Vestbo et al. 1996), level of lung function (Burrows et al.

1987), and bronchial hyperresponsiveness (Kanner et al. 1994; Paoletti et al. 1995; Rijcken et al. 1995; Villar et al. 1995). Among cigarette smokers, bronchial hyperresponsiveness to a variety of stimuli (e.g., histamine and methacholine) was associated with an accelerated rate of decline in $FEV_1$. Rijcken and colleagues (1995) analyzed the results of histamine challenge tests and longitudinal spirometric data obtained between 1965 and 1990 from 698 women and 921 men in two communities in the Netherlands. The average annual rate of $FEV_1$ decline was -33.1 mL/year among women who smoked during the entire study period and who had bronchial hyperresponsiveness; the rate among consistent smokers who did not have bronchial hyperresponsiveness was -27.3 mL/year. A similar pattern was observed among men. Tashkin and colleagues (1996) examined the relationship between bronchial hyperreactivity to methacholine and $FEV_1$ decline among 5,733 smokers, 35 through 60 years of age, with mild COPD (mean $FEV_1$/FVC, 65 percent; predicted $FEV_1$, 78 percent). After adjustment for age, gender, baseline smoking history, changes in smoking status, and baseline level of lung function, the investigators found that airway hyperreactivity during the five-year follow-up was a strong predictor of change in $FEV_1$ percent predicted. The greatest average decline of 2.2 percent predicted was among women who had the highest degree of hyperreactivity and who continued to smoke; the corresponding value among men was 1.7 percent predicted. In two cross-sectional analyses (Kanner et al. 1994; Paoletti et al. 1995), prevalence of bronchial hyperresponsiveness was higher among women smokers than among men smokers.

Cross-sectional and longitudinal investigations of decline in lung function among cigarette smokers provided conflicting results about the relative rate of decline among women compared with men (Xu et al. 1994). Xu and colleagues (1994) suggested that women may have a higher rate of $FEV_1$ decline. They hypothesized that gender differences in the distribution of unhealthy subjects in nonsmoking reference groups may explain conflicting results in studies that compared rates of $FEV_1$ decline among women and men.

Other study factors that may modify the effects of smoking and contribute to differences in study findings by gender include the year of birth of study participants (birth cohort) and the time period of a study (Samet and Lange 1996). In the Vlagtwedde-Vlaardingen study, Xu and colleagues (1995) reported a significant interaction between age and birth cohort in relation to decline in $FEV_1$ among women but not among men. The modifying effects of birth cohort may partly reflect changes in smoking behaviors.

Some studies have reported that sustained abstinence from smoking among former smokers slowed the decline in pulmonary function to that of women and men who had never smoked (USDHHS 1990) (Table 3.27). As suggested by the conceptual model for the development of COPD, age at the start of smoking cessation may substantially influence the level of lung function associated with aging, and recent evidence suggested that the benefits of smoking cessation are greatest for persons who stop smoking at younger ages (Camilli et al. 1987; Sherrill et al. 1994; Xu et al. 1994; Frette et al. 1996).

Among 147 women aged 18 years or older at entry in the prospective Tucson Epidemiological Study of Airways Obstructive Disease, Sherrill and colleagues (1994) found that, on average, smoking cessation was associated with a 4.3-percent improvement in $FEV_1$ at age 20 years and a 2.5-percent improvement at age 80 years. During 24 years of follow-up in the Dutch Vlagtwedde-Vlaardingen study that included 3,092 women aged 15 through 54 years at entry, Xu and associates (1994) found that mean $FEV_1$ loss was 20 mL/year less among women who had stopped smoking before age 45 years but only 5.4 mL/year less among women who had stopped smoking at age 45 years or older than among women who continued to smoke. As part of the Rancho Bernardo (California) Heart and Chronic Disease Study, 826 women and 571 men aged 51 through 95 years had spirometry testing in 1988–1991 (Frette et al. 1996). Among women former smokers who had stopped smoking before 40 years of age, $FEV_1$ was similar to that among women who had never smoked (2.09 and 2.13 L, respectively). Average $FEV_1$ among women who had stopped smoking at 40 through 60 years of age was 2.02 L, which was intermediate between that among women nonsmokers (2.13 L) and that among women current smokers (1.71 L). Women who had stopped smoking after 60 years of age had $FEV_1$ similar to that among current smokers (1.72 and 1.71 L, respectively). The same pattern of $FEV_1$ level in relation to age at smoking cessation was found among men.

Within the first year of smoking cessation, a small improvement in $FEV_1$ and a slowing in the rate of decline in $FEV_1$ are seen among former smokers compared with continuing smokers. In the Lung Health Study, Anthonisen and colleagues (1994) enrolled 5,887 women (37 percent) and men (63 percent) aged 35 through 60 years who were current smokers with mild COPD. During the first five years of follow-up,

**Table 3.27. Rate of decline in forced expiratory volume in 1 second ($FEV_1$) among women and men, by smoking status, population-based studies, 1984–1996**

| Study | Population | Period of study/follow-up | $FEV_1$ change | Type of study or comments |
|---|---|---|---|---|
| Tashkin et al. 1984 | 1,309 women, 1,092 men<br>Aged 25–64 years<br>Southern California | Baseline 1973–1975<br>Follow-up 1978–1980 | Women<br>Continuing smokers: -54 mL/year<br>Former smokers: -38 mL /year<br>Never smoked: -41 mL/year<br><br>Men<br>Continuing smokers: -70 mL/year<br>Former smokers: -52 mL/year<br>Never smoked: -56 mL/year | Longitudinal study |
| Krzyzanowski et al. 1986 | 1,065 women, 759 men<br>Aged 19–70 years<br>Kraków, Poland | Baseline 1968<br>Follow-up 1981 | Women<br>Continuing smokers: -42 mL/year<br>Former smokers: -38 mL/year<br>Never smoked: -38 mL/year<br><br>Men<br>Continuing smokers: -59 mL/year<br>Former smokers: -63 mL/year<br>Never smoked: -47 mL/year | Longitudinal study |
| Camilli et al. 1987 | 970 women, 735 men<br>Aged 20–90 years<br>Tucson, Arizona | Baseline 1972–1973<br>Mean follow-up 9.4 years | Women*<br>Current smokers: -7.38 mL/year†<br>Former smokers: -0.73 mL/year<br>Never smoked: -0.42 mL/year<br><br>Men‡<br>Current smokers: -19.03 mL/year†<br>Former smokers: -4.06 mL/year<br>Never smoked: -6.13 mL/year | Longitudinal study<br>Smoking cessation at age <35 years resulted in greatest improvement in $FEV_1$ |
| Dockery et al. 1988 | 4,477 women, 3,714 men<br>Aged 25–27 years<br>6 U.S. cities | 1974–1977 | Women<br>Lifetime smoking: -4.4 mL/pack-year§<br>Additional affect of current smoking: -107.1 mL/pack/day (current)<br>Men<br>Lifetime smoking: -7.4 mL/pack-year§<br>Additional affect of current smoking: -123.3 mL/pack/day (current) | Cross-sectional study |
| Tager et al. 1988 | 1,814 females, 1,767 males<br>Aged ≥5 years<br>East Boston, Massachusetts | Baseline 1975<br>Follow-up 10 years | Women<br>Current smokers: -20 to -30 mL/year<br>Nonsmokers: -10 to -35 mL/year<br><br>Men<br>Current smokers: -25 to -40 mL/year<br>Nonsmokers: -20 to -35 mL/year | Longitudinal study |

*$FEV_1$ decline >100 mL/year, 0.6%.
†Observed/expected ≥ $FEV_1$ for subjects aged <70 years, adjusted for age and height.
‡$FEV_1$ decline >100 mL/year, 4.2%.
§$FEV_1$ adjusted for height.

**Table 3.27. Continued**

| Study | Population | Period of study/follow-up | $FEV_1$ change | Type of study or comments |
|---|---|---|---|---|
| Lange et al. 1990a | 4,986 women, 3,139 men<br>Aged ≥20 years<br>Copenhagen, Denmark | Baseline 1976–1978<br>Follow-up 1981–1983 | Women<br>Plain cigarettes: -34 mL/year<br>Filter-tipped cigarettes: -28 mL/year<br>Nonsmokers: -25 mL/year<br><br>Men<br>Plain cigarettes: -40 mL/year<br>Filter-tipped cigarettes: -42 mL/year<br>Nonsmokers: -30 mL/year | Longitudinal study<br>No significant difference in rate of decline for smokers of plain or filter-tipped cigarettes<br>Inconsistent association of inhalation with rate of decline |
| Peat et al. 1990 | 634 women, 350 men<br>Population-based sample<br>Brusselton, Australia | Baseline 1966<br>Follow-up every 3 years through 1984 | | Longitudinal study<br>Slope of $FEV_1$ decline greater for smokers than for nonsmokers; slope increased with age<br>No significant difference in slope for women and men<br>Rate of decline associated with current number of cigarettes smoked |
| Chen et al. 1991 | 605 women, 544 men<br>Aged 25–59 years<br>Rural Saskatchewan, Alberta, Canada | 1977 | Women: -6.2 mL/pack-year[Δ¶]<br>Men: -2.0 mL/pack-year[Δ] | Cross-sectional study |
| Xu et al. 1992 | 6,643 women, 5,437 men<br>Aged 25–78 years<br>6 U.S. cities | Follow-up 6 years<br>3 examinations | Women<br>Continuing smokers: -38.0 mL/year**<br><15 cigarettes/day: -31.2 mL/year**<br>15–24 cigarettes/day: -42.0 mL/year<br>≥25 cigarettes/day: -38.9 mL/year<br>Former smokers: -29.6 mL/year<br>Never smoked: -29.0 mL/year<br><br>Men<br>Continuing smokers: -52.9 mL/year**<br><15 cigarettes/day: -37.4 mL/year<br>15–24 cigarettes/day: -47.2 mL/year<br>≥25 cigarettes/day: -59.9 mL/year<br>Former smokers: -34.3 mL/year<br>Never smoked: -37.8 mL/year | Longitudinal study |

[Δ]$FEV_1$ adjusted for age, height, and weight.
[¶]Pack-years = Average number of packs smoked/day x number of years of smoking.
**Age-adjusted average rate.

**Table 3.27. Continued**

| Study | Population | Period of study/follow-up | $FEV_1$ change | Type of study or comments |
|---|---|---|---|---|
| Xu et al. 1994 | 3,092 women,<br>3,294 men<br>Aged 15–75 years<br>Vlaardingen, The Netherlands | Baseline<br>1965–1969<br>Follow-up<br>every 3 years<br>through 1990 | Women<br>Continuing smokers<br><15 cigarettes/day: -15.0 mL/year<br>15–24 cigarettes/day: -20.4 mL/year<br>≥25 cigarettes/day: -30.1 mL/year<br>Former smokers: -19.2 mL/year<br>Never smoked: -14.8 mL/year<br><br>Men<br>Continuing smokers<br><15 cigarettes/day: -18.8 mL/year<br>15–24 cigarettes/day: -26.3 mL/year<br>≥25 cigarettes/day: -33.2 mL/year<br>Former smokers: -20.0 mL/year<br>Never smoked: -5.8 mL/year | Longitudinal study |
| Frette et al. 1996 | 826 women,<br>571 men<br>Aged 51–95 years<br>Rancho Bernardo, California | 1988–1991 | Women<br>Current smokers<br>Aged <70 years: -49 mL/year<br>Aged 70–79 years: -74 mL/year<br>Aged ≥80 years: -112 mL/year<br><br>Former smokers<br>Aged <70 years: -44 mL/year<br>Aged 70–79 years: -28 mL/year<br>Aged ≥80 years: -20 mL/year<br><br>Never smoked<br>Aged <70 years: -37 mL/year<br>Aged 70–79: -23 mL/year<br>Aged ≥80 years: -35 mL/year<br><br>Men<br>Current smokers<br>Aged <70 years: -70 mL/year<br>Aged 70–79 years: -91 mL/year<br>Aged ≥80 years: 367 mL/year<br><br>Former smokers<br>Aged <70 years: -53 mL/year<br>Aged 70–79 years: -27 mL/year<br>Aged ≥80 years: -14 mL/year<br><br>Never smoked<br>Aged <70 years: -10 mL/year<br>Aged 70–79 years: -28 mL/year<br>Aged ≥80 years: -37 mL/year | Cross-sectional study |

**Table 3.27. Continued**

| Study | Population | Period of study/follow-up | $FEV_1$ change | Type of study or comments |
|---|---|---|---|---|
| Vestbo et al. 1996 | 5,354 women, 4,081 men<br>Aged 30–79 years<br>Copenhagen, Denmark | Baseline 1976–1978<br>Follow-up 1981–1983 | Women<br>1–14 g tobacco/day: -7.2 mL/year††<br>15–24 g tobacco/day: -7.8 mL/year††<br>≥25 g tobacco/day: -24.8 mL/year††<br>Chronic hypersecretion of mucus: -11.3 mL/year‡‡<br><br>Men<br>1–14 g/day: -3.3 mL/year††<br>15–24 g/day: -12.4 mL/year††<br>≥25 g/day: -14.1 mL/year††<br>Chronic hypersecretion of mucus: -23.0 mL/year‡‡ | Longitudinal study |
| Prescott et al. 1997 | 5,020 women, 4,063 men<br>Aged ≥20 years<br>Copenhagen, Denmark | Baseline 1976–1978 | Women<br>Smoke inhalers: -7.4 mL/pack-year<br>Noninhalers: -2.6 mL/pack-year<br><br>Men<br>Smoke inhalers: -6.3 mL/pack-year<br>Noninhalers: -1.0 mL/pack-year | Longitudinal studies |
| | 2,383 women, 2,431 men<br>Glostrup, Denmark | Baseline 1964<br>Follow-up 7–16 years | Women<br>Smoke inhalers: -10.5 mL/pack-year<br>Noninhalers: -12.4 mL/pack-year<br><br>Men<br>Smoke inhalers: -8.1 mL/pack-year<br>Noninhalers: -4.7 mL/pack-year | |

††In excess of nonsmokers at baseline survey.
‡‡In excess of subjects without chronic hypersecretion of mucus at any survey.

persons who sustained abstinence from smoking experienced an increase in postbronchodilator $FEV_1$ for the first two years of follow-up and then a decline, whereas continuing smokers had a persistent decline in $FEV_1$. Among persons who had stopped smoking by the one-year follow-up, $FEV_1$ had increased an average of 57 mL. In contrast, among those who continued to smoke, $FEV_1$ declined an average of 38 mL in the first year of follow-up. During the entire five-year follow-up, the average rate of decline in $FEV_1$ was 34 mL/year among those with sustained abstinence and 63 mL/year among continuing smokers. Results for women and men were combined in this analysis. Tashkin and colleagues (1996) found that the greatest improvements of $FEV_1$ occurred during the first year of cessation among women and men with the highest levels of airway reactivity.

## Prevalence of Chronic Obstructive Pulmonary Disease

In the United States, the major national databases on prevalence of COPD include NHIS, the National Hospital Discharge Survey, and the National Hospital Ambulatory Medical Care Survey. Mortality data are derived from the National Vital Statistics System.

Overall, nationwide data suggested that the prevalence of COPD increased among women aged 55 through 84 years over the period 1979–1985 (Feinleib et al. 1989). In NHIS, the age-adjusted prevalence of self-reported COPD among women increased from 8.8 percent in 1979 to 11.9 percent in 1985. The prevalence of COPD increased with age and peaked at ages 65 through 74 years. Data from the National Hospital Ambulatory Medical Care Survey showed that 11.4

**Table 3.28. Prevalence of airflow limitation as measured by forced expiratory volume in 1 second ($FEV_1$) among women and men, population-based, cross-sectional studies, 1989–1994**

| Study | Population | Measure |
|---|---|---|
| Lange et al. 1989 | 4,905 women, 4,001 men<br>Random, age-stratified sample<br>Aged 20–90 years<br>Denmark | $FEV_1$ <60%<br>$FEV_1$/FVC* <0.7 |
| Peat et al. 1990 | 634 women, 350 men<br>Population-based sample<br>Australia | $FEV_1$ <65% predicted on ≥ 2 occasions<br>$FEV_1$/FVC <0.65 |
| Bang 1993 | 328 black women, 243 black men<br>Aged 25–75 years<br>Spirometry testing in first National Health and Nutrition Examination Survey<br>United States | $FEV_1$ <65% |
| Higgins et al. 1993 | 2,869 women, 2,198 men<br>Population-based sample<br>Aged ≥65 years<br>United States | $FEV_1$ <5th percentile for healthy women and men |
| Isoaho et al. 1994 | 708 women, 488 men<br>Population sample<br>Aged ≥64 years<br>Finland | $FEV_1$/FVC ≥0.65 |
| Sherrill et al. 1994 | 891 women,[§] 633 men[§]<br>Population sample<br>Aged ≥55 years at 1st survey<br>United States | $FEV_1$ <75% |

*FVC = Forced vital capacity.
[†]Never smoked.
[‡]Current and former smokers.
[§]Survivors at 9th or 10th survey, spanning a period of ≤14 years.

percent of office visits by women in 1979 and 12.2 percent in 1985 were for COPD. In the National Hospital Discharge Survey, 0.8 percent of hospitalizations among women in 1979 and 0.9 percent in 1985 were for COPD.

Reported prevalence of COPD among women in Manitoba, Canada, also increased (Manfreda et al. 1993) between 1983–1984 and 1987–1988. The investigators used data from the Manitoba Health Services Commission, a registry of the entire Manitoba population and their use of inpatient and outpatient physician services. Prevalences of physician-diagnosed COPD and asthma were estimated for these two periods. Among women aged 55 years or older, COPD increased 23.3 percent—from 163.8 cases per 10,000 in 1983–1984 to 202 cases per 10,000 in 1987–1988. Larger increases were reported for combinations of diagnoses, including COPD and asthma (28.8 percent), COPD and bronchitis (29.5 percent), and COPD and asthmatic bronchitis (45.5 percent).

In population-based, cross-sectional studies conducted worldwide (Table 3.28), prevalence estimates for COPD among women, based on spirometric data, varied widely. The estimates ranged from

| Prevalence (%) | | | | |
|---|---|---|---|---|
| | | | Smokers | |
| Nonsmokers | Former smokers | Current smokers | <15 (g/day) | ≥15 (g/day) |
| Women: 1.6<br>Men: 2.6 | Women: 3.1<br>Men: 4.4 | | Women: 6.2<br>Men: 6.4 | Women: 37.1<br>Men: 7.7 |
| Women: 7.6<br>Men: 5.2 | | Women: 17.8<br>Men: 23.6 | | |
| Women: 8.4[†]<br>Men: 0.0[†] | | Women: 5.0[‡]<br>Men: 5.4[‡] | | |
| Women: 13.6[†]<br>Men: 7.3[†] | Women: 28.2<br>Men: 18.5 | Women: 47.4<br>Men: 45.1 | | |
| Women: 1.9[†]<br>Men: 2.0[†] | Women: 14.3<br>Men: 12.3 | Women: 12.5<br>Men: 34.7 | | |
| Women: 5.9<br>Men: 8.0 | Women: 17.9<br>Men: 13.8 | Women: 29.6<br>Men: 36.4 | | |

approximately 2 percent among nonsmokers aged 40 years or older (Lange et al. 1989) to 47 percent among current smokers aged 65 years or older (Higgins et al. 1993). The wide variation in the prevalence of COPD may be the result of many factors, including differences in spirometric criteria for the diagnosis and differences in age distribution and exposure among populations. Regardless of the criteria for diagnosing COPD, prevalence was lowest among nonsmokers (Table 3.28). One exception to this pattern was reported by Bang (1993): black women who had never smoked (8.4 percent) had a higher prevalence of $FEV_1$ impairment than did current smokers and former smokers combined (5.0 percent). Although few recent analyses examined the relationship between dose or duration of smoking and the prevalence of COPD (Table 3.28), an inverse dose-response relationship between cigarette smoking and level of lung function is firmly established (USDHHS 1984).

## Mortality from Chronic Obstructive Pulmonary Disease

Since the late 1970s, COPD has been the fifth-leading cause of death in the United States. In 1992, 85,415 deaths were attributed to COPD (*ICD-9* items 491, 492, and 496), and 44 percent of these deaths occurred among women (NCHS 1996). Cigarette smoking is the most important cause of COPD among both women and men (USDHHS 1984).

Mortality from COPD has steadily increased in the United States during the twentieth century as the full impact of widespread cigarette smoking that began early in the century has taken effect (Speizer 1989). During 1979–1985, the annual age-adjusted death rates for COPD among women 55 years or older increased by 73 percent, from 46.6 per 100,000 to 80.7 per 100,000. Although the death rates for COPD among men were higher, the percent increase during 1979–1985 among men was only 16 percent, from 169.2 per 100,000 to 196.4 per 100,000.

According to NCHS (1995), the steep rise in mortality from COPD among women in the United States continued during 1980–1992 and was similar among white women and African American women (Figure 3.9). The age-adjusted death rates increased 75 percent among white women and 78 percent among African American women. In 1992, COPD mortality was 44 percent higher among white women than among African American women. During the same period, the age-adjusted death rate for men increased only 0.4 percent among whites and 19 percent among African Americans. In 1992, the overall age-adjusted death rates were 1.67 times higher among white men than among white women and 2.21 times higher among African American men than among African American women.

The prospective studies of ACS (CPS-I and CPS-II) provided further evidence for a marked increase in mortality from COPD among women (Thun et al. 1995, 1997a). Using CPS-I data, Thun and colleagues (1995) examined death rates during the period 1959–1965 among 298,687 current smokers and 487,700 nonsmokers. Age-adjusted death rates among women were 17.6 per 100,000 person-years for current smokers and 2.6 per 100,000 person-years for nonsmokers (RR, 6.7). The corresponding figures among men were 73.6 per 100,000 person-years and 8.0 per 100,000 person-years (RR, 9.3). In CPS-II, 228,682 current smokers and 482,681 nonsmokers were followed up in 1982–1988. In CPS-II, the death rate among women current smokers (61.6 per 100,000 person-years) was three times higher than that among women current smokers in CPS-I. The RR for mortality was 12.8 among women current smokers compared with women who had never smoked. Among men current smokers in CPS-II, the death rate (103.9 per 100,000 person-years) was 41 percent higher than that among men current smokers in CPS-I. The RR for mortality was 11.7 among men current smokers compared with men who had never smoked.

Using CPS-I and CPS-II data on RR for COPD mortality, Thun and colleagues (1997a,c) calculated the percentage of COPD deaths attributable to cigarette smoking. Among women in CPS-I, 85.0 percent of COPD deaths were attributable to smoking; this proportion increased to 92.2 percent in CPS-II. The corresponding values among men were 89.2 and 91.4 percent.

**Figure 3.9. Age-adjusted death rates for chronic obstructive pulmonary disease, by gender and race, United States, 1980–1992**

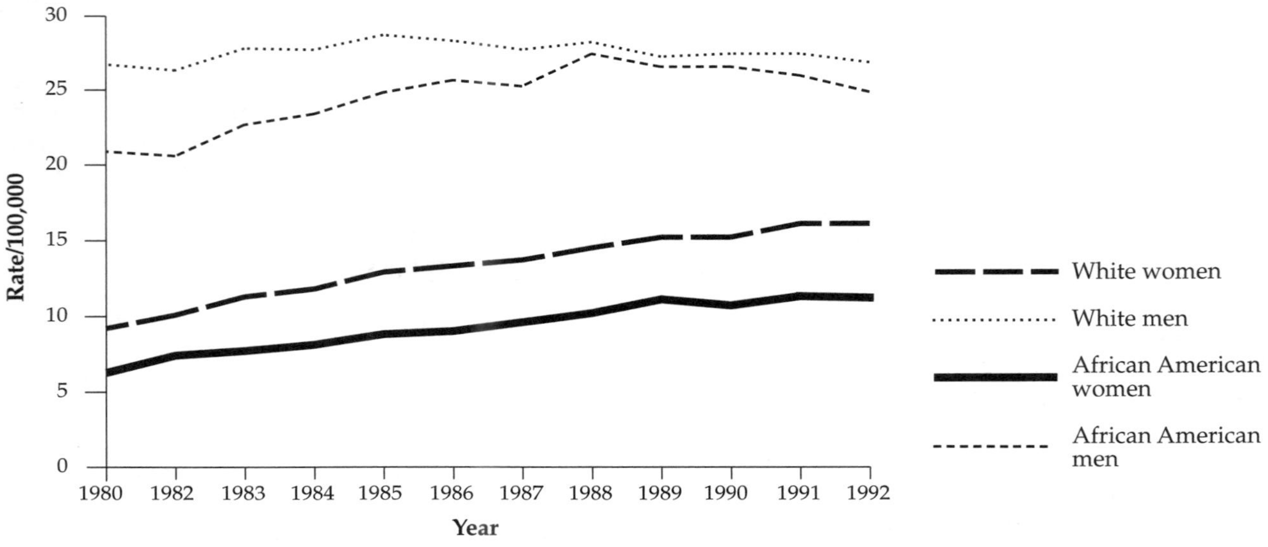

Source: National Center for Health Statistics 1995.

As in the United States, COPD mortality has increased among women worldwide (Brown et al. 1994a; Crockett et al. 1994; Guidotti and Jhangri 1994). For the period 1979–1988, Brown and colleagues (1994a) reported that COPD death rates among women increased in 16 of 31 countries they studied, remained constant in 9, and declined in 6. Increasing mortality from COPD among women was also reported from Alberta, Canada (Guidotti and Jhangri 1994), and from Australia (Crockett et al. 1994). During 1964–1990, age-standardized COPD mortality rates increased 2.6-fold among women in Australia (Crockett et al. 1994). It is difficult to correlate data on COPD trends with smoking patterns because of differences over time in the diagnostic coding of COPD from death certificates and because of scant longitudinal data on the prevalence of current smoking for many of the countries studied.

Several longitudinal studies specifically examined risk factors for mortality from COPD among women (Doll et al. 1980; USDHHS 1984, 1990; Speizer et al. 1989; Tockman and Comstock 1989; Lange et al. 1990b; Thun et al. 1995, 1997c; Friedman et al. 1997). Speizer and colleagues (1989) studied predictors of COPD mortality among 4,617 women and 3,806 men who were followed up for 9 through 12 years in the Harvard Six Cities Study of the effects of ambient air pollution on health. During the follow-up period, only 19 women and 26 men had died, but the ratio of observed-to-expected deaths from COPD generally appeared to increase with lifetime pack-years of smoking among both women and men. In the Copenhagen City Heart Study, Lange and colleagues (1990b) enrolled 7,420 women and 6,336 men from 1976 through 1978 and performed follow-ups through 1987. During this period, 47 women and 117 men died with obstructive lung disease as the underlying or contributory cause of death. Among women, with nonsmokers as the reference group, the RR for COPD-related death increased with lifetime pack-years of smoking: a RR of 6.7 (95 percent CI, 1.5 to 31) among smokers who inhaled and had less than 35 pack-years of smoking and a RR of 18.0 (95 percent CI, 1.3 to 94) among smokers who inhaled and had 35 or more pack-years of smoking. Self-report of inhalation of cigarette smoke was associated with a higher risk for COPD-related mortality among both women and men. Overall, the proportion of COPD-related mortality attributable to tobacco smoking was 90 percent among women and 78 percent among men.

Thun and colleagues (1997c) presented mortality rates for COPD in CPS-II in relation to the number of cigarettes currently smoked at baseline. The RR for death increased with the number of cigarettes smoked per day: 5.6 for 1 to 9 cigarettes per day, 7.9 for 10 to 19 cigarettes per day, 23.3 for 20 cigarettes per day, 22.9 for 21 to 39 cigarettes per day, and 25.2 for 40 cigarettes per day, all among women current smokers compared with women who had never smoked. The corresponding RRs among men current smokers compared with men who had never smoked were 8.8, 8.9, 10.4, 16.5, and 9.3.

Investigators determined mortality through 1987 in a cohort of 60,838 members of the Kaiser Permanente Medical Care Program aged 35 years or older between 1979 and 1986 (Friedman et al. 1997). The RRs for COPD mortality among women current smokers compared with women who had never smoked increased with the amount smoked, from 5.4 for 19 or fewer cigarettes per day to 13.9 for 20 or more cigarettes per day. The RRs among men were 9.2 and 10.9, respectively.

Limited data are available on the effects of smoking cessation on COPD mortality among women (USDHHS 1990). In the 22-year follow-up of 6,194 women in the British doctors' study, Doll and colleagues (1980) reported a standardized mortality ratio of 5 for chronic bronchitis and emphysema among women former smokers and a ratio of more than 10 among women current smokers. Similar overall results were found in CPS-II (USDHHS 1990). Even after 16 or more years of smoking cessation, mortality rates for COPD were higher among women who had stopped smoking than among women who had never smoked.

## Conclusions

1. Cigarette smoking is a primary cause of COPD among women, and the risk increases with the amount and duration of smoking. Approximately 90 percent of mortality from COPD among women in the United States can be attributed to cigarette smoking.
2. In utero exposure to maternal smoking is associated with reduced lung function among infants, and exposure to environmental tobacco smoke during childhood and adolescence may be associated with impaired lung function among girls.
3. Adolescent girls who smoke have reduced rates of lung growth, and adult women who smoke experience a premature decline of lung function.

4. The rate of decline in lung function is slower among women who stop smoking than among women who continue to smoke.
5. Mortality rates for COPD have increased among women over the past 20 to 30 years.
6. Although data for women are limited, former smokers appear to have a lower risk for dying from COPD than do current smokers.

# Sex Hormones, Thyroid Disorders, and Diabetes Mellitus

## Sex Hormones

Many studies have reported findings that indicate an effect of smoking on estrogen-related disorders among women (Baron et al. 1990). Women who smoke have an increased risk for disorders associated with estrogen deficiency and a decreased risk for some diseases associated with estrogen excess. Together, these patterns suggested that smoking has an "antiestrogenic" effect (Baron et al. 1990). The effects of smoking on hormone-related events (e.g., endometrial cancer) seem to be more common among postmenopausal women than among premenopausal women (Baron et al. 1990). The mechanisms underlying this effect are not clear. As discussed later in this section, it is unlikely that smoking-related changes in estrogen levels can explain this effect.

Changes in plasma levels of endogenous estradiol and estrone have not been associated with smoking among either premenopausal or postmenopausal women (Jensen et al. 1985; Friedman et al. 1987; Khaw et al. 1988; Longcope and Johnston 1988; Baron et al. 1990; Barrett-Connor 1990; Key et al. 1991; Berta et al. 1992; Cassidenti et al. 1992; Austin et al. 1993; Law et al. 1997a). In general, adjustment for weight has not altered the relationship between smoking and estrogen levels (Khaw et al. 1988; Baron et al. 1990).

Comparisons of urinary estrogen excretion among smokers and nonsmokers have not been entirely consistent. Among premenopausal women, excretion of some estrogens may be lower for smokers (MacMahon et al. 1982; Michnovicz et al. 1988; Berta et al. 1992; Westhoff et al. 1996), but details of the excretion patterns have varied among studies, and one investigation found no differences (Berta et al. 1992). One study of postmenopausal women found no association between smoking and urinary estrogen excretion (Trichopoulous et al. 1987).

Smoking clearly has effects on estrogen levels during pregnancy. Smokers have lower circulating levels of estriol (Targett et al. 1973; Mochizuki et al. 1984) and estradiol than do nonsmokers (Bernstein et al. 1989; Cuckle et al. 1990b; Petridou et al. 1990). Moreover, the conversion of dehydroepiandrosterone sulfate (DHEAS) to estradiol among pregnant smokers may be impaired (Mochizuki et al. 1984).

Jensen and colleagues (1985) showed that, among postmenopausal women taking oral estrogens and progestins for at least one year, levels of serum estrone and estradiol were lower for smokers than for nonsmokers. The results of this study, confirmed by Cassidenti and colleagues (1990), provided evidence that postmenopausal smokers who receive oral HRT have lower estradiol and estrone levels than do comparable nonsmokers. These results suggested that smoking affects the gastrointestinal absorption, distribution, or metabolism of these hormones.

Michnovicz and colleagues (1986) reported that smokers and nonsmokers metabolize estrogens differently. They found that, compared with female nonsmokers, women who smoked had a higher rate of formation of 2-hydroxyestradiol, which has virtually no estrogenic activity. In contrast, nonsmokers formed relatively more estriol, which has weak agonist properties. These findings could indicate that nonsmokers had more circulating active estrogens than did smokers. They are consistent with the increased activity of 2-hydroxylation and 4-hydroxylation in placental tissues of smokers (Chao et al. 1981; Juchau et al. 1982) and with reduced urinary excretion of estriol (Michnovicz et al. 1986, 1988; Key et al. 1996; Westhoff et al. 1996).

Data on plasma levels of testosterone among women have been inconclusive. Friedman and colleagues (1987) reported that serum testosterone concentrations were significantly higher among postmenopausal smokers than among postmenopausal nonsmokers. However, other investigators reported no association of smoking with serum levels of testosterone among postmenopausal women (Khaw et al. 1988; Cauley et al. 1989).

## Thyroid Disorders

For unknown reasons, most thyroid disorders are more common among women than among men (Larsen and Ingbar 1992). Enlargement of the thyroid gland (goiter) can occur because of inflammation, the metabolic stress of maintaining adequate thyroid hormone levels, or masses such as cysts or neoplasms. A relatively common cause of hyperthyroidism is Graves' disease, a systemic condition that typically includes hyperthyroidism with a diffuse goiter.

Several studies investigated the relationship between cigarette smoking and clinically apparent goiter, but findings have varied. Two population-based surveys of patients with a clinical diagnosis of goiter reported that the prevalence of goiter was 50 to 100 percent higher among women smokers than among women nonsmokers (Christensen et al. 1984; Ericsson and Lindgärde 1991). A study of hospital employees found that the prevalence of goiter among cigarette smokers was 10 times that among nonsmokers (30 vs. 3 percent; $p < 0.001$ for analysis of combined data for women and men) (Hegedüs et al. 1985). Other studies of women (Petersen et al. 1991) and studies in which data for women and men were combined (Bartalena et al. 1989; Prummel and Wiersinga 1993) did not find an association between smoking and goiter.

One investigation that used ultrasonography to measure thyroid volume among female smokers and nonsmokers reported that thyroid glands among smokers were 75 percent larger than those among nonsmokers (25 vs. 14 mL; $p < 0.001$) (Hegedüs et al. 1985). A small study of women and men confirmed these findings (Hegedüs et al. 1992). Another small study with a combined analysis of women and men did not find a difference between smokers and nonsmokers, but there was no adjustment for age or gender (Berghout et al. 1987).

A series of studies, mostly clinic based, have reported that cigarette smokers have a higher risk for Graves' disease with ophthalmopathy (eye involvement) than do nonsmokers (Hägg and Asplund 1987; Bartalena et al. 1989; Shine et al. 1990; Tellez et al. 1992; Prummel and Wiersinga 1993; Winsa et al. 1993). Various analyses were presented in these studies, and some made no adjustment for age and gender. Nonetheless, these findings consistently suggest that smoking modestly increases the risk for Graves' hyperthyroidism and greatly increases the risk for Graves' disease with ophthalmopathy. Only one of the studies reported results for women alone (Bartalena et al. 1989), but in most of the other investigations, at least three-fourths of the study participants were women. The data reported by Prummel and Wiersinga (1993) were analyzed in the most detail. Patients with Graves' disease who were attending an endocrinology clinic were compared with a control group selected from patients attending an ophthalmology clinic and persons accompanying patients to the endocrinology clinic. Cigarette smoking conferred a RR of 1.9 (95 percent CI, 1.1 to 3.2) for Graves' disease without ophthalmopathy and a RR of 7.7 (95 percent CI, 4.3 to 13.7) for Graves' disease with ophthalmopathy.

Data on the association of smoking with other thyroid disorders are limited. Available data have suggested, however, that smoking is not strongly associated with hypothyroidism, autoimmune thyroiditis, or autoimmune hypothyroidism (Bartalena et al. 1989; Ericsson and Lindgärde 1991; Petersen et al. 1991; Nyström et al. 1993; Prummel and Wiersinga 1993).

Comparison of the levels of the major thyroid hormones (triiodothyronine [$T_3$] and thyroxine [$T_4$]) among smokers and nonsmokers has not revealed a consistent pattern. Different investigations reported higher, lower, or equivalent hormone levels among smokers and nonsmokers (Bertelsen and Hegedüs 1994). However, in most studies, levels of thyroid-stimulating hormone (TSH) have been lower among smokers than among nonsmokers (Bertelsen and Hegedüs 1994).

These diverse effects of smoking on the thyroid gland are difficult to explain with a single mechanism. A higher prevalence of goiter among smokers than among nonsmokers would suggest that cigarette smoking impairs the synthesis or secretion of thyroid hormones. Indeed, cigarette smoke contains several substances, in particular thiocyanate, that may have such an effect (Sepkovic et al. 1984; Karakaya et al. 1987). However, evidence that TSH levels may be lower among smokers than among nonsmokers does not support such an interference with thyroid function, since TSH levels rise when patients become hypothryoid through effects on the thyroid gland. It is possible that goitrogenic effects of smoking are combined with thyroid-stimulating effects, for example, through the catecholamine release associated with smoking. The manner in which smoking increases the risk for Graves' ophthalmopathy is also not clear. Study findings suggested that thyroid-stimulating antibodies, the hallmark of this disease, are not increased among smokers (Hegedüs et al. 1992; Winsa et al. 1993).

## Diabetes Mellitus

Diabetes mellitus is a heterogeneous group of disorders, all characterized by high levels of blood glucose. The main types of diabetes have been defined as follows: type 1 (previously known as insulin-dependent diabetes mellitus), type 2 (previously known as non-insulin-dependent diabetes mellitus), gestational diabetes, and other specific types of diabetes (Expert Committee on the Diagnosis and Classification of Diabetes Mellitus 1997). Type 2 diabetes accounted for 90 to 95 percent of the estimated 5.6 million cases of diabetes diagnosed among U.S. women older than 20 years of age in 1997, and the number of undiagnosed cases of diabetes among women was estimated at 2.5 million (Harris et al. 1998). The total prevalence of diabetes (diagnosed and undiagnosed combined) is similar among women and men, and little evidence exists that suggests the risk for type 2 diabetes differs by gender (Rewers and Hamman 1995; Harris et al. 1998). The detrimental effects of smoking on diabetic complications, particularly nephropathy and macrovascular morbidity and mortality, are well established (Moy et al. 1990; Muhlhauser 1994), but only a few studies have investigated cigarette smoking as a cause of diabetes.

Type 1 diabetes often occurs among children and young adolescents, for whom smoking is uncommon. Although no studies have investigated the relationship between smoking and type 1 diabetes, three have investigated the effect of parental smoking on the risk for type 1 diabetes among children. None of them showed an association (Siemiatycki et al. 1989; Virtanen et al. 1994; Wadsworth et al. 1997). However, maternal smoking during pregnancy has been associated with the development of microalbuminuria and macroalbuminuria among term offspring who later develop type 1 diabetes (Rudberg et al. 1998).

Data on the effect of active smoking on the risk for type 2 diabetes have been conflicting. A positive association was reported among women in the U.S. Nurses' Health Study (Rimm et al. 1993) but not among women in the Tecumseh (Butler et al. 1982), Nauru (Balkau et al. 1985), or Framingham (Wilson et al. 1986) studies or among Pima Indian women (Hanson et al. 1995).

The U.S. Nurses' Health Study (Rimm et al. 1993) was the largest and most rigorous of these studies. Self-reported information on cigarette smoking, other behavioral risk factors, and diagnosis of diabetes was updated every 2 years during 12 years of follow-up. Supplementary questionnaires elicited information on diabetes symptoms, blood glucose levels, and the use of hypoglycemic medications. The data were used to apply established criteria to confirm reported diabetes. The investigators reviewed medical records for a random sample of women who reported a diagnosis of diabetes and judged the validity of the confirmation of diabetes to be high. After adjustment for age, BMI, family history of diabetes, menopausal status, hormone use, alcohol intake, and physical activity, the RR for diabetes among smokers compared with nonsmokers was 1.0 (95 percent CI, 0.8 to 1.2) for women who smoked 1 to 14 cigarettes per day, 1.2 (95 percent CI, 0.99 to 1.4) for women who smoked 15 to 24 cigarettes per day, and 1.4 (95 percent CI, 1.2 to 1.7) for women who smoked more than 25 cigarettes per day. Tests for trends across the three levels of current cigarette consumption were statistically significant ($p < 0.01$) in all analyses. The RR for diabetes among women former smokers compared with women who had never smoked was 1.1 (95 percent CI, 1.0 to 1.2). Further adjustment for hypertension; total caloric intake; and intakes of vegetable fat, potassium, calcium, and magnesium did not alter the estimates. Moreover, heightened detection of diabetes among smokers did not explain the relationship observed: the number of physician visits did not differ between women current smokers and women who had never smoked, and restriction of the model to women with symptoms of diabetes did not alter the results.

In contrast, none of the other follow-up studies of women (Butler et al. 1982; Balkau et al. 1985; Wilson et al. 1986; McPhillips et al. 1990; Hanson et al. 1995) found a significant association between cigarette smoking and the risk for type 2 diabetes. Not all studies, however, adequately controlled for diabetes risk factors. For example, the lack of adjustment for alcohol intake in the Framingham study (Wilson et al. 1986) may have masked the relationship between smoking and type 2 diabetes, because alcohol intake is correlated with smoking and may be negatively associated with type 2 diabetes (Stampfer et al. 1988a; Rimm et al. 1995). Nonetheless, smoking did not predict progression to diabetes, even after multiple covariates were controlled for, in two studies of women and men with impaired glucose tolerance (Keen et al. 1982; King et al. 1984). In one of these studies, smoking status was also not related to reversion to normoglycemia (Keen et al. 1982). Findings from studies examining the relationship between smoking and diabetes among men are similarly conflicting (Medalie et al. 1975; Butler et al. 1982; Balkau et al. 1985; Wilson et al. 1986; Ohlson et al. 1988; Feskens and Kromhout 1989; Shaten et al. 1993; Hanson et al. 1995; Perry et al. 1995; Rimm et al. 1995; Kawakami et al. 1997).

Data on the relationship between gestational diabetes and cigarette smoking have also not been consistent. In one study, more than 10,000 pregnant women in New York City underwent screening for glucose intolerance. They were given 50 g of glucose, and blood glucose was measured one hour later. Those with a blood glucose level higher than 135 mg/dL were further evaluated with a three-hour glucose tolerance test. Cigarette smoking during pregnancy was determined from a computer database drawn from medical records. Smoking was unrelated to gestational diabetes (RR, 0.8; 95 percent CI, 0.5 to 1.2) (Berkowitz et al. 1992). In a population-based study using birth certificate data abstracted from medical records, no association was found between smoking and a clinical diagnosis of gestational diabetes (Heckbert et al. 1988). Finally, in a cohort study of 116,000 female nurses aged 25 through 42 years, the multivariate RR for diagnosis of gestational diabetes during follow-up was 1.4 (95 percent CI, 1.1 to 1.8) among current smokers and 0.9 (95 percent CI, 0.8 to 1.1) among former smokers (Solomon et al. 1997).

Smoking appears to be associated with metabolic processes related to diabetes, including glucose homeostasis, hyperinsulinemia, and insulin resistance. Among both women and men with normal glucose tolerance, levels of hemoglobin $A_{1c}$, which reflect glucose levels in the previous few months, have been reported to be higher among smokers than among nonsmokers (Modan et al. 1988). In one study of 40 persons without diabetes (28 women and 12 men), a higher proportion of smokers than nonsmokers had hyperinsulinemia in response to a glucose tolerance test challenge (75 g of glucose given orally) (Facchini et al. 1992). Also, smokers have been found to be more insulin resistant than nonsmokers in response to a continuous infusion of glucose, insulin, and somatostatin (Modan et al. 1988). Other studies reported similar findings (Boyle et al. 1989; Eliasson et al. 1994; Zavaroni et al. 1994; Frati et al. 1996), although contradictory results have also been published (Nilsson et al. 1995; Mooy et al. 1998). The degree of insulin resistance may be related to the number of cigarettes smoked. In a study of 57 middle-aged male smokers, insulin resistance increased with increasing daily cigarette consumption (Eliasson et al. 1994).

The mechanisms that underlie these findings are not clear. Smoking may directly affect pancreatic insulin secretion, or the association of smoking with increased circulating levels of counterregulatory hormones, such as cortisol and catecholamines, may play a role. Moreover, higher levels of androstenedione and DHEAS have been observed among women who smoke. Hyperandrogenicity has been associated with a higher risk for type 2 diabetes (Lindstedt et al. 1991; Haffner et al. 1993; Andersson et al. 1994; Goodman-Gruen and Barrett-Connor 1997), but it is not known whether insulin resistance precedes or follows androgen excess. Smoking has been associated with upper-body fat distribution (see "Body Weight and Fat Distribution" later in this chapter), which is related to increased basal levels of insulin (Wing et al. 1991), two-hour postload plasma glucose (Wing et al. 1991; Mooy et al. 1995), two-hour postload insulin (Wing et al. 1991), and increased risk for type 2 diabetes (Björntorp 1988; Kaye et al. 1990; Carey et al. 1997).

## Conclusions

1. Women who smoke have an increased risk for estrogen-deficiency disorders and a decreased risk for estrogen-dependent disorders, but circulating levels of the major endogenous estrogens are not altered among women smokers.
2. Although consistent effects of smoking on thyroid hormone levels have not been noted, cigarette smokers may have an increased risk for Graves' ophthalmopathy, a thyroid-related disease.
3. Smoking appears to affect glucose regulation and related metabolic processes, but conflicting data exist on the relationship of smoking and the development of type 2 diabetes mellitus and gestational diabetes among women.

# Menstrual Function, Menopause, and Benign Gynecologic Conditions

Menstruation and menopause are normal aspects of female physiology, but they can affect a woman's well-being and quality of life (Daly et al. 1993; Jarrett et al. 1995). The effects of menopause on health go beyond cessation of menses. Many U.S. women now live one-half of their adult lives after menopause; the accompanying hormonal changes may result in symptoms and may also adversely affect the risk for disorders such as osteoporosis.

Menstrual disturbances and menopause are difficult to describe and study. No generally accepted definitions exist for dysmenorrhea (pain and discomfort during menstruation), menstrual irregularity (variable duration of the menstrual cycle), or amenorrhea (absence of menses). Moreover, some hormonal disturbances of menopause may precede the cessation of menstruation by several years. Menstrual symptoms and the timing of menses vary, and the point at which normal variation is exceeded and a true disorder exists may be difficult to define. Secondary amenorrhea (amenorrhea among women who have ever menstruated) also includes a continuum of menstrual irregularity, and sometimes the distinction between secondary amenorrhea and early menopause is difficult. The duration of amenorrhea required for menopause has varied in the literature. Currently, 12 months of amenorrhea is generally accepted as the definition of menopause (McKinlay 1996).

This presentation summarizes research on the relationship between cigarette smoking and several aspects of menstrual function, including dysmenorrhea, menstrual irregularity, secondary amenorrhea, and natural menopause.

## Menstrual Function and Menstrual Symptoms

Studies have investigated the relationship between smoking and dysmenorrhea (Table 3.29) or amenorrhea (Table 3.30). Some of these were cross-sectional investigations that could not directly address whether smoking led to the menstrual symptoms or whether the menstrual symptoms led to smoking. The proportion of women who reported dysmenorrhea varied widely across studies; these differences may be due to several other factors, including variation in the age of the participants and in the definitions of dysmenorrhea or amenorrhea. Except for a survey of 19-year-old women (Andersch and Milsom 1982), most studies found the prevalence of dysmenorrhea to be higher among current smokers than among former smokers or women who had never smoked (Kauraniemi 1969; Wood 1978; Wood et al. 1979; Sloss and Frerichs 1983; Brown et al. 1988; Pullon et al. 1988; Teperi and Rimpelä 1989; Sundell et al. 1990; Parazzini et al. 1994) (Table 3.29). The majority of studies did not report RRs, but the findings suggested that the prevalence of self-reported amenorrhea tends to be about 50 percent higher among smokers than among nonsmokers.

One survey found a weak trend of increasing prevalence of dysmenorrhea with increasing amount smoked (Wood et al. 1979) (Table 3.29). In a case-control study of women seeking care for pelvic symptoms at a clinic in Italy, smokers of 1 to 9 cigarettes daily were no more likely than nonsmokers to have dysmenorrhea, but the adjusted RR was 1.9 (95 percent CI, 0.8 to 5.0) among women who smoked 10 or more cigarettes daily (Parazzini et al. 1994). The adjusted RR was particularly high (3.4; 95 percent CI, 1.3 to 8.9) among long-term smokers (9 to 20 years). A follow-up study found that the mean duration of menstrual pain was 0.4 days longer among smokers than among nonsmokers (Hornsby et al. 1998). Other surveys also reported increasing risk for dysmenorrhea with increasing numbers of cigarettes smoked but did not present details (Pullon et al. 1988; Sundell et al. 1990).

Four studies of smoking and dysmenorrhea took into account the possible effects of multiple covariates, such as age, alcohol intake, and use of OCs (Table 3.29). A study from New Zealand found an independent effect of smoking on dysmenorrhea, but no estimate of RR was given (Pullon et al. 1988). In the study of clinic patients in Italy, the effect of smoking persisted after adjustment for multiple factors (Parazzini et al. 1994), but a Finnish investigation reported that the statistical significance of the effect of smoking was lost after adjustment for alcohol use, physical activity, gynecologic history, and health practices (Teperi and Rimpelä 1989). In a U.S. study, women who smoked reported about a half-day more pain with menses than did nonsmokers (Hornsby et al. 1998) (Table 3.29).

Data on menstrual irregularity and secondary amenorrhea are less extensive (Table 3.30). In a few surveys, the proportion of current smokers who reported menstrual irregularity and intermenstrual

**Table 3.29. Findings regarding smoking and dysmenorrhea**

| Study | Study type/ population | Findings | Comment |
|---|---|---|---|
| Kauraniemi 1969 | Population survey<br>Aged 25–60 years<br>Finland | Prevalence of dysmenorrhea<br>2,446 never smoked: 7.2%<br>258 former smokers: 9.7%<br>786 current smokers: 13.4% | |
| Wood et al. 1979 | Clinic survey<br>Aged 15–59 years<br>Australia | Prevalence of dysmenorrhea<br>227 never smoked: 37%<br>72 former smokers: 43%<br>227 current smokers: 60% | Weak trend of increasing prevalence of dysmenorrhea with increasing amount smoked |
| Andersch and Milsom 1982 | Population survey<br>Aged 19 years<br>Sweden | 573 participants<br>Statistically significant inverse association between dysmenorrhea score and smoking | |
| Brown et al. 1988 | Medical practice-based survey<br>Aged 18–49 years<br>England | Prevalence of dysmenorrhea<br>1,006 never smoked: 30.5%<br>458 former smokers: 32.1%<br>628 current smokers: 36.0% | |
| Pullon et al. 1988 | Medical practice-based survey<br>Aged 16–54 years<br>New Zealand | 1,826 participants<br>Higher prevalence of dysmenorrhea among smokers than among nonsmokers<br>Apparent dose-response pattern | |
| Teperi and Rimpelä 1989 | Population sample<br>Aged 12–18 years<br>Finland | Prevalence of dysmenorrhea<br>546 nonsmokers: 19%<br>221 occasional smokers: 25%<br>253 daily smokers: 31% | Association with smoking not statistically significant after adjustment for alcohol use, physical activity, gynecologic history, health practices |
| Sundell et al. 1990 | Population survey<br>Aged 19 years at start of 5-year follow-up<br>Sweden | Prevalence of dysmenorrhea<br>269 nonsmokers: 25.7%<br>198 current smokers: 40.4% | Dose-response pattern found |
| Parazzini et al. 1994 | Case-control study<br>Clinic patients<br>Aged 15–44 years<br>Italy | Relative risk for dysmenorrhea for current smokers of 10–30 cigarettes/day: 1.9 (95% confidence interval, 0.9–4.2) | Findings similar after adjustment for education, alcohol use, menstrual flow |
| Hornsby et al. 1998 | Follow-up study<br>Aged 37–39 years<br>United States | Mean duration of pain with menses<br>275 nonsmokers: 2 days<br>83 smokers: 2.5 days | |

**Table 3.30. Findings regarding smoking and menstrual irregularity or secondary amenorrhea**

| Study | Study type/ population | Findings | |
|---|---|---|---|
| | | Menstrual irregularity | Secondary amenorrhea |
| Hammond 1961 | Cohort study<br>Aged 30–39 years<br>United States | Prevalence<br>1,050 never smoked: 16.3%*<br>842 current smokers: 18.2%* | |
| Pettersson et al. 1973 | Population survey<br>Aged 18–45 years<br>Sweden | | Prevalence<br>824 never smoked: 3.7%<br>262 former smokers: 5.9%<br>773 current smokers: 4.8% |
| Brown et al. 1988 | Medical practice-based survey<br>Aged 18–49 years<br>England | Prevalence<br>1,006 never smoked: 8.9%<br>458 former smokers: 9.0%<br>628 current smokers: 14.6% | |
| Davies et al. 1990 | Case-control study<br>Clinic patients<br>Aged 16–40 years<br>England | | Unadjusted relative risk for ever smoking and amenorrhea = 2.1† |
| Johnson and Whitaker 1992 | Population survey<br>High school students<br>United States | | Adjusted relative risk for smokers of ≥1 pack/day: 2.0 (95% confidence interval, 1.2–3.1) |
| Hornsby et al. 1998 | Follow-up study<br>Aged 37–39 years<br>United States | Standard deviation of cycle length<br>275 nonsmokers: 2.1 days<br>83 smokers: 2.5 days | |

*Amenorrhea among women who ever had menstrual periods.
†Computed from data presented in report.

bleeding was modestly higher than that of nonsmokers (Hammond 1961; Wood 1978; Sloss and Frerichs 1983; Brown et al. 1988). The menstrual cycle length of smokers seems to be more variable than that of nonsmokers (Hornsby et al. 1998; Windham et al. 1999b). Smokers also appear to have shorter cycles on average (Zumoff et al. 1990; Hornsby et al. 1998; Windham et al. 1999b). Some studies have found that smoking was associated with an increased prevalence of secondary amenorrhea (Davies et al. 1990; Johnson and Whitaker 1992). For example, 2,544 high school girls were asked about their menstrual patterns and use of cigarettes (Johnson and Whitaker 1992). The RR for having missed three or more menstrual cycles was 2.0 (95 percent CI, 1.2 to 3.1) among girls who smoked one or more packs of cigarettes per day compared with nonsmokers, after multiple covariates were controlled for. The results of other investigations, however, did not suggest such an effect. In a study from Sweden, no substantial differences were found between smokers and nonsmokers after adjustment for the effects of age, OC use, and other factors (Pettersson et al. 1973). In another study, the unadjusted RR for secondary amenorrhea among women who had ever smoked was less than 1.0 (Gold et al. 1994).

## Age at Natural Menopause

The age at which menopause naturally occurs varies considerably among women. The factors that determine this variation are not well understood, and smoking is the only factor consistently associated with age at natural menopause.

Three cohort studies have reported relevant data (Table 3.31). In the Framingham study (McNamara et al. 1978), the mean age at menopause was about 0.8 years earlier among smokers than among nonsmokers.

In the U.S. Nurses' Health Study (Willett et al. 1983), the effect of smoking was greater: the median age at menopause among women who smoked 35 or more cigarettes per day was 2.0 years earlier than that among women who had never smoked. The RR for the occurrence of natural menopause was higher among smokers in all age categories, but the RRs tended to decrease with increasing age. Thus, among women aged 40 through 44 years, the RR for menopause (adjusted for weight) was 2.1 (95 percent CI, 1.7 to 2.7) for current smokers compared with women who had never smoked. Among women aged 50 through 55 years, the RR was 1.2 (95 percent CI, 1.1 to 1.3). The risk for menopause among former smokers was similar to that among women who had never smoked. In a follow-up study, the RR for menopause among current smokers compared with nonsmokers was 2.3 (McKinlay et al. 1992).

In a case-control study in Scotland, smoking strongly increased the risk for menopause among women aged 45 through 49 years, and a dose-response relationship with pack-years of smoking was demonstrated (Torgerson et al. 1994). Multivariate-adjusted RR estimates were similar with menopause defined as 6 and as 12 months of amenorrhea—2.3 and 2.7, respectively, among women with more than 20 pack-years of smoking compared with women who had never smoked. A case-control study of women hospitalized in Milan, Italy, found that smokers were less likely than nonsmokers to have menstrual periods at age 52 years (Parazzini et al. 1992b), and another case-control study found that women who had ever smoked had a higher risk for early menopause (age <47 years) than did nonsmokers (Cramer et al. 1995).

In a pooled analysis of findings from several cross-sectional surveys, the RR for being postmenopausal was 1.9 (95 percent CI, 1.7 to 2.2) among current smokers compared with women who had never smoked; risk increased with increasing amount smoked (Midgette and Baron 1990). The RR among former smokers was 1.3 (95 percent CI, 1.0 to 1.7), which suggested either that former smokers had not used tobacco as heavily as current smokers did or that the effect of smoking is largely reversible with cessation.

Numerous studies summarized the relationship between smoking and age at natural menopause by reporting the mean or median age at menopause among smokers and nonsmokers (Table 3.31). These data have been quite consistent: menopause occurs one or two years earlier among smokers than among nonsmokers. In several reports, the median or mean age at menopause was earlier among heavy smokers than among light smokers (McNamara et al. 1978; Adena and Gallagher 1982; McKinlay et al. 1985), but formal dose-response analyses were not conducted. Among former smokers, age at menopause was between that of women who had never smoked and that of current smokers (Adena and Gallagher 1982).

The mechanisms by which cigarette smoking might lead to an early menopause are not clear, but several possibilities have been advanced (Midgette and Baron 1990). Components of cigarette smoke, possibly PAHs, are toxic to ovaries in animals (Mattison 1980; Magers et al. 1995). In rodents, prolonged exposure to cigarette smoke seems to be associated with follicular atresia. Effects of nicotine on regulation of gonadotropins or sex hormone metabolism could also contribute to a detrimental effect of cigarette smoking on ovarian function (Midgette and Baron 1990).

## Menopausal Symptoms

Although data on the association between smoking and symptoms of menopause are limited, at least some menopausal symptoms appear to be more common among smokers. One survey of postmenopausal women found no overall association between cigarette smoking and hot flashes during menopause, but among thin women (BMI <24.3 $kg/m^2$), smokers reported this symptom significantly more often than did nonsmokers (Schwingl et al. 1994). In a population sample of perimenopausal women, smoking was associated with vasomotor symptoms, largely hot flashes (Collins and Landgren 1995). Similarly, surveys from Australia and England also reported that smokers were more likely than nonsmokers to have menopausal symptoms (Greenberg et al. 1987; Dennerstein et al. 1993). Women who smoke also have been reported to have increased risk for hot flashes after hysterectomy and oophorectomy (Langenberg et al. 1997). Smokers also may tend to have a shorter perimenopausal period than do nonsmokers (McKinlay et al. 1992).

## Endometriosis

Endometriosis, the presence of endometrial tissue outside the uterus, most commonly in the pelvis, is classically associated with dysmenorrhea, dyspareunia, and infertility. The prevalence of endometriosis has been difficult to assess in population-based studies because the disorder may be asymptomatic or may have nonspecific symptoms. Thus, its diagnosis may require invasive investigation (Houston et al. 1988). The best available estimate of incidence derives

**Table 3.31. Smoking and age at natural menopause**

| Study | Population | Duration of amenorrhea before menopause | Smoking status comparison | Decrease in mean or median age at menopause (years) |
|---|---|---|---|---|
| Bailey et al. 1977 | 475 participants in health screening program<br>United Kingdom | NR* | Current vs. former and never | 1.3† |
| Jick et al. 1977 | 1,842 hospital patients<br>1,253 hospital patients<br>United States | NR<br>NR | Current vs. never<br>Current vs. never | 1.7†<br>1.3† |
| McNamara et al. 1978 | 926 from general population<br>United States | 12 months | Current vs. never and former | 0.8‡ |
| Lindquist and Bengtsson 1979 | 873 from population sample<br>Sweden | 5 months | Current vs. never and former | 1.2† |
| Kaufman et al. 1980 | 656 hospital patients<br>United States | NR | Current vs. never<br>Former vs. never | 1.7§<br>0.2§ |
| Adena and Gallagher 1982 | 10,995 participants in multiphasic health screening program<br>Australia | 6 months | Current vs. never<br>Former vs. never | 1.0†<br>0.4‡ |
| Andersen et al. 1982b | 5,645 from population sample<br>Denmark | 6 months | Current vs. never and former | 1.0‡ |

*NR = Value not specified in report of study.
†Difference in mean ages.
‡Difference in median ages.
§Difference in ages at menopause computed by Adena and Gallagher (1982).

from a study of white women in Rochester, Minnesota (Houston et al. 1987). The findings suggested that each year approximately 0.3 percent of women aged 15 through 49 years receive a new diagnosis of endometriosis.

The association between endometriosis and smoking has been examined in numerous case-control studies (Cramer et al. 1986; FitzSimmons et al. 1987; Phipps et al. 1987; Parazzini et al. 1989; Darrow et al. 1993; Matorras et al. 1995; Sangi-Haghpeykar and Poindexter 1995; Signorello et al. 1997; Bérubé et al. 1998). Five of these studies included only cases associated with infertility (Cramer et al. 1986; FitzSimmons et al. 1987; Matorras et al. 1995; Signorello et al. 1997; Bérubé et al. 1998). All the studies except one (FitzSimmons et al. 1987) adjusted for potential confounding factors. The RRs for endometriosis associated with smoking were generally less than 1.0, typically approximately 0.7 (Cramer et al. 1986; FitzSimmons et al. 1987; Phipps et al. 1987; Darrow et al. 1993; Matorras et al. 1995; Sangi-Haghpeykar and Poindexter 1995), but in none of the studies was the inverse association statistically significant. In contrast to these findings, one study reported that women who had ever smoked had a nonsignificant increase in risk for endometriosis (Signorello et al. 1997), and two others found no association (Parazzini et al. 1989; Bérubé et al. 1998).

Endometriosis is considered an estrogen-dependent condition. Because of the antiestrogenic effect of smoking (Baron et al. 1990), it is plausible that smoking might lower the risk for this disorder. The available data are consistent with a protective effect, but no RR

**Table 3.31. Continued**

| Study | Population | Duration of amenorrhea before menopause | Smoking status comparison | Decrease in mean or median age at menopause (years) |
|---|---|---|---|---|
| Willett et al. 1983 | 66,663 nurses<br>United States | NR | Current (15–25 cigarettes/ day) vs. never | 1.4‡ |
| McKinlay et al. 1985 | 5,350 from population sample<br>United States | 12 months | Current vs. never and former | 1.7‡ |
| Everson et al. 1986 | 261 controls<br>United States | NR | Current vs. never | 1.1‡ |
| Hiatt and Fireman 1986 | 5,346 health maintenance organization members with multiphasic health examination<br>United States | NR | Current vs. never<br>Former vs. never | 0.9†<br>0.5† |
| Stanford et al. 1987a | 1,472 participants in mammography screening program<br>United States | 3 months | Ever vs. never | 0.3‡ |
| McKinlay et al. 1992 | 2,570 from population sample<br>United States | 12 months | Current vs. never and former | 1.8‡ |
| Luoto et al. 1994 | 1,505 from population sample<br>Finland | NR | Current vs. never and former | 1.6‡ |

†Difference in mean ages.
‡Difference in median ages.

estimate in published studies was significantly different from 1.0.

## Uterine Fibroids

Uterine fibroids (leiomyomas) are benign tumors of the uterine musculature that are believed to be estrogen dependent. Leiomyomas are typically diagnosed by clinical examination and ultrasonography. Because they may be asymptomatic, the prevalence of these tumors in the population is difficult to assess. Leiomyomas may affect fecundity, possibly by inhibiting conception or affecting implantation or completion of pregnancy (Buttram and Reiter 1981; Vollenhoven et al. 1990).

Four case-control studies (Ross et al. 1986; Parazzini et al. 1988, 1997; Samadi et al. 1996) and two cohort studies (Wyshak et al. 1986; Marshall et al. 1998) investigated the epidemiology of leiomyomas in detail. These studies reported evidence of a protective effect of smoking against leiomyomas; RRs generally ranged from 0.5 among heavy smokers to 0.8 among all smokers. In three investigations, risk decreased with increasing number of cigarettes smoked per day (Ross et al. 1986; Parazzini et al. 1988, 1997). In the Walnut Creek cohort study, Ramcharan and colleagues (1981) also reported a slightly decreased risk for uterine leiomyomas among heavy smokers but did not provide RR estimates. In contrast, Matsunaga and Shiota (1980) found less smoking among Japanese women who had undergone hysterectomy for leiomyomas during pregnancy than among women who had normal pregnancies or induced abortion, but the difference was not statistically significant. In one investigation, no protective effect was found against leiomyomas among former smokers (Parazzini et al. 1988). This finding suggested that the protective effect is reversible, but the duration of smoking cessation was not defined in the study. Another investigation of premenopausal women reported only weak evidence of an inverse association between smoking and uterine leiomyomas (Marshall et al. 1998).

Because of the antiestrogenic effect of cigarette smoking (Baron et al. 1990), a protective effect for uterine leiomyomas is biologically plausible, but this mechanism has not been examined extensively.

### Ovarian Cysts

Two studies reported a higher risk for ovarian cysts among women who smoked cigarettes than among nonsmokers (Wyshak et al. 1988; Holt et al. 1994). In one of these studies, both current and former smokers had a higher risk than nonsmokers, but information on the type of cysts was not well documented (Wyshak et al. 1988). The other study showed an association between current smoking and the occurrence of functional ovarian cysts (Holt et al. 1994). An Italian study, however, did not find an association between smoking and the development of serous, mucinous, or endometrial ovarian cysts (Parazzini et al. 1989).

### Conclusions

1. Some studies suggest that cigarette smoking may alter menstrual function by increasing the risks for dysmenorrhea (painful menstruation), secondary amenorrhea (lack of menses among women who ever had menstrual periods), and menstrual irregularity.
2. Women smokers have a younger age at natural menopause than do nonsmokers and may experience more menopausal symptoms.
3. Women who smoke may have decreased risk for uterine fibroids.

## Reproductive Outcomes

Cigarette smoking has clinically significant effects on many aspects of reproduction. Recent research has clarified the effects of smoking on fertility, maternal conditions, pregnancy, birth outcomes, breastfeeding, and risk for sudden infant death syndrome (SIDS).

### Delayed Conception and Infertility

The 1988 National Survey of Family Growth (Mosher and Pratt 1990) estimated that more than two million married couples in the United States are affected by fertility problems. Delayed conception results from a low probability of conception per menstrual cycle (Baird et al. 1986); infertility is commonly defined as the failure to conceive after unprotected sexual intercourse over a period of 12 months (Marchbanks et al. 1989). In primary infertility a woman has had no previous conception, whereas in secondary infertility at least one previous conception has occurred. Because smoking is associated with early spontaneous abortion (see "Spontaneous Abortion" later in this section), a distinction also should be made between absence of conception and very early pregnancy loss. These conditions represent two separate causes of impairment of fertility—inability to conceive and inability to carry a pregnancy to live birth.

The way in which smoking is analyzed may affect the results of studies of fertility. As noted later in this section, several investigations suggested that some effects of smoking on reproduction do not occur among former smokers. Thus, estimates for RR for infertility or conception delay among current and former smokers considered together (as ever smokers) are likely to be lower than those among current smokers. Also, several potential confounding variables need to be considered in analyses of smoking and reproductive outcomes. Maternal age is especially important because it strongly influences a woman's ability to conceive and because it is also related to the likelihood of smoking (see "Cigarette Smoking Among Pregnant Women and Girls" in Chapter 2).

### Delayed Conception

Several cohort studies have evaluated the effect of smoking on pregnancy rates through follow-up among women who were attempting to become pregnant and have assessed the experiences of women who were already pregnant (Tables 3.32 and 3.33).

Almost all of these investigations found that women who smoked became pregnant less quickly than did nonsmokers. Over defined periods of time, the pregnancy rates among smokers were typically only 60 to 90 percent of those among nonsmokers (Baird and Wilcox 1985; Howe et al. 1985; de Mouzon et al. 1988; Weinberg et al. 1989; Joesoef et al. 1993; Joffe and Li 1994; Bolumar et al. 1996; Curtis et al. 1997; Spinelli et al. 1997). Several studies reported trends of increasing time to conception with increasing amount smoked (Howe et al. 1985; Bolumar et al. 1996; Curtis et al. 1997; Hull et al. 2000). Other studies examined risk factors for conception delays; most of these investigations found maternal smoking to be associated with an increased risk for delay (Olsen et al. 1983; Harlap and Baras 1984; Suonio et al. 1990; Olsen 1991; Laurent et al. 1992; Alderete et al. 1995; Bolumar et al. 1996). The effect of cigarette smoking appears to be reversible: several investigators have found similar conception rates among former smokers and those who had never smoked (Howe et al. 1985; Laurent et al. 1992; Joesoef et al. 1993; Curtis et al. 1997).

## Infertility

A series of case-control studies have found current cigarette smoking to be associated with an increased risk for both primary and secondary infertility (Olsen et al. 1983; Cramer et al. 1985; Daling et al. 1987; Phipps et al. 1987; Joesoef et al. 1993; Tzonou et al. 1993) (Table 3.34). Infertility attributable to disease of the fallopian tubes in particular has repeatedly been reported among smokers (Cramer et al. 1985; Daling et al. 1987; Phipps et al. 1987). Like the cohort studies of delayed conception, no case-control study found an excess risk for infertility among former smokers (Daling et al. 1987; Phipps et al. 1987; Joesoef et al. 1993).

At least 10 investigations have compared the experience of smoking and nonsmoking women who underwent assisted reproduction such as in vitro fertilization (Trapp et al. 1986; Harrison et al. 1990; Elenbogen et al. 1991; Pattinson et al. 1991; Hughes et al. 1992; Rosevear et al. 1992; Rowlands et al. 1992; Sharara et al. 1994; Hughes and Brennan 1996; Sterzik et al. 1996; Van Voorhis et al. 1996). Some of those investigations reported findings consistent with an effect of smoking on the physiology of reproduction: lower peak serum estradiol levels during ovarian stimulation among smokers than among nonsmokers (Elenbogen et al. 1991; Gustafson et al. 1996; Sterzik et al. 1996; Van Voorhis et al. 1996) and lower concentrations of estradiol in follicular fluid among smokers (Elenbogen et al. 1991; Van Voorhis et al. 1992; Gustafson et al. 1996). Although the number of oocytes retrieved during assisted reproduction depends strongly on a woman's age, only one study adjusted for age in reporting associations with smoking (Van Voorhis et al. 1992). This study found an inverse relationship between pack-years of smoking and the number of oocytes retrieved. The largest relevant study (Harrison et al. 1990) did not adjust for age but did stratify by the number of cigarettes smoked per day. A nonsignificant trend toward fewer retrieved oocytes was noted with increasing number of cigarettes smoked. Further evidence of ovarian pathology derives from findings that smokers have a poor ovarian response to the clomiphene citrate challenge test (Navot et al. 1987).

The effect of smoking on fertilization and pregnancy rates during in vitro fertilization has varied widely in different investigations, but some studies indicated that smoking by women who were attempting to become pregnant may be detrimental (Hughes and Brennan 1996; Feichtinger et al. 1997). Only two of these analyses formally adjusted for age (Hughes et al. 1994; Van Voorhis et al. 1996), so it is possible that differences in age between smokers and nonsmokers may have affected these findings. Three studies reported that smokers had a significantly lower fertilization rate than did nonsmokers (Elenbogen et al. 1991; Rosevear et al. 1992; Rowlands et al. 1992); other investigations reported significantly fewer clinical pregnancies (Harrison et al. 1990; Gustafson et al. 1996; Van Voorhis et al. 1996; Chung et al. 1997) or nonsignificantly lower pregnancy rates (Trapp et al. 1986; Elenbogen et al. 1991) among women who smoked. In one investigation, smokers had modestly lower fertilization and implantation rates and an increased tendency for spontaneous abortion (Pattinson et al. 1991). Together, these factors resulted in a lower rate of successful delivery. However, other studies reported similar fertilization and pregnancy rates among smokers and nonsmokers (Hughes et al. 1994; Sharara et al. 1994; Sterzik et al. 1996).

Several reviews have provided useful summaries of clinical and laboratory data on the mechanisms by which smoking may affect female fertility (Stillman et al. 1986; Gindoff and Tidey 1989; Mattison et al. 1989a; Yeh and Barbieri 1989; Baron et al. 1990). Animal studies have found adverse effects of nicotine, cigarette smoke, and PAHs on the release of gonadotropins, formation of corpora lutea, gamete interaction, tubal function, and implantation of fertilized ova (Gindoff and Tidey 1989; Mattison et al. 1989b).

**Table 3.32. Relative risks for conception among women smokers**

| Study | Study type | Population | Study period | Smoking status | Relative conception rate (95% confidence interval) |
|---|---|---|---|---|---|
| Baird and Wilcox 1985 | Retrospective survey | 678 pregnant women United States | 1983 | Nonsmokers | 1.0 |
| | | | | Smokers | 0.7 (0.6–0.9) |
| | | | | ≤20 cigarettes/day | 0.8 (0.6–0.9) |
| | | | | >20 cigarettes/day | 0.6 (0.4–0.9) |
| Howe et al. 1985 | Cohort | 6,199 episodes of attempted conception United Kingdom | 1968–1983 | Never smoked | 1.0 |
| | | | | Former smokers | 1.0 (0.9–1.1) |
| | | | | Current smokers | |
| | | | | 1–5 cigarettes/day | 1.0 (0.9–1.1) |
| | | | | 6–10 cigarettes/day | 1.0 (0.9–1.1) |
| | | | | 11–15 cigarettes/day | 0.9 (0.8–1.0) |
| | | | | 16–20 cigarettes/day | 0.8 (0.7–0.9) |
| | | | | ≥21 cigarettes/day | 0.8 (0.6–1.0) |
| de Mouzon et al. 1988 | Cohort | 1,887 women with planned pregnancies France | 1977–1982 | Nonsmokers | 1.0 |
| | | | | Smokers | 0.9 (0.6–1.2) |
| Weinberg et al. 1989 | Cohort | 221 women with planned pregnancies United States | 1983–1985 | Nonsmokers | 1.0 |
| | | | | Smokers | 0.6 (0.3–1.0) |
| Joesoef et al. 1993 | Survey on deliveries | 2,817 women with planned pregnancies United States | 1981–1983 | Never smoked | 1.0 |
| | | | | Former smokers | 1.0 (0.9–1.1) |
| | | | | Current smokers | 0.9 (0.8–1.0) |
| Florack et al. 1994 | Cohort | 259 women planning pregnancy The Netherlands | 1987–1989 | Nonsmokers | 1.0 |
| | | | | Smokers | |
| | | | | 1–10 cigarettes/day | 1.4 (0.9–2.2) |
| | | | | >10 cigarettes/day | 0.8 (0.5–1.3) |
| Joffe and Li 1994 | Retrospective cohort | 2,942 women enrolled at birth of infant United Kingdom | 1991 | Nonsmokers | 1.0 |
| | | | | Smokers | 0.9 (0.8–1.0) |
| Curtis et al. 1997 | Retrospective cohort | 2,607 women with planned pregnancies Canada | 1986 | Nonsmokers | 1.0 |
| | | | | Former smokers | 1.0 (0.8–1.1) |
| | | | | Smokers | 0.9 (0.8–1.0) |
| | | | | 1–5 cigarettes/day | 1.1 (0.9–1.3) |
| | | | | 6–10 cigarettes/day | 1.0 (0.9–1.2) |
| | | | | 11–20 cigarettes/day | 0.9 (0.8–1.0) |
| | | | | >20 cigarettes/day | 0.7 (0.6–0.9) |
| Spinelli et al. 1997 | Survey on deliveries | 662 women with planned pregnancies Italy | 1993 | Nonsmokers | 1.0 |
| | | | | Smokers | 0.8 (0.7–1.0) |

*Note:* Relative conception rate compares probability of conception among smokers and nonsmokers; values <1.0 indicate impairment of fecundity.

| Adjustment factors |
|---|
| Maternal: age, body mass index, parity, previous infertility, frequency of sexual intercourse, last contraception method used, recent pregnancy, maternal alcohol consumption<br>Paternal: smoking |
| Contraception (results not altered by further adjustment for social class, maternal age at marriage, parity) |
| Maternal: contraception use, attempt to conceive before study entry, previous delivery, social class<br>Paternal: smoking |
| Education, body mass index, weight, gravidity, oral contraceptive use, induced and spontaneous abortions, previous pregnancy outcomes, termination of recent pregnancy, alcohol consumption, caffeine consumption, marijuana use, childhood exposure to cigarette smoke |
| Maternal: age, body mass index, education, age at menarche, gravidity, frequency of sexual intercourse, number of previous miscarriages, alcohol use, marijuana use, cocaine use |
| None |
| Maternal: age, education<br>Paternal: smoking, education |
| Maternal: age, spousal smoking, recent oral contraceptive use |
| Maternal: working hours, shift work, use of video display terminal, industrial occupation, noisy workplace, exposure to solvents, physical stress, job decision latitude, job demands, stress from lack of support, coffee consumption, tea consumption, alcohol intake, age, parity<br>Paternal: industrial occupation, exposure to solvents, exposure to fumes, smoking, frequency of sexual intercourse |

**Table 3.33. Relative risks for conception delay among women smokers**

| Study | Study type | Population | Study period | End point |
|---|---|---|---|---|
| Linn et al. 1982 | Survey on deliveries | 3,214 married nondiabetic women who gave birth after planned pregnancy<br>United States | 1977–1979 | Relative risk for conception delay ≥3 months |
| Olsen et al. 1983 | Case-control | Cases: 228 women attempting first pregnancy for ≥1 year<br>Controls: 1,400 parous women who achieved first pregnancy in <1 year<br>Denmark | 1977–1980 | Relative risk for conception delay ≥12 months (first pregnancy) |
| | | Cases: 195 parous women attempting pregnancy for ≥ 1 year<br>Controls: 1,800 parous women who achieved pregnancy in <1 year<br>Denmark | | Relative risk for conception delay ≥12 months (second or later pregnancy) |
| Suonio et al. 1990 | Survey of pregnant women | 2,198 pregnant women who conceived in ≤12 months<br>Finland | 1983 | Relative risk for conception delay ≥6 months |
| Olsen 1991 | Survey | 10,886 pregnant women<br>Denmark | 1984–1987 | Relative risk for conception delay ≥12 months |

*Note:* Relative risk for conception delay compares risks of waiting longer than a specified time; values >1.0 indicate impairment of fecundity.

Among smokers, all these effects could lead to dysfunction of the fallopian tubes, delay of conception, infertility, spontaneous abortion, or ectopic pregnancy. Evidence has also indicated that cigarette smoking has an antiestrogenic effect among women, which could impair the fertility of female smokers (Baron et al. 1990) (see "Menstrual Function, Menopause, and Benign Gynecologic Disorders" earlier in this chapter). Women who smoke may also have an increased risk for infertility because of tubal dysfunction attributable to pelvic inflammatory disease (PID). The high rates of PID could be related to immune impairment among smokers or to sexual patterns among smokers that predispose them to STDs.

Thus, a consistent association between cigarette smoking and impairment of female fertility has been found in both case-control and cohort epidemiologic studies (Hughes and Brennan 1996; Augood et al. 1998). In addition, some investigations have reported more pronounced effects in association with higher levels of smoking. Clinical and laboratory studies have suggested plausible biological mechanisms for these associations, particularly tubal defects. Former smokers appear to have little excess risk for infertility—an observation that suggested either that the effects of smoking are reversible or that former smokers did not smoke heavily enough or long enough for adverse events to occur.

| Smoking status | Relative risk (95% confidence interval) | Adjustment factors |
|---|---|---|
| Nonsmokers<br>Smokers | 1.0<br>1.0 (0.9–1.2) | Maternal: contraception use, age, history of spontaneous abortion, use of diethylstilbestrol (DES) by woman's mother, body mass index, marijuana use, age at menarche, race, religion, history of pelvic inflammatory disease, history of induced abortion or ectopic pregnancy, gravidity, education, welfare status |
| Nonsmokers<br>Smokers | 1.0<br>1.8 (1.3–2.5) | Maternal: age, education, parity, oral contraceptive use, alcohol consumption, residence |
| Nonsmokers<br>Smokers | 1.0<br>1.3 (1.0–1.8) | |
| Nonsmokers<br>Smokers | 1.0<br>1.5 (1.3–1.8) | Maternal: age, gravidity, spontaneous abortion, induced abortion, maternal alcohol consumption, occupation, working time, strain of work<br>Paternal: smoking, alcohol consumption |
| Smokers | | Maternal: number of pregnancies, education, shift work, age, alcohol intake, coffee intake<br>Paternal: age, smoking |
| 1–4 cigarettes/day | 1.0 | |
| 5–9 cigarettes/day | 1.8 (1.3–2.6) | |
| 10–14 cigarettes/day | 1.8 (1.3–2.6) | |
| 15–19 cigarettes/day | 1.8 (1.2–2.5) | |
| ≥20 cigarettes/day | 1.7 (1.2–2.5) | |

## Maternal Conditions

### Ectopic Pregnancy

Ectopic pregnancy results from the implantation of a fertilized ovum outside the uterus, usually in the fallopian tubes. The growth of the fetus in an abnormal location results in significant morbidity, and ectopic pregnancy has emerged as the leading cause of maternal death during the first trimester of pregnancy (Atrash et al. 1986). Between 1970 and 1989, the ectopic pregnancy rate in the United States increased almost fourfold, from 4.5 to 16.1 per 1,000 reported pregnancies (CDC 1992). An important risk factor for ectopic pregnancy is PID, which may result in anatomic abnormalities that increase the risk for ectopic pregnancy (Phipps et al. 1987; Coste et al. 1991b; Kalandidi et al. 1991). Other risk factors for ectopic pregnancy are STDs (which may lead to PID), previous ectopic pregnancy, pelvic surgery, and previous use of an intrauterine device (Coste et al. 1991b). Use of OCs or an intrauterine device at the time of conception is also a risk factor, probably because these contraceptives prevent intrauterine pregnancy but not necessarily fertilization of an ovum (Chow et al. 1987; Coste et al. 1991b).

Cigarette smoking has been associated with increased risk for ectopic pregnancy even after adjustment for factors such as previous abdominal surgery and a history of PID or STDs; adjusted RRs have typically been between 1.5 and 2.5 (Chow et al. 1988; Handler et al. 1989; Coste et al. 1991a; Tuomivaara and Ronnberg 1991; Phillips et al. 1992; Saraiya et al. 1998;

**Table 3.33. Continued**

| Study | Study type | Population | Study period | End point |
|---|---|---|---|---|
| Laurent et al. 1992 | Case-control | Cases: 483 women with history of conception delay ≥24 months<br>Controls: 2,231 women without conception delay ≥24 months<br>United States | 1980–1983 | Relative risk for conception delay ≥24 months |
| Bolumar et al. 1996 | Population survey of pregnancy history | 3,187 women with planned pregnancy<br>Europe | 1991–1993 | Relative risk for conception delay >9.5 months for first pregnancy |
| | Prenatal survey | 2,587 pregnant women with planned pregnancy<br>Europe | 1991–1993 | Relative risk for conception delay >9.5 months for first pregnancy |
| Hull et al. 2000 | Population-based survey | 14,182 pregnant women who reached 24 weeks' gestation<br>England | 1991–1992 | Relative risk for conception delay of >6 months* |

*Conception delay of >12 months was also examined, and results were similar.

Castles et al. 1999). Some investigations have reported an increasing risk for ectopic pregnancy with an increasing number of cigarettes smoked (Handler et al. 1989; Coste et al. 1991a; Saraiya et al. 1998). However, this association was not observed in two other studies (Phillips et al. 1992; Parazzini et al. 1992c), and biases or confounding remain a concern in other investigations (Matsunaga and Shiota 1980; Levin et al. 1982; Kalandidi et al. 1991; Stergachis et al. 1991; Tuomivaara and Ronnberg 1991).

Thus, women who smoke may have an increased risk for ectopic pregnancy. The mechanisms that might explain such an association are not clear, but smoking can impair tubal transport and delay entry of the ovum into the uterus. These factors predispose a woman who smokes to ectopic pregnancy (Phipps et al. 1987; Mattison et al. 1989a; Stergachis et al. 1991; Phillips et al. 1992). As noted earlier in this section, smoking is also associated with PID, possibly through impairment of immune function (Holt 1987) or because of confounding by factors related to sexual experience.

**Preterm Premature Rupture of Membranes**

Premature rupture of the membranes (PROM) is generally defined as the leakage of amniotic fluid more than one hour before the onset of labor. Preterm PROM (PPROM) is premature leakage occurring before 37 weeks' gestation; it occurs in approximately 20 to 40 percent of premature deliveries (Spinillo et al. 1994d). In some instances, PPROM is associated with increased risk for transmission of human immunodeficiency virus (HIV) from the mother to the infant (Burns et al. 1994). Risk factors for PPROM include bleeding during pregnancy, previous preterm delivery, infection, cervical incompetence, and decreased maternal levels of certain nutrients such as ascorbic acid and zinc (Hadley et al. 1990; Harger et al. 1990; Ekwo et al. 1992, 1993; Williams et al. 1992; Spinillo et al. 1994d).

Early studies produced conflicting results regarding the relationship between smoking and PPROM (Underwood et al. 1965; Naeye 1982). These studies were limited, however, by small numbers of participants or by lack of control for potential

| Smoking status | Relative risk (95% confidence interval) | Adjustment factors |
|---|---|---|
| Nonsmokers | 1.0 | Maternal: age, age at first sexual intercourse, education, ethnicity, history of benign ovarian disease |
| Smokers | | |
| 1–4 cigarettes/day | 1.0 (1.0–1.0) | |
| 5–9 cigarettes/day | 1.1 (1.0–1.1) | |
| 10–19 cigarettes/day | 1.2 (1.1–1.3) | |
| ≥20 cigarettes/day | 1.4 (1.1–1.6) | |
| Nonsmokers | 1.0 | Maternal: age, education, recent oral contraceptive use, frequency of sexual intercourse, paid work, alcohol consumption, coffee consumption |
| Smokers | | |
| 1–10 cigarettes/day | 1.4 (1.1–1.7) | |
| ≥11 cigarettes/day | 1.7 (1.3–2.1) | |
| Nonsmokers | 1.0 | |
| Smokers | | |
| 1–10 cigarettes/day | 1.4 (1.0–1.8) | |
| ≥11 cigarettes/day | 1.7 (1.3–2.3) | |
| Nonsmokers | | Maternal: age, education, duration of oral contraceptive use, alcohol consumption, housing tenure and type, overcrowding<br>Paternal: age, education, alcohol consumption |
| Smokers | | |
| 1–4 cigarettes/day | 1.0 | |
| 5–9 cigarettes/day | 1.2 (0.9–1.6) | |
| 10–14 cigarettes/day | 1.2 (0.9-11.6) | |
| 15-19 cigarettes/day | 1.5 (1.2-1.9) | |
| ≥20 cigarettes/day | 1.6 (1.3–2.0) | |

confounding factors (Harger et al. 1990). In more recent studies, smoking has been consistently associated with PPROM (Castles et al. 1999) (Table 3.35). The RR estimates reported have varied from approximately 2 to 5 among smokers compared with nonsmokers, depending on the control groups under study. When women with PPROM were compared with pregnant women of the same gestational duration, the RRs among smokers were between 2.0 and 3.0 (Hadley et al. 1990; Harger et al. 1990). When the comparison included women who had term deliveries without PROM, some of the adjusted RRs were over 4.0 (Ekwo et al. 1993; Spinillo et al. 1994d). In the two studies that examined whether risk increased with the amount smoked, findings were mixed (Williams et al. 1992; Spinillo et al. 1994d) (Table 3.35). Women who had stopped smoking during pregnancy were at lower risk for PPROM than were those who continued to smoke (Harger et al. 1990; Williams et al. 1992).

Thus, women who smoke have an increased risk for PPROM. The underlying biological mechanism for the association is not known. Through its vasoconstrictive effects, smoking may disrupt the mechanical integrity of the fetal membranes, and it may affect general maternal nutritional status by impairing protein metabolism and by reducing circulating levels of amino acids, vitamin $B_{12}$, and ascorbic acid (Hadley et al. 1990). Smoking may also impair maternal immunity, possibly increasing susceptibility to infections that may precipitate PROM (Holt 1987). The studies cited in Table 3.35 controlled for variables such as maternal ascorbic acid level (Hadley et al. 1990), cervicovaginal infection (Spinillo et al. 1994d), and bleeding during pregnancy (Williams et al. 1992; Spinillo et al. 1994d) and observed a relationship between smoking and PPROM. Thus, those factors cannot explain the association.

### Placental Complications of Pregnancy

#### *Abruptio Placentae*

Abruptio placentae is premature separation of the normally implanted placenta from the uterine wall. A leading cause of maternal and perinatal morbidity and mortality, abruptio placentae is estimated to cause 15 to 25 percent of perinatal deaths (Naeye 1980; Krohn et al. 1987; Raymond and Mills 1993;

**Table 3.34. Relative risks for infertility among women smokers, case-control studies**

| Study | Population | Study period | End point | Smoking status | Relative risk (95% confidence interval) | Adjustment factors |
|---|---|---|---|---|---|---|
| Olsen et al. 1983 | Cases: 213 women with primary infertility<br>Controls: 1,296 fertile women<br>Denmark | 1977–1980 | Primary infertility | Nonsmokers<br>Smokers | 1.0<br>1.6 (1.1–2.2) | Maternal age, parity, education, oral contraceptive use, alcohol consumption, residence |
| | Cases: 65 women with secondary infertility<br>Controls: 1,651 fertile women<br>Denmark | 1977–1980 | Secondary infertility | Nonsmokers<br>Smokers | 1.0<br>2.1 (1.3–3.6) | Maternal age, parity, education, oral contraceptive use, alcohol consumption, residence |
| Daling et al. 1987 | Cases: 170 women with primary tubal infertility<br>Controls: 170 fertile women never previously pregnant<br>United States | 1979–1981 | | Never smoked<br>Former smokers<br>Current smokers | 1.0<br>1.1 (0.5–2.5)<br>2.7 (1.4–5.3) | Matched for race, census tract of residence, age |
| Phipps et al. 1987 | Cases: 1,390 infertile women<br>Controls: 1,264 women after delivery<br>United States and Canada | 1981–1983 | Primary infertility | Nonsmokers<br>Smokers, infertility thought primarily due to:<br>Cervical factor<br>Tubal disease<br>Ovulatory factor<br>Endometriosis | 1.0<br><br><br>1.7 (1.0–2.7)<br>1.6 (1.1–2.2)<br>1.0 (0.8–1.4)<br>0.9 (0.6–1.3) | Maternal age, religion, contraception use, time since menarche, number of sexual partners, education |
| Joesoef et al. 1993 | Cases: 1,815 infertile women<br>Controls: 1,760 primiparous fertile women<br>United States | 1981–1983 | Primary infertility | Never smoked<br>Former smokers<br>Current smokers | 1.0<br>0.6 (0.5–0.8)<br>1.9 (1.5–2.3) | Maternal age, body mass index, education, age at menarche, gravidity, frequency of sexual intercourse, number of previous miscarriages, use of marijuana, use of cocaine, consumption of alcohol |
| Tzonou et al. 1993 | Cases: 84 infertile women<br>Controls: 168 pregnant women<br>Greece | 1987–1988 | Secondary infertility | Never smoked<br>Ever smoked | 1.0<br>2.6 (1.2–6.0) | Maternal age, gravidity, education, residence, |

Spinillo et al. 1994a). Risk factors for abruption include hypertension, abdominal trauma, intravenous drug use, previous preterm birth, stillbirth or spontaneous abortion, advanced maternal age, and residence at high altitude during pregnancy (Williams et al. 1991a,c; Raymond and Mills 1993; Spinillo 1994a).

Abruptio placentae has repeatedly been associated with maternal cigarette smoking (Karegard and Gennser 1986; Voigt et al. 1990; Saftlas et al. 1991; Williams et al. 1991a,c; Raymond and Mills 1993; Spinillo et al. 1994a; Ananth et al. 1996; Cnattingius et al. 1997; Ananth et al. 1999; Castles et al. 1999). In studies that controlled for multiple covariates, the RRs were 1.4 to 2.4 for maternal smoking (Table 3.36). The risk for abruptio placentae has been found to increase with the number of cigarettes smoked (Williams et al. 1991a; Raymond and Mills 1993; Ananth et al. 1996; Cnattingius et al. 1997). In one study, women who had stopped smoking during pregnancy had a lower risk than did women who continued to smoke throughout pregnancy (Naeye 1980).

Because of the complicated interrelationships of smoking, PPROM, preeclampsia, and abruptio placentae, the independent effects of smoking on each of these outcomes may be difficult to assess. Since prolonged PPROM may be associated with an increased risk for abruptio placentae (Nelson et al. 1986; Vintzileos et al. 1987; Gonen et al. 1989; Spinillo et al. 1994a), smoking may increase the risk for abruptio placentae in part through its association with PPROM. Other biological mechanisms could also explain the association between smoking and separation of the placenta from the uterine wall. For example, carboxyhemoglobinemia and vasoconstriction associated with smoking can lead to local hypoxia, which in turn could lead to premature placental separation (Voigt et al. 1990; Williams et al. 1991a).

#### *Placenta Previa*

Placenta previa occurs when the placenta either partially or totally obstructs the cervical os, thus increasing the risks for hemorrhage and preterm birth—outcomes with considerable morbidity and mortality for both mother and infant. Women with placenta previa also experience increased risks for cesarean section, fetal malpresentation, and postpartum hemorrhage. One study reported that placenta previa complicates nearly 5 per 1,000 deliveries annually (Iyasu et al. 1993). Risk factors for placenta previa include increasing parity, increasing maternal age, previous abortion or cesarean section, and pregnancy during residence at high altitude (Williams et al. 1991b).

Cigarette smoking has repeatedly been associated with placenta previa (Castles et al. 1999) (Table 3.36). The RR is typically between 1.5 and 3.0 among women who smoke during pregnancy compared with those who do not (Meyer et al. 1976; Meyer and Tonascia 1977; Kramer et al. 1991; Williams et al. 1991b; Zhang and Fried 1992; Handler et al. 1994; Monica and Lilja 1995; Ananth et al. 1996; Chelmow et al. 1996; McMahon et al. 1997). Adjustment for covariates such as maternal age, parity, and previous cesarean section has had little effect on the strength of the association. Significant trends of increasing risk for placenta previa with increasing number of cigarettes smoked have been found in some studies (Handler et al. 1994; Monica and Lilja 1995; McMahon et al. 1997) but not in others (Williams et al. 1991b; Ananth et al. 1996).

Smoking might lead to placenta previa through chronic hypoxia, which results in placental enlargement and extension of the placenta over the cervical os (Williams et al. 1991b). The vascular effects of smoking might also be involved (Meyer and Tonascia 1977; Zhang and Fried 1992).

### Spontaneous Abortion

Spontaneous abortion (miscarriage) is usually defined as the involuntary termination of an intrauterine pregnancy before 28 weeks' (sometimes 20 weeks') gestation. The rate of spontaneous abortion usually cannot be completely ascertained, because some women may not receive medical care for a spontaneous abortion and may not even be aware of the pregnancy and its loss. Approximately 10 to 15 percent of pregnancies end in clinically recognized spontaneous abortion; measurement of human chorionic gonadotropin hormone in the urine of sexually active women has suggested that the total rate of fetal loss after implantation of a fertilized ovum may be as high as 50 percent (Wilcox et al. 1988; Eskenazi et al. 1995a). The risk for spontaneous abortion increases with maternal age and is higher among women who have had a previous miscarriage. Other purported risk factors are alcohol consumption, fever, various forms of contraception, social class, and race (Kline et al. 1989). Some spontaneous abortions involve a fetus that has chromosomal or structural abnormalities; in others, the fetus is normal. The causes of and risk factors for spontaneous abortion may differ accordingly.

An association between spontaneous abortion and maternal cigarette smoking has been suspected since the early 1960s (DiFranza and Lew 1995), but early epidemiologic studies provided inconsistent

**Table 3.35. Relative risks for preterm premature rupture of membranes (PPROM) among women smokers, case-control studies**

| Study | Population | Study period | Smoking status | Relative risk (95% confidence interval) |
|---|---|---|---|---|
| Hadley et al. 1990 | Black women with singleton pregnancies<br>Cases: 133 women with PPROM<br>Controls: 133 pregnant women (not "high risk")<br>United States | Not reported | Nonsmokers<br>Smokers (>10 cigarettes/day) | 1.0<br>2.6 (1.6–4.5) |
| Harger et al. 1990 | Cases: 341 women with singleton pregnancies and PPROM<br>Controls: 253 pregnant women with intact membranes at 37 weeks' gestation<br>United States | 1982–1983 | Nonsmokers<br>Stopped smoking during pregnancy<br>Continuing smokers | 1.0<br>1.6 (0.8–3.3)<br>2.1 (1.4–3.1) |
| Williams et al. 1992 | Cases: 307 women with singleton pregnancies and PPROM<br>Controls: 2,252 women with term deliveries and no PROM<br>United States | 1977–1980 | Never smoked<br>Stopped smoking before conception<br>Stopped smoking during first trimester<br>Nonsmokers during pregnancy<br>Smokers throughout pregnancy<br>Smokers at some time during pregnancy<br>1–9 cigarettes/day<br>10–19 cigarettes/day<br>≥20 cigarettes/day | 1.0<br>1.4 (0.9–2.0)<br>1.6 (0.8–2.9)<br>1.0<br>2.2 (1.4–3.5)<br>1.6 (1.1–2.4)<br>1.8 (1.1–2.8)<br>1.5 (0.9–2.4)<br>1.7 (1.0–2.6) |
| Ekwo et al. 1993 | Cases: 184 women with PPROM<br>Controls: 184 pregnant women<br>United States | 1985–1990 | No smoke exposure<br>Passive smokers only<br>Active smokers only<br>Active and passive smokers | 1.0<br>1.0 (0.6–1.8)<br>4.2 (1.8–10.0)<br>2.1 (1.2–3.5) |
| Spinillo et al. 1994d | Cases: 138 women with PPROM (24–35 weeks' gestation)<br>Controls: 267 women with term pregnancies<br>Italy | 1988–1992 | Nonsmokers<br>Smokers<br>≤10 cigarettes/day<br>>10 cigarettes/day | 1.0<br>1.9 (1.1–3.2)<br>1.1 (0.5–2.2)<br>4.0 (1.9–8.8) |

findings (USDHHS 1980). These inconsistencies may have been due to the limitations of small sample size, inadequate control for covariates, and differences in ascertainment of smoking among case subjects and control subjects (Stillman et al. 1986).

Major studies published since 1975 that reported RRs for the association between smoking and spontaneous abortion are summarized in Table 3.37. Some studies found an increase in risk among smokers (Kline et al. 1977; Himmelberger et al. 1978; Armstrong et al. 1992; Dominguez-Rojas et al. 1994), whereas others reported no association or only a weak relationship (Hemminki et al. 1983; Sandahl 1989; Windham et al. 1992). Although the few studies that included both clinically recognized and unrecognized fetal losses were small, they provided some evidence that the risk for spontaneous abortion is higher among current smokers than among nonsmokers (Wilcox et al. 1990; Eskenazi et al. 1995a). Another study found that the risk among former smokers was similar to that among nonsmokers (Stein et al. 1981).

Two studies showed a clear dose-response relationship between smoking and spontaneous abortion; noticeable effects were seen among women who

| Adjustment factors |
|---|
| Matched for maternal age, parity, gestational age<br>Adjustment for previous PPROM, fundal placental location |
| None |
| Race, education, age, welfare status, martial status, marijuana and alcohol use, parity, previous spontaneous or therapeutic abortion, cervical incompetence, bleeding during pregnancy, body mass index, coffee consumption |
| Matched for maternal age, parity, race |
| Previous term and preterm deliveries, social class, prepregnancy body mass index, bleeding during pregnancy, incompetent cervix, preeclampsia, low hematocrit on hospital admission for delivery, documented cervicovaginal infection during pregnancy |

smoked more than 10 cigarettes per day (Armstrong et al. 1992; Dominguez-Rojas et al. 1994). In their study population, Armstrong and colleagues (1992) estimated that cigarette smoking accounted for 11 percent of all spontaneous abortions and could have explained 40 percent of spontaneous abortions among women smoking 20 or more cigarettes per day. In a small case-control study of habitual abortion (two or more spontaneous abortions), current smokers had a RR of 1.4 compared with women who had never smoked (95 percent CI, 0.8 to 2.9); risk increased with the number of cigarettes smoked per day (Parazzini et al. 1991a).

Only a few studies separately investigated spontaneous abortions of chromosomally normal and abnormal fetuses. Kline and colleagues (1989) reported an association between cigarette smoking during pregnancy and spontaneous abortion of a chromosomally normal fetus or abortion of a fetus with nontrisomic chromosomal aberration. A French study found that among women younger than 30 years old, the proportion of spontaneous abortions that were chromosomally normal was higher in smokers who inhaled than in noninhalers or nonsmokers (Boué et al. 1975). No such association was found among women aged 30 years or older. Yet another study reported that the proportion of losses of a chromosomally normal fetus increased with the number of cigarettes smoked during pregnancy (Alberman et al. 1976). Kline and colleagues (1995) later reported the findings on all 2,305 karyotyped cases of spontaneous abortion and 4,076 control pregnancies studied over a decade in public and private facilities of three New York City hospitals. Compared with nonsmokers, women who smoked 14 or more cigarettes per day at the time of conception had a significantly higher risk for spontaneous abortion of a chromosomally normal fetus (adjusted RR, 1.3; 95 percent CI, 1.1 to 1.7) and a nonsignificantly higher risk for spontaneous abortion of a fetus with nontrisomic chromosomal aberration (adjusted RR, 1.2; 95 percent CI, 0.8 to 1.8). The association was not evident among former smokers, and maternal age did not affect the findings. There was no association with loss of a fetus with trisomic chromosomal aberration.

In summary, the available data have been somewhat mixed but have suggested a modest association between cigarette smoking and spontaneous abortion (Hughes and Brennan 1996). The mechanisms underlying the putative association are not known, but they likely involve factors that interfere with normal implantation of a fertilized ovum (Gindoff and Tidey 1989), as discussed previously with regard to ectopic pregnancy (see "Maternal Conditions" earlier in this section). Also, several constituents of cigarette smoke (e.g., nicotine and carbon monoxide [CO]) are toxic for the developing fetus (Lambers and Clark 1996).

### Hypertensive Disorders of Pregnancy

Pregnancy-induced hypertensive disorders range from isolated hypertension during pregnancy (gestational hypertension) to preeclampsia (hypertension with proteinuria and edema) and eclampsia

**Table 3.36. Relative risks for placental disorders among women smokers**

| Study | Study type | Population | Study period | Adjustment factors |
|---|---|---|---|---|
| Voigt et al. 1990 | Case-control (population-based) | 1,089 women with singleton births with abruption<br>2,323 women with singleton births without abruption<br>United States | 1984–1986 | Maternal age, race, marital status, gravidity, income of census tract |
| Eriksen et al. 1991 | Case-control | 87 women with singleton births with abruption<br>5,697 women with singleton births without abruption<br>Denmark | 1980–1985 | Maternal age, social class, standing at work, congenital malformation, amniocentesis, small-for-gestational-age infant, preeclampsia, hemorrhage |
| Kramer et al. 1991 | Case-control (population-based) | 598 women with singleton births with placenta previa<br>2,422 women with singleton births without placenta previa<br>United States | 1984–1987 | Maternal age |
| Williams et al. 1991a,b | Case-control | 143 women with singleton births with abruption<br>1,257 women with singleton births without abruption | 1977–1980 | Placental abruption: diabetes, late prenatal registration, alcohol intake, cervical incompetence, marijuana use, previous spontaneous or induced abortion, stillbirth, prepregnancy body mass index <18; no adjustment for detailed abruption data |
| | | 69 women with singleton births with placenta previa<br>12,351 women with singleton births without placenta previa<br>United States | | Placenta previa: maternal age, payment status, parity, previous spontaneous abortion, previous cesarean section (placenta previa only), previous in utero exposure to diethylstilbestrol (DES), coffee consumption, alcohol intake |
| Williams et al. 1991c | Case-control | 943 women with singleton births with abruption<br>10,648 women with singleton births without abruption<br>United States | 1987–1988 | Previous stillbirth, chronic hypertension, maternal age, cervical incompetence, payment status, diabetes, multiparity, education, marital status |
| Zhang and Fried 1992 | Case-control (population-based) | 766 women with births with placenta previa<br>178,953 women with births without placenta previa<br>Both groups without pregnancy-induced hypertension<br>United States | 1988–1989 | Maternal age, race, gravidity, parity, previous pregnancy termination, previous cesarean section, gestational age |

| Abruptio placentae | | Placenta previa | |
|---|---|---|---|
| **Smoking status** | **Relative risk (95% confidence interval)** | **Smoking status** | **Relative risk (95% confidence interval)** |
| Nonsmokers | 1.0 | | |
| Smokers | 1.6 (1.3–1.8) | | |
| Nonsmokers | 1.0 | | |
| Smokers | 2.5 (1.2–5.1) | | |
| | | Nonsmokers | 1.0 |
| | | Smokers | 2.1 (1.7–2.5) |
| Nonsmokers | 1.0 | Nonsmokers | 1.0 |
| Smokers | 1.5 (1.0–2.2) | Smokers | 2.6 (1.3–5.5) |
| | | 1–9 cigarettes/day | 3.1 (1.4–6.6) |
| | | ≥10 cigarettes/day | 2.2 (0.9–5.1) |
| | | Never smoked | 1.0 |
| | | Stopped smoking before conception | 1.3 (0.5–3.3) |
| | | Stopped smoking during first trimester | 1.9 (0.6–6.7) |
| | | Smoked throughout pregnancy | 3.1 (1.2–8.1) |
| Nonsmokers | 1.0 | | |
| Smokers | 1.7 (1.5–2.0) | | |
| | | Nonsmokers | 1.0 |
| | | Smokers | 1.3 (1.1–1.6) |
| | | 1–9 cigarettes/day | 1.1 (0.8–1.6) |
| | | 10–19 cigarettes/day | 1.3 (1.0–1.8) |
| | | ≥20 cigarettes/day | 1.4 (1.0–1.9) |

**Table 3.36. Continued**

| Study | Study type | Population | Study period | Adjustment factors |
|---|---|---|---|---|
| Raymond and Mills 1993 | Cohort | 30,681 women with singleton births<br>307 women with births with abruption<br>United States | 1974–1977 | Maternal age, education, parity |
| Handler et al. 1994 | Case-control | 304 women with singleton births with placenta previa<br>2,732 women with singleton births without placenta previa<br>United States | 1988–1990 | Maternal age, parity, previous cesarean section, previous spontaneous abortion, previous induced abortion |
| Spinillo et al. 1994a | Case-control | 55 women with births with abruption (24–36 weeks' gestation)<br>726 women with births without abruption (24–36 weeks' gestation)<br>Italy | 1985–1991 | Maternal age, gestational age, number of clinic visits, abdominal trauma, intravenous drug abuse, hypertension, preeclampsia, diabetes |
| Monica and Lilja 1995 | Case-control | 2,345 women with births with placenta previa<br>825,856 women with births without placenta previa<br>Sweden | 1983–1990 | Maternal age, year of birth, parity |
| Ananth et al. 1996 | Cohort | 87,184 singleton births in 61,667 women<br>808 women with births with abruption<br>290 women with births with placenta previa<br>Canada | 1986–1993 | Hospital type, year of delivery, marital status, maternal age, parity, hypertension, preeclampsia |
| Chelmow et al. 1996 | Case-control | 32 women with births with placenta previa at >24 weeks' gestation<br>96 women with births without placenta previa at >24 weeks' gestation<br>United States | 1992–1994 | Referral source, maternal age |
| Cnattingius et al. 1997 | Cohort | 317,652 women ≤ 34 years old with singleton pregnancies, previously nulliparous | 1987–1993 | Maternal age, education, country of birth, cohabitating with infant's father |
| McMahon et al. 1997 | Case-control (population-based) | 342 women with singleton births with placenta previa<br>1,082 women with singleton births without placenta previa<br>United States | 1990 | Maternal age, race, previous spontaneous or induced abortion |

| Abruptio placentae | | Placenta previa | |
|---|---|---|---|
| **Smoking status** | **Relative risk (95% confidence interval)** | **Smoking status** | **Relative risk (95% confidence interval)** |
| Nonsmokers | 1.0 | | |
| Smokers | 1.4* (1.1–1.8) | | |
| | | Nonsmokers | 1.0 |
| | | Smokers | 1.7 (1.3–2.2) |
| | | 1–9 cigarettes/day | 0.8 (0.5–1.6) |
| | | 10–19 cigarettes/day | 1.2 (0.7–5.4) |
| | | 20–29 cigarettes/day | 2.3 (1.4–3.7) |
| | | 30–39 cigarettes/day | 1.9 (0.6–6.1) |
| | | 40–49 cigarettes/day | 3.1 (0.9–10.8) |
| Nonsmokers | 1.0 | | |
| Smokers | 2.4 (1.3–4.3) | | |
| Stopped smoking during pregnancy | 3.6 (1.3–10.1) | | |
| <10 cigarettes/day | 2.3 (1.0–4.8) | | |
| ≥10 cigarettes/day | 2.4 (1.1–5.3) | | |
| | | Nonsmokers | 1.0 |
| | | Smokers | 1.5 (1.4–1.7) |
| | | <10 cigarettes/day | 1.4 (1.3–1.6) |
| | | ≥10 cigarettes/day | 1.7 (1.5–1.9) |
| Nonsmokers | 1.0 | Nonsmokers | 1.0 |
| Smokers | 2.1 (1.8–2.4) | Smokers | 1.4 (1.0–1.8) |
| 1–5 cigarettes/day | 1.8 (1.3–2.5) | 1–5 cigarettes/day | 1.5 (0.8–2.7) |
| 6–10 cigarettes/day | 1.9 (1.5–2.5) | 6–10 cigarettes/day | 1.3 (0.8–2.1) |
| 11–15 cigarettes/day | 2.2 (1.8–2.8) | 11–15 cigarettes/day | 1.3 (0.8–2.0) |
| 16–20 cigarettes/day | 2.1 (1.5–2.9) | 16–20 cigarettes/day | 1.8 (1.1–3.1) |
| ≥21 cigarettes/day | 2.2 (1.8–2.7) | ≥21 cigarettes/day | 1.3 (0.8–2.0) |
| | | Nonsmokers | 1.0 |
| | | Smokers | 4.4 (1.4–14.1) |
| Nonsmokers | 1.0 | | |
| Smokers | | | |
| 1–9 cigarettes/day | 2.0 (1.9–2.1) | | |
| ≥10 cigarettes/day | 2.4 (2.3–2.6) | | |
| | | Nonsmokers | 1.0 |
| | | Smokers | |
| | | 1–10 cigarettes/day | 1.3 (0.9–1.9) |
| | | 11–20 cigarettes/day | 1.8 (1.2–2.8) |
| | | >20 cigarettes/day | 2.0 (0.8–4.8) |

**Table 3.37. Relative risks for spontaneous abortion among women smokers**

| Study | Study type | Population | Study period | Smoking status | Relative risk (95% confidence interval) | Adjustment factors |
|---|---|---|---|---|---|---|
| Kline et al. 1977 | Case-control | 574 cases with spontaneous abortion<br>320 controls delivering after ≥ 28 weeks' gestation<br>United States | 1974–1976 | Nonsmokers<br>Smokers | 1.0<br>1.8 (1.3–2.5) | Age at last menses, history of abortion and live births |
| Ericson and Källén 1986 | Case-control | 219 cases with spontaneous abortion<br>1,032 controls with live-born infant without major malformation<br>Sweden | 1980–1981 | Nonsmokers<br>Smokers | 1.0<br>1.0 (0.6–1.5) | Video screen use, stress |
| Sandahl 1989 | Case-control | 610 cases with spontaneous abortion<br>1,337 controls delivering infant<br>Sweden | 1980–1985 | Nonsmokers<br>Smokers<br>Any smoking<br>>10 cigarettes/day | 1.0<br><br>0.9 (0.8–1.0)<br>0.9 (0.7–1.0) | Maternal age, parity |
| Armstrong et al. 1992 | Cohort | 47,146 pregnant women<br>10,191 women with spontaneous abortion<br>Canada | 1982–1984 | Nonsmokers<br>Smokers<br>1–9 cigarettes/day<br>10–19 cigarettes/day<br>≥20 cigarettes/day | 1.0<br><br>1.1 (1.0–1.2)<br>1.2 (1.1–1.3)<br>1.7 (1.6–1.8) | Maternal age, education, ethnicity, employment during pregnancy |
| Windham et al. 1992 | Case-control | 626 cases with spontaneous abortion at ≤ 20 weeks' gestation<br>1,300 controls delivering live infant<br>United States | 1986–1987 | Nonsmokers<br>Smokers<br>1–10 cigarettes/day<br>>10 cigarettes/day | 1.0<br><br>0.9 (0.7–1.2)<br>1.1 (0.8–1.6) | Maternal age, previous fetal loss, marital status, insurance, alcohol intake, intake of bottled water |

(hypertension with proteinuria, edema, and seizures). Distinguishing between hypertensive disorders of pregnancy and chronic hypertension is difficult, and accepted classification systems for hypertensive disorders of pregnancy were not established until the late 1980s (Davey and MacGillivray 1988). Gestational hypertension is the most common hypertensive disorder of pregnancy. However, preeclampsia is associated with much greater risks for morbidity and mortality: it is a leading cause of maternal mortality (Berg et al. 1996) and a major contributor to fetal growth retardation and preterm birth (Heffner et al. 1993; Kleigman 1997). Risk factors for preeclampsia include chronic hypertension, multiple fetuses, nulliparity, previous preeclampsia or eclampsia, type 1 diabetes mellitus, previous adverse pregnancy outcomes, high prepregnancy weight and high pregnancy weight gain, working during pregnancy, and black race (Eskenazi et al. 1991).

Smoking has repeatedly been found to be inversely related to the risk for preeclampsia (Marcoux et al. 1989; Eskenazi et al. 1991; Klonoff-Cohen et al.

**Table 3.37. Continued**

| Study | Study type | Population | Study period | Smoking status | Relative risk (95% confidence interval) | Adjustment factors |
|---|---|---|---|---|---|---|
| Dominguez-Rojas et al. 1994 | Cohort | 711 women with ≥1 pregnancy<br>169 women with spontaneous abortion<br>Spain | 1989–1991 | Nonsmokers<br>Smokers<br>1–10 cigarettes/day<br>≥11 cigarettes/day | 1.0<br><br>1.0 (0.6–1.5)<br>3.4 (1.7–6.9) | Maternal age, age at menarche, previous spontaneous abortion, marital status |
| Chatenoud et al. 1998 | Case-control | 782 cases with spontaneous abortion at ≤12 weeks' gestation admitted to hospital<br>1,543 controls delivering healthy term infants<br>Italy | 1990–1997 | Never smoked<br>Former smokers<br>Smokers before pregnancy<br>Smokers before and during pregnancy | 1.0<br>0.9 (0.7–1.2)<br>0.7 (0.5–1.0)<br>1.3 (1.0–1.6) | Maternal age, education, marital status, history of spontaneous abortion or miscarriage, nausea, alcohol or coffee intake in first trimester |
| Ness et al. 1999 | Case-control | 570 cases with spontaneous abortion presenting in hospital emergency department<br>United States | 1995–1997 | Never smoked<br>Former smokers<br>Current smokers | 1.0<br>0.9 (0.6–1.3)<br>1.4 (1.0–1.9) | None |
| Windham et al. 1999b | Cohort | 5,342 pregnant women<br>499 women with spontaneous abortion<br>United States | 1990–1991 | Nonsmokers<br>Smokers<br>1–4 cigarettes/day<br>>5 cigarettes/day | 1.0<br><br>0.9 (0.6–1.5)<br>1.3 (0.9–1.9) | Maternal age, prior fetal loss, alcohol intake, caffeine intake, gestational age at interview |

1993; Spinillo et al. 1994b; Sibai et al. 1995; Mittendorf et al. 1996; Ros et al. 1998; Castles et al. 1999). This finding has persisted even in studies with rigorous diagnostic criteria, adequate adjustment for covariates, and careful assessment of smoking history (Marcoux et al. 1989; Klonoff-Cohen et al. 1993; Sibai et al. 1995; Mittendorf et al. 1996). In one study, the risk for preeclampsia decreased with increasing amount smoked (Marcoux et al. 1989), although in three other studies, no dose-response relationship was observed (Klonoff-Cohen et al. 1993; Spinillo et al. 1994b; Cnattingius et al. 1997; Ros et al. 1998). One investigation reported that the protective effect tended to be confined to women who continued smoking after 20 weeks' gestation (Marcoux et al. 1989); another study reported that the lowest risk for preeclampsia was among women who had stopped smoking at the start of pregnancy (Sibai et al. 1995).

Data on the relationship between cigarette smoking and gestational hypertension or eclampsia have been limited. In one large study, smoking was associated with a moderate reduction in risk for hypertensive disorders of pregnancy as a whole (RR, 0.7; 95 percent CI, 0.6 to 0.8) (Savitz and Zhang 1992). In another investigation, cigarette smoking conferred a modest reduction in risk for gestational hypertension (RR, 0.8; 95 percent CI, 0.5 to 1.1) and a more pronounced inverse association with preeclampsia (RR, 0.5; 95 percent CI, 0.3 to 0.8) (Marcoux et al. 1989). Other studies have also found that smoking during pregnancy was associated with a reduction in the risk for gestational hypertension (Misra and Kiely 1995;

Wong and Bauman 1997). A large, well-conducted study in Sweden found similar inverse associations between smoking and gestational hypertension, preeclampsia, and eclampsia (Cnattingius et al. 1997; Ros et al. 1998). In contrast, smoking was unrelated to eclampsia in one report (Abi-Said et al. 1995).

Thus, epidemiologic evidence has indicated that smoking is inversely related to hypertensive disorders of pregnancy. Little is known, however, about how smoking might exert such an effect (Ros et al. 1998). Despite this apparently beneficial association, other adverse effects make the net impact of smoking strongly detrimental for pregnant women. In a study of 317,652 births, smoking was associated with particularly increased risks in perinatal mortality, abruption, and infants who are small for gestational age (SGA) among women with severe preeclampsia (Cnattingius et al. 1997).

## Birth Outcomes

Previous reports of the Surgeon General have provided comprehensive reviews of the association between maternal smoking and fetal, neonatal, and perinatal mortality and morbidity (USDHHS 1980, 1989b). This section describes recent work highlighting the relationship between smoking and those outcomes as well as low birth weight (LBW), SGA (due to intrauterine growth retardation [IUGR]), preterm delivery, birth defects, and SIDS.

### Preterm Delivery

Preterm delivery (birth at <37 weeks' gestation) is strongly associated with increased risks for fetal, neonatal, and perinatal mortality. Preterm delivery may spontaneously follow PROM or may occur because of maternal bleeding, preeclampsia, multiple gestation, uterine anomalies, or urinary tract infection (Heffner et al. 1993). The 1979 Surgeon General's report on smoking and health concluded that smoking during pregnancy increases the risk for preterm delivery and that this risk increases with the quantity of cigarettes smoked (USDHEW 1979). The report estimated that 11 to 14 percent of preterm births are attributable to smoking during pregnancy.

Epidemiologic studies have continued to provide evidence for the association between smoking and preterm delivery (Table 3.38). The RRs among smokers compared with nonsmokers have ranged from 1.2 to more than 2.0 after multivariate adjustment (Shiono et al. 1986b; CDC 1990; Ferraz et al. 1990; Wen et al. 1990b; McDonald et al. 1992; Heffner et al. 1993; Olsén et al. 1995). One study showed that smokers had a higher risk for delivery before 32 weeks' gestation than did nonsmokers (RR, 1.9; 95 percent CI, 1.3 to 2.9) but no higher risk for delivery at 32 through 36 weeks' gestation (RR, 0.8; 95 percent CI, 0.6 to 1.2) (Peacock et al. 1995). Shiono and colleagues (1986b) also reported a stronger association between smoking and preterm delivery before 33 weeks' gestation than between smoking and later preterm delivery. A few studies have failed to find any association between smoking and preterm delivery after adjustment for factors such as race (Zhang and Bracken 1995) and other psychosocial indicators (Nordentoft et al. 1996).

Smoking may be associated with premature delivery only in certain circumstances. One investigation found that the RR for smoking was particularly high among women with no other risk factors for premature delivery (Heffner et al. 1993). Two other studies demonstrated a clear involvement of smoking among women whose spontaneous preterm delivery was primarily due to PPROM (see "Preterm Premature Rupture of Membranes" earlier in this section) (Shiono et al. 1986b; Meis et al. 1995).

The association between smoking and preterm birth may differ according to maternal characteristics. For example, the effect of smoking on the risk for premature birth may be more pronounced among older women than among those younger than 20 years old (Cornelius et al. 1995; Olsén et al. 1995). Three studies found that the RR for preterm delivery among smokers compared with nonsmokers increased with maternal age; the association was particularly strong among women older than age 35 years (Wen et al. 1990a; Cnattingius et al. 1993; Olsén et al. 1995). Wen and associates (1990a) reported a mean difference of one-half week in gestational age between infants of smoking and nonsmoking women 35 years old or younger. The mean difference for infants of smokers and nonsmokers older than 35 years was one week. Wisborg and colleagues (1996) did not confirm this pattern of increasing smoking-related risks with increasing maternal age. In one study, the age-related trend in RRs became less significant after an interaction of smoking with parity was included (Cnattingius et al. 1993).

Although most studies have demonstrated an association between maternal smoking and premature delivery, a pattern of increasing risk with increasing amount smoked has not consistently been found. Some studies have demonstrated a clear dose-response relationship between smoking and premature delivery in at least some subpopulations, such as women who consume high amounts of caffeine (Wisborg et al. 1996) or mothers of infants with placental abnormalities (Shiono et al. 1986b). However, other investigations failed to find a clear dose-response relationship after adjustment for potential confounding factors (McDonald et al. 1992; Cnattingius et al. 1993; Peacock et al. 1995).

Smoking cessation during pregnancy seems to reduce the risk for preterm delivery. In a randomized trial of the effect of smoking cessation on birth weight and gestational age, infants of women who had stopped smoking had a longer gestation than did infants of women who smoked throughout pregnancy (Li et al. 1993). (Smoking cessation was validated by determining salivary cotinine concentrations.) After adjustment for maternal age, race, height, and weight at entry into prenatal care, the mean gestational age was 39.2 weeks among infants delivered to women who had stopped smoking but 38.3 weeks among infants of women who continued to smoke (p = 0.07). The risk for preterm delivery among women who had stopped smoking during pregnancy was similar to that among women who had never smoked: the RR was 0.9 (95 percent CI, 0.4 to 2.2). However, simply reducing the amount smoked seemed to have no beneficial effect. According to NHIS data, women who discontinued smoking during the first trimester of pregnancy reduced the risk for preterm delivery to that of nonsmoking women (Mainous and Hueston 1994b). Compared with nonsmokers, women who had stopped smoking during the first trimester had a RR of 0.9 (95 percent CI, 0.6 to 1.5), and women who smoked after the first trimester had a RR of 1.6 (95 percent CI, 1.2 to 2.1).

The association between smoking and preterm delivery is biologically plausible, because nicotine-induced vasoconstriction in the placenta could initiate delivery (Lindblad et al. 1988; Bruner and Forouzan 1991; Wisborg et al. 1996). Furthermore, smoking may cause higher levels of circulating catecholamines that could precipitate premature labor (USDHHS 1980).

#### Stillbirth

Stillbirth (fetal death after 28 weeks' gestation) is a fairly rare occurrence in developed nations. In the United States, rates of stillbirth are estimated at 3.3 per 1,000 births among white women and 5.5 per 1,000 births among black women (Guyer et al. 1996). A number of risk factors have been identified. Advanced maternal age, nulliparity, previous fetal loss, race, multiple births, and higher maternal BMI all confer increased risks (Kiely et al. 1986; Cnattingius et al. 1988; Ferraz and Gray 1991; Cnattingius et al. 1992; Little and Weinberg 1993; Raymond et al. 1994).

In the past 15 years, cigarette smoking has been repeatedly associated with an increased risk for stillbirth. In early studies, investigators (Lowe 1959; Underwood et al. 1967) examined the effect of cigarette smoking but did not always find a positive relationship. This lack of association may have occurred because these studies were often statistically underpowered or did not control for known risk factors (DiFranza et al. 1995).

More recent studies have found an increased risk for stillbirth among women who smoked during pregnancy (Table 3.39). In one study of 281,808 pregnancies in Sweden, the RR for stillbirth among smokers compared with nonsmokers was 1.4 (95 percent CI, 1.2 to 1.6), after adjustment for maternal age, parity, and type of birth (single vs. multiple) (Cnattingius et al. 1988). Another investigation found that the effect of smoking on stillbirth decreased as gestational age increased but never reached the lower level of stillbirth among nonsmoking women (Raymond et al. 1994). The RRs among women who smoked were 1.6 (95 percent CI, 1.3 to 2.0) at 28 to 31 weeks' gestation and 1.1 (95 percent CI, 0.7 to 1.8) at 42 to 45 weeks' gestation.

A moderate increase in risk for stillbirth has been found with increasing cigarette consumption (Ahlborg and Bodin 1991; Cnattingius et al. 1992; Little and Weinberg 1993; Raymond et al. 1994; Cnattingius and Nordstrom 1996). One large study found that the rate of stillbirth among nonsmokers was 3.5 deaths per 1,000 births (Cnattingius et al. 1992). The rate was 4.4 deaths per 1,000 births among those who smoked 1 to 9 cigarettes per day and 4.9 deaths per 100,000 births among those who smoked more than 9 cigarettes per day. Similarly, another study reported that the RR for stillbirth among women who smoked 1 to 9 cigarettes per day compared with nonsmokers was 1.2 (95 percent CI, 1.02 to 1.4); the RR increased to 1.6 (95 percent CI, 1.4 to 1.8) among women who smoked 10 or more cigarettes per day (Raymond et al. 1994).

Recently, some studies have investigated ways to reduce the risk for stillbirth among women smokers. For example, in one report, the use of multivitamin and mineral supplements significantly reduced the rate of stillbirth among women who smoked (Wu et al. 1998). Schramm (1997) compared smoking patterns in successive pregnancies. Smoking during both the first and second pregnancies was associated with a significant RR for fetal death; however, women who

**Table 3.38. Relative risks for preterm delivery among women smokers**

| Study | Study type | Population | Study period | Smoking status | Relative risk (95% confidence interval) | Adjustment factors |
|---|---|---|---|---|---|---|
| Shiono et al. 1986b | Cohort | 30,596 women with preterm births at <37 weeks' gestation United States | 1974–1977 | Delivery at <37 weeks' gestation | | Maternal age, education, ethnicity, marital status, employment, gravidity, induced or spontaneous abortion, gender of infant, time prenatal care began, major malformation of infant, preeclampsia, alcohol use |
| | | | | Nonsmokers | 1.0 | |
| | | | | Smokers | | |
| | | | | <1 pack/day | 1.1 (0.9–1.2) | |
| | | | | ≥1 pack/day | 1.2 (1.1–1.4) | |
| | | | | Delivery at <33 weeks' gestation | | |
| | | | | Nonsmokers | 1.0 | |
| | | | | Smokers | | |
| | | | | <1 pack/day | 1.1 (0.8–1.5) | |
| | | | | ≥1 pack/day | 1.6 (1.2–2.3) | |
| Centers for Disease Control 1990 | Survey of pregnancy history | 74,139 women with singleton pregnancies United States | 1989 | Nonsmokers | 1.0 | Maternal age, race, prepregnancy weight, weight gain, alcohol use, infant's birth order, education, month prenatal care began, previous termination of pregnancy |
| | | | | Smokers | 1.3* | |
| Ferraz et al. 1990 | Case-control | 429 women with preterm births 2,555 controls Brazil | 1984–1986 | Nonsmokers | 1.0 | Adjustment factors in final model not stated |
| | | | | Smokers | 1.5 (1.2–2.0) | |
| Wen et al. 1990b | Cohort | 15,539 women with singleton preterm births at <37 weeks' gestation United States | 1983–1988 | Nonsmokers | 1.0 | Maternal race, marital status, prepregnancy weight, weight gain, parity, alcohol use |
| | | | | Smokers | | |
| | | | | Aged ≤16 years | 1.2 (0.7–2.2) | |
| | | | | Aged 17–19 years | 1.2 (0.9–1.6) | |
| | | | | Aged 20–25 years | 1.1 (0.9–1.3) | |
| | | | | Aged 26–30 years | 1.4 (1.1–1.8) | |
| | | | | Aged 31–35 years | 1.6 (1.0–2.4) | |
| | | | | Aged ≥36 years | 2.0 (0.7–6.3) | |
| McDonald et al. 1992 | Survey | 40,445 women with singleton births (7.0% delivered at <37 weeks' gestation) Canada | 1982–1984 | Nonsmokers | 1.0 | Maternal age, education, pregnancy order, previous spontaneous abortion, previous low-birth-weight infant, prepregnancy weight, ethnic group (white, French, or English), employment at start of pregnancy |
| | | | | Smokers | | |
| | | | | <10 cigarettes/day | 1.2 (1.1–1.4) | |
| | | | | 10–19 cigarettes/day | 1.4 (1.3–1.6) | |
| | | | | ≥20 cigarettes/day | 1.3 (1.2–1.5) | |

*95% confidence interval was not reported.

**Table 3.38. Continued**

| Study | Study type | Population | Study period | Smoking status | Relative risk (95% confidence interval) | Adjustment factors |
|---|---|---|---|---|---|---|
| Cnattingius et al. 1993 | Cohort | 538,829 women with singleton births<br>29,937 births at ≤36 weeks' gestation<br>Sweden | 1983–1988 | Nonsmokers | | Maternal age, parity |
| | | | | Multiparas | | |
| | | | | Aged 20–24 years | 1.0 | |
| | | | | Aged 25–29 years | 0.9 (0.8–0.9) | |
| | | | | Aged 30–34 years | 1.0 (0.9–1.0) | |
| | | | | Aged ≥35 years | 1.4 (1.3–1.5) | |
| | | | | Nulliparas | | |
| | | | | Aged 20–24 years | 1.5 (1.4–1.6) | |
| | | | | Aged 25–29 years | 1.5 (1.4–1.5) | |
| | | | | Aged 30–34 years | 1.6 (1.5–1.7) | |
| | | | | Aged ≥35 years | 2.1 (1.9–2.2) | |
| | | | | Smokers | | |
| | | | | Multiparas | | |
| | | | | Aged 20–24 years | 1.6 (1.6–1.7) | |
| | | | | Aged 25–29 years | 1.4 (1.3–1.5) | |
| | | | | Aged 30–34 years | 1.6 (1.5–1.7) | |
| | | | | Aged ≥ 35 years | 2.3 (2.1–2.4) | |
| | | | | Nulliparas | | |
| | | | | Aged 20–24 years | 1.7 (1.6–1.8) | |
| | | | | Aged 25–29 years | 1.6 (1.5–1.7) | |
| | | | | Aged 30–34 years | 1.8 (1.6–1.9) | |
| | | | | Aged ≥35 years | 2.3 (2.1–2.5) | |
| Heffner et al. 1993 | Case-control | Women aged 25–35 years<br>266 cases with birth at 20–26 weeks' gestation<br>512 controls with term birth<br>United States | 1988–1990 | Nonsmokers | 1.0 | Maternal age, race, gravidity, parity, income, third trimester bleeding, placental abruption, multiple gestation, previous preterm delivery, first or second trimester vaginal bleeding, chorioamnionitis, diethylstilbestrol exposure, uterine anomaly |
| | | | | Smokers | 2.0 (1.3–3.2) | |
| Li et al. 1993 | Clinical trial | 1,277 women with singleton live births and prenatal care at ≤ 32 weeks' gestation[†]<br>United States | 1986–1991 | Never smoked | 1.0 | Maternal weight, race |
| | | | | Stopped smoking | 1.0 (0.4–2.2) | |
| | | | | Reduced smoking | 1.6 (0.9–2.8) | |
| | | | | Did not change smoking habits | 1.3 (0.8–2.0) | |

[†]Preterm birth defined as <37 weeks' gestation.

**Table 3.38. Continued**

| Study | Study type | Population | Study period | Smoking status | Relative risk (95% confidence interval) | Adjustment factors |
|---|---|---|---|---|---|---|
| Mainous and Hueston 1994b | Case-control analysis of survey of pregnancy history | 305 women with deliveries at ≤ 36 weeks' gestation<br>4,766 women with term births<br>United States | 1988 | Nonsmokers<br>Smoked after first trimester<br>Stopped smoking in first trimester | 1.0<br>1.6 (1.2–2.1)<br>1.0 (0.6–1.5) | Maternal age, race, parity, family income |
| Meis et al. 1995 | Case-control analysis of survey of pregnancy history | 26,205 women with singleton births of infant >500 g<br>1,134 women with births at <257 days' gestation<br>Wales | 1970–1979 | Induced preterm delivery<br>Nonsmokers<br>Smokers<br>1–9 cigarettes/day<br>≥10 cigarettes/day<br>Spontaneous preterm delivery (including PPROM‡)<br>Nonsmokers<br>Smokers<br>1–9 cigarettes/day<br>≥10 cigarettes/day | <br>1.0<br><br>1.0 (0.8–1.4)<br>1.2 (1.0–1.5)<br><br>1.0<br><br>1.1 (0.9–1.4)<br>1.3 (1.1–1.6) | Maternal age, height, weight, parity, social class, employment during pregnancy, previous stillbirth or abortion, maternal hemoglobin at first visit, bacteriuria, bleeding early in pregnancy |
| Olsén et al. 1995 | Cohort | 20,363 women with singleton births<br>1,474 women with births at <37 weeks' gestation<br>Finland | 1966, 1985–1986 | Nonsmokers<br>Smokers | 1.0<br>1.3 (1.1–1.5) | Maternal age, height, body mass index, rural vs. urban residence, education level, employment status, socioeconomic state, desire for pregnancy, gravidity, previous spontaneous abortion |

‡PPROM = Preterm premature rupture of membranes.

smoked during the first pregnancy but not the second had lower rates of fetal death. These results suggested that smoking cessation may reduce the risk for stillbirth.

Although the causes of stillbirth are not completely understood, much of the increased risk is believed to be caused by IUGR, placental complications, or both (Raymond et al. 1994; Cnattingius and Nordstrom 1996; Wong and Bauman 1997). Another etiologic possibility is that nicotine induces a change in central respiratory control mechanism that may elicit fetal hypoxia-ischemia and lead to stillbirth (Slotkin 1998).

### Neonatal Mortality

Neonatal death (within 28 days of birth) occurs in about 4.8 of 1,000 live births in the United States (Guyer et al. 1996). The rate of neonatal death has dropped steadily since the early 1970s. However, significant racial differences in neonatal mortality continue to exist between black women and white women: 9.6 deaths per 1,000 live births among black women and 4.0 deaths per 1,000 live births among white women (Guyer et al. 1996). Racial differences in neonatal mortality likely reflect the higher percentage of LBW babies born to black women. Other risk factors for neonatal mortality include advanced maternal

**Table 3.38. Continued**

| Study | Study type | Population | Study period | Smoking status | Relative risk (95% confidence interval) | Adjustment factors |
|---|---|---|---|---|---|---|
| Peacock et al. 1995 | Cohort | 1,513 white women<br>113 women with births at <37 weeks' gestation<br>United Kingdom | 1982–1984 | Delivery at <32 weeks' gestation<br>Nonsmokers<br>Smokers<br><br>Delivery at 32–36 weeks' gestation<br>Nonsmokers<br>Smokers | <br><br>1.0<br>2.0 (1.3–2.9)<br><br><br>1.0<br>0.8 (0.6–1.2) | None |
| Zhang and Bracken 1995 | Cohort | 3,861 women with singleton live births<br>205 women with births at <37 weeks' gestation<br>United States | 1980–1982 | Nonsmokers<br>Smokers (>2 cigarettes/day) | 1.0<br>1.4[§] (1.0–1.9) | None |
| Nordentoft et al. 1996 | Cohort | 2,432 women with singleton pregnancies<br>212 women with deliveries at <37 weeks' gestation<br>Denmark | 1990–1992 | Nonsmokers<br>Smokers<br>1–9 cigarettes/day<br>10–15 cigarettes/day<br>>15 cigarettes/day | 1.0<br><br>1.1 (0.7–1.7)<br>1.1 (0.7–1.9)<br>0.5 (0.2–1.4) | Maternal age, education, cohabitation |
| Wisborg et al. 1996 | Cohort | 4,111 nulliparous women with singleton births<br>178 women with deliveries at <37 weeks' gestation<br>Denmark | 1989–1991 | Nonsmokers<br>Smokers<br>1–5 cigarettes/day<br>6–10 cigarettes/day<br>≥11 cigaretes/day | 1.0<br>1.4 (1.2–1.9)<br>1.0 (0.6–1.7)<br>1.5 (1.2–1.9)<br>1.8 (1.1–3.0) | Maternal age, education, marital status, weight, height, occupational status, alcohol abuse |

[§]Tree-based factor analysis. Relative risk was not significant after stratification by race.

age, previous fetal loss, nulliparity, multiple births, greater body mass, and high or low maternal education (Kiely et al. 1986; Cnattingius et al. 1988, 1992; Malloy et al. 1988; Haglund et al. 1993).

In the past decade, the detrimental effects of smoking on neonatal mortality have been well documented (Cnattingius et al. 1988, 1992; Malloy et al. 1988; Walsh 1994; Schramm 1997) (Table 3.39). In an investigation of 305,730 singleton white live births, the multivariate RR for neonatal deaths among smokers compared with nonsmokers was 1.2 (95 percent CI, 1.1 to 1.3) (Malloy et al. 1988). Another study (Cnattingius et al. 1988) reported a RR of 1.2 (95 percent CI, 1.0 to 1.4). Unlike the association of smoking with stillbirth, the dose-dependent effect of smoking on neonatal mortality is not clear (Cnattingius et al. 1992).

Smoking cessation appears to reduce the excess risk for adverse neonatal events. One investigation that compared the RR for neonatal deaths in first and second pregnancies found a significantly higher risk among women who smoked more in the second

**Table 3.39. Relative risks for stillbirth or neonatal death among women smokers, cohort studies**

| Study | Country | Number of pregnancies | Relative risk (95% confidence interval) | | | |
|---|---|---|---|---|---|---|
| | | | Stillbirth | | Neonatal death | |
| Cnattingius et al. 1988 | Sweden | 281,808 | Nonsmokers<br>Smokers | 1.0<br>1.4 (1.2–1.6) | Nonsmokers<br>Smokers | 1.0<br>1.2 (1.0–1.4) |
| Malloy et al. 1988 | United States | 305,730 | | | Nonsmokers<br>Smokers | 1.0<br>1.2 (1.1–1.3) |
| Raymond et al. 1994 | Sweden | 638,242 | Nonsmokers<br>Smokers | 1.0<br>1.4 (1.2–1.5) | | |
| Schramm 1997 | United States | 176,843 | Nonsmokers<br>Smokers | 1.0<br>1.2* | Nonsmokers<br>Smokers | 1.0<br>1.4* |

*p < 0.05.

pregnancy than in the first (Schramm 1997). The study also found a nonsignificant decrease in RR among women who smoked in the first pregnancy but not the second. Another study found that cessation of smoking reduced neonatal morbidity (Ahlsten et al. 1993). Specifically, the authors found that admission for hospital care occurred in 11.4 percent of infants born to mothers who smoked and 8.8 percent of infants born to mothers who did not smoke ($p < 0.05$). The mean birth weight and perinatal morbidity rates among infants of mothers who had stopped smoking during the pregnancy were almost identical to those among infants of nonsmokers.

### Perinatal Mortality

Although smoking may have different effects on the risks for stillbirth and neonatal mortality, in many studies the combined end point of perinatal mortality was presented. A meta-analysis of 25 studies of the effects of smoking on perinatal mortality revealed pooled RRs of 1.3 (95 percent CI, 1.2 to 1.3) in cohort studies and 1.2 (95 percent CI, 1.1 to 1.4) in case-control studies (DiFranza and Lew 1995). The authors estimated that 3.4 to 8.4 percent of perinatal deaths could be attributed to maternal smoking during pregnancy. Similarly, others have estimated that elimination of maternal smoking might lead to a 10-percent reduction in all infant deaths and a 12-percent reduction in death from perinatal conditions (Malloy et al. 1988). Not surprisingly, similar results of the effects of maternal smoking have been reported for the combined measure of perinatal mortality (Sachs 1989; Wilcox 1993).

### Birth Weight

Because LBW is associated with increased risks for neonatal, perinatal, and infant morbidity and mortality, birth weight has been studied extensively and used as a basic indicator of fetal health. The definition of LBW has varied among studies, but weight less than 2,500 g is a commonly accepted criterion for LBW at term. An SGA infant is one whose weight falls below a defined criterion for gestational age, such as two standard deviations or more below the population mean, or less than the 3rd or 10th percentile of weight (USDHHS 1988; Fanaroff and Martin 1992).

For more than 40 years, it has been known that babies born to mothers who smoke weigh less than babies born to mothers who do not smoke (USDHHS 1980). The effect of smoking is independent of other factors influencing birth weight, including gestational age and gender of the baby and maternal characteristics (e.g., age, parity, race, prepregnancy weight or body mass, socioeconomic status, and prenatal care). More than a dozen studies in the past decade have confirmed that the average difference in birth weight between infants born to smokers and those born to nonsmokers is about 250 g and that the difference increases with the amount smoked (Table 3.40). In a study of 257,698 births, infants of women who smoked were an average of 320 g lighter than infants born to women who did not smoke (Wilcox 1993).

Estimates of adjusted RRs for LBW associated with smoking during pregnancy have ranged from about 1.5 to 3.5, and those for SGA have ranged from about 1.5 to more than 10.0, depending on the amount smoked and other modifying factors (Table 3.41).

**Table 3.40. Difference in birth weight between infants born to women nonsmokers and those born to women smokers**

| Study | Study type | Population | Study period | Number of births | Smoking status | Difference in mean birth weight (g) | |
|---|---|---|---|---|---|---|---|
| Mathai et al. 1990 | Cohort | United Kingdom | 1987 | 285 | Nonsmokers/smokers | -66 | |
| Ahlsten et al. 1993 | Cohort | Sweden | 1987 | 3,476 | Nonsmokers/smokers | -211 | |
| Aronson et al. 1993 | Cohort | United States | 1991 | 1,282 | Nonsmokers/smokers | -258 | |
| Backe 1993 | Cohort | Norway | 1988–1989 | 1,827 | Nonsmokers/smokers | -182 | |
| | | | | | 1–5 cigarettes/day | -120 | |
| | | | | | 6–10 cigarettes/day | -201 | |
| | | | | | 11–15 cigarettes/day | -278 | |
| | | | | | 16–20 cigarettes/day | -347 | |
| | | | | | >20 cigarettes/day | +70 | |
| Castro et al. 1993 | Cohort | United States | 1986–1990 | 7,741 | Nonsmokers/smokers | -150 | |
| Li et al. 1993 | Intervention | United States | 1986–1991 | 803 | Smokers* | Blacks | Whites |
| | | | | | 101–200 ng/mL | -150 | -103 |
| | | | | | >200 ng/mL | -76 | -63 |
| Wilcox 1993 | Cohort | United States | 1980–1984 | 257,698 | Nonsmokers/smokers | -320 | |
| English et al. 1994 | Cohort | United States | 1959–1966 | 3,343 | Nonsmokers/smokers | Blacks | Whites |
| | | | | | <10 cigarettes/day | -211 | -131 |
| | | | | | 10–20 cigarettes/day | -215 | -151 |
| | | | | | >20 cigarettes/day | -277 | -207 |
| Muscati et al. 1994 | Cohort | Canada | 1979–1989 | 1,330 | Nonsmokers/smokers | -305 | |
| Cliver et al. 1995 | Cohort | United States | 1985–1988 | 1,205 | Nonsmokers/smokers | -130 | |
| Conter et al. 1995 | Cross-sectional | Italy | 1973–1981 | 12,987 | Nonsmokers/smokers | Girls | Boys |
| | | | | | 1–9 cigarettes/day | -88 | -107 |
| | | | | | ≥ 10 cigarettes/day | -168 | -247 |
| Eskenazi et al. 1995b | Cohort | United States | 1964–1967 | 3,529 | Nonsmokers/smokers† | | |
| | | | | | 0–78 ng/mL | -78 | |
| | | | | | 79–165 ng/mL | -191 | |
| | | | | | >165 ng/mL | -233 | |
| Murphy et al. 1996 | Cohort | Alaska Natives | 1989–1991 | 8,994 | Nonsmokers/smokers | | |
| | | | | | 1–5 cigarettes/day | -142 | |
| | | | | | 6–10 cigarettes/day | -239 | |
| | | | | | >10 cigarettes/day | -311 | |
| Zaren et al. 1996 | Cohort | Norway and Sweden | 1986–1988 | 933 | Nonsmokers/smokers | -231 | |
| | | | | | 1–9 cigarettes/day | -178 | |
| | | | | | ≥ 10 cigarettes/day | -263 | |

*Smokers with serum levels of cotinine <100 ng/mL after 32 weeks' gestation were compared with smokers who had higher levels.

†Smokers in each category of serum cotinine level were compared with nonsmokers.

**Table 3.41. Relative risks for infants with low birth weight (LBW) or small for gestational age (SGA) among women smokers**

| Study | Study type | Population | Study period | Number of births | Smoking status |
|---|---|---|---|---|---|
| Tenovuo et al. 1988 | Case-control | Finland | 1985 | 236 | Nonsmokers<br>Smokers<br>1–9 cigarettes/day<br>≥10 cigarettes/day |
| Cnattingius 1989 | Cohort | Sweden | 1983–1985 | 280,809 | Nonsmokers<br>Smokers<br>1–9 cigarettes/day<br>≥10 cigarettes/day |
| Alameda County Low Birth Weight Study Group 1990 | Case-control | United States | 1987 | 1,149 | Nonsmokers<br>Smokers |
| Centers for Disease Control 1990 | Survey | United States | 1989 | 74,139 | Nonsmokers<br>Smokers<br><10 cigarettes/day<br>10–20 cigarettes/day<br>>20 cigarettes/day |
| Ferraz et al. 1990 | Case-control | Brazil | 1984–1986 | 3,406 | Nonsmokers<br>Smokers |
| Wen et al. 1990b | Cohort | United States | 1983–1988 | 17,149 | Nonsmokers<br>Smokers<br>Aged ≤16 years<br>Aged 17–19 years<br>Aged 20–25 years<br>Aged 26–30 years<br>Aged 31–35 years<br>Aged ≥36 years |
| McDonald et al. 1992 | Survey | Canada | 1982–1984 | 40,445 | Nonsmokers<br>Smokers<br><10 cigarettes/day<br>10–19 cigarettes/day<br>≥20 cigarettes/day |
| Backe 1993 | Cohort | Norway | 1988–1989 | 1,827 | Nonsmokers<br>Smokers<br>Aged <25 years<br>Aged 25–34 years<br>Aged ≥35 years |

*LBW defined as birth weight <2,500 g or ≤ 2,500 g.
†95% confidence interval was not reported.
‡SGA defined as birth weight ≤ 2.5th percentile for gestational age.
§SGA defined as birth weight <5th percentile for gestational age.
ΔSGA defined as birth weight <10th percentile for gestational age.

| Relative risk (95% confidence interval) | | |
|---|---|---|
| **LBW*** | **SGA** | **Adjustment factors** |
| | 1.0<br>1.6[†‡]<br>3.4[†‡] | Matching on gestational age and mode of delivery, adjustment for previous SGA infant, low social class, low prepregnancy weight |
| | Single births: 1.0<br>2.0 (1.9–2.1)[§]<br>2.5 (2.4–2.6)[§]<br>Multiple births: 1.0<br>1.5 (1.3–1.6)[§]<br>1.8 (1.6–2.0)[§] | Maternal age, parity, relationship with father |
| Whites: 1.0<br>3.0 (1.7–5.3)<br>Blacks: 1.0<br>3.6 (2.4–5.6) | | Maternal age, parity, low prepregnancy weight, low socioeconomic status, alcohol intake, prior LBW infant, prenatal care |
| 1.0[†]<br>1.8[†]<br>2.2[†]<br>2.4[†] | | Maternal education, maternal age, prepregnancy weight, weight gain, alcohol consumption, infant's birth order, month prenatal care began, previous pregnancy terminations |
| | 1.0<br>1.5 (1.1–2.0)[Δ] | Adjustment factors in final model not stated |
| | 1.0<br>1.6 (0.7–3.4)[Δ]<br>2.0 (1.3–3.1)[Δ]<br>2.4 (1.9–3.2)[Δ]<br>2.4 (1.7–3.3)[Δ]<br>2.3 (1.3–4.0)[Δ]<br>5.1 (1.3–20.5)[Δ] | Race, parity, marital status, weight, weight gain, alcohol use |
| 1.0<br>1.6 (1.4–1.9)<br>2.4 (2.1–2.7)<br>2.9 (2.5–3.2) | 1.0<br>2.0 (1.7–2.3)[§]<br>2.6 (2.3–2.9)[§]<br>3.2 (2.8–3.6)[§] | Age, ethnic group, education, pregnancy order, previous spontaneous abortion or LBW infant, prepregnancy weight, employment, alcohol consumption, coffee consumption |
| | 1.0<br>1.3 (0.8–2.0)[Δ]<br>1.6 (1.1–2.3)[Δ]<br>3.8 (1.4–10.2)[Δ] | None |

**Table 3.41. Continued**

| Study | Study type | Population | Study period | Number of births | Smoking status |
|---|---|---|---|---|---|
| Bakketeig et al. 1993 | Cohort | Norway and Sweden | 1986–1988 | 5,722 | No other risk factors |
| | | | | | Nonsmokers |
| | | | | | Smokers |
| | | | | | Previous LBW infant |
| | | | | | Nonsmokers |
| | | | | | Smokers |
| | | | | | Maternal weight <50 kg |
| | | | | | Nonsmokers |
| | | | | | Smokers |
| | | | | | Previous LBW infant and maternal weight <50 kg |
| | | | | | Nonsmokers |
| | | | | | Smokers |
| Castro et al. 1993 | Cohort | United States | 1986–1990 | 7,741 | Nonsmokers |
| | | | | | Smokers |
| Lieberman et al. 1994 | Cohort | United States | 1977–1980 | 11,177 | Nonsmokers |
| | | | | | Smokers |
| | | | | | 1–5 cigarettes/day |
| | | | | | 6–10 cigarettes/day |
| | | | | | >10 cigarettes/day |
| Spinillo et al. 1994c | Case-control | Italy | 1988–1993 | 1,041 | Nonsmokers |
| | | | | | Smokers |
| | | | | | 1–10 cigarettes/day |
| | | | | | 11–20 cigarettes/day |
| | | | | | >20 cigarettes/day |
| Cornelius et al. 1995 | Cohort | Black adolescents United States | 1990–1993 | 310 | Nonsmokers |
| | | | | | Smokers |
| Eskenazi et al. 1995b | Cohort | United States | 1964–1967 | 3,529 | Nonsmokers (0–1.9 ng/mL) |
| | | | | | Smokers[¶] |
| | | | | | 0–78 ng/mL |
| | | | | | 79–165 ng/mL |
| | | | | | >165 ng/mL |
| Zhang and Bracken 1995 | Cohort | United States | 1980–1982 | 3,861 | Nonsmokers |
| | | | | | Smokers |
| Nordentoft et al. 1996 | Cohort | Denmark | 1990–1992 | 2,432 | Nonsmokers |
| | | | | | Smokers |
| | | | | | 0–9 cigarettes/day |
| | | | | | 10–15 cigarettes/day |
| | | | | | >15 cigarettes/day |
| Cnattingius 1997 | Cohort | Sweden | 1983–1992 | 1,057,711 | Nonsmokers |
| | | | | | Smokers |
| | | | | | 1–9 cigarettes/day |
| | | | | | ≥10 cigarettes/day |

*LBW defined as birth weight <2,500 g or ≤2,500 g.
[Δ]SGA defined as birth weight <10th percentile for gestational age.
[¶]Smokers in each category of serum cotinine concentration were compared with nonsmokers.

| Relative risk (95% confidence interval) | | |
|---|---|---|
| **LBW*** | **SGA** | **Adjustment factors** |
| | 1.0<br>1.8 (1.4–2.3)[Δ]<br><br>2.5 (1.7–3.8)[Δ]<br>6.9 (5.1–9.4)[Δ]<br><br>1.3 (0.6–2.6)[Δ]<br>4.7 (3.2–6.9)[Δ]<br><br>2.6 (0.6–10.4)[Δ]<br>8.8 (4.9–16.0)[Δ] | Adjustment factors not stated |
| | 1.0<br>2.0 (1.5–2.7)[Δ] | Race and ethnicity, nulliparity, insurance status, marital status |
| | 1.0<br><br>1.7 (1.3–2.1)[Δ]<br>2.2 (1.7–2.7)[Δ]<br>2.5 (2.1–3.0)[Δ] | Maternal age, education, race, marital status, body mass index, height, weight gain, late prenatal care, parity, exposure to diethylstilbestrol, hypertension, urinary tract infection, payment source |
| | 1.0<br>2.9 (2.1–3.9)[Δ]<br>1.5 (0.99–2.3)[Δ]<br>4.1 (2.7–6.3)[Δ]<br>9.9 (4.0–24.4)[Δ] | Maternal age, marital status, nulliparity, low prepregnancy weight, body mass index <20 kg/m², weight gain <5 kg, previous LBW infant, female infant, first trimester hemorrhage, hypertension, hypertensive disorders of pregnancy, maternal education <6th grade, manual (nonskilled) social class, alcohol consumption, coffee consumption |
| 1.0<br>3.1 (1.2–8.0) | | Adjustment factors in final model not stated |
| 1.0<br><br>1.2 (0.7–1.9)<br>1.6 (1.1–2.4)<br>3.3 (2.4–4.6) | | None |
| | Whites** / Blacks**<br>1.0 / 1.0<br>2.0 (1.2–3.0) / 1.5 (1.0–2.4) | None |
| | 1.0<br><br>2.4 (1.5–3.8)[Δ]<br>2.7 (1.5–4.7)[Δ]<br>2.9 (1.4–6.1)[Δ] | Maternal age, education, social network, psychosocial stress |
| | 1.0<br><br>2.1 (2.1–2.2)[††]<br>2.7 (2.6–2.8)[††] | Parity, maternal cohabitation with infant's father |

**SGA defined as in Brenner et al. 1976.
[††]SGA defined as birth weight ≤2 standard deviations below mean for gestational age.

Twenty percent or more of the incidence of LBW and SGA can be attributed to cigarette smoking (Alameda County Low Birth Weight Study Group 1990; CDC 1990; Backe 1993; Roquer et al. 1995; Muscati et al. 1996; Cnattingius 1997). Numerous studies have demonstrated a statistically significant dose-response relationship between the number of cigarettes smoked by the mother and higher RRs for LBW or SGA (Kleinman and Madans 1985; Bell and Lumley 1989; Brooke et al. 1989; CDC 1990; McDonald et al. 1992; Lieberman et al. 1994; Spinillo et al. 1994c). In most of these studies, adverse effects of smoking were apparent even among the lightest smokers (e.g., less than one-half pack of cigarettes per day). In a study examining the type of cigarettes smoked, Peacock and colleagues (1991) compared birth weights of infants born to women who smoked low-yield cigarettes (<12 mg of CO per cigarette) with those born to women who smoked high-yield cigarettes. They reported that women who smoked a low number (<15 cigarettes per day) of low-yield cigarettes had infants with birth weights comparable to those of nonsmokers' infants. However, women who smoked a low number of high-yield cigarettes had infants with an average birth weight 8 percent lower than that of nonsmokers' infants.

Studies that used cotinine or other nicotine metabolites as a measure of exposure to cigarette smoke also showed an increased risk for LBW among infants of smokers, as shown in Table 3.40 (Mathai et al. 1990; Li et al. 1993; Eskenazi et al. 1995b), in Table 3.41 (Eskenazi et al. 1995b), and in other studies (Bardy et al. 1993; English et al. 1994; Ellard et al. 1996; Wang et al. 1997b; Peacock et al. 1998). These studies are especially important because some women who smoke may report themselves as nonsmokers. This misreporting results in misclassification of smokers and nonsmokers and underestimation of the true effect of smoking (Bardy et al. 1993). Among 3,529 pregnant women who had serum cotinine concentration measured at approximately 27 weeks' gestation, smokers had infants weighing an average of 78, 191, and 233 g less than infants of nonsmokers for the first, second, and third tertiles of increasing cotinine concentration, respectively (Eskenazi et al. 1995b). Similar trends of decreasing birth weight with increasing urine cotinine concentration were found in several other studies (Mathai et al. 1990; Bardy et al. 1993; Ellard et al. 1996; Wang et al. 1997b; Peacock et al. 1998).

A number of investigations have found that the effects of smoking on birth weight become more pronounced as maternal age increases (Cnattingius et al. 1985, 1993; Cnattingius 1989; Wen et al. 1990a; Aronson et al. 1993; Backe 1993; Fox et al. 1994). For example, in a large study from Sweden, the RRs for delivering an SGA infant among women who smoked 10 or more cigarettes per day compared with nonsmokers were 1.9 (95 percent CI, 1.7 to 2.1) for mothers 15 through 19 years old and 3.4 (95 percent CI, 3.0 to 3.8) for mothers 40 through 44 years old (Cnattingius 1989). The reasons for this pattern of findings are not clear (Fox et al. 1994). The smoking-related risks for LBW and SGA may be higher among women who have had no live births than among those who have had at least one live birth (Cnattingius et al. 1993).

The effects of smoking on birth weight appear to be similar among various racial groups in the United States (e.g., whites and blacks) (Alameda County Low Birth Weight Study Group 1990; CDC 1990; Castro et al. 1993; USDHHS 1998), but the findings from one study suggested stronger effects among black women than among white women (English et al. 1994). Lower average birth weight has also been reported among infants of Alaska Native smokers (Murphy et al. 1996) and Mexican American smokers (Wolff et al. 1993) compared with nonsmokers of the same race or ethnicity. However, in these studies, no comparisons were made with other racial or ethnic groups.

Cliver and colleagues (1995) found that birth weight, crown-to-heel length, and chest circumference were significantly less affected among infants whose mothers had stopped smoking during pregnancy than among infants born to women who continued to smoke. It is unclear exactly how early in pregnancy smoking cessation must occur to avoid the adverse effects of smoking on fetal growth. The longer the mother smokes during pregnancy, the greater the effect on the infant's birth weight (Adriaanse et al. 1996). Most studies suggested that infants of women who stop smoking by the first trimester have weight and body measurements comparable to those of nonsmokers' infants and that smoking in the third trimester is particularly detrimental (MacArthur and Knox 1988; Frank et al. 1994; Lieberman et al. 1994; Mainous and Hueston 1994a; Zaren et al. 1996). In one study, even women who were heavy smokers in the first trimester but who had stopped smoking before the second trimester had only an insignificantly higher risk for delivering an LBW infant than did women nonsmokers (RR, 1.2; 95 percent CI, 0.7 to 2.1) (McDonald et al. 1992). Reducing the amount smoked by the mother seems to be associated with infant birth weights higher than those among infants of mothers who do not reduce the amount smoked, but the benefits are considerably smaller than for complete smoking cessation (McDonald et al. 1992; Li et al. 1993). Women nonsmokers who smoked during a previous pregnancy seem to have babies whose birth weights and risks for LBW and SGA are comparable to those of infants born to women who had never smoked (Nordstrom and Cnattingius 1994; Schramm 1997).

In principle, the apparent benefit of smoking cessation in observational studies could simply reflect other differences between women who stop smoking and those who continue to smoke. For example, women who stop smoking tend to be lighter smokers than those who continue to smoke (Lieberman et al. 1994; Nordstrom and Cnattingius 1994). However, the reported effects of cessation are probably not due to uncontrolled confounding. Even after consideration of the numbers of cigarettes smoked, cessation confers a benefit over continued smoking (McDonald et al. 1992; Li et al. 1993; Frank et al. 1994; Lieberman et al. 1994; Adriaanse et al. 1996). Randomized clinical trials of smoking cessation programs provided even stronger evidence of the benefit of cessation with regard to birth weight (Dolan-Mullen et al. 1994).

Smoking may lower birth weight by causing premature birth at less than 37 weeks' gestation (see "Preterm Delivery" earlier in this section), fetal growth retardation, or both. The nicotine and CO in cigarette smoke could cause fetal growth retardation (USDHHS 1988; Lambers and Clark 1996). Impairment of uteroplacental circulation, caused by the vasoconstrictive effect of nicotine, results in fetal hypoxia and impaired fetal nutrition, both of which may disrupt normal growth (Nash and Persaud 1988). Fetal hypoxia due to elevated carboxyhemoglobin levels from the CO in cigarette smoke may also retard fetal growth. Another mechanism contributing to the reduced birth weight associated with maternal smoking may be that pregnant women who smoke gain less weight than do nonsmokers (Ellard et al. 1996; Muscati et al. 1996). A study of more than 3,000 women reported that smokers gained an average of 9.9 kg (21.8 pounds) during pregnancy and that nonsmokers gained an average of 11.6 kg (25.5 pounds) (Ellard et al. 1996). The lower weight gain among women who smoke during pregnancy and the lower birth weight among their infants may not be explained by lower energy intake: in one investigation, smokers consumed significantly more calories per day than did nonsmokers but gained less weight (Muscati et al. 1996). Increased weight gain during pregnancy and higher prepregnancy weight among women who smoke may partially mitigate the negative effects of smoking on fetal growth (Muscati et al. 1996), but even after adjustment for pregnancy weight gain, maternal smoking is associated with SGA (Wen et al. 1990b; Lieberman et al. 1994; Spinillo et al. 1994c; Zaren et al. 1997).

### Congenital Malformations

Congenital malformations (birth defects) encompass a wide variety of structural malformations that occur during gestation. Common categories of birth defects include central nervous system (CNS) malformations, such as neural tube defects, circulatory and respiratory (e.g., cardiac) anomalies, chromosomal anomalies, gastrointestinal malformations, musculoskeletal and integumental anomalies (e.g., oral clefts and limb reductions), and urogenital malformations. Risk factors for congenital malformations are difficult to assess as a group, because different defects have distinct etiologies. However, in general, advanced maternal age, previous perinatal death, and radiation (Seidman et al. 1990; Pradat 1992) confer an increased risk for birth defects to the developing fetus. Folic acid intake appears to reduce the risk for some malformations, particularly neural tube defects (Medical Research Council Vitamin Study Research Group 1991; Shaw et al. 1991). In this section, recent literature highlighting the relationship between smoking and risk for congenital malformations is reviewed.

#### *Overall Risk*

To date, most studies have found no association between cigarette smoking during pregnancy and the overall risk for birth defects (Shiono et al. 1986a; Malloy et al. 1989; Seidman et al. 1990; Van den Eeden et al. 1990; McDonald et al. 1992; Werler 1997) (Table 3.42). For example, one study of 33,434 live births in California found a RR of 1.0 (95 percent CI, 0.8 to 1.2) for "major" malformations among smokers compared with nonsmokers (Shiono et al. 1986a). The risk among smokers for "minor" malformations was lower than that among nonsmokers (RR, 0.9; 95 percent CI, 0.8 to 0.9). Similarly, in a case-control study among 3,284 singleton live births with at least one malformation and 4,500 controls, RR was 1.0 (95 percent CI, 0.9 to 1.1) among smokers (Van den Eeden 1990). These results suggested that, as a whole, maternal cigarette smoking during pregnancy does not have teratogenic effects on live-born infants. Some investigators have suggested that this lack of effect on the risk for birth defects can be explained by the increased risk

**Table 3.42. Relative risks for congenital malformations among infants of women smokers**

| Study | Study type | Country | Number of infants | Relative risk (95% confidence interval) of malformations | |
|---|---|---|---|---|---|
| Shiono et al. 1986a | Cohort | United States | 33,434 | Nonsmokers | 1.0 |
| | | | | Smokers | |
| | | | | Major malformation of infant | 1.0 (0.8–1.2) |
| | | | | Minor malformation of infant | 0.9 (0.8–0.9) |
| Malloy et al. 1989 | Cohort | United States | 288,067 | Nonsmokers | 1.0 |
| | | | | Smokers | |
| | | | | All birth defects | 0.98 (0.94–1.03) |
| Seidman et al. 1990 | Cohort | Israel | 17,152 | Nonsmokers | 1.0 |
| | | | | Smokers | |
| | | | | Major malformation of infant | 0.9 (0.6–1.4) |
| | | | | Minor malformation of infant | 1.1 (0.9–1.3) |
| Van den Eeden et al. 1990 | Case-control | United States | 3,284 cases<br>4,500 controls | Nonsmokers | 1.0 |
| | | | | Smokers | |
| | | | | Any birth defect | 1.0 (0.9–1.1) |

for spontaneous abortion, stillbirth, or both among smokers (Shiono et al. 1986a; Van den Eeden et al. 1990; Li et al. 1996; Källén 1998). These outcomes would prevent a deformed fetus from being born alive and recognized as having a birth defect. Nonetheless, smoking may be modestly related to an increased risk for certain birth defects, such as oral clefts, limb reductions, and urogenital or gastrointestinal defects (see below). CO and nicotine from the cigarette smoke may increase the risks for fetal hypoxia and vascular disruption, which can cause birth defects (Czeizel et al. 1994; Li et al. 1996; Werler 1996). Other possible mechanisms by which cigarette smoke may produce birth defects include toxic effects on the fetus from metabolites present in the smoke (Li et al. 1996), decreased use of folate (Alderman et al. 1994), or mutagenic effects (Seidman et al. 1990).

*Central Nervous System Malformations*

CNS defects occur at a rate of about 100 per 100,000 live births (Ventura et al. 1997). Neural tube defects (anencephaly, spina bifida, and encephalocele) are the most common form of neurologic malformations (Werler 1997). Several studies have shown that maternal smoking during pregnancy is not related to an increased risk for neural tube defects (Van den Eeden et al. 1990; Wassermann et al. 1996; Källén 1998). After adjusting for year of birth, maternal age, parity, education level, and other possible risk factors, an investigator in Sweden found a protective effect of smoking for all neural tube defects (RR, 0.8; 95 percent CI, 0.6 to 0.9) (Källén 1998). On the other hand, some findings suggested a positive association of smoking with other CNS malformations (e.g., microcephaly) (Van den Eeden et al. 1990).

Craniosynostosis (premature closure of one or more suture joints in the skull) is not primarily a CNS defect, but it does have implications for the CNS. In one study, maternal smoking was found to confer an increased risk for craniosynostosis (Alderman et al. 1994).

*Cardiac Defects*

Heart malformations are relatively common birth defects and occur in about 124 of 100,000 live births (Ventura et al. 1997). No strong evidence has appeared for an association between maternal smoking and the risk for cardiac malformation (Malloy et al. 1989; Van den Eeden et al. 1990; Pradat 1992). A case-control study of major congenital heart defects found a RR of 0.9 (95 percent CI, 0.8 to 1.1) among women smokers compared with nonsmokers (Pradat 1992). However, another study that examined the effect of smoking on conotruncal malformations found a higher risk when both parents smoked than when neither parent smoked (RR, 1.9; 95 percent CI, 1.2 to 3.1) (Wassermann et al. 1996). No effect was found for maternal smoking only.

*Oral Clefts*

Oral clefts are estimated to occur in 82 of 100,000 live births (Ventura et al. 1997) and are categorized as cleft lip (with or without cleft palate) and cleft palate (Wyszynski et al. 1997). These defects have been the subject of several epidemiological investigations. For cleft lip with or without cleft palate, one investigation found a RR of 1.5 (95 percent CI, 1.0 to 2.1) among smokers after adjustment for maternal age and parity (Van den Eeden et al. 1990). In three large studies (Shaw et al. 1996; Christensen et al. 1999; Lorente et al. 2000), investigators noted an increasing risk for cleft lip with or without cleft palate with increasing amount of maternal smoking. However, a third large study did not find a dose-effect relationship (Werler et al. 1990).

For cleft palate only, one investigation found a RR of 1.4 (95 percent CI, 1.1 to 1.6) among smokers (Källén 1997b). Others found the risk for cleft palate to be increased among women who smoked 20 or more cigarettes per day (RR, 2.2; 95 percent CI, 1.1 to 4.5) (Shaw et al. 1996). No effect of smoking was found among women who smoked fewer than 20 cigarettes per day. Other investigators reported no effect of smoking on the risk for cleft palate (Van den Eeden 1990; Werler et al. 1990; Christensen et al. 1999). A meta-analysis reported an overall RR of 1.3 (95 percent CI, 1.2 to 1.4) for cleft lip with or without cleft palate and an overall RR of 1.3 (95 percent CI, 1.1 to 1.6) for cleft palate (Wyszynski et al. 1997). This association does not appear to be due to confounding by alcohol intake (Källén 1997b).

Recent evidence suggested that the inconsistency among reports may be, in part, explained by an interaction between smoking and genetic factors (Hwang et al. 1995; Shaw et al. 1996; Werler 1997). Two studies (Hwang et al. 1995; Shaw et al. 1996) reported that women with the uncommon allele for transforming growth factor alpha and who smoke during pregnancy are at significantly greater risk for delivering an infant with cleft lip with or without cleft palate or an infant with cleft palate than are nonsmoking women with the common allele.

*Limb Reductions*

Limb reductions (the absence or severe underdevelopment of proximal or distal limbs) are reported to occur in 60 per 100,000 live births (Källén 1997c). Most studies have found no effect of maternal smoking on the risk for overall limb reductions (Shiono et al. 1986a; Van den Eeden et al. 1990; McDonald et al. 1992; Wassermann et al. 1996), although a case-control study among Swedish infants found a RR of 1.3 (95 percent CI, 1.1 to 1.5) for any maternal smoking and the risk for limb reduction (Källén 1997c).

Two studies reported significant associations between certain limb reductions and maternal smoking. Källén (1997c) reported a RR of 1.3 (95 percent CI, 1.01 to 1.6) for transverse reductions. Other investigators found RRs of 2.1 (95 percent CI, 1.3 to 3.6) for terminal transverse deficiencies among infants of smokers compared with infants of nonsmokers; a significant dose-response relationship was found after multivariate adjustment (Czeizel et al. 1994). The association between transverse limb reductions and maternal smoking is biologically plausible, because these defects are believed to result from vascular interruption (Werler 1997).

*Down Syndrome*

Down syndrome affects about 45 per 100,000 live births (Ventura et al. 1997), and the risk increases sharply among older women (Chard and Macintosh 1995). A few studies have found a protective effect of maternal smoking on the risk for giving birth to a child with Down syndrome (Hook and Cross 1985, 1988; Shiono et al. 1986a). Most investigations, however, have reported no effect of smoking (Cuckle et al. 1990a; Seidman et al. 1990; Van den Eeden 1990; Källén 1997a), particularly after careful control for maternal age (Chen et al. 1999).

*Digestive and Urinary Tract Malformations*

Urogenital abnormalities have been reported to occur at a rate of 121 per 100,000 live births (Ventura et al. 1997). Three large case-control studies found no effect of smoking on the risk to the offspring for developing urogenital anomalies (Shiono et al. 1986a; Seidman et al. 1990; Van den Eeden et al. 1990). More recent investigations that have examined individual defects have reported cases of smoking-related malformations of urinary organs. For example, one study reported a weak association (RR, 1.2; 95 percent CI, 1.0 to 1.5) between maternal smoking and kidney malformations (Källén 1997d). Smoking was also found to be a risk factor for congenital urinary tract abnormalities (RR, 2.3; 95 percent CI, 1.2 to 4.5), but no dose-response relationship could be substantiated (Li et al. 1996).

Gastrointestinal abnormalities are much less frequent and occur in about 82 per 100,000 live births (Ventura et al. 1997). Maternal smoking during pregnancy has sometimes been associated with increased risks for gastroschisis (Werler et al. 1992; Torfs et al. 1994) and anal atresia (Yuan et al. 1995). However, three case-control studies did not find any affect of smoking on the risk for gastrointestinal abnormalities (Shiono et al. 1986a; Seidman et al. 1990; Van den Eeden et al. 1990).

## Breastfeeding

Breastfeeding is widely recognized to have nutritional benefits and preventive effects against infectious diseases, such as respiratory tract infections and diarrhea, among infants (Victora et al. 1987). These conditions are the leading causes of death among infants in developing countries, where infant mortality is high. Duration of lactation differs among societies, but studies have generally shown a positive association with maternal age, education, and socioeconomic class (Andersen et al. 1982a).

Because the definitions of breastfeeding, weaning, and smoking differ greatly among studies, summarizing information about the relationship between smoking and breastfeeding is difficult. Nevertheless, studies have consistently shown that women who smoke are less likely to start breastfeeding than are nonsmokers (Yeung et al. 1981) and tend to wean an infant earlier than do nonsmokers (Lyon 1983; Counsilman and Mackay 1985; Feinstein et al. 1986; Woodward 1988; Matheson and Rivrud 1989; Rutishauser and Carlin 1992; Ever-Hadani et al. 1994). Maternal milk production of smokers is more than 250 mL/day less than that of nonsmokers (Vio et al. 1991; Hopkinson et al. 1992); the number of cigarettes smoked per day and the duration of breastfeeding are negatively associated (Horta et al. 1997). In most epidemiologic studies, these associations are evident even after careful adjustment for indicators of social class (Lyon 1983; Nylander and Matheson 1989; Horta et al. 1997). A study from southern Brazil is typical: 28 percent of mothers who smoked at least 20 cigarettes per day were still breastfeeding at 6 months after delivery, whereas 40 percent of mothers who did not smoke were still breastfeeding then (Horta et al. 1997). Findings from this study have also suggested that exposure to ETS may be associated with shorter duration of breastfeeding.

Initiation and maintenance of lactation require maternal secretion of the hormone prolactin (Akre 1989). One group of investigators found that among lactating women, basal prolactin levels were lower for smokers than for nonsmokers (Andersen and Schiöler 1982; Andersen et al. 1982a). This effect could provide a physiologic basis for an association between smoking and early weaning. Several studies of men and nonlactating women also reported lower prolactin levels among smokers than among nonsmokers (Andersen and Schiöler 1982; Andersen et al. 1984; Baron et al. 1986a; Fuxe et al. 1989), but other studies have not found this pattern (Wilkins et al. 1982; Jernström et al. 1992). These discrepancies may relate to differences across studies in the pattern of smoking before blood sampling. In rats, isolated exposure to nicotine has increased prolactin levels (Sharp and Beyer 1986), whereas repeated exposure has inhibited secretion (Terkel et al. 1973; Andersson et al. 1985; Fuxe et al. 1989).

## Sudden Infant Death Syndrome

Sudden infant death syndrome (SIDS) is the sudden death of an infant younger than 1 year of age that remains unexplained after a thorough investigation, including a complete autopsy, examination of the death scene, and a review of the clinical history (Willinger et al. 1991). In the United States, SIDS is the leading cause of death among infants 1 to 12 months of age and affects more than 0.1 percent of live births. Although the causes of SIDS are unknown, several risk factors have been identified. Black infants and American Indian infants have SIDS mortality rates two to three times higher than do white infants. Prone sleeping position and not having been breastfed are also associated with increased risk (Willinger et al. 1994).

In many studies, maternal smoking during pregnancy has been associated with SIDS (Bergman and Wiesner 1976; Avery and Frantz 1983; Malloy et al. 1988, 1992; Kraus et al. 1989; McGlashan 1989; Bulterys et al. 1990; Haglund and Cnattingius 1990; Li and Daling 1991; Mitchell et al. 1991; Schoendorf and Kiely 1992; Scragg et al. 1993; DiFranza and Lew 1995; Klonoff-Cohen et al. 1995; Golding 1997; MacDorman et al. 1997). The association has persisted after adjustment for covariates such as infant sleeping position, birth weight, and race as well as maternal age, marital status, education, and parity (Malloy et al. 1988; Bulterys et al. 1990; Li and Daling 1991; Schoendorf and Kiely 1992; Scragg et al. 1993). However, because smoking during and after pregnancy are highly correlated, it is difficult to separate the effects of these two exposures (Spiers 1999).

Few studies of SIDS obtained data to distinguish between the effects of maternal smoking during pregnancy and the effects of passive smoking on the infant after delivery. Schoendorf and Kiely (1992) compared the risk for SIDS among infants of mothers who did not smoke, infants of mothers who smoked during pregnancy and after delivery, and infants of mothers who smoked only after delivery. After adjustment for demographic risk factors, infants whose mothers smoked both during pregnancy and after delivery had three times the risk for SIDS as infants born to mothers who did not smoke. Among infants of mothers who smoked only after delivery, the adjusted RR for SIDS was about 2.0. A case-control study from southern California also reported an independent effect of passive exposure to smoke after delivery on the risk for SIDS (Klonoff-Cohen et al. 1995).

Several case-control and cohort studies reported a dose-response relationship between the number of cigarettes smoked during pregnancy and the risk for SIDS (Kraus et al. 1989; Bulterys et al. 1990; Haglund and Cnattingius 1990; Malloy et al. 1992; Scragg et al. 1993; Klonoff-Cohen et al. 1995; MacDorman et al. 1997). For example, in a study that included 636 infants who died of SIDS, the RR for SIDS among infants whose mothers smoked less than one pack of cigarettes per day was 2.0 (95 percent CI, 1.6 to 2.4), and the RR among infants whose mothers smoked at least one pack per day was 2.9 (95 percent CI, 2.3 to 3.5) (Malloy et al. 1992).

In summary, maternal smoking during pregnancy has been repeatedly associated with SIDS, and the risk increases with the number of cigarettes smoked daily. A meta-analysis of studies that compared the incidence of SIDS among the offspring of women who smoked during pregnancy and those who did not yielded a pooled RR of 3.0 (95 percent CI, 2.5 to 3.5) (DiFranza and Lew 1995). The mechanism by which smoking affects the risk for SIDS is not clear. One possibility is that tobacco smoke interferes with neuroregulation of breathing and causes apneic spells that lead to sudden infant death (Avery and Frantz 1983).

### Conclusions

1. Women who smoke have increased risks for conception delay and for both primary and secondary infertility.
2. Women who smoke may have a modest increase in risks for ectopic pregnancy and spontaneous abortion.
3. Smoking during pregnancy is associated with increased risks for preterm premature rupture of membranes, abruptio placentae, and placenta previa, and with a modest increase in risk for preterm delivery.
4. Women who smoke during pregnancy have a decreased risk for preeclampsia.
5. The risk for perinatal mortality—both stillbirth and neonatal deaths—and the risk for sudden infant death syndrome (SIDS) are increased among the offspring of women who smoke during pregnancy.
6. Infants born to women who smoke during pregnancy have a lower average birth weight and are more likely to be small for gestational age than are infants born to women who do not smoke.
7. Smoking does not appear to affect the overall risk for congenital malformations.
8. Women smokers are less likely to breastfeed their infants than are women nonsmokers.
9. Women who quit smoking before or during pregnancy reduce the risk for adverse reproductive outcomes, including conception delay, infertility, preterm premature rupture of membranes, preterm delivery, and low birth weight.

## Body Weight and Fat Distribution

### Body Weight

The term "obesity" is most often understood to refer to a high body weight in relation to height. BMI is the most commonly used measure of body size and is defined as weight (in kilograms) divided by the square of height (in meters) (Bray 1998). Beside the effects on health, body weight may be a focus of concern about attractiveness and body image. The association between smoking and low body weight has been recognized by the lay public (USDHHS 1988, 1990; Klesges et al. 1989), and concern about weight may encourage smoking initiation and impede cessation (see "Factors Influencing Initiation of Smoking" in Chapter 4 and "Weight Control" in Chapter 5). Smoking cessation may result in weight gain, yet smoking may promote a harmful pattern of body fat distribution. These aspects of the relationship between smoking and weight are discussed here.

Cross-sectional studies generally have found that smokers weigh less than former smokers and those who had never smoked (Klesges et al. 1989; Grunberg 1990). The weight differences increase with age—a finding that suggested smoking may inhibit weight gain over relatively long periods of time (Klesges et al. 1989, 1991a). Among current smokers, there tends to be a U-shaped curve for the relationship between smoking and body mass: typically, moderate smokers (approximately 10 to 20 cigarettes per day) weigh less than light smokers (<10 cigarettes per day), and heavy smokers (≥ 20 cigarettes per day) weigh more than moderate smokers (Albanes et al. 1987; Klesges et al. 1989, 1991b; Klesges and Klesges 1993). Most of the data on this association have been generated by research among whites. One study, however, reported that this relationship was particularly pronounced among black women, in contrast to a regular inverse relationship in that study between the number of cigarettes smoked and weight among white women, white men, and black men who smoked (Klesges and Klesges 1993).

### Body Weight and Smoking Initiation

Because of the negative relationship between smoking and body weight and the common finding that weight gain occurs after smoking cessation, the public and several reviews of the literature (USDHHS 1988, 1990; Klesges et al. 1989) concluded, perhaps prematurely, that persons who start smoking lose weight. Concern about body weight appears to be related to smoking initiation (see "Other Issues" in Chapter 2 and "Concerns About Weight Control" in Chapter 4). Most adolescents believe that smoking controls body weight (Camp et al. 1993), and women, in particular, report that they smoke to keep body weight down (USDHHS 1988; Gritz et al. 1989; Grunberg 1990). However, more recent studies indicated that smoking initiation may not be related to short-term changes in body weight.

Only four prospective studies that included women examined changes in body weight after smoking initiation, and three of these were among women aged about 30 through 60 years, after the age of smoking initiation for most women. Results from these studies were conflicting. Data on more than 3,500 women (mean age at baseline, 38 years) showed that weight gain over two years did not differ significantly among women and men who started smoking or among those who did not (French et al. 1994). Similar results were reported for the 55,000 women in the U.S. Nurses' Health Study after eight years of follow-up (Colditz et al. 1992). The nurses who began smoking gained an average of 9.2 pounds over the eight years, whereas those who had never smoked gained 8.2 pounds on average. Among current smokers of 1 to 24 cigarettes per day, the mean weight gain was 11.2 pounds; that among women who currently smoked 25 or more cigarettes per day was 11.9 pounds. In contrast, in a cohort of women followed for an average of six years, the women who started smoking lost 0.37 BMI units and the women who had never smoked gained 0.62 BMI units ($p < 0.01$) (Lissner et al. 1992).

One prospective study examined the relationship between smoking initiation and body weight among adults aged 18 through 30 years (Klesges et al. 1998). The investigators evaluated 5,115 women and men at three time points during a seven-year period. Continuing smokers, persons who began smoking between the first and second evaluations, and those who had never smoked were compared with persons who had stopped smoking. Although persons in all groups gained weight, no significant differences in body weight among the groups emerged during the follow-up period; those who began smoking did not lose weight or have an attentuated weight gain. At least over a seven-year period, smoking initiation did not affect body weight and continued smoking did not have anorectic effects or suppress weight.

No prospective studies of smoking initiation and body weight have been conducted among adolescents, who are the most likely age group to start smoking (see "Smoking Initiation" in Chapter 2). Such studies should be a high priority for future research because concerns about body weight appear to be associated with smoking initiation among adolescents (see "Smoking Initiation" in Chapter 2). However, the anorectic effect of smoking is small, and smoking may affect body weight only after decades of smoking (Klesges et al. 1989). Because most cross-sectional studies of body weight differences between smokers and nonsmokers focused on middle-aged persons, the anorectic qualities of smoking may have been overestimated. For example, if the average weight difference between smokers and nonsmokers in middle age (e.g., 45 years of age) is about 5.5 pounds after about 30 years of smoking (Klesges et al. 1989), then on average, each year of smoking would contribute less than two-tenths of a pound to the weight difference.

### Body Weight and Smoking Cessation

Smoking cessation has been shown to result in weight gain among both women and men, but the magnitude of the gain and the mechanisms involved are not clear (Klesges et al. 1989; Williamson et al. 1991). In a review of 43 longitudinal studies that examined the effects of smoking cessation on body weight (USDHHS 1988), the average weight gain was 6.2 pounds (range, 1.8 to 18.1 pounds) during the first year after cessation. A 1990 review of the most methodologically rigorous studies (USDHHS 1990) showed that the weight gain among persons who had stopped smoking was greater than that among persons who continued to smoke (mean, 4.6 vs. 0.8 pounds). This summary also invalidated the commonly reported, but empirically unsupported, estimate that one-third of persons who stop smoking gain weight, one-third have stable weight, and one-third lose weight (USDHEW 1977). The 1990 review concluded that 79 percent (range, 58 to 87 percent) of persons who had stopped smoking gained weight and that 56 percent (33 to 62 percent) of persons who continued to smoke gained weight. A major weight gain (>10 pounds) also was found to be more common among persons who had stopped smoking (20.3 percent) than among persons who continued to smoke (0.8 percent).

Findings similar to those in the 1990 review were reported from a prospective study of 121,700 female nurses who had eight years of follow-up (Colditz et al. 1992). The mean weight gain attributable to smoking cessation was 3.1 pounds among women who had smoked fewer than 25 cigarettes daily and 6.2 pounds among women who had smoked 25 or more cigarettes daily. A weight gain of 11 pounds or more occurred within two years among 24.3 percent of women who had stopped smoking but among only 8.4 percent of women who continued to smoke. Weight gain after cessation was positively associated with the amount smoked before cessation, younger age, and lower initial weight.

The actual weight gain after smoking cessation may be greater than the 4 to 8 pounds suggested by the 1990 review (USDHHS 1990). Few studies were designed to prospectively assess the effects of smoking cessation on weight gain, and most relied on self-reported smoking status and weight (USDHHS 1990), which are subject to systematic error (bias). Weight is typically underreported (Klesges 1983; Crawley and Portides 1995), and smokers are more likely to state that they had stopped smoking than are nonsmokers to describe themselves as smokers (Klesges et al. 1992). Moreover, many of the estimates of weight changes were based on studies conducted during the 1970s and 1980s. Thus, women who have stopped smoking in more recent years may have been more nicotine dependent and may have smoked more cigarettes daily than did women who had stopped smoking in earlier decades. These two factors may increase the risk for postcessation weight gain (Williamson et al. 1991; Colditz et al. 1992). Investigators also have typically used point prevalence rather than sustained smoking cessation to determine smoking status, and sustained cessation may be associated with greater weight gain.

Large-scale follow-up studies have avoided several of these limitations (Williamson et al. 1991; O'Hara et al. 1998). More than 9,000 respondents in the first National Health and Nutrition Examination Survey (NHANES) were interviewed during 1971–1975 and reinterviewed during 1982–1984 (Williamson et al. 1991). Consistent with previous reports, women who had stopped smoking tended to gain more weight than did men who had stopped smoking. A major weight gain (>29 pounds) occurred among 13.4 percent of women and among 9.8 percent of men who sustained cessation for more than 1 year. The RR for major weight gain among women who had stopped smoking compared with those who continued to smoke was 5.8 (95 percent CI, 3.7 to 9.1). Risk for major weight gain was higher among women who were initially underweight, younger (25 to 54 years vs. 55 to 74 years), physically inactive, and parous. Average weight gains were 12.1 pounds among women who had stopped smoking for more than 1 year and 3.7 pounds among women who continued to smoke. The average weight gain attributable to smoking cessation was greater among both women and men than that in previous reviews (USDHHS 1988, 1990). This finding was possibly due to the longer follow-up period (10 years). Despite the high overall weight gain among these women, the mean body weight of women former smokers after follow-up was similar to that of women who had never smoked. Similarly, in the Lung Health Study (O'Hara et al. 1998), women who sustained cessation for 5 years gained an average of 19.1 pounds during that interval, whereas women who continued to smoke gained an average of 4.3 pounds. During the first year of cessation, weight gain was strongly associated with the number of cigarettes formerly smoked. In subsequent years, weight gain was less strongly associated with baseline smoking.

Other studies have also suggested that the magnitude of postcessation weight gain is higher than previous estimates. In one investigation, sustained smoking cessation resulted in a weight gain almost double the average reported in earlier studies of women (11.7 pounds at 1-year follow-up) (Nides et al. 1994). Another analysis examined self-reported weight change in the previous 10 years among participants in the third NHANES, which was conducted from 1988 through 1991 (Flegal et al. 1995). The age-adjusted increase in weight during the previous 10 years was 8.46 ± 0.91 kg (18.6 pounds) among women who had quit smoking during that 10-year period, 4.75 ± 1.20 kg (10.5 pounds) among those who had quit smoking 10 or more years before, 2.96 ± 0.61 kg (6.5 pounds) among current smokers, and 3.75 ± 0.41 kg (8.3 pounds) among those who had never smoked. When the difference in weight gain between those who had quit smoking and continuing smokers was taken into account and when age and other factors were adjusted for, the estimated weight gain due to smoking cessation was 5.0 kg (95 percent CI, 2.0 to 8.0 kg) (11.0 pounds) among women and 4.4 kg (95 percent CI, 2.5 to 6.3 kg) (9.7 pounds) among men. In another study, women abstinent at 1-year follow-up, but not abstinent at one or more of the previous follow-ups, had gained an average of 6.7 pounds, a figure similar to previous estimates. However, women who achieved sustained abstinence had gained almost twice this amount—13.0 pounds (Klesges et al. 1997).

Weight gain after smoking cessation occurs largely in the first few years of abstinence. Thereafter, the rate of excess weight gain slows. In the follow-up of the first NHANES (Williamson et al. 1991), the RR for major weight gain (>29 pounds) did not increase as a function of duration of cessation. In the U.S. Nurses' Health Study, women who had stopped smoking within the past two years gained 4.7 pounds more than did continuing smokers. This excess weight gain fell to 1.2 pounds during subsequent two-year intervals (Colditz et al. 1992). In the Lung Health Study, women who sustained smoking cessation for five years gained more weight in the first year of abstinence than in the next four years (O'Hara et al. 1998).

Thus, more recent estimates of RR indicated that weight gain may be higher than previous estimates, but the health benefits of smoking cessation still far outweigh the health risk from the extra body weight, unless the weight gain is extraordinarily large (USDHHS 1990).

## Distribution of Body Fat and Smoking

Abdominal obesity refers to a pattern of body fat distribution characterized by excess subcutaneous or visceral fat in the abdominal region. This pattern is sometimes referred to as a male pattern, whereas gluteal obesity (excess fat in the hips and buttocks) is more typical of women. However, abdominal obesity can occur among both women and men (Tarui et al. 1991). This type of obesity is a risk factor for several conditions, including type 2 diabetes mellitus (Hartz et al. 1984; Ohlson et al. 1985; Cassano et al. 1992), dyslipidemia or hyperinsulinemia (Kissebah et al. 1982; Krotkiewski et al. 1983; Evans et al. 1984; Marti et al. 1989; Landsberg et al. 1991; Ward et al. 1994), sympathetic overactivity and hypertension (Evans et al. 1984; Hartz et al. 1984; Cassano et al. 1990; Landsberg et al. 1991; Ward et al. 1994), stroke (Lapidus et al. 1984; Larsson et al. 1984), coronary artery disease (Lapidus et al. 1984; Larsson et al. 1984; Donahue et al. 1987; Terry et al. 1992), and possibly breast cancer (Folsom et al. 1990). Abdominal obesity is also associated with increased total mortality among both women and men (Lapidus et al. 1984; Larsson et al. 1984; Stevens et al. 1992a,b; Folsom et al. 1993), possibly because of its association with such metabolic abnormalities.

Because overall obesity is positively associated with abdominal obesity (Haffner et al. 1987), smokers might be expected to have less abdominal fat than do nonsmokers. However, many studies reported a positive association of smoking with a high waist-to-hip ratio (WHR) among women (Table 3.43). The relationship between smoking and WHR may be stronger among women than among men. Barrett-Connor and Khaw (1989) reported that among women, WHR was 2.9 percent higher for current smokers than for those who had never smoked, but only 1.8 percent higher among men. In another study, WHR among white women was 2.3 percent higher among current smokers than among those who had never smoked and 2.0 percent higher among comparable groups of black women (Kaye et al. 1993). WHR was also higher among current smokers than among those who had never smoked, for women and men, black or white (Duncan et al. 1995). However, the difference in WHR for current smokers and those who had never smoked was one-third higher among white women than among white men and twice as high among black women as among black men.

The mechanisms underlying the positive relationship between smoking and increased WHR are unknown, but at least two plausible explanations exist. First, smoking may not directly influence WHR but may be part of several adverse health behaviors that together directly increase WHR. Several studies have documented that WHR is positively associated with physical inactivity and with increased intake of total calories, alcohol, and fat (Troisi et al. 1991; Rodin 1992; Slattery et al. 1992; Randrianjohany et al. 1993; Duncan et al. 1995). Because cigarette smoking has been associated with all these behaviors, the observed relationship between smoking and WHR could be due to these factors. No study has investigated whether this is the case.

Second, smoking could directly promote deposition of fat in the abdominal area by increasing the relative balance of androgenic and estrogenic sex hormones. Patterns of fat deposition among both women and men are known to be determined partly by sex steroid hormones (Kirschner et al. 1990; Bouchard et al. 1993). These hormones are involved in the regulation of lipoprotein lipase (LPL) in adipose tissue, the key enzyme regulating deposition of triglyceride in fat cells (Bouchard et al. 1993). Before menopause, when estrogen levels are high, LPL activity is higher in femoral fat depots than in abdominal depots, which promotes deposition of femoral fat (Rebuffé-Scrive et al. 1985). After menopause, when the ovarian production of sex hormones slows or ceases, LPL activity decreases in the femoral region and becomes similar to activity in the abdominal depots, which promotes deposition of abdominal fat. Compared with women with femoral obesity, premenopausal and postmenopausal women who develop high WHR have elevated production rates and serum levels of testosterone, as well as lower levels of sex hormone-binding globulin. These findings suggested that increased androgenicity promotes high WHR among women (Evans et al. 1983; Seidell et al. 1989; Kirschner et al. 1990; Kirschner and Samojlik 1991). The antiestrogenic effect of smoking, together with the increases in adrenal androgens seen among smokers, could thus contribute to their high WHR.

### Conclusions

1. Initiation of cigarette smoking does not appear to be associated with weight loss, but smoking does appear to attenuate weight gain over time.
2. The average weight of women who are current smokers is modestly lower than that of women who have never smoked or who are long-term former smokers.
3. Smoking cessation among women typically is associated with a weight gain of about 6 to 12 pounds in the year after they quit smoking.
4. Women smokers have a more masculine pattern of body fat distribution (i.e., a higher waist-to-hip ratio) than do women who have never smoked.

## Bone Density and Fracture Risk

Bone fractures are a common health problem among women: about 16 percent of 50-year-old white women and 5.5 percent of 50-year-old black women will have a hip fracture in their remaining lifetime (Cummings et al. 1989). Risk rises steeply with age (Melton 1988); most patients who sustain a hip fracture are older than 70 years. The mortality after hip fracture is also high; more than 10 percent of patients die within six months of injury (Magaziner et al. 1989; Lu-Yao et al. 1994). Some of the mortality after hip fracture seems to be due to the debilitated state of the patient sustaining the fracture (Poór et al. 1995). Nonetheless, the event often is devastating, and the fracture imposes a significant burden of morbidity and mortality.

Compared with men, women are at increased risk for virtually all types of fractures; among women older than 65 years, the risk for fracture at most anatomic sites is about twice the risk among men the same age (Griffin et al. 1992; Baron et al. 1994a, 1996a). The incidence of fracture of the vertebrae or distal forearm increases among women around the time of menopause; among women younger than about age 70 years, both types of fractures occur more frequently than do hip fractures. Fractures of the ankle are fairly common among middle-aged women but appear to become less common later in life (Griffin et al. 1992; Baron et al. 1994a).

Osteoporosis, the state of having low bone density, impairs the structural integrity of the bone and heightens its susceptibility to trauma. Low bone density (measured at the wrist) is associated with an increased risk for fracture at most bone sites (Seeley et al. 1991). Data on the relationships between smoking and bone density and between smoking and fracture risk are presented here.

**Table 3.43. Findings regarding the relationship between smoking and abdominal obesity as measured by waist-to-hip ratio (WHR)**

| Study | Population | Smoking status | Relationship with WHR | Covariate adjustment factors |
|---|---|---|---|---|
| Haffner et al. 1986 | 388 women, 563 men<br>Aged 25–64 years | Cigarettes/day | Positive association for both women and men | BMI,* age, physical activity level, alcohol intake, ethnicity |
| Barrett-Connor and Khaw 1989 | 1,112 women, 836 men<br>Aged 50–79 years | Never smoked<br>Former smokers<br>Current smokers | Positive linear trend across smoking categories for both women and men<br>Positive linear trend for women within BMI tertiles<br>Nonsignificant positive trend for men within BMI tertiles | Age, BMI |
| den Tonkelaar et al. 1989 | 152 premenopausal women, 300 postmenopausal women<br>Aged 41–75 years | Nonsmokers<br>Current smokers | WHR higher for smokers than for nonsmokers among premenopausal women only | BMI |
| Lapidus et al. 1989 | 1,462 women<br>Aged 38–60 years | Cigarettes/day | Positive association | Age, BMI |
| den Tonkelaar et al. 1990 | 5,923 premenopausal women, 3,568 postmenopausal women<br>Aged 40–73 years | Never smoked<br>Former smokers, >20 cigarettes/day<br>Current smokers, <10, 10–20, or >20 cigarettes/day | Positive linear trend across categories of number of cigarettes smoked for both premenopausal and postmenopausal women<br>Positive linear trend within BMI tertiles for current smokers | BMI, $BMI^2$, age |
| Kaye et al. 1990 | 40,980 postmenopausal women<br>Aged 55–69 years | Never smoked<br>Former smokers<br>Current smokers | Positive linear trend across smoking categories | Age, BMI |

*BMI = Body mass index.

## Smoking and Bone Density

The technology of bone density measurement is evolving rapidly, and several radiographic techniques were used to generate the data summarized here. Single photon absorptiometry was used in many studies of the peripheral skeleton, generally the radius (forearm) or the calcaneus (heel). Dual photon absorptiometry can be used for assessing those sites, as well as the hip and the axial skeleton, generally the spine. Dual X-ray absorptiometry, a refinement of the dual photon technique, offers higher resolution, shorter scanning times, and increased precision (Mazess and Barden 1989).

The growth of the skeleton continues until peak bone mass is reached, probably before age 30 years (Sowers and Galuska 1993). A slow decrease in bone density then begins and accelerates for several years after menopause (Riggs and Melton 1986; Resnick and Greenspan 1989). Because of these age-related patterns, studies of bone density are considered here by menopausal status of participants. Cross-sectional studies reporting mean bone density for at least 100 smokers and nonsmokers are summarized in Tables 3.44 and 3.45.

It is not clear whether environmental factors such as smoking affect bone differently at different anatomic sites. One large study reported similar effects of

**Table 3.43. Continued**

| Study | Population | Smoking status | Relationship with WHR | Covariate adjustment factors |
|---|---|---|---|---|
| Marti et al. 1991 | 2,756 women, 2,526 men<br>Aged 25–64 years | 7-point scale<br>1 = never smoked<br>7 = current smokers of ≥25 cigarettes/day | No statistically significant independent association across smoking index in women or men | Age, education, heart rate, dietary fat, alcohol consumption, exercise |
| Wing et al. 1991 | 487 women<br>Aged 42–50 years | Never smoked<br>Former smokers<br>Current smokers | Positive linear trend across smoking groups<br>Positive association with number of cigarettes smoked | BMI |
| Daniel et al. 1992 | 56 women<br>Aged 20–35 years | Nonsmokers<br>Never smoked<br>Former smokers<br>Current smokers | WHR higher for smokers than for nonsmokers | None |
| Armellini et al. 1993 | 307 women, 294 men<br>Outpatients<br>Aged 20–60 years | Never smoked<br>Current smokers, <10, 10–15, or >15 cigarettes/day | WHR and number of cigarettes smoked not significantly associated for women or men | Age, BMI, alcohol intake, physical activity level, menopausal status |
| Kaye et al. 1993 | 1,464 black women, 1,142 black men<br>1,300 white women, 1,159 white men<br>Aged 18–30 years | Never smoked<br>Former smokers<br>Current smokers | Positive linear trend across smoking categories for both genders and races | Age, BMI |
| Duncan et al. 1995 | 2,366 black women, 1,444 black men<br>5,872 white women, 5,293 white men<br>Aged 45–64 years | Never smoked<br>Former smokers<br>Current smokers | WHR higher for current smokers than for those who never smoked for both genders and races | Age, education, BMI, physical activity, menopausal status, alcohol intake |

smoking at the radius and the calcaneus (Bauer et al. 1993). However, another large investigation found more pronounced effects for measurements at the hip than at the spine or radius (Hollenbach et al. 1993). Several investigators also reported greater differences in bone density between smokers and nonsmokers at the hip than at other sites (Hansen et al. 1991; Nguyen et al. 1994; Ortego-Centeno et al. 1994), but others reported more marked effects at the radius (Krall and Dawson-Hughes 1991; Bauer et al. 1993; Kiel et al. 1996; Orwoll et al. 1996).

### Cross-Sectional Studies

Some studies of premenopausal women have suggested a lower bone density at various sites among smokers than among nonsmokers (Stevenson et al. 1989; McCulloch et al. 1990; Mazess and Barden 1991; Ortego-Centeno et al. 1994; Jones and Scott 1999) (Table 3.44). However, other investigations did not find a substantial effect (Sowers et al. 1985a,b; Bilbrey et al. 1988; Picard et al. 1988; Davies et al. 1990; Cox et al. 1991; Laitinen et al. 1991; Turner et al. 1992; Hansen 1994; Välimäki et al. 1994; Daniel and Martin 1995;

**Table 3.44. Relative bone density among premenopausal women, for smokers compared with nonsmokers, cross-sectional studies**

| Study | Population | Smoking status | Relative bone density* (%) |
|---|---|---|---|
| Davies et al. 1990 | Patients with amenorrhea<br>Aged 16–40 years<br>England | 39 current smokers<br>93 never smoked | Lumbar spine: -3.4 |
| McCulloch et al. 1990 | Hospital employees<br>Mean age 28.5 years<br>Canada | 25 daily smokers<br>76 nondaily smokers | Calcaneus: -6.7 |
| Mazess and Barden 1991 | Volunteers<br>Aged 20–39 years<br>United States | 39 smokers<br>261 nonsmokers | Lumbar spine: -3.9† <br>Mid-radius: -1.4<br>Distal radius: 0.0<br>Femoral neck: -4.0 |
| Daniel et al. 1992 | Volunteers<br>Aged 20–35 years<br>Canada | 25 smokers<br>27 nonsmokers | Lumbar spine: +2.3<br>Femoral neck: +3.8<br>Trochanter: +3.2<br>Ward's triangle: +3.3 |
| Ortego-Centeno et al. 1994 | Healthy volunteers<br>Mean age 28.2 years<br>Spain | 47 current smokers<br>54 former smokers or never smoked | Lumbar spine: -1.3<br>Femoral neck: -5.0‡<br>Trochanter: -3.8<br>Ward's triangle: -5.6‡ |
| Law et al. 1997a | Healthy volunteers<br>Aged ≥35 years<br>England | 142 current smokers<br>350 never smokers | Distal radius: +1.0 |
| Jones and Scott 1999 | Participants in follow-up study<br>Mean age 32.7 years for smokers, 34.0 years for nonsmokers<br>Australia | 118 smokers<br>158 nonsmokers | Lumbar spine: -3.7<br>Femoral neck: -4.7 |

*Relative bone density = (bone density in smokers – bone density in nonsmokers)/bone density in nonsmokers, based on unadjusted bone density means.
†Statistically significant at $p < 0.05$.
‡Statistically significant, but statistical significance lost after adjustment for age and weight.

McKnight et al. 1995; Franceschi et al. 1996; Law et al. 1997a; Fujita et al. 1999), and one study from China reported a statistically significant trend of increasing bone density with number of cigarettes smoked (Hu et al. 1994). In many of these studies, no adjustment was made for potentially important covariates such as age and body weight, which hampered interpretation of the findings.

Results from cross-sectional studies of perimenopausal women have been similar to findings from studies of premenopausal women: an effect of smoking on bone density was not consistently seen (Johnell and Nilsson 1984; Jensen and Christiansen 1988; Elders et al. 1989; Slemenda et al. 1989; Cheng et al. 1991; Spector et al. 1992; Kröger et al. 1994; Leino et al. 1994; McKnight et al. 1995).

Among postmenopausal women, an association of lower bone density with smoking has generally been reported (Law and Hackshaw 1997). The majority of cross-sectional studies found a lower bone mass among smokers (Table 3.45) (Holló et al. 1979; Rundgren and Mellström 1984; Jensen 1986; Hansen et al. 1991; Krall and Dawson-Hughes 1991; Bauer et al. 1993; Cheng et al. 1993; Johansson et al. 1993; Nguyen et al. 1994; Ward et al. 1995; Orwoll et al. 1996; Grainge et al. 1998). Nonetheless, several other such studies reported no substantial effect (Sowers et al. 1985a,b; Nordin and Polley 1987; Bilbrey et al. 1988; Cauley et al. 1988; Hunt et al. 1989; Stevenson et al. 1989; Ho et al. 1995), and a study from China reported a positive correlation between cigarette smoking and bone mass (Hu et al. 1994). In the Framingham study, bone density was lower only among smokers who took oral estrogen (Kiel et al. 1996). Findings among men in cross-sectional studies have not been entirely consistent, but men who smoke seem to have lower bone density than do nonsmokers, with a reduction in bone mass similar to that reported among postmenopausal women smokers (Holló et al. 1979; Suominen et al. 1984; Johansson et al. 1992; Kröger and Laitinen 1992; Cheng et al. 1993; Hollenbach et al. 1993; May et al. 1994; Kiel et al. 1996).

### Longitudinal and Twin Studies

Few substantial differences in bone loss between smokers and nonsmokers have emerged among premenopausal women (Mazess and Barden 1991; Sowers et al. 1992) or perimenopausal women (Slemenda et al. 1989; Spector et al. 1992) who were studied longitudinally. Some studies of postmenopausal women have also reported statistically similar bone loss among smokers and nonsmokers (Aloia et al. 1983; Hansen et al. 1991; Jones et al. 1994), but most investigations of these women reported a higher rate of bone loss among smokers (Lindsay 1981; Krall and Dawson-Hughes 1991; Writing Group for the PEPI Trial 1996; Burger et al. 1998). One longitudinal study of male twins supported an association between smoking and bone loss (Slemenda et al. 1992), but another longitudinal study of men found no differences in bone loss between smokers and nonsmokers (Jones et al. 1994). All these longitudinal studies faced substantial statistical impediments. Changes in bone density over a few years are small, and the analyses typically have only limited statistical power to detect differences that would be substantial if cumulated over a longer period.

A potentially important aspect of the relationship between smoking and bone density among perimenopausal women emerged from studies in Denmark. Among women receiving oral estrogen, bone loss was more rapid for smokers than for nonsmokers (Jensen and Christiansen 1988). In contrast, smoking had no effect among women who were not taking estrogens or who were taking them percutaneously. This estrogen-related variation in the effect of smoking on bone density mirrors the variation in fracture risk found in one cohort study of hip fracture (Kiel et al. 1992). In one clinical trial, however, HRT affected the change in bone density similarly among smokers and nonsmokers (Writing Group for the PEPI Trial 1996).

Studies of twins provided additional information on the relationship between smoking and bone density. In these studies, adjustment can be made for known and unknown genetic factors, as well as early-life exposures such as diet. In the largest of these studies of adults, 41 pairs of twins discordant for amount of smoking had measurements of bone density at several anatomic locations, including the lumbar spine, the femoral neck, and the femoral shaft (Hopper and Seeman 1994). At each site, bone density was lower for the heavier smoker. Similar findings were reported from an earlier, smaller analysis (Pocock et al. 1989). A study of female twins aged 10 to 26 years showed no differences in bone mass by smoking status, but the analysis lacked statistical power (Young et al. 1995).

### Effects of Covariates

Only a few studies presented both adjusted and unadjusted data from analyses of smoking and bone density (Lindsay 1981; Rundgren and Mellström 1984; Bauer et al. 1993; Nguyen et al. 1994; Ortego-Centeno et al. 1994; Välimäki et al. 1994). In general, any association found was shown both in crude analyses (or those adjusted for age only) and in those adjusted for factors such as body weight and exercise. However, adjustment, particularly for weight, lowers the magnitude of the association. For example, in the Study of Osteoporotic Fractures, the age-adjusted bone mass was 5.8 percent (95 percent CI, 5.0 to 7.7 percent) lower among current smokers than among nonsmokers (Bauer et al. 1993). After further adjustment for multiple factors, including weight, WHR, age at menopause, calcium intake, lifetime activity, and estrogen use, the reduction was 2.1 percent (95 percent CI, 0.2 to 4.0 percent).

Data on the effect of smoking cessation on bone density are scant. In most studies, bone density of women former smokers was intermediate between that of women current smokers and women who had never smoked (Rundgren and Mellström 1984; Davies et al. 1990; Bauer et al. 1993; Cheng et al. 1993; Hollenbach et al. 1993).

**Table 3.45. Relative bone density among postmenopausal women for smokers compared with nonsmokers, cross-sectional studies**

| Study | Population | Smoking status | Relative bone density* (%) | Comments |
|---|---|---|---|---|
| Holló et al. 1979 | Volunteers<br>Aged 61–75 years<br>Hungary‡ | 41 smokers<br>125 nonsmokers | Radius: -6.0† | |
| Rundgren and Mellström 1984 | Population sample<br>Aged 70, 75, 79 years<br>Sweden | 111 current smokers<br>825 never smoked | Calcaneus: -13.6 to -31.4†§ | |
| Sowers et al. 1985b | Population sample<br>Aged 55–80 years<br>United States | 72 ever smoked<br>252 never smoked | Distal radius: +1.6 | Adjustment for age, muscle mass |
| Jensen 1986 | Population sample<br>Aged 70 years<br>Denmark§ | 77 current smokers<br>103 never smoked | Radius: -5.2 | |
| Jensen and Christiansen 1988 | Clinical trial participants<br>Aged 45–54 years<br>Denmark§ | 56 smokers<br>54 nonsmokers | Distal forearm: -1.3 | |
| Hansen et al. 1991 | Clinical trial participants<br>Menopause in past 3 years<br>Denmark | 61 current smokers<br>117 nonsmokers | Lumbar spine: -3.4<br>Radius: +1.0<br>Femoral neck: -5.8†<br>Trochanter: -8.1†<br>Ward's triangle: -8.2† | Findings similar after adjustment for multiple factors |
| Krall and Dawson-Hughes 1991 | Clinical trial participants<br>Low-to-moderate calcium intake<br>Aged 40–70 years<br>United States§ | 35 current smokers<br>285 nonsmokers | Lumbar spine: +0.4<br>Radius: -0.5<br>Femoral neck: -0.8<br>Calcaneus: -2.4 | Multiple regression: pack-years significant predictor of bone density of radius |
| Bauer et al. 1993; Orwoll et al. 1996 | Volunteers<br>Aged ≥65 years<br>United States | 970 current smokers<br>8,734 nonsmokers | Distal radius: -5.8†<br>Femoral neck: -4.5† | Age-adjusted estimates<br>Multivariate-adjusted estimate for radius, -2.1%<br>Age- and weight-adjusted estimate for hip, -1.9%† |
| Cheng et al. 1993 | Responders to population survey<br>Aged 75 years<br>Finland | 10 current smokers<br>161 nonsmokers | Calcaneus: -15 | Estimate adjusted for body mass<br>Analysis of variance: statistically significant differences among former and current smokers and persons who never smoked |

*Relative bone density = (bone density in smokers – bone density in nonsmokers)/bone density in nonsmokers, based on unadjusted bone density means, unless otherwise noted in comments.

†Statistically significant at $p < 0.05$.

‡Dates of subject recruitment not stated.

§Different age groups.

**Table 3.45. Continued**

| Study | Population | Smoking status | Relative bone density* (%) | Comments |
|---|---|---|---|---|
| Hollenbach et al. 1993 | Responders to population survey<br>Aged 60–100 years<br>United States | 181 current smokers<br>573 nonsmokers | Lumbar spine: -0.3<br>Mid-radius: -2.6<br>Ultradistal radius: -1.3<br>Total hip: -5.0† | Estimates adjusted for multiple factors |
| Nguyen et al. 1994 | Responders to population survey<br>Australia | 1,080 participants | Lumbar spine: -5.9†<br>Femoral neck: -7.6† | Estimates adjusted for age, weight |
| Egger et al. 1996 | Responders to study of long-term residents<br>Aged 63–73 years<br>England | 23 current smokers<br>99 never smoked | Lumbar spine: -8.2<br>Femoral neck: -3.9 | Estimates adjusted for multiple factors |
| Kiel et al. 1996 | Participants in cohort study<br>Aged ≥ 70 years<br>United States | 51 current smokers<br>222 never smoked | Never used menopausal estrogen<br>Radial shaft: 0<br>Ultradistal radius: -5.8<br>Femoral neck: -0.7<br>Trochanter: -2.4<br>Ward's area: -3.4<br>L2–L4 spine: +4.1 | Estimates adjusted for multiple factors |
| | | | Ever used menopausal estrogen<br>Radial shaft: -4.4<br>Ultradistal radius: -19.0†<br>Femoral neck: -3.2<br>Trochanter: -8.0†<br>Ward's area: -7.3<br>L2–L4 spine: +2.2 | Estimates adjusted for multiple factors |
| Law et al. 1997a | Healthy volunteers<br>Aged <65 years<br>England | 105 current smokers<br>288 never smokers | Distal radius: 0 | |

*Relative bone density = (bone density in smokers – bone density in nonsmokers)/bone density in nonsmokers, based on unadjusted bone density means, unless otherwise noted in comments.
†Statistically significant at $p < 0.05$.

### Mechanisms

Smoking could affect osteoporosis and osteoporotic fractures through several mechanisms (Law and Hackshaw 1997). A lower bone density in smokers may partially explain associations of smoking with fracture risk. If smoking increases the risk for trauma, it could be a risk factor for fractures through other mechanisms as well.

Body weight tends to be lower among smokers than among nonsmokers (see "Body Weight and Fat Distribution" earlier in this chapter), and this weight difference may itself lead to lower bone density and higher risk for fracture (Cummings et al. 1995). In several analyses, weight explains much of the increased risk associated with smoking (e.g., Lindsay 1981; Bauer et al. 1993). This effect may be derived from lower estrogen production in relatively thin postmenopausal women; reduced padding of bones, which results in less protection from fracture during falls; and decreased physical loading of weight-bearing bones, which reduces the stimulus for bone growth. The antiestrogenic effect of smoking may also contribute to osteoporosis among women (see "Sex Hormones" earlier in this chapter).

Clinical evidence is consistent with the hypothesis that smoking is associated with increased bone resorption. Levels of parathyroid hormone and 25-hydroxy vitamin $D_3$ are lower among smokers than among nonsmokers (Gudmundsson et al. 1987; Mellström et al. 1993; Hopper and Seeman 1994), an expected consequence of increased release of calcium from resorbed bone. Perhaps because of this hormonal milieu, smoking leads to decreased absorption of calcium or decreased retention of calcium in the gut (Aloia et al. 1983; Krall and Dawson-Hughes 1991; Clement and Fung 1995).

Other possible mechanisms have been proposed but remain to be confirmed. Vascular effects of smoking may adversely affect bone (Daftari et al. 1994), and the excess exposure to cadmium associated with smoking may be deleterious (Bhattacharyya et al. 1988). A smoking-related resistance to calcitonin has also been described (Holló et al. 1979), but smoking seems to lead to increased calcitonin levels (Tabassian et al. 1988; Eliasson et al. 1993). Finally, smoking probably results in a modest chronic elevation of cortisol levels (Baron et al. 1994a), which may adversely affect bone, and nicotine may have direct effects on osteoblasts (Fang et al. 1991).

## Smoking and Fracture Risk

The relationship between smoking and risk for bone fracture has been investigated intensively for fracture of the hip (Law and Hackshaw 1997). A few studies have also addressed fractures of the vertebrae, distal forearm, proximal humerus, ankle, and foot.

### Hip Fracture

Six cohort studies that included at least 50 women with hip fracture reported the effect of smoking (Table 3.46). Most of these studies focused on white women, and most of the fractures were observed at older ages, although one investigation from Norway included only middle-aged women (Meyer et al. 1993). In these studies, the age-adjusted RR was consistently elevated, although often only modestly; among current smokers compared with women who had never smoked, the age-adjusted RR varied between 1.2 and 2.1. Risk estimates adjusted for multiple covariates were lower than those adjusted for age only. One study found no overall effect (RR, 1.2) but reported a substantially increased risk associated with smoking among women who took menopausal estrogen (Kiel et al. 1992). Other studies, however, did not find a similar interaction of smoking with estrogen use (Williams et al. 1982; Cauley et al. 1995).

In several cohort studies, the risk for hip fracture was higher among heavy smokers than among light smokers, but statistical tests for trend by amount smoked were not reported (Kiel et al. 1992; Meyer et al. 1993). In the one study that considered the effect of duration of smoking, the number of years of smoking did not affect risk for hip fracture (Meyer et al. 1993). In the cohort studies, the risk among women former smokers was not substantially higher than that among women who had never smoked (Paganini-Hill et al. 1991; Kiel et al. 1992; Meyer et al. 1993; Forsén et al. 1998).

Ten case-control studies that included at least 75 women with hip fracture reported the effect of smoking (Table 3.47). Again, most of the studies focused on older white women. The RRs were fairly consistent: generally elevated but less than 2.0 after adjustment for age, and 1.0 to 1.5 after adjustment for body mass and other factors. Few of the RR estimates were statistically significant. The risk for hip fracture among former smokers was about the same as that among current smokers (La Vecchia et al. 1991b; Grisso et al. 1994; Michaëlsson et al. 1995). In one large multicenter study, however, the RR was lower among women former smokers than among women who had never smoked, after adjustment for age, BMI, and center (0.8; 95 percent CI, 0.6 to 0.97) (Johnell et al. 1995).

The epidemiology of fractures has been more extensively studied among women than among men, probably because of the greater susceptibility of women to fractures. Two cohort studies showed similar relationships between smoking and risk for hip fracture among women and men (Paganini-Hill et al. 1991; Meyer et al. 1993), and one small case-control study reported an effect of smoking on risk for hip fracture among men (Grisso et al. 1991). In contrast, one cohort study and one case-control study of hip fracture—both with limited statistical power—found no association among men (Felson et al. 1988; Hemenway et al. 1994).

In the literature as a whole, the age-adjusted RR for current smoking and hip fracture among women appears to be between 1.5 and 2.0. Adjustment for the lower body weight or BMI of smokers tends to reduce

**Table 3.46. Relative risks for hip fracture among women, among current smokers, cohort studies**

| Study | Study description | Population | Age-adjusted relative risk (95% confidence interval) | Multivariate analysis | |
|---|---|---|---|---|---|
| | | | | Relative risk (95% confidence interval) | Adjustment factors |
| Paganini-Hill et al. 1991 | 281 cases over 7 years | Retirement community residents<br>Median age 73 years<br>United States | 1.8 (1.3–2.0) | 1.6 (1.2–2.3) | Age at menarche, parity, body mass, exercise |
| Kiel et al. 1992 | 207 cases over 38 years | Framingham study participants<br>Aged 28–62 years<br>United States | 1.2 (0.8–1.7) | 1.2 (0.8–2.0) | Age, body mass, alcohol use, estrogen use |
| Scott et al. 1992 | 218 cases over 6 years | Population sample<br>Aged ≥ 65 years<br>United States | Not reported | 1.9 | Estrogen use, residence, disability, milk consumption, use of sleeping pills |
| Meyer et al. 1993 | 146 cases over 13 years | Population sample<br>Aged 35–49 years<br>Norway | 1.5 (0.8–2.6)* | 1.4 (0.8–2.5) | Multiple factors, including body mass, height, physical activity |
| Forsén et al. 1994 | 421 fractures over 4 years | Population sample<br>Aged >20 years<br>Norway | Not reported | 1.8 (1.2–2.6) | Body mass, physical activity, self-reported health status |
| Cummings et al. 1995 | 192 fractures over 4.1 years (mean) | White volunteers<br>Aged ≥ 65 years<br>United States | 2.1 (1.4–3.3) | 1.4 (0.9–2.3) | Multiple factors, including weight change, health status |

*Current smoking was defined as smoking ≥ 15 cigarettes/day.

the magnitude of the effect of smoking. This finding suggested that the effect of smoking on hip fracture may act at least partly through the association of smoking with reduced body weight (see "Body Weight and Fat Distribution" earlier in this chapter).

### Other Fractures

Some studies have reported an increased prevalence of vertebral fractures among women who smoke (Aloia et al. 1985; Spector et al. 1993), but other investigations have reported no association (Kleerekoper et al. 1989; Cooper et al. 1991; Santavirta et al. 1992) (Table 3.48). Santavirta and colleagues (1992) conducted a large-scale, population-based investigation—by far the largest published survey of the prevalence of vertebral fractures. Among the 27,278 females aged 15 years or older, only 105 had fractures of the thoracic spine. Because no separate risk estimate was given for postmenopausal women, the lack of an effect of smoking in these data does not provide much evidence against an association between smoking and osteoporotic vertebral fractures among older women. Findings in three studies suggested that male smokers are at increased risk for fractures of the vertebrae (Seeman et al. 1983; Santavirta et al. 1992; Scane et al. 1999).

Data are also sparse on the association of smoking with the risk for fractures at other sites among women. The one published study of fractures of the proximal humerus found no association of risk with

**Table 3.47. Relative risks for hip fracture among women smokers, case-control studies**

| Study | Population | Smoking status | Age-adjusted relative risk (95% confidence interval) | Multivariate analysis | |
|---|---|---|---|---|---|
| | | | | Relative risk (95% confidence interval) | Adjustment factors |
| Paganini-Hill et al. 1981 | 83 community cases, 166 community controls<br>Postmenopausal, aged <80 years | Postmenopausal smokers<br>1–10 cigarettes/day<br>≥11 cigarettes/day | <br><br>0.9*<br>1.7* | <br><br>1.1*<br>2.0* | Age, estrogen use, oophorectomy |
| Williams et al. 1982 | 160 hospital cases, 567 community controls<br>Aged 50–74 years | | Risk elevated in smokers | | |
| Kreiger and Hilditch 1986 | 98 hospital cases, 884 hospital controls<br>Aged 45–74 years | Ever smoked | 1.5†<br>1.8* | 1.3†<br>1.3* | Age, body mass, lactation, ovariectomy, estrogen use |
| La Vecchia et al. 1991b | 209 hospital cases, 1,449 hospital controls<br>Median age 62 years | Current smokers | 1.6 (1.0–2.3) | 1.5 (1.0–2.1) | Age, body mass, education, menopausal status, estrogen use, alcohol use |
| Kreiger et al. 1992 | 102 hospital cases, 277 hospital controls<br>Mean age 74 years | Current smokers | 2.7 (1.5–4.8) | 1.7 (0.9–3.3) | Age, body mass, ovariectomy, estrogen use |
| Jaglal et al. 1993 | 381 hospital cases, 1,138 controls from population<br>Aged 55–84 years | ≥ 60 pack-years | 1.4 (0.7–2.8)† | 1.2 (0.6–2.5) | Multiple variables, including age, body mass, estrogen use, physical activity |
| Yamamoto et al. 1993 | 100 cases, 100 controls<br>Population sample<br>Aged ≥35 years | Habitual smokers | 1.5 (0.5–4.7) | | |
| Grisso et al. 1994 | 144 hospital cases, 218 controls from population<br>Aged ≥45 years | Current smokers | Not reported | 1.3 (0.7–2.6) | Age, body mass, residence area |
| Johnell et al. 1995 | 2,086 cases from population, 3,532 controls from population or neighbors<br>Mean age 78 years | Current smokers | 0.9 (0.7–1.2) | 1.1 (0.8–1.5) | Body mass; mental score; intake of tea, coffee, alcohol, calcium; physical activity |
| Michaëlsson et al. 1995 | 247 cases, 893 controls<br>Population sample | Current smokers, >20 pack-years | 1.8 (1.0–3.2)‡ | 1.6 (0.9–3.0) | Multiple variables, including body mass, height, estrogen use, physical activity |

*95% confidence interval was not reported.
†Two control groups.
‡Not adjusted for age.

smoking (Kelsey et al. 1992) (Table 3.48). The same investigation showed that smoking was also unrelated to risk for ankle or foot fractures (Seeley et al. 1996). Another study, based on a one-time survey of fractures during the previous 10 years, did not find a significant association between smoking and wrist fractures but did report that smoking was associated with increased risk for ankle fractures (Honkanen et al. 1998). The data on fracture of the distal forearm also indicated that the relationship with smoking is modest at most (Table 3.48). No association with cigarette smoking was found in the only study of distal forearm fractures among men (Hemenway et al. 1994).

### Conclusions

1. Postmenopausal women who currently smoke have lower bone density than do women who do not smoke.
2. Women who currently smoke have an increased risk for hip fracture compared with women who do not smoke.
3. The relationship among women between smoking and the risk for bone fracture at sites other than the hip is not clear.

## Gastrointestinal Disease

### Gallbladder Disease

Gallstones are common in most Western countries. In the United States, autopsy series showed gallstones in 20 percent of women and 8 percent of men older than age 40 years (Johnston and Kaplan 1993). Risk for gallstones increases with age and is higher among women than among men (Johnston and Kaplan 1993). Weight gain and obesity increase risk; alcohol intake appears to be protective (Friedman et al. 1966; Maclure et al. 1989). Because smoking is associated with low body mass (see "Body Weight" earlier in this chapter) and alcohol use (Schoenborn and Benson 1988; Willard and Schoenborn 1995), it is necessary to consider these factors in studies of the relationship between smoking and gallstones.

Several population surveys presented information on the association of cigarette smoking and gallbladder disease. In a sample of 3,418 women and men aged 30, 40, 50, or 60 years who lived in western Copenhagen County, Denmark, ultrasonography of the gallbladder showed a higher prevalence of gallstones among smokers than among persons who had never smoked, particularly men. After adjustment for other risk factors, including family history, BMI, and alcohol intake, the RR for gallstones among women smokers was 1.2 ($p > 0.20$) (Jorgensen 1989) and the RR among male smokers was 1.9 ($p > 0.10$). Among 70-year-olds, the RR was 3.3 among men and 1.6 among women (both $p > 0.05$) (Jorgensen et al. 1990). Ultrasonography of pregnant women in Ireland also showed a positive relationship between smoking and gallstones (Basso et al. 1992). An Italian survey found that the prevalence of gallstones increased with the number of cigarettes smoked per day among men but not among women (Rome Group for Epidemiology and Prevention of Cholelithiasis 1988). No statistically significant overall association was observed between smoking and the presence of gallstones. A survey from Germany found an increased risk among smokers that was not statistically significant (Kratzer et al. 1997).

Several cohort studies reported an association between smoking and gallbladder disease. The Oxford Family Planning Contraceptive Study, which followed up more than 17,000 women and observed 227 cases, found an increased risk for hospitalization for gallstones or cholecystectomy among smokers (Layde et al. 1982). The RR was 1.6 among women who smoked fewer than 15 cigarettes per day and 1.4 among women who smoked 15 or more cigarettes per day. Results were controlled for multiple factors, including age, parity, and BMI. These findings remained unchanged after additional follow-up (Vessey and Painter 1994). In a second British follow-up study of 46,000 women, 1,087 reported a first episode of symptomatic cholelithiasis (Murray et al. 1994). In a comparison of all smokers with nonsmokers, the RR was 1.2 (95 percent CI, 1.1 to 1.3) after adjustment for age, socioeconomic level, and parity. Risk increased with the number of cigarettes smoked per day.

**Table 3.48. Relative risks for fractures other than hip fractures among women smokers**

| Site of fracture/study | Study type | Population | Results (95% confidence interval) |
|---|---|---|---|
| **Vertebrae** | | | |
| Aloia et al. 1985 | Age-matched, case-control study | 58 cases, 58 controls<br>Volunteer women<br>Mean age 64 years<br>United States | Percentage of smokers; $p < 0.01$<br>Cases: 59%<br>Controls: 30% |
| Kleerekoper et al. 1989 | Case-control study | 266 cases, 263 controls<br>Postmenopausal women screened for osteoporosis trial<br>Aged 45–75 years<br>United States | Percentage of current smokers; $p > 0.05$<br>Cases: 27%<br>Controls: 20% |
| Cooper et al. 1991 | Survey of general practice patients | 1,012 women<br>79 fractures<br>Aged 48–81 years<br>United Kingdom | Smoking >10 cigarettes/day for >10 years not related to fracture risk |
| Santavirta et al. 1992 | Population-based survey | 27,278 girls and women<br>105 fractures<br>Aged ≥15 years<br>Finland | RR* = 1.1 (0.6–2.0) for current smokers<br>Adjusted for age, history of trauma, tuberculosis, peptic ulcer, BMI,† occupation |
| **Distal forearm** | | | |
| Williams et al. 1982 | Population-based, case-control study | 184 cases, 567 controls<br>Aged 50–74 years<br>United States | Higher fracture risk in women smokers using estrogens |
| Kelsey et al. 1992 | Cohort study | 9,704 women<br>171 fractures over 2.2 years (mean)<br>Aged ≥65 years<br>United States | RR = 1.0 (0.96–1.0) for current smokers (10 cigarettes/day) vs. never smoked |
| Kreiger et al. 1992 | Hospital case-control study | 54 fractures<br>Aged 50–84 years<br>Canada | RR = 1.5 (0.9–2.6) for current smokers vs. former smokers or never smoked<br>Adjusted for age, BMI |

*RR = Relative risk.
†BMI = Body mass index.

In the U.S. Nurses' Health Study II, 425 of the 96,211 women (aged 25 through 42 years) who were followed up for two years had a diagnosis of gallstones (Grodstein et al. 1994). After adjustment for established risk factors, current cigarette smokers were at a slightly higher risk for gallstones than were nonsmokers (RR, 1.3; 95 percent CI, 1.0 to 1.7). No evidence was found for a dose-response relationship. Former smokers were not at higher risk than those who had never smoked. In a more detailed analysis of incident cases of symptomatic gallstones and of cholecystectomies during six years of follow-up of the U.S. Nurses' Health Study cohort, Stampfer and colleagues (1992) observed an increase in risk with increasing number of cigarettes smoked per day. Women who smoked 25 to 34 cigarettes per day had a RR of 1.3 (95 percent CI, 1.1 to 1.6) compared with women who had never smoked; those who smoked 35 or more cigarettes per day had a RR of 1.5 (95 percent CI, 1.2 to 1.9). These results are consistent with findings from a study of 868 female twins; the RR among smokers compared with persons who had never smoked was 1.8 (95 percent CI, 1.0 to 3.3) (Petitti et al. 1981). Smoking was also a risk factor for the

Table 3.48. Continued

| Site of fracture/study | Study type | Population | Results (95% confidence interval) |
|---|---|---|---|
| Mallmin et al. 1994 | Population-based, case-control study | 385 cases, 385 controls<br>Aged 40–80 years<br>Sweden | RR = 0.9 (0.5–1.6) for current smokers<br>Adjusted for multiple factors, including age, BMI, physical activity, hormone use |
| Honkanen et al. 1998 | Retrospective survey | 12,192 women<br>345 fractures<br>Aged 47–56 years<br>Finland | Current smoking<br>RR = 0.9 (0.6–1.4)<br>Any smoking<br>RR = 0.6 (0.3–1.1) for 1–10 cigarettes/day<br>RR = 1.4 (0.9–2.3) for >10 cigarettes/day<br>Adjusted for age, BMI, menopausal status, chronic health disorders |
| **Proximal humerus** | | | |
| Kelsey et al. 1992 | Cohort study | 9,704 women<br>79 fractures over 2.2 years (mean)<br>Aged ≥65 years<br>United States | RR = 1.2 (0.9–1.6) for current smokers (10 cigarettes/day) |
| **Ankle** | | | |
| Seeley et al. 1996 | Cohort study | 9,704 women<br>191 fractures over 5.9 years (mean)<br>Aged ≥65 years | No association for current smokers |
| Honkanen et al. 1998 | Retrospective survey | 12,192 women<br>210 fractures<br>Aged 47–56 years<br>Finland | Current smoking<br>RR = 2.2 (1.6–3.2)<br>Any smoking<br>RR = 1.6 (0.9–2.8) for 1–10 cigarettes/day<br>RR = 3.0 (1.9–4.6) for >10 cigarettes/day<br>Adjusted for age, BMI, menopausal status, chronic health disorders |
| **Foot** | | | |
| Seeley et al. 1996 | Cohort study | 9,704 women<br>204 fractures over 5.9 years (mean)<br>Aged ≥65 years | No association for current smokers |

development of gallstones among women and men in a population followed up with repeat ultrasonography (Misciagna et al. 1996). Finally, an Australian case-control study suggested an adverse effect of smoking on the risk for gallbladder disease among women younger than age 35 years (McMichael et al. 1992).

In contrast with these positive findings, another cohort study reported no relationship between smoking and gallbladder disease among 1,303 women in a California retirement community (Mohr et al. 1991). A case-control study from Italy also found no substantial association between smoking and surgery for gallstone disease among women and men (La Vecchia et al. 1991a). Data from the Framingham study suggested lower risk for cholelithiasis or cholecystitis among female smokers than among female nonsmokers, but the difference in risk was not statistically significant and no adjustment was made for alcohol intake (Friedman et al. 1966). Unadjusted analyses from a small population survey in Italy also suggested an inverse association between smoking and gallbladder disease among women and men (Okolicsanyi et al. 1995), as did a small case-control study in Greece (Pastides et al. 1990). Another retrospective study also showed that smoking was associated with a lower risk for symptomatic gallbladder disease among both women and men (Rhodes and Venables 1991). However, the low response rate for cases (62 percent) and the procedures for selection of the control subjects raise concerns about the validity of these findings.

## Peptic Ulcer Disease

Peptic ulcer disease comprises a group of chronic ulcerative conditions that primarily affect the proximal duodenum and the gastric mucosa. The 1979 Surgeon General's report on smoking and health noted a strong association between peptic ulcer and smoking (USDHEW 1979). This conclusion was reaffirmed in the 1990 Surgeon General's report on the health benefits of smoking cessation, which also concluded that smoking impairs the healing of ulcers and causes an increased risk for recurrence that decreases after smoking cessation (USDHHS 1990).

Several studies have demonstrated an increased prevalence of peptic ulcers among women who smoke compared with women who do not smoke (Higgins and Kjelsberg 1967; Alp et al. 1970; Friedman et al. 1974). In a Norwegian case-control study of patients with radiographic diagnosis of a first gastric or duodenal ulcer and no family history of peptic disease, the RR among women smokers compared with women nonsmokers was 2.0 for duodenal ulcers and 1.3 for gastric ulcers (no CIs were provided). A population survey in Göteborg, Sweden, reported similar findings (Schöön et al. 1991). Women former smokers tended to have RRs between those among women current smokers and women who had never smoked. Women who smoked also had an increased risk for incident ulcers.

Prospective studies provided strong support for a relationship between smoking and incident peptic ulcer among women. The NHANES Epidemiologic Followup Study (Anda et al. 1990b) found 140 incident cases of peptic ulcer during 12.5 years of followup among 2,851 women. After adjustment for age, education, regular use of aspirin, number of cups of coffee or tea consumed per day, and alcohol use, the RR among current smokers was 1.8 (95 percent CI, 1.2 to 2.6). The RR increased with the number of cigarettes smoked per day. Among former smokers, the RR was 1.3 (95 percent CI, 0.7 to 2.9). An estimated 20 percent of incident cases of peptic ulcer during the study period was attributable to current smoking.

A prospective study from Norway also found an elevated risk for incident peptic ulcer among women who smoked; effects were similar for gastric and duodenal ulcers and were similar among women and men (Johnsen et al. 1994). Likewise, in a large cohort study in the United Kingdom, women who smoked had an increased risk for reported gastric and duodenal ulcers (Vessey et al. 1992). However, in a Finnish twin study, smoking was a clear risk factor for incident peptic ulcer disease only among men; risks were not significantly elevated among women smokers (Räihä et al. 1998).

Thus, data for women—like data for men—support a relationship between smoking and the incidence of peptic ulcer. At comparable levels of smoking, the mortality from this disorder is equivalent for women and men (Kurata et al. 1986). In a meta-analysis, the RR for peptic ulcer among women smokers compared with women nonsmokers was 2.3 (95 percent CI, 1.9 to 2.7); about 23 percent of the peptic ulcers in the populations studied could be attributed to smoking (Kurata and Nogawa 1997).

Little research has been conducted on the effects of smoking or smoking cessation on the healing or recurrence of peptic ulcer among women. Breuer-Katschinski and associates (1995) reported findings on the influence of smoking patterns on relapse of duodenal ulcers among female and male patients taking ranitidine. They observed that 18.0 percent of patients who had never smoked and 23.4 percent of patients who were smoking at the start of the trial had relapse of duodenal ulcers during the two-year study period. Patients who had stopped smoking had significantly fewer relapses than did continuing smokers ($p < 0.001$), and those who had stopped smoking before study entry had relapse significantly more often than did those who had never smoked ($p < 0.001$). In an earlier double-blind trial of the effects of cimetidine and ranitidine on the healing and relapse of peptic ulcer, women who smoked (42 percent) tended to have lower healing rates than did women nonsmokers (83 percent); no p value was given (Peden et al. 1981). Similar findings among women and men combined have also documented the deleterious effects of smoking on ulcer relapse (Berndt and Gütz 1981; Sonnenberg et al. 1981; Korman et al. 1983; Kratochvil and Brandstätter 1983; Lee et al. 1984; Sontag et al. 1984; Bertschinger et al. 1987; Van Deventer et al.

1989). One study of self-reported peptic ulcers that was based on data from a national survey found a strong association of smoking with chronic ulcers but no association with incident ulcers (Everhart et al. 1998). No gender-specific results were presented.

These findings emphasize the importance of smoking in perpetuating ulcers that develop, at least with treatment regimens used in the early 1990s. However, in studies conducted largely among men, smoking has not been a risk factor for ulcer recurrence after eradication of *Helicobacter pylori* (Borody et al. 1992; Graham et al. 1992; Bardhan et al. 1997; Chan et al. 1997). Smoking may thus have a smaller impact on ulcer healing under newer treatment regimens.

## Inflammatory Bowel Disease

Inflammatory bowel disease (IBD) includes three chronic gastrointestinal diseases: ulcerative colitis, ulcerative proctitis, and Crohn's disease. These three diseases affect about 1 per 1,000 persons in the United States (Everhart 1994).

### Ulcerative Colitis and Ulcerative Proctitis

The first published investigation of the relationship between smoking and IBD demonstrated a much lower prevalence of smoking among patients with ulcerative colitis than among control subjects (Harries et al. 1982). Since then, both case-control and prospective studies have addressed the relationship between smoking and risk for ulcerative colitis. The results are summarized in Table 3.49. All except one of the studies in the table reported decreased risk associated with current smoking compared with never smoking, and all studies except one showed increased risk with former smoking.

The relationship between smoking and ulcerative colitis appears to be present among both genders. Seven studies reported RRs separately for women and men and found similar results among both genders (Gyde et al. 1984; Logan et al. 1984; Benoni and Nilsson 1987; Franceschi et al. 1987; Tobin et al. 1987; Persson et al. 1990; Nakamura et al. 1994). Moreover, the cohort studies that included women only reported findings similar to those of the case-control studies that included both women and men (Vessey et al. 1986; Logan and Kay 1989).

Two relatively small, randomized controlled trials of transdermal administration of nicotine as treatment for active ulcerative colitis symptoms showed benefit after four weeks (Sandborn et al. 1997) and six weeks (Pullan et al. 1994) of treatment. One of these studies reported that effects were similar among women and men (Pullan et al. 1994).

### Crohn's Disease

In contrast to the risk for ulcerative colitis, the risk for Crohn's disease seems to be increased by cigarette smoking (Table 3.50). Both case-control and cohort studies found higher risks among current smokers and, less markedly, among former smokers than among persons who had never smoked. Of the five studies that presented gender-specific results, all showed higher RRs for current smoking among women than among women and men combined (Table 3.50).

For several reasons, the clinical course of Crohn's disease in relation to smoking has been studied more successfully than that of ulcerative colitis. The higher prevalence of smoking among patients with Crohn's disease facilitates the study of its effects on the clinical severity of the disease. Also, because severe Crohn's disease often leads to surgical resection, the number and extent of surgical resections provide a convenient proxy measure for disease severity.

Five retrospective studies and one prospective study examined the association between smoking and severity of Crohn's disease; the findings were fairly consistent. Patients who smoked tended to have more frequent hospital admissions (Holdstock et al. 1984), early treatment with surgery rather than drugs alone (Lindberg et al. 1992), and repeated surgical treatment (Sutherland et al. 1990; Lindberg et al. 1992). Moreover, smokers have a higher risk for disease recurrence than do nonsmokers, and they tend to need immunosuppressive therapy more often (Duffy et al. 1990; Cottone et al. 1994; Cosnes et al. 1996; Timmer et al. 1998).

## Conclusions

1. Some studies suggest that women who smoke have an increased risk for gallbladder disease (gallstones and cholecystitis), but the evidence is inconsistent.
2. Women who smoke have an increased risk for peptic ulcers.
3. Women who currently smoke have a decreased risk for ulcerative colitis, but former smokers have an increased risk—possibly because smoking suppresses symptoms of the disease.
4. Women who smoke appear to have an increased risk for Crohn's disease, and smokers with Crohn's disease have a worse prognosis than do nonsmokers.

**Table 3.49. Relative risks for ulcerative colitis among former and current smokers, case-control and cohort studies**

| Study | Number of cases | Time in relation to diagnosis | Relative risk (95% confidence interval)* | |
|---|---|---|---|---|
| | | | Former smokers | Current smokers |
| **Case-control** | | | | |
| Harries et al. 1982 | 230 | A[†] | Increased risk | Decreased risk |
| Jick and Walker 1983 | 239 | A | 1.2 (0.8–1.8) | 0.3 (0.2–0.4) |
| Gyde et al. 1984 | 74 | A | Decreased risk[‡] | Decreased risk[§] |
| | 31[Δ] | A | Decreased risk[‡] | Decreased risk[§] |
| Logan et al. 1984[¶] | 120 | D** | NR[††] | Decreased risk[‡‡] |
| | 64[Δ] | D | NR | Decreased risk[‡‡] |
| Thornton et al. 1985 | 30 | D | Increased risk[§] | Decreased risk[§] |
| Burns 1986 | 63 | A | Increased risk[§] | Decreased risk[‡‡] |
| Benoni and Nilsson 1987[¶] | 173 | D | 1.6 | 0.3[§] |
| | 80[Δ] | D | 1.8 | 0.3[§] |
| Boyko et al. 1987[¶] | 212 | D | 1.9 (1.1–3.5) | 0.6 (0.4–1.0) |
| Franceschi et al. 1987 | 124 | D | 2.7 (1.5–4.9) | 0.5 (0.3–1.0) |
| | 49[Δ] | D | 2.6 (1.0–7.2) | 1.1 (0.4–2.2) |
| Tobin et al. 1987 | 143 | D | 1.5 (0.8–2.8) | 0.2 (0.1–0.3)[‡‡] |
| | 81[Δ] | D | NR | Decreased risk |
| Lindberg et al. 1988[¶] | 258 | D | 2.3 (1.4–3.9) | 0.7 (0.4–1.0) |
| Lorusso et al. 1989 | 84 | D | 3.0 (0.9–10.3) | Decreased risk[‡] |
| Persson et al. 1990[¶] | 145 | D | 2.2 (0.9–5.0) | 0.8 (0.5–1.3) |
| | 63 | D | 1.6 (0.6–4.2) | 0.7 (0.4–1.4) |
| Samuelsson et al. 1991 | 167 | A | 1.1 (0.6–2.3) | 0.5 (0.3–0.9) |
| Epidemiology Group of the Research Committee of Inflammatory Bowel Disease in Japan 1994 | 76 | D | 2.4 (1.0–6.0) | 0.7 (0.2–2.0)[§§] |

*Compared with those who never smoked, unless otherwise indicated.
[†]A = Smoking status ascertained after diagnosis.
[‡]Statistically significant differences in relative risk by smoking status, $p < 0.05$.
[§]Percentage of smokers differed significantly between cases and controls; $p < 0.05$.
[Δ]Number of women.
[¶]Population-based study.
**D = Smoking status ascertained before or soon after diagnosis.
[††]NR = Not reported.
[‡‡]Compared with former smokers and those who never smoked.
[§§]≥20 cigarettes/day.

Table 3.49. Continued

| Study | Number of cases | Time in relation to diagnosis | Relative risk (95% confidence interval)* | |
|---|---|---|---|---|
| | | | Former smokers | Current smokers |
| **Case-control (continued)** | | | | |
| Nakamura and Labarthe 1994; | 384[Δ] | D | 1.7 (1.0–2.9) | 0.3 (0.2–0.5) |
| Nakamura et al. 1994 | 199 | | 2.3 (0.9–5.7) | 0.4 (0.2–1.0) |
| Rutgeerts et al. 1994 | 174 | A | NR | Decreased risk[‡‡] |
| Silverstein et al. 1994 | 100 | D | 1.2 (0.5–3.0) | 0.1 (0.1–0.4) |
| Reif et al. 1995 | 54 | A | No difference | No difference |
| Corrao et al. 1998 | 594 | D | 3.0 (2.1–4.3) | 0.9 (0.7–1.2) |
| **Cohort** | | | | |
| Vessey et al. 1986 | 24[Δ] | D | Increased risk | Decreased risk[‡‡] |
| Logan and Kay 1989 | 78 | D | NR | Decreased risk[‡‡] |

*Compared with those who never smoked, unless otherwise indicated.
ΔNumber of women.
‡‡Compared with former smokers and those who never smoked.

# Arthritis

Arthritic diseases are a diverse group of disorders that can lead to considerable morbidity among women (Lawrence et al. 1989b). These disorders prominently affect the joints but may also affect other organs. In this section, the three most common arthritic disorders are discussed: rheumatoid arthritis (RA), osteoarthritis (OA), and systemic lupus erythematosus (SLE). RA and SLE are systemic immune diseases characterized by the production of antibodies that participate in the disease process (Firestein 1997; Lahita 1997). OA, on the other hand, is largely a degenerative joint disorder (Solomon 1997). RA and SLE are more common among women than among men; OA occurs with similar frequency in both genders (Firestein 1997; Harris 1997; Lahita 1997; Solomon 1997).

## Rheumatoid Arthritis

The prevalence of RA in the United States is approximately 1 percent, and it is three times higher among women than among men. Characteristic clinical features include bilateral symmetric inflammation of small and large joints in both upper and lower extremities.

Several cohort studies reported findings on the relationship between smoking and RA. In a study of 17,000 women recruited from family-planning clinics in the United Kingdom, the age-adjusted risk for RA among women who smoked was significantly increased (Vessey et al. 1987). Those who smoked 15 or more cigarettes per day had more than twice the risk among nonsmokers. The analysis was based on only 78 cases, however, and few details were provided. In contrast to these findings, data from the U.S. Nurses' Health Study cohort suggested no relationship between smoking and RA (Hernandez-Avila et al. 1990), and a study of 24,445 women in Finland found that women who smoked 1 to 14 cigarettes per day did not have an increased risk for either seropositive or seronegative RA compared with nonsmokers (Heliovaara et al. 1993).

**Table 3.50. Relative risks for Crohn's disease among former and current smokers, case-control and cohort studies**

| Study | Number of cases | Time in relation to diagnosis | Relative risk (95% confidence interval)* | |
|---|---|---|---|---|
| | | | Former smokers | Current smokers |
| **Case-control** | | | | |
| Somerville et al. 1984[†] | 81 | D[‡] | NR[§] | 4.8 (2.4–9.7)[Δ¶] |
| | 52** | D | NR | 8.2 (2.8–24.0)[Δ¶] |
| Thornton et al. 1985 | 30 | D | Increased risk | Increased risk[††] |
| Burns 1986 | 25 | A[‡‡] | Decreased risk | Increased risk[††] |
| Benoni and Nilsson 1987 | 155 | D | 0.7 | 2.2[‡] |
| | 90** | D | 0.2 | 2.7[‡] |
| Franceschi et al. 1987 | 109 | D | 3.5 (1.5–8.0) | 4.2 (2.3–7.7) |
| | 49** | D | 3.0 (0.9–10.6) | 4.8 (2.0–11.3) |
| Tobin et al. 1987 | 132** | D | 1.6 (0.6–4.1) | 3.1 (1.6–6.0)[¶] |
| | | | NR | |
| Lindberg et al. 1988[†] | 144 | D | 1.9 (0.8–4.3) | 2.0 (1.3–3.1) |
| Silverstein et al. 1989 | 115 | | 1.5 (0.7–2.9) | 3.7 (1.9–7.1) |
| Persson et al. 1990[†] | 60 | D | 1.2 (0.5–3.1) | 1.3 (0.7–2.6) |
| | 89** | D | 1.0 (0.3–4.0) | 5.0 (2.7–9.2) |
| Katschinski et al. 1993 | 83 | D | 1.1 (0.3–4.3) | 3.8 (1.5–9.5) |
| Reif et al. 1995 | 33 | A | Increased risk | Decreased risk[††] |
| Corrao et al. 1998 | 225 | D | 1.7 (0.9–3.3) | 1.7 (1.1–2.6) |
| **Cohort** | | | | |
| Vessey et al. 1986 | 18** | D | Decreased risk[§§] | Increased risk[††] |
| Logan and Kay 1989 | 42** | D | NR | Increased risk[¶] |

*Compared with those who never smoked, unless otherwise indicated.
[†]Population-based study.
[‡]D = Smoking status ascertained before or soon after diagnosis.
[§]NR = Not reported.
[Δ]$p < 0.05$.
[¶]Compared with former smokers and those who never smoked.
**Number of women.
[††]Percentage of smokers differed significantly between cases and controls; $p < 0.05$.
[‡‡]A = Smoking status ascertained after diagnosis.
[§§]$p > 0.05$.

Several case-control studies addressed the relationship between smoking and risk for RA. Voigt and colleagues (1994) identified 349 patients with RA through Group Health Cooperative of Puget Sound, Washington. The investigators reported a RR of 1.5 (95 percent CI, 1.0 to 2.0) among women with 20 or more pack-years of smoking compared with women who had never smoked. RRs were similar in premenopausal and postmenopausal groups. In a case-control analysis of 120 female twins, current smokers were at much higher risk than were nonsmokers for developing RA (RR, 3.8; 95 percent CI, 1.4 to 13.0) (Silman et al. 1996). The RR among males was similar. A population-based study from England also reported findings consistent with an increased risk among smokers (Symmons et al. 1997). A study from Norway suggested an increased risk for seronegative RA among women who smoked (RR, 1.5; 95 percent CI, 0.99 to 2.4), but no association was found for seropositive RA (RR, 0.7; 95 percent CI, 0.4 to 1.2) (Uhlig et al. 1999). The RRs among men were higher. In contrast to these reports, a clinic-based, case-control study found a reduced risk for RA among women smokers compared with nonsmokers (Hazes et al. 1990). The use of controls drawn from rheumatology outpatient clinics may account for the discrepancy between these results and those from other published studies.

## Osteoarthritis

Osteoarthritis, a degenerative joint disease, is the most common form of arthritis and the leading cause of rheumatic disability in the United States (Lawrence et al. 1989b). Body weight, which is lower among smokers, must be taken into account when interpreting epidemiologic data on smoking and OA.

Cross-sectional data from the first NHANES showed an inverse relationship between cigarette smoking and the risk for OA of the knee, as diagnosed by radiography among 2,765 women. In age-adjusted analyses, the RR among female smokers compared with nonsmokers was 0.7 (95 percent CI, 0.5 to 0.99); the association was similar after adjustment for BMI and other risk factors, although not statistically significant (Anderson and Felson 1988). The RRs among men were similar. Extending this work, the investigators analyzed follow-up data from the Framingham Heart Study (Felson et al. 1989) and reported an inverse association between smoking and the prevalence of radiographically diagnosed OA of the knee. The RR per 20 cigarettes smoked per day was 0.7 (95 percent CI, 0.6 to 0.95). This association persisted after adjustment for age, gender, weight, physical activity, and participation in sports. These investigators confirmed this finding in a subsequent longitudinal analysis (Felson et al. 1997), in which women smokers had reduced risk for incident OA diagnosed by radiography. Similarly, in a survey conducted in North Carolina, female and male smokers had a lower prevalence of OA of the knee diagnosed by radiography, even after adjustment for factors such as obesity and race (RR, 0.7; 95 percent CI, 0.6 to 0.9) (Jordan et al. 1995).

An inverse association between smoking and clinical OA of the knee was also observed in a British clinic-based study of women: for ever smoking, the RR was 0.3 (95 percent CI, 0.1 to 0.6) (Samanta et al. 1993). Also, in a Swedish radiographic survey of 79-year-old women and men, RR was 0.7 (95 percent CI, 0.4 to 0.7) for current smoking compared with never smoking, after adjustment for gender and BMI (Bagge et al. 1991). However, findings in a detailed British study of OA among 985 women were contrary (Hart and Spector 1993). After adjustment for age and BMI, no reduction in risk for OA of the knee was found among smokers compared with nonsmokers, but the number of cases was small and the CIs for the estimated RRs were wide.

Data on OA of the hip have not consistently suggested a relationship with cigarette smoking. One study reported that women who smoked had a lower prevalence of hip OA than did those who did not smoke (Samanta et al. 1993); another investigation found a lower risk among men who smoked than among those who did not, but no association was found among women (Cooper et al. 1998). Other studies reported no association of hip OA with smoking among women and men (Jordan et al. 1995) or even suggested an increased risk among women who smoked (Vingard et al. 1997). Small-joint OA (e.g., of the hand) appears to be unrelated to smoking (Bagge et al. 1993; Hart and Spector 1993).

## Systemic Lupus Erythematosus

Systemic lupus erythematosus (SLE) is a multisystemic autoimmune disease characterized by disturbances of the immune system that lead to increased production of antibodies, formation of immune complexes, and tissue injury.

Some studies suggested an increased risk for SLE among women who smoke, but overall the data on smoking and SLE have been somewhat inconsistent. In a case-control study that included 50 female patients, the RR among current smokers compared with women who had never smoked was 2.0 (95 percent CI, 0.5 to 4.8) (Benoni et al. 1990). In a larger Japanese case-control study of SLE among women, the RR for SLE among current smokers compared with those who had never smoked was 2.3 (95 percent CI, 1.3 to 4.0) (Nagata et al. 1995). In a case-control study in England with 150 women and men with SLE, risk among current smokers was increased compared with those who had never smoked (RR, 2.0; 95 percent CI, 1.1 to 3.3) (Hardy et al. 1998). However, the prospective U.S. Nurses' Health Study found no significant relationship between smoking and the risk for SLE (Sanchez-Guerrero et al. 1996). On the basis of data from 85 cases of SLE that met established criteria for diagnosis, the age-adjusted RR was 1.1 (95 percent CI, 0.7 to 1.8) among women current smokers compared with women who had never smoked. Furthermore, no substantial relationship was observed between the number of cigarettes smoked per day and risk for SLE among current smokers.

### Conclusions

1. Some but not all studies suggest that women who smoke may have a modestly elevated risk for rheumatoid arthritis.
2. Women who smoke have a modestly reduced risk for osteoarthritis of the knee; data regarding osteoarthritis of the hip are inconsistent.
3. The data on the risk for systemic lupus erythematosus among women who smoke are inconsistent.

## Eye Disease

### Cataract

Cataract (opacity in the lens of the eye) is a major health concern among older adults in the United States. However, only a few studies have specifically addressed the relationship between smoking and the risk for cataract among women. In the Beaver Dam (Wisconsin) Eye Study, a cross-sectional analysis of 2,762 women showed a strong relationship between smoking and cataract (Klein et al. 1993b). The age-adjusted RR for each 10 pack-years of smoking was significantly elevated for nuclear sclerosis (RR, 1.1; 95 percent CI, 1.0 to 1.2), posterior subcapsular cataract (RR, 1.1; 95 percent CI, 0.98 to 1.1), and a history of cataract surgery (RR, 1.1; 95 percent CI, 1.03 to 1.2) but not for cortical opacity (RR, 1.02; 95 percent CI, 0.96 to 1.1).

Prospective data from the U.S. Nurses' Health Study also showed a strong relationship between smoking and cataract extraction (Hankinson et al. 1992). A total of 493 cases were reported in the cohort of 121,700 women who were followed up since 1976. The multivariate RR was 1.6 (95 percent CI, 1.2 to 2.3) among women with more than 65 pack-years of smoking compared with women who had never smoked. Risk was generally lower among women former smokers than among women who continued to smoke, although those who had formerly smoked more than 35 cigarettes per day had a higher risk than did those who had never smoked (RR, 1.7; 95 percent CI, 1.0 to 2.7).

Several studies that included both women and men reported a relationship between smoking and risk for cataract (Klein et al. 1985; Flaye et al. 1989; Leske et al. 1991; Cumming and Mitchell 1997; Hiller et al. 1997; Leske et al. 1998), but others found no significant association after adjustment for other factors (Bochow et al. 1989; Mohan et al. 1989; Italian-American Cataract Study Group 1991). In studies of this association among men, findings were generally similar to those reported among women (West et al. 1989; Christen et al. 1992; Klein et al. 1993b).

### Age-Related Macular Degeneration

Age-related macular degeneration is a relatively common disorder among older adults. In its mildest forms, it may affect more than one-fourth of the U.S. population older than 75 years. Advanced macular degeneration is an important cause of visual impairment and blindness (Klein and Klein 1996).

In a cohort study of more than 30,000 women, smoking was associated with an increased risk for macular degeneration (Seddon et al. 1996). Women who smoked 25 or more cigarettes daily were 2.4 times as likely to have macular degeneration (adjusted RR of 2.4; 95 percent CI, 1.4 to 4.0) as were women who had never smoked. The RR increased with the number of pack-years of smoking and did not decline even after 15 years of cessation. In a related cohort investigation, similar findings were reported among men (Christen et al. 1996).

A population-based, cross-sectional analysis reported a higher risk for exudative age-related macular degeneration among women current smokers than among women who had never smoked (RR, 2.5; 95 percent CI, 1.0 to 6.2) (Klein et al. 1993c). The RR among men smokers was similar. However, no association was found between smoking and less advanced age-related maculopathy among either women or men. In the follow-up phase of the study, current smoking at baseline was associated with an increased risk for some lesions associated with early, age-related macular degeneration and with progression to advanced disease. In general, the associations were stronger among men than among women (Klein et al. 1993c). Another investigation reported that men smokers had an increased risk for macular degeneration with visual impairment, but no association was found among women smokers (Hyman et al. 1983). In contrast, a similar study from Australia found risk to be increased among both women and men who smoked (Smith et al. 1996): women current smokers were 5.4 times as likely as women who had never smoked to have macular degeneration (RR of 5.4; 95 percent CI, 2.4 to 12.4). Studies in which data for women and men were combined have generally reported that smoking is a risk factor for macular degeneration or that smokers with a diagnosis of this condition have a worse prognosis than do nonsmokers (Macular Photocoagulation Study Group 1986; Eye Disease Case-Control Study Group 1992; Tsang et al. 1992; Vinding et al. 1992; Holz et al. 1994; Hirvelä et al. 1996).

### Open-Angle Glaucoma

Open-angle glaucoma is a progressive optic neuropathy often associated with high intraocular pressure (ocular hypertension). A series of population surveys have investigated the relationship between cigarette smoking and the risk for open-angle glaucoma. All reported that smoking was unrelated to this disease (Klein et al. 1993a; Ponte et al. 1994; Stewart et al. 1994; Leske et al. 1995).

### Conclusions

1. Women who smoke have an increased risk for cataract.
2. Women who smoke may have an increased risk for age-related macular degeneration.
3. Studies show no consistent association between smoking and open-angle glaucoma.

## HIV Disease

Smoking has been associated with infection with human immunodeficiency virus type 1 (HIV-1) among women, but it is unclear whether this association is due to an underlying relationship between smoking and high-risk sexual behavior, biological effects of smoking, or both. An association between smoking and increased risk for HIV-1 infection among women was first identified in a longitudinal study of pregnant women in Haiti (Boulos et al. 1990). The association persisted after adjustment for marital status, age, number of sexual partners in the year before pregnancy, and serologic evidence of syphilis. The risk for HIV-1 infection also appeared to increase with the number of cigarettes smoked. A nested case-control study was subsequently performed in the same population to more fully assess the contribution of sexual practices, other substance use, parenteral exposures, and other potential confounders (Halsey et al. 1992). This study also reported an independent association between smoking and HIV-1 infection.

Smoking also has been associated with HIV-1 infection among homosexual and heterosexual men (Newell et al. 1985; Burns et al. 1991; Penkower et al. 1991; Siraprapasiri et al. 1996) and with other STDs among both women and men (Daling et al. 1986; Aral and Holmes 1990; Willmott 1992). Whether these associations are causal or a coincidence of high-risk sexual behavior is unclear (Aral and Holmes 1990). The influence of smoking on progression of HIV-1 infection and on survival among women has not been examined in cohorts sufficiently large for meaningful interpretation.

### Conclusion

1. Limited data suggest that women smokers may be at higher risk for HIV-1 infection than are nonsmokers.

# Facial Wrinkling

Wrinkling of the facial skin occurs with age and with long-term exposure to sunlight. Except for these two recognized factors, little is known about the causes of wrinkling. Four studies reported that smoking is associated with prominent skin wrinkling, particularly in the lateral periorbital "crow's foot" area of the face. Ippen and Ippen (1965) defined "cigarette skin" as pale, grayish, and wrinkled, especially on the cheeks, and thickened between the wrinkles. In a study of women 35 through 84 years old, 66 of 84 smokers (79 percent) and 27 of 140 nonsmokers (19 percent) had cigarette skin. Because no adjustment was made for differences between smokers and nonsmokers in age or sun exposure, the independent effect of smoking in that study cannot be assessed (Ippen and Ippen 1965).

One researcher examined facial wrinkles and smoking status among 589 women aged 30 through 70 years (Daniell 1971). Skin wrinkling was assessed in the crow's foot area and the adjacent forehead and cheeks and was graded in six categories of increasing severity. Ratings of 4 to 6 (more severe wrinkling) were more prevalent among smokers than among nonsmokers and were also more common with increasing age and sun exposure. According to calculations from the published data, smokers were significantly more likely than nonsmokers to be evaluated as having prominent wrinkling (categories 4 to 6 vs. categories 1 to 3). All women with ratings in the most severe wrinkling category were smokers. Severity of wrinkling increased with duration of smoking and number of cigarettes smoked daily. The occurrence of prominent wrinkling was as common among women smokers aged 40 through 49 years as among women nonsmokers 20 years older. The association of smoking with prominent wrinkling was found in each age, sex, and sun-exposure group. Although these findings suggested that smoking is associated with skin wrinkling among women, the measurement of wrinkling was not precise. An attempt was made to use a blinded procedure in the assessment of wrinkling, but participants were patients and friends of the investigator, who may have known the smoking status of many of them.

Two subsequent studies of the effect of smoking on facial wrinkling and other facial changes did not provide adequate data to assess the effect among women (Allen et al. 1973; Model 1985). In another study, Kadunce and colleagues (1991) used Daniell's categories of wrinkling in a blinded procedure to evaluate wrinkling shown in standardized photographs of the right temple area of the face for 59 white women aged 35 through 59 years. After adjustment for age, sun exposure, and skin pigmentation, smoking was associated with an increased risk for prominent wrinkling of the temple area of the face, but the study included only 12 nonsmokers and the result was not statistically significant (RR, 4.7; 95 percent CI, 0.2 to 89.1).

Other investigators studied 463 white women aged 40 through 69 years enrolled in an HMO in northern California (Ernster et al. 1995). Smoking status, pack-years of smoking, age, and sun exposure were assessed by questionnaire. Examiners who were blinded to the smoking status of the women visually evaluated several areas of the face by using standardized procedures. The examiners determined facial wrinkle category, a dichotomous variable, and facial wrinkle score, a continuous variable based on number, length, and depth of wrinkles. Adjustment for age, sun exposure, and BMI indicated that women current smokers were three times as likely as women who had never smoked to have moderate or severe facial wrinkling (RR, 3.1; 95 percent CI, 1.6 to 5.9). Former smokers were also more likely to have moderate or severe wrinkling than were women who had never smoked (RR, 1.8; 95 percent CI, 1.0 to 3.1). Risk for wrinkling increased with pack-years of smoking.

Smoking has been shown to produce short-term decreases in capillary and arteriolar blood flow in the skin (Reus et al. 1984; Richardson 1987) and in oxygen tension in subcutaneous wound tissue (Jensen et al. 1991). These findings suggest that chronic ischemia of the dermis may contribute to wrinkling. In the lung, cigarette smoke damages collagen and elastin, which are connective tissue elements that help to maintain the integrity of the skin. Facial wrinkling may also be promoted by chronic squinting caused by the irritating effects of smoke on the nostrils and eyes.

## Conclusion

1. Limited but consistent data suggest that women smokers have more facial wrinkling than do nonsmokers.

# Depression and Other Psychiatric Disorders

Depression, anxiety disorders, and bulimia and binge eating are considerably more prevalent among women than among men (Halmi et al. 1981; Pyle et al. 1983; Killen et al. 1987; Patton et al. 1990; Timmerman et al. 1990; Weissman et al. 1991; Johnson et al. 1992). Thus, these psychiatric disorders, in their own right, constitute a public health problem among women and take a large toll in terms of lost productivity and diminished quality of life. To the extent that they are associated with an increased likelihood of smoking or greater difficulty in stopping, the health-related consequences of these disorders are magnified. A recent analysis of data from the National Comorbidity Survey, a nationally representative study conducted from 1991 through 1992, compared smoking prevalence among respondents with no mental illness (22.5 percent), those who had been mentally ill at any time in their lives (34.8 percent), and those with active mental illness in the past month (41.0 percent) (Lasser et al. 2000). The RR for being a current smoker among those with mental illness in the past month, adjusted for age, sex, and region of the country, was 2.7 (95 percent CI, 2.3 to 3.1). The mental illness category grouped together many of the psychiatric disorders considered individually below, and gender-specific results were not presented. Still, the authors estimated that persons with a diagnosable mental disorder in the past month consume nearly half of the cigarettes smoked in the United States, and they underscored the importance of addressing smoking prevention and cessation efforts to the mentally ill.

## Smoking and Depression

Hughes and associates (1986) reported an excess of both female and male smokers among psychiatric outpatients with major depression compared with local and national population-based samples. Glassman and colleagues (1988) observed that 61 percent of the 71 participants in a smoking cessation trial had a history of clinical depression, even though they were not currently depressed. Subsequently, in analyses of a community database, Glassman and colleagues (1990) confirmed their clinical observation of an excess of depressed persons among smokers. Using the St. Louis, Missouri, node of the Epidemiological Catchment Area survey, they obtained information on psychiatric diagnosis and smoking for 3,213 respondents. The lifetime prevalence of major depressive disorder (MDD) among smokers (6.6 percent) was more than double that among nonsmokers (2.9 percent), and smokers with a lifetime history of clinical depression (14.0 percent) were one-half as likely as smokers without such a history (28.0 percent) to succeed in attempts to stop smoking.

Since 1990, the relationship between smoking and depression or dysphoric mood has been confirmed in numerous clinical studies and population-based surveys (e.g., Anda et al. 1990a; Breslau et al. 1991, 1992; Hall et al. 1991; Lee and Markides 1991; Kendler et al. 1993). In one study the association was found among girls throughout the teenage years, but only among younger teenage boys (Patton et al. 1996). Some studies among adults also suggested that the relationship may be even stronger for women than for men (Anda et al. 1990a; Glassman et al. 1990; Pérez-Stable et al. 1990), but a stronger link between smoking and depression among women has not been universally observed (Breslau 1995; Breslau et al. 1998). (See also "Beliefs About Mood Control and Depression" in Chapter 4, and "Depression" in Chapter 5.)

Inferential evidence supports the hypothesis that persons with depression smoke as a form of self-medication. Nicotine has been described as having antidepressant effects (Rausch et al. 1989; Balfour 1991). It is known to have important effects on several neurotransmitter systems in the CNS (Pomerleau and Pomerleau 1984) that contribute to depression (Janowsky and Risch 1987; Siever 1987) and to affect brain regions that influence mood and well-being (Gilbert and Spielberger 1987; Carmody 1989; Pomerleau and Rosecrans 1989). Studies found that smoking a single cigarette can cause mood elevations and transient pleasurable effects among smokers (Jasinski et al. 1984; Henningfield et al. 1987). Investigators also have reported that these effects were more intense after abstinence from smoking than during smoking ad libitum and were more pronounced as nicotine dose increased (Pomerleau and Pomerleau 1992).

Studies of the effects of nicotine replacement products in reducing postcessation dysphoric mood have produced inconsistent results; some studies showed a reduction in dysphoric mood (see West 1984; Fagerström et al. 1993), but others did not (see

Fiore et al. 1994). A study by Kinnunen and colleagues (1996), showing a significant reduction in depressive symptoms only among depressed smokers, suggested a possible explanation for these discrepancies and raises the possibility that depressed smokers are particularly sensitive to the mood-enhancing effects of nicotine.

Because several large studies suggested that smoking precedes the onset of depression or that the relationship is bidirectional, self-medication is clearly not an exhaustive explanation for the link. Choi and colleagues (1997) found that cigarette smoking was the strongest predictor of the development of depressive symptoms among adolescents and that the effect was more pronounced among girls than among boys. A longitudinal study by Breslau and colleagues (1998) among 1,007 young adults showed that a history of daily smoking at study entry significantly increased the risk for major depression five years later and that a history of major depression at baseline increased risk for progression to daily smoking; no interaction with gender was detected. Patton and colleagues (1998) showed that depression and anxiety symptoms among adolescents are associated with a higher risk for smoking initiation through increased susceptibility to the influence of peer smoking. This effect was significant among both girls and boys when most peers smoked but only among girls when some peers smoked. A study of 1,731 young persons aged 8 through 14 years in Atlanta, who were assessed at least twice from 1989 through 1994, found that previous smoking was associated with an increased risk for subsequent depressed mood but that previous depressed mood was not associated with risk for subsequent smoking initiation (Wu and Anthony 1999). Findings were not presented separately by gender. Finally, in an analysis of data from the National Longitudinal Study of Adolescent Health, Goodman and Capitman (2000) found, in a sample of 8,704 adolescents who were not depressed at baseline, that current cigarette smoking was the strongest predictor of developing high depressive symptoms at one-year follow-up. However, in a companion analysis of 6,947 teens from the same study who were not smokers at baseline, high depressive symptoms at baseline did not predict moderate-to-heavy smoking (≥ 1 pack per week) at follow-up in multivariate analysis. Results were not presented separately by gender.

Hughes (1988) proposed that there may be a common predisposition to both smoking and depression, either because of cognitive factors such as low self-efficacy and low self-esteem or because of a common genetic defect. Kendler and associates (1993) likewise minimized the causal element, arguing that the strong association they observed between smoking and major depression among women was most likely the result of inherited, neurobiological factors that predispose to both conditions. The researchers based this hypothesis on the best-fitting bivariate twin model in an elegant study of 1,566 dizygotic and monozygotic female twin pairs who were either concordant or discordant for a history of depression or for smoking.

Finally, in an early molecular genetic study of smoking, Lerman and associates (1998) reported an interaction of the gene for the $D_4$ dopamine receptor (*DRD4*) and depression. They suggested that self-medication of depression may occur—but only in a subgroup of smokers with depression who are homozygous for the short alleles of the gene *DRD4*.

Antidepressant drugs have been tested with some success as adjuncts to smoking cessation therapy in clinical trials, but the explanation for their effects in promoting smoking cessation is unclear (Benowitz 1997). In a placebo-controlled trial of sustained-release bupropion, investigators reported significantly higher rates of abstinence among bupropion-treated smokers with or without a history of depression, but treatment-related effects were noted for postcessation depression (Hurt et al. 1997). In another study, nortriptyline produced significantly higher abstinence rates than the placebo, regardless of history of depression. Postcessation increases in negative affect also were alleviated by nortriptyline (Hall et al. 1998). Even though improvement in symptoms has been demonstrated, it remains to be determined whether treatment of depression improves the outcome of smoking cessation treatment among persons with current depression or with a history of depression (e.g., Dalack et al. 1995). (See "Depression" in Chapter 5).

## Psychiatric Disorders Other than Depression

### Anxiety Disorders, Bulimia Nervosa, and Attention Deficit Disorder

Hughes and associates (1986) observed increased smoking prevalence among patients with anxiety disorders, and these findings have been supported by a number of other investigations. Breslau and associates (1991) studied a sample of more than 1,000 young adults and reported a relationship between anxiety disorders and severity of nicotine dependence based on *Diagnostic and Statistical Manual of Mental Disorders,* third edition (revised) criteria (American Psychiatric Association [APA] 1987). This relationship was noted after adjustment for gender. Similar findings among children and adolescents were reported by Kandel and colleagues (1997), who observed that effects were more pronounced among girls than among boys. Covey and colleagues (1994) showed an association of smoking with generalized anxiety disorder among both women and men. Women with anxiety disorders, however, were more likely than men with anxiety disorders to stop or reduce smoking. Pohl and associates (1992) noted a higher prevalence of smoking among women with panic disorder (40 vs. 25 percent in control group) but not among men. Thus, although study findings support a relationship between smoking and anxiety disorders, the evidence is less consistent than that for depression (Glassman 1997).

A high prevalence of smoking has been observed among patients with bulimia nervosa (Weiss and Ebert 1983; Bulik et al. 1992; Welch and Fairburn 1998) and among dieters and binge eaters in school- and community-based populations (Killen et al. 1986; Krahn et al. 1992; Pomerleau and Krahn 1993). In contrast, no association has been observed between smoking and anorexia nervosa (Bulik et al. 1992; Wiederman and Pryor 1996).

Attention deficit disorder (ADD), an impairment in "the capacity to receive, hold, scan, and selectively screen out stimuli in a sequential order" (Clements and Peters 1962, p. 20), has been studied extensively as a disorder of childhood and adolescence (Barkley 1990). Although prevalence of adult ADD is higher among men than among women and most available data on smoking are largely based on samples of men, the validity of the diagnosis also has been supported for women, and little evidence exists of gender-specific differences in the expression of adult ADD or in the distribution of subtypes (Biederman et al. 1994). Both children and adults with ADD are significantly more likely to be smokers than are non-ADD controls (Borland and Heckman 1976; Hartsough and Lambert 1987; Barkley et al. 1990; Pomerleau et al. 1995).

### Schizophrenia

Smoking is highly prevalent and, in some studies, close to universal among persons with schizophrenia (O'Farrell et al. 1983; Masterson and O'Shea 1984; Hughes et al. 1986; Goff et al. 1992; Lohr and Flynn 1992), more so than other types of substance dependence (Schneier and Siris 1987). Moreover, persons with schizophrenia are extremely heavy smokers and show higher levels of cotinine (a metabolite of nicotine) than do those in control groups with similar smoking patterns (Olincy et al. 1997). The mechanism for this association is unknown, but dopaminergic effects of nicotine in the brain have frequently been implicated (Lohr and Flynn 1992). Although evidence is mixed, case reports suggested that nicotine withdrawal leads to exacerbation of both negative and positive symptoms of schizophrenia (Dalack and Meador-Woodruff 1996) and that smoking reduces negative symptoms (Lohr and Flynn 1992).

Although the occurrence of schizophrenia is generally thought to be about equal among women and men, especially as evidenced in community-based surveys (APA 1994), marked gender-specific differences in the presentation and course of this disorder do exist. Women are likely to have later onset of schizophrenia (median age in late 20s for women and early 20s for men), more prominent mood symptoms, and more favorable prognosis (APA 1994). Although conflicting evidence exists (e.g., Hughes et al. 1986), smoking prevalence may also be lower among women than among men with schizophrenia (de Leon et al. 1995).

### Dependence on Alcohol and Other Drugs

The high prevalence of smoking among persons with alcoholism has long been recognized (Istvan and Matarazzo 1984) and is similar among women and men (Bobo 1989). Possible mechanisms for this relationship are that nicotine may increase tolerance to the deleterious effects of alcohol on behavior, may directly enhance the reinforcing effects of alcohol, or may act in both ways (Pomerleau 1995). Because of the high rate of comorbidity of alcohol dependence and major depression (Weissman and Myers 1980; Helzer et al. 1988; Ross et al. 1988; Merikangas and Gelernter 1990; Regier et al. 1990), coexisting depression may contribute to or mediate the association between alcohol dependence and smoking. In a study of women and men smokers with a history of alcohol dependence, those who currently consumed alcohol had significantly higher self-ratings of depression than those who did not consume alcohol (Pomerleau et al. 1997). Another study showed that the occurrence of depression together with alcohol dependence exerted a detrimental effect on the ability to stop smoking among men but not among women (Covey et al. 1993).

## Conclusions

1. Smokers are more likely to be depressed than are nonsmokers, a finding that may reflect an effect of smoking on the risk for depression, the use of smoking for self-medication, or the influence of common genetic or other factors on both smoking and depression. The association of smoking and depression is particularly important among women because they are more likely to be diagnosed with depression than are men.
2. The prevalence of smoking generally has been found to be higher among patients with anxiety disorders, bulimia, attention deficit disorder, and alcoholism than among individuals without these conditions; the mechanisms underlying these associations are not yet understood.
3. The prevalence of smoking is very high among patients with schizophrenia, but the mechanisms underlying this association are not yet understood.
4. Smoking may be used by some persons who would otherwise manifest psychiatric symptoms to manage those symptoms; for such persons, cessation of smoking may lead to the emergence of depression or other dysphoric mood states.

# Neurologic Diseases

## Parkinson's Disease

Parkinson's disease (PD), an idiopathic neurodegenerative disorder, is characterized clinically by muscular rigidity, slowness of movement, and a characteristic tremor (Yahr 1985). A major cause of disability in the United States, PD may affect half a million to one million people nationally; it has been estimated that as many as 50,000 new cases occur each year (Yahr 1985). The incidence of PD among both women and men increases exponentially with age after about 55 years until about age 75 years. The incidence among women and men is generally similar, but some data have suggested a higher incidence of PD among men (Zhang and Román 1993).

Cigarette smoking is inversely related to the development of PD (Baron 1986; Morens et al. 1995). This association was first observed in follow-up studies of mortality in two cohorts of men. The standardized mortality ratio (SMR) was 0.23 among men current smokers in the study by Kahn (1966) and 0.72 among men who had ever smoked in the study by Hammond (1966). Similar inverse associations were also noted in prospective mortality studies of men in England (SMR, 0.43) (Doll and Peto 1976) and of women and men in Japan (SMR, 0.57) (Hirayama 1985). Results of prospective cohort studies by investigators who actively sought incident cases of PD (Wolf et al. 1991; Grandinetti et al. 1994) support these findings. Numerous case-control studies have also found that PD occurs less often among smokers than among persons who had never smoked (Baron 1986; Morens et al. 1995).

The inverse association between PD and smoking appears to be present among both women and men. In the only cohort study with data for both genders, Hirayama (1985) reported similarly reduced risks for PD mortality among women and men. Case-control studies that presented data separately for women and men are summarized in Table 3.51. These findings showed similar inverse associations among women and men. Thus, no compelling evidence exists that gender modifies the relationship between smoking and development of PD.

## Alzheimer's Disease

Alzheimer's disease (AD) is a neurodegenerative disorder characterized by progressive cognitive impairment and shortened life expectancy (for review, see Terry et al. 1994). An estimated four million U.S. residents have AD (National Institute on Aging 1992). Because age is a strong risk factor for AD and women have a longer life expectancy than do men, more women than men develop this disease. Even after adjustment for age, however, many studies found the prevalence of AD to be higher among women (e.g., Jorm et al. 1987; Rocca et al. 1991; Bachman et al. 1992; Canadian Study of Health and Aging Working Group 1994). Reports of longer survival among women with AD than among affected men (e.g., Heyman et al.

**Table 3.51. Relative risks for Parkinson's disease among smokers, women and men, case-control studies**

| Study | Smoking status | Relative risk | | Comments |
|---|---|---|---|---|
| | | Women | Men | |
| Kessler and Diamond 1971 | Ever vs. never smoked | 0.7 | 0.6* | |
| | | 0.7 | 0.7* | Adjusted for hospitalization diagnoses |
| Kessler 1972 | Ever vs. never smoked | 0.6 | 0.4† | Adjusted for age |
| Haack et al. 1981 | Ever vs. never smoked | 0.2‡ | 0.7 | |
| Godwin-Austen et al. 1982 | | 0.6* | 0.5* | |
| Ogawa et al. 1984 | Smokers vs. nonsmokers | 0.5§ | 0.3* | Hospital control (adjusted) |
| | | 0.6§ | 0.4 | Neighborhood control (adjusted) |
| Hofman et al. 1989 | Ever vs. never smoked | 0.3§ | 0.8 | |
| Hellenbrand et al. 1997 | Ever vs. never smoked | 0.6§ | 0.4§ | |

*$p < 0.01$.
†$p < 0.001$.
‡$p < 0.0001$.
§$p < 0.05$.

1996; Kokmen et al. 1996) suggested another reason that prevalence is higher among women. Differences in the incidence of AD by gender are less clear. Some studies reported the incidence of AD to be similar among women and men after adjustment for age (Schoenberg et al. 1987; Bachman et al. 1993; Letenneur et al. 1994a). In other studies, however, incidence was substantially higher among women, although the differences were not statistically significant (Brayne et al. 1995; Yoshitake et al. 1995; Aevarsson and Skoog 1996). One study reported that age-specific incidence rates were consistently higher among women, significantly so in one age group (Fratiglioni et al. 1997). Another report found a higher age-adjusted incidence among women than among men (RR, 1.7; 95 percent CI, 1.0 to 2.6) (Ott et al. 1998a).

Although results are inconsistent, many studies have found an inverse association between smoking and AD. This association is evident in the meta-analyses by Graves and associates (1991) and by van Duijn and Hofman (1992). The RRs for AD decreased with increasing number of pack-years of smoking, from 0.7 (95 percent CI, 0.5 to 1.1) for less than 15.5 pack-years to 0.6 (95 percent CI, 0.4 to 0.95) for 15.5 to 37.0 pack-years and to 0.5 (95 percent CI, 0.3 to 0.8) for more than 37.0 pack-years.

The inverse relationship between smoking and AD reported in these studies and meta-analyses needs to be interpreted in the light of the potential limitations discussed here. For example, a significant protective effect of smoking shown in one study disappeared after adjustment for appropriate confounding factors (Tyas 1998). This pattern was consistent with that of another investigation (Letenneur et al. 1994b) and suggested that failure to adjust for confounders may have contributed to the variation in the findings for the effects of smoking on AD (Tyas 1998). In another example, a protective association reported in one case-control study was based on unadjusted analyses of data obtained from proxy respondents for case subjects but not for control subjects (Ferini-Strambi et al. 1990).

Another meta-analysis included data from 19 investigations, primarily case-control studies, of the relationship between AD and smoking (Lee 1994). Of the 19 studies analyzed, 4 showed a statistically significant protective effect of smoking, 11 showed a nonsignificantly lower risk for AD among smokers, 3 reported a nonsignificantly increased risk among smokers, and 1 found no significant effect and did not describe the direction of the association. Case-control studies published after the meta-analyses by Graves and colleagues (1991), van Duijn and Hofman (1992), and Lee (1994) have reported statistically significant inverse associations (Brenner et al. 1993; van Duijn et al. 1995; Callahan et al. 1996) or no association (Canadian Study of Health and Aging Workshop 1994; Letenneur et al. 1994b; Forster et al. 1995; Wang et al. 1997a).

Cohort studies have been less supportive of an inverse association. Katzman and colleagues (1989) noted that persons who developed AD were less likely to have been smokers than were those who did not have AD. Other investigators reported a nonsignificantly reduced risk for incident AD among smokers (Hebert et al. 1992; Yoshitake et al. 1995), no association (Wang et al. 1999), or an increased risk (Ott et al. 1998b; Launer et al. 1999). A significant protective effect of smoking was reported in a case-control study (Mayeux and Tang 1993), but a significantly higher risk for AD was reported among smokers in an associated cohort study (Merchant et al. 1999). Failure to adequately adjust for confounders and other methodological problems may have contributed to some of the variation in the findings across studies (Tyas 1998).

Because smokers are more likely than nonsmokers to die before developing AD, the issue of selective mortality has been used to argue against a causal protective association between smoking and AD (Riggs 1993; Graves and Mortimer 1994). The higher mortality among smokers compared with nonsmokers would create an apparent lower risk for AD among smokers if those who died were more likely than nonsmokers to have developed AD if they had lived. Some researchers have argued against such an explanation (e.g., Plassman et al. 1995; van Duijn et al. 1995). Nonetheless, the possibility that a protective effect of smoking could be attributable to survival bias is plausible, particularly when prevalent cases are studied (Wang et al. 1999).

Most studies have not presented findings on cigarette smoking and AD separately for women and men. Those that have examined the interaction between gender and smoking on AD have reported inconsistent results (Ferini-Strambi et al. 1990; Graves et al. 1991; Hebert et al. 1992; Letenneur et al. 1994a; Salib and Hillier 1997; Launer et al. 1999).

### Conclusions

1. Women who smoke have a decreased risk for Parkinson's disease.
2. Data regarding the association between smoking and Alzheimer's disease are inconsistent.

## Nicotine Pharmacology and Addiction

The 1988 Surgeon General's report on the health consequences of smoking focused on nicotine addiction (USDHHS 1988). The report concluded that cigarettes and other tobacco products are addicting and that nicotine causes the addiction. Primary criteria for addiction included (1) psychoactive effects that involve alterations in mood, behavior, and/or cognition; (2) reinforcing effects that maintain self-administration of the drug; and (3) highly controlled or compulsive use driven by strong urges to use the drug. Additional criteria included (4) development of physical dependence on the drug, which is characterized by tolerance and withdrawal symptoms; (5) continued use despite negative consequences; (6) difficulty in maintaining abstinence or in reducing the quantity consumed; and (7) recurrent cravings for the drug (*British Journal of Addiction* 1982; APA 1994).

USDHHS (1995) summarized studies documenting addiction among smokers. The report indicated that approximately 90 percent of cigarette smokers smoke daily. Of those who smoke one pack of cigarettes per day, 80 percent have unsuccessfully tried to reduce the number of cigarettes smoked. About 50 percent of those who stop smoking experience nicotine withdrawal syndrome. Of those making a serious attempt to stop, fewer than 3 percent have long-term success. Data from the 1991 and 1992 National Household Survey on Drug Abuse showed that three-fourths of women current smokers reported feeling dependent on cigarettes; about 80 percent reported experiencing at least one of four indicators of nicotine addiction (CDC 1995) (see "Nicotine Dependence Among Women and Girls" in Chapter 2).

The pharmacology of nicotine was discussed in depth in the 1988 Surgeon General's report on smoking and health (USDHHS 1988) and in several subsequent reviews (Le Houezec and Benowitz 1991; Benowitz 1992; Henningfield et al. 1995). This discussion emphasizes those aspects for which gender-specific differences have been explored. The pharmacologic processes relevant to drug addiction include absorption, distribution, elimination, and dosing of nicotine in the body (pharmacokinetics); pharmacologic effects on target organs (pharmacodynamics); and behavorial manifestations of the pharmacologic effects.

## Absorption, Distribution, and Metabolism of Nicotine

When tobacco burns during smoking, nicotine is distilled and carried into the lungs, where it is absorbed rapidly through the pulmonary alveoli. After absorption, nicotine is distributed to various body tissues. Evidence from animal studies showed that tissues with the highest affinity for nicotine are the kidney, liver, lung, brain, and heart, in that order. Skeletal muscle has moderate affinity for nicotine, and adipose tissue has the lowest affinity (Benowitz et al. 1990). Women in general have a higher percentage of fat than do men (average, 34 percent vs. 20 percent of total body weight) (Watson et al. 1980). Because nicotine has a relatively low affinity for fat, it is largely distributed in lean tissues. The lower lean body weight of women might then suggest that, for a nicotine dose normalized to total weight, women would have higher concentrations in blood and other organs than would men. Animal studies have reported gender-specific differences in nicotine concentrations in the brain, and these differences support the hypothesis that there are differences in nicotine distribution among females and males (Rosecrans 1972; Rosecrans and Schechter 1972; Hatchell and Collins 1980). Such differences have not been investigated in clinical studies with humans.

Nicotine is broken down to several metabolites in the liver. Beckett and associates (1971) suggested that the extent of nicotine metabolism is different among women and men, reporting that women nonsmokers excreted more nicotine and less cotinine in urine than did men nonsmokers. This early study involved a small number of participants and was based on 24-hour urine collections, but 24 hours is an insufficient period for complete excretion of metabolites. Gender-specific patterns of urinary excretion of nicotine metabolites have not been described in more recent research. Indeed, a study involving administration of labeled nicotine and cotinine, which permits quantification of nicotine metabolic pathways, found essentially identical conversion of nicotine to cotinine (72 to 73 percent) among 10 women and 10 men (Benowitz and Jacob 1994).

In a study of men, Armitage and colleagues (1975) used $^{14}C$-labeled nicotine to measure absorption of nicotine from cigarette smoke. Regular smokers generally absorbed 80 to 90 percent of the nicotine that was inhaled. Comparisons between women and men were not made. However, a study of nicotine absorption from ETS among nonsmoking women compared the nicotine content of inspired versus expired air (Iwase et al. 1991). On average, 71 percent (range, 60 to 80 percent) of the nicotine inhaled was absorbed.

Studies of gender-specific differences in nicotine clearance among humans have shown varying results. An early study reported that the total clearance of nicotine, when normalized for body weight, was significantly greater among 11 men than among 11 age-matched women ($20.5 \pm 5.0$ vs. $15.7 \pm 4.7$ mL/[min × kg]) (Benowitz and Jacob 1984). However, a more recent study of 10 women and 10 men found no difference in normalized clearance (Benowitz and Jacob 1994). Thus, it is not known whether drug metabolic activity, expressed as clearance per kilogram of body weight, differs between women and men. Nonetheless, because men tend to weigh more than do women, total body clearance (body weight × clearance normalized by body weight) is consistently greater among men than among women. One study compared the clearance of cotinine among women and men (Benowitz and Jacob 1994). Both total clearance of cotinine and clearance normalized for body weight tended to be higher among men than among women, but the differences were not statistically significant.

## Nicotine Levels and Dosing

The daily dose of nicotine from cigarette smoking is strongly related to the number of cigarettes smoked per day but only weakly related to the machine-determined nicotine yield of cigarettes (Benowitz et al. 1983; Gori and Lynch 1985; Höfer et al. 1991a). The dose of nicotine from a cigarette also depends on the efficiency of systemic absorption and how the cigarette is smoked (i.e., number of puffs, intensity of puffing, volume of smoke inhaled, and whether the filter holes are blocked). No data are available on gender-specific differences in the efficiency of pulmonary absorption of nicotine, but cigarette-puffing behavior has been studied by using cigarette-holder flowmeter devices. The results of such studies must be interpreted with caution, because in general, single cigarettes are tested in laboratory settings with unfamiliar cigarette holders, which could influence a smoker's puffing behavior.

Several investigators testing in such a laboratory setting found gender-specific differences in smoking behavior. One study reported that among hospitalized smokers, men took puffs of larger volume and longer duration than did women but that the number of puffs taken per cigarette was similar (Moody 1980). Bättig and coworkers (1982) also observed that men had larger puff volume and longer puff duration than did women but that women tended to have a greater increase in expired CO after smoking a cigarette. Women took an average of one extra puff per cigarette, which partially offset the difference in volume per puff. Höfer and colleagues (1991a) reported similar results and noted that the increase in plasma nicotine levels after smoking a cigarette was greater among men than among women. Epstein and coworkers (1982) found that men had greater total puff duration than did women, but no significant differences were found in the number of puffs taken per cigarette or in puff volume. Because men generally inhale more smoke from each cigarette, the increase in plasma nicotine concentration and the amount of nicotine absorbed after smoking would be expected to be greater among men than among women. These predictions have been confirmed in two laboratory studies (Höfer et al. 1991a; Benowitz and Jacob 1994). However, comparison of the increase in plasma nicotine concentration after dosing with nicotine nasal spray showed no gender-specific difference (Perkins et al. 1995).

With regular use of tobacco in any form, blood nicotine concentrations are determined by the dose of nicotine delivered and by the rates of absorption and clearance. Some studies reported that concentrations of nicotine and cotinine in plasma during smoking ad libitum were similar among women and men, even though women, on average, smoked fewer cigarettes than did men (Russell et al. 1980, 1986; Höfer et al. 1991a). These data suggested that the lower daily dose of nicotine from cigarettes among women may be balanced by their lower total body clearance and may result in similar average concentrations of plasma nicotine. In several more recent studies, women smokers had lower salivary or serum concentrations of cotinine than did men smokers, as might be expected from the lower number of cigarettes smoked by women (Wagenknecht et al. 1990; Woodward and Tunstall-Pedoe 1993; Bjornson et al. 1995). These findings suggested that the number of cigarettes smoked per day is the major determinant of nicotine exposure and that, in general, women are exposed to less nicotine than are men because they smoke fewer cigarettes per day (Benowitz and Hatsukami 1998).

## Psychoactive and Rewarding Effects of Nicotine

Nicotine produces a variety of subjective, cognitive, and physiologic effects in humans. Gender-specific differences in these effects can be determined by comparing the extent of nicotine self-administration, the ability to discriminate nicotine as a stimulus, and responsiveness to the rewarding effects of nicotine.

Nicotine self-administration has been demonstrated among both animals and humans, providing evidence that nicotine is itself reinforcing (USDHHS 1988). Few studies have closely examined differences by gender in the self-administration of nicotine. In general, women smoke fewer cigarettes and inhale less than do men (Grunberg et al. 1991; Perkins 1996), but as previously noted, the circulating concentrations of nicotine may be the same among both genders. In a laboratory study that examined the reinforcing value of smoking, women and men had a similar response pattern in working for puffs on a cigarette (Perkins et al. 1994b). In another experimental study, however, women self-administered nicotine nasal spray at a lower rate than did men, even when the dose was corrected for body weight (Perkins et al. 1996a). Lower concentrations of plasma nicotine reflected this lower rate of nicotine self-administration among women. Furthermore, men self-administered nicotine nasal spray to a greater extent than a placebo spray, whereas no difference was observed among women in self-administration of nicotine versus placebo. These results suggested that nicotine administered via nasal spray is reinforcing among men but not among women. Whether this difference in self-administration reflects reduced reinforcement from nicotine as a result of differential sensitivity to nicotine is not known.

The limited data available suggested that women are less effective than men in maintaining a particular concentration of nicotine in the body by changing nicotine self-administration (Benowitz and Hatsukami 1998). For example, studies of male smokers reported significant declines in the number of cigarettes smoked after self-administration of nicotine, whereas studies that showed little or no compensation in smoking in response to nicotine self-administration predominantly involved women (Perkins 1996). Only one study directly compared smoking behavior of women and men after self-administration of various doses of nicotine via nasal spray (Perkins et al. 1992). In this study, women did not compensate for nicotine self-administration to the same extent by smoking less as did men. Further evidence for less-effective nicotine regulation among women was provided by a study that observed women to have increasing serum cotinine and alveolar CO with use of cigarette brands with higher nicotine yields, whereas men had similar CO and cotinine levels regardless of machine-determined yield (Woodward and Tunstall-Pedoe 1993). This finding suggested that men smoked cigarettes to obtain the same dose of nicotine from all brands, whereas women smoked different cigarettes in a similar fashion, irrespective of nicotine delivery. However, an earlier study provided contradictory findings; it showed better nicotine regulation among women than among men (Bättig et al. 1982). Less effective nicotine regulation among women is consistent with data indicating that women are less able than men to distinguish nicotine from placebo or to distinguish different doses of nicotine in blind comparisons (Perkins 1995; Perkins et al. 1996b; Benowitz and Hatsukami 1998).

Nicotine produces variable effects on mood. Depending on the dose and the state (withdrawal or tolerance) or initial mood of the individual, nicotine can enhance arousal and alertness or can relax and calm (USDHHS 1998; Parrott 1994). Few data on gender-specific differences in nicotine's mood-altering effects have been available. Most studies showed no differences between women and men in subjective responses to nicotine (Perkins et al. 1993, 1994c). However, one investigation reported more dizziness among women than among men after smoking cigarettes (Perkins et al. 1994a), and another found that women reported greater increase in comfort and relaxation after smoking (Perkins et al. 1994d). No such differences by gender were observed across doses of nicotine delivered via nasal spray. Because no gender-specific differences in response to nicotine were found (Perkins 1996), these results indicated that influences independent of nicotine may be more important determinants of mood responses to smoking among women than among men.

An important area in understanding the reinforcing influence of nicotine is its effect among smokers who are confronted with a stressful situation or who are experiencing negative affect. Smokers report a greater desire for cigarettes (Perkins and Grobe 1992) and demonstrate increased intensity of smoking during periods of stress (e.g., Schachter 1978; Dobbs et al. 1981; Rose et al. 1983; Pomerleau and Pomerleau 1987, 1989). It is more common for women than for men to smoke in response to negative affect or stress (Frith 1971; Ikard and Tomkins 1973; Karasek et al. 1987; Sorensen and Pechacek 1987; Livson and Leino 1988; Bjornson et al. 1995), and women report smoking for sedative effects (Russell et al. 1974). In contrast, men report that they smoke more for stimulation (Gilbert 1995). Even in an adolescent population, smoking to relax or cope with stress or depression was significantly more common among girls than among boys (Oakley et al. 1992). For example, young women who reported on a questionnaire that they needed more information about how to cope with stress or depression were more likely to be smokers than were young men who reported needing this information. It is possible that women have a greater propensity to smoke in a state of negative affect or stress because they have fewer coping strategies or that women more commonly use strategies that alter emotional arousal without addressing the source of stress (Pomerleau et al. 1991; Solomon and Flynn 1993). Another explanation may be that nicotine has a greater effect on stress or negative affect among women than among men, which would increase the potential for nicotine to be reinforcing among women.

Nicotine may have beneficial effects on several aspects of human performance, including improved attention, learning and memory functioning, and enhanced sensory and motor performance (Levin 1992; Heishman et al. 1994). No study has demonstrated gender-specific differences in such effects. Studies have shown the same enhancement of performance among women as among men or a combination of women and men, particularly during smoking deprivation (Heishman et al. 1994).

Much of the research examining gender-specific differences in the reinforcing effects of nicotine has been related to weight (see "Body Weight and Fat Distribution" earlier in this chapter, "Concerns About Weight Control" in Chapter 4, and "Weight Control" in Chapter 5). Tobacco use is inversely related to body weight, and women in particular report that they smoke to keep body weight down (USDHHS 1988; Gritz et al. 1989; Grunberg 1990; Camp et al. 1993) (see "Body Weight and Fat Distribution" earlier in this chapter). The difference in weight between smokers and nonsmokers is greater among women than among men (Klesges et al. 1989). After cessation of smoking, women are more likely to gain more weight than are men (e.g., Williamson et al. 1991), and among women but not among men, dose-related effects of nicotine gum appear to limit weight gain after smoking cessation (Leischow et al. 1992). These data indicated that the weight-related reinforcing effects of nicotine and cigarette smoking are stronger among women than among men.

## Physical Dependence on Nicotine

Physical dependence refers to the development of withdrawal symptoms after cessation of drug use. Withdrawal symptoms are associated with the development of tolerance, a decreased effect after repeated exposure to a drug, or the need for increased drug dose to obtain a specific effect. Some retrospective studies showed that symptoms of cigarette withdrawal are more severe among women than among men (Shiffman 1979), but results in other retrospective studies (Breslau et al. 1992) and prospective studies (Svikis et al. 1986; Hughes et al. 1991; Hughes 1992; Tate et al. 1993; Pomerleau et al. 1994) indicated that women and men have similar types and severity of withdrawal symptoms. Gender-specific differences observed in retrospective studies could be due to the finding that men tend to minimize cigarette withdrawal symptoms when asked to recall their experience (Pomerleau et al. 1994).

Nicotine addiction is also supported by stimuli that become associated with tobacco use through learning or conditioning. These cues include environmental and internal stimuli and sensory aspects of tobacco use. Stimuli that are repeatedly paired with abstinence from tobacco (e.g., being in locations where smoking is prohibited) can elicit withdrawal-like responses (Wikler 1965) that oppose or compensate for the effects of nicotine (Siegel 1983). Similarly, stimuli that are repeatedly paired with tobacco use (e.g., sight of ashtrays) can lead to states like those elicited by the drug itself (Stewart et al. 1984).

In particular, sensory aspects of smoking may also have a role in the maintenance of smoking. Cues such as the smell and taste of cigarette smoking, as well as irritation of the mouth, throat, and respiratory tree, may become conditioned reinforcers (Stolerman et al. 1973; Rose and Levin 1991). Blocking the sensory aspects of smoking attenuates the effects of inhaled nicotine on craving for cigarettes (Rose et al. 1985). Similarly, the administration of aerosols that mimic the sensory aspects of smoking (e.g., irritant effects on the respiratory tract) reduces craving (Rose and Hickman 1987; Behm et al. 1990, 1993; Rose and Behm 1994; Westman et al. 1995). The magnitude of reduction was similar to that produced by smoking of high-nicotine cigarettes (Rose et al. 1993). The aerosols also reduce smoking (Rose and Behm 1987; Rose et al. 1993) and enhance short-term smoking cessation rates (Levin et al. 1990; Behm et al. 1993; Westman et al. 1995).

Some investigations have shown that women are particularly sensitive to the sensory aspects of smoking (Hasenfratz et al. 1993; Baldinger et al. 1995) and may be more responsive to their effects than are men (Höfer et al. 1991b). Consequently, the presence of sensory cues associated with smoking in the absence of nicotine may cause greater discomfort among women smokers than among men smokers (Perkins et al. 1994d).

Results from studies of gender-specific differences in the efficacy of nicotine replacement therapy for tobacco withdrawal have varied. No such differences were found for the effects of 2-mg nicotine polacrilex gum (Schneider et al. 1984) or of the 21-mg transdermal nicotine system (Repsher 1994) on composite scores for symptoms of tobacco withdrawal. However, other studies of smoking cessation using nicotine replacement agents showed that such treatment tends to be less effective among women than among men (Perkins et al. 1996b). After cessation of use of nicotine polacrilex gum, withdrawal symptoms were observed to be more severe among women than among men—a difference seen for 2-mg doses of nicotine but not for 4-mg doses (Hatsukami et al. 1995). This finding suggested that women may have more severe withdrawal symptoms at lower doses of nicotine than do men. A similar finding was observed in another investigation with 2-mg polacrilex nicotine gum: women had no reduction in craving for cigarettes when they used active nicotine gum compared with placebo, but men did have a significant reduction (Killen et al. 1990).

## Conclusions

1. Nicotine pharmacology and the behavioral processes that determine nicotine addiction appear generally similar among women and men; when standardized for the number of cigarettes smoked, the blood concentration of cotinine (the main metabolite of nicotine) is similar among women and men.
2. Women's regulation of nicotine intake may be less precise than men's. Factors other than nicotine (e.g., sensory cues) may play a greater role in determining smoking behavior among women.

# Environmental Tobacco Smoke

During 1988–1991, 37 percent of adult non-tobacco users in the United States lived in a home with at least one smoker or reported exposure to ETS at work; the proportion reporting ETS exposure was somewhat lower among women (32.9 percent) than among men (43.5 percent) (Pirkle et al. 1996). Three major outcomes of ETS exposure are considered in this section—lung cancer, CHD, and reproductive effects. ETS exposure is also discussed briefly in "Breast Cancer" and "Cervical Cancer" earlier in this chapter. These are by no means the only conditions of importance to women's health potentially affected by exposure to ETS, but they are the outcomes that have been most studied to date.

## Environmental Tobacco Smoke and Lung Cancer

### Previous Reviews

In 1986, two major reviews of the data on exposure to ETS and its potential health effects, including lung cancer, were published (NRC 1986; USDHHS 1986b). In the NRC review (1986), the estimate of overall (summary) RR for lung cancer among women nonsmokers who lived with a spouse who smoked was 1.3 (95 percent CI, 1.2 to 1.5); the estimated RR among men, which was based on much smaller numbers of nonsmokers with lung cancer, was 1.6 (95 percent CI, 0.99 to 2.6). Among both genders combined, the estimated RR was 1.3 (95 percent CI, 1.2 to 1.5). Two additional analyses, which corrected RR estimates for two types of systematic errors, were provided in the NRC report. The first analysis incorporated plausible assumptions about misclassification of former smokers as "never smokers" and about the tendency for spouses to have similar smoking habits. The conclusions were that the observed overall RR of 1.3 could reflect an underlying true RR of no less than 1.2 and, more likely, 1.3, and that, under reasonable assumptions, this type of misclassification could not account for all the increased risk for lung cancer reported from these epidemiologic studies. The second analysis evaluated the effect of incorrectly classifying some nonsmokers as "unexposed" because of sole consideration of household exposure. The risk among a group of nonsmokers married to nonsmokers, but nevertheless exposed to ETS, was estimated to be at least 8 percent higher than the risk among nonsmokers who were never exposed to ETS. The overall adjusted RR estimate, corrected for both possible misclassification of smokers and background ETS exposure, was 1.4 (range, 1.2 to 1.6).

The 1986 Surgeon General's report (USDHHS 1986b) included a review of the same 13 epidemiologic studies (Garfinkel 1981; Hirayama 1981, 1984a; Chan and Fung 1982; Correa et al. 1983; Trichopoulos et al. 1983; Buffler et al. 1984; Gillis et al. 1984; Kabat and Wynder 1984; Koo et al. 1984; Garfinkel et al. 1985; Akiba et al. 1986; Lee et al. 1986; Pershagen et al. 1987) as well as an assessment of ETS chemistry, deposition, and absorption of specific constituents and determination of their carcinogenicity. This review focused on qualitative assessments of the studies and concluded that involuntary (passive) smoking is a cause of disease, including lung cancer, among healthy nonsmokers.

An international ETS working group met in 1985, and its findings were summarized in two monographs from IARC (1986, 1987). The 1986 IARC monograph stated that,

> The observations on nonsmokers that have been made so far are compatible with either an increased risk from "passive" smoking or an absence of risk. Knowledge of the nature of sidestream and mainstream smoke, of the materials absorbed during "passive" smoking, and of the quantitative relationships between dose and effect that are commonly observed from exposure to carcinogens, however, leads to the conclusion that passive smoking gives rise to some risk of [lung] cancer (IARC 1986, p. 314).

In an assessment of ETS in the workplace and its relationship to lung cancer, the National Institute for Occupational Safety and Health (NIOSH 1991) reviewed the same 13 studies considered in the NRC report and the Surgeon General's report, plus 8 additional epidemiologic studies that were published in 1987–1990 (Brownson et al. 1987; Gao et al. 1987; Humble et al. 1987a; Lam et al. 1987; Geng et al. 1988; Shimizu et al. 1988; Hole et al. 1989; Janerich et al. 1990). NIOSH concluded that the results of these epidemiologic studies supported and reinforced the 1986 findings of the reports of NRC and the Surgeon

General, demonstrating an excess risk for lung cancer of about 30 percent among nonsmokers who live with a smoker compared with nonsmokers who live with a nonsmoker. The data on which NIOSH based the conclusion that ETS is potentially carcinogenic to occupationally exposed workers were not gathered in occupational settings but on the surrogate measure of "lived with a smoker."

In 1992, EPA produced a comprehensive review of the association between ETS and lung cancer among women nonsmokers (EPA 1992). EPA concluded that ETS is a human lung carcinogen. This conclusion was based on a "weight-of-the-evidence" analysis that included, but was not limited to, data from reports of 31 epidemiologic studies of lung cancer among women nonsmokers that were published in 1981–1991 (Garfinkel 1981; Trichopoulos et al. 1981, 1983; Chan and Fung 1982; Correa et al. 1983; Buffler et al. 1984; Hirayama 1984b; Kabat and Wynder 1984; Garfinkel et al. 1985; Lam 1985; Wu et al. 1985; Akiba et al. 1986; Lee et al. 1986; Brownson et al. 1987; Gao et al. 1987; Humble et al. 1987a; Koo et al. 1987; Lam et al. 1987; Pershagen et al. 1987; Butler 1988; Geng et al. 1988; Inoue and Hirayama 1988; Shimizu et al. 1988; Hole et al. 1989; Svensson et al. 1989; Janerich et al. 1990; Kalandidi et al. 1990; Sobue et al. 1990; Wu-Williams et al. 1990; Fontham et al. 1991; Liu et al. 1991).

In the EPA report, summary RRs were estimated by using meta-analysis, which included an assessment of the various study designs and an adjustment for possible misclassification of smokers. Exposure was defined as having lived with a spouse who smoked. Among women nonsmokers in the United States, the estimate of RR was 1.2 (90 percent CI, 1.04 to 1.4) for those who were ever exposed to ETS and 1.4 (90 percent CI, 1.1 to 1.7) at the highest exposure level. The summary RR estimate for the highest exposure level worldwide was 1.8 (90 percent CI, 1.6 to 2.1). The weight-of-the-evidence approach used by EPA in its determination that ETS is a human carcinogen included an assessment of biochemical and toxicologic data as well as data from epidemiologic studies.

The California Environmental Protection Agency (CEPA) published a report on the health effects of ETS (NCI 1999) that updated the EPA report. Eight additional epidemiologic studies were reviewed in addition to the 31 included in the EPA report (Brownson et al. 1992a; Stockwell et al. 1992; Liu et al. 1993; Fontham et al. 1994; Kabat et al. 1995; Schwartz et al. 1996; Cardenas et al. 1997; Ko et al. 1997). The report concluded that the studies subsequent to the EPA report provided additional evidence that ETS exposure is causally associated with lung cancer and that findings of recent studies and the EPA meta-analysis indicated about a 20-percent increased risk for lung cancer among nonsmokers.

Beside these comprehensive reviews, numerous meta-analyses have been published. Hackshaw and associates (1997) analyzed the 37 published studies on women and found a pooled RR of 1.2 (95 percent CI, 1.1 to 1.4). Tests of heterogeneity indicated that RR estimates for lung cancer and ETS exposure did not significantly differ between women and men, by geographic region, by year of publication, or between cohort and case-control studies. The pooled RR estimates were virtually identical each year from 1990 through 1997, indicating that the pooled RR was not materially influenced by the more recent larger studies.

In the year 2000, USDHHS released the ninth edition of the Report on Carcinogens, which identifies substances that are "known" or "reasonably anticipated" to cause cancer and to which a significant number of persons in the United States are exposed (USDHHS 2000). ETS was among the substances included on the list of known human carcinogens.

#### Epidemiologic Studies 1992–1998

Nine studies of the relationship between exposure to ETS and lung cancer (one cohort study and eight case-control studies) published since 1992 are summarized in Table 3.52.

*Cohort Study*

Cardenas and associates (1997) used data from the CPS-II cohort to evaluate the relationship between ETS and lung cancer deaths among 192,234 women and 96,542 men who had never smoked, with follow-up during 1982–1989. ETS exposure was defined as smoking status of the current spouse at enrollment in the study. Duration of exposure was defined as the number of years in the current marriage, intensity of exposure was defined as the number of cigarettes smoked per day by the spouse, and pack-years were estimated in this study as the product of the duration of marriage and the intensity of exposure to ETS. RRs were adjusted for age, race, years of education, blue-collar employment, occupational exposure to asbestos, weekly servings of vegetables and citrus fruit, total dietary fat, and self-reported history of chronic lung disease. The adjusted lung cancer death rate was 20 percent higher among women whose husband had ever smoked during their current marriage than among those married to a nonsmoker. At the highest level of cigarettes per day smoked by a spouse ($\geq 40$), the RR was 1.9 (95 percent CI, 1.0 to 3.6; p for trend

= 0.03). RRs were generally higher among women whose husband continued to smoke (1.2; 95 percent CI, 0.8 to 1.8), smoked cigars or pipes (1.5; 95 percent CI, 0.6 to 2.8), or exceeded 35 pack-years of smoking (1.5; 95 percent CI, 0.8 to 2.9). Although only one estimate of risk was statistically significant, the statistical power in this study was low. The authors concluded that their results were consistent with the EPA summary estimate that spousal smoking increases the risk for lung cancer by about 20 percent among women nonsmokers.

*Case-Control Studies*

Brownson and associates (1992a) reported findings from a population-based, case-control study of white women nonsmokers in Missouri aged 30 through 84 years. Age and previous lung disease were shown to confound the risk estimates and RRs were, therefore, adjusted for these two factors. No increased risk for lung cancer was associated with childhood ETS exposure in the study sample, but the validity of the data on childhood exposure is questionable because of the high proportion of proxy respondents. Qualitative indicators of exposure were associated with some increased risk: "moderate" exposure (RR, 1.7; 95 percent CI, 1.1 to 2.5) and "heavy" exposure (RR, 2.4; 95 percent CI, 1.3 to 4.7). The RR for lung cancer among women who were ever exposed to spousal ETS was 1.1 (95 percent CI, 0.8 to 1.3). Adulthood ETS exposure was associated with an increased risk at high levels of exposure (>40 pack-years): the RRs were 1.3 (95 percent CI, 1.0 to 1.7) for exposure from a spouse only and 1.3 (95 percent CI, 1.0 to 1.8) for exposure from all household members combined, including a spouse. The qualitative estimates of ETS exposure during adulthood indicated an increased risk associated with heavy exposure (RR, 1.8; 95 percent CI, 1.1 to 2.9).

Stockwell and associates (1992) conducted a population-based, case-control study in central Florida. ETS exposure was defined as any exposure to ETS from specific persons living in the household and was measured as smoke-years of exposure from household sources, and RRs were adjusted for age, race, and education. The RR for lung cancer among women who lived with a spouse who smoked was 1.6 (95 percent CI, 0.8 to 3.0) (Table 3.52). Other estimates of RR among women who were ever exposed to ETS from a specific source were similar: mother (RR, 1.6; 95 percent CI, 0.6 to 4.3), father (RR, 1.2; 95 percent CI, 0.6 to 2.3), and siblings and others (RR, 1.7; 95 percent CI, 0.8 to 3.9). Increasing risks were observed with increasing duration of ETS exposure, and statistically significant trends were found for adulthood household exposures (p = 0.025) and lifetime household exposures (p = 0.004).

Liu and associates (1993) conducted a hospital-based, case-control study in Quangzhou, China. The study included 38 women with lung cancer and 69 women in the control group who were lifetime nonsmokers. Among the nonsmokers, women who lived with a husband who smoked 20 or more cigarettes per day had a significantly higher risk for lung cancer than did women whose husband did not smoke (RR, 2.9; 95 percent CI, 1.2 to 7.3; p for trend = 0.03) (Table 3.52).

In a report of a five-year multicenter study of ETS and lung cancer among women who did not smoke, Fontham and colleagues (1994) extended the findings of an earlier three-year report (Fontham et al. 1991). At the home interview, a urine sample was obtained from consenting study participants—81 percent of the living patients with lung cancer (54 percent of the case group) and 83 percent of the control group. Test results from the urine sample were used to screen for misclassification of current smoking status. RRs were adjusted for age, race, study area, education, intake of fruits and vegetables and supplemental vitamins, dietary cholesterol, family history of lung cancer, and employment in potentially high-risk occupations for five years or more. The increased risk for lung cancer among women who lived with a spouse who smoked tobacco was about 30 percent (RR, 1.3; 95 percent CI, 1.04 to 1.6) (Table 3.52). An increasing risk for lung cancer was observed with increasing pack-years of smoking by a spouse (p for trend = 0.03). At the highest level of pack-years (≥ 80), the RR was 1.8 (95 percent CI, 0.99 to 3.3). Elevated RRs indicated an association between reported ETS exposure in the household (RR, 1.2; 95 percent CI, 0.96 to 1.6), in the workplace (RR, 1.4; 95 percent CI, 1.1 to 1.7), and in social settings (RR, 1.5; 95 percent CI, 1.2 to 1.9). A cumulative measure of ETS exposure in all three settings during adult life demonstrated increasing risk with increasing duration of exposure (p for trend = 0.0001) and an estimated RR of 1.7 (95 percent CI, 1.1 to 2.7) at the highest level of exposure (≥ 48 smoke-years). No significant association was found between exposure during childhood and lung cancer risk.

Wang and associates (1994a) conducted a matched-pair, case-control study of lung cancer in Harbin, China. Patients and controls were matched for age, residential area, and lifetime nonsmoking status. Information on indoor smoking was collected for each residence in which a participant lived for at least three years, and RR was assessed by age at the time of exposure to ETS. In this study, no increased risk for lung

**Table 3.52. Epidemiologic studies of environmental tobacco smoke (ETS) and lung cancer published during 1992–1998**

| Factor | Brownson et al. (1992a) | Stockwell et al. (1992) | Liu et al. (1993) | Fontham et al. (1994) |
|---|---|---|---|---|
| Study design | Population-based, case-control study | Population-based, case-control study | Hospital-based, case-control study | Population-based, case-control study |
| Country | United States | United States | China | United States |
| Number of cases (women nonsmokers) | 432 | 210 | 38 | 653 |
| Type of interview | Telephone | In-person, in home<br>41% of cases<br>54% of controls<br>Telephone<br>51% of cases<br>46% of controls<br>Mail<br>8% of cases<br>0.3% of controls | In-person | In-person, in home |
| Respondent type | Cases: 35% self<br>65% proxy<br>Controls: 100% self | Cases: 33% self<br>67% proxy<br>Controls: 100% self | Cases: 100% self<br>Controls: 100% self | Cases: 63% self<br>37% proxy<br>Controls: 100% self |
| Pathologic confirmation | 100% | 100% | 32% | 100% |
| Percentage with independent slide review | 76% | Not done | Not done | 85% |
| Adjustment factors | Age, previous lung disease (dietary beta-carotene and fat also evaluated) | Age, race, education | Education, occupation, living area | Age, race, study area, education, family history of lung cancer, employment in high-risk occupation, dietary cholesterol, fruits, vegetables, supplemental vitamins (previous lung disease, dietary beta-carotene, vitamin C, vitamin E also evaluated) |

*Lung cancer deaths.

cancer was observed for household exposures that occurred during adult life, but estimates of RR from childhood exposure to ETS were relatively high (>3.0).

Kabat and associates (1995) conducted a U.S. hospital-based, case-control study that included 69 women as case subjects and 187 women as control subjects. RRs were adjusted for age, education, and the type of hospital. Exposure to ETS in childhood was associated with a borderline increase in risk for lung cancer (RR, 1.6; 95 percent CI, 0.95 to 2.8) (Table 3.52). Risk was significantly elevated for the highest tertile of smoke-years for childhood exposure (RR, 2.2; 95 percent CI, 1.1 to 4.5), and the linear trend was statistically significant ($p = 0.02$). No increased risk

| Wang et al. (1994a) | Kabat et al. (1995) | Cardenas et al. (1997) | Boffetta et al. (1998) | Jöckel et al. (1998) |
|---|---|---|---|---|
| Hospital-based, case-control study | Hospital-based, case-control study | Prospective cohort study | Mixed hospital and population-based, case-control study | Population-based, case-control study |
| China | United States | United States | 7 European countries | Germany |
| 55 | 69 | 150* | 509 | 53 |
| In person | In-person, in hospital | Questionnaire self-administered by spouse of nonsmoker | | |
| Cases: 100% self<br>Controls: 100% self | Cases: 100% self<br>Controls: 100% self | Cohort: 100% self | Cases: 100% self<br>Controls: 100% self | Cases: 100% self<br>Controls: 100% self |
| 100% | 100% | Death certificate only | 96.5% | 100% |
| Not done | Not done | Not done | Not done | Not done |
| None | Age, education, type of hospital | Age, race, education, weekly vegetable and citrus fruit intake, dietary fat, self-reported history of chronic lung disease, occupational exposure to asbestos, blue-collar employment | Age, interaction between sex and study center | Age, sex, region |

was observed for home exposure in adulthood (RR, 0.95; 95 percent CI, 0.5 to 1.7); the RR among women who reported having a husband who smoked was 1.1 (95 percent CI, 0.5 to 1.7).

Schwartz and associates (1996) conducted a population-based study of lung cancer among nonsmokers in metropolitan Detroit, Michigan. Control subjects were frequency-matched to cases by age group, sex, race, and county of residence. Participants were described as "non-cigarette smoking," and cigar and pipe smokers were later excluded from analyses. Of the participants, 72 percent of case subjects and 64 percent of control subjects were women, but no gender-specific risk estimates were provided. Estimates of RR for lung cancer for ETS exposure were reported for two sources, exposure at home (RR, 1.1;

**Table 3.52. Continued**

| Factor | Brownson et al. (1992a) | Stockwell et al. (1992) | Liu et al. (1993) | Fontham et al. (1994) |
|---|---|---|---|---|
| Estimated relative risk (95% confidence interval) for lung cancer | | | | |
| ETS exposure through spouse | Ever: 1.1 (0.8–1.3)<br>>40 pack-years:[†‡]<br>1.3 (1.0–1.7) | Ever: 1.6 (0.8–3.0) | ≥20 cigarettes/day:[†]<br>2.9 (1.2–7.3)<br>p for trend = 0.03 | Ever: 1.3 (1.04–1.6)<br>≥80 pack-years:[†]<br>1.8 (0.99–3.3)<br>p for trend = 0.03 |
| Other measures of ETS exposure | Adult household exposure (>40 pack-years vs. no exposure):<br>1.3 (1.0–1.8)<br>Childhood exposure to parental smoking:<br>0.7 (0.5–0.9)<br>Adult workplace exposure (highest quartile):<br>1.2 (0.9–1.7) | Adult household exposure (≥40 smoke-years[§] vs. no exposure):<br>2.4 (1.1–5.3)<br>Lifetime household exposure (≥40 smoke-years):<br>2.3 (1.1–4.6)<br>Childhood/adolescent household exposure (≥22 smoke-years):<br>2.4 (1.1–5.4)<br>Adult workplace exposure:<br>no increased risk (data not shown)<br>Adult social exposure:<br>no increased risk (data not shown) | | Childhood household exposure: 0.9 (0.7–1.1)<br>Adult household exposure:<br>Ever, 1.2 (0.96–1.6)<br>High,[Δ] 1.2 (0.9–1.7)<br>Adult workplace exposure:<br>Ever, 1.4 (1.1–1.7)<br>High, 1.9 (1.2–2.8)<br>Adult societal exposure:<br>Ever, 1.5 (1.2–1.9)<br>High, 1.5 (0.9–2.5) |
| Power to detect relative risk = 1.2 ($\alpha$ = 0.05) for ETS exposure through spouse (%) | 24 | 13 | <5 | 34 |

[†]Highest level of ETS exposure examined.
[‡]Pack-years = number of years of smoking multiplied by the number of packs of cigarettes smoked.
[§]Sum of reported years of exposure to ETS from variety of sources; does not represent years per se, because these exposures may occur concurrently.
[Δ]>30 years.

95 percent CI, 0.8 to 1.6) and exposure at work (RR, 1.5; 95 percent CI, 1.0 to 2.2).

The first large multicenter study of ETS and lung cancer from Europe was published in 1998 (Boffetta et al. 1998). This study did not employ a single protocol but had a core of common questions used by all centers. The selection of controls varied by center: five centers were hospital based, one center was hospital and community based, and six centers were community based. Control subjects were individually matched to case subjects by gender and age in some centers, and frequency matching was performed in

| Wang et al. (1994a) | Kabat et al. (1995) | Cardenas et al. (1997) | Boffetta et al. (1998) | Jöckel et al. (1998) |
|---|---|---|---|---|
| | Ever: 1.1 (0.6–1.9)<br>≥11 cigarettes/day:†<br>1.1 (0.5–2.3) | Ever: 1.2 (0.8–1.6)<br>≥40 cigarettes/day:†<br>1.9 (1.0–3.6)<br>p for trend = 0.03 | Ever: 1.1 (0.9–1.4)<br>High (years x hours/day):<br>1.7 (1.1–2.8) | Ever : 1.1 (0.5–2.3)<br>High: 1.9 (0.5–7.7) |
| Residential exposure, risk by age at exposure:<br>0–6 years, 3.6 (1.2–13.3)<br>7–14 years, 3.4 (1.1–12.7)<br>15–22 years, 2.4 (0.9–7.3)<br>23–30 years, 0.9 (0.4–2.3)<br>31–69 years, 0.9 (0.3–2.5) | Childhood household exposure:<br>Any, 1.6 (0.95–2.8)<br>High, 2.2 (1.1–4.5)<br>Adult household exposure:<br>Any, 0.95 (0.5–1.7)<br>High, 1.1 (0.6–2.3)<br>Adult workplace exposure:<br>Any, 1.2 (0.6–2.1)<br>High, 1.4 (0.6–2.8) | | Childhood household exposure:<br>Ever, 0.8 (0.6–0.96)<br>High, 1.1 (0.7–1.9)<br>Adult workplace exposure:<br>Ever, 1.2 (0.9–1.5)<br>High (years), 1.2 (0.7–2.3)<br>High (years × hours/day × level of smokiness), 1.9 (1.1–3.2) | Childhood household exposure:<br>High, 2.0 (0.6–6.8)<br>Adulthood other sources:<br>High, 3.1 (1.1–8.6)<br>Total cumulative exposure:<br>High, 3.2 (1.4–7.3) |
| <5 | 5 | 15 | <30 | <5 |

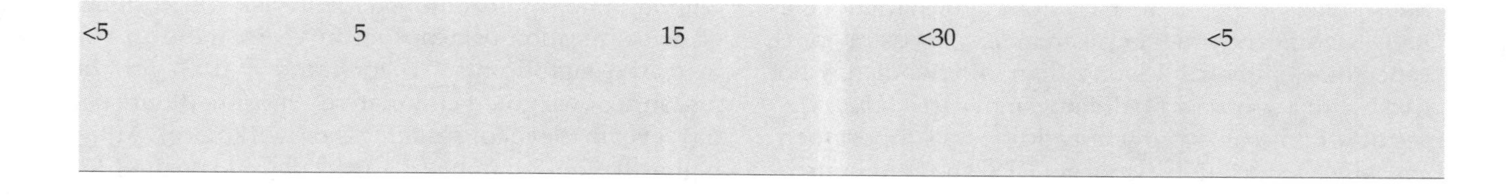

the others. Nonsmoking status was defined as never having smoked more than 400 cigarettes over one's lifetime. The overall RR associated with ever having been exposed to ETS in childhood was 0.8 (95 percent CI, 0.6 to 0.96) (Table 3.52). Among women who were ever married, a RR of 1.2 (95 percent CI, 0.9 to 1.6) was found for any exposure to spousal ETS. No significant trend was associated with duration of ETS exposure from husbands, in years, but the cumulative measure of hours per day times years of exposure demonstrated a significant positive trend ($p = 0.03$). The RR at the highest level of cumulative dose related to spousal ETS was 1.7 (95 percent CI, 1.1 to 2.8).

The authors noted that exposure to ETS in a large number of subjects had ended several years before the study and hypothesized that the somewhat lower estimates of risk in this study compared with other European studies may, in part, reflect risk reduction after cessation of exposure.

Findings from one of the participating European centers, in northwestern Germany, were reported separately by Jöckel and colleagues (1998). The nonsmokers in this study included occasional smokers, but data for the subgroup of persons who had never smoked were also examined separately. However, results were not reported by gender. Total ETS exposure was estimated by a variable that included cumulative duration of exposure during childhood and from spouse and other sources during adult life. The RRs were 2.1 (95 percent CI, 1.02 to 4.3) among nonsmokers and 3.2 (95 percent CI, 1.4 to 7.3) among persons who had never smoked, for the highest total ETS exposure from all sources; 1.5 (95 percent CI, 0.4 to 5.9) and 1.9 (95 percent CI, 0.5 to 7.7) for high level of exposure to spousal ETS; 1.3 (95 percent CI, 0.5 to 3.8) and 2.0 (95 percent CI, 0.6 to 6.8) for high childhood exposure; and 2.3 (95 percent CI, 0.9 to 5.9) and 3.1 (95 percent CI, 1.1 to 8.6) for high exposure to other ETS sources during adulthood (workplace, public transportation, and other public places). Because of small numbers, this study had limited statistical power.

Another epidemiologic study, by Trichopoulos and coworkers (1992), focused on the association of ETS exposure and pathologic indicators of lung cancer risk. In this autopsy-based study, lung specimens taken within four hours of death from 400 persons aged 35 years or older were evaluated. Specimens were examined and scored for basal cell hyperplasia, squamous cell metaplasia, cell atypia, and mucous cell metaplasia; an index of epithelial lesions that were possibly precancerous was generated. Included in the study were 17 women nonsmokers whose husband smoked at some time and 13 women nonsmokers whose husband had never smoked. Women nonsmokers exposed to ETS from spousal smoking had a significantly higher mean index of possibly precancerous epithelial lesions than did women who lived with a spouse who did not smoke ($p = 0.02$). The results of this study provided additional support for a causative association between ETS and pulmonary carcinogenesis.

Thus, the results of recent epidemiologic studies of ETS support the findings of the EPA's 1992 detailed assessment, which concluded that ETS is causally associated with lung cancer among persons who have never smoked.

### Workplace Exposure to Environmental Tobacco Smoke

Assessments of lung cancer risk associated with ETS exposure among women smokers have primarily focused on exposure from the spouse because this indicator can be consistently defined (NRC 1986; USDHHS 1986b; NIOSH 1991; EPA 1992). Table 3.53 lists studies that specifically assessed workplace exposure; several of these studies are also included among the studies of ETS exposure conducted since 1992 shown in Table 3.52. Although the results of nine U.S. studies have been reported, the data in one study related only to current work exposure. Of the remaining eight studies, five showed RRs of 1.2 to 1.9, primarily at high exposure levels (Wu et al. 1985; Butler 1988; Brownson et al. 1992a; Fontham et al. 1994; Kabat et al. 1995), although results were statistically significant only in the largest study (Fontham et al. 1994). Two studies showed RRs less than 1.0 (Garfinkel et al. 1985; Janerich et al. 1990), and one study did not provide risk estimates but reported no association (Stockwell et al. 1992). The largest U.S. study (Fontham et al. 1994) showed an increasing risk for lung cancer with increasing years of exposure in the workplace. RRs were 1.3 (95 percent CI, 1.01 to 1.7) for 1 through 15 years, 1.4 (95 percent CI, 1.04 to 1.9) for 16 through 30 years, and 1.9 (95 percent CI, 1.2 to 2.8) for more than 30 years (p for trend = 0.001). A later analysis of these data, reported by Reynolds and associates (1996), was restricted to women who were ever employed outside the home for six months or more, and values were adjusted for sources of ETS exposure other than the workplace during adult life. The resulting RRs were slightly higher than those reported in the study by Fontham and colleagues (1994), and the trend remained statistically significant.

Workplace exposure was also examined in the European multicenter study of ETS and lung cancer (Boffetta et al. 1998). Among women who were ever exposed to ETS, RR was 1.2 (95 percent CI, 0.9 to 1.5). Although no significant increase in risk was correlated with duration of exposure in years, trend in risk increased significantly (p for trend = 0.03) for the measure of weighted cumulative exposure (hours per day × years × level of smokiness of workplace). At the highest level of cumulative workplace exposure, RR was 1.9 (95 percent CI, 1.1 to 3.2).

### Conclusion

1. Exposure to ETS is a cause of lung cancer among women who have never smoked.

## Environmental Tobacco Smoke and Coronary Heart Disease

### Previous Reviews

Approximately 20 reports of epidemiologic studies that investigated the association between ETS and risk for CHD among nonsmokers have been

**Table 3.53. Relative risks for lung cancer associated with workplace exposure to environmental tobacco smoke among women who never smoked**

| Study | Country | Workplace exposure indicator | Relative risk (95% confidence interval) |
|---|---|---|---|
| Kabat and Wynder 1984 | United States | Current regular exposure | 0.7 (0.3–1.5) |
| Koo et al. 1984 | Hong Kong | Exposure at work or work and home* | 1.4 (0.5–3.7) |
| Garfinkel et al. 1985 | United States | Exposure at work for last 25 years | 0.9 (0.7–1.2) |
| Wu et al. 1985 | United States | Exposure at work | 1.3 (0.5–3.3) |
| Lee et al. 1986 | England | Exposure at work | 0.6 (0.2–2.3) |
| Butler 1988 | United States | Exposure at work for ≥ 11 years | 1.5 (0.2–14.1) |
| Shimizu et al. 1988 | Japan | Exposure at work | 1.2 (0.7–2.0) |
| Janerich et al. 1990 | United States | Exposure at work, 150 person-years | 0.9 (0.8–1.04)† |
| Kalandidi et al. 1990 | Greece | Highest level of exposure | 1.1 (0.2–1.9) |
| Wu-Williams et al. 1990 | China | Exposure at work | 1.1 (0.9–1.6) |
| Brownson et al. 1992a | United States | Any exposure<br>Highest level of exposure | No association<br>1.2 (0.9–1.7) |
| Stockwell et al. 1992 | United States | Not specified | No association |
| Fontham et al. 1994 | United States | Any exposure<br>Highest level of exposure | 1.4 (1.1–1.7)<br>1.9 (1.2–2.8) |
| Kabat et al. 1995 | United States | Any exposure<br>Highest level of exposure | 1.2 (0.6–2.1)<br>1.4 (0.6–2.8) |
| Boffetta et al. 1998 | 7 European countries | Any exposure<br>Highest level of exposure | 1.2 (0.9–1.5)<br>1.9 (1.1–3.2) |
| Jöckel et al. 1998 | Germany | Highest level of exposure | 2.7 (0.7–9.7)† |

*Total exposure was as follows: 2,121 hours over 2.0 years for cases; 1,681 hours over 1.2 years for controls.
†Includes women and men study participants. No separate data reported for women.

published. Several reviews (Table 3.54), a position paper from the American Heart Association (Taylor et al. 1992), and commentaries on methodologic issues of concern (Glantz and Parmley 1996; Kawachi and Colditz 1996) were also published on this topic. The reviews included qualitative evaluation of the studies, meta-analyses deriving a pooled estimate of the RR for CHD in relation to ETS exposure, and risk assessments estimating the number of CHD deaths among nonsmokers that were attributable to ETS exposure. These reviews concluded that ETS exposure significantly increases the risk for CHD among nonsmokers. The pooled estimates for CHD mortality and morbidity reported in the different reviews were similar.

*Cohort Studies*

Cohort studies that examined the relationship between ETS and the risk for CHD among nonsmokers, including deaths and nonfatal events, are listed in Table 3.55. Of the eight studies that provided data for women, seven showed higher risk for CHD

**Table 3.54. Associations between risk for coronary heart disease (CHD) mortality or morbidity and exposure to environmental tobacco smoke among persons who never smoked, reviews**

| Review | References* | Qualitative review | Population | Pooled relative risk (95% confidence interval) | Estimated number of deaths from CHD/year among women and men combined |
|---|---|---|---|---|---|
| National Research Council 1986 | 1–4 | Yes | NR[†] | NR | NR |
| U.S. Department of Health and Human Services 1986b | 1–4 | Yes | NR | NR | NR |
| Wells 1988, 1989 | 1–6 | No | Women<br>Men | 1.2 (1.1–1.4)[‡]<br>1.3 (1.1–1.6)[‡] | 31,900 |
| Wu-Williams and Samet 1990 | 1–6 | Yes | NR | NR | NR |
| Glantz and Parmley 1991 | 1–10 | Yes | Women<br>Men<br>Women and men | 1.3 (1.2–1.4)[‡]<br>1.3 (1.1–1.6)[‡]<br>1.3 (1.2–1.4)[‡] | 37,000 |
| Steenland 1992 | 1, 3–9, 11 | Yes | NR | NR | 28,026 |
| Wells 1994 | 1, 3–5, 7–14, 15 | Yes | Women<br>Women<br>Men<br>Men<br>Women and men<br>Women and men | 1.2 (1.1–1.4)[§]<br>1.5 (1.2–2.0)[Δ]<br>1.3 (1.03–1.5)[§]<br>1.3 (0.9–1.8)[Δ]<br>1.2 (1.1–1.4)[§]<br>1.4 (1.1–1.8)[Δ] | 61,912 |
| Law et al. 1997b | 1, 3–5, 7–9, 11–13, 15–20 | Yes | Women and men | 1.3 (1.2–1.3)[‡] | |
| Wells 1998 | 1, 3–5, 7–20 | Yes | Women<br>Women<br>Men<br>Men<br>Women and men<br>Women and men | 2.8 (0.95–8.3)[§]<br>1.9 (1.3–3.0)[Δ]<br>1.1 (0.2–5.2)[§]<br>2.7 (0.6–12.1)[Δ]<br>1.2 (1.1–1.3)[§]<br>1.5 (1.3–1.8)[Δ] | |
| He et al. 1999 | 1, 3–5, 7–19 | Yes | Women<br>Men | 1.2 (1.2–1.3)[‡]<br>1.2 (1.1–1.4)[‡] | NR |

*References included Hirayama 1984b (1), Gillis et al. 1984 (2), Garland et al. 1985 (3), Lee et al. 1986 (4), Svendsen et al. 1987 (5), Helsing et al. 1988 (6), He et al. 1989 (7), Hole et al. 1989 (8), Humble et al. 1990 (9), Butler 1988 (10), Dobson et al. 1991b (11), He et al. 1994 (12), La Vecchia et al. 1993a (13), Jackson 1989 (14), Sandler et al. 1989 (15), Muscat and Wynder 1995a (16), Steenland et al. 1996 (17), Kawachi et al. 1997a (18), Ciruzzi et al. 1998 (19), Tunstall-Pedoe et al. 1995 (20). References 2 and 8 described the same study population; references 6 and 15 described the same study population.

[†]NR = Data not calculated or not reported.

[‡]CHD mortality and morbidity.

[§]CHD mortality.

[Δ]CHD morbidity.

among women whose husband was a smoker than among women whose husband was a nonsmoker (Hirayama 1984a; Garland et al. 1985; Butler 1988; Helsing et al. 1988; Humble et al. 1990; Steenland et al. 1996; Kawachi et al. 1997a) (Table 3.55 and Figure 3.10). Three of five studies that included data for men also showed higher risk for CHD associated with wives' smoking (Svendsen et al. 1987; Helsing et al. 1988; Steenland et al. 1996) (Table 3.55 and Figure 3.10). One cohort analysis that used CPS-I and CPS-II data showed no association between the risk for CHD mortality and spousal smoking among either women or men (LeVois and Layard 1995). However, this conclusion was based on any ETS exposure (i.e., former or current) from the spouse, and the effect of the spouse's current smoking on the risk for CHD was not reported separately. A more careful and complete analysis of the CPS-II data was conducted by Steenland and coworkers (1996). Their analysis showed that exposure to the spouse's current smoking was associated with an increased risk for CHD among both women and men. The U.S. Nurses' Health Study (Kawachi et al. 1997a) also demonstrated that ETS exposure at home and at work separately or in combination was associated with an increased risk for both nonfatal MI and fatal CHD.

*Case-Control Studies*

Almost all of the 10 case-control studies that examined the association between exposure to ETS and CHD risk were small, hospital-based studies with direct interviews about relevant sources of ETS exposure among both case subjects and control subjects (Table 3.56). Only 1 study (Layard 1995) relied exclusively on mailed responses provided by next of kin for persons who had died of CHD or unspecified causes not related to smoking. In 7 studies, risk for CHD was elevated among persons with a spouse who smoked (He 1989; Jackson 1989; La Vecchia et al. 1993a; He et al. 1994; Muscat and Wynder 1995a; Ciruzzi et al. 1998) or among persons who were exposed to unspecified sources of ETS (Tunstall-Pedoe et al. 1995). In 2 other studies, associations were reported either among women (Dobson et al. 1991b) or among men (Lee et al. 1986) but not among both genders (Figure 3.11). In 1 study (Layard 1995), no association was found between spousal smoking and risk for CHD. However, the quality of information on ETS exposure in this study was questionable. It is not known whether spousal ETS exposure was current or former exposure or whether it was from a current or previous marriage. All respondents for both case and control groups were next of kin, and 18 percent of respondents were not even first-degree relatives. Approximately one-half of all available CHD deaths in this study were also excluded from the analysis because of missing information on marital status, smoking behavior of the spouse, or both factors.

**Dose-Response Relationship**

More than one-half of the studies shown in Tables 3.55 and 3.56 investigated whether a dose-response relationship exists between exposure to ETS from spousal smoking and risk for CHD among nonsmokers. Some studies determined risk among nonsmokers whose spouse was a former or current smoker and among nonsmokers whose spouse had never smoked (Garland et al. 1985; Butler 1988; La Vecchia et al. 1993a; Steenland et al. 1996). Three of these studies reported that the risk was higher among nonsmokers married to a current smoker than among nonsmokers married to a former smoker (Butler 1988; La Vecchia et al. 1993a; Steenland et al. 1996). Several studies also investigated the intensity of ETS exposure by examining the number of cigarettes smoked by the spouse of nonsmokers (Hirayama 1984a, 1990; He 1989; La Vecchia et al. 1993a; Layard 1995; LeVois and Layard 1995; Ciruzzi et al. 1998), the number of years of smoking (Butler 1988; Muscat and Wynder 1995a; Kawachi et al. 1997a), the number of pack-years of smoking (Steenland et al. 1996), a cumulative index of ETS exposure from the spouse and coworkers (He et al. 1994; Kawachi et al. 1997a), a score representing household exposure (Helsing et al. 1988), and a qualitative assessment of level of exposure (Tunstall-Pedoe et al. 1995). More intense ETS exposure was associated with a higher risk for CHD in some of these studies, but the differences in risk between levels of ETS exposure were not large (Hirayama 1984b; Butler 1988; Helsing et al. 1988; He 1989; La Vecchia et al. 1993a; He et al. 1994; Tunstall-Pedoe et al. 1995; Steenland et al. 1996; Kawachi et al. 1997a).

**Sources of Exposure Other than Spousal Smoking**

Several case-control and cohort studies collected information on exposure to ETS from sources other than the spouse (Lee et al. 1986; Svendsen et al. 1987; Butler 1988; Dobson et al. 1991b; He et al. 1994; Muscat and Wynder 1995a; Steenland et al. 1996; Kawachi et al. 1997a; Ciruzzi et al. 1998). One study specifically assessed ETS exposure from children of index subjects and reported an increase of 80 percent in

**Table 3.55. Associations between adult exposure to environmental tobacco smoke (ETS) from spouses or household members or in the workplace and relative risks for mortality or morbidity from coronary heart disease (CHD), among persons who never smoked, cohort studies**

| Study | Population | Year study began/average length of follow-up | Number of CHD events | Relative risk (95% confidence interval) | Adjustment factors |
|---|---|---|---|---|---|
| Hirayama 1984b | 91,540 married women<br>Japan | 1966<br>16 years | 494 deaths | 1.3 (1.1–1.6)* | Age, spouse's occupation |
| Garland et al. 1985 | 695 married women<br>San Diego, California | 1972<br>10 years | 10 deaths | 2.7† | Age, systolic blood pressure, plasma cholesterol level, obesity, years of marriage |
| Svendsen et al. 1987 | 1,245 married men<br>18 U.S. cities | 1973<br>7 years | 13 deaths<br>69 fatal and nonfatal events | 2.2 (0.7–6.9)‡<br>1.6 (1.0–2.7)‡ | Age, blood pressure, cholesterol level, weight, alcohol use, education |
| Butler 1988 | 9,785 women (from spouse pairs)<br>Loma Linda, California | 1976<br>6 years | 87 deaths | 1.4 (0.5–3.8)§ | Body mass index, history of hypertension and diabetes, exercise |
| | 3,488 women, 1,489 men<br>Adventist Health Smog Study<br>Loma Linda, California | 1976<br>6 years | Women: 70 deaths<br>Men: 76 deaths | 1.5 (0.9–2.5)Δ<br>0.6 (0.3–1.2)Δ | Age |
| Helsing et al. 1988 | 12,348 women, 3,454 men<br>Western Maryland | 1963 | Women: 988 deaths<br>Men: 370 deaths | 1.2 (1.1–1.4)¶<br>1.3 (1.1–1.6)¶ | Education, marital status, age, housing quality |
| Hole et al. 1989 | 2,455 women and men<br>Scotland | 1972<br>11.5 years | 84 deaths | 2.0 (1.2–3.4)** | Age, gender, social class, diastolic blood pressure, serum cholesterol level, body mass index |
| Humble et al. 1990 | 513 married women<br>Evans County, Georgia | 1960<br>20 years | 76 deaths | 1.6 (1.0–2.6)‡ | Age, blood pressure, cholesterol level, body mass index |

*Spouse smoked >20 cigarettes/day vs. spouse never smoked.
†Spouse was current or former smoker vs. spouse did not smoke; the confidence interval was not provided, but the p value was reported to be ≤ 0.10.
‡Spouse smoked vs. spouse did not smoke.
§Spouse was current smoker vs. spouse never smoked.
ΔLived with a smoker for >11 years vs. no ETS exposure at home.
¶Score for household ETS >1 vs. 0.
**Any passive smoking vs. none.

**Table 3.55. Continued**

| Study | Population | Year study began/average length of follow-up | Number of CHD events | Relative risk (95% confidence interval) | Adjustment factors |
|---|---|---|---|---|---|
| LeVois and Layard 1995 | 247,412 women, 88,458 men CPS-I[††] | 1960 13 years | Women and men: 14,901 deaths | 1.00 (0.97–1.04)[‡] | Age, race |
| | | | Women: 7,133 deaths | 1.03 (0.98–1.1)[‡] | |
| | | | Men: 7,768 deaths | 0.97 (0.9–1.1)[‡] | |
| | 226,067 women, 108,772 men CPS-II[‡‡] | 1983 6 years | Women: 1,099 deaths | 1.0 (0.98–1.1)[‡] | |
| | | | Men: 1,966 deaths | 0.97 (0.9–1.1)[‡] | |
| Steenland et al. 1996 | 208,372 women, 101,227 men CPS-II | 1982 7 years | Women: 1,325 deaths | 1.1 (0.96–1.3)[§] | Age; history of heart disease, hypertension, arthritis; body mass index; alcohol use; use of aspirin and diuretics; employment status; exercise; estrogen use in women |
| | | | Men: 2,494 deaths | 1.2 (1.1–1.4)[§] | |
| Kawachi et al. 1997a | 32,046 women Nurses' Health Study | 1982 10 years | 152 total events | 1.7 (1.03–2.8)[§§] | Alcohol use; body mass index; history of hypertension, diabetes, hypercholesterolemia, infarctions; menopausal status; use of hormones; physical activity; intake of vitamin E and fat; aspirin use; family history |
| | | | 127 nonfatal myocardial infarctions | 1.7 (0.99–3.0)[§§] | |
| | | | 25 deaths | 1.9 (0.6–8.2)[§§] | |

[‡]Spouse smoked vs. spouse did not smoke.
[§]Spouse was current smoker vs. spouse did not smoke.
[††]CPS-I = Cancer Prevention Study I; American Cancer Society cohort.
[‡‡]CPS-II = Cancer Prevention Study II; American Cancer Society cohort.
[§§]Any ETS exposure at home or at work vs. none.

association with such exposure (Ciruzzi et al. 1998). The strongest evidence of ETS exposure in the workplace associated with CHD was observed in a case-control study from China (He et al. 1994) and a cohort study of nurses in the United States—the U.S. Nurses' Health Study (Kawachi et al. 1997a). He and colleagues (1994) reported that the risk for CHD was higher among women who had more hours of ETS exposure per day in the workplace, were exposed to a greater number of smokers, were exposed for more years, or had a higher cumulative exposure (number of cigarettes per day × duration). However, a smooth dose-response trend for years of exposure at work was not observed. In the U.S. Nurses' Health Study (Kawachi et al. 1997a), the multivariate RRs for total CHD (fatal and nonfatal events combined) among women who had never smoked and who were exposed to ETS only at work were 1.5 (95 percent CI, 0.7 to 3.1) for occasional exposure and 1.9 (95 percent CI, 0.9 to 4.2) for regular exposure. Weaker effects associated with ETS exposure at work were reported in other U.S. studies (Svendsen et al. 1987; Butler 1988; Steenland et al. 1996).

**Figure 3.10. Exposure to environmental tobacco smoke from spouses' smoking and relative risks for mortality or morbidity from coronary heart disease (CHD), cohort studies**

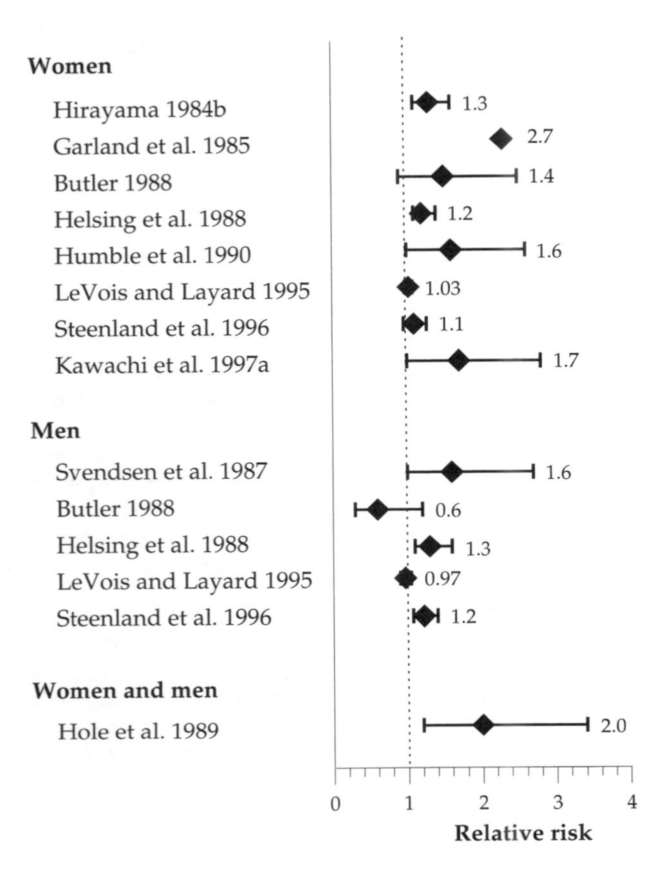


*The confidence interval was not provided, but the p value was reported to be ≤0.10.

### Mortality, Morbidity, and Symptoms

ETS exposure is associated with risk for CHD mortality (fatal events), morbidity (nonfatal events), and symptoms. Most of the data on the association with mortality were from cohort studies, but most of the data on the association with morbidity were from case-control investigations. Nonetheless, the magnitude of association is similar in both sets of results. The risk for CHD morbidity and mortality from ETS exposure could be directly compared within two studies (Svendsen et al. 1987; Hole et al. 1989). These comparisons suggested that the effect of ETS may be stronger for CHD mortality than for CHD morbidity. In one study (Hole et al. 1989), the RR for CHD mortality was 2.0 (95 percent CI, 1.2 to 3.4) (Table 3.55), but for angina or major abnormalities shown by electrocardiography, the RRs were 1.1 (95 percent CI, 0.7 to 1.7) and 1.3 (95 percent CI, 0.5 to 3.4), respectively. In another study (Svendsen et al. 1987), the RR for CHD mortality was 2.2 (95 percent CI, 0.7 to 6.9), but the RR for mortality and morbidity combined was 1.6 (95 percent CI, 1.0 to 2.7) (Table 3.55).

In summary, data from cohort and case-control studies for diverse populations of women and men support a causal association between ETS exposure and CHD mortality and morbidity among nonsmokers. Although few of the risk estimates in individual studies were statistically significant, pooled estimates from meta-analyses showed a significant, 30-percent increase in risk for CHD in relation to ETS exposure. More than one-half of the studies were cohort studies, and the information on smoking status and exposure to ETS was obtained at study entry, thus minimizing recall and misclassification bias. Estimates of risk were determined after adjustment for demographic factors and often for other factors related to CHD that may confound the association.

### Effects on Markers of Cardiovascular Function

Studies of mechanisms through which exposure to ETS increases the risk for CHD among nonsmokers have been reviewed (Glantz and Parmley 1991, 1995; National Cancer Institute 1999). Evidence suggested that exposure to ETS has acute effects on cardiovascular function among healthy nonsmokers and among those at risk for CHD. These deleterious effects include thickening of the carotid artery wall, dysfunction of endothelium, compromised exercise performance, change in lipoprotein distribution, increased plasma fibrinogen, and increased platelet aggregation—conditions that may account for both short-term and long-term effects of ETS on the heart.

### Conclusion

1. Epidemiologic and other data support a causal relationship between ETS exposure from the spouse and coronary heart disease mortality among women nonsmokers.

## Environmental Tobacco Smoke and Reproductive Outcomes

Active smoking has been causally associated with various adverse reproductive outcomes, including LBW and early age at menopause (see "Reproductive Outcomes" earlier in this chapter). This section summarizes studies published between 1966 and early 1999 that examined the relationship between exposure to ETS and developmental and reproductive outcomes. Several previous reviews have been published, the most comprehensive of which is the one by CEPA and the California Department of Health Services (CEPA 1997; Hood 1990; Seidman and Mashiach 1991; Ahlborg 1994). Two meta-analyses have also been conducted (Peacock et al. 1998; Windham et al. 1999a).

### Perinatal Effects

Three categories of adverse pregnancy outcomes are reviewed here in relation to ETS exposure during pregnancy: fetal growth, including LBW and IUGR; fetal loss, including spontaneous abortion and perinatal mortality; and congenital malformations. Emphasis is on fetal growth, the outcome for which the most epidemiologic data have been collected.

#### *Fetal Growth*

More than 25 epidemiologic studies of the relationship between fetal growth and ETS exposure have been published. Some studies included fetal length (Karakostov 1985; Schwartz-Bickenbach et al. 1987; Lazzaroni et al. 1990; Roquer et al. 1995; Luciano et al. 1998), which was slightly lower with ETS exposure (0.3 to 1.1 cm). In three of these studies, however, results were not adjusted for covariates. The findings of these studies on fetal length are not considered further here.

When fetal growth is examined, several covariables should be considered. These covariables include maternal age, race, parity or previous reproductive history, and socioeconomic status or access to prenatal care. Few studies have information on maternal stature or weight gain, but these data are also important determinants of fetal weight, as are certain maternal illnesses, complications of pregnancy, and the gender of the infant. However, only if these factors were also related to ETS exposure would they be confounders. Gestational age at delivery, the strongest predictor of birth weight, was taken into account in some but not all studies.

#### *Mean Birth Weight*

Studies that examined mean birth weight and reported a measure of variability generally also reported lower birth weights in association with ETS exposure, although some of the differences in weight were small (Figure 3.12). Four studies (Haddow et al. 1988; Eskenazi et al. 1995b; Rebagliato et al. 1995; Peacock et al. 1998) measured cotinine, a biomarker of ETS exposure, and adjusted differences in mean birth weight for covariates (Table 3.57 and Figure 3.12, bottom). Haddow and colleagues (1988) found an average weight deficit of 104 g among the offspring of women who had a cotinine level of 1 to 10 ng/mL compared with women who had a level of less than 0.5 ng/mL.

Eskenazi and coworkers (1995b) reported an adjusted weight decrement of 45 g among infants of mothers who had a cotinine level of 2 to 10 ng/mL compared with mothers who had a level of less than 2 ng/mL (defined as unexposed). However, the proportion of women categorized as exposed to ETS (5 percent) was smaller than that in other studies, and 50 percent of the women whose cotinine level indicated nonexposure reported having a husband who smoked. The detection limit of the cotinine assay was high (2 ng/mL) and samples were stored for 25 years, which may indicate that persons in the unexposed group may be misclassified.

In the study by Rebagliato and coworkers (1995), mean infant birth weight was decreased 87.3 g at the highest quintile of maternal cotinine level (>1.7 ng/mL) among nonsmokers, but the dose-response trend was inconsistent in a multiple regression model. When the categories were combined, the estimated crude decrement in birth weight at a cotinine level higher than 0.5 ng/mL was 34.5 g. Peacock and colleagues (1998) also examined mean birth weight in relation to quintiles of serum cotinine level less than 15 ng/mL among white, nonsmoking pregnant women. A statistically significant trend toward lower mean birth weight was noted across increasing cotinine level; however, the decrement of 73 g in the highest quintile group (≥ 0.796 ng/mL) compared with the lowest quintile group (≤ 0.18 ng/mL) was not statistically significant. After adjustment for gestational age and other covariates, the birth weight ratio (observed to expected based on an external standard) indicated a nonsignificant weight decrement of only 0.2 percent for ETS exposure compared with 5 percent for active smoking. Thus, the results from the more recent studies were in the direction of findings in the study of Haddow and colleagues (1988) but showed weaker effects. Adjustment for gestational age (e.g., Eskenazi et al. 1995b; Peacock et al. 1998) may represent overcontrolling because gestational age is a determinant of birth weight, but the adjustment was performed in an attempt to separate effects of gestational age from effects of growth retardation.

**Table 3.56. Relative risks for coronary heart disease (CHD) associated with adult exposure to environmental tobacco smoke (ETS) among persons who never smoked or nonsmokers, case-control studies**

| Study | Population* | Source: Cases | Source: Controls | Relative risk[†] (95% confidence interval) | Adjustment factors |
|---|---|---|---|---|---|
| Lee et al. 1986 | Women<br>77 cases<br>318 controls<br>Men<br>41 cases<br>133 controls<br>United Kingdom | Hospital | Hospital | Women:<br>0.9 (0.6–1.7)<br>0.4 (0.1–1.4)[‡]<br>Men:<br>1.2 (0.6–2.8)<br>0.8 (0.2–2.0)[‡] | Not available |
| He 1989 | Women[§]<br>34 cases<br>68 controls<br>China | Hospital | Hospital and population | Women: 1.5 (1.3–1.8) | Alcohol use; exercise; personal and family history of CHD, hypertension, hyperlipidemia |
| Jackson 1989 | Women[Δ]<br>22 cases<br>174 controls<br>Men[Δ]<br>44 cases<br>84 controls<br>New Zealand | Hospital<br>Myocardial infarction<br><br>Death from CHD | Hospital | Women: 2.7 (0.6–12.3)[¶]<br>Men: 1.0 (0.3–3.0)[¶]<br><br>Women: 5.8 (1.0–35.2)[¶]<br>Men: 1.1 (0.2–5.3)[¶] | Age, social status, history of CHD |
| Dobson et al. 1991b | Women[Δ]<br>160 cases<br>532 controls<br>Men[Δ]<br>183 cases<br>293 controls<br>Australia | Hospital deaths from myocardial infarction and CHD | Community-based survey of risk | Women: 2.5 (1.5–4.1)[¶]<br>Men: 1.0 (0.5–1.8)[¶] | Age, history of myocardial infarction |
| La Vecchia et al. 1993a | Women<br>43 cases<br>56 controls<br>Men<br>64 cases<br>161 controls<br>Italy | Hospital | Hospital | Women and men:<br>1.2 (0.6–2.5)** | Gender, age, coffee intake, body mass index, cholesterol level, diabetes, hypertension, family history of myocardial infarction |

*Unless otherwise specified, study population never smoked.
†Unless otherwise specified, relative risk from any exposure to ETS from spouse vs. no exposure.
‡ETS score 5–12 vs. 0–1, including ETS exposure at home, work, travel, and leisure.
§Nonsmokers.
ΔNonsmokers, but unclear whether population never smoked.
¶For any exposure to ETS at home vs. no exposure.
**Spouse was current smoker vs. spouse did not smoke.

**Table 3.56. Continued**

| Study | Population* | Source: Cases | Source: Controls | Relative risk† (95% confidence interval) | Adjustment factors |
|---|---|---|---|---|---|
| He et al. 1994 | Women<br>59 cases<br>126 controls<br>China | Hospital | Hospital<br>Population | Women:<br>1.2 (0.6–1.8)<br>1.9 (0.9–4.0)†† | Age, type A personality, total and high-density lipoprotein cholesterol levels, history of hypertension |
| Layard 1995 | Women<br>914 cases<br>969 controls<br>Men<br>475 cases<br>998 controls<br>National Mortality Follow-back Survey<br>United States | Deaths from ischemic heart disease identified in survey | Deaths from unspecified causes not related to smoking | Women: 1.0 (0.8–1.2)<br>Men: 1.0 (0.7–1.3) | Age, race |
| Muscat and Wynder 1995a | Women<br>46 cases<br>50 controls<br>Men<br>68 cases<br>108 controls<br>4 U.S. cities | Hospital | Hospital | Women and men:<br>1.5 (0.9–2.6)‡‡<br>Women: 1.3 (0.7–2.4)‡‡<br>Men: 1.7 (0.7–3.7)‡‡ | Age, education, hypertension |
| Tunstall-Pedoe et al. 1995 | Women and men<br>70 cases<br>2,278 controls<br>Scotland | General practitioner list; self-report of a diagnosed CHD | General practitioner list; self-report of a diagnosed CHD | Women and men:<br>2.4 (1.1–4.8)§§ | Age, housing, tenure, cholesterol level, diastolic blood pressure |
| Ciruzzi et al. 1998 | Women<br>180 cases<br>218 controls<br>Men<br>156 cases<br>228 controls<br>10 South American countries | Hospital | Hospital | Women: 1.5 (0.95–2.5)ΔΔ<br>Men: 1.9 (1.1–3.2) | Age, cholesterol level, diabetes, hypertension, body mass index, education, socioeconomic status, exercise, family history of myocardial infarction |

*Unless otherwise specified, study population never smoked.
†Unless otherwise specified, relative risk from any exposure to ETS from spouse vs. no exposure.
††For any ETS exposure at work vs. no exposure.
‡‡For any ETS exposure including spouse, work, transportation, and other vs. no exposure.
§§Any exposure to ETS from someone else in last 3 days.
ΔΔOne or more relatives smoking.

**Figure 3.11. Exposure to environmental tobacco smoke from spouses' smoking and risk of coronary heart disease (CHD), case-control studies**

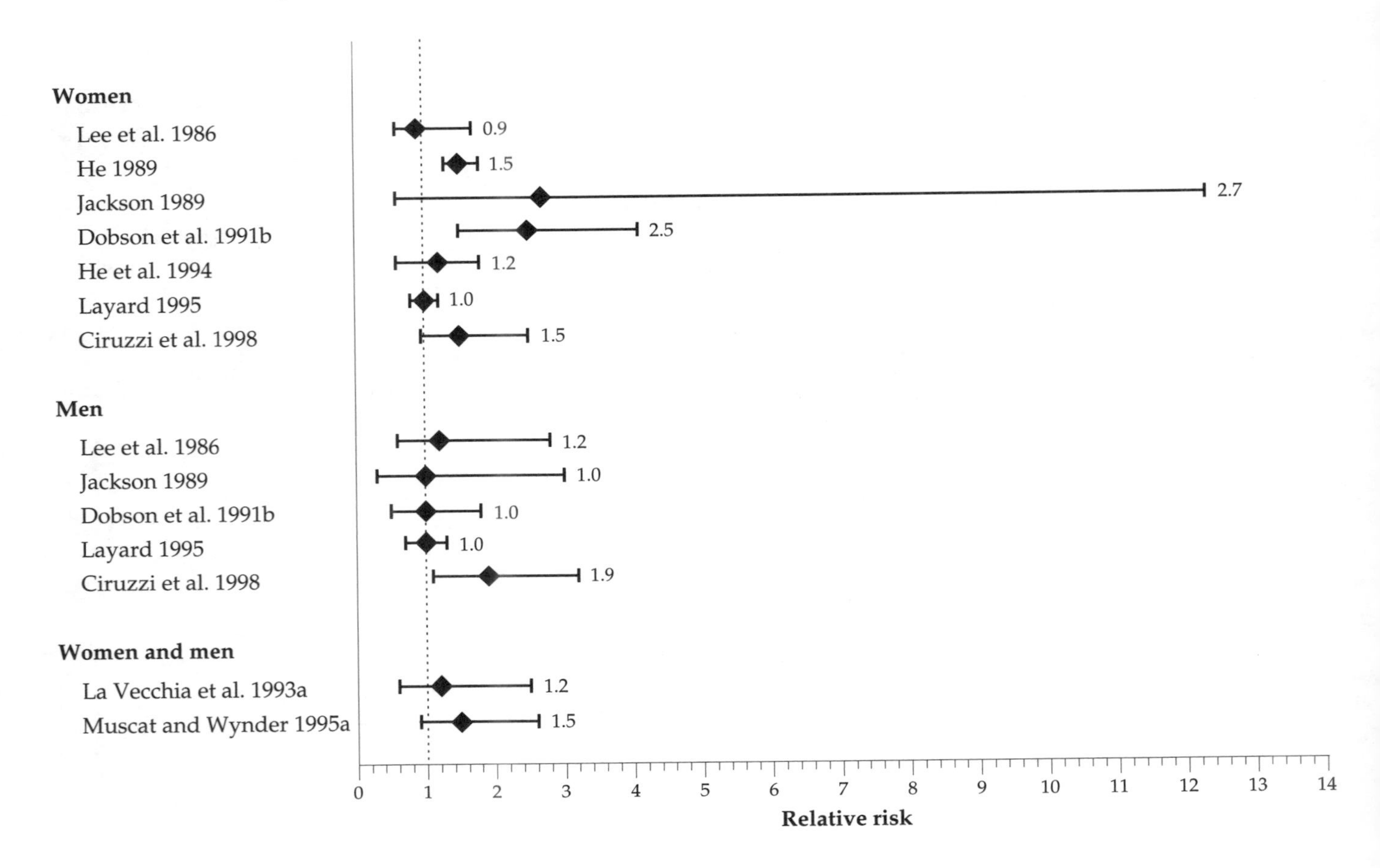


Studies that attempted to ascertain total ETS exposure from multiple sources by self-report provided further evidence of an effect of ETS exposure (Figure 3.12, bottom). After adjustment for potential confounders, most of the studies (Figure 3.12, bottom) showed small-to-moderate decrements in mean birth weight (10 to 90 g) associated with ETS exposure. Ogawa and associates (1991) provided an adjusted estimate of a 10.8-g decrement, but because no CI was provided, it is not included in Figure 3.12. The studies were not, however, comparable in their definition of exposure, and the reference groups may have included some women whose exposure was low (particularly Ahlborg and Bodin 1991; Ogawa et al. 1991). Some studies examined term births only (Martin and Bracken 1986; Lazzaroni et al. 1990; Ogawa et al. 1991; Luciano et al. 1998); weight differences for term births tended to be less variable than those for all births. Findings of the prospective studies (Martin and Bracken 1986; Ahlborg and Bodin 1991; Rebagliato et al. 1995) were not consistently different from those of other studies. Two European studies found large weight decrements in relation to high exposure, that is, among infants of mothers exposed to the equivalent of one pack of cigarettes per day at home or work, but results were not adjusted for potential confounding factors (Roquer et al. 1995; Luciano et al. 1998).

Several of these studies provided information on level of exposure to ETS. Mainous and Hueston (1994a) found a weight decrement among infants of mothers in the highest category of exposure only (e.g., mothers who were always in contact with persons who smoked), whereas Rebagliato and colleagues (1995) found a decrement for all quintiles of total hours of exposure but no consistent gradient with increasing exposure. Lazzaroni and coworkers (1990) reported evidence of greater weight decrements with greater exposure, and the mean birth weight among infants of women who were exposed five or more

**Figure 3.12. Differences in mean birth weight (and 95% confidence interval) among infants of mothers exposed to environmental tobacco smoke (ETS) compared with infants of mothers not exposed to ETS**

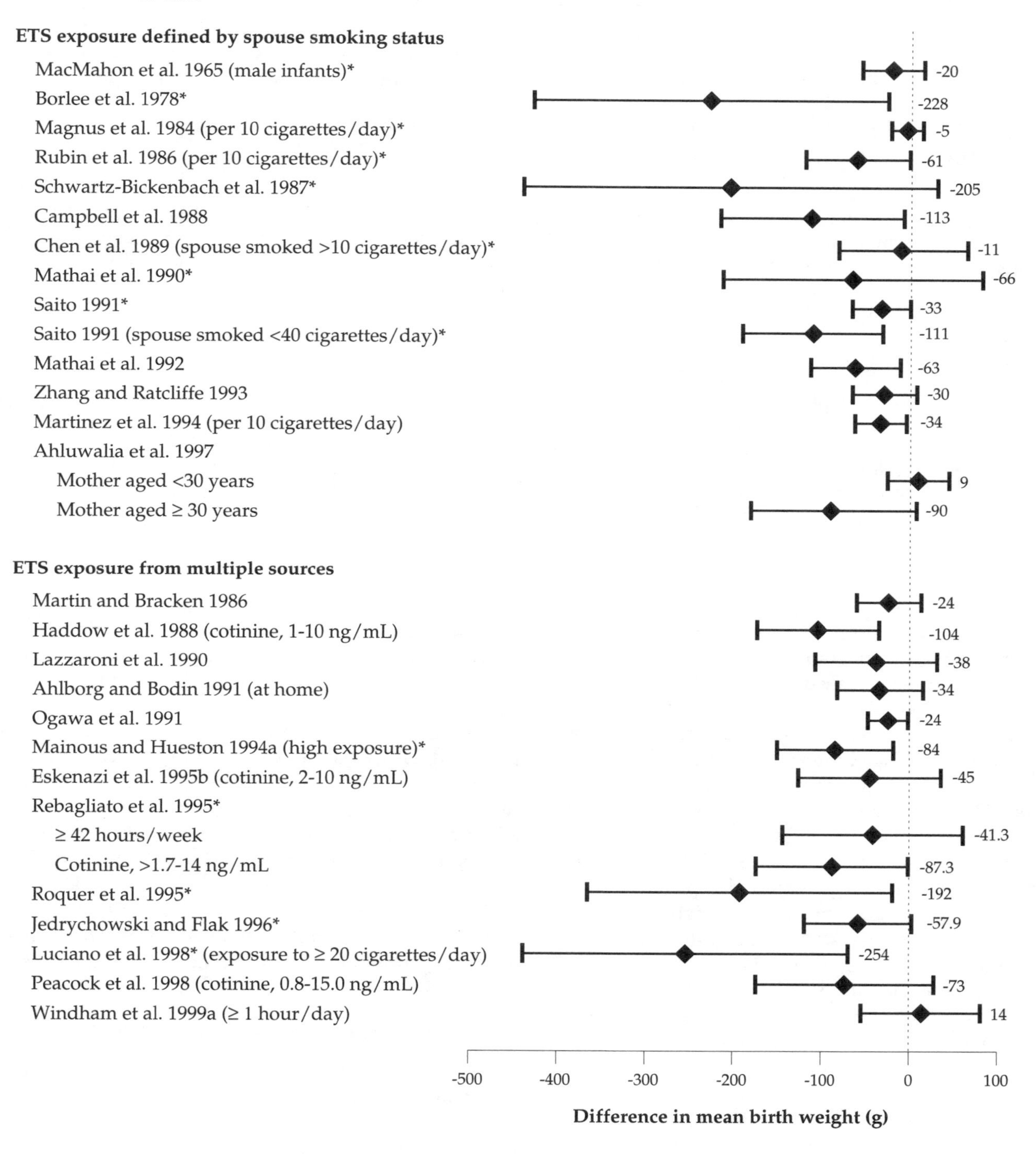


*Differences and confidence intervals calculated by using data from published report of study.
†Study includes maternal smokers; results adjusted for maternal smoking.
‡Adjusted for various confounders, depending on study.

**Table 3.57. Differences in birth weight between infants of nonsmoking mothers exposed to environmental tobacco smoke (ETS) and infants of mothers not exposed to ETS, based on measurement of biomarkers**

| Study (location) | Number of samples | Cotinine level defining exposure (% of mothers exposed) | Difference in mean birth weight between exposed and unexposed (95% confidence interval) | Results for low birth weight |
|---|---|---|---|---|
| Haddow et al. 1988 (Maine) | 1,231 serum samples obtained in second trimester | 1–10 ng/mL (3.4%) | -104 g (-173 to 35 g) | 29% increase in rate* |
| Eskenazi et al. 1995b (California) | 2,243 serum samples obtained in second trimester | 2–10 ng/mL (5%) | -45 g (-125.6 to 36.0 g) | Relative risk = 1.4 (95% confidence interval, 0.6–3.0) |
| Rebagliato et al. 1995 (Spain) | 690 saliva samples obtained in third trimester | >1.7–14 ng/mL (19%) | -87.3 g (-173.5 to -1.1 g) | Not given |
| Peacock et al. 1998 (United Kingdom) | Serum samples from 827 nonsmokers<br>Mean of two or three serum cotinine levels | Quintiles<br>Lowest: 0–0.18 ng/mL<br>Highest: 0.796–15 ng/mL | -73 g (-174 to 28 g)<br>Unadjusted mean difference between infants of women in highest and lowest quintiles; significant dose trend | Not given |

*No statistical test.

hours per day was similar to that among infants of women who were light smokers.

A few studies examined sources of exposure separately. In Sweden, Ahlborg and Bodin (1991) found a slight decrement in infant weight in relation to maternal exposure to ETS at home (-34 g; 95 percent CI, -82 to 15 g) and a slight increment in relation to exposure at work (20 g; 95 percent CI, -37 to 77 g), but neither estimate was statistically significant. In Spain, Rebagliato and associates (1995) found birth weight decrements at all levels of maternal exposure to ETS at work and other public places but a slight increment with exposure at home; statistical significance varied by type and level of exposure. Workplace exposure may differ from that at home because of the number of smokers contributing to ETS and the influence of environmental conditions (e.g., rates of air exchange, temperature, and room size).

Thus, minor inconsistencies related to dose and source of exposure emerge from studies of multiple sources of exposure. On average, however, the infants of women exposed to ETS during pregnancy appear to have a weight decrement in the range of 40 to 50 g. Furthermore, the decrease in birth weight may be greatest among infants of women with the highest exposure to ETS.

The weight differences among infants that were reported from studies based only on maternal exposure to ETS from spousal or household smokers vary greatly—from a decrement of 5 g to a decrement of more than 200 g. (See Figure 3.12, top, for studies that provided CIs or data to calculate them.) The studies were difficult to compare because of their many differences, including when they were conducted over a 25-year span, the location and nationality of study populations, the sample size and selection, the extent to which confounders were controlled, and the analytic methods used. Some of these earlier studies included maternal smokers but adjusted for that variable (Magnus et al. 1984; Rubin et al. 1986; Campbell et al. 1988).

*Low Birth Weight and Intrauterine Growth Retardation*

Most studies that have reported RRs for LBW or IUGR in relation to ETS exposure found a slightly elevated risk for these conditions among infants of mothers exposed to ETS (Table 3.57 and Figure 3.13). The area of overlap for all the CIs is consistent with up to a 1.4- or 1.5-fold higher risk for small fetal size, but is also consistent with no association. One study that used cotinine to assess ETS exposure (Eskenazi et

**Figure 3.13. Relative risks (95% confidence interval) for low birth weight (LBW) or intrauterine growth retardation (IUGR) among infants of mothers exposed to environmental tobacco smoke (ETS) compared with infants of mothers not exposed to ETS**

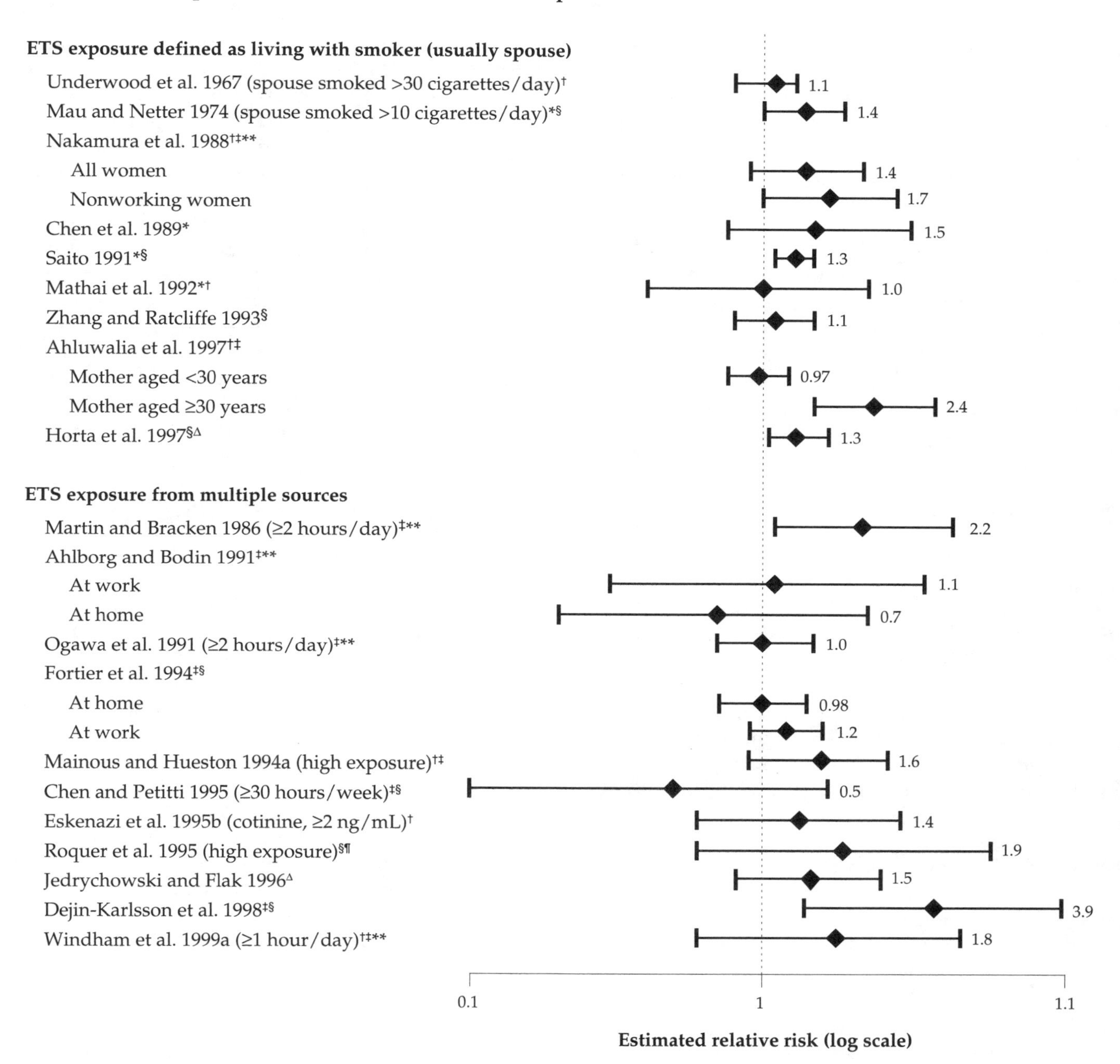


*Relative risks and confidence intervals calculated by using data from published report of study.
†Examined LBW, usually defined as <2,500 g, but Mathai et al. (1992) defined it as <2,000 g.
‡Adjusted for various confounders, depending on study.
§Examined IUGR, usually defined as <10th percentile of weight for gestational age, but Saito et al. (1991) defined it as <1.5 standard deviations of the mean for gestational age, and Dejin-Karlsson (1998) defined it as <2 standard deviations below the mean.
ΔStudy includes maternal smokers; results adjusted for maternal smoking.
¶High exposure at work or home, based on 1 smoker of >1 pack/day or ≥2 smokers of 10 cigarettes/day.
**Based on low birth weight at term.

al. 1995b) found a slight and nonsignificant elevation in risk for LBW. The comparison group may have included women who were exposed to ETS, as discussed earlier in this section, which would dilute the estimated effect. Another study that used cotinine measurement reported a 29-percent increase in risk, but did not adjust for potential confounders nor provide a CI for its finding on LBW (Haddow et al. 1988) (Table 3.57). A recent small, case-control study of IUGR found an association with detectable nicotine level in infant hair samples (RR, 2.6; 95 percent CI, 0.9 to 8.1) and with detectable maternal hair nicotine level among nonsmokers (Nafstad et al. 1998). The reported results were not adjusted for confounders, although the authors stated that several potential confounders had no effect.

Except for a small case-control study (Chen and Petitti 1995), the studies of LBW or IUGR that assessed maternal exposure to ETS from multiple sources (Figure 3.13, bottom) also reported slightly or highly elevated risks for LBW or IUGR. Findings from only two of the studies achieved statistical significance (Martin and Bracken 1986; Dejin-Karlsson et al. 1998). The studies that separately examined ETS exposure at work and home generally reported slightly higher risk from exposure at work than at home (Ahlborg and Bodin 1991; Fortier et al. 1994; Chen and Petitti 1995), but the CIs overlapped considerably. The first two of these studies also found evidence of a slight dose-response trend with increasing level of ETS exposure in the workplace. A study of LBW found a moderate increase in risk with the highest maternal exposure to ETS (RR, 1.6) and some evidence of a dose-response trend (Mainous and Hueston 1994a).

The studies of exposure to paternal or household ETS (Figure 3.13, top) showed RR estimates that were only slightly lower than those in the studies of ETS exposure from multiple sources described earlier. The best and the most recent of these studies, which were conducted since the late 1980s, were consistent in showing a slight increase in the risk for LBW or IUGR (RRs, 1.1 to 1.7). Two of these studies showed no indication of a greater effect at higher exposure levels (Chen et al. 1989; Zhang and Ratcliffe 1993), but two others suggested a greater effect (Nakamura et al. 1988; Saito 1991). The large U.S. study of low-income women, which was stratified by maternal age, found increased risks for LBW (RR, 2.4; 95 percent CI, 1.5 to 3.9) and preterm birth (RR, 1.9; 95 percent CI, 1.2 to 2.9) only among infants of women aged 30 years or older (Ahluwalia et al. 1997).

The biological plausibility of the findings from epidemiologic studies is supported by the well-established relationships between active smoking and IUGR among humans and between constituents of tobacco smoke (e.g., nicotine, CO, toluene, or cadmium) and fetal growth retardation among animals (Longo 1977; Baranski 1985; Ungváry and Tátrai 1985; Seidenberg et al. 1986; Donald et al. 1991). A primary mechanism of the effects of nicotine and CO is thought to be fetal hypoxia, because CO binds to hemoglobin and nicotine has vasoconstrictive properties.

Thus, in numerous epidemiologic studies, maternal exposure to ETS is associated with a slight decrement in birth weight and increases in LBW and IUGR. A meta-analysis of studies conducted before mid-1995 reported a weighted-average decrement in mean birth weight of -28 g (95 percent CI, -41 to -16 g) among the offspring of women nonsmokers exposed to ETS and a summary RR of 1.2 (95 percent CI, 1.1 to 1.3) for IUGR or LBW at term among these offspring (Windham et al. 1999a). Greater decrements were found in the three studies that measured cotinine. A subsequent analysis (Peacock et al. 1998) reported a pooled weight decrement of -31 g (95 percent CI, -44 to -19), which was very similar to that reported by Windham and associates (1999a). A small effect (e.g., 25 to 50 g) may not be clinically significant for an otherwise healthy infant, but such a decrement may put infants who are already compromised by other health conditions or risk factors at even higher risk. An increased risk of even 20 percent for LBW or IUGR with maternal exposure to ETS would affect many infants nationwide, because household ETS exposure is common.

Residual confounding or misclassification may be difficult to rule out in studies reporting weakly elevated RRs. Nevertheless, the studies reviewed here have consistently found an association, and some have found evidence of dose-response effects. Studies with better data on ETS exposure, including biochemical measures of exposure, are needed, but maternal exposure to ETS appears to be causally associated with detrimental effects on fetal growth.

#### *Fetal Loss and Neonatal Mortality*

Few studies have addressed whether maternal exposure to ETS affects the risk for stillbirth. Some studies examined the effect of ETS exposure on spontaneous abortion or miscarriage, which affects 10 to 15 percent of recognized pregnancies (Kline and Stein 1984) and is now commonly defined as fetal loss in the first 20 weeks of gestation.

Results of several early studies that examined neonatal mortality (Comstock and Lundin 1967) and perinatal mortality rates (Mau and Netter 1974) or spontaneous abortion (Koo et al. 1988; Lindbohm et al. 1991) by paternal smoking status suggested an increased risk of up to 50 percent from ETS exposure, but interpretation of these studies is hampered by lack of control for confounding factors, lack of restriction of analysis to nonsmokers, or insufficient presentation of data.

Two studies of fetal loss and maternal exposure to ETS (Ahlborg and Bodin 1991; Windham et al. 1992) that assessed self-reported exposure at home, at work, or both reported about a 50-percent increase in risk. In the Swedish study (Ahlborg and Bodin 1991), an increase associated with exposure at work was observed only for early losses (≤ 12 weeks) (Table 3.58). In the California study (Windham et al. 1992), risk was increased among women who reported any exposure of an hour or more per day; work exposure could not be assessed separately, although the study examined paternal smoking separately and found RRs across categories of amount smoked by the father that were all close to unity. The California study found a greater association with spontaneous abortion in the second trimester than in the first trimester. Some of the estimates of association between ETS exposure and spontaneous abortion reported in these two studies are as high as those found for active smoking (see "Reproductive Outcomes" earlier in this chapter), which seems biologically implausible.

In contrast, a large prospective study in California based on more detailed questions about hours of exposure at home and work did not confirm previous findings (Windham et al. 1999c) (Table 3.58). The adjusted RR for spontaneous abortion was slightly greater than 1.0 for home exposure and slightly less than 1.0 for work exposure, and no trend was found with increasing hours of exposure.

In clinical studies and animal studies, very high levels of several components of tobacco smoke, including CO (Singh and Scott 1984; Koren et al. 1991), toluene (Ungváry and Tátrai 1985; Ng et al. 1992), and cadmium (Baranski et al. 1982; Wardell et al. 1982; Kaur 1989) were associated with fetal death. Some but not all studies in humans have suggested that active smoking contributes to neonatal mortality and late spontaneous abortion (Kline et al. 1977; Kleinman et al. 1988) (see "Reproductive Outcomes" earlier in this chapter).

There are few studies of ETS exposure during pregnancy in relation to spontaneous abortion and perinatal mortality and few studies of the effect of prenatal, as distinct from postnatal, ETS exposure on risk for SIDS. Results of these studies have been inconsistent, and further work in these areas would be useful.

**Table 3.58. Relative risks for spontaneous abortion among nonsmokers exposed to environmental tobacco smoke (ETS) compared with nonsmokers not exposed to ETS**

| Study (location) | Study design | Population | Measure of exposure to ETS | Relative risk (95% confidence interval) |
|---|---|---|---|---|
| Ahlborg and Bodin 1991 (Sweden) | Prospective study<br>Self-administered questionnaire | 2,936 nonsmokers | Living with smoker<br>Spending most time at work around smokers | 1.0 (0.7–1.5) for exposure at home*<br>1.5 (1.0–2.4) for exposure at workplace*<br>1.1 (0.8–1.5) for any exposure* |
| Windham et al. 1992 (California) | Case-control study<br>Telephone interview | 626 cases<br>1,300 controls | Spending ≥ 1 hour/day at home or work around smokers<br>Number of cigarettes smoked by father | 1.6 (1.2–2.1) for any exposure ≥ 1 hour/day†<br>1.0 (0.8–1.3) for any paternal smoking†<br>No dose-response effect |
| Windham et al. 1999c (California) | Prospective study<br>Telephone interview | 5,144 pregnancies<br>4,209 nonsmokers | Hours/day at home and/or work<br>Amount smoked by spouse or partner | 1.0 (0.8–1.3)‡ for any ETS; no dose-response effect |

*Adjusted relative risk for spontaneous abortions and stillbirths combined.
†Adjusted relative risk for spontaneous abortion at ≤20 weeks' gestation.
‡Adjusted for age, prior spontaneous abortion, alcohol and caffeine consumption, and gestational age at interview.

*Congenital Malformations*

Congenital malformations include a wide variety of diagnoses, such as neural tube defects (e.g., anencephaly and spina bifida), orofacial clefts, and defects of the genitourinary and cardiovascular systems. Because of potential differences in causality, lumping all defects may obscure specific associations. The few studies that provided data on effects of prenatal exposure to ETS on congenital malformations (Table 3.59) were not all designed to examine this issue, so several based exposure assessment solely on paternal smoking status. In these types of studies, a direct effect of active smoking on the genetic material in the sperm cannot be ruled out as a mechanism for any association observed.

The findings of these studies suggested that paternal smoking results in a slight risk for severe congenital malformations (RR, 1.2 to 1.4), for all malformations combined, or for major malformations (Table 3.59). Several studies found a greater risk for specific defects, but these defects differed across studies, suggesting that some of these associations may have occurred by chance. The findings were most consistent for cleft lip, cleft palate, or both. Two studies reported indications of a dose-response trend for at least some diagnoses (Savitz et al. 1991; Zhang et al. 1992), but these results were based on small numbers of cases and were not adjusted for confounders.

A case-control study of orofacial clefts examined maternal and paternal smoking and various sources of ETS exposure (Shaw et al. 1996). Paternal smoking in the months surrounding conception was not an independent risk factor, but women nonsmokers exposed to ETS at home at least once a week and with exposure that occurred at close range (within 6 feet) were at increased risk for having offspring with orofacial cleft malformations, particularly isolated cleft lip or cleft palate (RR, 2.0; 95 percent CI, 1.2 to 3.4). The investigators reported slightly increased but nonsignificant risks from workplace exposure to ETS, but neither RRs nor raw data were presented for that association. Among infants born to women nonsmokers, risks associated with ETS exposure were higher for infants with the less common genotype of an allele (*A2*) for transforming growth factor alpha, a secretory protein.

Another study (Wasserman et al. 1996) examined ETS exposure of maternal nonsmokers during early pregnancy in relation to three types of birth defects (Table 3.59). Maternal exposure to ETS, particularly at work, was associated with conotruncal heart defects and limb-reduction defects, with particularly high risk for a subset of heart defects—tetralogy of Fallot (for ETS at work, RR, 2.9; 95 percent CI, 1.3 to 6.6). Paternal smoking of one or more packs of cigarettes per day was also associated with increases of 60 to 110 percent in these two categories of major congenital defects, but maternal smokers were included in the analysis. When the mother was a nonsmoker, any paternal smoking, regardless of the amount, was not associated with the heart defects but was slightly associated with the limb-reduction defects (RR, 1.4; 95 percent CI, 0.9 to 2.2). The RRs presented were not adjusted for other variables, but the authors noted that little change occurred in any estimates when results were adjusted for race, gravidity, alcohol use, or vitamin use.

Thus, several studies showed associations between paternal smoking and congenital malformations among offspring, but whether these are due to maternal exposure to paternal smoking or to direct effects of paternal smoking or other factors is unclear.

Because results on the effects of active smoking on perinatal development have been inconsistent (see "Reproductive Outcomes" earlier in this chapter), it would be premature to draw conclusions about the risks associated with ETS exposure. Detecting a weak teratogen with rare outcomes such as birth defects is difficult. A few studies suggested associations, but further studies with adequate power to examine specific defects and with more comprehensive assessments of exposure would be necessary to determine the relationship of ETS exposure with the occurrence of birth defects.

**Fertility and Fecundity**

The epidemiologic data on whether ETS exposure may be associated with reduced fertility have been limited and inconsistent. If delayed conception is found when exposure is defined as spousal smoking, the results may be due to effects of ETS exposure per se or to direct effects of paternal smoking on male reproductive parameters (e.g., semen quality). One study in Denmark (Olsen 1991) found a slight but significant increase in risk for delay of 6 to 12 months in conception, but a more rigorous U.S. study did not find an increased risk (Baird and Wilcox 1985). A recent study from Denmark (Jensen et al. 1998) also found reduced fecundity with male partner's smoking. Two additional studies, one in Scandinavia and one in the Netherlands (Suonio et al. 1990; Florack et al. 1994), examined the relationship between delay to conception and partner smoking. The Scandanavian study reported an effect similar to that of the Danish

**Table 3.59. Relative risks for congenital malformations among infants with prenatal exposure to environmental tobacco smoke (ETS)**

| Study (location) | Study design | Population | Relative risk (95% confidence interval) |
|---|---|---|---|
| Seidman et al. 1990[†‡] (Israel) | Cross-sectional study<br>Postpartum interview | 14,477 infants of nonsmokers | 1.5 (0.7–2.8) for major birth defects*<br>1.1 (0.9–1.5) for minor birth defects* |
| Savitz et al. 1991[†‡§] (California) | Prospective cohort of health maintenance organization members | 14,685 infants of nonsmokers and smokers | 2.4 (0.6–9.3) for hydrocephalus<br>2.0 (0.9–4.3) for ventricular septal defect<br>2.0 (0.6–6.4) for urethral stenosis<br>1.7 (0.5–6.0) for cleft lip and/or palate<br>0.6 (0.2–2.5) for neural tube defects<br>(All results adjusted for smoking) |
| Zhang et al. 1992[†‡] (China) | Case-control study<br>Interview in hospital | Infants of nonsmokers<br>1,012 cases<br>1,012 controls | 1.2 (1.0–1.5) for all birth defects<br>1.6 for cleft palate[Δ]<br><1.5 for hydrocephalus[Δ]<br><1.0 for ventricular septal defect[Δ]<br>2.0 (1.1–3.7) for neural tube defects |
| Shaw et al. 1996[¶**] (California) | Case-control study of orofacial clefts | Infants of nonsmokers<br>487 cases<br>554 controls | 2.0 (1.2–3.4) for isolated cleft lip and/or palate, for home exposure to ETS[††]<br>9.8 (1.1–218.0) for isolated cleft lip and/or palate with A2 allele for transforming growth factor alpha, for any ETS exposure |
| Wasserman et al. 1996[‡‡] (California) | Case-control study of three types of birth defects | 207 infants with conotruncal heart defects<br>264 infants with neural tube defects<br>178 infants with limb-reduction defects<br>481 control infants | 1.3 (0.8–2.1) for conotruncal defects, for ETS at home<br>1.7 (0.9–3.0) for conotruncal defects, for ETS at work<br>1.2 (0.8–1.9) for neural tube defects, for ETS at home or work<br>1.3 (0.8–2.1) for limb-reduction defects, for ETS at home<br>1.4 (0.7–2.5) for limb-reduction defects, for ETS at work |

*Adjustment did not change relative risk.

[†]Confidence intervals were calculated by using data from the published report of the study.

[‡]For Seidman et al. 1990, ETS exposure was defined as paternal smoking of >30 cigarettes/day. For Savitz et al. 1991 and Zhang et al. 1992, ETS exposure was defined as any paternal smoking.

[§]Included maternal smokers. Results are adjusted for maternal smoking.

[Δ]Not significant ($p > 0.05$).

[¶]Besides paternal smoking, other sources of ETS exposure were examined, including exposure of mothers at home and at work.

**ETS exposure at home was defined as at least weekly tobacco smoking in the home within 6 feet of the mother, during the period from 1 month before to 3 months after conception.

[††]Risk of orofacial clefts was slightly but not significantly elevated with paternal smoking around the time of conception and with ETS exposure at work.

[‡‡]ETS exposure was defined as others smoking at home, work, and/or other places and was assessed in maternal nonsmokers. Paternal smoking was evaluated separately.

study (Jensen et al. 1998), but the Dutch study did not show evidence of an adverse effect. A large population-based study of pregnant women in England found that, after adjustment for multiple factors, the RR for conception delay of more than 6 months among nonsmokers exposed to ETS was 1.17 (95 percent CI, 1.02 to 1.37); the RR for conception delay of more than 12 months was 1.14 (95 percent CI, 0.92 to 1.42) (Hull et al. 2000).

Four studies investigated childhood exposure to ETS and fecundity (Weinberg et al. 1989; Wilcox et al. 1989; Schwingl 1992; Jensen et al. 1998). The same investigators conducted two of the studies in different populations (Weinberg et al. 1989; Wilcox et al. 1989). They reported that such exposure tended to increase the adjusted fecundity ratio, that is, the relative probability of conceiving in a given cycle among exposed women compared with unexposed women. The two other studies found little association between fecundity and exposure to ETS as a child. Problems with these studies include the potential unreliability of self-reported recall of exposure and the lack of ascertainment of possible confounders associated with childhood exposure to ETS.

### Conclusions

1. Infants born to women who are exposed to ETS during pregnancy may have a small decrement in birth weight and a slightly increased risk for intrauterine growth retardation compared with infants born to women who are not exposed; both effects are quite variable across studies.
2. Studies of ETS exposure and the risks for delay in conception, spontaneous abortion, and perinatal mortality are few, and the results are inconsistent.

## Conclusions

### *Total Mortality*

1. Cigarette smoking plays a major role in the mortality of U.S. women.
2. The excess risk for death from all causes among current smokers compared with persons who have never smoked increases with both the number of years of smoking and the number of cigarettes smoked per day.
3. Among women who smoke, the percentage of deaths attributable to smoking has increased over the past several decades, largely because of increases in the quantity of cigarettes smoked and the duration of smoking.
4. Cohort studies with follow-up data analyzed in the 1980s show that the annual risk for death from all causes is 80 to 90 percent greater among women who smoke cigarettes than among women who have never smoked. A woman's annual risk for death more than doubles among continuing smokers compared with persons who have never smoked in every age group from 45 through 74 years.
5. In 1997, approximately 165,000 U.S. women died prematurely from a smoking-related disease. Since 1980, approximately three million U.S. women have died prematurely from a smoking-related disease.
6. U.S. females lost an estimated 2.1 million years of life each year during the 1990s as a result of smoking-related deaths due to neoplastic, cardiovascular, respiratory, and pediatric diseases as well as from burns caused by cigarettes. For every smoking attributable death, an average of 14 years of life was lost.
7. Women who stop smoking greatly reduce their risk for dying prematurely. The relative benefits of smoking cessation are greater when women stop smoking at younger ages, but smoking cessation is beneficial at all ages.

### *Lung Cancer*

8. Cigarette smoking is the major cause of lung cancer among women. About 90 percent of all lung cancer deaths among U.S. women smokers are attributable to smoking.
9. The risk for lung cancer increases with quantity, duration, and intensity of smoking. The risk for dying of lung cancer is 20 times higher among

women who smoke two or more packs of cigarettes per day than among women who do not smoke.

10. Lung cancer mortality rates among U.S. women have increased about 600 percent since 1950. In 1987, lung cancer surpassed breast cancer to become the leading cause of cancer death among U.S. women. Overall age-adjusted incidence rates for lung cancer among women appear to have peaked in the mid-1990s.
11. In the past, men who smoked appeared to have a higher relative risk for lung cancer than did women who smoked, but recent data suggest that such differences have narrowed considerably. Earlier findings largely reflect past gender-specific differences in duration and amount of cigarette smoking.
12. Former smokers have a lower risk for lung cancer than do current smokers, and risk declines with the number of years of smoking cessation.

*International Trends in Female Lung Cancer*

13. International lung cancer death rates among women vary dramatically. This variation reflects historical differences in the adoption of cigarette smoking by women in different countries. In 1990, lung cancer accounted for about 10 percent of all cancer deaths among women worldwide and more than 20 percent of cancer deaths among women in some developed countries.

*Female Cancers*

14. The totality of the evidence does not support an association between smoking and risk for breast cancer.
15. Several studies suggest that exposure to environmental tobacco smoke is associated with an increased risk for breast cancer, but this association remains uncertain.
16. Current smoking is associated with a reduced risk for endometrial cancer, but the effect is probably limited to postmenopausal disease. The risk for this cancer among former smokers generally appears more similar to that of women who have never smoked.
17. Smoking does not appear to be associated with risk for ovarian cancer.
18. Smoking has been consistently associated with an increased risk for cervical cancer. The extent to which this association is independent of human papillomavirus infection is uncertain.
19. Smoking may be associated with an increased risk for vulvar cancer, but the extent to which the association is independent of human papillomavirus infection is uncertain.

*Other Cancers*

20. Smoking is a major cause of cancers of the oropharynx and bladder among women. Evidence is also strong that women who smoke have increased risks for cancers of the pancreas and kidney. For cancers of the larynx and esophagus, evidence among women is more limited but consistent with large increases in risk.
21. Women who smoke may have increased risks for liver cancer and colorectal cancer.
22. Data on smoking and cancer of the stomach among women are inconsistent.
23. Smoking may be associated with an increased risk for acute myeloid leukemia among women but does not appear to be associated with other lymphoproliferative or hematologic cancers.
24. Women who smoke may have a decreased risk for thyroid cancer.
25. Women who use smokeless tobacco have an increased risk for oral cancer.

*Cardiovascular Disease*

26. Smoking is a major cause of coronary heart disease among women. For women younger than 50 years, the majority of coronary heart disease is attributable to smoking. Risk increases with the number of cigarettes smoked and the duration of smoking.
27. The risk for coronary heart disease among women is substantially reduced within 1 or 2 years of smoking cessation. This immediate benefit is followed by a continuing but more gradual reduction in risk to that among nonsmokers by 10 to 15 or more years after cessation.
28. Women who use oral contraceptives have a particularly elevated risk of coronary heart disease if they smoke. Currently evidence is conflicting as to whether the effect of hormone replacement therapy on coronary heart disease risk differs between smokers and nonsmokers.
29. Women who smoke have an increased risk for ischemic stroke and subarachnoid hemorrhage. Evidence is inconsistent concerning the association between smoking and primary intracerebral hemorrhage.
30. In most studies that include women, the increased risk for stroke associated with smoking

is reversible after smoking cessation; after 5 to 15 years of abstinence, the risk approaches that of women who have never smoked.

31. Conflicting evidence exists regarding the level of the risk for stroke among women who both smoke and use either the oral contraceptives commonly prescribed in the United States today or hormone replacement therapy.
32. Smoking is a strong predictor of the progression and severity of carotid atherosclerosis among women. Smoking cessation appears to slow the rate of progression of carotid atherosclerosis.
33. Women who are current smokers have an increased risk for peripheral vascular atherosclerosis. Smoking cessation is associated with improvements in symptoms, prognosis, and survival.
34. Women who smoke have an increased risk for death from ruptured abdominal aortic aneurysm.

***Chronic Obstructive Pulmonary Disease (COPD) and Lung Function***

35. Cigarette smoking is a primary cause of COPD among women, and the risk increases with the amount and duration of smoking. Approximately 90 percent of mortality from COPD among women in the United States can be attributed to cigarette smoking.
36. In utero exposure to maternal smoking is associated with reduced lung function among infants, and exposure to environmental tobacco smoke during childhood and adolescence may be associated with impaired lung function among girls.
37. Adolescent girls who smoke have reduced rates of lung growth, and adult women who smoke experience a premature decline of lung function.
38. The rate of decline in lung function is slower among women who stop smoking than among women who continue to smoke.
39. Mortality rates for COPD have increased among women over the past 20 to 30 years.
40. Although data for women are limited, former smokers appear to have a lower risk for dying from COPD than do current smokers.

***Sex Hormones, Thyroid Disease, and Diabetes Mellitus***

41. Women who smoke have an increased risk for estrogen-deficiency disorders and a decreased risk for estrogen-dependent disorders, but circulating levels of the major endogenous estrogens are not altered among women smokers.
42. Although consistent effects of smoking on thyroid hormone levels have not been noted, cigarette smokers may have an increased risk for Graves' ophthalmopathy, a thyroid-related disease.
43. Smoking appears to affect glucose regulation and related metabolic processes, but conflicting data exist on the relationship of smoking and the development of type 2 diabetes mellitus and gestational diabetes among women.

***Menstrual Function, Menopause, and Benign Gynecologic Conditions***

44. Some studies suggest that cigarette smoking may alter menstrual function by increasing the risks for dysmenorrhea (painful menstruation), secondary amenorrhea (lack of menses among women who ever had menstrual periods), and menstrual irregularity.
45. Women smokers have a younger age at natural menopause than do nonsmokers and may experience more menopausal symptoms.
46. Women who smoke may have decreased risk for uterine fibroids.

***Reproductive Outcomes***

47. Women who smoke have increased risks for conception delay and for both primary and secondary infertility.
48. Women who smoke may have a modest increase in risks for ectopic pregnancy and spontaneous abortion.
49. Smoking during pregnancy is associated with increased risks for preterm premature rupture of membranes, abruptio placentae, and placenta previa, and with a modest increase in risk for preterm delivery.
50. Women who smoke during pregnancy have a decreased risk for preeclampsia.
51. The risk for perinatal mortality—both stillbirth and neonatal deaths—and the risk for sudden infant death syndrome (SIDS) are increased among the offspring of women who smoke during pregnancy.
52. Infants born to women who smoke during pregnancy have a lower average birth weight and are more likely to be small for gestational age than are infants born to women who do not smoke.

53. Smoking does not appear to affect the overall risk for congenital malformations.
54. Women smokers are less likely to breastfeed their infants than are women nonsmokers.
55. Women who quit smoking before or during pregnancy reduce the risk for adverse reproductive outcomes, including conception delay, infertility, preterm premature rupture of membranes, preterm delivery, and low birth weight.

*Body Weight and Fat Distribution*

56. Initiation of cigarette smoking does not appear to be associated with weight loss, but smoking does appear to attenuate weight gain over time.
57. The average weight of women who are current smokers is modestly lower than that of women who have never smoked or who are long-term former smokers.
58. Smoking cessation among women typically is associated with a weight gain of about 6 to 12 pounds in the year after they quit smoking.
59. Women smokers have a more masculine pattern of body fat distribution (i.e., a higher waist-to-hip ratio) than do women who have never smoked.

*Bone Density and Fracture Risk*

60. Postmenopausal women who currently smoke have lower bone density than do women who do not smoke.
61. Women who currently smoke have an increased risk for hip fracture compared with women who do not smoke.
62. The relationship among women between smoking and the risk for bone fracture at sites other than the hip is not clear.

*Gastrointestinal Diseases*

63. Some studies suggest that women who smoke have an increased risk for gallbladder disease (gallstones and cholecystitis), but the evidence is inconsistent.
64. Women who smoke have an increased risk for peptic ulcers.
65. Women who currently smoke have a decreased risk for ulcerative colitis, but former smokers have an increased risk—possibly because smoking suppresses symptoms of the disease.
66. Women who smoke appear to have an increased risk for Crohn's disease, and smokers with Crohn's disease have a worse prognosis than do nonsmokers.

*Arthritis*

67. Some but not all studies suggest that women who smoke may have a modestly elevated risk for rheumatoid arthritis.
68. Women who smoke have a modestly reduced risk for osteoarthritis of the knee; data regarding osteoarthritis of the hip are inconsistent.
69. The data on the risk for systemic lupus erythematosus among women who smoke are inconsistent.

*Eye Disease*

70. Women who smoke have an increased risk for cataract.
71. Women who smoke may have an increased risk for age-related macular degeneration.
72. Studies show no consistent association between smoking and open-angle glaucoma.

*Human Immunodeficiency Virus (HIV) Disease*

73. Limited data suggest that women smokers may be at higher risk for HIV-1 infection than are nonsmokers.

*Facial Wrinkling*

74. Limited but consistent data suggest that women smokers have more facial wrinkling than do nonsmokers.

*Depression and Other Psychiatric Disorders*

75. Smokers are more likely to be depressed than are nonsmokers, a finding that may reflect an effect of smoking on the risk for depression, the use of smoking for self-medication, or the influence of common genetic or other factors on both smoking and depression. The association of smoking and depression is particularly important among women because they are more likely to be diagnosed with depression than are men.
76. The prevalence of smoking generally has been found to be higher among patients with anxiety disorders, bulimia, attention deficit disorder, and alcoholism than among individuals without these conditions; the mechanisms underlying these associations are not yet understood.
77. The prevalence of smoking is very high among patients with schizophrenia, but the mechanisms underlying this association are not yet understood.

78. Smoking may be used by some persons who would otherwise manifest psychiatric symptoms to manage those symptoms; for such persons, cessation of smoking may lead to the emergence of depression or other dysphoric mood states.

*Neurologic Diseases*

79. Women who smoke have a decreased risk for Parkinson's disease.
80. Data regarding the association between smoking and Alzheimer's disease are inconsistent.

*Nicotine Pharmacology and Addiction*

81. Nicotine pharmacology and the behavioral processes that determine nicotine addiction appear generally similar among women and men; when standardized for the number of cigarettes smoked, the blood concentration of cotinine (the main metabolite of nicotine) is similar among women and men.
82. Women's regulation of nicotine intake may be less precise than men's. Factors other than nicotine (e.g., sensory cues) may play a greater role in determining smoking behavior among women.

*Environmental Tobacco Smoke (ETS) and Lung Cancer*

83. Exposure to ETS is a cause of lung cancer among women who have never smoked.

*ETS and Coronary Heart Disease*

84. Epidemiologic and other data support a causal relationship between ETS exposure from the spouse and coronary heart disease mortality among women nonsmokers.

*ETS and Reproductive Outcomes*

85. Infants born to women who are exposed to ETS during pregnancy may have a small decrement in birth weight and a slightly increased risk for intrauterine growth retardation compared with infants born to women who are not exposed; both effects are quite variable across studies.
86. Studies of ETS exposure and the risks for delay in conception, spontaneous abortion, and perinatal mortality are few, and the results are inconsistent.

# Appendix. Description of Epidemiologic Studies Relating to Total Mortality

## Studies Measuring Death Rates

### American Cancer Society Cancer Prevention Studies

The American Cancer Society (ACS) Cancer Prevention Studies I and II (CPS-I and CPS-II) are the largest prospective studies of smoking and mortality among women (Table 3.1). Because the two studies were similar with respect to selection and follow-up (Garfinkel 1985; Stellman and Garfinkel 1986; Garfinkel and Stellman 1988), they provide a longitudinal perspective on how smoking attributable risk changed among U.S. women from the late 1950s through the 1980s (U.S. Department of Health and Human Services [USDHHS] 1989b; Thun et al. 1995, 1997a). CPS-I covered 25 states (Hammond 1966); CPS-II was nationwide. Participants were recruited by ACS volunteers in the fall of 1959 and in the fall of 1982, respectively. Volunteers sought to recruit participants from among their friends, neighbors, and acquaintances and to interview all adults aged 30 years or older in the households. Compared with the general U.S. population, participants were older, had more years of education, and were more likely to be married and to be in the middle class. Whites made up 97 and 93 percent of CPS-I and CPS-II participants, respectively. At the start of the study, CPS-I included 391,748 women who had never smoked cigarettes and 152,228 who were current smokers. During the six years of follow-up, 28,922 deaths occurred (Table 3.1). Women in CPS-II included 355,518 women who had never smoked cigarettes (15,450 deaths), 126,794 current smokers (6,232 deaths), and 121,802 former smokers (4,663 deaths). During the six years of follow-up, 26,345 deaths occurred.

### British Doctors' Study

The British doctors' study was a landmark prospective study of tobacco smoking and mortality (Doll and Hill 1966; Doll et al. 1980, 1994). In 1951, the British Medical Association mailed to all British physicians a questionnaire inquiring about smoking and other lifestyle habits; 6,194 female physicians and 34,439 male physicians responded to the survey. The women in this study represented 60 percent of female British physicians at the time. Updated information was obtained in 1961 and again in 1973 on all but 1.8 and 4.1 percent, respectively, of the surviving female physicians. Results from 1973, reflecting 22 years of follow-up, have been published (Doll et al. 1980); 1,094 deaths had occurred among the women (Table 3.1). Four of these deaths were excluded from the analyses because the participants smoked tobacco products other than cigarettes. Of the data from the 40-year follow-up, results for the men physicians have been published (Doll et al. 1994), but results for the women physicians have not been published.

### Japanese Study of 29 Health Districts

In late 1965, 142,857 women and 122,261 men aged 40 years or older in Japan were enrolled in the Japanese study of 29 health districts (Hirayama 1990) (Table 3.1). Participants represented a range of 91 to 99 percent of adults in this age group in these districts. Information on tobacco smoking was obtained by a self-administered questionnaire at enrollment. After 6 years, reinterview of 3,728 randomly selected women showed that the percentage of smokers had decreased only slightly (from 10.4 to 9.7 percent). During 17 years of follow-up (through 1982), 23,544 deaths among women occurred (Table 3.1). This is the only large prospective study of smoking and mortality in a non-Western culture.

### U.S. Nurses' Health Study

In 1976, in the U.S. Nurses' Health Study, 121,700 female registered nurses aged 30 through 55 years completed and returned a mailed questionnaire requesting information on current and past smoking habits (Kawachi et al. 1993a, 1997b). Follow-up questionnaires were subsequently mailed every 2 years to update information on smoking behavior, other cardiovascular risk factors, and development of major illnesses. During the first 12 years of follow-up (through April 30, 1988), deaths occurred among 2,847 of the 117,001 female nurses who, at the start of the study, were free from manifest coronary heart disease, stroke, and cancer (except nonmelanoma skin cancer) (Table 3.1) (Kawachi et al. 1993a, 1997b). Of the 2,847 nurses who died, 933 had never smoked, 799 were former smokers, and 1,115 were current smokers. The U.S. Nurses' Health Study is one of five prospective studies of smoking among women that have been started since 1975.

### Kaiser Permanente Medical Care Program Study

Between 1979 and 1986, the Kaiser Permanente Medical Care Program obtained baseline information about tobacco smoking from 36,035 women and 24,803 men aged 35 years or older (Table 3.1) (Friedman et al. 1997). Participants in the program make up about 30 percent of the population in the areas it serves. Follow-up through 1987 identified 1,098 deaths among all women (308 current smokers, 165 former smokers, and 625 women who had never smoked). This study provides the only published data on premature death associated with cigarette smoking among African American women.

### Leisure World Cohort Study

Information on tobacco use and other factors was collected in 1981 from questionnaires that were mailed and returned by 8,869 women and 4,999 men who lived in the affluent Leisure World Retirement community in southern California (Paganini-Hill and Hsu 1994). Participants who completed the questionnaire (61 percent of the community) had a median age of 73 years at the start of the study. During 9.5 years of follow-up (through December 1990), 1,987 deaths occurred among women and 2,015 among men (Table 3.1). This is one of two prospective studies of a population consisting primarily of older adults.

### Study of Three U.S. Communities

From 1981 through 1983, 4,469 women and 2,709 men aged 65 years or older were enrolled in a study at three sites: East Boston, Massachusetts; rural Iowa; and New Haven, Connecticut (LaCroix et al. 1991). The participants were interviewed by telephone annually during the five years of follow-up, which was completed in 1988. Approximately 82 percent of the target population were enrolled in the study. There were 1,442 deaths from all causes, but the number among women was not specified. One objective of the study was to measure the impact of continued smoking on death rates among older adults.

## Studies Measuring Probability of Death

### Framingham Study

The Framingham study began in 1948 with a cohort of 5,209 white adults (2,873 women and 2,336 men) aged 30 through 62 years when they were first examined in Framingham, Massachusetts, between 1948 and 1952 (Freund et al. 1993). Information on smoking was obtained at the first examination. Surviving members of the original sample and volunteers were generally reexamined and reinterviewed about smoking at 2-year intervals. Deaths were identified from interviews with next of kin and death certificates. Results over the first 18 years of follow-up (through 1966) were expressed as cumulative incidence or probability of death (Table 3.1 and Figure 3.4) (Shurtleff 1974). During that time, 296 deaths occurred among women participants. Subsequent analyses of pooled biennial data were undertaken to determine annual death rates (Cupples and D'Agostino 1987; Freund et al. 1993). However, investigators could not control for the changing background cardiovascular death rates, and, therefore, data from those analyses are not included here.

### Canadian Pensioners' Study

Beginning in 1955, the Department of National Health and Welfare, Canada, enrolled 14,226 women (mostly widows of veterans) and 77,541 men (veterans on pension) younger than age 30 years to over age 80 years in the Canadian pensioners' study—a study of smoking-related mortality (Best et al. 1961). During the six years of follow-up, 9,491 of the men and 1,794 of the women died. The association between smoking and all-cause mortality among women that is shown in Figure 3.4 is from the final report of this study (Canadian Department of National Health and Welfare 1966).

### British-Norwegian Migrant Study

In October 1962, questionnaires on morbidity requesting information on personal and demographic characteristics, including cigarette smoking and symptoms of cardiorespiratory disease, were sent to approximately 32,000 British migrants and 18,000 Norwegian migrants to the United States. At that time, three-fourths of the British and Norwegian immigrants to the United States resided in 12 states

(Pearl et al. 1966). The questionnaires were sent to all British and Norwegian migrants, who made up a 25-percent random sample of all residents of those states for whom country of birth was recorded in the 1960 U.S. Census. The response rate was 86 percent. The respondents then were followed up for survival and cause of death for five years, from January 1, 1963, through December 31, 1967. Responses to the questionnaire were received from 9,057 female British migrants and 5,337 female Norwegian migrants (Table 3.1). During the five-year follow-up, 588 female British migrants and 354 female Norwegian migrants died. The cumulative probability ratios shown in Figure 3.4 were obtained from the 1980 Surgeon General's report on the health consequences of smoking among women (USDHHS 1980). The raw data are no longer available to calculate 95 percent confidence intervals.

**Swedish Study**

In 1963, questionnaires about smoking were mailed to a national probability sample of 55,000 Swedish adults (27,732 women) aged 18 through 69 years (Cederlöf et al. 1975). The response rate was 89 percent. On the basis of information about smoking status in 1963 and linkage with national death registries over the ensuing 10 years, RR for death was estimated among women who currently or formerly smoked cigarettes compared with women who had never smoked. The results for 10 years of follow-up were published in 1975 (Table 3.1).

## References


Abi-Said D, Annegers JF, Combs-Cantrell D, Frankowski RF, Willmore LJ. Case-control study of the risk factors for eclampsia. *American Journal of Epidemiology* 1995; 142(4):437–41.

Adami H-O, Lund E, Bergstrom R, Meirik O. Cigarette smoking, alcohol consumption and risk of breast cancer in young women. *British Journal of Cancer* 1988;58(6):832–7.

Adami J, Nyren O, Bergstrom R, Ekborn A, Enghom A, Enghom G, Englund A, Glimelius B. Smoking and the risk of leukemia, lymphoma, and multiple myeloma (Sweden). *Cancer Causes and Control* 1998; 9(1):49–56.

Adena MA, Gallagher HG. Cigarette smoking and the age at menopause. *Annals of Human Biology* 1982; 9(2):121–30.

Adriaanse HP, Knottnerus JA, Delgado LR, Cox HH, Essed GGM. Smoking in Dutch pregnant women and birth weight. *Patient Education and Counseling* 1996;28(1):25–30.

Aevarsson O, Skoog I. A population-based study on the incidence of dementia disorders between 85 and 88 years of age. *Journal of the American Geriatrics Society* 1996;44(12):1455–60.

Aguayo SM. Determinants of susceptibility to cigarette smoke: potential roles for neuroendocrine cells and neuropeptides in airway inflammation, airway wall remodeling, and chronic airflow obstruction. *American Journal of Respiratory and Critical Care Medicine* 1994;149(6):1692–8.

Ahlborg G Jr. Health effects of environmental tobacco smoke on the offspring of non-smoking women. *Journal of Smoking-Related Disorders* 1994;5(Suppl 1): 107–12.

Ahlborg G Jr, Bodin L. Tobacco smoke exposure and pregnancy outcome among working women: a prospective study at prenatal care centers in Örebro County, Sweden. *American Journal of Epidemiology* 1991;133(4):338–47.

Ahlsten G, Cnattingius S, Lindmark G. Cessation of smoking during pregnancy improves foetal growth and reduces infant morbidity in the neonatal period. A population-based prospective study. *Acta Paediatrica* 1993;82(2):177–81.

Ahluwalia IB, Grummer-Strawn L, Scanlon KS. Exposure to environmental tobacco smoke and birth outcome: increased effects on pregnant women aged 30 years or older. *American Journal of Epidemiology* 1997;146(1):42–7.

Akiba S, Hirayama T. Cigarette smoking and cancer mortality risk in Japanese men and women: results from reanalysis of the six-prefecture cohort study data. *Environmental Health Perspectives* 1990; 87:19–26.

Akiba S, Kato H, Blot WJ. Passive smoking and lung cancer among Japanese women. *Cancer Research* 1986;46(9):4804–7.

Akre J, editor. Infant feeding. The physiological basis. *Bulletin of the World Health Organization* 1989;67 (Suppl):1–108.

Alameda County Low Birth Weight Study Group. Cigarette smoking and the risk of low birth weight: a comparison in black and white women. *Epidemiology* 1990;1(3):201–5.

Alavanja MCR, Brown CC, Swanson C, Brownson RC. Saturated fat intake and lung cancer risk among nonsmoking women in Missouri. *Journal of the National Cancer Institute* 1993;85(23):1906–16.

Albanes D, Jones DY, Micozzi MS, Mattson ME. Associations between smoking and body weight in the US population: analysis of NHANES II. *American Journal of Public Health* 1987;77(4):439–44.

Alberman E, Creasy M, Elliott M, Spicer C. Maternal factors associated with fetal chromosomal anomalies in spontaneous abortions. *British Journal of Obstetrics and Gynaecology* 1976;83(8):621–7.

Alderete E, Eskenazi B, Sholtz R. Effect of cigarette smoking and coffee drinking on time to conception. *Epidemiology* 1995;6(4):403–8.

Alderman BW, Bradley CM, Greene C, Fernbach SK, Baron AE. Increased risk of craniosynostosis with maternal cigarette smoking during pregnancy. *Teratology* 1994;50(1):13–8.

Alexander FE, Roberts MM. The menopause and breast cancer. *Journal of Epidemiology and Community Health* 1987;41(2):94–100.

Allen HB, Johnson BL, Diamond SM. Smoker's wrinkles? *Journal of the American Medical Association* 1973;225(9):1067–9.

Aloia JF, Cohn SH, Vaswani A, Yeh JK, Yuen K, Ellis K. Risk factors for postmenopausal osteoporosis. *American Journal of Medicine* 1985;78(1):95–100.

Aloia JF, Vaswani AN, Yeh JK, Ross P, Ellis K, Cohn SH. Determinants of bone mass in postmenopausal women. *Archives of Internal Medicine* 1983; 143(9):1700–4.

Alp MH, Hislop IG, Grant AK. Gastric ulcer in South Australia 1954–1963. I. Epidemiological factors. *Medical Journal of Australia* 1970;2(24):1128–32.

Alpha-Tocopherol Beta-Carotene Cancer Prevention Study Group. The effect of vitamin E and beta carotene on the incidence of lung cancer and other cancers in male smokers. *New England Journal of Medicine* 1994;330(15):1029–35.

Ambrosone CB, Freudenheim JL, Graham S, Marshall JR, Vena JE, Brasure JR, Laughlin R, Nemoto T, Michalek AM, Harrington A, Ford TD, Shields PG. Cytochrome P4501A1 and glutathione *S*-transferase (M1) genetic polymorphisms and postmenopausal breast cancer risk. *Cancer Research* 1995;55(16):3483–5.

Ambrosone CB, Freudenheim JL, Graham S, Marshall JR, Vena JE, Brasure JR, Michalek AM, Laughlin R, Nemoto T, Gillenwater KA, Shields PG. Cigarette smoking, *N*-acetyltransferase 2 genetic polymorphisms, and breast cancer risk. *Journal of the American Medical Association* 1996;276(18):1494–501.

American Psychiatric Association. *Diagnostic and Statistical Manual of Mental Disorders, 3rd ed., Revised. DSM-III-R.* Washington: American Psychiatric Association, 1987.

American Psychiatric Association. *Diagnostic and Statistical Manual of Mental Disorders, 4th ed. DSM-IV*. Washington: American Psychiatric Association, 1994.

American Thoracic Society. Standards for the diagnosis and care of patients with chronic obstructive pulmonary disease (COPD) and asthma. *American Review of Respiratory Disease* 1987;136(1):225–44.

Amos CI, Caporaso NE, Weston A. Host factors in lung cancer risk: a review of interdisciplinary studies. *Cancer Epidemiology, Biomarkers and Prevention* 1992;1(6):505–13.

Ananth CV, Savitz DA, Luther ER. Maternal cigarette smoking as a risk factor for placental abruption, placenta previa, and uterine bleeding in pregnancy. *American Journal of Epidemiology* 1996;144(9): 881–9.

Ananth CV, Smulian JC, Vintzileos AM. Incidence of placental abruption in relation to cigarette smoking and hypertensive disorders during pregnancy: a meta-analysis of observational studies. *Obstetrics and Gynecology* 1999;93(4):622–8.

Anda RF, Williamson DF, Escobedo LG, Mast EE, Giovino GA, Remington PL. Depression and the dynamics of smoking: a national perspective. *Journal of the American Medical Association* 1990a; 264(12):1541–5.

Anda RF, Williamson DF, Escobedo LG, Remington PL. Smoking and the risk of peptic ulcer disease among women in the United States. *Archives of Internal Medicine* 1990b;150(7):1437–41.

Andersch B, Milsom I. An epidemiologic study of young women with dysmenorrhea. *American Journal of Obstetrics and Gynecology* 1982;144(6): 655–60.

Andersen AN, Lund-Andersen C, Larsen JF, Christensen NJ, Legros JJ, Louis F, Angelo H, Molin J. Suppressed prolactin but normal neurophysin levels in cigarette-smoking breast-feeding women. *Clinical Endocrinology* 1982a;17(4):363–8.

Andersen AN, Schiöler V. Influence of breast-feeding pattern on pituitary-ovarian axis of women in an industrialized community. *American Journal of Obstetrics and Gynecology* 1982;143(6):673–7.

Andersen AN, Semczuk M, Tabor A. Prolactin and pituitary-gonadal function in cigarette smoking infertile patients. *Andrologia* 1984;16(5):391–6.

Andersen FS, Transbøl I, Christiansen C. Is cigarette smoking a promoter of the menopause? *Acta Medica Scandinavica* 1982b;212(3):137–9.

Andersen RA, Kasperbauer MJ, Burton HR, Hamilton JI, Yoder EE. Changes in chemical composition of homogenized leaf-cured and air-cured burley tobacco stored in controlled environments. *Journal of Agricultural and Food Chemistry* 1982c;30(4):663–8.

Andersen WA, Franquemont DW, Williams J, Taylor PT, Crum CP. Vulvar squamous cell carcinoma and papillomaviruses: two separate entities? *American Journal of Obstetrics and Gynecology* 1991; 165(2):329–36.

Anderson JJ, Felson DT. Factors associated with osteoarthritis of the knee in the first National Health and Nutrition Examination Survey (HANES 1): evidence for an association with overweight, race, and physical demands of work. *American Journal of Epidemiology* 1988;128(1):179–89.

Andersson B, Marin P, Lissner L, Vermeulen A, Björntorp P. Testosterone concentrations in women and men with NIDDM. *Diabetes Care* 1994;17(5):405–11.

Andersson K, Eneroth P, Fuxe K, Mascagni F, Agnati LF. Effects of chronic exposure to cigarette smoke on amine levels and turnover in various hypothalamic catecholamine nerve terminal systems and on the secretion of pituitary hormones in the male rat. *Neuroendocrinology* 1985;41(6):462–6.

Anthonisen NR, Connett JE, Kiley JP, Altose MD, Bailey WC, Buist AS, Conway WA Jr, Enright PL, Kanner RE, O'Hara P, Owens GR, Scanlon PD, Tashkin DP, Wise RA. Effects of smoking intervention and the use of an inhaled anticholinergic bronchodilator on the rate of decline of $FEV_1$. *Journal of the American Medical Association* 1994; 272(19):1497–505.

Aral SO, Holmes KK. Epidemiology of sexual behavior and sexually transmitted diseases. In: Holmes KK, Mardh P-A, Sparling PF, Wiesner PJ, editors. *Sexually Transmitted Diseases.* 2nd ed. New York: McGraw-Hill, 1990:19–36.

Armellini F, Zamboni M, Frigo L, Mandragona R, Robbi R, Micciolo R, Bosello O. Alcohol consumption, smoking habits and body fat distribution in Italian men and women aged 20–60 years. *European Journal of Clinical Nutrition* 1993;47(1):52–60.

Armitage AK, Dollery CT, George CF, Houseman TH, Lewis PJ, Turner DM. Absorption and metabolism of nicotine from cigarettes. *British Medical Journal* 1975;4(5992):313–6.

Armstrong BG, McDonald AD, Sloan M. Cigarette, alcohol, and coffee consumption and spontaneous abortion. *American Journal of Public Health* 1992; 82(1):85–7.

Aronson RA, Uttech S, Soref M. The effect of maternal cigarette smoking on low birth weight and preterm birth in Wisconsin, 1991. *Wisconsin Medical Journal* 1993;92(11):613–7.

Atrash HK, Hughes JM, Hogue CJ. Ectopic pregnancy in the United States, 1970–1983. *Morbidity and Mortality Weekly Report* 1986;35(SS-2):2955–3755.

Auerbach O, Garfinkel L. The changing pattern of lung carcinoma. *Cancer* 1991;68(9):1973–7.

Augood C, Duckitt K, Templeton AA. Smoking and female infertility: a systematic review and meta-analysis. *Human Reproduction* 1998;13(6):1532–9.

Austin DF, Reynolds P. Laryngeal cancer. In: Schottenfeld D, Fraumeni JF, editors. *Cancer Epidemiology and Prevention.* 2nd ed. New York: Oxford University Press, 1996:619–36.

Austin H, Drews C, Partridge EE. A case-control study of endometrial cancer in relation to cigarette smoking, serum estrogen levels, and alcohol use. *American Journal of Obstetrics and Gynecology* 1993;169(5):1086–91.

Avery ME, Frantz ID III. To breathe or not to breathe—what have we learned about apneic spells and sudden infant death? *New England Journal of Medicine* 1983;309(2):107–8.

Bachman DL, Wolf PA, Linn R, Knoefel JE, Cobb J, Belanger A, D'Agostino RB, White LR. Prevalence of dementia and probable senile dementia of the Alzheimer type in the Framingham Study. *Neurology* 1992;42(1):115–9.

Bachman DL, Wolf PA, Linn RT, Knoefel JE, Cobb JL, Belanger AJ, White LR, D'Agostino RB. Incidence of dementia and probable Alzheimer's disease in a general population: the Framingham Study. *Neurology* 1993;43(3 Pt 1):515–9.

Backe B. Maternal smoking and age: effect on birthweight and risk for small-for-gestational age births. *Acta Obstetricia et Gynecologica Scandinavica* 1993; 72(3):172–6.

Bagge E, Bjelle A, Edén S, Svanborg A. Factors associated with radiographic osteoarthritis: results from the population study of 70-year-old people in Göteborg. *Journal of Rheumatology* 1991;18(8): 1218–22.

Bagge E, Eden S, Rosen T, Bengtsson BA. The prevalence of radiographic osteoarthritis is low in elderly patients with growth hormone deficiency. *Acta Endocrinologica (Copenhagen)* 1993;129(4):296–300.

Bailey A, Robinson D, Vessey M. Smoking and age of natural menopause [letter]. *Lancet* 1977;2(8040): 722.

Baird DD, Wilcox AJ. Cigarette smoking associated with delayed conception. *Journal of the American Medical Association* 1985;253(20):2979–83.

Baird DD, Wilcox AJ, Weinberg CR. Use of time to pregnancy to study environmental exposures. *American Journal of Epidemiology* 1986;124(3): 470–80.

Bakketeig LS, Jacobsen G, Hoffman HJ, Lindmark G, Bergsjo P, Molne K, Rodsten J. Pre-pregnancy risk factors of small-for-gestational age births among parous women in Scandinavia. *Acta Obstetricia et Gynecologica Scandinavica* 1993;72(4):273–9.

Baldinger B, Hasenfratz M, Bättig K. Switching to ultralow nicotine cigarettes: effects of different tar yields and blocking of olfactory cues. *Pharmacology, Biochemistry and Behavior* 1995;50(2):233–9.

Balfour DJ. The influence of stress on psychopharmacological responses to nicotine. *British Journal of Addiction* 1991;86(5):489–93.

Balkau B, King H, Zimmet P, Raper LR. Factors associated with the development of diabetes in the Micronesian population of Nauru. *American Journal of Epidemiology* 1985;122(4):594–605.

Bang KM. Prevalence of chronic obstructive pulmonary disease in blacks. *Journal of the National Medical Association* 1993;85(1):51–5.

Baranski B. Effect of exposure of pregnant rats to cadmium on prenatal and postnatal development of the young. *Journal of Hygiene, Epidemiology, Microbiology and Immunology* 1985;29(3):253–62.

Baranski B, Stetkiewicz I, Trzcinka-Ochocka M, Sitarek K, Szymczak W. Teratogenicity, fetal toxicity and tissue concentration of cadmium administered to female rats during organogenesis. *Journal of Applied Toxicology* 1982;2(5):255–9.

Bardhan KD, Graham DY, Hunt RH, O'Morain CA. Effects of smoking on cure of Helicobacter pylori infection and duodenal ulcer recurrence in patients treated with clarithromycin and omeprazole. *Helicobacter* 1997;2(1):27–31.

Bardy AH, Seppälä T, Lillsunde P, Kataja JM, Koskela P, Pikkarainen J, Hiilesmaa VK. Objectively measured tobacco exposure during pregnancy: neonatal effects and relation to maternal smoking. *British Journal of Obstetrics and Gynaecology* 1993; 100(8):721–6.

Barkley RA. *Attention-Deficit Hyperactivity Disorder: A Handbook for Diagnosis and Treatment*. New York: Guilford Press, 1990.

Barkley RA, Fischer M, Edelbrock CS, Smallish L. The adolescent outcome of hyperactive children diagnosed by research criteria: I. An 8-year prospective follow-up study. *Journal of the American Academy of Child and Adolescent Psychiatry* 1990;29(4):546–57.

Baron JA. Cigarette smoking and Parkinson's disease. *Neurology* 1986;36(11):1490–6.

Baron JA, Barrett J, Malenka D, Fisher E, Kniffin W, Bubolz T, Tosteson T. Racial differences in fracture risk. *Epidemiology* 1994a;5(1):42–7.

Baron JA, Bulbrook RD, Wang DY, Kwa HG. Cigarette smoking and prolactin in women. *British Medical Journal* 1986a;293(6545):482–3.

Baron JA, Byers T, Greenberg ER, Cummings KM, Swanson M. Cigarette smoking in women with cancers of the breast and reproductive organs. *Journal of the National Cancer Institute* 1986b;77(3): 677–80.

Baron JA, Gerhardsson deVerdier M, Ekbom A. Coffee, tea, tobacco, and cancer of the large bowel. *Cancer Epidemiology, Biomarkers and Prevention* 1994b; 3(7):565–70.

Baron JA, Karagas M, Barrett J, Kniffin W, Malenka D, Mayor M, Keller RB. Basic epidemiology of fractures of the upper and lower limb among Americans over 65 years of age. *Epidemiology* 1996a;7(6): 612–8.

Baron JA, La Vecchia C, Levi F. The antiestrogenic effect of cigarette smoking in women. *American Journal of Obstetrics and Gynecology* 1990;162(2):502–14.

Baron JA, Newcomb PA, Longnecker MP, Mittendorf R, Storer BE, Clapp RW, Bogdan G, Yuen J. Cigarette smoking and breast cancer. *Cancer Epidemiology, Biomarkers and Prevention* 1996b;5(5):399–403.

Barrett-Connor E. Smoking and endogenous sex hormones in men and women. In: Wald N, Baron JA, editors. *Smoking and Hormone-Related Disorders*. New York: Oxford University Press, 1990:183–96.

Barrett-Connor E, Khaw K-T. Cigarette smoking and increased central adiposity. *Annals of Internal Medicine* 1989;111(10):783–7.

Barrett-Connor E, Khaw KT, Wingard DL. A ten-year prospective study of coronary heart disease mortality among Rancho Bernardo women. In: Eaker ED, Packard B, Wenger NK, Clarkson TB, Tyroler HA, editors. *Coronary Heart Disease in Women. Proceedings of an N.I.H. Workshop*. New York: Haymarket Doyma, 1987:117–21.

Barsky SH, Cameron R, Osann KE, Tomita D, Holmes EC. Rising incidence of bronchioloalveolar lung carcinoma and its unique clinicopathologic features. *Cancer* 1994;73(4):1163–70.

Bartalena L, Martino E, Marcocci C, Bogazzi F, Panicucci M, Velluzzi F, Loviselli A, Pinchera A. More on smoking habits and Graves' ophthalmopathy. *Journal of Endocrinological Investigation* 1989;12(10): 733–7.

Barton SE, Maddox PH, Jenkins D, Edwards R, Cuzick J, Singer A. Effect of cigarette smoking on cervical epithelial immunity: a mechanism for neoplastic change? *Lancet* 1988;2(8612):652–4.

Basso L, McCollum PT, Darling MR, Tocchi A, Tanner WA. A descriptive study of pregnant women with gallstones. Relation to dietary and social habits, education, physical activity, height, and weight. *European Journal of Epidemiology* 1992;8(5):629–33.

Bättig K, Buzzi R, Nil R. Smoke yield of cigarettes and puffing behavior in men and women. *Psychopharmacology (Berlin)* 1982;76(2):139–48.

Bauer DC, Browner WS, Cauley JA, Orwoll ES, Scott JC, Black DM, Tao JL, Cummings SR. Factors associated with appendicular bone mass in older women. *Annals of Internal Medicine* 1993;118(9): 657–65.

Becker TM, Wheeler CM, McGough NS, Parmenter CA, Stidley CA, Jamison SF, Jordan SW. Cigarette smoking and other risk factors for cervical dysplasia in southwestern Hispanic and non-Hispanic white women. *Cancer Epidemiology, Biomarkers and Prevention* 1994;3(2):113–9.

Beckett AH, Gorrod JW, Jenner P. The effect of smoking on nicotine metabolism *in vivo* in man. *Journal of Pharmacy and Pharmacology* 1971;23(Suppl): 62S–67S.

Behm FM, Levin ED, Lee YK, Rose JE. Low-nicotine regenerated smoke aerosol reduces desire for cigarettes. *Journal of Substance Abuse* 1990;2(2):237–47.

Behm FM, Schur C, Levin ED, Tashkin DP, Rose JE. Clinical evaluation of a citric acid inhaler for smoking cessation. *Drug and Alcohol Dependence* 1993;31(2):131–8.

Bell BA, Ambrose J. Smoking and the risk of a stroke. *Acta Neurochirurgica* 1982;64(1–2):1–7.

Bell R, Lumley J. Alcohol consumption, cigarette smoking and fetal outcome in Victoria, 1985. *Community Health Studies* 1989;13(4):484–91.

Benhamou E, Benhamou S, Flamant R. Lung cancer and women: results of a French case-control study. *British Journal of Cancer* 1987;55(1):91–5.

Benhamou S, Benhamou E. The effect of age at smoking initiation on lung cancer risk [letter]. *Epidemiology* 1994;5(5):560.

Bennett WP, Hussain SP, Vahakangas KH, Khan MA, Shields PG, Harris CC. Molecular epidemiology of human cancer risk: gene-environment interactions and *p53* mutation spectrum in human lung cancer. *Journal of Pathology* 1999;187(1):8–18.

Bennicke K, Conrad C, Sabroe S, Sorensen HT. Cigarette smoking and breast cancer. *British Medical Journal* 1995;310(6992):1431–3.

Benoni C, Nilsson Å. Smoking habits in patients with inflammatory bowel disease. A case-control study. Scandinavian *Journal of Gastroenterology* 1987;22(9): 1130–6.

Benoni C, Nilsson Å, Nived O. Smoking and inflammatory bowel disease: comparison with systemic lupus erythematosus. A case-control study. *Scandinavian Journal of Gastroenterology* 1990;25(7):751–5.

Benowitz NL. Cigarette smoking and nicotine addiction. *Medical Clinics of North America* 1992;76(2): 415–37.

Benowitz NL. Treating tobacco addiction—nicotine or no nicotine? *New England Journal of Medicine* 1997; 337(17):1230–1.

Benowitz NL, Hall SM, Herning RI, Jacob P III, Jones RT, Osman A-L. Smokers of low-yield cigarettes do not consume less nicotine. *New England Journal of Medicine* 1983;309(3):139–42.

Benowitz NL, Hatsukami D. Gender differences in the pharmacology of nicotine addiction. *Addiction Biology* 1998;3:383–404.

Benowitz NL, Jacob P III. Daily intake of nicotine during cigarette smoking. *Clinical Pharmacology and Therapeutics* 1984;35(4):499–504.

Benowitz NL, Jacob P III. Metabolism of nicotine to cotinine studied by a dual stable isotope method. *Clinical Pharmacology and Therapeutics* 1994;56(5): 483–93.

Benowitz NL, Porchet H, Jacob P III. Pharmacokinetics, metabolism, and pharmacodynamics of nicotine. In: Wonnacott S, Russell MAH, Stolerman IP, editors. *Nicotine Psychopharmacology: Molecular, Cellular and Behavioural Aspects*. Oxford: Oxford University Press, 1990:112–57.

Berg CJ, Atrash HK, Koonin LM, Tucker M. Pregnancy-related mortality in the United States, 1987–1990. *Obstetrics and Gynecology* 1996;88(2):161–7.

Berggren C, Sjostedt S. Preinvasive carcinoma of the cervix uteri and smoking. *Acta Obstetrica et Gynecologica Scandinavica* 1983;62(6):593–8.

Berghout A, Wiersinga WM, Smits NJ, Touber JL. Determinants of thyroid volume as measured by ultrasonography in healthy adults in a non-iodine deficient area. *Clinical Endocrinology* 1987;26(3): 273–80.

Bergman AB, Wiesner LA. Relationship of passive cigarette-smoking to sudden infant death syndrome. *Pediatrics* 1976;58(5):665–8.

Berkowitz GS, Canny PF, Livolsi VA, Merino MJ, O'Connor TZ, Kelsey JL. Cigarette smoking and benign breast disease. *Journal of Epidemiology and Community Health* 1985;39(4):308–13.

Berkowitz GS, Lapinski RH, Wein R, Lee D. Race/ethnicity and other risk factors for gestational diabetes. *American Journal of Epidemiology* 1992;135(9): 965–73.

Berlin I, Cournot A, Renout P, Duchier J, Safar M. Peripheral haemodynamic effects of smoking in habitual smokers: a methodological study. *European Journal of Clinical Pharmacology* 1990;38(1): 57–60.

Berndt VH, Gütz H-J. Versuche zur langzeittherapie mit carbenoxolon beim ulcus duodeni. *Deutsche Zeitschrift fuer Verdauungsund Stoffwechselkrankheiten* 1981;41:98–102.

Bernstein L, Pike MC, Lobo RA, Depue RH, Ross RK, Henderson BE. Cigarette smoking in pregnancy results in marked decrease in maternal hCG and oestradiol levels. *British Journal of Obstetrics and Gynaecology* 1989;96(1):92–6.

Bernstein L, Ross RK. Endogenous hormones and breast cancer risk. *Epidemiologic Reviews* 1993;15(1): 48–65.

Berta L, Fortunati N, Gennari P, Appendino P, Casella M, Frairia R. Influence of cigarette smoking on pituitary and sex hormone balance in healthy premenopausal women. *Fertility and Sterility* 1991; 56(4):788–9.

Berta L, Frairia R, Fortunati N, Fazzari A, Gaidano G. Smoking effects on the hormonal balance of fertile women. *Hormone Research* 1992;37(1–2):45–8.

Bertelsen JB, Hegedüs L. Cigarette smoking and the thyroid. *Thyroid* 1994;4(3):327–31.

Bertschinger P, Lacher G, Aenishänslin W, Baerlocher C, Bernoulli R, Egger G, Eisner M, Fasel F, Fehr H-R, Fumagalli I, Gassmann R, Güller R, Kobler E, Leuthold E, Nuesch H-J, Pace F, Pelloni S,

Plancherel P, Realini S, Seiler P, Stocker H, Vetter D, Schmid P, Simonian B, Vogel E, Blum AL. Presenting characteristics of patients with duodenal ulcer and outcome of medical treatment in controlled clinical trials using cimetidine and diethylamine persilate to treat ulcer attack and diethylamine persilate and placebo to prevent relapses. *Digestion* 1987;36(3):148–61.

Bérubé S, Marcoux S, Maheux R, Canadian Collaborative Group on Endometriosis. Characteristics related to the prevalence of minimal or mild endometriosis in infertile women. *Epidemiology* 1998; 9(5):504–10.

Best EWR, Josie GH, Walker CB. A Canadian study of mortality in relation to smoking habits: a preliminary report. *Canadian Journal of Public Health* 1961; 52(3):99–106.

Bhattacharyya MH, Whelton BD, Stern PH, Peterson DP. Cadmium accelerates bone loss in ovariectomized mice and fetal rat limb bones in culture. *Proceedings of the National Academy of Sciences of the United States of America* 1988;85(22):8761–5.

Biederman J, Faraone SV, Spencer T, Wilens T, Mick E, Lapey K. Gender differences in a sample of adults with attention deficit hyperactivity disorder. *Psychiatry Research* 1994;53(1):13–29.

Bilbrey GL, Weix J, Kaplan GD. Value of single photon absorptiometry in osteoporosis screening. *Clinical Nuclear Medicine* 1988;13(1):7–12.

Bjornson W, Rand C, Connett JE, Lindgren P, Nides M, Pope F, Buist AS, Hoppe-Ryan C, O'Hara P. Gender differences in smoking cessation after 3 years in the Lung Health Study. *American Journal of Public Health* 1995;85(2):223–30.

Björntorp P. Abdominal obesity and the development of noninsulin-dependent diabetes mellitus. *Diabetes/Metabolism Reviews* 1988;4(6):615–22.

Blanchard JF. Epidemiology of abdominal aortic aneurysms. *Epidemiologic Reviews* 1999;21(2):207–21.

Bloss JD, Liao S-Y, Wilczynski SP, Macri C, Walker J, Peake M, Berman ML. Clinical and histologic features of vulvar carcinomas analyzed for human papillomavirus status: evidence that squamous cell carcinoma of the vulva has more than one etiology. *Human Pathology* 1991;22(7):711–8.

Blot WJ. Esophageal cancer trends and risk factors. *Seminars in Oncology* 1994;21(4):403–10.

Blot WJ, Devesa SS, Kneller RW, Fraumeni JF Jr. Rising incidence of adenocarcinoma of the esophagus and gastric cardia. *Journal of the American Medical Association* 1991;265(10):1287–9.

Blot WJ, McLaughlin JK, Devesa SS, Fraumeni JF Jr. Cancers of the oral cavity and pharynx. In: Schottenfeld D, Fraumeni JF Jr, editors. *Cancer Epidemiology and Prevention.* 2nd ed. New York: Oxford University Press, 1996:666–80.

Blot WJ, McLaughlin JK, Winn DM, Austin DF, Greenberg RS, Preston-Martin S, Bernstein L, Schoenberg JB, Stemhagen A, Fraumeni JF Jr. Smoking and drinking in relation to oral and pharyngeal cancer. *Cancer Research* 1988;48(11):3282–7.

Bobo JK. Nicotine dependence and alcoholism epidemiology and treatment. *Journal of Psychoactive Drugs* 1989;21(3):323–9.

Bochow TW, West SK, Azar A, Munoz B, Sommer A, Taylor HR. Ultraviolet light exposure and risk of posterior subcapsular cataracts. *Archives of Ophthalmology* 1989;107(3):369–72.

Boffetta P, Agudo A, Ahrens W, Benhamou E, Benhamou S, Darby SC, Ferro G, Fortes C, Gonzalez CA, Jöckel KH, Krauss M, Kreienbrock L, Kreuzer M, Mendes A, Merletti F, Nyberg F, Pershagen G, Pohlabeln H, Riboli E, Schmid G, Simonato L, Trédaniel J, Whitley E, Wickman HE, Winck C, Zambon P, Saracci R. Multicenter case-control study of exposure to environmental tobacco smoke and lung cancer in Europe. *Journal of the National Cancer Institute* 1998;90(19):1440–50.

Boffetta P, Stellman SD, Garfinkel L. A case-control study of multiple myeloma nested in the American Cancer Society prospective study. *International Journal of Cancer* 1989;43(4):554–9.

Bolumar F, Olsen J, Boldsen J. Smoking reduces fecundity: a European multicenter study on infertility and subfecundity. The European Study Group on Infertility and Subfecundity. *American Journal of Epidemiology* 1996;143(6):578–87.

Bonithon-Kopp C, Jouven X, Taquet A, Touboul P-J, Guize L, Scarabin P-Y. Early carotid atherosclerosis in healthy middle-aged women: a follow-up study. *Stroke* 1993;24(12):1837–43.

Borland BL, Heckman HK. Hyperactive boys and their brothers: a 25-year follow-up study. *Archives of General Psychiatry* 1976;33(6):669–75.

Borlee I, Bouckaert A, Lechat MF, Misson CB. Smoking patterns during and before pregnancy: weight, length and head circumference of progeny. *European Journal of Obstetrics Gynecology and Reproductive Biology* 1978;8(4):171–7.

Borody TJ, George LL, Brandl S, Andrews P, Jankiewicz E, Ostapowicz N. Smoking does not contribute to duodenal ulcer relapse after *Helicobacter pylori* eradication. *American Journal of Gastroenterology* 1992;87(10):1390–3.

Bosch FX, Manos MM, Munoz N, Sherman M, Jansen AM, Peto J, Schiffman MH, Moreno V, Kurman R, Shah KV. Prevalence of human papillomavirus in cervical cancer: a worldwide perspective. *Journal of the National Cancer Institute* 1995;87(1):796–802.

Bosch FX, Munoz N, de Sanjose S, Izarzugaza I, Gili M, Viladiu P, Tormo MJ, Moreo P, Ascunce N, Gonzalez LC, Tafur L, Kaldor JM, Guerrero E, Aristizabal N, Santamaria M, de Ruiz PA, Shah K. Risk factors for cervical cancer in Colombia and Spain. *International Journal of Cancer* 1992;52(5):750–8.

Bosken CH, Wiggs BR, Pare PD, Hogg JC. Small airway dimensions in smokers with obstruction to airflow. *American Review of Respiratory Disease* 1990; 142(3):563–70.

Bouchard C, Després J-P, Mauriège P. Genetic and nongenetic determinants of regional fat distribution. *Endocrine Reviews* 1993;14(1):72–93.

Boué J, Boué A, Lazar P. Retrospective and prospective epidemiological studies of 1500 karyotyped spontaneous human abortions. *Teratology* 1975; 12(1):11–26.

Boulos R, Halsey NA, Holt E, Ruff A, Brutus J-R, Quinn TC, Adrien M, Boulos C. HIV-1 in Haitian women 1982–1988. *Journal of Acquired Immune Deficiency Syndromes* 1990;3(7):721–8.

Boutron M-C, Faivre J, Dop M-C, Quipourt V, Senesse P. Tobacco, alcohol, and colorectal tumors: a multistep process. *American Journal of Epidemiology* 1995; 141(11):1038–46.

Boyko EJ, Koepsell TD, Perera DR, Inui TS. Risk of ulcerative colitis among former and current cigarette smokers. *New England Journal of Medicine* 1987;316(12):707–10.

Boyle P, Hsieh CC, Maisonneuve P, La Vecchia C, Macfarlane GJ, Walker AM, Trichopoulos D. Epidemiology of pancreas cancer (1988). *International Journal of Pancreatology* 1989;5(4):327–46.

Braga C, Negri E, La Vecchia C, Filiberti R, Franceschi S. Cigarette smoking and the risk of breast cancer. *European Journal of Cancer Prevention* 1996;5(3): 159–64.

Bray GA. Obesity: a time bomb to be defused [commentary]. *Lancet* 1998;352(9123):160–1.

Brayne C, Gill C, Huppert FA, Barkley C, Gehlhaar E, Girling DM, O'Connor DW, Paykel ES. Incidence of clinically diagnosed subtypes of dementia in an elderly population: Cambridge Project for Later Life. *British Journal of Psychiatry* 1995;167(2): 255–62.

Brenner DE, Kukull WA, van Belle G, Bowen JD, McCormick WC, Teri L, Larson EB. Relationship between cigarette smoking and Alzheimer's disease in a population-based case-control study. *Neurology* 1993;43(2):293–300.

Brenner WE, Edelman DA, Hendricks CH. A standard of fetal growth for the United States of America. *American Journal of Obstetrics and Gynecology* 1976; 126(5):555–64.

Breslau N. Psychiatric comorbidity of smoking and nicotine dependence. *Behavior Genetics* 1995;25(2): 95–101.

Breslau N, Kilbey MM, Andreski P. Nicotine dependence, major depression, and anxiety in young adults. *Archives of General Psychiatry* 1991;48(12): 1069–74.

Breslau N, Kilbey MM, Andreski P. Nicotine withdrawal symptoms and psychiatric disorders: findings from an epidemiologic study of young adults. *American Journal of Psychiatry* 1992;149(4):464–9.

Breslau N, Peterson EL, Schultz LR, Chilcoat HD, Andreski P. Major depression and stages of smoking. A longitudinal investigation. *Archives of General Psychiatry* 1998;55(2):161–6.

Breuer-Katschinski BD, Armstrong D, Goebell H, Arnold R, Classen M, Fischer M, Blum AL. Smoking as a risk factor for duodenal ulcer relapse. *Zeitschrift fuer Gastroenterologie* 1995;33(9):509–12.

Brinton LA, Barrett RJ, Berman ML, Mortel R, Twiggs LB, Wilbanks GD. Cigarette smoking and the risk of endometrial cancer. *American Journal of Epidemiology* 1993;137(3):281–91.

Brinton LA, Nasca PC, Mallin K, Baptiste MS, Wilbanks GD, Richart RM. Case-control study of cancer of the vulva. *Obstetrics and Gynecology* 1990; 75(5):859–66.

Brinton LA, Schairer C, Haenszel W, Stolley P, Lehman HF, Levine R, Savitz DA. Cigarette smoking and invasive cervical cancer. *Journal of the American Medical Association* 1986a;255(23):3265–9.

Brinton LA, Schairer C, Stanford JL, Hoover RN. Cigarette smoking and breast cancer. *American Journal of Epidemiology* 1986b;123(4):614–22.

*British Journal of Addiction*. Nomenclature and classification of drug- and alcohol-related problems: a shortened version of a WHO memorandum. *British Journal of Addiction* 1982;77(1):3–20.

Brock KE, Berry G, Mock PA, MacLennan R, Truswell AS, Brinton LA. Nutrients in diet and plasma and risk of *in situ* cervical cancer. *Journal of the National Cancer Institute* 1988;80(8):580–5.

Brock KE, MacLennan R, Brinton LA, Melnick JL, Adam E, Mock PA, Berry G. Smoking and infectious agents and risk of *in situ* cervical cancer in Sydney, Australia. *Cancer Research* 1989;49(17): 4925–8.

Bromen K, Pohlabeln H, Jahn I, Ahrens W, Jöckel K-H. Aggregation of lung cancer in families: results from a population-based case-control study in Germany. *American Journal of Epidemiology* 2000; 152(6):497–505.

Brooke OG, Anderson HR, Bland JM, Peacock JL, Stewart CM. Effects on birth weight of smoking, alcohol, caffeine, socioeconomic factors, and psychosocial stress. *British Medical Journal* 1989; 298(6676):795–801.

Brown CA, Crombie IK, Tunstall-Pedoe H. Failure of cigarette smoking to explain international differences in mortality from chronic obstructive pulmonary disease. *Journal of Epidemiology and Community Health* 1994a;48(2):134–9.

Brown CC, Kessler LG. Projections of lung cancer mortality in the United States: 1985–2025. *Journal of the National Cancer Institute* 1988;80(1):43–51.

Brown LM, Everett GD, Gibson R, Burmeister LF, Schuman LM, Blair A. Smoking and risk of non-Hodgkin's lymphoma and multiple myeloma. *Cancer Causes and Control* 1992;3(1):49–55.

Brown LM, Silverman DT, Pottern LM, Schoenberg JB, Greenberg RS, Swanson GM, Liff JM, Schwartz AG, Hayes RB, Blot WJ, Hoover RN. Adenocarcinoma of the esophagus and esophagogastric junction in white men in the United States: alcohol, tobacco, and socioeconomic factors. *Cancer Causes and Control* 1994b;5(4):333–40.

Brown S, Vessey M, Stratton I. The influence of method of contraception and cigarette smoking on menstrual patterns. *British Journal of Obstetrics and Gynaecology* 1988;95(9):905–10.

Brownson RC. Cigarette smoking and risk of myeloma [letter]. *Journal of the National Cancer Institute* 1991;83(14):1036–7.

Brownson RC, Alavanja MCR, Hock ET, Loy TS. Passive smoking and lung cancer in nonsmoking women. *American Journal of Public Health* 1992a; 82(11):1525–30.

Brownson RC, Blackwell CW, Pearson DK, Reynolds RD, Richens JW Jr, Papermaster BW. Risk of breast cancer in relation to cigarette smoking. *Archives of Internal Medicine* 1988;148(1):140–4.

Brownson RC, Chang JC, Davis JR. Cigarette smoking and risk of adult leukemia. *American Journal of Epidemiology* 1991;134(9):938–41.

Brownson RC, Chang JC, Davis JR. Gender and histologic type variations in smoking-related risk of lung cancer. *Epidemiology* 1992b;3(1):61–4.

Brownson RC, Loy TS, Ingram E, Myers JL, Alavanja MCR, Sharp DJ, Chang JC. Lung cancer in nonsmoking women. *Cancer* 1995;75(1):29–33.

Brownson RC, Novotny TE, Perry MC. Cigarette smoking and adult leukemia: a meta-analysis. *Archives of Internal Medicine* 1993;153(4):469–75.

Brownson RC, Reif JS, Keefe TJ, Ferguson SW, Pritzl JA. Risk factors for adenocarcinoma of the lung. *American Journal of Epidemiology* 1987;125(1):25–34.

Bruner JP, Forouzan I. Smoking and buccally administered nicotine. Acute effect on uterine and umbilical artery Doppler flow velocity waveforms. *Journal of Reproductive Medicine* 1991;36(6):435–40.

Brunet J-S, Ghadirian P, Rebbeck TR, Lerman C, Garber JE, Tonin PN, Abrahamson J, Foulkes WD, Daly M, Wagner-Costalas J, Godwin A, Olopade OI, Moslehi R, Liede A, Futreal PA, Weber BL, Lenoir GM, Lynch HT, Narod SA. Effect of smoking on breast cancer in carriers of mutant BRCA1 or BRCA2 genes. *Journal of the National Cancer Institute* 1998;90(10):761–6.

Buckley JD, Harris RWC, Doll R, Vessey MP, Williams PT. Case-control study of the husbands of women with dysplasia or carcinoma of the cervix uteri. *Lancet* 1981;2(8254):1010–5.

Buffler PA, Pickle LW, Mason TJ, Contant C. The causes of lung cancer in Texas. In: Mizell M, Correa P, editors. *Lung Cancer: Causes and Prevention*. Deerfield Beach (FL): Verlag Chemie International, 1984: 83–99.

Buiatti E, Palli D, Decarli A, Amadori D, Avellini C, Bianchi S, Biserni R, Cipriani F, Cocco P, Giacosa A, Marubini E, Puntoni R, Vindigni C, Fraumeni J Jr, Blot W. A case-control study of gastric cancer and diet in Italy. *International Journal of Cancer* 1989;44(4):611–6.

Bulik CM, Sullivan PF, Epstein LH, McKee M, Kaye WH, Dahl RE, Weltzin TE. Drug use in women with anorexia and bulimia nervosa. *International Journal of Eating Disorders* 1992;11(3):213–25.

Bulterys MG, Greenland S, Kraus JF. Chronic fetal hypoxia and sudden infant death syndrome: interaction between maternal smoking and low hematocrit during pregnancy. *Pediatrics* 1990;86(4): 535–40.

Burch JD, Rohan TE, Howe GR, Risch HA, Hill GB, Steele R, Miller AB. Risk of bladder cancer by source and type of tobacco exposure: a case-control study. *International Journal of Cancer* 1989; 44(4):622–8.

Burger H, de Laet CE, van Daele PL, Weel AE, Witteman JC, Hofman A, Pols HA. Risk factors for increased bone loss in elderly population: the Rotterdam Study. *American Journal of Epidemiology* 1998; 147(9):871–9.

Burger MPM, Hollema H, Gouw ASH, Pieters WJLM, Quint WGV. Cigarette smoking and human papillomavirus in patients with reported cervical cytological abnormality. *British Medical Journal* 1993; 306(6880):749–52.

Burns DG. Smoking in inflammatory bowel disease and the irritable bowel syndrome. *South African Medical Journal* 1986;69(4):232–3.

Burns DM, Lee L, Shen LZ, Gilpin E, Tolley HD, Vaughn J, Shanks TG. Cigarette smoking behavior in the United States. In: Shopland DR, Burns DM, Garfinkel L, Samet JM, editors. *Changes in Cigarette-Related Disease Risks and Their Implication for Prevention and Control.* Smoking and Tobacco Control Monograph 8. Rockville (MD): U.S. Department of Health and Human Services, Public Health Service, National Institutes of Health, National Cancer Institute, 1997a:13–42. NIH Publication No. 97-4213.

Burns DM, Shanks TG, Choi W, Thun MJ, Heath CW Jr, Garfinkel L. The American Cancer Society Cancer Prevention Study I: 12-year followup of 1 million men and women. In: Shopland DR, Burns DM, Garfinkel L, Samet JM, editors. *Changes in Cigarette-Related Disease Risks and Their Implication for Prevention and Control.* Smoking and Tobacco Control Monograph 8. Rockville (MD): U.S. Department of Health and Human Services, Public Health Service, National Institutes of Health, National Cancer Institute, 1997b:113–304. NIH Publication No. 97-4213.

Burns DN, Kramer A, Yellin F, Fuchs D, Wachter H, DiGioia RA, Sanchez WC, Grossman RJ, Gordin FM, Biggar RJ, Goedert JJ. Cigarette smoking: a modifier of human immunodeficiency virus type 1 infection? *Journal of Acquired Immune Deficiency Syndromes* 1991;4(1):76–83.

Burns DN, Landesman S, Muenz LR, Nugent RP, Goedert JJ, Minkoff H, Walsh JH, Mendez H, Rubinstein A, Willoughby A. Cigarette smoking, premature rupture of membranes, and vertical transmission of HIV-1 among women with low CD4+ levels. *Journal of Acquired Immune Deficiency Syndromes* 1994;7(7):718–26.

Burns PB, Swanson GM. Risk of urinary bladder cancer among Blacks and Whites: the role of cigarette use and occupation. *Cancer Causes and Control* 1991;2(6):371–9.

Burns PB, Swanson GM. Stomach cancer risk among black and white men and women: the role of occupation and cigarette smoking. *Journal of Occupational and Environmental Medicine* 1995;37(10): 1218–23.

Burrows B, Knudson RJ, Camilli AE, Lyle SK, Lebowitz MD. The "horse-racing effect" and predicting decline in forced expiratory volume in one second from screening spirometry. *American Review of Respiratory Disease* 1987;135(4):788–93.

Burton HR, Childs GH Jr, Andersen RA, Fleming PD. Changes in chemical composition of burley tobacco during senescence and curing. 3. Tobacco-specific nitrosamines. *Journal of Agricultural and Food Chemistry* 1989;37(2):426–30.

Bush TL, Criqui MH, Cowan LD, Barrett-Connor E, Wallace RB, Tyroler HA, Suchindran CM, Cohn R, Rifkind BM. Cardiovascular disease mortality in women: results from the Lipid Research Clinics Follow-up Study. In: Eaker ED, Packard B, Wenger NK, Clarkson TB, Tyroler HA, editors. *Coronary Heart Disease in Women. Proceedings of an N.I.H. Workshop.* New York: Haymarket Doyma, 1987: 106–11.

Butler TL. The Relationship of Passive Smoking to Various Health Outcomes Among Seventh-Day Adventists in California [dissertation]. Los Angeles: University of California, 1988.

Butler C, Samet JM, Humble CG, Sweeney ES. Histopathology of lung cancer in New Mexico, 1970–1972 and 1980–1981. *Journal of the National Cancer Institute* 1987;78(1):85–90.

Butler WJ, Ostrander LD Jr, Carman WJ, Lamphiear DE. Diabetes mellitus in Tecumseh, Michigan: prevalence, incidence, and associated conditions. *American Journal of Epidemiology* 1982;116(6):971–80.

Buttram VC Jr, Reiter RC. Uterine leiomyomata: etiology, symptomatology, and management. *Fertility and Sterility* 1981;36(4):433–5.

Byers T, Marshall J, Graham S, Mettlin C, Swanson M. A case-control study of dietary and nondietary factors in ovarian cancer. *Journal of the National Cancer Institute* 1983;71(4):681–6.

Byers TE, Graham S, Haughey BP, Marshall JR, Swanson MK. Diet and lung cancer risk: findings from the Western New York Diet Study. *American Journal of Epidemiology* 1987;125(3):351–63.

California Environmental Protection Agency. *Health Effects of Exposure to Environmental Tobacco Smoke.* Sacramento (CA): California Environmental Protection Agency, Office of Environmental Health Hazard Assessment, Reproductive and Cancer Hazard Assessment Section and Air Toxicology and Epidemiology Section, 1997.

Callahan CM, Hall KS, Hui SL, Musick BS, Unverzagt FW, Hendrie HC. Relationship of age, education, and occupation with dementia among a community-based sample of African Americans. *Archives of Neurology* 1996;53(2):134–40.

Calle EE, Miracle-McMahill HL, Thun MJ, Heath CW Jr. Cigarette smoking and risk of fatal breast cancer. *American Journal of Epidemiology* 1994;139(10): 1001–7.

Camilli AE, Burrows B, Knudson RJ, Lyle SK, Lebowitz MD. Longitudinal changes in forced expiratory volume in one second in adults: effects of smoking and smoking cessation. *American Review of Respiratory Disease* 1987;135(4):794–9.

Camilli AE, Robbins DR, Lebowitz MD. Death certificate reporting of confirmed airways obstructive disease. *American Journal of Epidemiology* 1991; 133(8):795–800.

Camp DE, Klesges RC, Relyea G. The relationship between body weight concerns and adolescent smoking. *Health Psychology* 1993;12(1):24–32.

Campbell MJ, Lewry J, Wailoo M. Further evidence for the effect of passive smoking on neonates. *Postgraduate Medical Journal* 1988;64(755):663–5.

Canadian Department of National Health and Welfare. *A Canadian Study of Smoking and Health.* Canada: Department of National Health and Welfare, 1966.

Canadian Study of Health and Aging Working Group. Canadian Study of Health and Aging: study methods and prevalence of dementia. *Canadian Medical Association Journal* 1994;150(6): 899–913.

Cardenas VM, Thun MJ, Austin H, Lally CA, Clark WS, Greenberg RS, Heath CW Jr. Environmental tobacco smoke and lung cancer mortality in the American Cancer Society's Cancer Prevention Study II. *Cancer Causes and Control* 1997;8(1):57–64.

Carey VJ, Walters EE, Colditz GA, Solomon CG, Willett WC, Rosner BA, Speizer FE, Manson JE. Body fat distribution and risk of non-insulin-dependent diabetes mellitus in women. The Nurses' Health Study. *American Journal of Epidemiology* 1997;145(7): 614–9.

Carmody TP. Affect regulation, nicotine addiction, and smoking cessation. *Journal of Psychoactive Drugs* 1989;21(3):331–42.

Cassano PA, Rosner B, Vokonas PS, Weiss ST. Obesity and body fat distribution in relation to the incidence of non-insulin-dependent diabetes mellitus: a prospective cohort study of men in the Normative Aging Study. *American Journal of Epidemiology* 1992;136(12):1474–86.

Cassano PA, Segal MR, Vokonas PS, Weiss ST. Body fat distribution, blood pressure, and hypertension: a prospective cohort study of men in the Normative Aging Study. *Annals of Epidemiology* 1990;1(1): 33–48.

Cassidenti DL, Pike MC, Vijod AG, Stanczyk FZ, Lobo RA. A reevaluation of estrogen status in postmenopausal women who smoke. *American Journal of Obstetrics and Gynecology* 1992;166(5):1444–8.

Cassidenti DL, Vijod AG, Vijod MA, Stanczyk FZ, Lobo RA. Short-term effects of smoking on the pharmacokinetic profiles of micronized estradiol in postmenopausal women. *American Journal of Obstetrics and Gynecology* 1990;163(6 Pt 1):1953–60.

Castles A, Adams EK, Melvin CL, Kelsch C, Boulton ML. Effects of smoking during pregnancy: five meta-analyses. *American Journal of Preventive Medicine* 1999;16(3):208–15.

Castro LC, Azen C, Hobel CJ, Platt LD. Maternal tobacco use and substance abuse: reported prevalence rates and associations with the delivery of small for gestational age neonates. *Obstetrics and Gynecology* 1993;81(3):396–401.

Cauley JA, Gutai JP, Kuller LH, LeDonne D, Powell JG. The epidemiology of serum sex hormones in postmenopausal women. *American Journal of Epidemiology* 1989;129(6):1120–31.

Cauley JA, Gutai JP, Kuller LH, LeDonne D, Sandler RB, Sashin D, Powell JG. Endogenous estrogen levels and calcium intakes in postmenopausal women. *Journal of the American Medical Association* 1988;260(21):3150–5.

Cauley JA, Seeley DG, Ensrud K, Ettinger B, Black D, Cummings SR. Estrogen replacement therapy and fractures in older women. *Annals of Internal Medicine* 1995;122(1):9–16.

Cederlöf R, Friberg L, Hrubec Z, Lorich U. *The Relationship of Smoking and Some Social Covariables to Mortality and Cancer Morbidity: A Ten Year Follow-up in a Probability Sample of 55,000 Swedish Subjects Age 18 to 69*. Stockholm: Karolinska Institute, Department of Environmental Hygiene, 1975.

Centers for Disease Control. Effects of maternal cigarette smoking on birth weight and preterm birth—Ohio, 1989. *Morbidity and Mortality Weekly Report* 1990;39(38):662–5.

Centers for Disease Control. Ectopic pregnancy—United States, 1988–1989. *Morbidity and Mortality Weekly Report* 1992;41(32):591–94.

Centers for Disease Control and Prevention. Indicators of nicotine addiction among women—United States, 1991–1992. *Morbidity and Mortality Weekly Report* 1995;44(6):102–5.

Centers for Disease Control and Prevention. Smoking-attributable mortality and years of potential life lost—United States, 1984. *Morbidity and Mortality Weekly Report* 1997;46(20):444–51.

Chan FK, Sung JJ, Lee YT, Leung WK, Chan LY, Yung MY, Chung SC. Does smoking predispose to peptic ulcer relapse after eradication of *Helicobacter pylori*? *American Journal of Gastroenterology* 1997; 92(3):442–5.

Chan WC, Fung SC. Lung cancer in nonsmokers in Hong Kong. In: Grundmann E, Clemmesen J, Muir CS, editors. *Geographical Pathology in Cancer Epidemiology. Cancer Campaign.* Vol. 6. New York: Gustav Fischer Verlag, 1982:199–202.

Chao A, Thun MJ, Jacobs EJ, Henley SJ, Rodriguez C, Calle EE. Cigarette smoking and colorectal cancer mortality in the Cancer Prevention Study II. *Journal of the National Cancer Institute* 2000;92(23): 1888–96.

Chao ST, Omiecinski CJ, Namkung MJ, Nelson SD, Dvorchik BH, Juchau MR. Catechol estrogen formation in placental and fetal tissues of humans, macaques, rats and rabbits. *Developmental Pharmacology and Therapeutics* 1981;2(1):1–16.

Chard T, MacIntosh MC. Screening for Down's syndrome [review]. *Journal of Perinatal Medicine* 1995; 23(6):421–36.

Chatenoud L, Parazzini F, di Cintio E, Zanconato G, Benzi G, Bortolus R, La Vecchia C. Paternal and maternal smoking habits before conception and during the first trimester: relation to spontaneous abortion. *Annals of Epidemiology* 1998;8(8):520–6.

Chelmow D, Andrew DE, Baker ER. Maternal cigarette smoking and placenta previa. *Obstetrics and Gynecology* 1996;87(5 Pt 1):703–6.

Chen CL, Gilbert TJ, Daling JR. Maternal smoking and Down syndrome: the confounding effect of maternal age. *American Journal of Epidemiology* 1999; 149(5):442–6.

Chen LH, Petitti DB. Case-control study of passive smoking and the risk of small-for-gestational-age at term. *American Journal of Epidemiology* 1995; 142(2):158–65.

Chen Y, Horne SL, Dosman JA. Increased susceptibility to lung dysfunction in female smokers. *American Review of Respiratory Disease* 1991;143(6): 1224–30.

Chen Y, Pederson LL, Lefcoe NM. Passive smoking and low birthweight [letter]. *Lancet* 1989;2(8653): 54–5.

Cheng S, Suominen H, Heikkinen E. Bone mineral density in relation to anthropometric properties, physical activity and smoking in 75-year-old men and women. *Aging—Clinical and Experimental Research* 1993;5(1):55–62.

Cheng S, Suominen H, Rantanen T, Parkatti T, Heikkinen E. Bone mineral density and physical activity in 50–60-year-old women. *Bone and Mineral* 1991; 12(2):123–32.

Choi WS, Patten CA, Gillin JC, Kaplan RB, Pierce JP. Cigarette smoking predicts development of depressive symptoms among U.S. adolescents. *Annals of Behavioral Medicine* 1997;19(1):42–50.

Chow WH, Daling JR, Cates W Jr, Greenberg RS. Epidemiology of ectopic pregnancy. *Epidemiologic Reviews* 1987;9:70–94.

Chow WH, Daling JR, Weiss NS, Voigt LF. Maternal cigarette smoking and tubal pregnancy. *Obstetrics and Gynecology* 1988;71(2):167–70.

Chow W-H, McLaughlin JK, Menck HR, Mack TM. Risk factors for extrahepatic bile duct cancers: Los Angeles County, California (USA). *Cancer Causes and Control* 1994;5(3):267–72.

Chow WH, Swanson CA, Lissowska J, Groves FD, Sobin LH, Nasierowska-Guttmejer A, Radziszewski J, Regula J, Hsing AW, Jagannatha S, Zatonski W, Blot WJ. Risk of stomach cancer in relation to consumption of cigarettes, alcohol, tea and coffee in Warsaw, Poland. *International Journal of Cancer* 1999;81(6):871–6.

Christen WG, Glynn RJ, Manson JE, Ajani UA, Buring JE. A prospective study of cigarette smoking and risk of age-related macular degeneration in men. *Journal of the American Medical Association* 1996; 276(14):1147–51.

Christen WG, Manson JE, Seddon JM, Glynn RJ, Buring JE, Rosner B, Hennekens CH. A prospective study of cigarette smoking and risk of cataract in men. *Journal of the American Medical Association* 1992;268(8):989–93.

Christensen K, Olsen J, Norgaard-Pedersen B, Basso O, Stovring H, Milhollin-Johnson L, Murray JC. Oral clefts, transforming growth factor alpha gene variants, and maternal smoking: a population-based case-control study in Denmark, 1991–1994. *American Journal of Epidemiology* 1999;149(3): 248–55.

Christensen SB, Ericsson U-B, Janzon L, Tibblin S, Melander A. Influence of cigarette smoking on goiter formation, thyroglobulin, and thyroid hormone levels in women. *Journal of Clinical Endocrinology and Metabolism* 1984;58(4):615–8.

Chu SY, Stroup NE, Wingo PA, Lee NC, Peterson HB, Gwinn ML. Cigarette smoking and the risk of breast cancer. *American Journal of Epidemiology* 1990; 131(2):244–53.

Chung PH, Yeko TR, Mayer JC, Clark B, Welden SW, Maroulis GB. Gamete intrafallopian transfer. Does smoking play a role? *Journal of Reproductive Medicine* 1997;42(2):65–70.

Churg A. Lung cancer cell type and occupational exposure. In: Samet JM, editor. *Epidemiology of Lung Cancer.* New York: Marcel Dekker, 1994.

Chute CG, Willett WC, Colditz GA, Stampfer MJ, Baron JA, Rosner B, Speizer FE. A prospective study of body mass, height, and smoking on the risk of colorectal cancer in women. *Cancer Causes and Control* 1991;2(2):117–24.

Ciruzzi M, Pramaro P, Esteban O, Rozlosnik J, Tartaglione J, Abecasis B, Cesar J, De Rosa J, Paterno C, Schargrodsky H. Case-control study of passive smoking at home and risk of acute myocardial infarction. *Journal of the American College of Cardiology* 1998;31(4):797–803.

Clarke EA, Hatcher J, McKeown-Eyssen GE, Lickrish GM. Cervical dysplasia: association with sexual behavior, smoking, and oral contraceptive use? *American Journal of Obstetrics and Gynecology* 1985; 151(5):612–6.

Clarke EA, Morgan RW, Newman AM. Smoking as a risk factor in cancer of the cervix: additional evidence from a case-control study. *American Journal of Epidemiology* 1982;115(1):59–66.

Clement BJA, Fung YK. Effect of nicotine administration on calcium absorption in rat duodenum. *Pharmaceutical Sciences* 1995;1(2):67–9.

Clements SD, Peters JE. Minimal brain dysfunctions in the school-aged child: diagnosis and treatment. *Archives of General Psychiatry* 1962;6(Mar):185–97.

Cliver SP, Goldenberg RL, Cutter GR, Hoffman HJ, Davis RO, Nelson KG. The effect of cigarette smoking on neonatal anthropometric measurements. *Obstetrics and Gynecology* 1995;85(4):625–30.

Cnattingius S. Does age potentiate the smoking-related risk of fetal growth retardation? *Early Human Development* 1989;20(3-4):203–11.

Cnattingius S. Maternal age modifies the effect of maternal smoking on intrauterine growth retardation but not on late fetal death and placental abruption. *American Journal of Epidemiology* 1997;145(4):319–23.

Cnattingius S, Axelsson O, Eklund G, Lindmark G. Smoking, maternal age, and fetal growth. *Obstetrics and Gynecology* 1985;66(4):449–52.

Cnattingius S, Forman MR, Berendes HW, Graubard BI, Isotalo L. Effect of age, parity, and smoking on pregnancy outcome: a population-based study. *American Journal of Obstetrics and Gynecology* 1993; 168(1 Pt 1):16–21.

Cnattingius S, Forman MR, Berendes HW, Isotalo L. Delayed childbearing and risk of adverse perinatal outcome. A population-based study. *Journal of the American Medical Association* 1992;268(7):886–90.

Cnattingius S, Haglund B, Meirik O. Cigarette smoking as risk factor for late fetal and early neonatal death. *British Medical Journal* 1988;297(6643):258–61.

Cnattingius S, Mills JL, Yuen J, Eriksson O, Salonen H. The paradoxical effect of smoking in preeclamptic pregnancies: smoking reduces the incidence but increases the rates of perinatal mortality, abruptio placentae, and intrauterine growth restriction. *American Journal of Obstetrics and Gynecology* 1997; 177(1):156–61.

Cnattingius S, Nordstrom ML. Maternal smoking and feto-infant mortality: biological pathways and public health significance. *Acta Paediatrica* 1996; 85(12):1400–2.

Coker AL, Rosenberg AJ, McCann MF, Hulka BS. Active and passive cigarette smoke exposure and cervical intraepithelial neoplasia. *Cancer Epidemiology, Biomarkers and Prevention* 1992;1(5):349–56.

Colditz GA, Segal MR, Myers AH, Stampfer MJ, Willett W, Speizer FE. Weight change in relation to smoking cessation among women. *Journal of Smoking-Related Disorders* 1992;3(2):145–53.

Colditz GA, Stampfer MJ, Willett WC. Diet and lung cancer: a review of the epidemiologic evidence in humans. *Archives of Internal Medicine* 1987;147(1): 157–60.

Collaborative Group for the Study of Stroke in Young Women. Oral contraceptives and stroke in young women: associated risk factors. *Journal of the American Medical Association* 1975;231(7):718–22.

Collins A, Landgren B-M. Reproductive health, use of estrogen and experience of symptoms in perimenopausal women: a population-based study. *Maturitas* 1995;20:101–11.

Comstock GW, Helzlsouer KJ, Bush TL. Prediagnostic serum levels of carotenoids and vitamin E as related to subsequent cancer in Washington County, Maryland. *American Journal of Clinical Nutrition* 1991;53(Suppl 1):260S–264S.

Comstock GW, Lundin FE Jr. Parental smoking and perinatal mortality. *American Journal of Obstetrics and Gynecology* 1967;98(5):708–18.

Conter V, Cortinovis I, Rogari P, Riva L. Weight growth in infants born to mothers who smoked during pregnancy. *British Medical Journal* 1995; 310(6982):768–71.

Cooper C, Inskip H, Croft P, Campbell L, Smith G, McLaren M, Coggon D. Individual risk factors for hip osteoarthritis: obesity, hip injury, and physical activity. *American Journal of Epidemiology* 1998; 147(6):516–22.

Cooper C, Shah S, Hand DJ, Adams J, Compston J, Davie M, Woolf A. Screening for vertebral osteoporosis using individual risk factors. *Osteoporosis International* 1991;2(1):48–53.

Cooper JA, Rohan TE, Cant ELM, Horsfall DJ, Tilley WD. Risk factors for breast cancer by oestrogen receptor status: a population-based case-control study. *British Journal of Cancer* 1989;59(1):119–25.

Cornelius MD, Taylor PM, Geva D, Day NL. Prenatal tobacco and marijuana use among adolescents: effects on offspring gestational age, growth, and morphology. *Pediatrics* 1995;95(5): 738–43.

Corrao G, Tragnone A, Caprilli R, Trallori G, Papi C, Andreoli A, Di Paolo M, Riegler G, Rigo G-P, Ferraù O, Mansi C, Ingrosso M, Valpiani D. Risk of inflamatory bowel disease attributable to smoking, oral contraception and breastfeeding in Italy: a nationwide case-control study. *International Journal of Epidemiology* 1998;27(3):397–404.

Correa P, Fontham E, Pickle LW, Lin Y, Haenszel W. Passive smoking and lung cancer. *Lancet* 1983; 2(8350):595–7.

Cosnes J, Carbonnel F, Beaugerie L, Le Quintrec Y, Gendre JP. Effects of cigarette smoking on the long-term course of Crohn's disease. *Gastroenterology* 1996;110(2):424–31.

Coste J, Job-Spira N, Fernandez H. Increased risk of ectopic pregnancy with maternal cigarette smoking. *American Journal of Public Health* 1991a;81(2): 199–201.

Coste J, Job-Spira N, Fernandez H, Papiernik E, Spira A. Risk factors for ectopic pregnancy: a case-control study in France, with special focus on infectious factors. *American Journal of Epidemiology* 1991b;133(9):839–49.

Cottone M, Rosselli M, Orlando A, Oliva L, Puleo A, Cappello M, Traina M, Tonelli F, Pagliaro L. Smoking habits and recurrence in Crohn's disease. *Gastroenterology* 1994;106(3):643–8.

Counsilman JJ, Mackay EV. Cigarette habits of pregnant women in Brisbane, Australia. *Australian and New Zealand Journal of Obstetrica and Gynaecology* 1985;25(4):244–7.

Covey LS, Glassman AH, Stetner F, Becker J. Effect of history of alcoholism or major depression on smoking cessation. *American Journal of Psychiatry* 1993;150(10):1546–7.

Covey LS, Hughes DC, Glassman AH, Blazer DG, George LK. Ever-smoking, quitting, and psychiatric disorders: evidence from the Durham, North Carolina, Epidemiologic Catchment Area. *Tobacco Control* 1994;3(3):222–7.

Cox ML, Khan SA, Gau DW, Cox SAL, Hodkinson HM. Determinants of forearm bone density in premenopausal women: a study in one general practice. *British Journal of General Practice* 1991; 41(346):194–6.

Cramer DW, Schiff I, Schoenbaum SC, Gibson M, Belisle S, Albrecht B, Stillman RJ, Berger MJ, Wilson E, Stadel BV, Seibel M. Tubal infertility and the intrauterine device. *New England Journal of Medicine* 1985;312(15):941–7.

Cramer DW, Wilson E, Stillman RJ, Berger MJ, Belisle S, Schiff I, Albrecht B, Gibson M, Stadel BV, Schoenbaum SC. The relation of endometriosis to menstrual characteristics, smoking, and exercise. *Journal of the American Medical Association* 1986; 255(14):1904–8.

Cramer DW, Xu H, Harlow BL. Does "incessant" ovulation increase risk for early menopause? *American Journal of Obstetrics and Gynecology* 1995; 172(2 Pt 1):568–73.

Crawley JF, Portides G. Self-reported versus measured height, weight, and body mass index amongst 16–17 year old British teenagers. *International Journal of Obesity and Related Metabolic Disorders* 1995;19(8):579–84.

Criqui MH, Langer RD, Fronek A, Feigelson HS, Klauber MR, McCann TJ, Browner D. Mortality over a period of 10 years in patients with peripheral arterial disease. *New England Journal of Medicine* 1992;326(6):381–6.

Criqui MH, Suarez L, Barrett-Connor E, McPhillips J, Wingard DL, Garland C. Postmenopausal estrogen use and mortality: results from a prospective study in a defined, homogeneous community. *American Journal of Epidemiology* 1988;128(3): 606–14.

Crockett AJ, Cranston JM, Moss JR, Alpers JH. Trends in chronic obstructive pulmonary disease mortality in Australia. *Medical Journal of Australia* 1994;161(10):600–3.

Croft P, Hannaford PC. Risk factors for acute myocardial infarction in women: evidence from the Royal College of General Practitioners' Oral Contraception Study. *British Medical Journal* 1989; 298(6667):165–8.

Cuckle HS, Alberman E, Wald NJ, Royston P, Knight G. Maternal smoking habits and Down's syndrome. *Prenatal Diagnosis* 1990a;10(9):561–7.

Cuckle HS, Wald NJ, Densem JW, Royston P, Knight GJ, Haddow JE, Palomaki GE, Canick JA. The effect of smoking in pregnancy on maternal serum alpha-fetoprotein, unconjugated oestriol, human chorionic gonadotrophin, progesterone and dehydroepiandrosterone sulphate levels. *British Journal of Obstetrics and Gynaecology* 1990b;97(3):272–4.

Cumming RG, Mitchell P. Alcohol, smoking, and cataracts: the Blue Mountains Eye Study. *Archives of Ophthalmology* 1997;115(10):1296–303.

Cummings SR, Black DM, Rubin SM. Lifetime risks of hip, Colles', or vertebral fracture and coronary heart disease among white postmenopausal women. *Archives of Internal Medicine* 1989;149(11): 2445–8.

Cummings SR, Nevitt MC, Browner WS, Stone K, Fox KM, Ensrud KE, Cauley J, Black D, Vogt TM. Risk factors for hip fracture in white women. *New England Journal of Medicine* 1995;332(12):767–73.

Cunningham J, Dockery DW, Gold DR, Speizer FE. Racial differences in the association between maternal smoking during pregnancy and lung function in children. *American Journal of Respiratory and Critical Care Medicine* 1995;152(2):565–9.

Cunningham J, Dockery DW, Speizer FE. Maternal smoking during pregnancy as a predictor of lung function in children. *American Journal of Epidemiology* 1994;139(12):1139–52.

Cupples LA, D'Agostino RB. Some risk factors related to the annual incidence of cardiovascular disease and death using pooled repeated biennial measurements: Framingham Heart Study, 30-year follow-up. Section 34. In: Kannel WB, Wolf PA, Garrison RJ, editors. *The Framingham Study: An Epidemiological Investigation of Cardiovascular Disease.* U.S. Department of Health and Human Services, Public Health Service, National Institutes of Health, National Heart, Lung, and Blood Institute, 1987. NIH Publication No. 87-2703.

Curtis KM, Savitz DA, Arbuckle TE. Effects of cigarette smoking, caffeine consumption, and alcohol intake on fecundability. *American Journal of Epidemiology* 1997;146(1):32–41.

Cuzick J, Babiker AG. Pancreatic cancer, alcohol, diabetes mellitus and gall-bladder disease. *International Journal of Cancer* 1989;43(3):415–21.

Czeizel AE, Kodaj I, Lenz W. Smoking during pregnancy and congenital limb deficiency. *British Medical Journal* 1994;308(6942):1473–6.

Daftari TK, Whitesides TE, Heller JG, Goodrich AC, McCarey BE, Hutton WC. Nicotine on the revascularization of bone graft. *Spine* 1994;19(8):904–11.

Dahlgren E, Friberg L-G, Johansson S, Lindstrom B, Oden A, Samsioe G, Janson PO. Endometrial carcinoma; ovarian dysfunction—a risk factor in young women. *European Journal of Obstetrics and Gynecology and Reproductive Biology* 1991;41(2): 143–50.

Dalack GW, Glassman AH, Rivelli S, Covey L, Stetner F. Mood, major depression, and fluoxetine response in cigarette smokers. *American Journal of Psychiatry* 1995;152(3):398–403.

Dalack GW, Meador-Woodruff JH. Smoking, smoking withdrawal and schizophrenia: case reports and a review of the literature. *Schizophrenia Research* 1996;22(2):133–41.

Daling J, Weiss N, Spadoni L, Moore DE, Voigt L. Cigarette smoking and primary tubal infertility. In: Rosenberg MJ, editor. *Smoking and Reproductive Health.* Littleton (MA): PSG Publishing, 1987: 40–6.

Daling JR, Madeleine MM, McKnight B, Carter JJ, Wipf GC, Ashley R, Schwartz SM, Beckmann AM, Hagensee ME, Mandelson MT, Galloway DA. The relationship of human papillomavirus-related cervical tumors to cigarette smoking, oral contraceptive use, and prior herpes simplex virus type 2 infection. *Cancer Epidemiology, Biomarkers and Prevention* 1996;5(7):541–8.

Daling JR, Sherman KJ, Weiss NS. Risk factors for condyloma acuminatum in women. *Sexually Transmitted Diseases* 1986;13(1):16–8.

Daly E, Gray A, Barlow D, McPherson K, Roche M, Vessey M. Measuring the impact of menopausal symptoms on quality of life. *British Medical Journal* 1993;307(6908):836–40.

Daniel M, Martin AD. Bone mineral density and adipose tissue distribution in young women: relationship to smoking status. *Annals of Human Biology* 1995;22(1):29–42.

Daniel M, Martin AD, Faiman C. Sex hormones and adipose tissue distribution in premenopausal cigarette smokers. *International Journal of Obesity* 1992;16(4):245–54.

Daniell HW. Smoker's wrinkles: a study in the epidemiology of "crow's feet." *Annals of Internal Medicine* 1971;75(6):873–80.

Daniell HW. Breast cancer and cigarette smoking [letter]. *New England Journal of Medicine* 1984; 310(23):1531.

Darrow SL, Vena J, Batt R, Zielezny M, Michalek A, Selman S. Menstrual cycle characteristics and the risk of endometriosis. *Epidemiology* 1993;4(2): 135–42.

D'Avanzo B, La Vecchia C, Franceschi S, Gallotti L, Talamini R. Cigarette smoking and colorectal cancer: a study of 1,584 cases and 2,879 controls. *Preventive Medicine* 1995a;24(6):571–9.

D'Avanzo B, La Vecchia C, Franceschi S, Negri E, Talamini R. History of thyroid diseases and subsequent thyroid cancer risk. *Cancer Epidemiology, Biomarkers and Prevention* 1995b;4(3):193–9.

D'Avanzo B, La Vecchia C, Negri E, Parazzini F, Franceschi S. Oral contraceptive use and risk of myocardial infarction: an Italian case-control study. *Journal of Epidemiology and Community Health* 1994; 48(3):342–5.

Davey DA, MacGillivray I. The classification and definition of the hypertensive disorders of pregnancy. *American Journal of Obstetrics and Gynecology* 1988; 158(4):882–8.

Davies MC, Hall ML, Jacobs HS. Bone mineral loss in young women with amenorrhoea. *British Medical Journal* 1990;301(6755):790–3.

De Cesaris R, Ranieri G, Filitti V, Bonfantino MV, Andriani A. Cardiovascular effects of cigarette smoking. *Cardiology* 1992;81(4–5):233–7.

de Leon J, Dadvand M, Canuso C, White AO, Stanilla JK, Simpson GM. Schizophrenia and smoking: an epidemiological survey in a state hospital. *American Journal of Psychiatry* 1995;152(3):453–5.

de Mouzon J, Spira A, Schwartz D. A prospective study of the relation between smoking and fertility. *International Journal of Epidemiology* 1988;17(2): 378–84.

De Stefani E, Fierro L, Barrios E, Ronco A. Tobacco, alcohol, diet and risk of non-Hodgkin's lymphoma: a case-control study in Uruguay. *Leukemia Research* 1998;22(5):445–52.

de Vet HCW, Sturmans F, Knipschild PG. The role of cigarette smoking in the etiology of cervical dysplasia. *Epidemiology* 1994;5(6):631–3.

Dejin-Karlsson E, Hanson BS, Ostergren PO, Sjèoberg NO, Marsal K. Does passive smoking in early pregnancy increase the risk of small-for-gestational-age infants? *American Journal of Public Health* 1998;88(10):1523–7.

den Tonkelaar I, Seidell JC, van Noord PAH, Baanders-van Halewijn EA, Jacobus JH, Bruning PF. Factors influencing waist/hip ratio in randomly selected pre- and post-menopausal women in the Dom-Project (preliminary results). *International Journal of Obesity* 1989;13(6):817–24.

den Tonkelaar I, Seidell JC, van Noord PAH, Baanders-van Halewijn EA, Ouwehand IJ. Fat distribution in relation to age, degree of obesity, smoking habits, parity and estrogen use: a cross-sectional study in 11,825 Dutch women participating in the Dom-Project. *International Journal of Obesity* 1990;14(9):753–61.

Dennerstein L, Smith AM, Morse C, Burger H, Green A, Hopper J, Ryan M. Menopausal symptoms in Australian women. *Medical Journal of Australia* 1993;159(4):232–6.

Devesa SS, Blot WJ, Stone BJ, Miller BA, Tarone RE, Fraumeni JF Jr. Recent cancer trends in the United States. *Journal of the National Cancer Institute* 1995; 87(3):175–82.

Devesa SS, Shaw GL, Blot WJ. Changing patterns of lung cancer incidence by histological type. *Cancer Epidemiology, Biomarkers and Prevention* 1991;1(1): 29–34.

Devesa SS, Silverman DT, McLaughlin JK, Brown CC, Connelly RR, Fraumeni JF Jr. Comparison of the descriptive epidemiology of urinary tract cancers. *Cancer Causes and Control* 1990;1(2):133–41.

DiFranza JR, Lew RA. Effect of maternal cigarette smoking on pregnancy complications and sudden infant death syndrome. *Journal of Family Practice* 1995;40(4):385–94.

Djordjevic MV, Stellman SD, Zang E. Doses of nicotine and lung carcinogens delivered to cigarette smokers. *Journal of the National Cancer Institute* 2000; 92(2):106–11.

Dobbs SD, Strickler DP, Maxwell WA. The effects of stress and relaxation in the presence of stress on urinary pH and smoking behaviors. *Addictive Behaviors* 1981;6(4):345–53.

Dobson AJ, Alexander HM, Heller RF, Lloyd DM. How soon after quitting smoking does risk of heart attack decline? *Journal of Clinical Epidemiology* 1991a;44(11):1247–53.

Dobson AJ, Alexander HM, Heller RF, Lloyd DM. Passive smoking and the risk of heart attack or coronary death. *Medical Journal of Australia* 1991b; 154(12):793–7.

Dockery DW, Speizer FE, Ferris BG Jr, Ware JH, Louis TA, Spiro A. Cumulative and reversible effects of lifetime smoking on simple tests of lung function in adults. *American Review of Respiratory Disease* 1988;137(2):286–92.

Dodds L, Davis S, Polissar L. Population-based study of lung cancer incidence trends by histologic type, 1974–1981. *Journal of the National Cancer Institute* 1986;76(1):21–9.

Dodge R, Cline MG, Burrows B. Comparisons of asthma, emphysema, and chronic bronchitis diagnoses in a general population sample. *American Review of Respiratory Disease* 1986;133(6):981–6.

Dolan-Mullen P, Ramírez G, Groff JY. A meta-analysis of randomized trials of prenatal smoking cessation interventions. *American Journal of Obstetrics and Gynecology* 1994;171(5):1328–34.

Doll R, Gray R, Hafner B, Peto R. Mortality in relation to smoking: 22 years' observations on female British doctors. *British Medical Journal* 1980; 280(6219):967–71.

Doll R, Hill AB. Mortality of British doctors in relation to smoking: observations on coronary thrombosis. In: Haenszel W, editor. *Epidemiological Approaches to the Study of Cancer and Other Chronic Diseases.* National Cancer Institute Monograph 19. Bethesda (MD): U.S. Department of Health, Education, and Welfare, Public Health Service, National Cancer Institute, 1966:205–68.

Doll R, Peto R. Mortality in relation to smoking: 20 years' observations on male British doctors. *British Medical Journal* 1976;2(6051):1525–36.

Doll R, Peto R. The causes of cancer: quantitative estimates of avoidable risks of cancer in the United States today. *Journal of the National Cancer Institute* 1981;66(6):1191–308.

Doll R, Peto R, Wheatley K, Gray R, Sutherland I. Mortality in relation to smoking: 40 years' observations on male British doctors. *British Medical Journal* 1994;309(6959):901–11.

Dominguez-Rojas V, de Juanes-Pardo JR, Astasio-Arbiza P, Ortega-Molina P, Gordillo-Florencio E. Spontaneous abortion in a hospital population: are tobacco and coffee intake risk factors? *European Journal of Epidemiology* 1994;10(6):665–8.

Donahue RP, Abbott RD, Bloom E, Reed DM, Yano K. Central obesity and coronary heart disease in men. *Lancet* 1987;1(8537):821–4.

Donald JM, Hooper K, Hopenhayn-Rich C. Reproductive and developmental toxicity of toluene: a review. *Environmental Health Perspectives* 1991;94: 237–44.

Donnan GA, McNeil JJ, Adena MA, Doyle AE, O'Malley HM, Neill GC. Smoking as a risk factor for cerebral ischaemia. *Lancet* 1989;2(8664):643–7.

Dorgan JF, Ziegler RG, Schoenberg JB, Hartge P, McAdams MJ, Falk RT, Wilcox HB, Shaw GL. Race and sex differences in associations of vegetables, fruits, and carotenoids with lung cancer risk in New Jersey (United States). *Cancer Causes and Control* 1993;4(3):273–81.

Duffy LC, Zielezny MA, Marshall JR, Weiser MM, Byers TE, Phillips JF, Ogra PL, Graham S. Cigarette smoking and risk of clinical relapse in patients with Crohn's disease. *American Journal of Preventive Medicine* 1990;6(3):161–6.

Duncan BB, Chambless LE, Schmidt MI, Szklo M, Folsom AR, Carpenter MA, Crouse JR III. Correlates of body fat distribution: variation across categories of race, sex, and body mass in the atherosclerosis risk in communities study. *Annals of Epidemiology* 1995;5(3):192–200.

Dunn N, Thorogood M, Faragher B, de Caestecker L, MacDonald TM, McCollum C, Thomas S, Mann R. Oral contraceptives and myocardial infarction: results of the MICA case-control study. *British Medical Journal* 1999;318(7198):1579–84.

Eaker ED, Chesebro JH, Sacks FM, Wenger NK, Whisnant JP, Winston M. Cardiovascular disease in women. *Circulation* 1993;88(4 Pt 1):1999–2009.

Egger P, Dugglesby S, Hobbs R, Fall C, Cooper C. Cigarette smoking and bone mineral density in the elderly. *Journal of Epidemiology and Community Health* 1996;50(1):47–50.

Ekwo EE, Gosselink CA, Moawad A. Unfavorable outcome in penultimate pregnancy and premature rupture of membranes in successive pregnancy. *Obstetrics and Gynecology* 1992;80(2):166–72.

Ekwo EE, Gosselink CA, Woolson R, Moawad A. Risks for premature rupture of amniotic membranes. *International Journal of Epidemiology* 1993; 22(3):495–503.

Elders PJM, Netelenbos JC, Lips P, Khoe E, van Ginkel FC, Hulshof KFAM, van der Stelt PF. Perimenopausal bone mass and risk factors. *Bone and Mineral* 1989;7(3):289–99.

Elenbogen A, Lipi tz S, Mashiach S, Dor J, Levran D, Ben-Rafael Z. The effect of smoking on the outcome of in-vitro fertilization—embryo transfer. *Human Reproduction* 1991;6(2):242–4.

Eliasson B, Attvall S, Taskinen M-R, Smith U. The insulin resistance syndrome in smokers is related to smoking habits. *Arteriosclerosis and Thrombosis* 1994;14(12):1946–50.

Eliasson M, Hägg E, Lundblad D, Karlsson R, Bucht E. Influence of smoking and snuff use on electrolytes, adrenal and calcium regulating hormones. *Acta Endrocrinologica* 1993;128(1):35–40.

Ellard GA, Johnstone FD, Prescott RJ, Ji-Xian W, Jian-Hua M. Smoking during pregnancy: the dose dependence of birthweight deficits. *British Journal of Obstetrics and Gynaecology* 1996;103(8):806–13.

el-Torky M, el-Zeky F, Hall JC. Significant changes in the distribution of histologic types of lung cancer. A review of 4,928 cases. *Cancer* 1990;65(10):2361–7.

Eluf-Neto J, Booth M, Munoz N, Bosch FX, Meijer CJLM, Walboomers JMM. Human papillomavirus and invasive cervical cancer in Brazil. *British Journal of Cancer* 1994;69(1):114–9.

Engeland A, Anderson A, Haldorsen T, Tretli S. Smoking habits and risks of cancers other than lung cancer: 28 years' follow-up of 26,000

Norwegian men and women. *Cancer Causes and Control* 1996;7(5):497–506.

English PB, Eskenazi B, Christianson RE. Black-white differences in serum cotinine levels among pregnant women and subsequent effects on infant birthweight. *American Journal of Public Health* 1994; 84(9):1439–43.

Environmental Protection Agency. *Respiratory Health Effects of Passive Smoking: Lung Cancer and Other Disorders.* Washington: U.S. Environmental Protection Agency, Office of Research and Development, Office of Air and Radiation, 1992. EPA/ 600/6-90.

Epidemiology Group of the Research Committee of Inflammatory Bowel Disease in Japan. Dietary and other risk factors of ulcerative colitis: a case-control study in Japan. *Journal of Clinical Gastroenterology* 1994;19(2):166–71.

Epstein LH, Dickson BE, Ossip DJ, Stiller R, Russell PO, Winter K. Relationships among measures of smoking topography. *Addictive Behaviors* 1982;7(3): 307–10.

Ericson A, Källén B. An epidemiological study of work with video screens and pregnancy outcome. II. A case-control study. *American Journal of Industrial Medicine* 1986;9(5):459–75.

Ericsson U-B, Lindgärde F. Effects of cigarette smoking on thyroid function and the prevalence of goitre, thyrotoxicosis and autoimmune thyroiditis. *Journal of Internal Medicine* 1991;229(1):67–71.

Eriksen G, Wohlert M, Ersbak V, Hvidman L, Hedegaard M, Skajaa K. Placental abruption. A case-control investigation. *British Journal of Obstetrics and Gynaecology* 1991;98(5):448–52.

Ernster VL. The epidemiology of lung cancer in women. *Annals of Epidemiology* 1994;4(2):102–10.

Ernster VL, Grady D, Miike R, Black D, Selby J, Kerlikowske K. Facial wrinkling in men and women, by smoking status. *American Journal of Public Health* 1995;85(1):78–82.

Eskenazi B, Fenster L, Sidney S. A multivariate analysis of risk factors for preeclampsia. *Journal of American Medical Association* 1991;266(2):237–41.

Eskenazi B, Gold EB, Lasley BL, Samuels SJ, Hammond SK, Wight S, O'Neill Rasor M, Hines CJ, Schenker MB. Prospective monitoring of early fetal loss and clinical spontaneous abortion among female semiconductor workers. *American Journal of Industrial Medicine* 1995a;28(6):833–46.

Eskenazi B, Prehn AW, Christianson RE. Passive and active maternal smoking as measured by serum cotinine: the effect on birthweight. *American Journal of Public Health* 1995b;85(3):395–8.

Evans DJ, Hoffmann RG, Kalkhoff RK, Kissebah AH. Relationship of androgenic activity to body fat topography, fat cell morphology, and metabolic aberrations in premenopausal women. *Journal of Clinical Endocrinology and Metabolism* 1983;57(2): 304–10.

Evans DJ, Hoffmann RG, Kalkhoff RK, Kissebah AH. Relationship of body fat topography to insulin sensitivity and metabolic profiles in premenopausal women. *Metabolism* 1984;33(1):68–75.

Ever-Hadani P, Seidman DS, Manor O, Harlap S. Breast feeding in Israel: maternal factors associated with choice and duration. *Journal of Epidemiology and Community Health* 1994;48(3):281–5.

Everhart JE. Overview. In: Everhart JE, editor. *Digestive Diseases in the United States: Epidemiology and Impact.* U.S. Department of Health and Human Services, Public Health Service, National Institutes of Health, National Institute of Diabetes and Digestive and Kidney Diseases, 1994. NIH Publication No. 94-1447.

Everhart JE, Byrd-Holt D, Sonnenberg A. Incidence and risk factors for self-reported peptic ulcer disease in the United States. *American Journal of Epidemiology* 1998;147(6):529–36.

Everson RB, Sandler DP, Wilcox AJ, Schreinemachers D, Shore DL, Weinberg C. Effect of passive exposure to smoking on age at natural menopause. *British Medical Journal* 1986;293(6550):792.

Ewertz M. Smoking and breast cancer risk in Denmark. *Cancer Causes and Control* 1990;1(1):31–7.

Expert Committee on the Diagnosis and Classification of Diabetes Mellitus. Report of the Expert Committee on the Diagnosis and Classification of Diabetes Mellitus. *Diabetes Care* 1997;20(7):1183–97.

Eye Disease Case-Control Study Group. Risk factors for neovascular age-related macular degeneration. *Archives of Ophthalmology* 1992;110(12):1701–8.

Facchini FS, Hollenbeck CB, Jeppesen J, Chen Y-DI, Reaven GM. Insulin resistance and cigarette smoking. *Lancet* 1992;339(8802):1128–30.

Fagerström KO, Schneider NG, Lunell E. Effectiveness of nicotine patch and nicotine gum as individual versus combined treatments for tobacco withdrawal symptoms. *Psychopharmacology (Berlin)* 1993;111(3):271–7.

Falk RT, Pickle LW, Brown LM, Mason TJ, Buffler PA, Fraumeni JF Jr. Effect of smoking and alcohol consumption on laryngeal cancer risk in coastal Texas. *Cancer Research* 1989;49(14):4024–9.

Fanaroff AA, Martin RF, editors. *Neonatal-Perinatal Medicine: Diseases of the Fetus and Infant.* 3rd ed. St. Louis (MO): Mosby, 1992:166–9.

Fang MA, Frost PJ, Iida-Klein A, Hahn TJ. Effects of nicotine on cellular function in UMR 106–01 osteoblast-like cells. *Bone* 1991;12(4):283–6.

Feichtinger W, Papalambrou K, Poehl M, Krischker U, Neumann K. Smoking and in vitro fertilization: a meta-analysis. *Journal of Assisted Reproduction and Genetics* 1997;14(10):596–9.

Feinleib M, Rosenberg HM, Collins JG, Delozier JE, Pokras R, Chevarley FM. Trends in COPD morbidity and mortality in the United States. *American Review of Respiratory Disease* 1989;140(3 Pt 2): S9–S18.

Feinstein JM, Berkelhamer JE, Gruszka ME, Wong CA, Carey AE. Factors related to early termination of breast-feeding in an urban population. *Pediatrics* 1986;78(2):210–5.

Felson DT, Anderson JJ, Naimark A, Hannan MT, Kannel WB, Meenan RF. Does smoking protect against osteoarthritis? *Arthritis and Rheumatism* 1989;32(2):166–72.

Felson DT, Kiel DP, Anderson JJ, Kannel WB. Alcohol consumption and hip fractures: the Framingham Study. *American Journal of Epidemiology* 1988; 128(5):1102–10.

Felson DT, Zhang Y, Hannan MT, Naimark A, Weissman B, Aliabadi P, Levy D. Risk factors for incident radiographic knee osteoarthritis in the elderly: the Framingham Study. *Arthritis and Rheumatism* 1997;40(4):728–33.

Ferini-Strambi L, Smirne S, Garancini P, Pinto P, Franceschi M. Clinical and epidemiological aspects of Alzheimer's disease with presenile onset: a case control study. *Neuroepidemiology* 1990;9(1):39–49.

Ferraz EM, Gray RH. A case-control study of stillbirths in northeast Brazil. *International Journal of Gynaecology and Obstetrics* 1991;34(1):13–9.

Ferraz EM, Gray RH, Cunha TM. Determinants of preterm delivery and intrauterine growth retardation in north-east Brazil. *International Journal of Epidemiology* 1990;19(1):101–8.

Ferrucci L, Izmirlian G, Leveille S, Phillips CL, Corti MC, Brock DB, Guralnik JM. Smoking, physical activity, and active life expectancy. *American Journal of Epidemiology* 1999;149(7):645–53.

Feskens EJM, Kromhout D. Cardiovascular risk factors and the 25-year incidence of diabetes mellitus in middle-aged men: the Zutphen Study. *American Journal of Epidemiology* 1989;130(6):1101–8.

Field NA, Baptiste MS, Nasca PC, Metzger BB. Cigarette smoking and breast cancer. *International Journal of Epidemiology* 1992;21(5):842–8.

Finucane FF, Madans JH, Bush TL, Wolf PH, Kleinman JC. Decreased risk of stroke among postmenopausal hormone users. Results from a national cohort. *Archives of Internal Medicine* 1993; 153(1):73–9.

Fiore MC, Kenford SL, Jorenby DE, Wetter DW, Smith SS, Baker TB. Two studies of the clinical effectiveness of the nicotine patch with different counseling treatments. *Chest* 1994;105(2):524–33.

Firestein GS. Etiology and pathogenesis of rheumatoid arthritis. In: Kelley WN, Ruddy S, Harris ED Jr, Sledge CB, editors. *Textbook of Rheumatology.* Vol. 1. 5th ed. Philadelphia: W.B. Saunders, 1997: 851–97.

Fischer S, Spiegelhalder B, Preussmann R. Preformed tobacco-specific nitrosamines in tobacco—role of nitrate and influence of tobacco type. *Carcinogenesis* 1989;10(8):1511–7.

Fisher B. Curing the TSNA problem. *Tobacco Reporter* 2000;August:51, 53, 55–6.

FitzSimmons J, Stahl R, Gocial B, Shapiro SS. Spontaneous abortion and endometriosis. *Fertility and Sterility* 1987;47(4):696–8.

Flaye DE, Sullivan KN, Cullinan TR, Silver JH, Whitelocke RAF. Cataracts and cigarette smoking: the City Eye Study. *Eye* 1989;3(Pt 4):379–84.

Flegal KM, Troiano RP, Pamuk ER, Kuczmarski RJ, Campbell SM. The influence of smoking cessation on the prevalence of overweight in the United States. *New England Journal of Medicine* 1995; 333(18): 1165–70.

Fletcher CM, Peto R, Tinker C, Speizer FE. *The Natural History of Chronic Bronchitis and Emphysema. An Eight-Year Study of Early Chronic Obstructive Lung Disease in Working Men in London.* New York: Oxford University Press, 1976.

Florack EIM, Zielhuis GA, Rolland R. Cigarette smoking, alcohol consumption, and caffeine intake and fecundability. *Preventive Medicine* 1994;23(2):175–80.

Folsom AR, Kaye SA, Prineas RJ, Potter JD, Gapstur SM, Wallace RB. Increased incidence of carcinoma of the breast associated with abdominal adiposity in postmenopausal women. *American Journal of Epidemiology* 1990;131(5):794–803.

Folsom AR, Kaye SA, Sellers TA, Hong C-P, Cerhan JR, Potter JD, Prineas RJ. Body fat distribution and 5-year risk of death in older women. *Journal of the American Medical Association* 1993;269(4):483–7.

Fontham ETH. Protective dietary factors and lung cancer. *International Journal of Epidemiology* 1990; 19(Suppl 1):S32–S42.

Fontham ETH, Correa P, Reynolds P, Wu-Williams A, Buffler PA, Greenberg RS, Chen VW, Alterman T, Boyd P, Austin DF, Liff J. Environmental tobacco smoke and lung cancer in nonsmoking women: a multicenter study. *Journal of the American Medical Association* 1994;271(22):1752–9.

Fontham ETH, Correa P, Wu-Williams A, Reynolds P, Greenberg RS, Buffler PA, Chen VW, Boyd P, Alterman T, Austin DF, Liff J, Greenberg SD. Lung cancer in nonsmoking women: a multicenter case-control study. *Cancer Epidemiology, Biomarkers and Prevention* 1991;1(1):35–43.

Fontham ETH, Pickle LW, Haenszel W, Correa P, Lin Y, Falk RT. Dietary vitamins A and C and lung cancer risk in Louisiana. *Cancer* 1988;62(10):2267–73.

Forsén L, Bjartveit K, Bjørndal A, Edna T-H, Meyer HE, Schei B. Ex-smokers and risk of hip fracture. *American Journal of Public Health* 1998;88(10):1481–3.

Forsén L, Bjørndal A, Bjartveit K, Edna T-H, Holmen J, Jessen V, Westberg G. Interaction between current smoking, leanness, and physical inactivity in the prediction of hip fracture. *Journal of Bone and Mineral Research* 1994;9(11):1671–8.

Forster DP, Newens AJ, Kay DW, Edwardson JA. Risk factors in clinically diagnosed presenile dementia of the Alzheimer type: a case-control study in northern England. *Journal of Epidemiology and Community Health* 1995;49(3):253–8.

Fortier I, Marcoux S, Brisson J. Passive smoking during pregnancy and the risk of delivering a small-for-gestational-age infant. *American Journal of Epidemiology* 1994;139(3):294–301.

Fowkes FG. Aetiology of peripheral atherosclerosis. *British Medical Journal* 1989;298(6671):405–6.

Fowkes FGR, Housley E, Riemersma RA, Macintyre CCA, Cawood EHH, Prescott RJ, Ruckley CV. Smoking, lipids, glucose intolerance, and blood pressure as risk factors for peripheral atherosclerosis compared with ischemic heart disease in the Edinburgh Artery Study. *American Journal of Epidemiology* 1992;135(4):331–40.

Fowkes FGR, Pell JP, Donnan PT, Housley E, Lowe GDO, Riemersma RA, Prescott RJ. Sex differences in susceptibility to etiologic factors for peripheral atherosclerosis: importance of plasma fibrinogen and blood viscosity. *Arteriosclerosis and Thrombosis* 1994;14(6):862–8.

Fox SH, Koepsell TD, Daling JR. Birth weight and smoking during pregnancy—effect modification by maternal age. *American Journal of Epidemiology* 1994;139(10):1008–115.

Franceschi S, Boyle P, Maisonneuve P, La Vecchia C, Burt AD, Kerr DJ, MacFarlane GJ. The epidemiology of thyroid carcinoma. *Critical Reviews in Oncogenesis* 1993;4(1):24–52.

Franceschi S, Fassina A, Talamini R, Mazzolini A, Vianello S, Bidolo E, Cizza G, La Vecchia C. The influence of reproductive and hormonal factors on thyroid cancer in women. *Revue d'Epidémiologie et de Santé Publique* 1990;38(1):27–34.

Franceschi S, Panza E, La Vecchia C, Parazzini F, Decarli A, Porro GB. Nonspecific inflammatory bowel disease and smoking. *American Journal of Epidemiology* 1987;125(3):445–52.

Franceschi S, Schinella D, Bidoli E, Dal Maso L, La Vecchia C, Parazzini F, Zecchin R. The influence of body size, smoking, and diet on bone density in pre- and postmenopausal women. *Epidemiology* 1996;7(4):411–4.

Franceschi S, Serraino D, Bidoli E, Talamini R, Tirelli U, Carbone A, La Vecchia C. The epidemiology of non-Hodgkin's lymphoma in the north-east of Italy: a hospital-based case-control study. *Leukemia Research* 1989;13(6):465–72.

Frank P, McNamee R, Hannaford PC, Kay CR. Effect of changes in maternal smoking habits in early pregnancy on infant birthweight. *British Journal of General Practice* 1994;44(379):57–9.

Franks AL, Kendrick JS, Tyler CW Jr. Postmenopausal smoking, estrogen replacement therapy, and the risk of endometrial cancer. *American Journal of Obstetrics and Gynecology* 1987a;156(1):20–3.

Franks AL, Lee NC, Kendrick JS, Rubin GL, Layde PM. Cigarette smoking and the risk of epithelial ovarian cancer. *American Journal of Epidemiology* 1987b;126(1):112–7.

Frati AC, Iniestra F, Ariza CR. Acute effect of cigarette smoking on glucose tolerance and other cardiovascular risk factors. *Diabetes Care* 1996;19(2):112–8.

Fratiglioni L, Viitanen M, von Strauss E, Tontodonati V, Herlitz A, Winblad B. Very old women at highest risk of dementia and Alzheimer's disease: incidence data from the Kungsholmen Project, Stockholm. *Neurology* 1997;48:132–8.

Fraumeni JF Jr, Devesa SS, McLaughlin JK, Stanford JL. Biliary tract cancer. In: Schottenfeld D, Fraumeni JF Jr, editors. *Cancer Epidemiology and Prevention.* 2nd ed. New York: Oxford University Press, 1996:794–805.

Freedman DS, Tolbert PE, Coates R, Brann EA, Kjeldsberg CR. Relation of cigarette smoking to non-Hodgkin's lymphoma among middle-aged men. *American Journal of Epidemiology* 1998;148(9):833–41.

Freestone S, Ramsay LE. Effect of coffee and cigarette smoking on the blood pressure of untreated and diuretic-treated hypertensive patients. *American Journal of Medicine* 1982;73(3):348–53.

French SA, Jeffery RW, Forster JL, McGovern PG, Kelder SH, Baxter JE. Predictors of weight change over two years among a population of working adults: the Healthy Worker Project. *International Journal of Obesity* 1994;18(3):145–54.

Frette C, Barrett-Connor E, Clausen JL. Effect of active and passive smoking on ventilatory function in elderly men and women. *American Journal of Epidemiology* 1996;143(8):757–65.

Freund KM, Belanger AJ, D'Agostino RB, Kannel WB. The health risks of smoking. The Framingham Study: 34 years of follow-up. *Annals of Epidemiology* 1993;3(4):417–24.

Friedman AJ, Ravnikar VA, Barbieri RL. Serum steroid hormone profiles in postmenopausal smokers and nonsmokers. *Fertility and Sterility* 1987;47(3):398–401.

Friedman GD. Cigarette smoking, leukemia, and multiple myeloma. *Annals of Epidemiology* 1993;3(4): 425–8.

Friedman GD, Kannel WB, Dawber TR. The epidemiology of gallbladder disease: observations in the Framingham Study. *Journal of Chronic Diseases* 1966; 19(3):273–92.

Friedman GD, Siegelaub AB, Seltzer CC. Cigarettes, alcohol, coffee and peptic ulcer. *New England Journal of Medicine* 1974;290(9):469–73.

Friedman GD, Tekawa I, Sadler M, Sidney S. Smoking and mortality: the Kaiser Permanente experience. In: Shopland DR, Burns DM, Garfinkel L, Samet J, editors. *Changes in Cigarette Related Disease Risks and Their Implication for Prevention and Control.* Smoking and Tobacco Control Monograph 8. Rockville (MD): U.S. Department of Health and Human Services, Public Health Service, National Institutes of Health, National Cancer Institute, 1997:477–99. NIH Publication No. 97-4213.

Frith CD. Smoking behaviour and its relation to the smoker's immediate experience. *British Journal of Social and Clinical Psychology* 1971;10(1):73–8.

Fuchs CS, Colditz GA, Stampfer MJ, Giovannucci EL, Hunter DJ, Rimm EB, Willett WC, Speizer FE. A prospective study of cigarette smoking and the risk of pancreatic cancer. *Archives of Internal Medicine* 1996;156(19):2255–60.

Fujita Y, Katsumata K, Unno A, Tawa T, Tokita A. Factors affecting peak bone density in Japanese women. *Calcified Tissue International* 1999;64(2):107–11.

Fuxe K, Andersson K, Eneroth P, Härfstrand A, Agnati L. Neuroendocrine actions of nicotine and of exposure to cigarette smoke: medical implications. *Psychoneuroendocrinology* 1989;14(1–2):19–41.

Galanti MR, Hansson L, Lund E, Bergström R, Grimelius L, Stalsberg H, Carlsen E, Baron JA, Persson I, Ekbom A. Reproductive history and cigarette smoking as risk factors for thyroid cancer in women: a population-based case-control study. *Cancer Epidemiology, Biomarkers and Prevention* 1996; 5(6):425–31.

Galanti MR, Lambe M, Ekbom A, Sparen P, Pettersson B. Parity and risk of thyroid cancer: a nested case-control study of a nationwide Swedish cohort. *Cancer Causes and Control* 1995a;6(1):37–44.

Galanti MR, Sparen P, Karlsson A, Grimelius L, Ekbom A. Is residence in areas of endemic goiter a risk factor for thyroid cancer? *International Journal of Cancer* 1995b;61(5):615–21.

Gammon MD, Hibshoosh H, Terry MB, Bose S, Schoenberg JB, Brinton LA, Bernstein JL, Thompson WD. Cigarette smoking and other risk factors in relation to p53 expression in breast cancer among young women. *Cancer Epidemiology, Biomarkers and Prevention* 1999;8(3):255–63.

Gammon MD, Schoenberg JB, Ahsan H, Risch HA, Vaughan TL, Chow WH, Rotterdam H, West AB, Dubrow R, Stanford JL, Mayne ST, Farrow DC, Niwa S, Blot WJ, Fraumeni JF Jr. Tobacco, alcohol, and socioeconomic status and adenocarcinomas of the esophagus and gastric cardia. *Journal of the National Cancer Institute* 1997;89(17):1277–84.

Gammon MD, Schoenberg JB, Teitelbaum SL, Brinton LA, Potischman N, Swanson CA, Brogan DJ, Coates RJ, Malone KE, Stanford JL. Cigarette smoking and breast cancer risk among young women (United States). *Cancers Causes and Control* 1998;9(6):583–90.

Gao Y-T, Blot WJ, Zheng W, Ershow AG, Hsu CW, Levin LI, Zhang R, Fraumeni JF Jr. Lung cancer among Chinese women. *International Journal of Cancer* 1987;40(5):604–9.

Garfinkel L. Cancer mortality in nonsmokers: prospective study by the American Cancer Society. *Journal of the National Cancer Institute* 1980;65(5): 1169–73.

Garfinkel L. Time trends in lung cancer mortality among nonsmokers and a note on passive smoking. *Journal of the National Cancer Institute* 1981; 66(6):1061–6.

Garfinkel L. Selection, follow-up, and analysis in the American Cancer Society prospective studies. *National Cancer Institute Monographs* 1985;67:49–52.

Garfinkel L, Auerbach O, Joubert L. Involuntary smoking and lung cancer: a case-control study. *Journal of the National Cancer Institute* 1985;75(3): 463–9.

Garfinkel L, Boffetta P. Association between smoking and leukemia in two American Cancer Society prospective studies. *Cancer* 1990;65(10):2356–60.

Garfinkel L, Stellman SD. Smoking and lung cancer in women: findings in a prospective study. *Cancer Research* 1988;48(23):6951–5.

Garland C, Barrett-Connor E, Suarez L, Criqui MH, Wingard DL. Effects of passive smoking on ischemic heart disease mortality of nonsmokers: a prospective study. *American Journal of Epidemiology* 1985;121(5):645–50. [See also erratum *American Journal of Epidemiology* 1985;122(6):1112.]

Gealy R, Zhang L, Siegfried JM, Luketich JD, Keohavong P. Comparison of mutations in the p53 and K-ras genes in lung carcinomas from smoking and nonsmoking women. *Cancer Epidemiology, Biomarkers and Prevention* 1999;8(4 Pt 1):297–302.

Geng G-Y, Liang ZH, Zhang A-Y, Wu GL. On the relationship between smoking and female lung cancer. In: Aoki M, Hisamichi S, Tominaga S, editors. *Smoking and Health* 1987. Proceedings of the 6th World Conference on Smoking and Health; 1987 Nov 9–12; Tokyo. Amsterdam: Elsevier Science, 1988:483–6.

Geyelin M. Philip Morris chemist says data destroyed. *Wall Street Journal* 1997 Feb 21;Sect B:6.

Ghadirian P, Simard A, Baillargeon J. A population-based case-control study of cancer of the bile ducts and gallbladder in Quebec, Canada. *Revue d'Épidémiologie et de Santé Publique* 1993;41(2):107–12.

Gilbert DG. *Smoking: Individual Differences, Psychopathology, and Emotion*. Philadelphia: Taylor and Francis, 1995.

Gilbert DG, Spielberger CD. Effects of smoking on heart rate, anxiety, and feelings of success during social interaction. *Journal of Behavioral Medicine* 1987;10(6):629–38.

Gill JS, Shipley MJ, Tsementzis SA, Hornby R, Gill SK, Hitchcock ER, Beevers DG. Cigarette smoking: a risk factor for hemorrhagic and nonhemorrhagic stroke. *Archives of Internal Medicine* 1989;149(9): 2053–7.

Gillis CR, Hole DJ, Hawthorne VM, Boyle P. Environmental tobacco smoke 3.6. The effect of environmental tobacco smoke in two urban communities in the west of Scotland. *European Journal of Respiratory Disease* 1984;65(Suppl 133):121S–126S.

Gindoff PR, Tidey GF. Effects of smoking on female fecundity and early pregnancy outcome. *Seminars in Reproductive Endocrinology* 1989;7(4):305–13.

Giovannucci E, Colditz GA, Stampfer MJ, Hunter D, Rosner BA, Willett WC, Speizer FE. A prospective study of cigarette smoking and risk of colorectal adenoma and colorectal cancer in U.S. women. *Journal of the National Cancer Institute* 1994a;86(3): 192–9.

Giovannucci E, Rimm EB, Stampfer MJ, Colditz GA, Ascherio A, Kearney J, Willett WC. A prospective study of cigarette smoking and risk of colorectal adenoma and colorectal cancer in U.S. men. *Journal of the National Cancer Institute* 1994b;86(3): 183–91.

Glantz SA, Parmley WW. Passive smoking and heart disease: epidemiology, physiology, and biochemistry. *Circulation* 1991;83(1):1–12.

Glantz SA, Parmley WW. Passive smoking and heart disease: mechanisms and risk. *Journal of the American Medical Association* 1995;273(13):1047–53.

Glantz SA, Parmley WW. Passive and active smoking: a problem for adults. *Circulation* 1996;94(4):596–8.

Glassman AH. Cigarette smoking and its comorbidity. In: Onken LS, Blaine JD, Genser S, Horton AM, editors. *National Institute on Drug Abuse. Treatment of Drug-Dependent Individuals with Comorbid Mental Disorders.* NIDA Research Monograph 172. Rockville (MD): U.S. Department of Health and Human Services, Public Health Service, National Institutes of Health, National Institute on Drug Abuse, 1997:52–60.

Glassman AH, Helzer JE, Covey LS, Cottler LB, Stetner F, Tipp JE, Johnson J. Smoking, smoking cessation, and major depression. *Journal of the American Medical Association* 1990;264(12):1546–9.

Glassman AH, Stetner F, Walsh BT, Raizman PS, Fleiss JL, Cooper TB, Covey LS. Heavy smokers, smoking cessation, and clonidine: results of a double-blind, randomized trial. *Journal of the American Medical Association* 1988;259(19):2863–6.

Godwin-Austen RB, Lee PN, Marmot MG, Stern GM. Smoking and Parkinson's disease. *Journal of Neurology, Neurosurgery, and Psychiatry* 1982;45(7): 577–81.

Goff DC, Henderson DC, Amico E. Cigarette smoking in schizophrenia: relationship to psychopathology and medication side effects. *American Journal of Psychiatry* 1992;149(9):1189–94.

Gofin R, Kark JD, Friedlander Y. Cigarette smoking, blood pressure and pulse rate in the Jerusalem Lipid Research Clinic Prevalence Study. *Israel Journal of Medical Sciences* 1982;18(12):1217–22.

Gold EB, Bush T, Chee E. Risk factors for secondary amenorrhea and galactorrhea. *International Journal of Fertility and Menopausal Studies* 1994;39(3):177–84.

Golding J. Sudden infant death syndrome and parental smoking—a literature review [Review]. *Paediatric and Perinatal Epidemiology* 1997;11(1): 67–77.

Gonen R, Hannah ME, Milligan JE. Does prolonged preterm premature rupture of the membranes predispose to abruptio placentae? *Obstetrics and Gynecology* 1989;74(3 Pt 1):347–50.

Goodman DS. Overview of current knowledge of metabolism of vitamin A and carotenoids. *Journal of the National Cancer Institute* 1984;73(6):1375–9.

Goodman E, Capitman J. Depressive symptoms and cigarette smoking among teens. *Pediatrics* 2000; 106(4):748–55.

Goodman MT, Kolonel LN, Wilkens LR. The association of body size, reproductive factors and thyroid cancer. *British Journal of Cancer* 1992;66(6):1180–4.

Goodman MT, Moriwaki H, Vaeth M, Akiba S, Hayabuchi H, Mabuchi K. Prospective cohort study of risk factors for primary liver cancer in Hiroshima and Nagasaki, Japan. *Epidemiology* 1995;6(1): 36–41.

Goodman-Gruen D, Barrett-Connor E. Sex hormone-binding globulin and glucose tolerance in postmenopausal women. The Rancho Bernardo Study. *Diabetes Care* 1997;20(4):645–9.

Gori GB, Lynch CJ. Analytical cigarette yields as predictors of smoke bioavailability. *Regulatory Toxicology and Pharmacology* 1985;5(3):314–26.

Graham DY, Lew GM, Klein PD, Evans DG, Evans DJ Jr, Saeed ZA, Malaty HM. Effect of treatment of *Helicobacter pylori* infection on the long-term recurrence of gastric or duodenal ulcer: a randomized, controlled study. *Annals of Internal Medicine* 1992; 116(9):705–8.

Grainge MJ, Coupland AC, Cliffe SJ, Chilvers CED, Hosking DJ. Cigarette smoking, alcohol and caffeine consumption, and bone mineral density in postmenopausal women. *Osteoporosis International* 1998;8(4):355–63.

Gram IT, Austin H, Stalsberg H. Cigarette smoking and the incidence of cervical intraepithelial neoplasia, grade III, and cancer of the cervix uteri. *American Journal of Epidemiology* 1992;135(4):341–6.

Grandinetti A, Morens DM, Reed D, MacEachern D. Prospective study of cigarette smoking and the risk of developing idiopathic Parkinson's disease. *American Journal of Epidemiology* 1994;139(12): 1129–38.

Graves AB, Mortimer JA. Does smoking reduce the risks of Parkinson's and Alzheimer's diseases? *Journal of Smoking-Related Disorders* 1994;5(Suppl 1):79–90.

Graves AB, van Duijn CM, Chandra V, Fratiglioni L, Heyman A, Jorm AF, Kokmen E, Kondo K, Mortimer JA, Rocca WA, Shalat SL, Soininen H, Hofman A. Alcohol and tobacco consumption as risk factors for Alzheimer's disease: a collaborative re-analysis of case-control studies. *International Journal of Epidemiology* 1991;20(2 Suppl 2):S48–S57.

Green MS, Jucha E, Luz Y. Blood pressure in smokers and nonsmokers: epidemiologic findings. *American Heart Journal* 1986;111(5):932–40.

Greenberg ER, Vessey M, McPherson K, Yeates D. Cigarette smoking and cancer of the uterine cervix. *British Journal of Cancer* 1985;51(1):139–41.

Greenberg G, Thompson SG, Meade TW. Relation between cigarette smoking and use of hormonal replacement therapy for menopausal symptoms. *Journal of Epidemiology and Community Health* 1987; 41(1):26–9.

Greene SB, Aavedal MJ, Tyroler HA, Davis CE, Hames CG. Smoking habits and blood pressure change: a seven-year follow-up. *Journal of Chronic Diseases* 1977;30(7):401–13.

Greenlee RT, Murray T, Bolden S, Wingo PA. Cancer Statistics, 2000. *CA: A Cancer Journal for Clinicians* 2000;50(1):7–33.

Griffin MR, Ray WA, Fought RL, Melton LJ III. Black-white differences in fracture rates. *American Journal of Epidemiology* 1992;136(11):1378–85.

Grisso JA, Chiu GY, Maislin G, Steinmann WC, Portale J. Risk factors for hip fractures in men: a preliminary study. *Journal of Bone and Mineral Research* 1991;6(8):865–8.

Grisso JA, Kelsey JL, Strom BL, O'Brien LA, Maislin G, LaPann K, Samelson L, Hoffman S. Risk factors for hip fracture in black women. *New England Journal of Medicine* 1994;330(22):1555–9.

Gritz ER, Klesges RC, Meyers AW. The smoking and body weight relationship: implications for intervention and postcessation weight control. *Society of Behavioral Medicine* 1989;11(4):144–53.

Grodstein F, Colditz GA, Hunter DJ, Manson JE, Willett WC, Stampfer MJ. A prospective study of symptomatic gallstones in women: relation with oral contraceptives and other risk factors. *Obstetrics and Gynecology* 1994;84(2):207–14.

Grodstein F, Stampfer MJ. Estrogen for women at varying risk of coronary disease. *Maturitas* 1998; 30(1):19–26.

Groppelli A, Giorgi DMA, Omboni S, Parati G, Mancia G. Persistent blood pressure increase induced by heavy smoking. *Journal of Hypertension* 1992; 10(5):495–9.

Grunberg NE. The inverse relationship between tobacco use and body weight. In: Kozlowski LT, Annis HM, Chappel HD, Glaser FB, Goodstadt MS, Israel Y, Kalant H, Sellers EM, Vingilis ER, editors. *Research Advances in Alcohol and Drug Problems.* Vol 10. New York: Plenum Press, 1990: 270–315.

Grunberg NE, Winders SE, Wewers ME. Gender differences in tobacco use. *Health Psychology* 1991; 10(2):143–53.

Gudmundsson JA, Ljunghall S, Bergquist C, Wide L, Nillius SJ. Increased bone turnover during gonadotropin-releasing hormone superagonist-induced ovulation inhibition. *Journal of Clinical Endocrinology and Metabolism* 1987;65(1):159–63.

Guidotti TL, Jhangri GS. Mortality from airways disorders in Alberta, 1927–1987: an expanding epidemic of COPD, but asthma shows little change. *Journal of Asthma* 1994;31(4):277–90.

Gustafson O, Nylund L, Carlstrom K. Does hyperandrogenism explain lower in vitro fertilization (IVF) success rates in smokers? *Acta Obstetricia et Gynecologica Scandinavica* 1996;75(2):149–56.

Guyer B, Strobino DM, Ventura SJ, MacDorman M, Martin JA. Annual Summary of Vital Statistics. *Pediatrics* 1996;98(6):1007–19.

Gyde SN, Prior P, Alexander F, Evans S, Taylor K, John WG, Waterhouse JAH, Allan RN. Ulcerative colitis: why is the mortality from cardiovascular disease reduced? *Quarterly Journal of Medicine* 1984;53(211):351–7.

Haack DG, Baumann RJ, McKean HE, Jameson HD, Turbek JA. Nicotine exposure and Parkinson disease. *American Journal of Epidemiology* 1981;114(2): 191–200.

Haapanen A, Koskenvuo M, Kaprio J, Kesäniemi YA, Heikkilä K. Carotid arteriosclerosis in identical twins discordant for cigarette smoking. *Circulation* 1989;80(1):10–6.

Hackshaw AK, Law MR, Wald NJ. The accumulated evidence on lung cancer and environmental tobacco smoke. *British Medical Journal* 1997;315(7114): 980–8.

Haddow JE, Knight GJ, Palomaki GE, McCarthy JE. Second-trimester serum cotinine levels in nonsmokers in relation to birth weight. *American Journal of Obstetrics and Gynecology* 1988;159(2):481–4.

Hadley CB, Main DM, Gabbe SG. Risk factors for preterm premature rupture of the fetal membranes. *American Journal of Perinatology* 1990;7(4): 374–9.

Haenszel W, Kurihara M, Segi M, Lee RKC. Stomach cancer among Japanese in Hawaii. *Journal of the National Cancer Institute* 1972;49(4):969–88.

Haffner SM, Stern MP, Hazuda HP, Pugh J, Patterson JK. Do upper-body and centralized adiposity measure different aspects of regional body-fat distribution? Relationship to non-insulin-dependent diabetes mellitus, lipids, and lipoproteins. *Diabetes* 1987;36(1):43–51.

Haffner SM, Stern MP, Hazuda HP, Pugh J, Patterson JK, Malina R. Upper body and centralized adiposity in Mexican Americans and non-Hispanic whites: relationship to body mass index and other behavioral and demographic variables. *International Journal of Obesity* 1986;10(6):493–502.

Haffner SM, Valdez RA, Morales PA, Hazuda HP, Stern MP. Decreased sex hormone-binding globulin predicts noninsulin-dependent diabetes mellitus in women but not in men. *Journal of Clinical Endocrinology and Metabolism* 1993;77(1):56–60.

Hägg E, Asplund K. Is endocrine ophthalmopathy related to smoking? *British Medical Journal* 1987; 295(6599):634–5.

Haglund B, Cnattingius S. Cigarette smoking as a risk factor for sudden infant death syndrome: a population-based study. *American Journal of Public Health* 1990;80(1):29–32.

Haglund B, Cnattingius S, Nordstrom ML. Social differences in late fetal death and infant mortality in Sweden 1985–86. *Paediatric and Perinatal Epidemiology* 1993;7(1):33–44.

Hall SM, Muñoz RF, Reus V. Smoking cessation, depression and dysphoria. *NIDA Research Monographs* 1991;105:312–3.

Hall SM, Reus VI, Muñoz RF, Sees KL, Humfleet G, Hartz DT, Frederick S, Triffleman E. Nortriptyline and cognitive-behavorial therapy in the treatment of cigarette smoking. *Archives of General Psychiatry* 1998;55(8):683–90.

Hallquist A, Hardell L, Degerman A, Boquist L. Thyroid cancer: reproductive factors, previous diseases, drug intake, family history and diet: a case-control study. *European Journal of Cancer Prevention* 1994;3(6):481–8.

Halmi KA, Falk JR, Schwartz E. Binge-eating and vomiting: a survey of a college population. *Psychological Medicine* 1981;11(4):697–706.

Halsey NA, Coberly JS, Holt E, Coreil J, Kissinger P, Moulton LH, Brutus J-R, Boulos R. Sexual behavior, smoking, and HIV-1 infection in Haitian women. *Journal of the American Medical Association* 1992;267(15):2062–6.

Hammond EC. Smoking in relation to physical complaints. *Archives of Environmental Health* 1961;3(2): 146–64.

Hammond EC. Smoking in relation to the death rates of one million men and women. In: Haenszel W, editor. *Epidemiological Approaches to the Study of Cancer and Other Chronic Diseases*. National Cancer Insitute Monograph 19. Bethesda (MD): U.S. Department of Health, Education, and Welfare, Public Health Service, National Cancer Institute, 1966: 127–204

Handler A, Davis F, Ferre C, Yeko T. The relationship of smoking and ectopic pregnancy. *American Journal of Public Health* 1989;79(9):1239–42.

Handler AS, Mason ED, Rosenberg DL, Davis FG. The relationship between exposure during pregnancy to cigarette smoking and cocaine use and placenta previa. *American Journal of Obstetrics and Gynecology* 1994;170(3):884–9.

Hankinson SE, Willett WC, Colditz GA, Seddon JM, Rosner B, Speizer FE, Stampfer MJ. A prospective study of cigarette smoking and risk of cataract surgery in women. *Journal of the American Medical Association* 1992;268(8):994–8.

Hannaford PC, Croft PR, Kay CR. Oral contraception and stroke: evidence from the Royal College of General Practitioners' Oral Contraception Study. *Stroke* 1994;25(5):935–42.

Hanrahan JP, Tager IB, Segal MR, Tosteson TD, Castile RG, Van Vunakis H, Weiss ST, Speizer FE. The effect of maternal smoking during pregnancy on early infant lung function. *American Review of Respiratory Disease* 1992;145(5):1129–35.

Hansen MA. Assessment of age and risk factors on bone density and bone turnover in healthy premenopausal women. *Osteoporosis International* 1994; 4(3):123–8.

Hansen MA, Overgaard K, Riis BJ, Christiansen C. Potential risk factors for development of postmenopausal osteoporosis—examined over a 12-year period. *Osteoporosis International* 1991;1(2): 95–102.

Hanson RL, Narayan KMV, McCance DR, Pettitt DJ, Jacobsson LTH, Bennett PH, Knowler WC. Rate of weight gain, weight fluctuation, and incidence of NIDDM. *Diabetes* 1995;44(3):261–6.

Hansson L-E, Baron J, Nyren O, Bergstrom R, Wolk A, Adami H-O. Tobacco, alcohol and the risk of gastric cancer: a population-based case-control study in Sweden. *International Journal of Cancer* 1994; 57(1):26–31.

Hardy CJ, Palmer BP, Muir KR, Sutton AJ, Powell RJ. Smoking history, alcohol consumption, and systemic lupus erythematosus: a case-control study. *Annals of the Rheumatic Diseases* 1998;57(8):451–5.

Harger JH, Hsing AW, Tuomala RE, Gibbs RS, Mead PB, Eschenbach DA, Knox GE, Polk BF. Risk factors for preterm premature rupture of fetal membranes: a multicenter case-control study. *American Journal of Obstetrics and Gynecology* 1990;163(1 Pt 1): 130–7.

Harlap S, Baras M. Conception-waits in fertile women after stopping oral contraceptives. *International Journal of Fertility* 1984;29(2):73–80.

Harnack LJ, Anderson KE, Zheng W, Folsom AR, Sellers TA, Kushi LH. Smoking, alcohol, coffee, and tea intake and incidence of cancer of the exocrine pancreas: the Iowa Women's Health Study. *Cancer Epidemiology, Biomarkers and Prevention* 1997;6(12): 1081–6.

Harries AD, Baird A, Rhodes J. Non-smoking: a feature of ulcerative colitis. *British Medical Journal* (Clinical Research Edition) 1982;284(6317):706.

Harris ED Jr. *Rheumatoid Arthritis*. Philadelphia: W.B. Saunders, 1997.

Harris JE. Cigarette smoking among successive birth cohorts of men and women in the United States during 1900–80. *Journal of the National Cancer Institute* 1983;71(3):473–9.

Harris MI, Flegal KM, Cowie CC, Eberhardt MS, Goldstein DE, Little RR, Wiedmeyer HM, Byrd-Holt DD. Prevalence of diabetes, impaired fasting glucose, and impaired glucose tolerance in U.S. adults. The Third National Health and Nutrition Examination Survey, 1988–1994. *Diabetes Care* 1998; 21(4):518–24.

Harris RE, Zang EA, Anderson JI, Wynder EL. Race and sex differences in lung cancer risk associated with cigarette smoking. *International Journal of Epidemiology* 1993;22(4):592–9.

Harris RWC, Brinton LA, Cowdell RH, Skegg DCG, Smith PG, Vessey MP, Doll R. Characteristics of women with dysplasia or carcinoma in situ of the cervix uteri. *British Journal of Cancer* 1980;42(3): 359–69.

Harrison KL, Breen TM, Hennessey JF. The effect of patient smoking habit on the outcome of IVF and GIFT treatment. *Australian and New Zealand Journal of Obstetrics and Gynaecology* 1990;30(4):340–2.

Hart DJ, Spector TD. Cigarette smoking and risk of osteoarthritis in women in the general population: the Chingford Study. *Annals of the Rheumatic Diseases* 1993;52(2):93–6.

Hartge P, Schiffman MH, Hoover R, McGowan L, Lesher L, Norris HJ. A case-control study of epithelial ovarian cancer. *American Journal of Obstetrics and Gynecology* 1989;161(1):10–6.

Hartge P, Silverman D, Hoover R, Schairer C, Altman R, Austin D, Cantor K, Child M, Key C, Marrett LD, Mason TJ, Meigs JW, Myers MH, Narayana A, Sullivan JW, Swanson GM, Thomas D, West D. Changing cigarette habits and bladder cancer risk: a case-control study. *Journal of the National Cancer Institute* 1987;78(6):1119–25.

Hartge P, Silverman DT, Schairer C, Hoover RN. Smoking and bladder cancer risk in blacks and whites in the United States. *Cancer Causes and Control* 1993;4(4):391–4.

Hartsough CS, Lambert NM. Pattern and progression of drug use among hyperactives and controls: a prospective short-term longitudinal study. *Journal of Child Psychology and Psychiatry* 1987;28(4):543–53.

Hartz AJ, Rupley DC, Rimm AA. The association of girth measurements with disease in 32,856 women. *American Journal of Epidemiology* 1984; 119(1):71–80.

Hasenfratz M, Baldinger B, Bättig K. Nicotine or tar titration in cigarette smoking behavior? *Psychopharmacology (Berlin)* 1993;112(2–3):253–8.

Hatchell PC, Collins AC. The influence of genotype and sex on behavioral sensitivity to nicotine in mice. *Psychopharmacology* 1980;71(1):45–9.

Hatsukami D, Skoog K, Allen S, Bliss R. Gender and the effects of different doses of nicotine gum on tobacco withdrawal symptoms. *Experimental and Clinical Psychopharmacology* 1995;3(2):163–73.

Hazes JMW, Dijkmans BAC, Vandenbroucke JP, de Vries RRP, Cats A. Lifestyle and the risk of rheumatoid arthritis: cigarette smoking and alcohol consumption. *Annals of the Rheumatic Diseases* 1990;49(12):980–2.

He Y. Women's passive smoking and coronary heart disease. *Chung-Hua Yu Fang I Hsueh Tsa Chih* [*Chinese Journal of Preventive Medicine*] 1989;23(1):19–22.

He J, Vupputuri S, Allen K, Prerost MR, Hughes J, Whelton PK. Passive smoking and the risk of coronary heart disease: a meta-analysis of epidemiologic studies. *New England Journal of Medicine* 1999;340(12):920–6.

He Y, Lam TH, Li LS, Du RY, Jia GL, Huang JY, Zheng JS. Passive smoking at work as a risk factor for coronary heart disease in Chinese women who have never smoked. *British Medical Journal* 1994; 308(6925):380–4.

He Y, Li L, Wan Z, Li L, Zheng X, Jia G. Women's passive smoking and coronary heart disease. *Chung-Hua Yu Fang I Hsueh Tsa Chih* [*Chinese Journal of Preventive Medicine*] 1989;23:19–22. (In Chinese)

Hebert LE, Scherr PA, Beckett LA, Funkenstein HH, Albert MS, Chown MJ, Evans DA. Relation of smoking and alcohol consumption to incident Alzheimer's disease. *American Journal of Epidemiology* 1992;135(4):347–55.

Heckbert SR, Stephens CR, Daling JR. Diabetes in pregnancy: maternal and infant outcome. *Paediatric and Perinatal Epidemiology* 1988;2(4):314–26.

Heffner LJ, Sherman CB, Speizer FE, Weiss ST. Clinical and environmental predictors of preterm labor. *Obstetrics and Gynecology* 1993;81(5 Pt 1):750–7.

Hegedüs L, Bliddal H, Karstrup S, Bech K. Thyroid stimulating immunoglobulins are not influenced by smoking in healthy subjects. *Thyroidology* 1992; 4(2):91–2.

Hegedüs L, Karstrup S, Veiergang D, Jacobsen B, Skovsted L, Feldt-Rasmussen U. High frequency of goitre in cigarette smokers. *Clinical Endocrinology* 1985;22(3):287–92.

Hegmann KT, Fraser AM, Keaney RP, Moser SE, Nilasena DS, Sedlars M, Higham-Gren L, Lyon JL. The effect of age at smoking initiation on lung cancer risk. *Epidemiology* 1993;4(5):444–8.

Heineman EF, Zahm SH, McLaughlin JK, Vaught JB. Increased risk of colorectal cancer among smokers: results of a 26-year follow-up of US veterans and a review. *International Journal of Cancer* 1994; 59(6):728–38.

Heineman EF, Zahm SH, McLaughlin JK, Vaught JB, Hrubec Z. A prospective study of tobacco use and multiple myeloma: evidence against an association. *Cancer Causes and Control* 1992;3(1):31–6.

Heishman SJ, Taylor RC, Henningfield JE. Nicotine and smoking: a review of effects on human performance. *Experimental and Clinical Psychopharmacology* 1994;2(4):345–95.

Heliovaara M, Aho K, Aromaa A, Knekt P, Reunanen A. Smoking and risk of rheumatoid arthritis. *Journal of Rheumatology* 1993;20(11):1830–5.

Hellberg D, Valentin J, Nilsson S. Smoking as risk factor in cervical neoplasia [letter]. *Lancet* 1983; 2(8365–6):1497.

Hellenbrand W, Seidler A, Robra B-P, Vieregge P, Oertel WH, Joerg J, Nischan P, Schneider E, Ulm G. Smoking and Parkinson's disease: a case-control study in Germany. *International Journal of Epidemiology* 1997;26(2):328–39.

Helms PJ. Lung growth: implications for the development of disease. *Thorax* 1994;49(5):440–1.

Helsing KJ, Sandler DP, Comstock GW, Chee E. Heart disease mortality in nonsmokers living with smokers. *American Journal of Epidemiology* 1988; 127(5):915–22.

Helzer JE, Canino GJ, Hwu H-G, Bland RC, Newman S, Yeh E-K. Alcoholism: a cross-national comparison of population surveys with the Diagnostic Interview Schedule. In: Rose RM, Barrett J, editors. *Alcoholism: Origins and Outcome.* New York: Raven Press, 1988:31–47.

Hemenway D, Azrael DR, Rimm EB, Feskanich D, Willett WC. Risk factors for wrist fracture: effect of age, cigarettes, alcohol, body height, relative weight, and handedness on the risk for distal forearm fractures in men. *American Journal of Epidemiology* 1994;140(4):361–7.

Hemminki K, Mutanen P, Saloniemi I. Smoking and the occurrence of congenital malformations and spontaneous abortions: multivariate analysis. *American Journal of Obstetrics and Gynecology* 1983; 145(1):61–6.

Henderson BE, Paganini-Hill A, Ross RK. Estrogen replacement therapy and protection from acute myocardial infarction. *American Journal of Obstetrics and Gynecology* 1988;159(2):312–7.

Hennekens CH, Buring JE. Smoking and coronary heart disease in women [editorial]. *Journal of the American Medical Association* 1985;253(20):3003–4.

Henningfield JE, London ED, Jaffe JH. Nicotine reward: studies of abuse liability and physical dependence potential. In: Engel J, Oreland L, editors. *Brain Reward Systems and Abuse.* New York: Raven Press, 1987:147–64.

Henningfield JE, Miyasato K, Jasinski DR. Abuse liability and pharmacodynamic characteristics of intravenous and inhaled nicotine. *Journal of Pharmacology and Experimental Therapeutics* 1985;234(1): 1–12.

Henningfield JE, Schuh LM, Jarvik ME. Pathophysiology of tobacco dependence. In: Bloom FE, Kupfer DJ, editors. *Psychopharmacology: The Fourth Generation of Progress.* New York: Raven Press, 1995: 1715–29.

Hernandez-Avila M, Liang MH, Willett WC, Stampfer MJ, Colditz GA, Rosner B, Roberts WN, Hennekens CH, Speizer FE. Reproductive factors, smoking, and the risk for rheumatoid arthritis. *Epidemiology* 1990;1(4):285–91.

Herrero R, Brinton LA, Reeves WC, Brenes MM, Tenorio F, de Britton RC, Gaitan E, Garcia M, Rawls WE. Invasive cervical cancer and smoking in Latin America. *Journal of the National Cancer Institute* 1989;81(3):205–11.

Herrinton LJ, Friedman GD. Cigarette smoking and risk of non-Hodgkin's lymphoma subtypes. *Cancer Epidemiology, Biomarkers and Prevention* 1998; 7(1):25–8.

Hertz-Picciotto I, Smith AH, Holtzman D, Lipsett M, Alexeeff G. Synergism between occupational arsenic exposure and smoking in the induction of lung cancer. *Epidemiology* 1992;3(1):23–31.

Heyman A, Peterson B, Fillenbaum G, Pieper C. Consortium to Establish a Registry for Alzheimer's Disease (CERAD). Part XIV: demographic and clinical predictors of survival in patients with Alzheimer's disease. *Neurology* 1996;46(3):656–60.

Hiatt RA, Fireman BH. Smoking, menopause, and breast cancer. *Journal of the National Cancer Institute* 1986;76(5):833–8.

Higgins M, Keller JB, Ostrander LD. Risk factors for coronary heart disease in women: Tecumseh Community Health Study, 1959 to 1980. In: Eaker ED, Packard B, Wenger NK, Clarkson TB, Tyroler HA, editors. *Coronary Heart Disease in Women. Proceedings of an N.I.H. Workshop.* New York: Haymarket Doyma, 1987:83–9.

Higgins MW, Enright PL, Kronmal RA, Schenker MB, Anton-Culver H, Lyles M. Smoking and lung function in elderly men and women: the Cardiovascular Health Study. *Journal of the American Medical Association* 1993;269(21):2741–8.

Higgins MW, Kjelsberg M. Characteristics of smokers and nonsmokers in Tecumseh, Michigan. II. The distribution of selected physical measurements and physiologic variables and the prevalence of certain diseases in smokers and nonsmokers. *American Journal of Epidemiology* 1967;86(1):60–77.

Hildesheim A, Gravitt P, Schiffman MH, Kurman RJ, Barnes W, Jones S, Tchabo J-G, Brinton LA, Copeland C, Epp J, Manos MM. Determinants of genital human papillomavirus infection in low-income women in Washington, D.C. *Sexually Transmitted Diseases* 1993;20(5):279–85.

Hiller R, Sperduto RD, Podgor MJ, Wilson PW, Ferris FL 3rd, Colton T, D'Agostino RB, Roseman JM, Stockman ME, Milton RC. Cigarette smoking and the risk of development of lens opacities. The Framingham Studies. *Archives of Ophthalmology* 1997;115(9):1113–8.

Himmelberger DU, Brown BW Jr, Cohen EN. Cigarette smoking during pregnancy and the occurrence of spontaneous abortion and congenital abnormality. *American Journal of Epidemiology* 1978;108(6):470–9.

Hinds MW, Kolonel LN, Hankin JH, Lee J. Dietary vitamin A, carotene, vitamin C and risk of lung cancer in Hawaii. *American Journal of Epidemiology* 1984;119(2):227–37.

Hirayama T. Non-smoking wives of heavy smokers have a higher risk of lung cancer: a study from Japan. *British Medical Journal* 1981;282(6259):183–5.

Hirayama T. Cancer mortality in nonsmoking women with smoking husbands based on a large-scale cohort study in Japan. *Preventive Medicine* 1984a; 13(6):680–90.

Hirayama T. Lung cancer in Japan: effects of nutrition and passive smoking. In: Mizell M, Correa P, editors. *Lung Cancer: Causes and Prevention.* Deerfield Beach (MA): Verlag Chemie International, 1984b:175–95.

Hirayama T. *Life-Style and Mortality: A Large-Scale Census-Based Cohort Study in Japan. Contributions to Epidemiology and Biostatistics.* Vol. 6. New York: Karger, 1990.

Hirayama Y. Epidemiological patterns of Parkinson's disease based on a cohort study [in Japanese]. In: *Epidemiology of Intractable Diseases Research Committee.* Tokyo: Japan Ministry of Health and Welfare 1985:219–27.

Hirvelä H, Luukinen H, Läärä E, Laatikainen L. Risk factors of age-related maculopathy in a population 70 years of age or older. *Ophthalmology* 1996;103(6): 871–7.

Hirvonen E, Idänpään-Heikkilä J. Cardiovascular death among women under 40 years of age using low-estrogen oral contraceptives and intrauterine devices in Finland from 1975 to 1984. *American Journal of Obstetrics and Gynecology* 1990;163(1 Pt 2): 281–4.

Ho GYF, Kadish AS, Burk RD, Basu J, Palan PR, Mikhail M, Romney SL. HPV 16 and cigarette smoking as risk factors for high-grade cervical intra-epithelial neoplasia. *International Journal of Cancer* 1998;78(3):281–5.

Ho SC, Chan SSG, Woo J, Leung PC, Lau J. Determinants of bone mass in the Chinese old-old population. *Osteoporosis International* 1995;5(3):161–6.

Hoar SK, Blair A, Holmes FF, Boysen CD, Robel RJ, Hoover R, Fraumeni JF Jr. Agricultural herbicide use and risk of lymphoma and soft-tissue sarcoma. *Journal of the American Medical Association* 1986;256(9):1141–7.

Höfer I, Nil R, Bättig K. Nicotine yield as determinant of smoke exposure indicators and puffing behavior. *Pharmacology, Biochemistry and Behavior* 1991a; 40(1):139–49.

Höfer I, Nil R, Bättig K. Ultralow-yield cigarettes and type of ventilation: the role of ventilation blocking. *Pharmacology, Biochemistry and Behavior* 1991b;40(4):907–14.

Hofman A, Collette HJA, Bartelds AIM. Incidence and risk factors of Parkinson's disease in The Netherlands. *Neuroepidemiology* 1989;8(6):296–9.

Holdstock G, Savage D, Harman M, Wright R. Should patients with inflammatory bowel disease smoke? *British Medical Journal (Clinical Research Edition)* 1984;288(6414):362.

Hole DJ, Gillis CR, Chopra C, Hawthorne VM. Passive smoking and cardiorespiratory health in a general population in the west of Scotland. *British Medical Journal* 1989;299(6696):423–7.

Hollenbach KA, Barrett-Connor E, Edelstein SL, Holbrook T. Cigarette smoking and bone mineral density in older men and women. *American Journal of Public Health* 1993;83(9):1265–70.

Holló I, Gergely I, Boross M. Influence of heavy smoking upon the bone mineral content of the radius of the aged and effect of tobacco smoke on the sensitivity to calcitonin of rats. *Aktuelle Gerontologie* 1979;9(8):365–8.

Holowaty EJ, Risch HA, Miller AB, Burch JD. Lung cancer in women in the Niagara region, Ontario: a case-control study. *Canadian Journal of Public Health* 1991;82(5):304–9.

Holt PG. Immune and inflammatory function in cigarette smokers. *Thorax* 1987;42(4):241–9.

Holt VL, Daling JR, McKnight B, Moore DE, Stergachis A, Weiss NS. Cigarette smoking and functional ovarian cysts. *American Journal of Epidemiology* 1994;139(8):781–6.

Holz FG, Wolfensberger TJ, Piquet B, Gross-Jendroska M, Wells JA, Minassin DC, Chisholm IH, Bird AC. Bilateral macular drusen in age-related macular degeneration: prognosis and risk factors. *Ophthalmology* 1994;101(9):1522–8.

Honkanen R, Tupparainen M, Kröger H, Alhava E, Saarikoski S. Relationships between risk factors and fractures differ by type of fracture: a population-based study of 12192 perimenopausal women. *Osteoporosis International* 1998;8(1):25–31.

Hood RD. An assessment of potential effects of environmental tobacco smoke on prenatal development and reproductive capacity. In: Ecobichon DJ, Wu JM, editors. *Environmental Tobacco Smoke. Proceedings of the International Symposium at McGill University, 1989.* Lexington (MA): Lexington Books, 1990:242–89.

Hook EB, Cross PK. Cigarette smoking and Down syndrome. *American Journal of Human Genetics* 1985; 37(6):1216–24.

Hook EB, Cross PK. Maternal cigarette smoking, Down syndrome in live births, and infant race. *American Journal of Human Genetics* 1988;42(3):482–9.

Hoover DR. Re: Are female smokers at higher risk for lung cancer than male smokers? a case-control analysis by histologic type [letter]. *American Journal of Epidemiology* 1994;140(2):186–7.

Hopkinson JM, Schanler RJ, Fraley JK, Garza C. Milk production by mothers of premature infants: influence of cigarette smoking. *Pediatrics* 1992; 90(6):934–8.

Hopper JL, Seeman E. The bone density of female twins discordant for tobacco use. *New England Journal of Medicine* 1994;330(6):387–92.

Horn-Ross PL, Ljung BM, Morrow M. Environmental factors and the risk of salivary gland cancer. *Epidemiology* 1997;8(4):414–9.

Hornsby PP, Wilcox AJ, Weinberg CR. Cigarette smoking and disturbance of menstrual function. *Epidemiology* 1998;9(2):193–8.

Horta BL, Victora CG, Menezes AM, Barros FC. Environmental tobacco smoking and breastfeeding duration. *American Journal of Epidemiology* 1997; 146(2):128–33.

Horton AW. Indoor tobacco smoke pollution: a major risk factor for both breast and lung cancer? *Cancer* 1988;62(1):6–14.

Horwitz RI, Smaldone LF, Viscoli CM. An ecogenetic hypothesis for lung cancer in women. *Archives of Internal Medicine* 1988;148(12):2609–12.

Houston DE, Noller KL, Melton LJ III, Selwyn BJ. The epidemiology of pelvic endometriosis. *Clinical Obstetrics and Gynecology* 1988;31(4):787–800.

Houston DE, Noller KL, Melton LJ III, Selwyn BJ, Hardy RJ. Incidence of pelvic endometriosis in Rochester, Minnesota, 1970–1979. *American Journal of Epidemiology* 1987;125(6):959–69.

Howard G, Wagenknecht LE, Burke GL, Diez-Roux A, Evans GW, McGovern P, Nieto J, Tell GS, for the ARIC Investigators. Cigarette smoking and progression of atherosclerosis: the Atherosclerosis Risk in Communities (ARIC) Study. *Journal of the American Medical Association* 1998;279(2):119–24.

Howe G, Westoff C, Vessey M, Yeates D. Effects of age, cigarette smoking, and other factors on fertility: findings in a large prospective study. *British Medical Journal* 1985:290(6483):1697–700.

Howe GR, Jain M, Burch JD, Miller AB. Cigarette smoking and cancer of the pancreas: evidence from a population-based case-control study in Toronto, Canada. *International Journal of Cancer* 1991;47(3):323–8.

Hu J-F, Zhao X-H, Chen J-S, Fitzpatrick J, Parpia B, Campbell TC. Bone density and lifestyle characteristics in premenopausal and postmenopausal Chinese women. *Osteoporosis International* 1994; 4(6):288–97.

Hughes JR. Clonidine, depression, and smoking cessation. *Journal of the American Medical Association* 1988;259(19):2901–2.

Hughes JR. Tobacco withdrawal in self-quitters. *Journal of Consulting and Clinical Psychology* 1992;60(5): 689–97.

Hughes DA, Haslam PL, Townsend PJ, Turner-Warwick M. Numerical and functional alterations in circulatory lymphocytes in cigarette smokers. *Clinical and Experimental Immunology* 1985;61(2): 459–66.

Hughes EG, Brennan BG. Does cigarette smoking impair natural or assisted fecundity? *Fertility and Sterility* 1996;66(5):679–89.

Hughes EG, Yeo J, Claman P, YoungLai EV, Sagle MA, Daya S, Collins JA. Cigarette smoking and the outcomes of in vitro fertilization: measurement of effect size and levels of action. *Fertility and Sterility* 1994;62(4):807–14.

Hughes EG, YoungLai EV, Ward SM. Cigarette smoking and outcomes of in-vitro fertilization and embryo transfer: a prospective cohort study. *Human Reproduction* 1992;7(3):358–61.

Hughes JR, Gust SW, Skoog K, Keenan RM, Fenwick JW. Symptoms of tobacco withdrawal: a replication and extension. *Archives of General Psychiatry* 1991;48(1):52–9.

Hughes JR, Hatsukami DK, Mitchell JE, Dahlgren LA. Prevalence of smoking among psychiatric outpatients. *American Journal of Psychiatry* 1986;143(8): 993–7.

Hull MGR, North K, Taylor H, Farrow A, Ford WCL, and the Avon Longitudinal Study of Pregnancy and Childhood Study Team. Delayed conception and active and passive smoking. *Fertility and Sterility* 2000;74(4):725–33.

Hulley S, Grady D, Bush T, Furberg C, Herrington D, Riggs B, Vittinghoff E, for the Heart and Estrogen/progestin Replacement Study (HERS) Research Group. Randomized trial of estrogen plus progestin for secondary prevention of coronary heart disease in postmenopausal women. *Journal of the American Medical Association* 1998;280(7): 605–13.

Humble C, Croft J, Gerber A, Casper M, Hames CG, Tyroler HA. Passive smoking and 20-year cardiovascular disease mortality among nonsmoking wives, Evans County, Georgia. *American Journal of Public Health* 1990;80(5):599–601.

Humble CG, Samet JM, Pathak DR. Marriage to a smoker and lung cancer risk. *American Journal of Public Health* 1987a;77(5):598–602.

Humble CG, Samet JM, Pathak DR, Skipper BJ. Cigarette smoking and lung cancer in 'Hispanic' whites and other whites in New Mexico. *American Journal of Public Health* 1985;75(2):145–8.

Humble CG, Samet JM, Skipper BE. Use of quantified and frequency indices of vitamin A intake in a case-control study of lung cancer. *International Journal of Epidemiology* 1987b;16(3):341–6.

Hunt IF, Murphy NJ, Henderson C, Clark VA, Jacobs RM, Johnston PK, Coulson AH. Bone mineral content in postmenopausal women: comparison of omnivores and vegetarians. *American Journal of Clinical Nutrition* 1989;50(3):517–23.

Hunter DJ, Hankinson SE, Hough H, Gertig DM, Garcia-Closas M, Spiegelman D, Manson JE, Colditz GA, Willett WC, Speizer FE, Kelsey K. A prospective study of NAT2 acetylation genotype, cigarette smoking, and risk of breast cancer. *Carcinogenesis* 1997;18(11):2127–32.

Hurt RD, Sachs DP, Glover ED, Offord KP, Johnston JA, Dale LC, Khayrallah MA, Schroeder DR, Glover PN, Sullivan CR, Croghan IT, Sullivan PM. A comparison of sustained-release bupropion and placebo for smoking cessation. *New England Journal of Medicine* 1997;337(17):1195–202.

Hwang SJ, Beaty TH, Panny SR, Street NA, Joseph JM, Gordon S, McIntosh I, Francomano CA. Association study of transforming growth factor alpha (TGF alpha) TaqI polymorphism and oral clefts: indication of gene-environment interaction in a population-based sample of infants with birth defects. *American Journal of Epidemiology* 1995; 141(7):629–36.

Hyman LG, Lilienfeld AM, Ferris FL III, Fine SL. Senile macular degeneration: a case-control study. *American Journal of Epidemiology* 1983;118(2):213–27.

Ikard FF, Tomkins S. The experience of affect as a determinant of smoking behavior: a series of validity studies. *Journal of Abnormal Psychology* 1973;81(2):172–81.

Ingall TJ, Homer D, Baker HL Jr, Kottke BA, O'Fallon WM, Whisnant JP. Predictors of intracranial carotid artery atherosclerosis: duration of cigarette smoking and hypertension are more powerful than serum lipid levels. *Archives of Neurology* 1991;48(7):687–91.

Inoue M, Tajima K, Hirose K, Hamajima N, Takezaki T, Hirai T, Kato T, Ohno Y. Subsite-specific risk factors for colorectal cancer: a hospital-based case-control study in Japan. *Cancer Causes and Control* 1995;6(1):14–22.

Inoue M, Tajima K, Yamamura Y, Hamajima N, Hirose K, Nakamura S, Kodera Y, Kito T, Tominaga S. Influence of habitual smoking on gastric cancer by histologic subtype. *International Journal of Cancer* 1999;81(1):39–43.

Inoue R, Hirayama T. Passive smoking and lung cancer in women. In: Aoki M, Hisamichi S, Tominaga S, editors. *Smoking and Health 1987.* Proceedings of the 6th World Conference on Smoking and Health; 1987 Nov 9–12; Tokyo. Amsterdam: Elsevier Science Publishers BV, 1988:283–5.

International Agency for Research on Cancer. *IARC Monographs on the Evaluation of the Carcinogenic Risk of Chemicals to Humans: Tobacco Habits Other Than Smoking; Betel-Quid and Areca-Nut Chewing and Some Related Nitrosamines.* Vol. 37. Lyon (France): World Health Organization, 1985.

International Agency for Research on Cancer. Tobacco Smoking. *IARC Monographs on the Evaluation of the Carcinogenic Risk of Chemicals to Humans.* Vol. 38. Lyon (France): International Agency for Research on Cancer, 1986.

International Agency for Research on Cancer. *Environmental Carcinogenesis: Methods of Analysis and Exposure Measurement. Vol. 9. Passive smoking.* Lyon (France): International Agency for Research on Cancer, 1987. IARC Scientific Publication No. 81.

International Agency for Research on Cancer. *IARC Monographs on the Evaluation of the Carcinogenic Risk of Chemicals to Humans: Alcohol Drinking; Epidemiological Studies of Cancer in Humans.* Vol. 44. Lyon (France): World Health Organization, 1988.

Ippen M, Ippen H. Approaches to a prophylaxis of skin aging. *Journal of the Society of Cosmetic Chemists* 1965;16:305–8.

Ishibe N, Hankinson SE, Colditz GA, Spiegelman D, Willett WC, Speizer FE, Kelsey KT, Hunter DJ. Cigarette smoking, cytochrome *P450 1A1* polymorphisms, and breast cancer risk in the Nurses' Health Study. *Cancer Research* 1998;58(4):667–71.

Isoaho R, Puolijoki H, Huhti E, Kivela SL, Laippala P, Tala E. Prevalence of chronic obstructive pulmonary disease in elderly Finns. *Respiratory Medicine* 1994;88(8):571–80.

Istvan J, Matarazzo JD. Tobacco, alcohol, and caffeine use: a review of their interrelationships. *Psychological Bulletin* 1984;95(2):301–26.

Istvan JA, Lee WW, Buist AS, Connett JE. Relation of salivary cotinine to blood pressure in middle-aged cigarette smokers. *American Heart Journal* 1999; 137(5):928–31.

Italian-American Cataract Study Group. Risk factors for age-related cortical, nuclear, and posterior subcapsular cataracts. *American Journal of Epidemiology* 1991;133(6):541–53.

Ives JC, Buffler PA, Selwyn BG, Hardy RJ, Decker M. Lung cancer mortality among women employed in high-risk industries and occupations in Harris County, Texas, 1977–1980. *American Journal of Epidemiology* 1988;127(1):65–74.

Iwase A, Aiba M, Kira S. Respiratory nicotine absorption in nonsmoking females during passive smoking. *International Archives of Occupational and Environmental Health* 1991;63(2):139–43.

Iyasu S, Saftlas AK, Rowley DL, Koonin LM, Lawson HW, Atrash HK. The epidemiology of placenta previa in the United States, 1979 through 1987. *American Journal of Obstetrics and Gynecology* 1993; 168(5):1424–9.

Jackson R. The Auckland Heart Study: a case-control study of coronary heart disease [dissertation]. Auckland (New Zealand): University of Auckland, 1989.

Jaglal SB, Kreiger N, Darlington G. Past and recent physical activity and risk of hip fracture. *American Journal of Epidemiology* 1993;138(2):107–18.

Jain M, Burch JD, Howe GR, Risch HA, Miller AB. Dietary factors and risk of lung cancer: results from a case-control study, Toronto, 1981–1985. *International Journal of Cancer* 1990;45(2):287–93.

Jamrozik K, Broadhurst RJ, Anderson CS, Stewart-Wynne EG. The role of lifestyle factors in the etiology of stroke. A population-based case-control study in Perth, Western Australia. *Stroke* 1994; 25(1):51–9.

Janerich DT, Thompson WD, Varela LR, Greenwald P, Chorost S, Tucci C, Zaman MB, Melamed MR, Kiely M, McKneally MF. Lung cancer and exposure to tobacco smoke in the household. *New England Journal of Medicine* 1990;323(10):632–6.

Janowsky DS, Risch SC. Role of acetylcholine mechanisms in the affective disorders. In: Meltzer HY, Coyle JT, Kopin IJ, Bunney WE Jr, Davis KL, Schuster CR, Shader RI, Simpson GM, editors. *Psychopharmacology: The Third Generation of Progress.* New York: Raven Press, 1987:527–33.

Jarrett M, Heitkemper MM, Shaver JF. Symptoms and self-care strategies in women with and without dysmenorrhea. *Health Care for Women International* 1995;16(2):167–78.

Jasinski DR, Boren JJ, Henningfield JE, Johnson RE, Lange WR, Lukas SE. Progress report from the NIDA Addiction Research Center. In: *Problems of Drug Dependence 1983: Proceedings of the 45th Annual Scientific Meeting. The Committee on Problems of Drug Dependence.* NIDA Research Monograph 49. U.S. Department of Health and Human Services, Public Health Service, Alcohol, Drug Abuse, and Mental Health Administration, National Institute on Drug Abuse, 1984:69–76.

Jedrychowski W, Becher H, Wahrendorf J, Basa-Cierpialek Z. A case-control study of lung cancer with special reference to the effect of air pollution in Poland. *Journal of Epidemiology and Community Health* 1990;44(2):114–20.

Jedrychowski W, Flak E. Confronting the prenatal effects of active and passive tobacco smoking on the birth weight of children. *Central European Journal of Public Health* 1996;4(3):201–5.

Jedrychowski W, Krzyzanowski M, Wysocki M. Are chronic wheezing and asthma-like attacks related to $FEV_1$ decline? the Cracow Study. *European Journal of Epidemiology* 1988;4(3):335–42.

Jensen GF. Osteoporosis of the slender smoker revisited by the epidemiologic approach. *European Journal of Clinical Investigation* 1986;16(3):239–42.

Jensen J, Christiansen C. Effects of smoking on serum lipoproteins and bone mineral content during postmenopausal hormone replacement therapy. *American Journal of Obstetrics and Gynecology* 1988; 159(4):820–5.

Jensen J, Christiansen C, Rodbro P. Cigarette smoking, serum estrogens and bone loss during hormone-replacement therapy early after menopause. *New England Journal of Medicine* 1985;313(16):973–5.

Jensen JA, Goodson WH, Hopf HW, Hunt TK. Cigarette smoking decreases tissue oxygen. *Archives of Surgery* 1991;126(9):1131–4.

Jensen OM, Knudsen JB, McLaughlin JK, Sørensen BL. The Copenhagen case-control study of renal pelvis and ureter cancer: role of smoking and occupational exposures. *International Journal of Cancer* 1988;41(4):557–61.

Jensen TK, Henriksen TB, Hjollund NH, Scheike T, Kolstad H, Giwercman A, Ernst E, Bonde JP, Skakkebæk NE, Olsen J. Adult and prenatal exposures to tobacco smoke as risk indicators of fertility among 430 Danish couples. *American Journal of Epidemiology* 1998;148(10):992–7.

Jernström H, Knutsson M, Taskila P, Olsson H. Plasma prolactin in relation to menstrual cycle phase, oral contraceptive use, arousal time and smoking habits. *Contraception* 1992;46(6):543–8.

Ji B-T, Chow W-H, Dai Q, McLaughlin JK, Benichou J, Hatch MC, Gao Y-T, Fraumeni JF Jr. Cigarette smoking and alcohol consumption and the risk of pancreatic cancer: a case-control study in Shanghai, China. *Cancer Causes and Control* 1995;6(4): 369–76.

Jick H, Porter J, Morrison AS. Relation between smoking and age of natural menopause. *Lancet* 1977; 1(8026):1354–5.

Jick H, Walker AM. Cigarette smoking and ulcerative colitis. *New England Journal of Medicine* 1983;308(5): 261–3.

Jöckel KH, Pohlabeln H, Ahrens W, Krauss M. Environmental tobacco smoke and lung cancer. *Epidemiology* 1998;9(6):672–5.

Joesoef MR, Beral V, Aral SO, Rolfs RT, Cramer DW. Fertility and use of cigarettes, alcohol, marijuana, and cocaine. *Annals of Epidemiology* 1993;3(6):592–4.

Joffe M, Li Z. Male and female factors in fertility. *American Journal of Epidemiology* 1994;140(10):921–9.

Johansson C, Mellström D, Lerner U, Österberg T. Coffee drinking: a minor risk factor for bone loss and fractures. *Age and Ageing* 1992;21(1):20–6.

Johansson C, Mellström D, Milsom I. Reproductive factors as predictors of bone density and fractures in women at the age of 70. *Maturitas* 1993;17(1): 39–50.

Johnell O, Gullberg B, Kanis JA, Allander E, Elffors L, Dequeker J, Dilsen G, Gennari C, Vaz AL, Lyritis G, Mazzuoli G, Miravet L, Passeri M, Cano RP, Rapado A, Ribot C. Risk factors for hip fracture in European women: the MEDOS Study. *Journal of Bone and Mineral Research* 1995;10(11):1802–15.

Johnell O, Nilsson BE. Life-style and bone mineral mass in perimenopausal women. *Calcified Tissue International* 1984;36(4):354–6.

Johnsen R, Forde OH, Straume B, Burhol PG. Aetiology of peptic ulcer: a prospective population study in Norway. *Journal of Epidemiology and Community Health* 1994;48(2):156–60.

Johnson J, Weissman MM, Klerman GL. Service utilization and social morbidity associated with depressive symptoms in the community. *Journal of the American Medical Association* 1992;267(11): 1478–83.

Johnson J, Whitaker AH. Adolescent smoking, weight changes, and binge-purge behavior: associations with secondary amenorrhea. *American Journal of Public Health* 1992;82(1):47–54.

Johnson KC, Hu J, Mao Y. The Canadian Cancer Registries Epidemiology Research Group. Passive and active smoking and breast cancer risk in Canada, 1994–97. *Cancer Causes and Control* 2000;11(3): 211–21.

Johnston DE, Kaplan MM. Pathogenesis and treatment of gallstones. *New England Journal of Medicine* 1993;328(6):412–21.

Jones G, Nguyen T, Sambrook P, Kelly PJ, Eisman JA. Progressive loss of bone in the femoral neck in elderly people: longitudinal findings from the Dubbo osteoporosis epidemiology study. *British Medical Journal* 1994;309(6956):691–5.

Jones G, Scott FS. A cross-sectional study of smoking and bone mineral density in premenopausal parous women: effect of body mass index, breastfeeding, and sports participation. *Journal of Bone and Mineral Research* 1999;14(9):1628–33.

Jordan JM, Renner JB, Fryer JG, Marcum SB, Woodard J, Helmick C. Smoking and osteoarthritis (OA) of the knee and hip. *Arthritis and Rheumatism* 1995; 38(9 Suppl):S342.

Jorgensen T. Gall stones in a Danish population: relation to weight, physical activity, smoking, coffee consumption, and diabetes mellitus. *Gut* 1989; 30(4):528–34.

Jorgensen T, Kay L, Schultz-Larsen K. The epidemiology of gallstones in a 70-year-old Danish population. *Scandinavian Journal of Gastroenterology* 1990; 25(4):335–40.

Jorm AF, Korten AE, Henderson AS. The prevalence of dementia: a quantitative integration of the literature. *Acta Psychiatrica Scandinavica* 1987;76(5): 465–79.

Juchau MR, Namkung J, Chao ST. Mono-oxygenase induction in the human placenta. Interrelationships among position-specific hydroxylations of 17 beta-estradiol and benzo[a]pyrene. *Drug Metabolism and Disposition* 1982;10(3):220–4.

Juvela S, Hillbom M, Numminen H, Koskinen P. Cigarette smoking and alcohol consumption as risk factors for aneurysmal subarachnoid hemorrhage. *Stroke* 1993;24(5):639–46.

Juvela S, Hillbom M, Palomaki H. Risk factors for spontaneous intracerebral hemorrhage. *Stroke* 1995; 26(9):1558–64.

Kabat GC. Recent developments in the epidemiology of lung cancer. *Seminars in Surgical Oncology* 1993; 9(2):73–9.

Kabat GC, Augustine A, Hebert JR. Re: Smoking and leukemia: evaluation of a causal hypothesis [letter]. *American Journal of Epidemiology* 1994a;139(8): 849–52.

Kabat GC, Chang CJ, Wynder EL. The role of tobacco, alcohol use, and body mass index in oral and pharyngeal cancer. *International Journal of Epidemiology* 1994b;23(6):1137–44.

Kabat GC, Stellman SD, Wynder EL. Relation between exposure to environmental tobacco smoke and lung cancer in lifetime nonsmokers. *American Journal of Epidemiology* 1995;142(2):141–8.

Kabat GC, Wynder EL. Lung cancer in nonsmokers. *Cancer* 1984;53(5):1214–21.

Kadunce DP, Burr R, Gress R, Kanner R, Lyon JL, Zone JT. Cigarette smoking: risk factor for premature facial wrinkling. *Annals of Internal Medicine* 1991;114(10):840–4.

Kahn HA. The Dorn study of smoking and mortality among U.S. veterans: report on eight and one-half years of observation. In: Haenszel W, editor. *Epidemiological Approaches to the Study of Cancer and Other Chronic Diseases.* National Cancer Institute Monograph 19. Bethesda (MD): U.S. Department of Health, Education, and Welfare, Public Health Service, National Cancer Institute, 1966:1–27.

Kalandidi A, Doulgerakis M, Tzonou A, Hsieh CC, Aravandinos D, Trichopoulos D. Induced abortions, contraceptive practices, and tobacco smoking as risk factors for ectopic pregnancy in Athens, Greece. *British Journal of Obstetrics and Gynaecology* 1991;98(2):207–13.

Kalandidi A, Katsouyanni K, Voropoulou N, Bastas G, Saracci R, Trichopoulos D. Passive smoking and diet in the etiology of lung cancer among nonsmokers. *Cancer Causes and Control* 1990;1(1):15–21.

Källén K. Down's syndrome and maternal smoking in early pregnancy. *Genetic Epidemiology* 1997a;14(1):77–84.

Källén K. Maternal smoking and orofacial clefts. *Cleft Palate-Craniofacial Journal* 1997b;34(1):11–6.

Källén K. Maternal smoking during pregnancy and limb reduction malformations in Sweden. *American Journal of Public Health* 1997c;87(1):29–32.

Källén K. Maternal smoking and urinary organ malformations. *International Journal of Epidemiology* 1997d;26(3):571–4.

Källén K. Maternal smoking, body mass index, and neural tube defects. *American Journal of Epidemiology* 1998;147(12):1103–11.

Kandel DB, Johnson JG, Bird HR, Canino G, Goodman SH, Lahey BB, Regier DA, Schwab-Stone M. Psychiatric disorders associated with substance use among children and adolescents: findings from the Methods for the Epidemiology of Child and Adolescent Mental Disorders (MECA) Study. *Journal of Abnormal Child Psychology* 1997;25(2):121–32.

Kanner RE, Connett JE, Altose MD, Buist AS, Lee WW, Tashkin DP, Wise RA. Gender difference in airway hyperresponsiveness in smokers with mild COPD: the Lung Health Study. *American Journal of Respiratory and Critical Care Medicine* 1994;150(4):956–61.

Karakaya A, Tunçel N, Alptuna G, Koçer Z, Erbay G. Influence of cigarette smoking on thyroid hormone levels. *Human Toxicology* 1987;6(6):507–9.

Karakostov K. Passive smoking among pregnant women and its effect on the weight and height of the newborn. *Akusherstvoi Ginekologiia (Sofiia)* 1985;24(2):28–31.

Karasek R, Gardell B, Lindell J. Work and nonwork correlates of illness and behavior in male and female Swedish white collar workers. *Journal of Occupational Behavior* 1987;8:187–207.

Karegard M, Gennser G. Incidence and recurrence rate of abruptio placentae in Sweden. *Obstetrics and Gynecology* 1986;67(4):523–8.

Kato I, Tominaga S, Ito Y, Kobayashi S, Yoshii Y, Matsuura A, Kameya A, Kano T. A comparative case-control analysis of stomach cancer and atrophic gastritis. *Cancer Research* 1990;50(20):6559–64.

Kato I, Tominaga S, Terao C. Alcohol consumption and cancers of hormone-related organs in females. *Japanese Journal of Clinical Oncology* 1989;19(3):202–7.

Katschinski B, Fingerle D, Scherbaum B, Goebell H. Oral contraceptive use and cigarette smoking in Crohn's disease. *Digestive Diseases and Sciences* 1993;38(9):1596–600.

Katsouyanni K, Trichopoulos D, Kalandidi A, Tomos P, Riboli E. A case-control study of air pollution and tobacco smoking in lung cancer among women in Athens. *Preventive Medicine* 1991;20(2):271–8.

Katzman R, Aronson M, Fuld P, Kawas C, Brown T, Morgenstern H, Frishman W, Gidez L, Eder H, Ooi WL. Development of dementing illnesses in an 80-year-old volunteer cohort. *Annals of Neurology* 1989;25(4):317–24.

Kaufman DW, Palmer JR, Rosenberg L, Stolley P, Warshauer E, Shapiro S. Tar content of cigarettes in relation to lung cancer. *American Journal of Epidemiology* 1989;129(4):703–11.

Kaufman DW, Slone D, Rosenberg L, Miettinen OS, Shapiro S. Cigarette smoking and age at natural menopause. *American Journal of Public Health* 1980;70(4):420–2.

Kaur S. Lead and cadmium in maternal blood, umbilical cord blood, amniotic fluid and placenta of cows and buffaloes after foetal death (abortion) and after normal parturition. *Science of the Total Environment* 1989;79(3):287–90.

Kauraniemi T. Gynecological health screening by means of questionnaire and cytology. *Acta Obstetrica et Gynecologica Scandinavica* 1969;(Suppl 4): 1–224.

Kawachi I, Colditz GA. Invited commentary: confounding, measurement error, and publication bias in studies of passive smoking. *American Journal of Epidemiology* 1996;144(10):909–15.

Kawachi I, Colditz GA, Speizer FE, Manson JE, Stampfer MJ, Willett WC, Hennekens CH. A prospective study of passive smoking and coronary heart disease. *Circulation* 1997a;95(10): 2374–479.

Kawachi I, Colditz GA, Stampfer MJ, Willett WC, Manson JE, Rosner B, Hunter DJ, Hennekens CH, Speizer FE. Smoking cessation in relation to total mortality rates in women: a prospective cohort study. *Annals of Internal Medicine* 1993a;119(10): 992–1000.

Kawachi I, Colditz GA, Stampfer MJ, Willett WC, Manson JE, Rosner B, Hunter DJ, Hennekens CH, Speizer FE. Smoking cessation and decreased risks of total mortality, stroke, and coronary heart disease incidence among women: a prospective cohort study. In: Shopland DR, Burns DM, Garfinkel L, Samet JM, editors. *Changes in Cigarette-Related Disease Risks and Their Implication for Prevention and Control.* Smoking and Tobacco Control Monograph 8. Rockville (MD): U.S. Department of Health and Human Services, Public Health Service, National Institutes of Health, National Cancer Institute, 1997b:531–64. NIH Publication No. 97-4213.

Kawachi I, Colditz GA, Stampfer MJ, Willett WC, Manson JE, Rosner B, Speizer FE, Hennekens CH. Smoking cessation and decreased risk of stroke in women. *Journal of the American Medical Association* 1993b;269(2):232–6.

Kawachi I, Colditz GA, Stampfer MJ, Willett WC, Manson JE, Rosner B, Speizer FE, Hennekens CH. Smoking cessation and time course of decreased risks of coronary heart disease in middle-aged women. *Archives of Internal Medicine* 1994;154(2): 169–75.

Kawakami N, Takatsuka N, Shimizu H, Ishibashi H. Effects of smoking on the incidence of non-insulin-dependent diabetes mellitus. Replication and extension in a Japanese cohort of male employees. *American Journal of Epidemiology* 1997; 145(2):103–9.

Kaye SA, Folsom AR, Jacobs DR Jr, Hughes GH, Flack JM. Psychosocial correlates of body fat distribution in black and white young adults. *International Journal of Obesity* 1993;17(5):271–7.

Kaye SA, Folsom AR, Prineas RJ, Potter JD, Gapstur SM. The association of body fat distribution with lifestyle and reproductive factors in a population study of postmenopausal women. *International Journal of Obesity* 1990;14(7):583–91.

Keen H, Jarrett RJ, McCartney P. The ten-year follow-up of the Bedford Survey (1962–1972): glucose tolerance and diabetes. *Diabetologia* 1982;22(2):73–8.

Kelsey JL, Browner WS, Seeley DG, Nevitt MC, Cummings SR. Risk factors for fractures of the distal forearm and proximal humerus. *American Journal of Epidemiology* 1992;135(5):477–89.

Kelsey KT, Hankinson SE, Colditz GA, Springer K, Garcia-Closas M, Spiegelman D, Manson JE, Garland M, Stampfer MJ, Willett WC, Speizer FE, Hunter DJ. Glutathione *S*-transferase class μ deletion polymorphism and breast cancer: results from prevalent versus incident cases. *Cancer Epidemiology, Biomarkers and Prevention* 1997;6(7):511–5.

Kendler KS, Neale MC, MacLean CJ, Heath AC, Eaves LJ, Kessler RC. Smoking and major depression: a causal analysis. *Archives of General Psychiatry* 1993; 50(1):36–43.

Kessler II. Epidemiologic studies of Parkinson's disease. III. A community-based survey. *American Journal of Epidemiology* 1972;96(4):242–54.

Kessler II, Diamond EL. Epidemiologic studies of Parkinson's disease. I. Smoking and Parkinson's disease: a survey and explanatory hypothesis. *American Journal of Epidemiology* 1971;94(1):16–25.

Key TJA, Pike MC, Baron JA, Moore JW, Wang DY, Thomas BS, Bulbrook RD. Cigarette smoking and steroid hormones in women. *Journal of Steroid Biochemistry and Molecular Biology* 1991;39(4A):529–34.

Key TJA, Pike MC, Brown JB, Hermon C, Allen DS, Wang DY. Cigarette smoking and urinary oestrogen excretion in premenopausal and postmenopausal women. *British Journal of Cancer* 1996; 74(8):1313–6.

Khaw K-T, Tazuke S, Barrett-Connor E. Cigarette smoking and levels of adrenal androgens in postmenopausal women. *New England Journal of Medicine* 1988;318(26):1705–9.

Kiel DP, Baron JA, Anderson JJ, Hannan MT, Felson DT. Smoking eliminates the protective effect of oral estrogens on the risk for hip fracture among women. *Annals of Internal Medicine* 1992;116(9): 716–21.

Kiel DP, Zhang Y, Hannan MT, Anderson JJ, Baron JA, Felson DT. The effect of smoking at different life stages on bone mineral density in elderly men and women. *Osteoporosis International* 1996;6(3):240–8.

Kiely J, Paneth N, Susser M. An assessment of the effects of maternal age and parity in different components of perinatal mortality. *American Journal of Epidemiology* 1986;123(3):444–53.

Kikendall JW, Bowen PE, Burgess MB, Magnetti C, Woodward J, Langenberg P. Cigarettes and alcohol as independent risk factors for colonic adenomas. *Gastroenterology* 1989;97(3):660–4.

Killen JD, Fortmann SP, Newman B, Varady A. Evaluation of a treatment approach combining nicotine gum with self-guided behavioral treatments for smoking relapse prevention. *Journal of Consulting and Clinical Psychology* 1990;58(1):85–92.

Killen JD, Taylor CB, Telch MJ, Robinson TN, Maron DJ, Saylor KE. Depressive symptoms and substance use among adolescent binge eaters and purgers: a defined population study. *American Journal of Public Health* 1987;77(12):1539–41.

Killen JD, Taylor CB, Telch MJ, Saylor KE, Maron DJ, Robinson TN. Self-induced vomiting and laxative and diuretic use among teenagers: precursors of the binge-purge syndrome? *Journal of the American Medical Association* 1986;255(11):1447–9.

King H, Zimmet P, Raper LR, Balkau B. The natural history of impaired glucose tolerance in the Micronesian population of Nauru: a six-year follow-up study. *Diabetologia* 1984;26(1):39–43.

Kinlen LJ, McPherson K. Pancreas cancer and coffee and tea consumption: a case-control study. *British Journal of Cancer* 1984;49(1):93–6.

Kinnunen T, Doherty K, Militello FS, Garvey AJ. Depression and smoking cessation: characteristics of depressed smokers and effects of nicotine replacement. *Journal of Consulting and Clinical Psychology* 1996;64(4):791–8.

Kirschner MA, Samojlik E. Sex hormone metabolism in upper and lower body obesity. *International Journal of Obesity* 1991;15(Suppl 2):101–8.

Kirschner MA, Samojlik E, Drejka M, Szmal E, Schneider G, Ertel N. Androgen-estrogen metabolism in women with upper body versus lower body obesity. *Journal of Clinical Endocrinology and Metabolism* 1990;70(2):473–9.

Kissebah AH, Vydelingum N, Murray R, Evans DJ, Hartz AJ, Kalkhoff RK, Adams PW. Relation of body fat distribution to metabolic complications of obesity. *Journal of Clinical Endocrinology and Metabolism* 1982;54(2):254–60.

Kiyohara Y, Ueda K, Fujishima M. Smoking and cardiovascular disease in the general population in Japan. *Journal of Hypertension* 1990;8(Suppl 5): S9–S15.

Kjaer SK, Engholm G, Dahl C, Bock JE. Case-control study of risk factors for cervical squamous cell neoplasia in Denmark. IV. Role of smoking habits. *European Journal of Cancer Prevention* 1996;5(5): 359–65.

Kleerekoper M, Peterson E, Nelson D, Tilley B, Phillips E, Schork MA, Kuder J. Identification of women at risk for developing postmenopausal osteoporosis with vertebral fractures: role of history and single photon absorptiometry. *Bone and Mineral* 1989;7(2):171–86.

Kleigman RM. Intrauterine growth retardation. In: Fanaroff AA, Martin RJ, editors. *Neonatal-Perinatal Medicine: Diseases of the Fetus and Infant.* 6th ed. St. Louis (MO): Mosby-Year Book, 1997:203–40.

Klein BEK, Klein R, Moss SE. Prevalence of cataracts in a population-based study of persons with diabetes mellitus. *Ophthalmology* 1985;92(9):1191–6.

Klein BEK, Klein R, Ritter LL. Relationship of drinking alcohol and smoking to prevalence of open-angle glaucoma. The Beaver Dam Eye Study. *Ophthalmology* 1993a;100(11):1609–13.

Klein BEK, Linton KLP, Klein R, Franke T. Cigarette smoking and lens opacities: the Beaver Dam Eye Study. *American Journal of Preventive Medicine* 1993b;9(1):27–30.

Klein R, Klein BEK. Smoke gets in your eyes too [editorial]. *Journal of the American Medical Association* 1996;276(14):1178–9.

Klein R, Klein BEK, Linton KLP, DeMets DL. The Beaver Dam Eye Study: the relation of age-related maculopathy to smoking. *American Journal of Epidemiology* 1993c;137(2):190–200.

Kleinbaum DG, Kupper LL, Morgenstern H. *Epidemiologic Research: Principles and Quantitative Methods.* Belmont (CA): Lifetime Learning Publications, 1982.

Kleinman JC, Madans JH. The effects of maternal smoking, physical stature, and educational attainment on the incidence of low birth weight. *American Journal of Epidemiology* 1985;121(6):843–55.

Kleinman JC, Pierre MB Jr, Madans JH, Land GH, Schramm WF. The effects of maternal smoking on fetal and infant mortality. *American Journal of Epidemiology* 1988;127(2):274–82.

Klesges RC. An analysis of body image distortions in a nonpatient population. *International Journal of Eating Disorders* 1983;2(2):35–41.

Klesges LM, Klesges RC, Cigrang JA. Discrepancies between self-reported smoking and carboxyhemoglobin: an analysis of the Second National Health and Nutrition Survey. *American Journal of Public Health* 1992;82(7):1026–9.

Klesges RC, DePue K, Audrain J, Klesges LM, Meyers AW. Metabolic effects of nicotine gum and cigarette smoking: potential implications for post-cessation weight gain? *Journal of Consulting and Clinical Psychology* 1991a;59(5):749–52.

Klesges RC, Klesges LM. The relationship between body mass and cigarette smoking using a biochemical index of smoking exposure. *International Journal of Obesity and Related Metabolic Disorders* 1993;17(10):585–91.

Klesges RC, Klesges LM, Meyers AW. Relationship of smoking status, energy balance, and body weight: analysis of the Second National Health and Nutrition Examination Survey. *Journal of Consulting and Clinical Psychology* 1991b;59(6):899–905.

Klesges RC, Meyers AW, Klesges LM, LaVasque ME. Smoking, body weight, and their effects on smoking behavior: a comprehensive review of the literature. *Psychological Bulletin* 1989;106(2):204–30.

Klesges RC, Ward KD, Ray JW, Cutter G, Jacobs DR, Wagenknecht LE. The prospective relationships between smoking, and weight in a young, biracial cohort: The CARDIA study. *Journal of Clinical Psychology* 1998;66(6):987–93.

Klesges RC, Winders SE, Meyers AW, Eck LH, Ward KD, Hultquist CM, Ray JW, Shadish WR. How much weight gain occurs following smoking cessation? A comparison of weight gain using both continuous and point prevalence abstinence. *Journal of Consulting and Clinical Psychology* 1997;65(2):286–91.

Kline J, Levin B, Kinney A, Stein Z, Susser M, Warburton D. Cigarette smoking and spontaneous abortion of known karyotype: precise data but uncertain inferences. *American Journal of Epidemiology* 1995;141(5):417–27.

Kline J, Stein Z. Spontaneous abortion. In: Bracken MB, editor. *Perinatal Epidemiology.* New York: Oxford University Press, 1984:23–51.

Kline J, Stein Z, Susser M. *Conception to Birth: Epidemiology of Prenatal Development. Monograph in Epidemiology and Biostatistics.* Vol. 14. New York: Oxford University Press, 1989.

Kline J, Stein ZA, Susser M, Warburton D. Smoking: a risk factor for spontaneous abortion. *New England Journal of Medicine* 1977;297(15):793–6.

Klonoff-Cohen H, Edelstein S, Savitz D. Cigarette smoking and preeclampsia. *Obstetrics and Gynecology* 1993;81(4):541–4.

Klonoff-Cohen HS, Edelstein SL, Lefkowitz ES, Srinivasan IP, Kaegi D, Chang JC, Wiley KJ. The effect of passive smoking and tobacco exposure through breast milk on sudden infant death syndrome. *Journal of the American Medical Association* 1995;273(10):795–8.

Knekt P, Hakama M, Jarvinen R, Pukkala E, Heliovaara M. Smoking and risk of colorectal cancer. *British Journal of Cancer* 1998;78(1):136–9.

Knekt P, Reunanen A, Aho K, Heliovaara M, Rissanen A, Aromaa A, Impivaara O. Risk factors for subarachnoid hemorrhage in a longitudinal population study. *Journal of Clinical Epidemiology* 1991;44(9):933–9.

Kneller RW, McLaughlin JK, Bjelke E, Schuman LM, Blot WJ, Wacholder S, Gridley G, CoChien HT, Fraumeni JF Jr. A cohort study of stomach cancers in a high-risk American population. *Cancer* 1991;68(3):672–8.

Ko YE, Lee CH, Chen MJ, Huang CC, Chang WY, Lin HJ, Wang HZ, Chang PY. Risk factors for primary lung cancer among non-smoking women in Taiwan. *International Journal of Epidemiology* 1997;26(1):24–31.

Kokmen E, Beard CM, O'Brien PC, Kurland LT. Epidemiology of dementia in Rochester, Minnesota. *Mayo Clinic Proceedings* 1996;71(3):275–82.

Kolata G. Estrogen use tied to slight increase in risks to heart. *The New York Times* 2000 Apr 5;Sect A:1 (col 3).

Kolonel LN, Hankin JH, Wilkens LR, Fukunaga FH, Hinds MW. An epidemiologic study of thyroid cancer in Hawaii. *Cancer Causes and Control* 1990;1(3):223–4.

Kono S, Ikeda M, Tokudome S, Kuratsune M. A case-control study of gastric cancer and diet in northern Kyushu, Japan. *Japanese Journal of Cancer Research* 1988;79(10):1067–74.

Koo LC. Dietary habits and lung cancer risk among Chinese females in Hong Kong who never smoked. *Nutrition and Cancer* 1988;11(3):155–72.

Koo LC, Ho JH-C, Rylander R. Life-history correlates of environmental tobacco smoke: a study on nonsmoking Hong Kong Chinese wives with smoking versus nonsmoking husbands. *Social Science and Medicine* 1988;26(7):751–60.

Koo LC, Ho JH-C, Saw D. Is passive smoking and [sic] added risk factor for lung cancer in Chinese women? *Journal of Experimental and Clinical Cancer Research* 1984;3(3):277–83.

Koo LC, Ho JH-C, Saw D, Ho C-Y. Measurements of passive smoking and estimates of lung cancer risk among non-smoking Chinese females. *International Journal of Cancer* 1987;39(2):162–9.

Koren G, Sharav T, Pastuszak A, Garrettson LK, Hill K, Samson I, Rorem M, King A, Dolgin JE. A multicenter, prospective study of fetal outcome following accidental carbon monoxide poisoning in pregnancy. *Reproductive Toxicology* 1991;5(5): 397–403.

Korman MG, Hansky J, Eaves ER, Schmidt GT. Influence of cigarette smoking on healing and relapse in duodenal ulcer disease. *Gastroenterology* 1983; 85(4):871–4.

Koumantaki Y, Tzonou A, Koumantakis E, Kaklamani E, Aravantinos D, Trichopoulos D. A case-control study of cancer of endometrium in Athens. *International Journal of Cancer* 1989;43(5):795–9.

Krahn D, Kurth C, Demitrack M, Drewnowski A. The relationship of dieting severity and bulimic behaviors to alcohol and other drug use in young women. *Journal of Substance Abuse* 1992;4(4): 341–53.

Krall EA, Dawson-Hughes B. Smoking and bone loss among postmenopausal women. *Journal of Bone and Mineral Research* 1991;6(4):331–8.

Kramer MD, Taylor V, Hickok DE, Daling JR, Vaughan TL, Hollenbach KA. Maternal smoking and placenta previa. *Epidemiology* 1991;2(3):221–3.

Kratochvil P, Brandstätter G. Results of two years of long-term prevention of duodenal ulcer with cimetidine. *Medizinische Welt* 1983;34(48):1380–2.

Kratzer W, Kachele V, Mason RA, Muche R, Hay B, Wiesneth M, Hill V, Beckh K, Adler G. Gallstone prevalence in relation to smoking, alcohol, coffee consumption, and nutrition. The Ulm Gallstone Study. *Scandinavian Journal of Gastroenterology* 1997;32(9):953–8.

Kraus JF, Greenland S, Bulterys M. Risk factors for sudden infant death syndrome in the US Collaborative Perinatal Project. *International Journal of Epidemiolology* 1989;18(1):113–20.

Kreiger N, Gross A, Hunter G. Dietary factors and fracture in postmenopausal women: a case-control study. *International Journal of Epidemiology* 1992;21(5):953–8.

Kreiger N, Hilditch S. Re: Cigarette smoking and estrogen-dependent diseases [letter]. *American Journal of Epidemiology* 1986;123(1):200.

Kreuzer M, Kreienbrock L, Gerken M, Heinrich J, Bruske-Hohlfeld I, Muller K-M, Wichmann HE. Risk factors for lung cancer in young adults. *American Journal of Epidemiology* 1998;147(11): 1028–37.

Kreyberg L. Histological lung cancer types: a morphological and biological correlation. *Acta Pathologica et Microbiologica Scandinavica* 1962;157(Suppl): 11–90.

Kröger H, Laitinen K. Bone mineral density measured by dual-energy X-ray absorptiometry in normal men. *European Journal of Clinical Investigation* 1992;22(7):454–60.

Kröger H, Tuppurainen M, Honkanen R, Alhava E, Saarikoski S. Bone mineral density and risk factors for osteoporosis—a population-based study of 1600 perimenopausal women. *Calcified Tissue International* 1994;55(1):1–7.

Krohn M, Voigt L, McKnight B, Daling JR, Starzyk P, Benedetti TJ. Correlates of placental abruption. *British Journal of Obstetrics and Gynaecology* 1987; 94(4):333–40.

Krotkiewski M, Björntorp P, Sjöström L, Smith U. Impact of obesity on metabolism in men and women: importance of regional adipose tissue distribution. *Journal of Clinical Investigation* 1983; 72(3):1150–62.

Krzyzanowski M, Jedrychowski W, Wysocki M. Factors associated with the change in ventilatory function and the development of chronic obstructive pulmonary disease in a 13-year follow-up of the Cracow Study. Risk of chronic obstructive pulmonary disease. *American Review of Respiratory Disease* 1986;134(5):1011–9.

Kuller L, Borhani N, Furberg C, Gardin J, Manolio T, O'Leary D, Psaty B, Robbins J. Prevalence of subclinical atherosclerosis and cardiovascular disease and association with risk factors in the Cardiovascular Health Study. *American Journal of Epidemiology* 1994;139(12):1164–79.

Kune GA, Kune S, Vitetta L, Watson LF. Smoking and colorectal cancer risk: data from the Melbourne colorectal cancer study and brief review of literature. *International Journal of Cancer* 1992;50(3): 369–72.

Kurata JH, Elashoff JD, Nogawa AN, Haile BM. Sex and smoking differences in duodenal ulcer mortality. *American Journal of Public Health* 1986;76(6): 700–2.

Kurata JH, Nogawa AN. Meta-analysis of risk factors for peptic ulcer. Nonsteroidal antiinflammatory drugs, *Helicobactor pylori,* and smoking. *Journal of Clinical Gastroenterology* 1997;24(1):2–17.

Kurman RJ, Kaminski PF, Norris HJ. The behavior of endometrial hyperplasia: a long-term study of "untreated" hyperplasia in 170 patients. *Cancer* 1985;56(2):403–12.

La Vecchia C, D'Avanzo B, Franzosi MG, Tognoni G. Passive smoking and the risk of acute myocardial infarction. *Lancet* 1993a:341(8843):505–6.

La Vecchia C, Decarli A, Fasoli M, Parazzini F, Franceschi S, Gentile A, Negri E. Dietary vitamin A and the risk of intraepithelial and invasive cervical neoplasia. *Gynecologic Oncology* 1988;30(2): 187–95.

La Vecchia C, Franceschi S, Decarli A, Fasoli M, Gentile A, Tognoni G. Cigarette smoking and the risk of cervical neoplasia. *American Journal of Epidemiology* 1986;123(1):22–9.

La Vecchia C, Negri E, D'Avanzo B, Franceschi S. Smoking and renal cell carcinoma. *Cancer Research* 1990;50(17):5231–3.

La Vecchia C, Negri E, D'Avanzo B, Franceschi S, Boyle P. Risk factors for gallstone disease requiring surgery. *International Journal of Epidemiology* 1991a;20(1):209–15.

La Vecchia C, Negri E, Franceschi S, Parazzini F. Long term impact of reproductive factors on cancer risk. *International Journal of Cancer* 1993b;53(2):215–9.

La Vecchia C, Negri E, Levi F, Baron JA. Cigarette smoking, body mass and other risk factors for fractures of the hip in women. *International Journal of Epidemiology* 1991b;20(3):671–7.

La Vecchia C, Talamini R, Bosetti C, Negri E, Franceschi S. Response: re: cancer of the oral cavity and pharynx in nonsmokers who drink alcohol and in nondrinkers who smoke tobacco [letter]. *Journal of the National Cancer Institute* 1999;91(15):1337–8.

LaCroix AZ, Lang J, Scherr P, Wallace RB, Cornoni-Huntley J, Berkman L, Curb JD, Evans D, Hennekens CH. Smoking and mortality among older men and women in three communities. *New England Journal of Medicine* 1991;324(23):1619–25.

Lahita RG. Effects of gender on the immune system. Implications for neuropsychiatric systemic lupus erythematosus. *Annals of the New York Academy of Science* 1997;823:247–51.

Laitinen K, Välimäki M, Keto P. Bone mineral density measured by dual-energy X-ray absorptiometry in healthy Finnish women. *Calcified Tissue International* 1991;48(4):224–31.

Lam WK. A clinical and epidemiological study of carcinoma of lung in Hong Kong [dissertation]. Hong Kong: University of Hong Kong, 1985.

Lam TH, Kung ITM, Wong CM, Lam WK, Kleevens JWL, Saw D, Hsu C, Seneviratne S, Lam SY, Lo KK, Chan WC. Smoking, passive smoking and histological types in lung cancer in Hong Kong Chinese women. *British Journal of Cancer* 1987; 56(5):673–8.

Lambers DS, Clark KE. The maternal and fetal physiologic effects of nicotine [review]. *Seminars in Perinatology* 1996;20(2):115–26.

Landis SH, Murray T, Bolden S, Wingo PA. Cancer statistics 1998. *CA: A Cancer Journal for Clinicians* 1999;49(1):8–31.

Landsberg L, Troisi R, Parker D, Young JB, Weiss ST. Obesity, blood pressure, and the sympathetic nervous system. *Annals of Epidemiology* 1991;1(4): 295–303.

Lange P, Groth S, Nyboe J, Appleyard M, Mortensen J, Jensen G, Schnohr P. Chronic obstructive lung disease in Copenhagen: cross-sectional epidemiological aspects. *Journal of Internal Medicine* 1989; 226(1):25–32.

Lange P, Groth S, Nyboe J, Mortensen J, Appleyard M, Jensen G, Schnohr P. Decline of the lung function related to the type of tobacco smoked and inhalation. *Thorax* 1990a;45(1):22–6.

Lange P, Nyboe J, Appleyard M, Jensen G, Schnohr P. Relation of ventilatory impairment and of chronic mucus hypersecretion to mortality from obstructive lung disease and from all causes. *Thorax* 1990b;45(8):579–85.

Langenberg P, Kjerulff KH, Stolley PD. Hormone replacement and menopausal symptoms following hysterectomy. *American Journal of Epidemiology* 1997;146(10):870–80.

Lapidus L, Bengtsson C, Hällström T, Björntorp P. Obesity, adipose tissue distribution and health in women—results from a population study in Gothenburg, Sweden. *Appetite* 1989;12(1):25–35.

Lapidus L, Bengtsson C, Larsson B, Pennert K, Rybo E, Sjöström L. Distribution of adipose tissue and risk of cardiovascular disease and death: a 12 year followup of participants in the population study of women in Gothenburg, Sweden. *British Medical Journal* 1984;289(6454):1257–61.

Larsen PR, Ingbar SH. The thyroid gland. In: Wilson JD, Foster DW, editors. *Williams Textbook of Endocrinology.* 8th ed. Philadelphia: W.B. Saunders, 1992:357–487.

Larsson B, Svärdsudd K, Welin L, Wilhelmsen L, Björntorp P, Tibblin G. Abdominal adipose tissue distribution, obesity, and risk of cardiovascular disease and death: a 13 year follow up of participants in the study of men born in 1913. *British Medical Journal* 1984;288(6428):1401–4.

Lash TL, Aschengrau A. Active and passive cigarette smoking and the occurrence of breast cancer. *American Journal of Epidemiology* 1999;149(1):5–12.

Lasser K, Boyd JW, Woolhandler S, Himmelstein DU, McCormick D, Bor DH. Smoking and mental illness: a population-based prevalence study. *Journal of the American Medical Association* 2000;284(20):2606–10.

Launer LJ, Andersen K, Dewey ME, Letenneur L, Ott A, Amaducci LA, Brayne C, Copeland JR, Dartigues JF, Kragh-Sorensen P, Lobo A, Martinez-Lage JM, Stijnen T, Hofman A. Rates and risk factors for dementia and Alzheimer's disease: results from EURODEM pooled analyses. *Neurology* 1999;52(1):78–84.

Laurent SL, Thompson SJ, Addy C, Garrison CZ, Moore EE. An epidemiologic study of smoking and primary infertility in women. *Fertility and Sterility* 1992;57(3):565–72.

Law MR, Cheng R, Hackshaw AK, Allaway S, Hale AK. Cigarette smoking, sex hormones and bone density in women. *European Journal of Epidemiology* 1997a;13(5):553–8.

Law MR, Hackshaw AK. A meta-analysis of cigarette smoking, bone mineral density and risk of fracture: recognition of a major effect. *British Medical Journal* 1997;315(7112):841–6.

Law MR, Morris JK, Wald NJ. Environmental tobacco smoke exposure and ischaemic heart disease: an evaluation of the evidence. *British Medical Journal* 1997b;315(7114):973–80.

Lawrence C, Tessaro I, Durgerian S, Caputo T, Richart R, Jacobson H, Greenwald P. Smoking, body weight, and early-stage endometrial cancer. *Cancer* 1987;59(9):1665–9.

Lawrence C, Tessaro I, Durgerian S, Caputo T, Richart RM, Greenwald P. Advanced-stage endometrial cancer: contributions of estrogen use, smoking, and other risk factors. *Gynecologic Oncology* 1989a;32(1):41–5.

Lawrence RC, Hochberg MC, Kelsey JL, McDuffie FC, Medsger TA Jr, Felts WR, Shulman LE. Estimates of the prevalence of selected arthritic and musculoskeletal diseases in the United States. *Journal of Rheumatology* 1989b;16(4):427–41.

Layard MW. Ischemic heart disease and spousal smoking in the National Mortality Followback Survey. *Regulatory Toxicology and Pharmacology* 1995;21(1):180–3.

Layde PM, Vessey MP, Yeates D. Risk factors for gall-bladder disease: a cohort study of young women attending family planning clinics. *Journal of Epidemiology and Community Health* 1982;36(4):274–8.

Lazzaroni F, Bonassi S, Manniello E, Morcaldi L, Repetto E, Ruocco A, Calvi A, Cotellessa G. Effect of passive smoking during pregnancy on selected perinatal parameters. *International Journal of Epidemiology* 1990;19(4):960–6.

Le Houezec J, Benowitz NL. Basic and clinical psychopharmacology of nicotine. *Clinics in Chest Medicine* 1991;12(4):681–99.

Le Marchand L, Wilkens LR, Kolonel LN. Ethnic differences in the lung cancer risk associated with smoking. *Cancer Epidemiology, Biomarkers and Prevention* 1992;1(2):103–7.

Le Marchand L, Wilkens LR, Kolonel LN, Hankin JH, Lyu LC. Associations of sedentary lifestyle, obesity, smoking, alcohol use, and diabetes with the risk of colorectal cancer. *Cancer Research* 1997;57(21):4787–94.

Le Marchand L, Yoshizawa CN, Kolonel LN, Hankin JH, Goodman MT. Vegetable consumption and lung cancer risk: a population-based case-control study in Hawaii. *Journal of the National Cancer Institute* 1989;81(15):1158–64.

Lee PN. Smoking and Alzheimer's disease: a review of the epidemiological evidence. *Neuroepidemology* 1994;13(4):131–44.

Lee DJ, Markides KS. Health behaviors, risk factors, and health indicators associated with cigarette use in Mexican Americans: results from the Hispanic HANES. *American Journal of Public Health* 1991;81(7):859–64.

Lee FI, Fielding JD, Holmes GK, Hine KR, Gibson JA, Lochee-Bayne E, Mackay C, Mitchell KG, Pickard WR, Orchard RT, Stone WD. Ranitidine: prophylaxis of duodenal ulcer recurrence. *Hepato-Gastroenterology* 1984;31(2):85–7.

Lee PN, Chamberlain J, Alderson MR. Relationship of passive smoking to risk of lung cancer and other smoking-associated diseases. *British Journal of Cancer* 1986;54(1):97–105.

Lee WC, Neugut AI, Garbowski GC, Forde KA, Treat MR, Waye JD, Fenoglio-Preiser C. Cigarettes, alcohol, coffee, and caffeine as risk factors for colorectal adenomatous polyps. *Annals of Epidemiology* 1993;3(3):239–44.

Leino A, Järvisalo J, Impivaara O, Kaitsaari M. Ovarian hormone status, life-style factors, and markers of bone metabolism in women aged 50 years. *Calcified Tissue International* 1994;54(4):262–7.

Leischow SJ, Sachs DPL, Bostrom AG, Hansen MD. Effects of differing nicotine-replacement doses on weight gain after smoking cessation. *Archives of Family Medicine* 1992;1(2):233–7.

Lerman C, Caporaso N, Main D, Audrain J, Boyd NR, Bowman ED, Shields PG. Depression and self-medication with nicotine: the modifying influence of the dopamine D4 receptor gene. *Health Psychology* 1998;17(1):56–62.

Leske MC, Chylack LT Jr, He Q, Wu SY, Schoenfeld E, Friend J, Wolfe J. Risk factors for nuclear opalescence in a longitudinal study. LSC Group. Longitudinal Study of Cataract. *American Journal of Epidemiology* 1998;147(1):36–41.

Leske MC, Chylack LT Jr, Wu S-Y. The Lens Opacities Case-Control Study: risk factors for cataract. *Archives of Ophthalmology* 1991;109(2):244–51.

Leske MC, Connell AM, Wu SY, Hyman LG, Schachat AP. Risk factors for open-angle glaucoma. The Barbados Eye Study. *Archives of Ophthalmology* 1995;113(7):918–24.

Lesko SM, Rosenberg L, Kaufman DW, Helmrich SP, Miller DR, Strom B, Schottenfeld D, Rosenshein NB, Knapp RC, Lewis J, Shapiro S. Cigarette smoking and the risk of endometrial cancer. *New England Journal of Medicine* 1985;313(10):593–6.

Letenneur L, Commenges D, Dartigues JF, Barberger-Gateau P. Incidence of dementia and Alzheimer's disease in elderly community residents of south-western France. *International Journal of Epidemiology* 1994a;23(6):1256–61.

Letenneur L, Dartigues J-F, Commenges D, Barberger-Gateau P, Tessier J-F, Orgogozo J-M. Tobacco consumption and cognitive impairment in elderly people: a population-based study. *Annals of Epidemiology* 1994b;4(6):449–54.

Levi F, Franceschi S, Gulie C, Negri E, La Vecchia C. Female thyroid cancer: the role of reproductive and hormonal factors in Switzerland. *Oncology* 1993;50(4):309–15.

Levi F, Franceschi S, La Vecchia C, Randimbison L, Te VC. Lung carcinoma trends by histologic type in Vaud and Neuchatel, Switzerland, 1974–1994. *Cancer* 1997;79(5):906–14.

Levi F, La Vecchia C, Decarli A. Cigarette smoking and the risk of endometrial cancer. *European Journal of Cancer and Clinical Oncology* 1987;23(7):1025–9.

Levin ED. Nicotinic systems and cognitive function. *Psychopharmacology (Berlin)* 1992;108(4):417–31.

Levin AA, Schoenbaum SC, Stubblefield PG, Zimicki S, Monson RR, Ryan KJ. Ectopic pregnancy and prior induced abortion. *American Journal of Public Health* 1982;72(3):253–6.

Levin ED, Behm F, Rose JE. The use of flavor in cigarette substitutes. *Drug and Alcohol Dependence* 1990;26(2):155–60.

LeVois ME, Layard MW. Publication bias in the environmental tobacco smoke/coronary heart disease epidemiologic literature. *Regulatory Toxicology and Pharmacology* 1995;21(1):184–91.

Lewis MA, Spitzer WO, Heinemann LAJ, MacRae KD, Bruppacher R, Thorogood M. Third generation oral contraceptives and risk of myocardial infarction: an international case-control study. *British Medical Journal* 1996;312(7023):88–90.

Li CQ, Windsor RA, Perkins L, Goldenberg RL, Lowe JB. The impact on infant birth weight and gestational age of cotinine-validated smoking reduction during pregnancy. *Journal of the American Medical Association* 1993;269(12):1519–24.

Li DK, Daling JR. Maternal smoking, low birth weight, and ethnicity in relation to sudden infant death syndrome. *American Journal of Epidemiology* 1991;134(9):958–64.

Li DK, Mueller BA, Hickok DE, Daling JR, Fantel AG, Checkoway HW, Weiss NS. Maternal smoking during pregnancy and the risk of congenital urinary tract anomalies. *American Journal of Public Health* 1996;86(2):249–53.

Licciardone JC, Wilkins JR III, Brownson RC, Chang JC. Cigarette smoking and alcohol consumption in the aetiology of uterine cervical cancer. *International Journal of Epidemiology* 1989;18(3):533–7.

Lidegaard Ø. Oral contraception and risk of a cerebral thromboembolic attack: results of a case-control study. *British Medical Journal* 1993;306(6883):956–63.

Lieberman E, Gremy I, Lang JM, Cohen AP. Low birthweight at term and the timing of fetal exposure to maternal smoking. *American Journal of Public Health* 1994;84(7):1127–31.

Lindberg E, Järnerot G, Huitfeldt B. Smoking in Crohn's disease: effect on localisation and clinical course. *Gut* 1992;33(6):779–82.

Lindberg E, Tysk C, Andersson K, Järnerot G. Smoking and inflammatory bowel disease: a case control study. *Gut* 1988;29(3):352–7.

Lindblad A, Marsal K, Andersson KE. Effect of nicotine on human fetal blood flow. *Obstetrics and Gynecology* 1988;72(3 Pt 1):371–82.

Lindbohm M-L, Sallmén M, Anttila A, Taskinen H, Hemminki K. Paternal occupational lead exposure and spontaneous abortion. *Scandinavian Journal of Work, Environment and Health* 1991;17(2):95–103.

Lindenstrøm E, Boysen G, Nyboe J. Lifestyle factors and risk of cerebrovascular disease in women: the Copenhagen City Heart Study. *Stroke* 1993;24(10):1468–72.

Lindquist O, Bengtsson C. Menopausal age in relation to smoking. *Acta Medica Scandinavica* 1979;205(1–2): 73–7.

Lindsay R. The influence of cigarette smoking on bone mass and bone loss. In: DeLuca HF, Frost HM, Jee WSS, Johnston CC Jr, Parfitt AM, editors. *Osteoporosis: Recent Advances in Pathogenesis and Treatment.* Baltimore: University Park Press, 1981: 481–2.

Lindstedt G, Lundberg PA, Lapidus L, Lundgren H, Bengtsson C, Björntorp P. Low sex-hormone-binding globulin concentration as independent risk factor for development of NIDDM. 12-yr follow-up of population study of women in Gothenburg, Sweden. *Diabetes* 1991;40(1):123–8.

Linet MS, McLaughlin JK, Hsing AW, Wacholder S, Co Chien HT, Schuman LM, Bjelke E, Blot WJ. Is cigarette smoking a risk factor for non-Hodgkin's lymphoma or multiple myeloma? Results from the Lutheran Brotherhood Cohort Study. *Leukemia Research* 1992;16(6–7):621–4.

Linn S, Schoenbaum SC, Monson RR, Rosner B, Ryan KJ. Delay in conception for former 'pill' users. *Journal of the American Medical Association* 1982; 247(5):629–32.

Lissner L, Bengtsson C, Lapidus L, Björkelund C. Smoking initiation and cessation in relation to body fat distribution based on data from a study of Swedish women. *American Journal of Public Health* 1992;82(2):273–5.

Little RE, Weinberg C. Risk factors for antepartum and intrapartum stillbirth. *American Journal of Epidemiology* 1993;137(11):1177–89.

Liu Q, Sasco AJ, Riboli E, Hu MX. Indoor air pollution and lung cancer in Guangzhou, People's Republic of China. *American Journal of Epidemiology* 1993; 137(2):145–54.

Liu ZY, He XZ, Chapman RS. Smoking and other risk factors for lung cancer in Xuanwei, China. *International Journal of Epidemiology* 1991;20(1):26–31.

Livson N, Leino EV. Cigarette smoking motives: factorial structure and gender differences in a longitudinal study. *International Journal of the Addictions* 1988;23(6):535–44.

Logan RFA, Edmond M, Somerville KW, Langman MJS. Smoking and ulcerative colitis. *British Medical Journal* 1984;288(6419):751–3.

Logan RFA, Kay CR. Oral contraception, smoking and inflammatory bowel disease—findings in the Royal College of General Practitioners Oral Contraception Study. *International Journal of Epidemiology* 1989;18(1):105–7.

Lohr JB, Flynn K. Smoking and schizophrenia. *Schizophrenia Research* 1992;8(2):93–102.

London SJ, Colditz GA, Stampfer MJ, Willett WC, Rosner BA, Speizer FE. Prospective study of smoking and the risk of breast cancer. *Journal of the National Cancer Institute* 1989;81(21):1625–31.

Longcope C, Johnston CC Jr. Androgen and estrogen dynamics in pre- and postmenopausal women: a comparison between smokers and nonsmokers. *Journal of Clinical Endocrinology and Metabolism* 1988;67(2):379–83.

Longo LD. The biological effects of carbon monoxide on the pregnant woman, fetus, and newborn infant. *American Journal of Obstetrics and Gynecology* 1977;129(1):69–103.

Longstreth WT Jr, Nelson LM, Koepsell TD, van Belle G. Cigarette smoking, alcohol use, and subarachnoid hemorrhage. *Stroke* 1992;23(9):1242–9.

Longstreth WT Jr, Nelson LM, Koepsell TD, van Belle G. Subarachnoid hemorrhage and hormonal factors in women: a population-based case-control study. *Annals of Internal Medicine* 1994;121(3): 168–73.

Lopez AD. The lung cancer epidemic in developed countries. In: Lopez AD, Caselli G, Valkonen T, editors. *Adult Mortality in Developed Countries: From Description to Explanation.* Oxford: Clarendon Press, 1995:111–34.

Lorente C, Cordier S, Goujard J, Aymé S, Bianchi F, Calzolari E, De Walle HEK, Knill-Jones R, and the Occupational Exposure and Congenital Malformation Working Group. *American Journal of Public Health* 2000;90(3):415–9.

Lorusso D, Leo S, Misciagna G, Guerra V. Cigarette smoking and ulcerative colitis: a case control study. *Hepato-Gastroenterology* 1989;36(4):202–4.

Lowe CR. Effects of mother's smoking habits on birth weight of their children. *British Medical Journal* 1959;2(1):673–6.

Lu AY, Kuntzman R, West S, Jacobson M, Conney AH. Reconstituted liver microsomal enzyme system that hydroxylates drugs, other foreign compounds, and endogenous substrates. II. Role of the cytochrome P-450 and P-448 fractions in drug and steriod hydroxylations. *Journal of Biological Chemistry* 1972;247(6):1727–34.

Lubin JH. Lung cancer and exposure to residential radon [commentary]. *American Journal of Epidemiology* 1994;140(4):323–32.

Lubin JH, Blot WJ. Assessment of lung cancer risk factors by histologic category. *Journal of the National Cancer Institute* 1984;73(2):383–9.

Lubin JH, Blot WJ, Berrino F, Flamant R, Gillis CR, Kunze M, Schmahl D, Visco G. Patterns of lung cancer risk according to type of cigarette smoked. *International Journal of Cancer* 1984;33(5):569–76.

Luciano A, Bolognani M, Biodani P, Ghizzi C, Zoppi G, Signori E. The influence of maternal passive and light active smoking on intrauterine growth and body composition of the newborn. *European Journal of Clinical Nutrition* 1998;52(10):760–3.

Lund E. Re: Smoking and estrogen-related disease [letter]. *American Journal of Epidemiology* 1985; 121(2):324–5.

Luoto R, Kaprio J, Uutela A. Age at natural menopause and sociodemographic status in Finland. *American Journal of Epidemiology* 1994;139(1):64–76.

Lu-Yao GL, Baron JA, Barrett JA, Fisher ES. Treatment and survival among elderly Americans with hip fractures: a population-based study. *American Journal of Public Health* 1994;84(8):1287–91.

Lynch HT, Kimberling WJ, Markvicka SE, Biscone KA, Lynch JF, Whorton E Jr, Mailliard J. Genetics and smoking-associated cancers: a study of 485 families. *Cancer* 1986;57(8):1640–6.

Lynch HT, Mulcahy GM, Harris RE, Guirgis HA, Lynch JF. Genetic and pathologic findings in a kindred with hereditary sarcoma, breast cancer, brain tumors, leukemia, lung, laryngeal, and adrenal cortical carcinoma. *Cancer* 1978;41(5):2055–64.

Lyon AJ. Effects of smoking on breast feeding. *Archives of Disease in Childhood* 1983;58(5):378–80.

Lyon JL, Gardner JW, West DW, Stanish WM, Hebertson RM. Smoking and carcinoma in situ of the uterine cervix. *American Journal of Public Health* 1983;73(5):558–62.

Mabuchi K, Bross DS, Kessler II. Epidemiology of cancer of the vulva: a case-control study. *Cancer* 1985;55(8):1843–8.

MacArthur C, Knox EG. Smoking in pregnancy: effects of stopping at different stages. *British Journal of Obstetrics and Gynaecology* 1988;95(6):551–5.

MacDorman MF, Cnattingius S, Hoffman HJ, Kramer MS, Haglund B. Sudden infant death syndrome and smoking in the United States and Sweden. *American Journal of Epidemiology* 1997;146(3):249–57.

Macfarlane GJ, Zheng T, Marshall JR, Boffetta P, Niu S, Brasure J, Merletti F, Boyle P. Alcohol, tobacco, diet and the risk of oral cancer: a pooled analysis of three case-control studies. *European Journal of Cancer Part B, Oral Oncology* 1995;31B(3):181–7.

Mack TM, Yu MC, Hanisch R, Henderson BE. Pancreas cancer and smoking, beverage consumption, and past medical history. *Journal of the National Cancer Institute* 1986;76(1):49–60.

Maclure KM, Hayes KC, Colditz GA, Stampfer MJ, Speizer FE, Willett WC. Weight, diet, and the risk of symptomatic gallstones in middle-aged women. *New England Journal of Medicine* 1989;321(9): 563–9.

MacMahon B, Alpert M, Salber EJ. Infant weight and parental smoking habits. *American Journal of Epidemiology* 1965;82(3):247–61.

MacMahon B, Trichopoulos D, Cole P, Brown J. Cigarette smoking and urinary estrogens. *New England Journal of Medicine* 1982;307(17):1062–5.

MacMahon B, Yen S, Trichopoulos D, Warren K, Nardi G. Coffee and cancer of the pancreas. *New England Journal of Medicine* 1981;304(11):630–3.

MacSweeney STR, Ellis M, Worrell PC, Greenhalgh RM, Powell JT. Smoking and growth rate of small abdominal aortic aneurysms. *Lancet* 1994;344(8923): 651–2.

Macular Photocoagulation Study Group. Recurrent choroidal neovascularization after argon laser photocoagulation for neovascular maculopathy. *Archives of Ophthalmology* 1986;104(4):503–12.

Magaziner J, Simonsick EM, Kashner TM, Hebel JR, Kenzora JE. Survival experience of aged hip fracture patients. *American Journal of Public Health* 1989;79(3):274–8.

Magers T, Talbot P, DiCarlantonio G, Knoll M, Demers D, Tsai I, Hoodbhoy T. Cigarette smoke inhalation affects the reproductive system of female hamsters. *Reproductive Toxicology* 1995;9(6):513–25.

Magnus P, Berg K, Bjerkedal T, Nance WE. Parental determinants of birth weight. *Clinical Genetics* 1984; 26(5):397–405.

Mainous AG, Hueston WJ. Passive smoke and low birth weight: evidence of a threshold effect. *Archives of Family Medicine* 1994a;3(10):875–8.

Mainous AG III, Hueston WJ. The effect of smoking cessation during pregnancy on preterm delivery and low birthweight. *Journal of Family Practice* 1994b;38(3):262–6.

Mallmin H, Ljunghall S, Persson I, Bergström R. Risk factors for fractures of the distal forearm: a population-based case-control study. *Osteoporosis International* 1994;4(6):298–304.

Malloy MH, Hoffman HJ, Peterson DR. Sudden infant death syndrome and maternal smoking. *American Journal of Public Health* 1992;82(10):1380–2.

Malloy MH, Kleinman JC, Bakewell JM, Schramm WF, Land GH. Maternal smoking during pregnancy: no association with congenital malformations in Missouri 1980–83. *American Journal of Public Health* 1989;79(9):1243–6.

Malloy MH, Kleinman JC, Land GH, Schramm WF. The association of maternal smoking with age and cause of infant death. *American Journal of Epidemiology* 1988;128(1):46–55.

Manfreda J, Becker AB, Wang P-Z, Roos LL, Anthonisen NR. Trends in physician-diagnosed asthma prevalence in Manitoba between 1980 and 1990. *Chest* 1993;103(1):151–7.

Mann RD, Lis Y, Chukwujindu J, Chanter DO. A study of the association between hormone replacement therapy, smoking, and the occurrence of myocardial infarction in women. *Journal of Clinical Epidemiology* 1994;47(3):307–12.

Mann SJ, James GD, Wang RS, Pickering TG. Elevation of ambulatory systolic blood pressure in hypertensive smokers: a case-control study. *Journal of the American Medical Association* 1991;265(17): 2226–8.

Mann SJ, Pickering TG, Alderman MH, Laragh JH. Assessment of the effects of alpha- and beta-blockade in hypertensive patients who smoke cigarettes. *American Journal of Medicine* 1989; 86(Suppl 1B):79–81.

Mant D, Villard-Mackintosh L, Vessey MP, Yeates D. Myocardial infarction and angina pectoris in young women. *Journal of Epidemiology and Community Health* 1987;41(3):215–9.

Marchbanks PA, Peterson HB, Rubin GL, Wingo PA. Research on infertility: definition makes a difference. The Cancer and Steroid Hormone Study Group. *American Journal of Epidemiology* 1989; 130(2):259–67.

Marcoux S, Brisson J, Fabia J. The effect of cigarette smoking on the risk of preeclampsia and gestational hypertension. *American Journal of Epidemiology* 1989;130(5):950–7.

Marshall JR, Graham S, Byers T, Swanson M, Brasure J. Diet and smoking in the epidemiology of cancer of the cervix. *Journal of the National Cancer Institute* 1983;70(5):847–51.

Marshall LM, Spiegelman D, Manson JE, Goldman MB, Barbieri RL, Stampfer MJ, Willett WC, Hunter DJ. Risk of uterine leiomyomata among premenopausal women in relation to body size and cigarette smoking. *Epidemiology* 1998;9(5):511–7.

Marti B, Suter E, Riesen WF, Tschopp A, Wanner H-U. Anthropometric and lifestyle correlates of serum lipoprotein and apolipoprotein levels among normal non-smoking men and women. *Atherosclerosis* 1989;75(2–3):111–22.

Marti B, Tuomilehto J, Salomaa V, Kartovaara L, Korhonen HJ, Pietinen P. Body fat distribution in the Finnish population: environmental determinants and predictive power for cardiovascular risk factor levels. *Journal of Epidemiology and Community Health* 1991;45(2):131–7.

Martin TR, Bracken MB. Association of low birth weight with passive smoke exposure in pregnancy. *American Journal of Epidemiology* 1986;124(4):633–42.

Martinez FD, Wright AL, Taussig LM. The effect of paternal smoking on the birth weight of newborns whose mothers did not smoke. *American Journal of Public Health* 1994;84(9):1489–91.

Masterson F, O'Shea B. Smoking and malignancy in schizophrenia. *British Journal of Psychiatry* 1984; 145:429–32.

Mathai M, Skinner A, Lawton K, Weindling AM. Maternal smoking, urinary cotinine levels and birth-weight. *Australian and New Zealand Journal of Obstetrics and Gynaecology* 1990;30(1):33–6.

Mathai M, Vijayasri R, Babu S, Jeyaseelan L. Passive maternal smoking and birthweight in a South Indian population. *British Journal of Obstetrics and Gynaecology* 1992;99(4):342–3.

Matheson I, Rivrud GN. The effect of smoking on lactation and infantile colic. *Journal of the American Medical Association* 1989;261(1):42–3.

Matorras R, Rodíquez F, Pijoan JI, Ramón O, Gutierrez de Terán G, Rodríguez-Escudero F. Epidemiology of endometriosis in infertile women. *Fertility and Sterility* 1995;63(1):34–8.

Matsunaga E, Shiota K. Ectopic pregnancy and myoma uteri: teratogenic effects and maternal characteristics. *Teratology* 1980;21(1):61–9.

Mattison DR. Morphology of oocyte and follicle destruction by polycyclic aromatic hydrocarbons in mice. *Toxicology and Applied Pharmacology* 1980; 53(2):249–59.

Mattison DR, Plowchalk DR, Meadows MJ, Miller MM, Malek A, London S. The effect of smoking on oogenesis, fertilization and implantation. *Seminars in Reproductive Endocrinology* 1989a;7(4):291–304.

Mattison DR, Singh H, Takizawa K, Thomford PJ. Ovarian toxicity of benzo(a)pyrene and metabolites in mice. *Reproductive Toxicology* 1989b;3(2): 115–25.

Mattison DR, Thorgeirsson SS. Smoking and industrial pollution, and their effects on menopause and ovarian cancer. *Lancet* 1978;1(8057):187–8.

Mau G, Netter P. The effects of paternal cigarette smoking on perinatal mortality and the incidence of malformations. *Deutsche Medizinische Wochenschrift* 1974;99(21):1113–8.

May H, Murphy S, Khaw K-T. Cigarette smoking and bone mineral density in older men. *Quarterly Journal of Medicine* 1994;87(10):625–30.

Mayberry RM. Cigarette smoking, herpes simplex virus type 2 infection, and cervical abnormalities. *American Journal of Public Health* 1985;75(6):676–8.

Mayeux R, Tang M-X. Smoking and Alzheimer's disease. *American Journal of Epidemiology* 1993;138(8): 645.

Mayne ST, Janerich DT, Greenwald P, Chorost S, Tucci C, Zaman MB, Melamed MR, Kiely M, McKneally MF. Dietary beta carotene and lung cancer risk in U.S. nonsmokers. *Journal of the National Cancer Institute* 1994;86(1):33–8.

Mazess RB, Barden HS. Bone densitometry for diagnosis and monitoring osteoporosis. *Proceedings of the Society for Experimental Biology and Medicine* 1989;191(3):261–71.

Mazess RB, Barden HS. Bone density in premenopausal women: effects of age, dietary intake, physical activity, smoking, and birth-control pills. *American Journal of Clinical Nutrition* 1991;53(1): 132–42.

McCann MF, Irwin DE, Walton LA, Hulka BS, Morton JL, Axelrad CM. Nicotine and cotinine in the cervical mucus of smokers, passive smokers, and nonsmokers. *Cancer Epidemiology, Biomarkers and Prevention* 1992;1(2):125–9.

McCredie M, Ford JM, Taylor JS, Stewart JH. Analgesics and cancer of the renal pelvis in New South Wales. *Cancer* 1982;49(12):2617–25.

McCredie M, Stewart JH. Risk factors for kidney cancer in New South Wales—I. Cigarette smoking. *European Journal of Cancer* 1992;28A(12):2050–4.

McCulloch RG, Bailey DA, Houston CS, Dodd BL. Effects of physical activity, dietary calcium intake and selected lifestyle factors on bone density in young women. *Canadian Medical Association Journal* 1990;142(3):221–7.

McDonald AD, Armstrong BG, Sloan M. Cigarette, alcohol, and coffee consumption and prematurity. *American Journal of Public Health* 1992;82(1):87–90.

McDuffie HH. Clustering of cancer in families of patients with primary lung cancer. *Journal of Clinical Epidemiology* 1991;44(1):69–76.

McDuffie HH, Klaassen DJ, Dosman JA. Men, women and primary lung cancer—a Saskatchewan personal interview study. *Journal of Clinical Epidemiology* 1991;44(6):537–44.

McGlashan ND. Sudden infant deaths in Tasmania, 1980–1986: a seven year prospective study. *Social Science and Medicine* 1989;29(8):1015–26.

McKinlay SM. The normal menopause transition: an overview. *Maturitas* 1996;23(2):137–45.

McKinlay SM, Bifano NL, McKinlay JB. Smoking and age at menopause in women. *Annals of Internal Medicine* 1985;103(3):350–6.

McKinlay SM, Brambilla DJ, Posner JG. The normal menopause transition. *Maturitas* 1992;14(2):103–15.

McKnight A, Steele K, Mills K, Gilchrist C, Taggart H. Bone mineral density in relation to medical and lifestyle risk factors for osteoporosis in premenopausal, menopausal and postmenopausal women in general practice. *British Journal of General Practice* 1995;45(395):317–20.

McLaughlin JK, Blot WJ, Devesa SS, Fraumeni JF Jr. Renal cancer. In: Schottenfeld D, Fraumeni JF Jr, editors. *Cancer Epidemiology and Prevention.* 2nd ed. New York: Oxford University Press, 1996: 1142–55.

McLaughlin JK, Hrubec Z, Blot WJ, Fraumeni JF Jr. Stomach cancer and cigarette smoking among U.S. veterans, 1954–1980 [letter]. *Cancer Research* 1990; 50(12):3804.

McLaughlin JK, Hrubec Z, Blot WJ, Fraumeni JF Jr. Smoking and cancer mortality among U.S. veterans: a 26-year follow-up. *International Journal of Cancer* 1995a;60(2):190–3.

McLaughlin JK, Lindblad P, Mellemgaard A, McCredie M, Mandel JS, Schlehofer B, Pommer W, Adami H-O. International Renal-Cell Cancer Study. I. Tobacco use. *International Journal of Cancer* 1995b;60(2):194–8.

McLaughlin JK, Mandel JS, Blot WJ, Schuman LM, Mehl ES, Fraumeni JF Jr. A population-based case-control study of renal cell carcinoma. *Journal of the National Cancer Institute* 1984;72(2):275–84.

McLaughlin JK, Silverman DT, Hsing AW, Ross RK, Schoenberg JB, Yu MC, Stemhagen A, Lynch CF, Blot WJ, Fraumeni JF Jr. Cigarette smoking and cancers of the renal pelvis and ureter. *Cancer Research* 1992;52(2):254–7.

McMahon MJ, Li R, Schenck AP, Olshan AF, Royce RA. Previous cesarean birth. A risk factor for placenta previa? *Journal of Reproductive Medicine* 1997; 42(7):409–12.

McMichael AJ, Baghurst PA, Scragg RKR. A case-control study of smoking and gallbladder disease: importance of examining time relations. *Epidemiology* 1992;3(6):519–22.

McNamara PM, Hjortland MC, Gordon T, Kannel WB. Natural history of menopause: the Framingham Study. *Journal of Continuing Education in Obstetrics and Gynecology* 1978;20:27–35.

McPhillips JB, Barrett-Connor E, Wingard DL. Cardiovascular disease risk factors prior to the diagnosis of impaired glucose tolerance and non-insulin-dependent diabetes mellitus in a community of older adults. *American Journal of Epidemiology* 1990;131(3):443–53.

McTiernan A, Thomas DB, Johnson LK, Roseman D. Risk factors for estrogen receptor-rich and estrogen receptor-poor breast cancers. *Journal of the National Cancer Institute* 1986;77(4):849–54.

McTiernan AM, Weiss NS, Daling JR. Incidence of thyroid cancer in women in relation to reproductive and hormonal factors. *American Journal of Epidemiology* 1984a;120(3):423–35.

McTiernan AM, Weiss NS, Daling JR. Incidence of thyroid cancer in women in relation to previous exposure to radiation therapy and history of thyroid disease. *Journal of the National Cancer Institute* 1984b;73(3):575–81.

Meara J, McPherson K, Roberts M, Jones L, Vessey M. Alcohol, cigarette smoking and breast cancer. *British Journal of Cancer* 1989;60(1):70–3.

Medalie JH, Papier CM, Goldbourt U, Herman JB. Major factors in the development of diabetes mellitus in 10,000 men. *Archives of Internal Medicine* 1975;135(6):811–7.

Medical Research Council Vitamin Study Research Group. Prevention of neural tube defects: results of the Medical Research Council vitamin study. *Lancet* 1991;338(8760):131–7.

Meis PJ, Michielutte R, Peters TJ, Wells HB, Sands RE, Coles EC, Johns KA. Factors associated with preterm birth in Cardiff, Wales. II. Indicated and spontaneous preterm birth. *American Journal of Obstetrics and Gynecology* 1995;173(2):597–602.

Mellström D, Johansson C, Johnell O, Lindstedt G, Lundberg P-A, Obrant K, Schoon I-M, Toss G, Ytterberg B-O. Osteoporosis, metabolic aberrations, and increased risk for vertebral fractures after partial gastrectomy. *Calcified Tissue International* 1993;53(6):370–7.

Melton LJ III. Epidemiology of fractures. In: Riggs BL, Melton LJ III, editors. *Osteoporosis: Etiology, Diagnosis, and Management.* New York: Raven Press, 1988:133–54.

Merchant C, Tang MX, Albert S, Manly J, Stern Y, Mayeux R. The influence of smoking on the risk of Alzheimer's disease. *Neurology* 1999;52(7):1408–12.

Merikangas KR, Gelernter CS. Comorbidity for alcoholism and depression. *Psychiatric Clinics of North America* 1990;13(4):613–32.

Meyer HE, Tverdal A, Falch JA. Risk factors for hip fracture in middle-aged Norwegian women and men. *American Journal of Epidemiology* 1993;137(11):1203–11.

Meyer MB, Jonas BS, Tonascia JA. Perinatal events associated with maternal smoking during pregnancy. *American Journal of Epidemiology* 1976;103(5):464–76.

Meyer MB, Tonascia JA. Maternal smoking, pregnancy complications, and perinatal mortality. *American Journal of Obstetrics and Gynecology* 1977;128(5):494–502.

Michaëlsson K, Holmberg L, Mallmin H, Sörensen S, Wolk A, Bergström R, Ljunghall S. Diet and hip fracture risk: a case-control study. *International Journal of Epidemiology* 1995;24(4):771–82.

Michnovicz JJ, Hershcopf RJ, Naganuma H, Bradlow HL, Fishman J. Increased 2-hydroxylation of estradiol as a possible mechanism for the antiestrogenic effect of cigarette smoking. *New England Journal of Medicine* 1986;315(21):1305–9.

Michnovicz JJ, Naganuma H, Hershcopf RJ, Bradlow HL, Fishman J. Increased urinary catechol estrogen excretion in female smokers. *Steroid* 1988;52(1–2):69–83.

Midgette AS, Baron JA. Cigarette smoking and the risk of natural menopause. *Epidemiology* 1990;1(6):474–80.

Mikkelsen KL, Wiinberg N, Hoegholm A, Christensen HR, Bang LE, Nielsen PE, Svendsen TL, Kampmann JP, Madsen NH, Bentzon MW. Smoking related to 24-h ambulatory blood pressure and heart rate: a study in 352 normotensive Danish subjects. *American Journal of Hypertension* 1997;10(5 Pt 1): 483–91.

Millikan RC, Pittman GS, Newman B, Tse CK, Selmin O, Rockhill B, Savitz D, Moorman PG, Bell DA. Cigarette smoking. *N*-acetyltransferases 1 and 2, and breast cancer risk. *Cancer Epidemiology, Biomarkers and Prevention* 1998;7(5):371–8.

Mills PK, Newell GR, Beeson WL, Fraser GE, Phillips RL. History of cigarette smoking and risk of leukemia and myeloma: results from the Adventist Health Study. *Journal of the National Cancer Institute* 1990;82(23):1832–6.

Mink PJ, Folsom AR, Sellers TA, Kushi LW. Physical activity, waist-to-hip ratio, and other risk factors for ovarian cancer: a follow-up study of older women. *Epidemiology* 1996;7(1):38–45.

Misciagna G, Leoci C, Guerra V, Chiloiro M, Elba S, Petruzzi J, Mossa A, Noviello MR, Coviello A, Minutolo MC, Mangini V, Messa C, Cavallini A, De Michele G, Giorgio I. Epidemiology of cholelithiasis in southern Italy. Part II: Risk factors. *European Journal of Gastroenterology and Hepatology* 1996;8(6):585–93.

Mishell DR Jr. Oral contraception: past, present, and future perspectives. *International Journal of Fertility* 1991;36(Suppl):7–18.

Misra DP, Kiely JL. The effect of smoking on the risk of gestational hypertension. *Early Human Development* 1995;40(2):95–107.

Mitchell EA, Scragg R, Stewart AW, Becroft DM, Taylor BJ, Ford RP, Hassall IB, Barry DM, Allen EM, Roberts AP. Results from the first year of the New Zealand cot death study. *New Zealand Medical Journal* 1991;104(906):71–6.

Mittendorf R, Lain KY, Williams MA, Walker CK. Preeclampsia. A nested, case-control study of risk factors and their interactions. *Journal of Reproductive Medicine* 1996;41(7):491–6.

Mochizuki M, Maruo T, Masuko K, Ohtsu T. Effects of smoking on fetoplacental-maternal system during pregnancy. *American Journal of Obstetrics and Gynecology* 1984;149(4):413–20.

Modan M, Meytes D, Rozeman P, Yosef SB, Sehayek E, Yosef NB, Lusky A, Halkin H. Significance of high $HbA_1$ levels in normal glucose tolerance. *Diabetes Care* 1988;11(5):422–8.

Model D. Smoker's face: an underrated clinical sign? *British Medical Journal* 1985;291(1755):1760–2.

Moerman CJ, Bueno de Mesquita HB, Runia S. Smoking, alcohol consumption and the risk of cancer of the biliary tract: a population-based case-control study in the Netherlands. *European Journal of Cancer Prevention* 1994;3(5):427–36.

Mohan M, Sperduto RD, Angra SK, Milton RC, Mathur RL, Underwood BA, Jaffery N, Pandya CB, Chhabra VK, Vajpayee RB, Kalra VK, Sharma YR. India-U.S. case-control study of age-related cataracts. *Archives of Ophthalmology* 1989;107(5):670–6.

Mohr GC, Kritz-Silverstein D, Barrett-Connor E. Plasma lipids and gallbladder disease. *American Journal of Epidemiology* 1991;134(1):78–85.

Monica G, Lilja C. Placenta previa, maternal smoking and recurrence risk. *Acta Obstetricia Gynecologica Scandinavica* 1995;74(5):341–5.

Moody PM. The relationships of quantified human smoking behavior and demographic variables. *Social Science and Medicine* 1980;14A(1):49–54.

Mooy JM, Grootenhuis PA, de Vries H, Bouter LM, Kostense PJ, Heine RJ. Determinants of specific serum insulin concentrations in a general Caucasian population aged 50 to 74 years (the Hoorn Study). *Diabetic Medicine* 1998;15(1):45–52.

Mooy JM, Grootenhuis PA, de Vries H, Valkenburg HA, Bouter LM, Kostense PJ, Heine RJ. Prevalence and determinants of glucose intolerance in a Dutch caucasian population. The Hoorn Study. *Diabetes Care* 1995;18(9):1270–3.

Morabia A, Bernstein M, Héritier S, Khatchatrian N. Relation of breast cancer with passive and active exposure to tobacco smoke. *American Journal of Epidemiology* 1996;143(9):918–28.

Morabia A, Bernstein M, Ruiz J, Héritier S, Diebold Berger S, Borisch B. Relation of smoking to breast cancer by estrogen receptor status. *International Journal of Cancer* 1998;75(3):339–42.

Morabia A, Bernstein MS, Bouchardy I, Kurtz J, Morris MA. Breast cancer and active and passive smoking: the role of the *N*-acetyltransferase 2 genotype. *American Journal of Epidemiology* 2000; 152(3):226–32.

Morabia A, Wynder EL. Cigarette smoking and lung cancer cell types. *Cancer* 1991;68(9):2074–8.

Morens DM, Grandinetti A, Reed D, White LR, Ross GW. Cigarette smoking and protection from Parkinson's disease: false association or etiologic clue? *Neurology* 1995;45(6):1041–51.

Mori M, Naito M, Watanabe H, Takeichi N, Dohi K, Ito A. Effects of sex difference, gonadectomy, and estrogen on *N*-methyl-*N*-nitrosourea induced rat thyroid tumors. *Cancer Research* 1990;50(23):7662–7.

Morris KM, Shaw MD, Foy PM. Smoking and subarachnoid haemorrhage: a case control study. *British Journal of Neurosurgery* 1992;6(5):429–32.

Morrison AS, Buring JE, Verhoek WG, Aoki K, Leck I, Ohno Y, Obata K. An international study of smoking and bladder cancer. *Journal of Urology* 1984; 131(4):650–4.

Mosher WD, Pratt WF. Fecundity and infertility in the United States, 1965–88. *Advance Data*. No. 192. Hyattsville (MD): U.S. Department of Health and Human Services, Public Health Service, Centers for Disease Control, National Center for Health Statistics, 1990.

Moy CS, LaPorte RE, Dorman JS, Songer TJ, Orchard TJ, Kuller LH, Becker DJ, Drash AL. Insulin-dependent diabetes mellitus mortality: the risk of cigarette smoking. *Circulation* 1990;82(1):37–43.

Mueller N. Hodgkin's disease. In: Schottenfeld D, Fraumeni JF Jr, editors. *Cancer Epidemiology and Prevention*. 2nd ed. New York: Oxford University Press, 1996:893–919.

Muhlhauser I. Cigarette smoking and diabetes: an update. *Diabetic Medicine* 1994;11(4):336–43.

Munoz N, Bosch FX, de Sanjose S, Vergara A, del Moral A, Munoz MT, Tafur L, Gili M, Izarzugaza I, Viladiu P, Navarro C, de Ruiz PA, Aristizabal N, Santamaria M, Orfila J, Daniel RW, Guerrero E, Shah KV. Risk factors for cervical intraepithelial neoplasia grade III carcinoma in situ in Spain and Colombia. *Cancer Epidemiology, Biomarkers and Prevention* 1993;2(5):423–31.

Murphy SL. Deaths: final data for 1998. *National Vital Statistics Reports* 2000;48(11):1–108.

Murphy NJ, Butler SW, Petersen KM, Heart V, Murphy CM. Tobacco erases 30 years of progress: preliminary analysis of the effect of tobacco smoking on Alaska Native birth weight. *Alaska Medicine* 1996;38(1):31–3.

Murray FE, Logan RFA, Hannaford PC, Kay CR. Cigarette smoking and parity as risk factors for the development of symptomatic gall bladder disease in women: results of the Royal College of General Practitioners' oral contraception study. *Gut* 1994;35(1):107–11.

Muscat JE, Richie JP Jr, Thompson S, Wynder EL. Gender differences in smoking and risk for oral cancer. *Cancer Research* 1996;56(22):5192–7.

Muscat JE, Stellman SD, Hoffmann D, Wynder EL. Smoking and pancreatic cancer in men and women. *Cancer Epidemiology, Biomarkers and Prevention* 1997;6(1):15–9.

Muscat JE, Wynder EL. Exposure to environmental tobacco smoke and the risk of heart attack. *International Journal of Epidemiology* 1995a;24(4):715–9.

Muscat JE, Wynder EL. Lung cancer pathology in smokers, ex-smokers and never smokers. *Cancer Letters* 1995b;88(1):1–5.

Muscati SK, Gray-Donald K, Newson EE. Interaction of smoking and maternal weight status in influencing infant size. *Canadian Journal of Public Health* 1994;85(6):407–12.

Muscati SK, Koski KG, Gray-Donald K. Increased energy intake in pregnant smokers does not prevent human fetal growth retardation. *Journal of Nutrition* 1996;126(12):2984–9.

Naeye RL. Abruptio placentae and placenta previa: frequency, perinatal mortality, and cigarette smoking. *Obstetrics and Gynecology* 1980;55(6):701–4.

Naeye RL. Factors that predispose to premature rupture of the fetal membrane. *Obstetrics and Gynecology* 1982;60(1):93–8.

Nafstad P, Fugelseth D, Qvigstad MD, Zahlsen K, Magnus P, Lindemann R. Nicotine concentration in the hair of nonsmoking mothers and size of offspring. *American Journal of Public Health* 1998;88(1):120–4.

Nagata C, Fujita S, Iwata H, Kurosawa Y, Kobayashi K, Kobayashi M, Motegi K, Omura T, Yamamoto M, Nose T. Systemic lupus erythematosus: a case-control epidemiologic study in Japan. *International Journal of Dermatology* 1995;34(5):333–7.

Nakamura M, Oshima A, Hiyama T, Kubota N, Wada K, Yano K. Effect of passive smoking during pregnancy on birth weight and gestation: a population-based prospective study in Japan. In: Aoki M, Hisamichi S, Tominaga S, editors. *Smoking and Health 1987*. Proceedings of the 6th World Conference on Smoking and Health, 1987 Nov 9–12; Tokyo. International Congress Series 780. Amsterdam: Excerpta Medica, 1988:267–9.

Nakamura Y, Kobayashi M, Nagai M, Iwata H, Nose T, Yamamoto M, Omura T, Motegi K, Kurosawa Y, Hossaka K, Nakamura K, Hashimoto T, Yanagawa H. A case-control study of ulcerative colitis in Japan. *Journal of Clinical Gastroenterology* 1994;18(1):72–9.

Nakamura Y, Labarthe DR. A case-control study of ulcerative colitis with relation to smoking habits and alcohol consumption in Japan. *American Journal of Epidemiology* 1994;140(10):902–11.

Nandakumar A, Thimmasetty KT, Sreeramareddy NM, Venugophal TC, Rajanna, Vinutha AT, Srinivas, Bhargava MK. A population-based case-control investigation of cancers of the oral cavity in Bangalore, India. *British Journal of Cancer* 1990;62(5):847–51.

Narkiewicz K, Maraglino G, Biasion T, Rossi G, Sanzuol F, Palatini P. Interactive effect of cigarettes and coffee on daytime systolic blood pressure in patients with mild essential hypertension. Harvest Study Group (Italy). Hypertension Ambulatory Recording VEnetia STudy. *Journal of Hypertension* 1995;13(0):965–70.

Nash JE, Persaud TVN. Embryopathic risks of cigarette smoking. *Experimental Pathology* 1988;33(2):65–73.

National Cancer Institute. *The FTC Cigarette Test Method for Determining Tar, Nicotine, and Carbon Monoxide Yields of U.S. Cigarettes. Report of the NCI Expert Committee.* Smoking and Tobacco Control Monograph 7. Bethesda (MD): U.S. Department of Health and Human Services, Public Health Service, National Institutes of Health, National Cancer Institute, 1996a. NIH Publication No. 96-4028.

National Cancer Institute. *Racial/Ethnic Patterns of Cancer in the United States, 1988–1992.* Bethesda (MD): U.S. Department of Health and Human Services, Public Health Service, National Institutes of Health, National Cancer Institute, Division of Cancer Prevention and Control, 1996b. NIH Publication No. 96-4104.

National Cancer Institute. *Changes in Cigarette-Related Disease Risks and Their Implication for Prevention and Control.* Smoking and Tobacco Control Monograph 8. Bethesda (MD): U.S. Department of Health and Human Services, Public Health Service, National Institutes of Health, National Cancer Institute, 1997. NIH Publication No. 97-4213.

National Cancer Institute. *Health Effects of Exposure to Environmental Tobacco Smoke: The Report of the California Environmental Protection Agency.* Smoking and Tobacco Control Monograph 10. Bethesda (MD): U.S. Department of Health and Human Services, National Institutes of Health, National Cancer Institute, 1999. NIH Publication No. 99-4645.

National Center for Health Statistics. *Health, United States, 1994.* Hyattsville (MD): U.S. Department of Health and Human Services, Public Health Service, Centers for Disease Control and Prevention, National Center for Health Statistics, 1995. DHHS Publication No. (PHS) 95-1232.

National Center for Health Statistics. *Vital Statistics of the United States, 1992. Vol II. Mortality, Part A.* Hyattsville (MD): U.S. Department of Health and Human Services, Public Health Service, Centers for Disease Control and Prevention, National Center for Health Statistics, 1996. DHHS Publication No. (PHS) 96-1101.

National Center for Health Statistics. *Health, United States, 1999 with Health and Aging Chartbook.* Hyattsville (MD): U.S. Department of Health and Human Services, Centers for Disease Control and Prevention, National Center for Health Statistics, 1999. DHHS Publication No. (PHS) 99-1232-1.

National Institute on Aging. *Alzheimer's Disease Currently Affects an Estimated 4 Million Americans: Progress Report on Alzheimer's Disease, 1992. Discoveries in Health for Aging Americans.* Rockville (MD): U.S. Department of Health and Human Services, Public Health Service, National Institutes of Health, and National Institute on Aging, 1992. NIH Publication No. 92-3409.

National Institute for Occupational Safety and Health. *Environmental Tobacco Smoke in the Workplace: Lung Cancer and Other Health Effects.* Current Intelligence Bulletin 54. Cincinnati (OH): U.S. Department of Health and Human Services, Public Health Service, Centers for Disease Control, National Institute for Occupational Safety and Health, 1991. DHHS (NIOSH) Publication No. 91-108.

National Research Council. *Environmental Tobacco Smoke: Measuring Exposures and Assessing Health Effects.* Washington: National Academy Press, 1986.

National Research Council. *Health Effects of Exposure to Radon: BEIR VI.* Washington: National Academy Press, 1999.

Navot D, Rosenwaks Z, Margalioth EJ. Prognostic assessment of female fecundity. *Lancet* 1987; 2(8560):645–7.

Negri E, La Vecchia C, D'Avanzo B, Nobili A, La Malfa RG. Acute myocardial infarction: association with time since stopping smoking in Italy. *Journal of Epidemiology and Community Health* 1994; 48(2):129–33.

Negri E, La Vecchia C, Franceschi S, Decarli A, Bruzzi P. Attributable risks for oesophageal cancer in Northern Italy. *European Journal of Cancer* 1992; 28A(6–7):1167–71.

Negri E, La Vecchia C, Franceschi S, Tavani A. Attributable risk for oral cancer in northern Italy. *Cancer Epidemiology, Biomarkers and Prevention* 1993; 2(3):189–93.

Nelson DM, Stempel LE, Zuspan FP. Association of prolonged preterm premature rupture of the membranes and abruptio placentae. *Journal of Reproductive Medicine* 1986;31(4):249–53.

Nelson RA, Levine AM, Marks G, Bernstein L. Alcohol, tobacco and recreational drug use and the risk of non-Hodgkin's lymphoma. *British Journal of Cancer* 1997;76(11):1532–7.

Ness RB, Grisso JA, Hirschinger N, Markovic N, Shaw LM, Day NL, Kline J. Cocaine and tobacco use and the risk of spontaneous abortion. *New England Journal of Medicine* 1999;340(5):333–9.

Neugut AI, Jacobson JS, DeVivo I. Epidemiology of colorectal adenomatous polyps. *Cancer Epidemiology, Biomarkers and Prevention* 1993;2(2):159–76.

Neugut AI, Murray T, Santos J, Amols H, Hayes MK, Flannery JT, Robinson E. Increased risk of lung cancer after breast cancer radiation therapy in cigarette smokers. *Cancer* 1994;73(6):1615–20.

Newcomb PA, Storer BE, Marcus PM. Cigarette smoking in relation to risk of large bowel cancer in women. *Cancer Research* 1995;55(21):4906–9.

Newcomb PA, Weiss NS, Daling JR. Incidence of vulvar carcinoma in relation to menstrual, reproductive, and medical factors. *Journal of the National Cancer Institute* 1984;73(2):391–6.

Newell GR, Mansell PWA, Wilson MB, Lynch HK, Spitz MR, Hersh EM. Risk factor analysis among men referred for possible acquired immune deficiency syndrome. *Preventive Medicine* 1985;14(1): 81–91.

Ng TP, Foo SC, Yoong T. Risk of spontaneous abortion in workers exposed to toluene. *British Journal of Industrial Medicine* 1992;49(11):804–8.

Nguyen TV, Kelly PJ, Sambrook PN, Gilbert C, Pocock NA, Eisman JA. Lifestyle factors and bone density in the elderly: implications for osteoporosis prevention. *Journal of Bone and Mineral Research* 1994;9(9):1339–46.

Nides M, Rand C, Dolce J, Murray R, O'Hara P, Voelker H, Connett J. Weight gain as a function of smoking cessation and 2-mg nicotine gum use among middle-aged smokers with mild lung impairment in the first 2 years of the Lung Health Study. *Health Psychology* 1994;13(4):354–61.

Nilsson PM, Lind L, Pollare T, Berne C, Lithell HO. Increased level of hemoglobin A1c, but not impaired insulin sensitivity, found in hypertensive and normotensive smokers. *Metabolism* 1995;44(5): 557–61.

Nischan P, Ebeling K, Schindler C. Smoking and invasive cervical cancer risk. Results from a case-control study. *American Journal of Epidemiology* 1988;128(1):74–7.

Njølstad I, Arnesen E, Lund-Larsen PG. Smoking, serum lipids, blood pressure, and sex differences in myocardial infarction. A 12-year follow-up of the Finnmark Study. *Circulation* 1996;93(3):450–6.

Nomura A. Stomach cancer. In: Schottenfeld D, Fraumeni JF Jr, editors. *Cancer Epidemiology and Prevention.* 2nd ed. New York: Oxford University Press, 1996:707–24.

Nomura A, Comstock GW, Tonascia JA. Epidemiologic characteristics of benign breast disease. *American Journal of Epidemiology* 1977;105(6):505–12.

Nordentoft M, Lou HC, Hansen D, Nim J, Pryds O, Rubin P, Hemmingsen R. Intrauterine growth retardation and premature delivery: the influence of maternal smoking and psychosocial factors. *American Journal of Public Health* 1996;86(3):347–54.

Nordin BEC, Polley KJ. Metabolic consequences of the menopause: a cross-sectional, longitudinal, and intervention study on 557 normal postmenopausal women. *Calcified Tissue International* 1987; 41(Suppl 1):S1–S59.

Nordlund LA, Carstensen JM, Pershagen G. Cancer incidence in female smokers: a 26-year follow-up. *International Journal of Cancer* 1997;73(5):625–8.

Nordstrom M-L, Cnattingius S. Smoking habits and birthweights in two successive births in Sweden. *Early Human Development* 1994;37(3):195–204.

Nylander G, Matheson I. Breast feeding. Effects of smoking and education [in Norwegian]. *Tidsskrift for den Norske Laegeforening* 1989;109(9):970–3.

Nyström E, Bengtsson C, Lapidus L, Petersen K, Lindstedt G. Smoking—a risk factor for hypothyroidism. *Journal of Endocrinological Investigation* 1993;16(2):129–31.

Oakley A, Brannen J, Dodd K. Young people, gender and smoking in the United Kingdom. *Health Promotion International* 1992;7(2):75–88.

O'Connell DL, Hulka BS, Chambless LE, Wilkinson WE, Deubner DC. Cigarette smoking, alcohol consumption, and breast cancer risk. *Journal of the National Cancer Institute* 1987;78(2):229–34.

O'Farrell TJ, Connors GJ, Upper D. Addictive behaviors among hospitalized psychiatric patients. *Addictive Behaviors* 1983;8(4):329–33.

Ogawa H, Tominaga S, Hori K, Noguchi K, Kanou I, Matsubara M. Passive smoking by pregnant women and fetal growth. *Journal of Epidemiology and Community Health* 1991;45(2):164–8.

Ogawa H, Tominaga S, Kubo N, Sasaki R, Hosoda Y, Aoki K, Uematsu M. A case-control study on Parkinson's disease—smoking and personality [Japanese; English abstract]. *Shinshin-Igaku* 1984; 24(6):467–77.

O'Hara P, Connett JE, Lee WW, Nides M, Murray R, Wise R. Early and late weight gain following smoking cessation in the Lung Health Study. *American Journal of Epidemiology* 1998;148(9): 821–30.

Ohlson LO, Larsson B, Björntorp P, Eriksson H, Svärdsudd K, Welin L, Tibblin G, Wilhelmsen L. Risk factors for type 2 (non-insulin-dependent) diabetes mellitus: thirteen and one-half years of follow-up of the participants in a study of Swedish men born in 1913. *Diabetologia* 1988;31(11):798–805.

Ohlson LO, Larsson B, Svärdsudd K, Welin L, Eriksson H, Wilhelmsen L, Björntorp P, Tibblin G. The influence of body fat distribution on the incidence of diabetes mellitus: 13.5 years of follow-up of the participants in the study of men born in 1913. *Diabetes* 1985;34(10):1055–8.

Okolicsanyi L, Passera D, Nassuato G, Lirussi F, Toso S, Crepaldi G. Epidemiology of gallstone disease in an older Italian population in Montegrotto Terme, Padua. *Journal of the American Geriatric Society* 1995;43(8):902–5.

Olincy A, Young DA, Freedman R. Increased levels of the nicotine metabolite cotinine in schizophrenic smokers compared to other smokers. *Biological Psychiatry* 1997;42(1):1–5.

Olsen J. Cigarette smoking, tea and coffee drinking, and subfecundity. *American Journal of Epidemiology* 1991;133(7):734–9.

Olsen J, Kronborg O. Coffee, tobacco and alcohol as risk factors for cancer and adenoma of the large intestine. *International Journal of Epidemiology* 1993; 22(3):398–402.

Olsen J, Rachootin P, Schiødt AV, Damsbo N. Tobacco use, alcohol consumption and infertility. *International Journal of Epidemiology* 1983;12(2):179–84.

Olsén P, Läärä E, Rantakallio P, Järvelin M-R, Sarpola A, Hartikainen AL. Epidemiology of preterm delivery in two birth cohorts with an interval of 20 years. *American Journal of Epidemiology* 1995; 142(11):1184–93.

Omenn GS, Anderson KW, Kronmal RA, Vlietstra RE. The temporal pattern of reduction of mortality risk after smoking cessation. *American Journal of Preventive Medicine* 1990;6(5):251–7.

Omenn GS, Goodman GE, Thornquist MD, Balmes J, Cullen MR, Glass A, Keogh JP, Meyskens FL Jr, Valanis B, Williams JH Jr, Barnhart S, Cherniack MG, Brodkin CA, Hammar S. Risk factors for lung cancer and for intervention effects in CARET, the Beta-Carotene and Retinol Efficacy Trial. *Journal of the National Cancer Institute* 1996;88(21):1550–9.

Ooi WL, Elston RC, Chen VW, Bailey-Wilson JE, Rothschild H. Increased familial risk for lung cancer. *Journal of the National Cancer Institute* 1986; 76(2):217–22.

Ortego-Centeno N, Munoz-Torres M, Hernandez-Quero J, Jurado-Duce A, de la Higuera Torres-Puchol J. Bone mineral density, sex steroids, and mineral metabolism in premenopausal smokers. *Calcified Tissue International* 1994;55(6):403–7.

Orwoll ES, Bauer DC, Vogt TM, Fox KM. Axial bone mass in older women. *Annals of Internal Medicine* 1996;124(2):187–96.

Osann KE. Lung cancer in women: the importance of smoking, family history of cancer, and medical history of respiratory disease. *Cancer Research* 1991;51(18):4893–7.

Osann KE, Anton-Culver H, Kurosaki T, Taylor T. Sex differences in lung cancer risk associated with cigarette smoking. *International Journal of Cancer* 1993;54(1):44–8.

Ostensen H, Gudmundsen TE, Ostensen M, Burhol PG, Bonnevie O. Smoking, alcohol, coffee, and familial factors: any associations with peptic ulcer disease? A clinically and radiologically prospective study. *Scandinavian Journal of Gastroenterology* 1985;20(10):1227–35.

Ott A, Bretelere MMB, van Harskamp F, Stijnen T, Hofman A. Incidence and risk of dementia: The Rotterdam Study. *American Journal of Epidemiology* 1998a;147(6):574–80.

Ott A, Slooter AJC, Hofman A, van Harskamp F, Witteman JCM, van Broeckhoven C, van Duijn CM, Breteler MMB. Smoking and risk of dementia and Alzheimer's disease in a population-based cohort study: the Rotterdam study. *Lancet* 1998b;351 (June):1840–3.

Paganini-Hill A, Chao A, Ross RK, Henderson BE. Exercise and other factors in the prevention of hip fracture: the Leisure World Study. *Epidemiology* 1991;2(1):16–25.

Paganini-Hill A, Hsu G. Smoking and mortality among residents of a California retirement community. *American Journal of Public Health* 1994;84(6): 992–5.

Paganini-Hill A, Ross RK, Gerkins VR, Henderson BE, Arthur M, Mack TM. Menopausal estrogen therapy and hip fractures. *Annals of Internal Medicine* 1981;95(1):28–31.

Paganini-Hill A, Ross RK, Henderson BE. Postmenopausal oestrogen treatment and stroke: a prospective study. *British Medical Journal* 1988;297(6647): 519–22.

Palmer JR, Rosenberg L. Cigarette smoking and the risk of breast cancer. *Epidemiologic Reviews* 1993; 15(1):145–56.

Palmer JR, Rosenberg L, Clarke EA, Stolley PD, Warshauer ME, Zauber AG, Shapiro S. Breast cancer and cigarette smoking: a hypothesis. *American Journal of Epidemiology* 1991;134(1):1–13.

Palmer JR, Rosenberg L, Shapiro S. Reproductive factors and risk of myocardial infarction. *American Journal of Epidemiology* 1992;136(4):408–16.

Paoff K, Preston-Martin S, Mack WJ, Monroe K. A case-control study of maternal risk factors for thyroid cancer in young women (California, United States). *Cancer Causes and Control* 1995;6(5):389–97.

Paoletti P, Carrozzi L, Viegi G, Modena P, Ballerin L, Di Pede F, Grado L, Baldacci S, Pedreschi M, Vellutini M, Paggiaro P, Mammini U, Fabbri L, Giuntini C. Distribution of bronchial responsiveness in a general population: effect of sex, age, smoking, and level of pulmonary function. *American Journal of Respiratory and Critical Care Medicine* 1995; 151(6):1770–7.

Parazzini F, Bocciolone L, Fedele L, Negri E, La Vecchia C, Acaia B. Risk factors for spontaneous abortion. *International Journal of Epidemiology* 1991a; 20(1):157–61.

Parazzini F, Ferraroni M, La Vecchia C, Baron JA, Levi F, Franceschi S, Decarli A. Smoking habits and risk of benign breast disease. *International Journal of Epidemiology* 1991b;20(2):430–4.

Parazzini F, La Vecchia C, Franceschi S, Negri E, Cecchetti G. Risk factors for endometrioid, mucinous and serous benign ovarian cysts. *International Journal of Epidemiology* 1989;18(1):108–12.

Parazzini F, La Vecchia C, Negri E, Cecchetti G, Fedele L. Epidemiologic characteristics of women with uterine fibroids: a case-control study. *Obstetrics and Gynecology* 1988;72(6):853–7.

Parazzini F, La Vecchia C, Negri E, Fedele L, Franceschi S, Gallotta L. Risk factors for cervical intraepithelial neoplasia. *Cancer* 1992a;69(9):2276–82.

Parazzini F, La Vecchia C, Negri E, Moroni S, Chatenoud L. Smoking and risk of endometrial cancer: results from an Italian case-control study. *Gynecologic Oncology* 1995;56(2):195–9.

Parazzini F, Negri E, La Vecchia C. Reproductive and general lifestyle determinants of age at menopause. *Maturitas* 1992b;15(2):141–9.

Parazzini F, Tozzi L, Ferraroni M, Bocciolone L, La Vecchia C, Fedele L. Risk factors for ectopic pregnancy: an Italian case-control study. *Obstetrics and Gynecology* 1992c;80(5):821–6.

Parazzini F, Tozzi L, Mezzopane R, Luchini L, Marchini M, Fedele L. Cigarette smoking, alcohol consumption, and risk of primary dysmenorrhea. *Epidemiology* 1994;5(4):469–72.

Parazzini F, Vercellini P, Panazza S, Chatenoud L, Oldani S, Crosignani PG. Risk factors for adenomyosis. *Human Reproduction* 1997;12(6):1275–9.

Parker SL, Tong T, Bolden S, Wingo PA. Cancer statistics, 1996. *CA—A Cancer Journal for Clinicians* 1996; 46(1):5–27.

Parkin DM, Muir CS, Whelan SL, Gao YT, Ferlay J, Powell J. *Cancer Incidence in Five Continents.* Vol. 6. Lyon (France): International Agency for Research on Cancer, 1992. IARC Scientific Publication No. 120.

Parkin DM, Pisani P, Ferlay J. Global cancer statistics. *CA: A Cancer Journal for Clinicians* 1999;49(1):33–64.

Parrott AC. Individual differences in stress and arousal during cigarette smoking. *Psychopharmacology (Berlin)* 1994;115(3):389–96.

Pasqualetti P, Festuccia V, Acitelli P, Collacciani A, Giusti A, Casale R. Tobacco smoking and risk of haematological malignancies in adults: a case-control study. *British Journal of Haematology* 1997; 97(3):659–62.

Pastides H, Najmar MA, Kelsey JL. Estrogen replacement therapy and fibrocystic breast disease. *American Journal of Preventive Medicine* 1987;3(5):282–6.

Pastides H, Tzonou A, Trichopoulos D, Katsouyanni K, Trichopoulou A, Kefalogiannis N, Manousos O. A case-control study of the relationship between smoking, diet, and gallbladder disease. *Archives of Internal Medicine* 1990;150(7):1409–12.

Pastorino U, Pisani P, Berrino F, Andreoli C, Barbieri A, Costa A, Mazzoleni C, Gramegna G, Marubini E. Vitamin A and female lung cancer: a case-control study on plasma and diet. *Nutrition and Cancer* 1987;10(4):171–9.

Pathak DR, Samet JM, Humble CG, Skipper BJ. Determinants of lung cancer risk in cigarette smokers in New Mexico. *Journal of the National Cancer Institute* 1986;76(4):597–604.

Pattinson HA, Taylor PJ, Pattinson MH. The effect of cigarette smoking on ovarian function and early pregnancy outcome of in vitro fertilization treatment. *Fertility and Sterility* 1991;55(4):780–3.

Patton GC, Carlin JB, Coffey C, Wolfe R, Hibbert M, Bowes G. Depression, anxiety, and smoking initiation: a prospective study over 3 years. *American Journal of Public Health* 1998;88(10):1518–22.

Patton GC, Hibbert M, Rosier MJ, Carlin JB, Caust J, Bowes G. Is smoking associated with depression and anxiety in teenagers? *American Journal of Public Health* 1996;86(2):225–30.

Patton GC, Johnson-Sabine E, Wood K, Mann AH, Wakeling A. Abnormal eating attitudes in London schoolgirls—a prospective epidemiological study: outcome at twelve month follow-up. *Psychological Medicine* 1990;20(2):383–94.

Paul SM, Bacharach B, Goepp C. A genetic influence on alveolar cell carcinoma. *Journal of Surgical Oncology* 1987;36(4):249–52.

Peacock JL, Bland JM, Anderson HR. Preterm delivery: effects of socioeconomic factors, psychological stress, smoking, alcohol, and caffeine. *British Medical Journal* 1995;311(7004):531–5.

Peacock JL, Bland JM, Anderson HR, Brooke OG. Cigarette smoking and birthweight: type of cigarette smoked and a possible threshold effect. *International Journal of Epidemiology* 1991;20(2):405–12.

Peacock JL, Cook DG, Carey IM, Ja MJ, Bland JM. Maternal cotinine level during pregnancy and birthweight for gestational age. *International Journal of Epidemiology* 1998;27(4):647–656.

Pearl RB, Levine DB, Gerson EJ. Studies of disease among migrants and native populations in Great Britain, Norway, and the United States. II. Conduct of field work in the United States. In: Haenszel W, editor. *Epidemiological Approaches to the Study of Cancer and Other Chronic Diseases.* National Cancer Institute Monograph 19. Bethesda (MD): U.S. Department of Health, Education and Welfare, Public Health Service, National Cancer Institute, 1966:301–20.

Peat JK, Woolcock AJ, Cullen K. Decline of lung function and development of chronic airflow limitation: a longitudinal study of non-smokers and smokers in Busselton, Western Australia. *Thorax* 1990;45(1):32–7.

Peden NR, Boyd EJS, Wormsley KG. Women and duodenal ulcer. *British Medical Journal (Clinical Research Edition)* 1981;282(6267):866.

Pedersen AT, Lidegaard O, Kreiner S, Ottesen B. Hormone replacement therapy and risk of non-fatal stroke. *Lancet* 1997;350(9087):1277–83.

Penkower L, Dew MA, Kingsley L, Becker JT, Satz P, Schaerf FW, Sheridan K. Behavioral, health and psychosocial factors and risk for HIV infection among sexually active homosexual men: the multicenter AIDS cohort study. *American Journal of Public Health* 1991;81(2):194–6.

Pérez-Stable EJ, Marín G, Marín BV, Katz MH. Depressive symptoms and cigarette smoking among Latinos in San Francisco. *American Journal of Public Health* 1990;80(12):1500–2.

Perkins KA. Individual variability in responses to nicotine. *Behavior Genetics* 1995;25(2):119–32.

Perkins KA. Sex differences in nicotine versus nonnicotine reinforcement as determinants of tobacco smoking. *Experimental and Clinical Psychopharmacology* 1996;4(2):166–77.

Perkins CI, Cohen R, Morris CR, Kwong AM, Schlag R, Wright WE. *Cancer in California: 1988–1995*. Sacramento (CA): California Department of Health Services, Cancer Surveillance Section, 1998.

Perkins KA, DiMarco A, Grobe J, Scierka A, Stiller RL. Nicotine discrimination in male and female smokers. *Psychopharmacology (Berlin)* 1994a;116(4):407–13.

Perkins KA, Epstein LH, Grobe J, Fonte C. Tobacco abstinence, smoking cues, and the reinforcing value of smoking. *Pharmacology, Biochemistry and Behavior* 1994b;47(1):107–12.

Perkins KA, Grobe JE. Increased desire to smoke during acute stress. *British Journal of Addiction* 1992;8 7(7):1037–40.

Perkins KA, Grobe JE, D'Amico D, Fonte C, Wilson AS, Stiller RL. Low-dose nicotine nasal spray use and effects during initial smoking cessation. *Experimental and Clinical Psychopharmacology* 1996a; 4(2):157–65.

Perkins KA, Grobe JE, D'Amico D, Sanders M, Scierka A, Stiller RL. Effect of training dose on nicotine discrimination in smokers. In: Harris LS, editor. *Problems of Drug Dependence 1995: Proceedings of the 57th Annual Scientific Meeting, the College on Problems of Drug Dependence.* NIDA Research Monograph 162. Rockville (MD): U.S. Department of Health and Human Services, National Institutes of Health, National Institute on Drug Abuse. 1996b:288.

Perkins KA, Grobe JE, Epstein LH, Caggiula A, Stiller RL, Jacob RG. Chronic and acute tolerance to subjective effects of nicotine. *Pharmacology, Biochemistry and Behavior* 1993;45(2):375–81.

Perkins KA, Grobe JE, Fonte C, Goettler J, Caggiula AR, Reynolds WA, Stiller RL, Scierka A, Jacob RG. Chronic and acute tolerance to subjective, behavioral and cardiovascular effects of nicotine in humans. *Journal of Pharmacology and Experimental Therapeutics* 1994c;270(2):628–38.

Perkins KA, Grobe JE, Stiller RL, Fonte C, Goettler J. Nasal spray nicotine replacement suppresses cigarette smoking desire and behavior. *Clinical Pharmacology and Therapeutics* 1992;52(6):627–34.

Perkins KA, Sexton JE, DiMarco A, Grobe JE, Scierka A, Stiller RL. Subjective and cardiovascular responses to nicotine combined with alcohol in male and female smokers. *Psychopharmacology (Berlin)* 1995;119(2):205–12.

Perkins KA, Sexton JE, Reynolds WA, Grobe JE, Fonte C, Stiller RL. Comparison of acute subjective heart rate effects of nicotine intake via tobacco smoking versus nasal spray. *Pharmacology, Biochemistry and Behavior* 1994d;47(2):295–9.

Perlman JA, Wolf PH, Ray R, Lieberknecht G. Cardiovascular risk factors, premature heart disease, and all-cause mortality in a cohort of Northern California women. *American Journal of Obstetrics and Gynecology* 1988;158(6 Pt 2):1568–74.

Perry IJ, Wannamethee SG, Walker MK, Thomson AG, Whincup PH, Shaper AG. Prospective study of risk factors for development of non-insulin dependent diabetes in middle aged British men. *British Medical Journal* 1995;310(6979):560–4.

Pershagen G, Hrubec Z, Svensson C. Passive smoking and lung cancer in Swedish women. *American Journal of Epidemiology* 1987;125(1):17–24.

Persson P-G, Ahlbom A, Hellers G. Inflammatory bowel disease and tobacco smoke—a case-control study. *Gut* 1990;31(12):1377–81.

Peters RK, Thomas D, Hagan DG, Mack TM, Henderson BE. Risk factors for invasive cervical cancer among Latinas and non-Latinas in Los Angeles County. *Journal of the National Cancer Institute* 1986; 77(5):1063–77.

Petersen K, Lindstedt G, Lundberg P-A, Bengtsson C, Lapidus L, Nyström E. Thyroid disease in middle-aged and elderly Swedish women: thyroid-related hormones, thyroid dysfunction and goitre in relation to age and smoking. *Journal of Internal Medicine* 1991;229(5):407–14.

Petitti DB, Friedman GD, Klatsky AL. Association of a history of gallbladder disease with a reduced concentration of high-density-lipoprotein cholesterol. *New England Journal of Medicine* 1981;304(23):1396–8.

Petitti DB, Sidney S, Bernstein A, Wolf S, Quesenberry C, Ziel HK. Stroke in users of low-dose oral contraceptives. *New England Journal of Medicine* 1996;335(1):8–15.

Petitti DB, Sidney S, Quesenberry CP Jr, Bernstein A. Ischemic stroke and use of estrogen and estrogen/progestrogen as hormone replacement therapy. *Stroke* 1998;29(1):23–8.

Petitti DB, Wingerd J. Use of oral contraceptives, cigarette smoking, and risk of subarachnoid haemorrhage. *Lancet* 1978;2(8083):234–6.

Peto R, Lopez AD, Boreham J, Thun M, Heath C Jr. *Mortality from Smoking in Developed Countries 1950–2000: Indirect Estimates from National Vital Statistics.* Oxford: Oxford University Press, 1994.

Petrakis NL, Gruenke LD, Beelen TC, Castagnoli N Jr, Craig JC. Nicotine in breast fluid of nonlactating women. *Science* 1978;199(4326):303–5.

Petridou E, Panagiotopoulou K, Katsouyanni K, Spanos E, Trichopoulos D. Tobacco smoking, pregnancy estrogens, and birth weight. *Epidemiology* 1990;1(3):247–50.

Pettersson F, Fries H, Nillius SJ. Epidemiology of secondary amenorrhea. I. Incidence and prevalence rates. *American Journal of Obstetrics and Gynecology* 1973;117(1):80–6.

Phillips AN, Smith GD. Cigarette smoking as a potential cause of cervical cancer: has confounding been controlled? *International Journal of Epidemiology* 1994;23(1):42–9.

Phillips RS, Tuomala RE, Feldblum PJ, Schachter J, Rosenberg MJ, Aronson MD. The effect of cigarette smoking. Chlamydia trachomatis infection, and vaginal douching on ectopic pregnancy. *Obstetrics and Gynecology* 1992;79(1):85–90.

Phipps WR, Cramer DW, Schiff I, Belisle S, Stillman R, Albrecht B, Gibson M, Berger MJ, Wilson E. The association between smoking and female infertility as influenced by cause of the infertility. *Fertility and Sterility* 1987;48(3):377–82.

Picard D, Ste-Marie LG, Coutu D, Carrier L, Chartrand R, Lepage R, Fugère P, D'Amour P. Premenopausal bone mineral content relates to height, weight and calcium intake during early adulthood. *Bone and Mineral* 1988;4(3):299–309.

Piper JM, Matanoski GM, Tonascia J. Bladder cancer in young women. *American Journal of Epidemiology* 1986;123(6):1033–42.

Pirkle JL, Flegal KM, Bernert JT, Brody DJ, Etzel RA, Maurer KR. Exposure of the US population to environmental tobacco smoke. The Third National Health and Nutrition Examination Survey 1988–1991. *Journal of the American Medical Association* 1996;275(16):1233–40.

Pisani P, Parkin DM, Bray F, Ferlay J. Estimates of the worldwide mortality from 25 cancers in 1990. *International Journal of Cancer* 1999;83(1):18–29.

Plassman BL, Helms MJ, Welsh KA, Saunders AM, Breitner JCS. Smoking, Alzheimer's disease, and confounding with genes [letter]. *Lancet* 1995; 345(8946):387.

Pocock NA, Eisman JA, Kelly PJ, Sambrook PN, Yeates MG. Effects of tobacco use on axial and appendicular bone mineral density. *Bone* 1989; 10(5):329–31.

Pohl R, Yeragani VK, Balon R, Lycaki H, McBride R. Smoking in patients with panic disorder. *Psychiatry Research* 1992;43(3):253–62.

Polychronopoulou A, Tzonou A, Hsieh C-C, Kaprinis G, Rebelakos A, Toupadaki N, Trichopoulos D. Reproductive variables, tobacco, ethanol, coffee and somatometry as risk factors for ovarian cancer. *International Journal of Cancer* 1993;55(3):402–7.

Pomerleau OF. Neurobiological interactions of alcohol and nicotine. In: Fertig JB, Allen JP, editors. *Alcohol and Tobacco: From Basic Science to Clinical Practice.* NIAAA Research Monograph 30. Bethesda (MD): National Institute on Alcohol Abuse and Alcoholism, 1995:145–58.

Pomerleau CS, Aubin HJ, Pomerleau OF. Self-reported alcohol use patterns in a sample of male and female heavy smokers. *Journal of Addictive Diseases* 1997;16(3):19–24.

Pomerleau CS, Krahn D. Smoking and eating disorders: a connection? *Journal of Addictive Diseases* 1993;12(4):169.

Pomerleau CS, Pomerleau OF. The effects of a psychological stressor on cigarette smoking and subsequent behavioral and physiological responses. *Psychophysiology* 1987;24(3):278–85.

Pomerleau CS, Pomerleau OF. Euphoriant effects of nicotine in smokers. *Psychopharmacology (Berlin)* 1992;108(4):460–5.

Pomerleau CS, Pomerleau OF, Garcia AW. Biobehavioral research on nicotine use in women. *British Journal of Addiction* 1991;86(5):527–31.

Pomerleau CS, Tate JC, Lumley MA, Pomerleau OF. Gender differences in prospectively versus retrospectively assessed smoking withdrawal symptoms. *Journal of Substance Abuse* 1994;6(4):433–40.

Pomerleau OF, Downey KK, Stelson FW, Pomerleau CS. Cigarette smoking in adult patients diagnosed with attention deficit hyperactivity disorder. *Journal of Substance Abuse* 1995;7(3):373–8.

Pomerleau OF, Pomerleau CS. Neuroregulators and the reinforcement of smoking: towards a biobehavioral explanation. *Neuroscience and Biobehavioral Reviews* 1984;8(4):503–13.

Pomerleau OF, Pomerleau CS. Stress, smoking and the cardiovascular system. *Journal of Substance Abuse* 1989;1(3):331–43.

Pomerleau OF, Rosecrans J. Neuroregulatory effects of nicotine. *Psychoneuroendocrinology* 1989;14(6): 407–23.

Ponte F, Giuffré G, Giammanco R, Dardanoni G. Risk factors of ocular hypertension and glaucoma. *Documenta Ophthalmologica* 1994;85(3):203–10.

Poór G, Atkinson EJ, O'Fallon WM, Melton LJ III. Determinants of reduced survival following hip fractures in men. *Clinical Orthopaedics and Related Research* 1995;319:260–5.

Porter JB, Jick H, Walker AM. Mortality among oral contraceptive users. *Obstetrics and Gynecology* 1987;70(1):29–32.

Potischman N, Brinton LA. Nutrition and cervical neoplasia. *Cancer Causes and Control* 1996;7(1):113–26.

Potter D, Pickle L, Mason T, Buffler P, Burau K. Smoking-related risk factors for lung cancer by cell type among women in Texas. *American Journal of Epidemiology* 1985;122(3):528.

Poulsen PL, Ebbehoj E, Hansen KW, Mogensen CE. Effects of smoking on 24-h ambulatory blood pressure and autonomic function in normalbuminuric insulin-dependent diabetes mellitus patients. *American Journal of Hypertension* 1998;11(9):1093–9.

Pradat P. A case-control study of major congenital heart defects in Sweden—1981–1986. *European Journal of Epidemiology* 1992;8(6):789–96.

Prentice RL, Yoshimoto Y, Mason MW. Relationship of cigarette smoking and radiation exposure to cancer mortality in Hiroshima and Nagasaki. *Journal of the National Cancer Institute* 1983;70(4):611–22.

Prescott E, Bjerg AM, Andersen PK, Lange P, Vestbo J. Gender difference in smoking effects on lung function and risk of hospitalization for COPD: results from a Danish longitudinal population study. *European Respiratory Journal* 1997;10(4):822–7.

Prescott E, Osler M, Andersen PK, Hein HO, Borch-Johnsen K, Lange P, Schnohr P, Vestbo J. Mortality in women and men in relation to smoking. *International Journal of Epidemiology* 1998a;27(1):27–32.

Prescott E, Osler M, Hein HO, Borch-Johnsen K, Lange P, Schnohr P, Vestbo J, and the Copenhagen Center for Prospective Population Studies. Gender and smoking-related risk of lung cancer. *Epidemiology* 1998b;9(1):79–83.

Preston-Martin S, Bernstein L, Pike MC, Maldonado AA, Henderson BE. Thyroid cancer among young women related to prior thyroid disease and pregnancy history. *British Journal of Cancer* 1987;55(2): 191–5.

Preston-Martin S, Jin F, Duda MJ, Mack WJ. A case-control study of thyroid cancer in women under age 55 in Shanghai (People's Republic of China). *Cancer Causes and Control* 1993;4(5):431–40.

Preston-Martin S, Thomas DC, White SC, Cohen D. Prior exposure to medical and dental X-rays related to tumors of the parotid gland. *Journal of the National Cancer Institute* 1988;80(12):943–9.

Prummel MF, Wiersinga WM. Smoking and risk of Graves' disease. *Journal of the American Medical Association* 1993;269(4):479–82.

Pullan RD, Rhodes J, Ganesh S, Mani V, Morris JS, Williams GT, Newcombe RG, Russell MAH, Feyerabend C, Thomas GAO, Säwe U. Transdermal nicotine for active ulcerative colitis. *New England Journal of Medicine* 1994;330(12):811–5.

Pullon S, Reinken J, Sparrow M. Prevalence of dysmenorrhoea in Wellington women. *New Zealand Medical Journal* 1988;101(839):52–4.

Pyle RL, Mitchell JE, Eckert ED, Halvorson PA, Neuman PA, Goff GM. The incidence of bulimia in freshman college students. *International Journal of Eating Disorders* 1983;2(3):75–85.

Räihä I, Kemppainen H, Kaprio J, Koskenvuo M, Sourander L. Lifestyle, stress, and genes in peptic ulcer disease: a nationwide twin cohort study. *Archives of Internal Medicine* 1998;158(7):698–704.

Ramcharan S, Pellegrin FA, Ray R, Hsu J-P, editors. *The Walnut Creek Contraceptive Drug Study. Vol. III. A Comparison of Disease Occurrence Leading to Hospitalization or Death in Users and Nonusers of Oral Contraceptives.* Bethesda (MD): National Institutes of Health, 1981. NIH Publication No. 81-564.

Randrianjohany A, Balkau B, Cubeau J, Ducimetière P, Warnet J-M, Eschwège E. The relationship between behavioural pattern, overall and central adiposity in a population of healthy French men. *International Journal of Obesity* 1993;17(11):651–5.

Ranocchia D, Minelli L, Modolo MA. Cigarette smoke and the hormonal receptors status in breast cancer. *European Journal of Epidemiology* 1991;7(4):389–95.

Rausch JL, Fefferman M, Ladisich-Rogers DG, Menard M. Effect of nicotine on human blood platelet serotonin uptake and efflux. *Progress in Neuro-Psychopharmacology and Biological Psychiatry* 1989;13(6):907–16.

Raymond E, Cnattingius S, Kiely J. Effects of maternal age, parity, and smoking on the risk of stillbirth. *British Journal of Obstetrics and Gynaecology* 1994; 101(4):301–6.

Raymond EG, Mills JL. Placental abruption. Maternal risk factors and associated fetal conditions. *Acta Obstetricia et Gynecologica Scandinavica* 1993;72(8): 633–9.

Rebagliato M, Florey C du V, Bolumar F. Exposure to environmental tobacco smoke in nonsmoking pregnant women in relation to birth weight. *American Journal of Epidemiology* 1995;142(5):531–7.

Rebuffé-Scrive M, Enk L, Crona N, Lönnroth P, Abrahamsson L, Smith U, Björntorp P. Fat cell metabolism in different regions in women. *Journal of Clinical Investigation* 1985;75(June):1973–6.

Regier DA, Farmer ME, Rae DS, Locke BZ, Keith SJ, Judd LL, Goodwin FK. Comorbidity of mental disorders with alcohol and other drug abuse: results from the Epidemiologic Catchment Area (ECA) Study. *Journal of the American Medical Association* 1990;264(19):2511–18.

Reif AE, Heeren T. Consensus on synergism between cigarette smoke and other environmental carcinogens in the causation of lung cancer. *Advances in Cancer Research* 1999;76:161–86.

Reif S, Klein I, Arber N, Gilat T. Lack of association between smoking and inflammatory bowel disease in Jewish patients in Israel. *Gastroenterology* 1995;108(6):1683–7.

Repsher LH. Smoking cessation by women and older persons: results from the Transdermal Nicotine Study Group. *Modern Medicine* 1994;62:34–8.

Resnick NM, Greenspan SL. 'Senile' osteoporosis reconsidered. *Journal of the American Medical Association* 1989;261(7):1025–9.

Reus WF, Robson MC, Zachary L, Heggers JP. Acute effects of tobacco smoking on blood flow in the cutaneous micro-circulation. *British Journal of Plastic Surgery* 1984;37(2):213–5.

Rewers M, Hamman RF. Risk factors for non-insulin-dependent diabetes. In: *Diabetes in America.* 2nd ed. U.S. Department of Health and Human Services, Public Health Service, National Institutes of Health, National Institute of Diabetes and Digestive and Kidney Diseases, 1995:179–220. NIH Publication No. 95-1468.

Reynolds P, Von Behren J, Fontham ET, Correa P, Wu A, Buffler PA, Greenberg RS. Occupational exposure to environmental tobacco smoke [letter]. *Journal of the American Medical Association* 1996;275(6): 441–2.

Rhodes M, Venables CW. Symptomatic gallstones—a disease of non-smokers? *Digestion* 1991;49(4):221–6.

Richardson D. Effects of tobacco smoke inhalation on capillary blood flow in human skin. *Archives of Environmental Health* 1987;42(1):19–25.

Rich-Edwards JW, Manson JE, Hennekens CH, Buring JE. The primary prevention of coronary heart disease in women. *New England Journal of Medicine* 1995;332(26):1758–66.

Ries LAG, Eisner MP, Kosary CL, Hankey BF, Miller BA, Clegg L, Edwards BK, editors. *SEER Cancer Statistics Review, 1973–1997.* Bethesda (MD): National Cancer Institute, 2000.

Riggs JE. Smoking and Alzheimer's disease: protective effect or differential survival bias? *Lancet* 1993; 342(8874):793–4.

Riggs BL, Melton LJ III. Involutional osteoporosis. *New England Journal of Medicine* 1986;314(26): 1676–86.

Rijcken B, Schouten JP, Xu X, Rosner B, Weiss ST. Airway hyperresponsiveness to histamine associated with accelerated decline in $FEV_1$. *American Journal of Respiratory and Critical Care Medicine* 1995;151(5): 1377–82.

Rimm EB, Chan J, Stampfer MJ, Colditz GA, Willett WC. Prospective study of cigarette smoking, alcohol use, and the risk of diabetes in men. *British Medical Journal* 1995;310(6979):555–9.

Rimm EB, Manson JE, Stampfer MJ, Colditz GA, Willett WC, Rosner B, Hennekens CH, Speizer FE. Cigarette smoking and the risk of diabetes in women. *American Journal of Public Health* 1993; 83(2):211–4.

Risch HA, Howe GR, Jain M, Burch JD, Holowaty EJ, Miller AB. Are female smokers at higher risk for lung cancer than male smokers? A case-control analysis by histologic type. *American Journal of Epidemiology* 1993;138(5):281–93.

Rocca WA, Hofman A, Brayne C, Breteler MMB, Clarke M, Copeland JRM, Dartigues J-F, Engedal K, Hagnell O, Heeren TJ, Jonker C, Lindesay J, Lobo A, Mann AH, Mölsä PK, Morgan K, O'Connor DW, da Silva Droux A, Sulkava R, Kay DWK, Amaducci L. Frequency and distribution of

Alzheimer's disease in Europe: a collaborative study of 1980–1990 prevalence findings. *Annals of Neurology* 1991;30(3):381–90.

Rodin J. Determinants of body fat localization and its implications for health. *Annals of Behavioral Medicine* 1992;14(4):275–81.

Rogers RG, Powell-Griner E. Life expectancies of cigarette smokers and nonsmokers in the United States. *Social Science and Medicine* 1991;32(10): 1151–9.

Rogers RL, Meyer JS, Judd BW, Mortel KF. Abstention from cigarette smoking improves cerebral perfusion among elderly chronic smokers. *Journal of the American Medical Association* 1985;253(20):2970–4.

Rogers RL, Meyer JS, Shaw TG, Mortel KF, Hardenberg JP, Zaid RR. Cigarette smoking decreases cerebral blood flow suggesting increased risk for stroke. *Journal of the American Medical Association* 1983;250(20):2796–800.

Rogot E, Murray JL. Smoking and causes of death among U.S. veterans: 16 years of observation. *Public Health Reports* 1980;95(3):213–22.

Rohan TE, Baron JA. Cigarette smoking and breast cancer. *American Journal of Epidemiology* 1989; 129(1):36–42.

Rohan TE, Cook MG, Baron JA. Cigarette smoking and benign proliferative epithelial disorders of the breast in women: a case-control study. *Journal of Epidemiology and Community Health* 1989;43(4):362–8.

Rome Group for Epidemiology and Prevention of Cholelithiasis. The epidemiology of gallstone disease in Rome, Italy. Part II. Factors associated with the disease. *Hepatology* 1988;8(4):907–13.

Ron E. Thyroid cancer. In: Schottenfeld D, Fraumeni JF, editors. *Cancer Epidemiology and Prevention.* 2nd ed. New York: Oxford University Press, 1996: 1000–21.

Ron E, Kleinermann RA, Boice JD Jr, Li Volsi VA, Flannery JT, Fraumeni JF Jr. A population-based case-control study of thyroid cancer. *Journal of the National Cancer Institute* 1987;79(1):1–12.

Roquer JM, Figueras J, Botet F, Jiménez R. Influence on fetal growth of exposure to tobacco smoke during pregnancy. *Acta Pediatrica* 1995;84(2):118–21.

Ros HS, Cnattingius S, Lipworth L. Comparison of risk factors for preeclampsia and gestational hypertension in a population-based cohort study. *American Journal of Epidemiology* 1998;147(11): 1062–70.

Rose JE, Ananda S, Jarvik ME. Cigarette smoking during anxiety-provoking and monotonous tasks. *Addictive Behaviors* 1983;8(4):353–9.

Rose JE, Behm F. Refined cigarette smoke as a method for reducing nicotine intake. *Pharmacology, Biochemistry and Behavior* 1987;28(2):305–10.

Rose JE, Behm FM. Inhalation of vapor from black pepper extract reduces smoking withdrawal symptoms. *Drug and Alcohol Dependence* 1994;34(3): 225–9.

Rose JE, Behm FM, Levin ED. Role of nicotine dose and sensory cues in the regulation of smoke intake. *Pharmacology, Biochemistry and Behavior* 1993;44(4):891–900.

Rose JE, Hickman CS. Citric acid aerosol as a potential smoking cessation aid. *Chest* 1987;92(6):1005–8.

Rose JE, Levin ED. Inter-relationships between conditioned and primary reinforcement in the maintenance of cigarette smoking. *British Journal of Addiction* 1991;86(5):605–9.

Rose JE, Tashkin DP, Ertle A, Zinser MC, Lafer R. Sensory blockade of smoking satisfaction. *Pharmacology, Biochemistry and Behavior* 1985;23(2):289–93.

Rosecrans JA. Brain area nicotine levels in male and female rats with different levels of spontaneous activity. *Neuropharmacology* 1972;11(6):863–70.

Rosecrans JA, Schechter MD. Brain area nicotine levels in male and female rats of two strains. *Archives Internationales de Pharmacodynamie et de Therapie* 1972;196(1):46–54.

Rosenberg L, Kaufman DW, Helmrich SP, Miller DR, Stolley PD, Shapiro S. Myocardial infarction and cigarette smoking in women younger than 50 years of age. *Journal of the American Medical Association* 1985;253(20):2965–9.

Rosenberg L, Palmer JR, Shapiro S. A case-control study of myocardial infarction in relation to use of estrogen supplements. *American Journal of Epidemiology* 1993;137(1):54–63.

Rosenberg L, Schwingl PJ, Kaufman DW, Miller DR, Helmrich SP, Stolley PD, Schottenfeld D, Shapiro S. Breast cancer and cigarette smoking. *New England Journal of Medicine* 1984;310(2):92–4.

Rosenberg L, Shapiro S, Kaufman DW, Slone D, Miettinen OS, Stolley PD. Cigarette smoking in relation to the risk of myocardial infarction in young women. Modifying influence of age and predisposing factors. *International Journal of Epidemiology* 1980a;9(1):57–63.

Rosenberg L, Slone D, Shapiro S, Kaufman D, Stolley PD, Miettinen OS. Noncontraceptive estrogens and myocardial infarction in young women. *Journal of the American Medical Association* 1980b;244(4): 339–42.

Rosevear SK, Holt DW, Lee TD, Ford WC, Wardle PG, Hull MG. Smoking and decreased fertilization rates in vitro. *Lancet* 1992;340(8829):1195–6.

Ross HE, Glaser FB, Germanson T. The prevalence of psychiatric disorders in patients with alcohol and other drug problems. *Archives of General Psychiatry* 1988;45(11):1023–31.

Ross RK, Mack TM, Paganini-Hill A, Arthur M, Henderson BE. Menopausal oestrogen therapy and protection from death from ischaemic heart disease. *Lancet* 1981;1(8225):858–60.

Ross RK, Paganini-Hill A, Landolph J, Gerkins V, Henderson BE. Analgesics, cigarette smoking, and other risk factors for cancer of the renal pelvis and ureter. *Cancer Research* 1989;49(4):1045–48.

Ross RK, Pike MC, Vessey MP, Bull D, Yeates D, Casagrande JT. Risk factors for uterine fibroids: reduced risk associated with oral contraceptives. *British Medical Journal* 1986;293(6543):359–62.

Rothman KJ. *Modern Epidemiology.* Boston: Little, Brown, 1986.

Rowlands DJ, McDermott A, Hull MG. Smoking and decreased fertilisation rates in vitro. *Lancet* 1992; 340(8832):1409–10.

Rubin DH, Krasilnikoff PA, Leventhal JM, Weile B, Berget A. Effect of passive smoking on birthweight. *Lancet* 1986;2(8504):415–7.

Rudberg S, Stattin EL, Dahlquist G. Familial and perinatal risk factors for micro- and macroalbuminuria in young IDDM patients. *Diabetes* 1998;47(7): 1121–6.

Rundgren A, Mellström D. The effect of tobacco smoking on the bone mineral content of the ageing skeleton. *Mechanisms of Ageing and Development* 1984;28(2–3):273–7.

Russell MAH, Jarvis M, Iyer R, Feyerabend C. Relation of nicotine yield of cigarettes to blood nicotine concentrations in smokers. *British Medical Journal* 1980;280(6219):972–6.

Russell MAH, Jarvis MJ, Feyerabend C, Saloojee Y. Reduction of tar, nicotine and carbon monoxide intake in low tar smokers. *Journal of Epidemiology and Community Health* 1986;40(1):80–5.

Russell MAH, Peto J, Patel UA. The classification of smoking by factorial structure of motives. *Journal of the Royal Statistical Society, Series A: General* 1974; 137(3):313–46.

Rutgeerts P, D'Haens G, Hiele M, Geboes K, Vantrappen G. Appendectomy protects against ulcerative colitis. *Gastroenterology* 1994;106(5):1251–3.

Rutishauser IH, Carlin JB. Body mass index and duration of breast feeding: a survival analysis during the first six months of life. *Journal of Epidemiology and Community Health* 1992;46(6):559–65.

Sachs BP. The effect of smoking on late pregnancy outcome. *Seminars in Reproductive Endocrinology* 1989;7(4):319–25.

Saftlas AF, Olson DR, Atrash HK, Rochat R, Rowley D. National trends in the incidence of abruptio placentae, 1979–1987. *Obstetrics and Gynecology* 1991;78(6):1081–6.

Saito R. The smoking habits of pregnant women and their husbands, and the effect on their infants. *Japan Journal of Public Health* 1991;38(2):124–31.

Salib E, Hillier V. A case-control study of smoking and Alzheimer's disease. *International Journal of Geriatric Psychiatry* 1997;12(3):295–300.

Salonen R, Salonen JT. Progression of carotid atherosclerosis and its determinants: a population-based ultrasonography study. *Atherosclerosis* 1990; 81(1):33–40.

Samadi AR, Lee NC, Flanders WD, Boring JR III, Parris EB. Risk factors for self-reported uterine fibroids: a case-control study. *American Journal of Public Health* 1996;86(6):858–62.

Samanta A, Jones A, Regan M, Wilson S, Doherty M. Is osteoarthritis in women affected by hormonal changes or smoking? *British Journal of Rheumatology* 1993;32(5):366–70.

Samet JM. Definitions and methodology in COPD research. In: Hensley MJ, Saunders NA, editors. *Clinical Epidemiology of Chronic Obstructive Pulmonary Disease.* New York: Marcel Dekker, 1989a: 1–22.

Samet JM. Radon and lung cancer. *Journal of the National Cancer Institute* 1989b;81(10):745–57.

Samet JM, Humble CG, Pathak DR. Personal and family history of respiratory disease and lung cancer risk. *American Review of Respiratory Disease* 1986; 134(3):466–70.

Samet JM, Humble CG, Skipper BE, Pathak DR. History of residence and lung cancer risk in New Mexico. *American Journal of Epidemiology* 1987; 125(5):800–11.

Samet JM, Lange P. Longitudinal studies of active and passive smoking. *American Journal of Respiratory and Critical Care Medicine* 1996;154(6 Pt 2):S257–S265.

Samet JM, Pathak DR, Morgan MV, Marbury MC, Key CR, Valdivia AA. Radon progeny exposure and lung cancer risk in New Mexico U miners: a case-control study. *Health Physics* 1989;56(4):415–21.

Samet JM, Skipper BJ, Humble CG, Pathak DR. Lung cancer risk and vitamin A consumption in New Mexico. *American Review of Respiratory Disease* 1985;131(2):198–202.

Samet JM, Tager IB, Speizer FE. The relationship between respiratory illness in childhood and chronic air-flow obstruction in adulthood. *American Review of Respiratory Disease* 1983;127(4):508–23.

Samuelsson S-M, Ekbom A, Zack M, Helmick CG, Adami H-O. Risk factors for extensive ulcerative colitis and ulcerative proctitis: a population based case-control study. *Gut* 1991;32(12):1526–30.

Sanchez-Guerrero J, Karlson EW, Colditz GA, Hunter DJ, Speizer FE, Liang MH. Hair dye use and the risk of developing systemic lupus erythematosus: a cohort study. *Arthritis and Rheumatism* 1996; 39(4):657–60.

Sandahl B. Smoking habits and spontaneous abortion. *European Journal of Obstetrics, Gynecology, and Reproductive Biology* 1989;31(1):23–31.

Sandborn WJ, Tremaine WJ, Offord KP, Lawson GM, Petersen BT, Batts KP, Croghan IT, Dale LC, Schroeder DR, Hurt RD. Transdermal nicotine for mildly to moderately active ulcerative colitis. A randomized, double-blind, placebo-controlled trial. *Annals of Internal Medicine* 1997;126(5):364–71.

Sanderson M, Williams MA, Malone KE, Stanford JL, Emanuel I, White E, Daling JR. Perinatal factors and risk of breast cancer. *Epidemiology* 1996;7(1): 34–7.

Sandler DP, Comstock GW, Helsing KJ, Shore DL. Deaths from all causes in non-smokers who lived with smokers. *American Journal of Public Health* 1989;79(2):163–7.

Sandler DP, Everson RB, Wilcox AJ. Passive smoking in adulthood and cancer risk. *American Journal of Epidemiology* 1985;121(1):37–48.

Sandler DP, Everson RB, Wilcox AJ. Cigarette smoking and breast cancer [letter]. *American Journal of Epidemiology* 1986;123(2):370–1.

Sandler RS, Sandler DP, Comstock GW, Helsing KJ, Shore DL. Cigarette smoking and the risk of colorectal cancer in women. *Journal of the National Cancer Institute* 1988;80(16):1329–33.

Sangi-Haghpeykar H, Poindexter AN III. Epidemiology of endometriosis among parous women [review]. *Obstetrics and Gynecology* 1995;85(6):983–92.

Sankaranarayanan R, Duffy SW, Day NE, Nair MK, Padmakumary G. A case-control investigation of cancer of the oral tongue and the floor of the mouth in southern India. *International Journal of Cancer* 1989a;60(4):617–21.

Sankaranarayanan R, Duffy SW, Padmakumary G, Day NE, Nair MK. Risk factors for cancer of the buccal and labial mucosa in Kerala, southern India. *Journal of Epidemiology and Community Health* 1990;44(4):286–92.

Sankaranarayanan R, Duffy SW, Padmakumary G, Day NE, Padmanabhan TK. Tobacco chewing, alcohol and nasal snuff in cancer of the gingiva in Kerala, India. *British Journal of Cancer* 1989b;60(4): 638–43.

Santavirta S, Konttinen YT, Heliövaara M, Knekt P, Lüthje P, Aromaa A. Determinants of osteoporotic-thoracic vertebral fracture. *Acta Orthopaedica Scandinavica* 1992;63(2):198–202.

Saracci R, Boffetta P. Interactions of tobacco smoking with other causes of lung cancer. In: Samet JM, editor. *Epidemiology of Lung Cancer.* New York: Marcel Dekker, 1994:465–93.

Saraiya M, Berg CJ, Kendrick JS, Strauss LT, Atrash HK, Ahn YW. Cigarette smoking as a risk factor for ectopic pregnancy. *American Journal of Obstetrics and Gynecology* 1998;178(3):493–8.

Sartwell PE, Stolley PD. Oral contraceptives and vascular disease. *Epidemiologic Reviews* 1982;4:95–109.

Sasson IM, Haley NJ, Hoffmann D, Wynder EL, Hellberg D, Nilsson S. Cigarette smoking and neoplasia of the uterine cervix: smoke constituents in cervical mucus [letter]. *New England Journal of Medicine* 1985;312(5):315–6.

Savitz DA, Schwingl PJ, Keels MA. Influence of paternal age, smoking, and alcohol consumption on congenital anomalies. *Teratology* 1991;44(4):429–40.

Savitz DA, Zhang J. Pregnancy-induced hypertension in North Carolina, 1988 and 1989. *American Journal of Public Health* 1992;82(5):675–9.

Scane AC, Francis RM, Sutcliffe AM, Francis MJ, Rawlings DJ, Chapple CL. Case-control study of the pathogenesis and sequelae of symptomatic vertebral fractures in men. *Osteoporosis International* 1999;9(1):91–7.

Schachter S. Pharmacological and psychological determinants of smoking: a New York University honors program lecture. *Annals of Internal Medicine* 1978;88(1):104–14.

Schechter MT, Miller AB, Howe GR. Cigarette smoking and breast cancer: a case-control study of screening program participants. *American Journal of Epidemiology* 1985;121(4):479–87.

Schechter MT, Miller AB, Howe GR, Baines CJ, Craib KJP, Wall C. Cigarette smoking and breast cancer: case-control studies of prevalent and incident cancer in the Canadian National Breast Screening

Study. *American Journal of Epidemiology* 1989;130(2): 213–20.

Schiff I, Bell WR, Davis V, Kessler CM, Meyers C, Nakajima S, Sexton BJ. Oral contraceptives and smoking, current considerations: recommendations of a consensus panel. *American Journal of Obstetrics and Gynecology* 1999;180(6 Pt 2):S383–4.

Schiffman MH, Bauer HM, Hoover RN, Glass AG, Cadell DM, Rush BB, Scott DR, Sherman ME, Kurman RJ, Wacholder S, Stanton CK, Manos MM. Epidemiologic evidence showing that human papillomavirus infection causes most cervical intraepithelial neoplasia. *Journal of the National Cancer Institute* 1993;85(12):958–64.

Schiffman MH, Haley NJ, Felton JS, Andrews AW, Kaslow RA, Lancaster WD, Kurman RJ, Brinton LA, Lannom LB, Hoffmann D. Biochemical epidemiology of cervical neoplasia: measuring cigarette smoke constituents in the cervix. *Cancer Research* 1987;47(14):3886–8.

Schneider NG, Jarvik ME, Forsythe AB. Nicotine versus placebo gum in the alleviation of withdrawal during smoking cessation. *Addictive Behaviors* 1984;9(2):149–56.

Schneier FR, Siris SG. A review of psychoactive substance use and abuse in schizophrenia. Patterns of drug choice. *Journal of Nervous and Mental Disease* 1987;175(11):641–52.

Schoenberg BS, Kokmen E, Okazaki H. Alzheimer's disease and other dementing illnesses in a defined United States population: incidence rates and clinical features. *Annals of Neurology* 1987;22(6):724–9.

Schoenberg JB, Wilcox HB, Mason TJ, Bill J, Stemhagen A. Variation in smoking-related risk among New Jersey women. *American Journal of Epidemiology* 1989;130(4):688–95.

Schoenborn CA, Benson V. Relationships between smoking and other unhealthy habits: United States, 1985. *Advance Data*. No. 154. Hyattsville (MD): U.S. Department of Health and Human Services, Public Health Service, Centers for Disease Control, National Center for Health Statistics, 1988.

Schoendorf KC, Kiely JL. Relationship of sudden infant death syndrome to maternal smoking during and after pregnancy. *Pediatrics* 1992;90(6):905–8.

Schöön I-M, Mellström D, Odén A, Ytterberg B-O. Peptic ulcer disease in older age groups in Gothenburg in 1985: the association with smoking. *Age and Ageing* 1991;20(5):371–6.

Schramm WF. Smoking during pregnancy: Missouri longitudinal study. *Paediatric and Perinatal Epidemiology* 1997;11(Suppl 1):73–83.

Schwartz AG, Yang G, Swanson GM. Familial risk of lung cancer among nonsmokers and their relatives. *American Journal of Epidemiology* 1996;144(6): 554–62.

Schwartz SM, Petitti DB, Siscovick DS, Longstreth WT Jr, Sidney S, Raghunathan TE, Quesenberry CP Jr, Kelaghan J. Stroke and use of low-dose oral contraceptives in young women: a pooled analysis of two U.S. studies. *Stroke* 1998;29(11):2277–84.

Schwartz-Bickenbach D, Schulte-Hobein B, Abt S, Plum C, Nau H. Smoking and passive smoking during pregnancy and early infancy: effects on birth weight, lactation period, and cotinine concentrations in mother's milk and infant's urine. *Toxicology Letters* 1987;35(1):73–81.

Schwingl PJ. Prenatal smoking exposure in relation to female adult fecundability [dissertation]. Chapel Hill (NC): University of North Carolina, 1992.

Schwingl PJ, Hulka BS, Harlow SD. Risk factors for menopausal hot flashes. *Obstetrics and Gynecology* 1994;84(1):29–34.

Scott J, Comstock GW, Hochberg M, Diamond E. Cigarette smoking and other risk factors for hip fracture in elderly women [abstract]. *American Journal of Epidemiology* 1992;special issue:977.

Scragg R, Mitchell EA, Taylor BJ, Stewart AW, Ford RP, Thompson JM, Allen EM, Becroft DM. Bed sharing, smoking, and alcohol in the sudden infant death syndrome. New Zealand Cot Death Study Group. *British Medical Journal* 1993;307(6915): 1312–8.

Seddon JM, Willett WC, Speizer FE, Hankinson SE. A prospective study of cigarette smoking and age-related macular degeneration in women. *Journal of the American Medical Association* 1996;276(14): 1141–6.

Seeley DG, Browner WS, Nevitt MC, Genant HK, Scott JC, Cummings SR. Which fractures are associated with low appendicular bone mass in elderly women? *Annals of Internal Medicine* 1991;115(11): 837–42.

Seeley DG, Kelsey J, Jergas M, Nevitt MC. Predictors of ankle and foot fractures in older women. *Journal of Bone and Mineral Research* 1996;11(9):1347–55.

Seeman E, Melton LJ III, O'Fallon WM, Riggs BL. Risk factors for spinal osteoporosis in men. *American Journal of Medicine* 1983;75(6):977–83.

Seidell JC, Cigolini M, Deurenberg P, Oosterlee A, Doornbos G. Fat distribution, androgens, and metabolism in nonobese women. *American Journal of Clinical Nutrition* 1989;50(2):269–73.

Seidenberg JM, Anderson DG, Becker RA. Validation of an in vivo developmental toxicity screen in the mouse. *Teratogenesis, Carcinogenesis, and Mutagenesis* 1986;6(5):361–74.

Seidman DS, Ever-Hadani P, Gale R. Effect of maternal smoking and age on congenital anomalies. *Obstetrics and Gynecology* 1990;76(6):1046–50.

Seidman DS, Mashiach S. Involuntary smoking and pregnancy. *European Journal of Obstetrics and Gynecology and Reproductive Biology* 1991;41(2):105–16.

Sellers TA, Bailey-Wilson JE, Elston RC, Wilson AF, Elston GZ, Ooi WL, Rothschild H. Evidence for Mendelian inheritance in the pathogenesis of lung cancer. *Journal of the National Cancer Institute* 1990;82(15):1272–9.

Sellers TA, Ooi WL, Elston RC, Chen VW, Bailey-Wilson JE, Rothschild H. Increased familial risk for non-lung cancer among relatives of lung cancer patients. *American Journal of Epidemiology* 1987; 126(2):237–46.

Sellers TA, Potter JD, Folsom AR. Association of incident lung cancer with family history of female reproductive cancers: the Iowa Women's Health Study. *Genetic Epidemiology* 1991;8(3):199–208.

Sepkovic DW, Haley NJ, Wynder EL. Thyroid activity in cigarette smokers. *Archives of Internal Medicine* 1984;144(3):501–3.

Severson RK, Davis S, Heuser L, Daling JR, Thomas DB. Cigarette smoking and acute nonlymphocytic leukemia. *American Journal of Epidemiology* 1990; 132(3):418–22.

Seyler LE Jr, Pomerleau OF, Fertig JB, Hunt D, Parker K. Pituitary hormone response to cigarette smoking. *Pharmacology, Biochemistry and Behavior* 1986; 24(1):159–62.

Shapiro S, Slone D, Rosenberg L, Kaufman DW, Stolley PD, Miettinen OS. Oral-contraceptive use in relation to myocardial infarction. *Lancet* 1979; 1(8119):743–7.

Sharara FI, Beatse SN, Leonardi MR, Navot D, Scott RT Jr. Cigarette smoking accelerates the development of diminished ovarian reserve as evidenced by the clomiphene citrate challenge test. *Fertility and Sterility* 1994;62(2):257–62.

Sharp BM, Beyer HS. Rapid desensitization of the acute stimulatory effects of nicotine on rat plasma adrencorticotropin and prolactin. *Journal of Pharmacology and Experimental Therapy* 1986;23(2): 486–91.

Shaten BJ, Smith GD, Kuller LH, Neaton JD. Risk factors for the development of type II diabetes among men enrolled in the usual care group of the Multiple Risk Factor Intervention Trial. *Diabetes Care* 1993; 16(10):1331–9.

Shaw GL, Falk RT, Pickle LW, Mason TJ, Buffler PA. Lung cancer risk associated with cancer in relatives. *Journal of Clinical Epidemiology* 1991;44(4–5): 429–37.

Shaw GM, Wasserman CR, Lammer EJ, O'Malley CD, Murray JC, Basart AM, Tolarova MM. Orofacial clefts, parental cigarette smoking, and transforming growth factor-alpha gene variants. *American Journal of Human Genetics* 1996;58(3):551–61.

Sherman CB, Xu X, Speizer FE, Ferris BG Jr, Weiss ST, Dockery DW. Longitudinal lung function decline in subjects with respiratory symptoms. *American Review of Respiratory Disease* 1992;146(4):855–9.

Sherrill DL, Holberg CJ, Enright PL, Lebowitz MD, Burrows B. Longitudinal analysis of the effects of smoking onset and cessation on pulmonary function. *American Journal of Respiratory and Critical Care Medicine* 1994;149(3 Pt 1):591–7.

Sherrill DL, Lebowitz MD, Knudson RJ, Burrows B. Smoking and symptom effects on the curves of lung function growth and decline. *American Review of Respiratory Disease* 1991;144(1):17–22.

Sherrill DL, Martinez FD, Lebowitz MD, Holdaway MD, Flannery EM, Herbison GP, Stanton WR, Silva PA, Sears MR. Longitudinal effects of passive smoking on pulmonary function in New Zealand children. *American Review of Respiratory Disease* 1992;145(5):1136–41.

Shiffman SM. The tobacco withdrawal syndrome. In: Krasnegor NA, editor. *Cigarette Smoking as a Dependence Process.* NIDA Research Monograph 23. Washington: U.S. Department of Health, Education and Welfare, Public Health Service, National Institutes of Health, National Institute on Drug Abuse, 1979:158–84.

Shimizu H, Morishita M, Mizuno K, Masuda T, Ogura Y, Santo M, Nishimura M, Kunishima K, Karasawa K, Nishiwaki K, Yamamoto M, Hisamichi S, Tominaga S. A case-control study of lung cancer in nonsmoking women. *Tohoku Journal of Experimental Medicine* 1988;154(4):389–97.

Shine B, Fells P, Edwards OM, Weetman AP. Association between Graves' ophthalmopathy and smoking. *Lancet* 1990;335(8700):1261–3.

Shinton R, Beevers G. Meta-analysis of relation between cigarette smoking and stroke. *British Medical Journal* 1989;298(6676):789–94.

Shiono PH, Klebanoff MA, Berendes HW. Congenital malformations and maternal smoking during pregnancy. *Teratology* 1986a;34(1):65–71.

Shiono PH, Klebanoff MA, Rhoads GG. Smoking and drinking during pregnancy: their effects on preterm birth. *Journal of the American Medical Association* 1986b;255(1):82–4.

Shopland DR. Tobacco use and its contribution to early cancer mortality with a special emphasis on cigarette smoking. *Environmental Health Perspectives* 1995;103(Suppl 8):131–41.

Shu XO, Brinton LA, Gao YT, Yuan JM. Population-based case-control study of ovarian cancer in Shanghai. *Cancer Research* 1989;49(13):3670–4.

Shurtleff D. Some characteristics related to the incidence of cardiovascular disease and death: Framingham Study, 18-year follow-up. In: Kannel WB, Gordon T, editors. *The Framingham Study: An Epidemiological Investigation of Cardiovascular Disease.* U.S. Department of Health, Education and Welfare, National Institutes of Health, 1974. DHEW Publication No. (NIH) 74-599.

Sibai BM, Gordon T, Thom E, Caritis SN, Klebanoff M, McNellis D, Paul RH. Risk factors for preeclampsia in healthy nulliparous women: a prospective multicenter study. The National Institute of Child Health and Human Development Network of Maternal-Fetal Medicine Units. *American Journal of Obstetrics and Gynecology* 1995;172(2 Pt 1):642–8.

Sidney S, Siscovick DS, Petitti DB, Schwartz SM, Quesenberry CP, Psaty BM, Raghunathan TE, Kelaghan J, Koepsell TD. Myocardial infarction and use of low-dose oral contraceptives: a pooled analysis of two U.S. studies. *Circulation* 1998; 98(11):1058–63.

Sidney S, Tekawa IS, Friedman GD. A prospective study of cigarette tar yield and lung cancer. *Cancer Causes and Control* 1993;4(1):3–10.

Siegel M. Smoking and leukemia: evaluation of a causal hypothesis. *American Journal of Epidemiology* 1983;138(1):1–9.

Siemiatycki J, Colle E, Campbell S, Dewar RA, Belmonte MM. Case-control study of IDDM. *Diabetes Care* 1989;12(3):209–16.

Siemiatycki J, Krewski D, Franco E, Kaiserman M. Associations between cigarette smoking and each of 21 types of cancer: a multi-site case-control study. *International Journal of Epidemiology* 1995; 24(3):504–14.

Siever LJ. Role of noradrenergic mechanisms in the etiology of the affective disorders. In: Meltzer HY, Coyle JT, Kopin IJ, Bunney WE Jr, Davis KL, Schuster CR, Shader RI, Simpson GM, editors. *Psychopharmacology: The Third Generation of Progress.* New York: Raven Press, 1987:493–504.

Signorello LB, Harlow BL, Cramer DW, Spiegelman D, Hill JA. Epidemiologic determinants of endometriosis: a hospital-based case-control study. *Annals of Epidemiology* 1997;7(4):267–741.

Siiteri PK. Adipose tissue as a source of hormones. *American Journal of Clinical Nutrition* 1987;45(1 Suppl):277–82.

Silman AJ, Newman J, MacGregor AJ. Cigarette smoking increases the risk of rheumatoid arthritis. Results from a nationwide study of disease-discordant twins. *Arthritis and Rheumatism* 1996; 39(5):732–5.

Sillman F, Stanek A, Sedlis A, Rosenthal J, Lanks KW, Buchhagen D, Nicastri A, Boyce J. The relationship between human papillomavirus and lower genital intraepithelial neoplasia in immunosuppressed women. *American Journal of Obstetrics and Gynecology* 1984;150(3):300–8.

Silverman DT, Dunn JA, Hoover RN, Schiffman M, Lillemoe KD, Schoenberg JB, Brown LM, Greenberg RS, Hayes RB, Swanson GM, Wacholder S, Schwartz AG, Liff JM, Pottern LM. Cigarette smoking and pancreas cancer: a case-control study based on direct interviews. *Journal of the National Cancer Institute* 1994;86(20):1510–6.

Silverman DT, Morrison AS, Devesa SS. Bladder cancer. In: Schottenfeld D, Fraumeni JF Jr, editors. *Cancer Epidemiology and Prevention.* 2nd ed. New York: Oxford University Press, 1996:1156–79.

Silverstein MD, Lashner BA, Hanauer SB. Cigarette smoking and ulcerative colitis: a case-control study. *Mayo Clinic Proceedings* 1994;69(5):425–9.

Silverstein MD, Lashner BA, Hanauer SB, Evans AA, Kirsner JB. Cigarette smoking in Crohn's disease. *American Journal of Gastroenterology* 1989;84(1):31–3.

Simons AM, van Herckenrode CM, Rodriguez JA, Maitland N, Anderson M, Phillips DH, Coleman DV. Demonstration of smoking-related DNA damage in cervical epithelium and correlation with human papillomavirus type 16, using exfoliated cervical cells. *British Journal of Cancer* 1995;71(2): 246–9.

Singh J, Scott LH. Threshold for carbon monoxide induced fetotoxicity. *Teratology* 1984;30(2):253–7.

Siraprapasiri T, Foy HM, Kreiss JK, Pruithitada N, Thongtub W. Frequency and risk of HIV infection among men attending a clinic for STD in Chiang Mai, Thailand. *Southeast Asian Journal of Tropical Medicine and Public Health* 1996;27(1):96–101.

Slattery ML, McDonald A, Bild DE, Caan BJ, Hilner JE, Jacobs DR Jr, Liu K. Associations of body fat and its distribution with dietary intake, physical activity, alcohol, and smoking in blacks and whites. *American Journal of Clinical Nutrition* 1992; 55(5):943–9.

Slattery ML, Potter JD, Friedman GD, Ma KN, Edwards S. Tobacco use and colon cancer. *International Journal of Cancer* 1997;70(3):259–64.

Slattery ML, Robison LM, Schuman KL, French TK, Abbott TM, Overall JC Jr, Gardner JW. Cigarette smoking and exposure to passive smoke are risk factors for cervical cancer. *Journal of the American Medical Association* 1989;261(11):1593–8.

Slemenda CW, Christian JC, Reed T, Reister TK, Williams CJ, Johnston CC. Long-term bone loss in men: effects of genetic and environmental factors. *Annals of Internal Medicine* 1992;117(4):286–91.

Slemenda CW, Hui SL, Longcope C, Johnston CC Jr. Cigarette smoking, obesity, and bone mass. *Journal of Bone and Mineral Research* 1989;4(5):737–41.

Slone D, Shapiro S, Rosenberg L, Kaufman DW, Hartz SC, Rossi AC, Stolley PD, Miettinen OS. Relation of cigarette smoking to myocardial infarction in young women. *New England Journal of Medicine* 1978;298(23):1273–6.

Sloss EM, Frerichs RR. Smoking and menstrual disorders. *International Journal of Epidemiology* 1983; 12(1):107–9.

Slotkin TA. Fetal nicotine or cocaine exposure: which one is worse? *Journal of Pharmacology and Experimental Therapeutics* 1998;285(3):931–45.

Smith EM, Sowers MF, Burns TL. Effects of smoking on the development of female reproductive cancers. *Journal of the National Cancer Institute* 1984; 73(2):371–6.

Smith SJ, Deacon JM, Chilvers CED. Alcohol, smoking, passive smoking and caffeine in relation to breast cancer risk in young women. *British Journal of Cancer* 1994;70(1):112–9.

Smith W, Mitchell P, Leeder SR. Smoking and age-related maculopathy: the Blue Mountains Eye Study. *Archives of Ophthalmology* 1996;114(12): 1518–23.

Sobue T, Suzuki T, Nakayama N, Inubushi T, Matsuda M, Doi O, Mori T, Furuse K, Fukuoka M, Yasumitsu T, Kuwabara O, Ichitani M, Kurata M, Kuwabari M, Nakahara K, Endo S, Hattori S. Association of indoor air pollution and passive smoking with lung cancer in Osaka, Japan [in Japanese]. *Gan No Rinsho* 1990;36(3):329–33.

Sokic SI, Adanja BJ, Vlajinac HD, Jankovic RR, Marinkovic JP, Zivaljevic VR. Risk factors for thyroid cancer. *Neoplasma* 1994;41(6):371–4.

Solomon L. Clinical features of osteoarthritis. In: Kelley WN, Ruddy S, Harris ED Jr, Sledge CB, editors. *Textbook of Rheumatology*. Vol. 2. 5th ed. Philadelphia: W.B. Saunders, 1997:1383–93.

Solomon CG, Willett WC, Carey VJ, Rich-Edwards J, Hunter DJ, Colditz GA, Stampfer MJ, Speizer FE, Spiegelman D, Manson JE. A prospective study of pregravid determinants of gestational diabetes mellitus. *Journal of the American Medical Association* 1997;278(13):1078–83.

Solomon LJ, Flynn BS. Women who smoke. In: Orleans C, Slade J, editors. *Nicotine Addiction: Principles and Management*. New York: Oxford University Press, 1993:339–49.

Somerville KW, Logan RFA, Edmond M, Langman MJS. Smoking and Crohn's disease. *British Medical Journal* 1984;289(6450):954–6.

Song S, Ashley DL. Supercritical fluid extraction and gas chromatography/mass spectrometry for the analysis of tobacco-specific nitrosamines in cigarettes. *Analytical Chemistry* 1999;71(7):1303–8.

Sonnenberg A, Muller-Lissner SA, Vogel E, Schmid P, Gonvers JJ, Peter P, Strohmeyer G, Blum AL. Predictors of duodenal ulcer healing and relapse. *Gastroenterology* 1981;81(6):1061–7.

Sontag S, Graham DY, Belsito A, Weiss J, Farley A, Grunt R, Cohen N, Kinnear D, Davis W, Archambault A, Achrod J, Thayer W, Gillies R, Sidorov J, Sabesin SM, Dyck W, Fleshler B, Cleator I, Wenger J, Opekun A Jr. Cimetidine, cigarette smoking and recurrence of duodenal ulcer. *New England Journal of Medicine* 1984;311(11):689–93.

Sorensen G, Pechacek TF. Attitudes toward smoking cessation among men and women. *Journal of Behavioral Medicine* 1987;10(2):129–37.

Sowers MR, Clark MK, Hollis B, Wallace RB, Jannausch M. Radial bone mineral density in pre- and perimenopausal women: a prospective study of rates and risk factors for loss. *Journal of Bone and Mineral Research* 1992;7(6):647–57.

Sowers MR, Galuska DA. Epidemiology of bone mass in premenopausal women. *Epidemiologic Reviews* 1993;15(2):374–98.

Sowers MR, Wallace RB, Lemke JH. Correlates of forearm bone mass among women during maximal bone mineralization. *Preventive Medicine* 1985a; 14(5):585–96.

Sowers MR, Wallace RB, Lemke JH. Correlates of midradius bone density among postmenopausal women: a community study. *American Journal of Clinical Nutrition* 1985b;41(5):1045–53.

Spector TD, Edwards AC, Thompson PW. Use of a risk factor and dietary calcium questionnaire in predicting bone density and subsequent bone loss at the menopause. *Annals of the Rheumatic Diseases* 1992;51(11):1252–3.

Spector TD, Hall GM, McCloskey EV, Kanis JA. Risk of vertebral fracture in women with rheumatoid arthritis. *British Medical Journal* 1993;306(6877):558.

Speizer FE. The rise in chronic obstructive pulmonary disease mortality: overview and summary. *American Review of Respiratory Disease* 1989;140(3 Pt 2): S106–S107.

Speizer FE, Fay ME, Dockery DW, Ferris BG Jr. Chronic obstructive pulmonary disease mortality in six U.S. cities. *American Review of Respiratory Disease* 1989;140(3 Pt 2):S49–S55.

Spiers PS. Disentangling the separate effects of prenatal and postnatal smoking on the risk of SIDS [comment]. *American Journal of Epidemiology* 1999; 149(7):603–7.

Spinelli A, Figa-Talamanca I, Osborn J. Time to pregnancy and occupation in a group of Italian women. *International Journal of Epidemiology* 1997; 26(3):601–9.

Spinillo A, Capuzzo E, Colonna L, Solerte L, Nicola S, Guaschino S. Factors associated with abruptio placentae in preterm deliveries. *Acta Obstetricia et Gynecologica Scandinavica* 1994a;73(4):307–12.

Spinillo A, Capuzzo E, Egbe TO, Nicola S, Piazzi G, Baltaro F. Cigarette smoking in pregnancy and risk of pre-eclampsia. *Journal of Human Hypertension* 1994b;8(10):771–5.

Spinillo A, Capuzzo E, Nicola SE, Colonna L, Egbe TO, Zara C. Factors potentiating the smoking-related risk of fetal growth retardation. *British Journal of Obstetrics and Gynaecology* 1994c;101(11):954–8.

Spinillo A, Nicola S, Piazzi G, Ghazal K, Colonna L, Baltaro F. Epidemiological correlates of preterm premature rupture of membranes. *International Journal of Gynaecology and Obstetrics* 1994d;47(1): 7–15.

Stadel BV. Oral contraceptives and cardiovascular disease. *New England Journal of Medicine* 1981; 305(11):612–8.

Stampfer MJ, Colditz GA. Estrogen replacement therapy and coronary heart disease: a quantitative assessment of epidemiologic evidence. *Preventive Medicine* 1991;20(1):47–63.

Stampfer MJ, Colditz GA, Willett WC, Manson JE, Arky RA, Hennekens CH, Speizer FE. A prospective study of moderate alcohol drinking and risk of diabetes in women. *American Journal of Epidemiology* 1988a;128(3):549–58.

Stampfer MJ, Colditz GA, Willett WC, Manson JE, Rosner B, Speizer FE, Hennekens CH. Postmenopausal estrogen therapy and cardiovascular disease. *New England Journal of Medicine* 1991; 325(11): 756–62.

Stampfer MJ, Hu FB, Manson JE, Rimm EB, Willett WC. Primary prevention of coronary heart disease in women through diet and lifestyle. *New England Journal of Medicine* 2000;343(1):16–22.

Stampfer MJ, Maclure KM, Colditz GA, Manson JE, Willett WC. Risk of symptomatic gallstones in women with severe obesity. *American Journal of Clinical Nutrition* 1992;55(3):652–8.

Stampfer MJ, Willett WC, Colditz GA, Speizer FE, Hennekens CH. A prospective study of past use of oral contraceptive agents and risk of cardiovascular diseases. *New England Journal of Medicine* 1988b;319(20):1313–7.

Stanford JL, Hartge P, Brinton LA, Hoover RN, Brookmeyer R. Factors influencing the age at natural menopause. *Journal of Chronic Diseases* 1987a; 40(11):995–1002.

Stanford JL, Szklo M, Boring CC, Brinton LA, Diamond EA, Greenberg RS, Hoover RN. A case-control study of breast cancer stratified by estrogen receptor status. *American Journal of Epidemiology* 1987b;125(2):184–94.

Steenland K. Passive smoking and the risk of heart disease. *Journal of the American Medical Association* 1992;267(1):94–9.

Steenland K, Thun M, Lally C, Heath C Jr. Environmental tobacco smoke and coronary heart disease in the American Cancer Society CPS-II cohort. *Circulation* 1996;94(4):622–8.

Stein Z, Kline J, Levin B, Susser M, Warburton D. Epidemiologic studies of environmental exposure in human reproduction. In: Berge CG, Maillie HD, editors. *Measurement of Risks*. New York: Plenum Press, 1981:163–83.

Steinmetz KA, Potter JD, Folsom AR. Vegetables, fruit, and lung cancer in the Iowa Women's Health Study. *Cancer Research* 1993;53(3):536–43.

Stellman SD, Garfinkel L. Smoking habits and tar levels in a new American Cancer Society prospective study of 1.2 million men and women. *Journal of the National Cancer Institute* 1986;76(6):1057–63.

Stellman SD, Muscat JE, Hoffman D, Wynder EL. Impact of filter cigarette smoking on lung cancer histology. *Preventive Medicine* 1997;26(4):451–6.

Stemhagen A, Slade J, Altman R, Bill J. Occupational risk factors and liver cancer: a retrospective case-control study of primary liver cancer in New

Jersey. *American Journal of Epidemiology* 1983; 117(4):443–54.

Stergachis A, Scholes D, Daling JR, Weiss NS, Chu J. Maternal cigarette smoking and the risk of tubal pregnancy. *American Journal of Epidemiology* 1991; 133(4):332–7.

Sterzik K, Strehler E, De Santo M, Trumpp N, Abt M, Rosenbusch B, Schneider A. Influence of smoking on fertility in women attending an in vitro fertilization program. *Fertility and Sterility* 1996;65(4): 810–4.

Stevens J, Keil JE, Rust PF, Tyroler HA, Davis CE, Gazes PC. Body mass index and body girths as predictors of mortality in black and white women. *Archives of Internal Medicine* 1992a;152(6):1257–62.

Stevens J, Keil JE, Rust PF, Verdugo RR, Davis CE, Tyroler HA, Gazes PC. Body mass index and body girths as predictors of mortality in black and white men. *American Journal of Epidemiology* 1992b; 135(10):1137–46.

Stevenson JC, Lees B, Devenport M, Cust MP, Ganger KF. Determinants of bone density in normal women: risk factors for future osteoporosis? *British Medical Journal* 1989;298(6678):924–8.

Stewart J, de Wit H, Eikelboom R. Role of unconditioned and conditioned drug effects in the self-administration of opiates and stimulants. *Psychological Reviews* 1984;91(2):251–68.

Stewart WC, Crinkley CMC, Murrell HP. Cigarette-smoking in normal subjects, ocular hypertensive, and chronic open-angle glaucoma patients. *American Journal of Ophthalmology* 1994;117(2):267–8.

Stillman RJ, Rosenberg MJ, Sachs BP. Smoking and reproduction. *Fertility and Sterility* 1986;46(4):545–66.

Stockwell HG, Goldman AL, Lyman GH, Noss CI, Armstrong AW, Pinkham PA, Candelora EC, Brusa MR. Environmental tobacco smoke and lung cancer risk in nonsmoking women. *Journal of the National Cancer Institute* 1992;84(18):1417–22.

Stockwell HG, Lyman GH. Cigarette smoking and the risk of female reproductive cancer. *American Journal of Obstetrics and Gynecology* 1987;157(1):35–40.

Stolerman IP, Goldfarb T, Fink R, Jarvik ME. Influencing cigarette smoking with nicotine antagonists. *Psychopharmacologia (Berlin)* 1973;28(3):247–59.

Stolley PD, Strom BL, Sartwell PE. Oral contraceptives and vascular disease. *Epidemiologic Reviews* 1989;11:241–3.

Sundell G, Milsom I, Andersch B. Factors influencing the prevalence and severity of dysmenorrhoea in young women. *British Journal of Obstetrics and Gynaecology* 1990;97(7):588–94.

Suominen H, Heikkinen E, Vainio P, Lahtinen T. Mineral density of calcaneus in men at different ages: a population study with special reference to life-style factors. *Age and Ageing* 1984;13(5):273–81.

Suonio S, Saarikoski S, Kauhanen O, Metsäpelto A, Terho J, Vohlonen I. Smoking does affect fecundity. *European Journal of Obstetrics, Gynecology, and Reproductive Biology* 1990;34(1–2):89–95.

Sutherland LR, Ramcharan S, Bryant H, Fick G. Effect of cigarette smoking on recurrence of Crohn's disease. *Gastroenterology* 1990;98(5 Pt 1):1123–8.

Svendsen KH, Kuller LH, Martin MJ, Ockene JK. Effects of passive smoking in the Multiple Risk Factor Intervention Trial. *American Journal of Epidemiology* 1987;126(5):783–95.

Svensson C, Pershagen G, Klominek J. Smoking and passive smoking in relation to lung cancer in women. *Acta Oncologica* 1989;28(5):623–9.

Svikis DS, Hatsukami DK, Hughes JR, Carroll KM, Pickens RW. Sex differences in tobacco withdrawal syndrome. *Addictive Behaviors* 1986;11(4):459–62.

Symmons DP, Bankhead CR, Harrison BJ, Brennan P, Barrett EM, Scott DG, Silman AJ. Blood transfusion, smoking, and obesity as risk factors for the development of rheumatoid arthritis: results from a primary care-based incident control study in Norfolk, England. *Arthritis and Rheumatism* 1997; 40(11):1955–61.

Tabassian AR, Nylen ES, Giron AE, Snider RH, Cassidy MM, Becker KL. Evidence for cigarette smoke-induced calcitonin secretion from lungs of man and hamster. *Life Sciences* 1988;42(23):2323–9.

Tager IB, Hanrahan JP, Tosteson TD, Castile RG, Brown RW, Weiss ST, Speizer FE. Lung function, pre- and post-natal smoke exposure, and wheezing in the first year of life. *American Review of Respiratory Disease* 1993;147(4):811–7.

Tager IB, Ngo L, Hanrahan JP. Maternal smoking during pregnancy: effects on lung function during the first 18 months of life. *American Journal of Respiratory and Critical Care Medicine* 1995;152(3):977–83.

Tager IB, Segal MR, Speizer FE, Weiss ST. The natural history of forced expiratory volumes: effect of cigarette smoking and respiratory symptoms. *American Review of Respiratory Disease* 1988;138(4): 837–49.

Talamini R, La Vecchia C, Levi F, Conti E, Favero A, Franceschi S. Cancer of the oral cavity and pharynx in nonsmokers who drink alcohol and in nondrinkers who smoke tobacco. *Journal of the National Cancer Institute* 1998;90(24):1901–3.

Tanaka K, Hirohata T, Fukuda K, Shibata A, Tsukuma H, Hiyama T. Risk factors for hepatocellular carcinoma among Japanese women. *Cancer Causes and Control* 1995;6(2):91–8.

Tanaka K, Hirohata T, Takeshita S, Hirohata I, Koga S, Sugimachi K, Kanematsu T, Ohryohji F, Ishibashi H. Hepatitis B virus, cigarette smoking and alcohol consumption in the development of hepatocellular carcinoma: a case-control study in Fukuoka, Japan. *International Journal of Cancer* 1992; 51(4):509–14.

Targett CS, Gunesee H, McBride F, Beischer NA. An evaluation of the effects of smoking on maternal oestriol excretion during pregnancy and on fetal outcome. *Journal of Obstetrics and Gynaecology of the British Commonwealth* 1973;80(9):815–21.

Tarui S, Tokunaga K, Fujioka S, Matsuzawa Y. Visceral fat obesity: anthropological and pathophysiological aspects. *International Journal of Obesity* 1991; 15(Suppl 2):1–8.

Tashkin DP, Altose MD, Connett JE, Kanner RE, Lee WW, Wise RA. Methacholine reactivity predicts changes in lung function over time in smokers with early chronic obstructive pulmonary disease. *American Journal of Respiratory and Critical Care Medicine* 1996;153(6 Pt 1):1802–11.

Tashkin DP, Clark VA, Coulson AH, Simmons M, Bourque LB, Reems C, Detels R, Sayre JW, Rokaw SN. The UCLA population studies of chronic obstructive respiratory disease. VIII. Effects of smoking cessation on lung function: a prospective study of a free-living population. *American Review of Respiratory Disease* 1984;130(5):707–15.

Tate JC, Pomerleau OF, Pomerleau CS. Temporal stability and within-subject consistency of nicotine withdrawal symptoms. *Journal of Substance Abuse* 1993;5(4):355–63.

Tavani A, Negri E, Franceschi S, Barbone F, La Vecchia C. Attributable risk for laryngeal cancer in northern Italy. *Cancer Epidemiology, Biomarkers and Prevention* 1994a;3(2):121–5.

Tavani A, Negri E, Franceschi S, La Vecchia C. Risk factors for esophageal cancer in women in northern Italy. *Cancer* 1993;72(9):2531–6.

Tavani A, Negri E, Franceschi S, Serraino D, La Vecchia C. Smoking habits and non-Hodgkin's lymphoma: a case-control study in northern Italy. *Preventive Medicine* 1994b;23(4):447–52.

Taylor AE, Johnson DC, Kazemi H. Environmental tobacco smoke and cardiovascular disease: a position paper from the Council on Cardiopulmonary and Critical Care, American Heart Association. *Circulation* 1992;86(2):699–702.

Tell GS, Howard G, McKinney WM, Toole JF. Cigarette smoking cessation and extracranial carotid atherosclerosis. *Journal of the American Medical Association* 1989;261(8):1178–80.

Tell GS, Polak JF, Ward BJ, Kittner SJ, Savage PJ, Robbins J. Relation of smoking with carotid artery wall thickness and stenosis in older adults: the Cardiovascular Health Study. *Circulation* 1994; 90(6):2905–8.

Tellez M, Cooper J, Edmonds C. Graves' ophthalmopathy in relation to cigarette smoking and ethnic origin. *Clinical Endocrinology* 1992;36(3):291–4.

Tenovuo AH, Kero PO, Korvenranta HJ, Erkkola RU, Klemi PJ, Tuominen J. Risk factors associated with severely small for gestational age neonates. *American Journal of Perinatology* 1988;5(3):267–71.

Teperi J, Rimpelä M. Menstrual pain, health and behaviour in girls. *Social Science and Medicine* 1989; 29(2):163–9.

Terkel J, Blake CA, Hoover V, Sawyer CH. Pup survival and prolactin levels in nicotine-treated lactating rats. *Proceedings of the Society for Experimental Biology and Medicine* 1973;143(4):1131–5.

Terry MB, Neugut AI. Cigarette smoking and the colorectal adenoma-carcinoma sequence: a hypothesis to explain the paradox. *American Journal of Epidemiology* 1998;147(10):903–10.

Terry RB, Page WF, Haskell WL. Waist/hip ratio, body mass index and premature cardiovascular disease mortality in US Army veterans during a twenty-three year follow-up study. *International Journal of Obesity* 1992;16(6):417–23.

Terry RD, Katzman R, Bick KL, editors. *Alzheimer Disease.* New York: Raven Press, 1994.

Thompson SG, Greenberg G, Meade TW. Risk factors for stroke and myocardial infarction in women in the United Kingdom as assessed in general practice: a case-control study. *British Heart Journal* 1989; 61(5):403–9.

Thornton JR, Emmett PM, Heaton KW. Smoking, sugar, and inflammatory bowel disease. *British Medical Journal* 1985;290(6484):1786–7.

Thorogood M, Mann J, Murphy M, Vessey M. Is oral contraceptive use still associated with an increased risk of fatal myocardial infarction? Report of a case-control study. *British Journal of Obstetrics and Gynaecology* 1991;98(12):1245–53.

Thorogood M, Mann J, Murphy M, Vessey M. Fatal stroke and use of oral contraceptives: findings from a case-control study. *American Journal of Epidemiology* 1992;136(1):35–45.

Thun MJ, Day-Lally C, Myers DG, Calle EE, Flanders WD, Zhu B-P, Namboodiri MM, Heath CW Jr.

Trends in tobacco smoking and mortality from cigarette use in Cancer Prevention Studies I (1959 through 1965) and II (1982 through 1988). In: Shopland DR, Burns DM, Garfinkel L, Samet JM, editors. *Changes in Cigarette-Related Disease Risks and Their Implication for Prevention and Control.* Smoking and Tobacco Control Monograph 8. Rockville (MD): U.S. Department of Health and Human Services, Public Health Service, National Institutes of Health, National Cancer Institute, 1997a:305–82. NIH Publication No. 97-4213.

Thun MJ, Day-Lally CA, Calle EE, Flanders WD, Heath CW Jr. Excess mortality among cigarette smokers: changes in a 20-year interval. *American Journal of Public Health* 1995;85(9):1223–30.

Thun MJ, Lally CA, Flannery JT, Calle EE, Flanders WD, Heath CW Jr. Cigarette smoking and changes in the histopathology of lung cancer. *Journal of the National Cancer Institute* 1997b;89:1580–6.

Thun MJ, Myers DG, Day-Lally C, Namboodiri MM, Calle EE, Flanders WD, Adams SL, Heath CW Jr. Age and the exposure-response relationships between cigarette smoking and premature death in Cancer Prevention Study II. In: Shopland DR, Burns DM, Garfinkel L, Samet JM, editors. *Changes in Cigarette-Related Disease Risks and Their Implication for Prevention and Control.* Smoking and Tobacco Control Monograph 8. Rockville (MD): U.S. Department of Health and Human Services, Public Health Service, National Institutes of Health, National Cancer Institute, 1997c:383–475. NIH Publication No. 97-4213.

Thurlbeck WM. Emphysema then and now. *Canadian Respiratory Journal* 1994;1(1):21–39.

Timmer A, Sutherland LR, Martin F. Oral contraceptive use and smoking are risk factors for relapse in Crohn's disease. The Canadian Mesalamine for Remission of Crohn's Disease Study Group. *Gastroenterology* 1998;114(6):1143–50.

Timmerman MG, Wells LA, Chen SP. Bulimia nervosa and associated alcohol abuse among secondary school students. *Journal of the American Academy of Child and Adolescent Psychiatry* 1990;29(1):118–22.

Tobin MV, Logan RFA, Langman MJS, McConnell RB, Gilmore IT. Cigarette smoking and inflammatory bowel disease. *Gastroenterology* 1987;93(2):316–21.

Tockman MS, Comstock GW. Respiratory risk factors and mortality: longitudinal studies in Washington County, Maryland. *American Review of Respiratory Disease* 1989;140(3 Pt 2):S56–S63.

Tokuhata GK. Smoking habits in lung-cancer proband families and comparable control families. *Journal of the National Cancer Institute* 1963;31(5):1153–71.

Tominaga K, Koyama Y, Sasagawa M, Hiroki M, Nagai M. A case-control study of stomach cancer and its genesis in relation to alcohol consumption, smoking, and familial cancer history. *Japanese Journal of Cancer Research* 1991;82(9):974–9.

Torfs CP, Velie EM, Oechsli FW, Bateson TF, Curry CJ. A population-based study of gastroschisis: Demographic pregnancy, and lifestyle risk factors. *Teratology* 1994:50(1):44–53.

Torgerson DJ, Avenell A, Russell IT, Reid DM. Factors associated with onset of menopause in women aged 45–9. *Maturitas* 1994;19(2):83–92.

Trapp M, Kemeter P, Feichtinger W. Smoking and in-vitro fertilization. *Human Reproduction* 1986; 1(6):357–8.

Travis WD, Travis LB, Devesa SS. Lung cancer. *Cancer* 1995;75(1 Suppl):191–202.

Trédaniel J, Boffetta P, Buiatti E, Saracci R, Hirsch A. Tobacco smoking and gastric cancer: review and meta-analysis. *International Journal of Cancer* 1997; 72(4):565–73.

Trevathan E, Layde P, Webster LA, Adams JB, Benigno BB, Ory H. Cigarette smoking and dysplasia and carcinoma in situ of the uterine cervix. *Journal of the American Medical Association* 1983;250(4): 499–502.

Trichopoulos D, Brown J, MacMahon B. Urine estrogens and breast cancer risk factors among postmenopausal women. *International Journal of Cancer* 1987;40(6):721–5.

Trichopoulos D, Kalandidi A, Sparros L. Lung cancer and passive smoking: conclusion of Greek study [letter]. *Lancet* 1983;2(8351):677–8.

Trichopoulos D, Kalandidi A, Sparros L, MacMahon B. Lung cancer and passive smoking. *International Journal of Cancer* 1981;27(1):1–4.

Trichopoulos D, MacMahon B, Sparros L, Merikas G. Smoking and hepatitis B-negative primary hepatocellular carcinoma. *Journal of the National Cancer Institute* 1980;65(1):111–4.

Trichopoulos D, Mollo F, Tomatis L, Agapitos E, Delsedime L, Zavitsanos X, Kalandidi A, Katsouyanni K, Riboli E, Saracci R. Active and passive smoking and pathological indicators of lung cancer risk in an autopsy study. *Journal of the American Medical Association* 1992;268(13):1697–701.

Troisi RJ, Heinold JW, Vokonas PS, Weiss ST. Cigarette smoking, dietary intake, and physical activity: effects on body fat distribution—the Normative Aging Study. *American Journal of Clinical Nutrition* 1991;53(5):1104–11.

Tsang NCK, Penfold PL, Snitch PJ, Billson F. Serum levels of antioxidants and age-related macular degeneration. *Documenta Ophthalmologica* 1992;81(4): 387–400.

Tsuda T, Babazono A, Yamamoto E, Kurumatani N, Mino Y, Ogawa T, Kishi Y, Aoyama H. Ingested arsenic and internal cancer: a historical cohort study followed for 33 years. *American Journal of Epidemiology* 1995;141(3):198–209.

Tsukuma H, Hiyama T, Oshima A, Sobue T, Fujimoto I, Kasugai H, Kojima J, Sasaki Y, Imaoka S, Horiuchi N, Okuda S. A case-control study of hepatocellular carcinoma in Osaka, Japan. *International Journal of Cancer* 1990;45(2):231–6.

Tulinius H, Sigfússon N, Sigvaldason H, Bjarnadóttir K, Tryggvadóttir L. Risk factors for malignant diseases: a cohort study on a population of 22,946 Icelanders. *Cancer Epidemiology, Biomarkers and Prevention* 1997;6(11):863–73.

Tunstall-Pedoe H, Brown CA, Woodward M, Tavendale R. Passive smoking by self report and serum cotinine and the prevalence of respiratory and coronary heart disease in the Scottish heart health study. *Journal of Epidemiology and Community Health* 1995;49(2):139–43.

Tuomivaara L, Ronnberg L. Ectopic pregnancy and infertility following treatment of infertile couples: a follow-up of 929 cases. *European Journal of Obstetrics, Gynecology, and Reproductive Biology* 1991;42(1):33–8.

Turner JG, Gilchrist NL, Ayling EM, Hassall AJ, Hooke EA, Sadler WA. Factors affecting bone mineral density in high school girls. *New Zealand Medical Journal* 1992;105(930):95–6.

Tuyns AJ, Estève J, Raymond L, Berrino F, Benhamou E, Blanchet F, Boffetta P, Crosignani P, del Moral A, Lehmann W, Merletti F, Péquignot G, Riboli E, Sancho-Garnier H, Terracini B, Zubiri A, Zubiri L. Cancer of the larynx/hypopharynx, tobacco and alcohol: IARC international case-control study in Turin and Varese (Italy), Zaragoza and Navarra (Spain), Geneva (Switzerland) and Calvados (France). *International Journal of Cancer* 1988;41(4): 483–91.

Tyas SL. Are tobacco and alcohol use related to Alzheimer's disease? Results from three Canadian data sets [dissertation]. London (Canada): The University of Western Ontario, 1998.

Tyler CW Jr, Webster LA, Ory HW, Rubin GL. Endometrial cancer: how does cigarette smoking influence the risk of women under age 55 years having this tumor? *American Journal of Obstetrics and Gynecology* 1985;151(7):899–905.

Tzonou A, Day NE, Trichopoulos D, Walker A, Saliaraki M, Papapostolou M, Polychronopoulou A. The epidemiology of ovarian cancer in Greece: a case-control study. *European Journal of Cancer and Clinical Oncology* 1984;20(8):1045–52.

Tzonou A, Hsieh CC, Trichopoulos D, Aravandinos D, Kalandidi A, Margaris D, Goldman M, Toupadaki N. Induced abortions, miscarriages, and tobacco smoking as risk factors for secondary infertility. *Journal of Epidemiology and Community Health* 1993;47(1):36–9.

Uhlig T, Hagen KB, Kvien TK. Current tobacco smoking, formal education, and the risk of rheumatoid arthritis. *Journal of Rheumatology* 1999;26(1):47–54.

Underwood P, Hester LL, Laffitte T Jr, Gregg KV. The relationship of smoking to the outcome of pregnancy. *American Journal of Obstetrics and Gynecology* 1965;91(2):270–6.

Underwood PB, Kesler KF, O'Lane JM, Callagan DA. Parental smoking empirically related to pregnancy outcome. *Obstetrics and Gynecology* 1967;29(1):1–8.

Ungváry G, Tátrai E. On the embryotoxic effects of benzene and its alkyl derivatives in mice, rats and rabbits. *Archives of Toxicology Supplement* 1985;8: 425–30.

U.S. Department of Health, Education, and Welfare. *Smoking and Health. Report of the Advisory Committee to the Surgeon General of the Public Health Service.* U.S. Department of Health, Education, and Welfare, Public Health Service, Communicable Disease Center, 1964. DHEW Publication No. 1103.

U.S. Department of Health, Education, and Welfare. *The Health Consequences of Smoking. A Report of the Surgeon General: 1971.* U.S. Department of Health, Education, and Welfare, Public Health Services and Mental Health Administration, 1971. DHEW Publication No. (HSM) 71-7513.

U.S. Department of Health, Education, and Welfare. *The Smoking Digest: Progress Report on a Nation Kicking the Habit.* Bethesda (MD): U.S. Department of Health, Education, and Welfare, Public Health Service, National Institutes of Health, Office of Cancer Communications, National Cancer Institute, 1977.

U.S. Department of Health, Education, and Welfare. *Smoking and Health. A Report of the Surgeon General.* Washington: U.S. Department of Health, Education, and Welfare, Public Health Service, Office of the Assistant Secretary for Health, Office on Smoking and Health, 1979. DHEW Publication No. (PHS) 79-50066.

U.S. Department of Health and Human Services. The *Health Consequences of Smoking for Women. A Report of the Surgeon General.* Washington: U.S. Department of Health and Human Services, Public Health Service, Office of the Assistant Secretary for Health, Office on Smoking and Health, 1980.

U.S. Department of Health and Human Services. *The Health Consequences of Smoking: Cancer. A Report of the Surgeon General.* Rockville (MD): U.S. Department of Health and Human Services, Public Health Service, Office on Smoking and Health, 1982. DHHS Publication No. (PHS) 82-50179.

U.S. Department of Health and Human Services. *The Health Consequences of Smoking: Cardiovascular Disease. A Report of the Surgeon General.* Rockville (MD): U.S. Department of Health and Human Services, Public Health Service, Office on Smoking and Health, 1983. DHHS Publication No. (PHS) 84-50204.

U.S. Department of Health and Human Services. *The Health Consequences of Smoking: Chronic Obstructive Lung Disease. A Report of the Surgeon General.* U.S. Department of Health and Human Services, Public Health Service, Office on Smoking and Health, 1984. DHHS Publication No. (PHS) 84-50205.

U.S. Department of Health and Human Services. *The Health Consequences of Using Smokeless Tobacco. A Report of the Advisory Committee to the Surgeon General.* Bethesda (MD): U.S. Department of Health and Human Services, Public Health Service, National Institutes of Health, 1986a. NIH Publication No. 86-2874.

U.S. Department of Health and Human Services. *The Health Consequences of Involuntary Smoking. A Report of the Surgeon General.* U.S. Department of Health and Human Services, Public Health Service, Centers for Disease Control, Center for Health Promotion and Education, Office on Smoking and Health, 1986b. DHHS Publication No. (CDC) 87-8398.

U.S. Department of Health and Human Services. *The Health Consequences of Smoking: Nicotine Addiction. A Report of the Surgeon General.* Atlanta: U.S Department of Health and Human Services, Public Health Service, Centers for Disease Control, Center for Health Promotion and Education, Office on Smoking and Health, 1988. DHHS Publication No. (CDC) 88-8406.

U.S. Department of Health and Human Services. *The International Classification of Diseases, 9th Revision, Clinical Modification. Vol. 1. Diseases: Tabular List.* 3rd ed. Rockville (MD): U.S. Department of Health and Human Services, Public Health Service, Health Care Financing Administration, 1989a. DHHS Publication No. 89-1260.

U.S. Department of Health and Human Services. *Reducing the Health Consequences of Smoking: 25 Years of Progress. A Report of the Surgeon General.* Rockville (MD): U.S. Department of Health and Human Services, Public Health Service, Centers for Disease Control, Center for Chronic Disease Prevention and Health Promotion, Office on Smoking and Health, 1989b. DHHS Publication No. (CDC) 89-8411.

U.S. Department of Health and Human Services. *The Health Benefits of Smoking Cessation. A Report of the Surgeon General.* Atlanta: U.S. Department of Health and Human Services, Public Health Service, Centers for Disease Control, Center for Chronic Disease Prevention and Health Promotion, Office on Smoking and Health, 1990. DHHS Publication No. (CDC) 90-8416.

U.S. Department of Health and Human Services. *Preventing Tobacco Use Among Young People: A Report of the Surgeon General.* Atlanta: U.S. Department of Health and Human Services, Public Health Service, Centers for Disease Control and Prevention, National Center for Chronic Disease Prevention and Health Promotion, Office on Smoking and Health, 1994.

U.S. Department of Health and Human Services. An Analysis Regarding the Food and Drug Administration's Jurisdiction Over Nicotine-Containing Cigarettes and Smokeless Tobacco Products, *60 Fed. Reg.* 41453 (1995).

U.S. Department of Health and Human Services. *SAMMEC 3.0. Smoking Attributable Mortality, Morbidity, and Economic Costs: Computer Software and Documentation.* U.S. Department of Health and Human Services, Public Health Service, Centers for Disease Control and Prevention, National Center for Chronic Disease Prevention and Health Promotion, Office on Smoking and Health, 1997.

U.S. Department of Health and Human Services. *Tobacco Use Among U.S. Racial/Ethnic Minority Groups—African Americans, American Indians and Alaska Natives, Asian Americans and Pacific Islanders, and Hispanics. A Report of the Surgeon General.* Atlanta: U.S. Department of Health and Human Services, Centers for Disease Control and Prevention, National Center for Chronic Disease Prevention and Health Promotion, Office on Smoking and Health, 1998.

U.S. Department of Health and Human Services. *9th Report on Carcinogens.* Research Triangle Park (NC): U.S. Department of Health and Human Services, Public Health Service, National Toxicology Program, 2000.

Välimäki MJ, Kärkkäinen M, Lamberg-Allardt C, Laitinen K, Alhava E, Heikkinen J, Impivaara O,

Mäkelä P, Palmgren J, Seppänen R, Vuori I. Exercise, smoking, and calcium intake during adolescence and early adulthood as determinants of peak bone mass. *British Medical Journal* 1994; 309(6949):228–35.

van den Brandt PA, Goldbohm A, van 't Veer P, Bode P, Dorant E, Hermus RJJ, Sturmans F. A prospective cohort study of selenium status and the risk of lung cancer. *Cancer Research* 1993;53(20):4860–5.

Van den Eeden SK, Karagas MR, Daling JR, Vaughan TL. A case-control study of maternal smoking and congenital malformations. *Paediatric and Perinatal Epidemiology* 1990;4(2):147–55.

Van Deventer GM, Elashoff JD, Reedy TJ, Schneidman D, Walsh JH. A randomized study of maintenance therapy with ranitidine to prevent the recurrence of duodenal ulcer. *New England Journal of Medicine* 1989;320(17):1113–9.

van Duijn CM, Havekes LM, Van Broeckhoven C, de Knijff P, Hofman A. Apolipoprotein E genotype and association between smoking and early onset Alzheimer's disease. *British Medical Journal* 1995; 310(6980):627–31.

van Duijn CM, Hofman A. Risk factors for Alzheimer's disease: the EURODEM collaborative reanalysis of case-control studies. *Neuroepidemiology* 1992;11(Suppl 1):106–13.

Van Voorhis BJ, Dawson JD, Stovall DW, Sparks AE, Syrop CH. The effects of smoking on ovarian function and fertility during assisted reproduction cycles. *Obstetrics and Gynecology* 1996;88(5):785–91.

Van Voorhis BJ, Syrop CH, Hammitt DG, Dunn MS, Snyder GD. Effects of smoking on ovulation induction for assisted reproductive techniques. *Fertility and Sterility* 1992;58(5):981–5.

Vatten LJ, Kvinnsland S. Cigarette smoking and risk of breast cancer: a prospective study of 24,329 Norwegian women. *European Journal of Cancer* 1990; 26(7):830–3.

Vaughan TL, Davis S, Kristal A, Thomas DB. Obesity, alcohol, and tobacco as risk factors for cancers of the esophagus and gastric cardia: adenocarcinoma versus squamous cell carcinoma. *Cancer Epidemiology, Biomarkers and Prevention* 1995;4(2):85–92.

Velema JP, Walker AM, Gold EB. Alcohol and pancreatic cancer: insufficient epidemiologic evidence for a causal relationship. *Epidemiologic Review* 1986; 8:28–41.

Ventura SJ, Martin JA, Curtin SC, Mathews TJ. Report of final natality statistics, 1995. *Monthly Vital Statistics Report* 1997;45(11 Suppl):1–57.

Verreault R, Chu J, Mandelson M, Shy K. A case-control study of diet and invasive cervical cancer. *International Journal of Cancer* 1989;43(6):1050–4.

Vessey M, Jewell D, Smith A, Yeates D, McPherson K. Chronic inflammatory bowel disease, cigarette smoking, and use of oral contraceptives: findings in a large cohort study of women of childbearing age. *British Medical Journal* 1986;292(6528):1101–3.

Vessey M, Painter R. Oral contraceptive use and benign gallbladder disease; revisited. *Contraception* 1994;50(2):167–73.

Vessey MP, Villard-Mackintosh L, Painter R. Oral contraceptives and pregnancy in relation to peptic ulcer. *Contraception* 1992;46(4):349–57.

Vessey MP, Villard-Mackintosh L, Yeates D. Oral contraceptives, cigarette smoking and other factors in relation to arthritis. *Contraception* 1987;35(5):457–64.

Vestbo J, Prescott E, Lange P. Association of chronic mucus hypersecretion with $FEV_1$ decline and chronic obstructive pulmonary disease morbidity. *American Journal of Respiratory Critical Care Medicine* 1996;153(5):1530–5.

Victora CG, Smith PG, Vaughan JP, Nobre LC, Lombardi C, Teixeira AM, Fuchs SM, Moreira LB, Gigante LP, Barros FC. Evidence for protection by breast-feeding against infant deaths from infectious diseases in Brazil. *Lancet* 1987;2(8554):319–22.

Villar MTA, Dow L, Coggon D, Lampe FC, Holgate ST. The influence of increased bronchial responsiveness, atopy, and serum IgE on decline in $FEV_1$: a longitudinal study in the elderly. *American Journal of Respiratory and Critical Care Medicine* 1995; 151(3):656–62.

Vinding T, Appleyard M, Nyboe J, Jensen G. Risk factor analysis for atrophic and exudative age-related macular degeneration: an epidemiological study of 1000 aged individuals. *Acta Ophthalmologica* 1992;70(1):66–72.

Vingard E, Alfredsson L, Malchau H. Lifestyle factors and hip arthrosis. A case referent study of body mass index, smoking and hormone therapy in 503 Swedish women. *Acta Orthopaedica Scandinavica* 1997;68(3):216–20.

Vintzileos AM, Campbell WA, Nochimson DJ, Weinbaum PJ. Preterm premature rupture of the membranes: a risk factor for the development of abruptio placentae. *American Journal of Obstetrics and Gynecology* 1987;56(5):1235–8.

Vio F, Salazar G, Infante C. Smoking during pregnancy and lactation and its effects on breast-milk volume. *American Journal of Clinical Nutrition* 1991; 54(6):1011–6.

Virtanen SM, Jaakkola L, Rasanen L, Ylonen K, Aro A, Lounamaa R, Akerblom HK, Tuomilehto J. Nitrate and nitrite intake and the risk for type 1 diabetes in Finnish children. Childhood Diabetes in Finland Study Group. *Diabetic Medicine* 1994;11(7):656–62.

Voigt LF, Hollenbach KA, Krohn MA, Daling JR, Hickok DE. The relationship of abruptio placentae with maternal smoking and small for gestational age infants. *Obstetrics and Gynecology* 1990;75(5):771–4.

Voigt LF, Koepsell TD, Nelson JL, Dugowson CE, Daling JR. Smoking, obesity, alcohol consumption, and the risk of rheumatoid arthritis. *Epidemiology* 1994;5(5):525–32.

Vollenhoven BJ, Lawrence AS, Healy DL. Uterine fibroids: a clinical review. *British Journal of Obstetrics and Gynaecology* 1990;97(4):285–98.

Wadsworth EJ, Shield JP, Hunt LP, Baum JD. A case-control study of environmental factors associated with diabetes in the under 5s. *Diabetic Medicine* 1997;14(5):390–6.

Wagenknecht LE, Cutter GR, Haley NJ, Sidney S, Manolio TA, Hughes GH, Jacobs DR. Racial differences in serum cotinine levels among smokers in the Coronary Artery Risk Development in (Young) Adults Study. *American Journal of Public Health* 1990;80(9):1053–6.

Walsh RA. Effects of maternal smoking on adverse pregnancy outcomes: examination of the criteria of causation. *Human Biology* 1994;66(6)1059–92.

Wang F-L, Love EJ, Liu N, Dai X-D. Childhood and adolescent passive smoking and the risk of female lung cancer. *International Journal of Epidemiology* 1994a;23(2):223–30.

Wang H-X, Fratiglioni L, Fisoni GB, Viitanen M, Winblad B. Smoking and the occurrence of Alzheimer's disease: cross-sectional and longitudinal data in a population-based study. *American Journal of Epidemiology* 1999;149(7):640–4.

Wang P-N, Wang S-J, Hong C-J, Liu T-T, Fuh J-L, Chi C-W, Lui C-Y, Liu H-C. Risk factors for Alzheimer's disease: a case-control study. *Neuroepidemiology* 1997a;16:234–40.

Wang X, Tager IB, Van Vunakis H, Speizer FE, Hanrahan JP. Maternal smoking during pregnancy, urine cotinine concentrations, and birth outcomes. A prospective cohort study. *International Journal of Epidemiology* 1997b;26(5):978–88.

Wang X, Wypij D, Gold DR, Speizer FE, Ware JH, Ferris BG Jr, Dockery DW. A longitudinal study of the effects of parental smoking on pulmonary function in children 6–18 years. *American Journal of Respiratory and Critical Care Medicine* 1994b;149(6):1420–5.

Wannamethee SG, Shaper AG, Whincup PH, Walker M. Smoking cessation and the risk of stroke in middle-aged men. *Journal of the American Medical Association* 1995;274(2):155–60.

Ward JA, Lord SR, Williams P, Anstey K, Zivanovic E. Physiologic, health and lifestyle factors associated with femoral neck bone density in older women. *Bone* 1995;16(4 Suppl):373S–378S.

Ward KD, Sparrow D, Vokonas PS, Willett WC, Landsberg L, Weiss ST. The relationships of abdominal obesity, hyperinsulinemia and saturated fat intake to serum lipid levels: the Normative Aging Study. *International Journal of Obesity* 1994;18(3):137–44.

Wardell RE, Seegmiller RE, Bradshaw WS. Induction of prenatal toxicity in the rat by diethylstilbestrol, zeranol, 3,4,3',4'-tetrachlorobiphenyl, cadmium, and lead. *Teratology* 1982;26(3):229–37.

Wartenberg D, Calle EE, Thun MJ, Heath CW Jr, Lally C, Woodruff T. Passive smoking exposure and female breast cancer mortality. *Journal of the National Cancer Institute* 2000;92(20)1666–73.

Wasserman CR, Shaw GM, O'Malley CD, Tolarova MM, Lammer EJ. Parental cigarette smoking and risk for congenital anomalies of the heart, neural tube, or limb. *Teratology* 1996;53(4):261–7.

Watson PE, Watson ID, Batt RD. Total body water volumes for adult males and females estimated from simple anthropometric measurements. *American Journal of Clinical Nutrition* 1980;33(1):27–39.

Weinberg CR, Wilcox AJ, Baird DD. Reduced fecundability in women with prenatal exposure to cigarette smoking. *American Journal of Epidemiology* 1989;129(5):1072–8.

Weir HK, Sloan M, Kreiger N. The relationship between cigarette smoking and the risk of endometrial neoplasms. *International Journal of Epidemiology* 1994;23(2):261–6.

Weiss NS, Farewell VT, Szekely DR, English DR, Kiviat N. Oestrogens and endometrial cancer: effect of other risk factors on the association. *Maturitas* 1980;2(3):185–90.

Weiss SR, Ebert MH. Psychological and behavioral characteristics of normal-weight bulimics and normal-weight controls. *Psychosomatic Medicine* 1983;45(4):293–303.

Weissman MM, Bruce ML, Leaf PJ, Florio LP, Holzer C III. Affective disorders. In: Robins LN, Regier DA, editors. *Psychiatric Disorders in America: the Epidemiologic Catchment Area Study*. New York: Free Press, 1991:53–80.

Weissman MM, Myers JK. Clinical depression in alcoholism. *American Journal of Psychiatry* 1980;137(3):372–3.

Welch SL, Fairburn CG. Smoking and bulimia nervosa. *International Journal of Eating Disorders* 1998;23(4):433–7.

Wells AJ. An estimate of adult mortality in the United States from passive smoking. *Environment International* 1988;14:249–65.

Wells AJ. Deadly smoke. *Occupational Health and Safety* 1989;58(10):20–2,44,69.

Wells AJ. Breast cancer, cigarette smoking, and passive smoking [letter]. *American Journal of Epidemiology* 1991;133(2):208–10.

Wells AJ. Passive smoking as a cause of heart disease. *Journal of the American College of Cardiology* 1994;24(2):546–54.

Wells AJ. Heart disease from passive smoking in the workplace. *Journal of the American College of Cardiology* 1998;31(1):1–9.

Wen SW, Goldenberg RL, Cutter GR, Hoffman HJ, Cliver SP. Intrauterine growth retardation and preterm delivery: prenatal risk factors in an indigent population. *American Journal of Obstetrics and Gynecology* 1990a;162(1):213–8.

Wen SW, Goldenberg RL, Cutter GR, Hoffman HJ, Cliver SP, Davis RO, Du Bard MB. Smoking, maternal age, fetal growth, and gestational age at delivery. *American Journal of Obstetrics and Gynecology* 1990b;162(1):53–8.

Werler MM. Teratogen update: smoking and reproductive outcomes. *Teratology* 1997;55(5):382–8.

Werler MM, Lammer EJ, Rosenberg L, Mitchell AA. Maternal cigarette smoking during pregnancy in relation to oral clefts. *American Journal of Epidemiology* 1990;132(5):926–32.

Werler MM, Louik C, Shapiro S, Mitchell AA. Prepregnant weight in relation to risk of neural tube defects. *Journal of the American Medical Association* 1996;275(14):1089–92.

Werler MM, Mitchell AA, Shapiro S. Demographic, reproductive, medical, and environmental factors in relation to gastroschisis. *Teratology* 1992;45(4):353–60.

West RJ. Psychology and pharmacology in cigarette withdrawal. *Journal of Psychosomatic Research* 1984;28(5):379–86.

West S, Munoz B, Emmett EA, Taylor HR. Cigarette smoking and risk of nuclear cataracts. *Archives of Ophthalmology* 1989;107(8):1166–9.

Westhoff C, Gentile G, Lee J, Zacur H, Helbig D. Predictors of ovarian steroid secretion in reproductive-age women. *American Journal of Epidemiology* 1996:144(4):381–8.

Westman EC, Behm FM, Rose JE. Airway sensory replacement combined with nicotine replacement for smoking cessation: a randomized, placebo-controlled trial using a citric acid inhaler. *Chest* 1995;107(5):1358–64.

Whisnant JP, Homer D, Ingall TJ, Baker HL Jr, O'Fallon WM, Wiebers DO. Duration of cigarette smoking is the strongest predictor of severe extracranial carotid artery atherosclerosis. *Stroke* 1990;21(5): 707–14.

Whittemore AS, Harris R, Itnyre J. Characteristics relating to ovarian cancer risk: collaborative analysis of 12 US case-control studies. IV. The pathogenesis of epithelial ovarian cancer. *American Journal of Epidemiology* 1992;136(10):1212–20.

WHO Collaborative Study of Cardiovascular Disease and Steroid Hormone Contraception. Ischaemic stroke and combined oral contraceptives: results of an international, multicentre, case-control study. *Lancet* 1996a;348(9026):498–505.

WHO Collaborative Study of Cardiovascular Disease and Steroid Hormone Contraception. Haemorrhagic stroke, overall stroke risk, and combined oral contraceptives: results of an international, multicentre, case-control study. *Lancet* 1996b;348(9026):505–10.

WHO Collaborative Study of Cardiovascular Disease and Steroid Hormone Contraception. Acute myocardial infarction and combined oral contraceptives: results of an international multi-centre case-control study. *Lancet* 1997;349(9060):1202–9.

Wiederman MW, Pryor T. Substance use and impulsive behaviors among adolescents with eating disorders. *Addictive Behaviors* 1996;21(2):269–72.

Wikler A. Conditioning factors in opiate addiction and relapse. In: Wilner DM, Kassebaum GG, editors. *Narcotics*. New York: McGraw-Hill, 1965:85–100.

Wilcox AJ. Birth weight and perinatal mortality: the effect of maternal smoking. *American Journal of Epidemiology* 1993;137(10):1098–104.

Wilcox AJ. Re: Are female smokers at higher risk for lung cancer than male smokers? A case-control analysis by histologic type [letter]. *American Journal of Epidemiology* 1994;140(2):186.

Wilcox AJ, Baird DD, Weinberg CR. Do women with childhood exposure to cigarette smoking have increased fecundability? *American Journal of Epidemiology* 1989;129(5):1079–83.

Wilcox AJ, Weinberg CR, Baird DD. Risk factors for early pregnancy loss. *Epidemiology* 1990;1(5):382–5.

Wilcox AJ, Weinberg CR, O'Connor JF, Baird DD, Schlatterer JP, Canfield RE, Armstrong EG, Nisula BC. Incidence of early loss of pregnancy. *New England Journal of Medicine* 1988;319(4):189–94.

Wilkins JN, Carlson HE, Van Vunakis H, Hill MA, Gritz E, Jarvik ME. Nicotine from cigarette smoking increases circulating levels of cortisol, growth hormone, and prolactin in male chronic smokers. *Psychopharmacology* 1982;78(4):305–8.

Willard JC, Schoenborn CA. Relationship between cigarette smoking and other unhealthy behaviors among our nation's youth: United States, 1992. *Advance Data* 1995;(263):1–11.

Willett WC. Vitamin A and lung cancer. *Nutrition Reviews* 1990;48(5):201–11.

Willett W, Stampfer MJ, Bain C, Lipnick R, Speizer FE, Rosner B, Cramer D, Hennekens CH. Cigarette smoking, relative weight, and menopause. *American Journal of Epidemiology* 1983;117(6):651–8.

Willett WC, Green A, Stampfer MJ, Speizer FE, Colditz GA, Rosner B, Monson RR, Stason W, Hennekens CH. Relative and absolute excess risks of coronary heart disease among women who smoke cigarettes. *New England Journal of Medicine* 1987;317(21):1303–9.

Williams AR, Weiss NS, Ure CL, Ballard J, Daling JR. Effect of weight, smoking, and estrogen use on the risk of hip and forearm fractures in postmenopausal women. *Obstetrics and Gynecology* 1982; 60(6):695–9.

Williams MA, Lieberman E, Mittendorf R, Monson RR, Schoenbaum SC. Risk factors for abruptio placentae. *American Journal of Epidemiology* 1991a; 134(9):965–72.

Williams MA, Mittendorf R, Lieberman E, Monson RR, Schoenbaum SC, Genest DR. Cigarette smoking during pregnancy in relation to placenta previa. *American Journal of Obstetrics and Gynecology* 1991b;165(1):28–32.

Williams MA, Mittendorf R, Monson RR. Chronic hypertension, cigarette smoking, and abruptio placentae. *Epidemiology* 1991c;2(6):450–3.

Williams MA, Mittendorf R, Stubblefield PG, Lieberman E, Schoenbaum SC, Monson RR. Cigarettes, coffee, and preterm premature rupture of the membranes. *American Journal of Epidemiology* 1992; 135(8):895–903.

Williams RR, Horm JW. Association of cancer sites with tobacco and alcohol consumption and socioeconomic status of patients: interview from the Third National Cancer Survey. *Journal of the National Cancer Institute* 1977;58(3):525–47.

Williamson DF, Madans J, Anda RF, Kleinman JC, Giovino GA, Byers T. Smoking cessation and severity of weight gain in a national cohort. *New England Journal of Medicine* 1991;324(11):739–45.

Willinger M, Hoffman HJ, Hartford RB. Infant sleep position and the risk for sudden infant death syndrome: report of meeting held January 13 and 14, 1994, National Institutes of Health, Bethesda, MD. *Pediatrics* 1994;93(5):814–9.

Willinger M, James LS, Catz C. Defining the sudden infant death syndrome (SIDS): deliberations of an expert panel convened by the National Institute of Child Health and Human Development. *Pediatric Pathology* 1991;11(5):677–84.

Willmott FE. Current smoking habits and genital infections in women. *International Journal of STD and AIDS* 1992;3(5):329–31.

Wilson PW, Heog JM, D'Agostino RB, Silbershatz H, Belanger AM, Poehlmann H, O'Leary D, Wolf PA. Cumulative effects of high cholesterol levels, high blood pressure and cigarette smoking on carotid stenosis. *New England Journal of Medicine* 1997; 337(8):516–22.

Wilson PWF, Anderson KM, Kannel WB. Epidemiology of diabetes mellitus in the elderly: the Framingham Study. *American Journal of Medicine* 1986; 80(Suppl 5A):3–9.

Wilson PWF, Garrison RJ, Castelli WP. Postmenopausal estrogen use, cigarette smoking, and cardiovascular morbidity in women over 50: the Framingham Study. *New England Journal of Medicine* 1985; 313(17):1038–43.

Windham GC, Eaton A, Hopkins B. Evidence for an association between environmental tobacco smoke exposure and birthweight: a meta-analysis and new data. *Paediatric and Perinatal Epidemiology* 1999a;13(1):35–57.

Windham GC, Elkin EP, Swan SH, Waller KO, Fenster L. Cigarette smoking and effects on menstrual function. *Obstetrics and Gynecology* 1999b;93(1): 59–65.

Windham GC, Swan SH, Fenster L. Parental cigarette smoking and the risk of spontaneous abortion. *American Journal of Epidemiology* 1992;135(12): 1394–403.

Windham GC, Von Behren J, Walker K, Fenster L. Exposure to environmental and mainstream tobacco smoke and risk of spontaneous abortion. *American Journal of Epidemiology* 1999c;149(3): 243–7.

Wing RR, Matthews KA, Kuller LH, Meilahn EN, Plantinga P. Waist to hip ratio in middle-aged women: associations with behavioral and psychosocial factors and with changes in cardiovascular risk factors. *Arteriosclerosis and Thrombosis* 1991; 11(5):1250–7.

Wingo PA, Ries LAG, Giovino GA, Miller DS, Rosenberg HM, Shopland DR, Thun MJ, Edwards BK. Annual report to the nation on the status of cancer, 1973–1996, with a special section on lung cancer and tobacco smoking. *Journal of the National Cancer Institute* 1999;91(8):675–90.

Winkelstein W Jr. Smoking and cancer of the uterine cervix: hypothesis. *American Journal of Epidemiology* 1977;106(4):257–9.

Winn DM, Blot WJ, Shy CM, Fraumeni JF Jr. Snuff dipping and oral cancer in the Southern United States. *New England Journal of Medicine* 1981; 304(13):745–9.

Winsa B, Mandahl A, Karlsson FA. Graves' disease, endocrine ophthalmopathy and smoking. *Acta Endocrinologica* 1993;128(2):156–60.

Wisborg K, Henriksen TB, Hedegaard M, Secher NJ. Smoking during pregnancy and preterm birth. *British Journal of Obstetrics and Gynaecology* 1996; 103(8):800–5.

Witteman JC, Grobbee DE, Valkenburg HA, van Hemert AM, Stijnen T, Hofman A. Cigarette smoking and the development and progression of aortic atherosclerosis: a 9-year population-based follow-up study in women. *Circulation* 1993;88(5 Pt 1):2156–62.

Wolf PA, D'Agostino RB, Kannel WB, Bonita R, Belanger AJ. Cigarette smoking as a risk factor for stroke: the Framingham Study. *Journal of the American Medical Association* 1988;259(7):1025–9.

Wolf PA, Feldman RG, Saint-Hilaire M, Kelly-Hayes M, Torres FJ, Mosback P, Kase CS. Precursors and natural history of Parkinson's disease: the Framingham Study. *Neurology* 1991;41(Suppl 1):371.

Wolff CB, Portis M, Wolff H. Birth weight and smoking practices during pregnancy among Mexican-American women. *Health Care for Women International* 1993;14(3):271–9.

Wong PP, Bauman A. How well does epidemiological evidence hold for the relationship between smoking and adverse obstetric outcomes in New South Wales? *Australian and New Zealand Journal of Obstetrics and Gynaecology* 1997;37(2):168–73.

Wood C. The association of psycho-social factors and gynaecological symptoms. *Australian Family Physician* 1978;7(4):471–8.

Wood C, Larsen L, Williams R. Social and psychological factors in relation to premenstrual tension and menstrual pain. *Australian and New Zealand Journal of Obstetrics and Gynaecology* 1979;19(2):111–5.

Woodward A. Smoking and reduced duration of breast-feeding. *Medical Journal of Australia* 1988; 148(9):477–8.

Woodward M, Tunstall-Pedoe H. Self-titration of nicotine: evidence from the Scottish Heart Health Study. *Addiction* 1993;88(6):821–30.

Wright JL. Small airways disease: its role in chronic airflow obstruction. *Seminars in Respiratory Medicine* 1992;13(2):72–84.

Writing Group for the PEPI Trial. Effects of hormone therapy on bone mineral density: results from the Postmenopausal Estrogen/Progestin Interventions (PEPI) Trial. *Journal of the American Medical Association* 1996;276(17):1389–96.

Wu AH, Henderson BE, Pike MC, Yu MC. Smoking and other risk factors for lung cancer in women. *Journal of the National Cancer Institute* 1985;74(4): 747–51.

Wu AH, Henderson BE, Thomas DC, Mack TM. Secular trends in histologic types of lung cancer. *Journal of the National Cancer Institute* 1986;77(1):53–6.

Wu AH, Yu MC, Thomas DC, Pike MC, Henderson BE. Personal and family history of lung disease as risk factors for adenocarcinoma of the lung. *Cancer Research* 1988;48(24):7279–84.

Wu L-T, Anthony JC. Tobacco smoking and depressed mood in late childhood and early adolescence. *American Journal of Public Health* 1999;89(12):1837–40.

Wu T, Buck G, Mendola P. Maternal cigarette smoking, regular use of multivitamin/mineral supplements, and risk of fetal death: the 1988 National Maternal and Infant Health Survey. *American Journal of Epidemiology* 1998;148(2):215–21.

Wu Y, Zheng W, Sellers TA, Kushi LH, Bostick RM, Potter JD. Dietary cholesterol, fat, and lung cancer incidence among older women: the Iowa Women's Health Study (United States). *Cancer Causes and Control* 1994;5(5):395–400.

Wu-Williams AH, Dai XD, Blot W, Xu ZY, Sun XW, Xiao HP, Stone BJ, Yu SF, Feng YP, Ershow AG, Sun J, Fraumeni JF Jr, Henderson BE. Lung cancer among women in north-east China. *British Journal of Cancer* 1990;62(6):982–7.

Wu-Williams AH, Samet JM. Environmental tobacco smoke: exposure-response relationships in epidemiologic studies. *Risk Analysis* 1990;10(1):39–48.

Wynder EL, Augustine A, Kabat GC, Hebert JR. Effect of the type of cigarette smoked on bladder cancer risk. *Cancer* 1988;61(3):622–7.

Wynder EL, Dieck GS, Hall NEL. Case-control study of decaffeinated coffee consumption and pancreatic cancer. *Cancer Research* 1986;46(10):5360–3.

Wynder EL, Hoffman D. Smoking and lung cancer: scientific challenges and opportunities. *Cancer Research* 1994;54(20):5284–95.

Wynder EL, Kabat GC. The effect of low-yield cigarette smoking on lung cancer risk. *Cancer* 1988; 62(6):1223–30.

Wynder EL, Stellman SD. Comparative epidemiology of tobacco-related cancers. *Cancer Research* 1977; 37(12):4608–22.

Wyshak G, Frisch RE, Albright NL, Albright TE, Schiff I. Lower prevalence of benign diseases of the breast and benign tumours of the reproductive system among former college athletes compared to non-athletes. *British Journal of Cancer* 1986;54(5): 841–5.

Wyshak G, Frisch RE, Albright TE, Albright NL, Schiff I. Smoking and cysts of the ovary. *International Journal of Fertility* 1988;33(6):398–404.

Wyszynski DF, Duffy DL, Beaty TH. Maternal cigarette smoking and oral clefts: a meta-analysis. *Cleft Palate-Craniofacial Journal* 1997;34(3):206–10.

Xu X, Dockery DW, Ware JH, Speizer FE, Ferris BG Jr. Effects of cigarette smoking on rate of loss of pulmonary function in adults: a longitudinal assessment. *American Review of Respiratory Disease* 1992; 146(5 Pt 1):1345–8.

Xu X, Laird N, Dockery DW, Schouten JP, Rijcken B, Weiss ST. Age, period, and cohort effects on pulmonary function in a 24-year longitudinal study. *American Journal of Epidemiology* 1995;141(6):554–66.

Xu X, Weiss ST, Rijcken B, Schouten JP. Smoking, changes in smoking habits, and rate of decline in $FEV_1$: new insight into gender differences. *European Respiratory Journal* 1994;7(6):1056–61.

Xu Z-Y, Blot WJ, Xiao H-P, Wu A, Feng Y-P, Stone BJ, Sun J, Ershow AG, Henderson BE, Fraumeni JF Jr. Smoking, air pollution, and the high rates of lung cancer in Shenyang, China. *Journal of the National Cancer Institute* 1989;81(23):1800–6.

Yahr MD. The Parkinsonian syndrome (paralysis agitans, shaking palsy). In: Conn RB, editor. *Current Diagnosis* 7. Philadelphia: W.B. Saunders, 1985: 179–82.

Yamamoto K, Nakamura T, Kishimoto H, Hagino H, Nose T. Risk factors for hip fracture in elderly Japanese women in Tottori Prefecture, Japan. *Osteoporosis International* 1993;3(Suppl 1):S48–S50.

Yang CP, Gallagher RP, Weiss NS, Band PR, Thomas DB, Russell DA. Differences in incidence rates of cancers of the respiratory tract by anatomic subsite and histologic type: an etiologic implication. *Journal of the National Cancer Institute* 1989;81(23): 1828–31.

Yeh J, Barbieri RL. Twenty-four-hour urinary-free cortisol in premenopausal cigarette smokers and nonsmokers. *Fertility and Sterility* 1989;52(6):1067–9.

Yen S, Hsieh C-C, MacMahon B. Extrahepatic bile duct cancer and smoking, beverage consumption, past medical history, and oral-contraceptive use. *Cancer* 1987;59(12):2112–6.

Yeung DL, Pennell MD, Leung M, Hall J. Breastfeeding: prevalence and influencing factors. *Canadian Journal of Public Health* 1981;72(5):323–30.

Ylitalo N, Sørensen P, Josefsson A, Frisch M, Sparén P, Pontén J, Gyllensten U, Melbye M, Adami H-O. Smoking and oral contraceptives as risk factors for cervical carcinoma in situ. *International Journal of Cancer* 1999;81(3):357–65.

Yoo K-Y, Tajima K, Miura S, Takeuchi T, Hirose K, Risch H, Dubrow R. Breast cancer risk factors according to combined estrogen and progesterone receptor status: a case-control analysis. *American Journal of Epidemiology* 1997;146(4):307–14.

Yoshitake T, Kiyohara Y, Kato I, Ohmura T, Iwamoto H, Nakayama K, Ohmori S, Nomiyama K, Kawano H, Ueda K, Sueishi K, Tsuneyoshi M, Fujishima M. Incidence and risk factors of vascular dementia and Alzheimer's disease in a defined elderly Japanese population: the Hisayama study. *Neurology* 1995;45(6):1161–8.

Young D, Hopper JL, Nowson CA, Green RM, Sherwin AJ, Kaymakci B, Smid M, Guest CS, Larkins RG, Wark JD. Determinants of bone mass in 10- to 26-year-old females: a twin study. *Journal of Bone and Mineral Research* 1995;10(4):558–67.

Young S, Le Souëf PN, Geelhoed GC, Stick SM, Turner KJ, Landau LI. The influence of a family history of asthma and parental smoking on airway responsiveness in early infancy. *New England Journal of Medicine* 1991;324(17):1168–73.

Yu GP, Ostroff JS, Zhang ZF, Tang J, Schantz SP. Smoking history and cancer patient survival: a hospital cancer registry study. *Cancer Detection and Prevention* 1997;21(6):497–509.

Yu H, Harris RE, Kabat GC, Wynder EL. Cigarette smoking, alcohol consumption and primary liver cancer: a case-control study in the USA. *International Journal of Cancer* 1988;42(3):325–8.

Yu H, Rohan TE, Cook MG, Howe GR, Miller AB. Risk factors for fibroadenoma: a case-control study in Australia. *American Journal of Epidemiology* 1992;135(3):247–58.

Yu MC, Tong MJ, Govindarajan S, Henderson BE. Nonviral risk factors for hepatocellular carcinoma in a low-risk population, the non-Asians of Los Angeles County, California. *Journal of the National Cancer Institute* 1991;83(24):1820–6.

Yuan JM, Castelao JE, Gago-Dominguez M, Yu MC, Ross RK. Tobacco use in relation to renal cell carcinoma. *Cancer Epidemiology, Biomarkers and Prevention* 1998;7(5):429–33.

Yuan P, Okazaki I, Kuroki Y. Anal atresia: effect of smoking and drinking habits during pregnancy. *Japanese Journal of Human Genetics* 1995;40(4):327–32.

Zahm SH, Weisenburger DD, Holmes FF, Cantor KP, Blair A. Tobacco and non-Hodgkin's lymphoma: combined analysis of three case-control studies (United States). *Cancer Causes and Control* 1997;8(2):159–66.

Zang EA, Wynder EL. Cumulative tar exposure: a new index for estimating lung cancer risk among cigarette smokers. *Cancer* 1992;70(1):69–76.

Zang EA, Wynder EL. Differences in lung cancer risk between men and women: examination of the evidence. *Journal of the National Cancer Institute* 1996;88(3/4):183–92.

Zaren B, Cnattingius S, Lindmark G. Fetal growth impairment from smoking—is it influenced by maternal anthropometry? *Acta Obstetricia et Gynecologica Scandinavica* 1997;165:30–4.

Zaren B, Lindmark G, Gebre-Medhin M. Maternal smoking and body composition of the newborn. *Acta Paediatrica* 1996;85(2):213–9.

Zavaroni I, Bonini L, Gasparini P, Dall'Aglio E, Passeri M, Reaven GM. Cigarette smokers are relatively glucose intolerant, hyperinsulinemic and dyslipidemic. *American Journal of Cardiology* 1994;73(12):904–5.

Zhang H, Bracken MB. Tree-based risk factor analysis of preterm delivery and small-for-gestational-age birth. *American Journal of Epidemiology* 1995;141(1):70–8.

Zhang J, Fried DB. Relationship of maternal smoking during pregnancy to placenta previa. *American Journal of Preventive Medicine* 1992;8(5):278–82.

Zhang J, Ratcliffe JM. Paternal smoking and birthweight in Shanghai. *American Journal of Public Health* 1993;83(2):207–10.

Zhang J, Savitz DA, Schwingl PJ, Cai W-W. A case-control study of paternal smoking and birth defects. *International Journal of Epidemiology* 1992;21(2):273–8.

Zhang Z-X, Román GC. Worldwide occurrence of Parkinson's disease: an updated review. *Neuroepidemiology* 1993;12(4):195–208.

Zheng T, Holford TR, Boyle P, Chen Y, Ward BA, Flannery J, Mayne ST. Time trend and the age-period-cohort effect on the incidence of histologic types of lung cancer in Connecticut, 1960–1989. *Cancer* 1994;74(5):1556–67.

Zheng W, Blot WJ, Shu XO, Gao YT, Ji BT, Ziegler RG, Fraumeni JF Jr. Diet and other risk factors for laryngeal cancer in Shanghai, China. *American Journal of Epidemiology* 1992;136(2):178–91.

Zheng W, Deitz AC, Campbell DR, Wen W-Q, Cerhan JR, Sellers TA, Folsom AR, Hein DW. *N*-acetyltransferase 1 genetic polymorphism, cigarette smoking, well-done meat intake, and breast cancer risk. *Cancer Epidemiology, Biomarkers and Prevention* 1999;8(3):233–9.

Zumoff B, Miller L, Levit CD, Miller EH, Heinz U, Kalin M, Denman H, Jandorek R, Rosenfeld RS. The effect of smoking on serum progesterone, estradiol, and luteinizing hormone levels over a menstrual cycle in normal women. *Steroids* 1990;55(11):507–11.

Zunzunegui MV, King M-C, Coria CF, Charlet J. Male influences on cervical cancer risk. *American Journal of Epidemiology* 1986;123(2):302–7.

Zur Hausen H. Human genital cancer: synergism between two virus infections or synergism between a virus infection and initiating events? *Lancet* 1982;2(8312):1370–2.

# Chapter 4. Factors Influencing Tobacco Use Among Women

# Introduction

The published work on smoking initiation, maintenance, and cessation, together with descriptive examinations of the trends and themes of cigarette marketing, has provided insights into why women start to smoke and why they continue. Numerous scholars (e.g., Magnusson 1981; Bandura 1986; Sadava 1987; Frankenhaeuser 1991; Jessor et al. 1991; DeKay and Buss 1992) have argued that a thorough understanding of any behavior must be based on a comprehensive analysis of the broad social environment or cultural milieu surrounding the behavior, the immediate social situation or context in which the behavior occurs, the characteristics or disposition of the person performing the behavior, the behavior itself and closely related behaviors, and the interaction of all these conditions. Research on the social, cultural, and personal factors that influence women's smoking has been based on the social and psychological theory of the past several decades, and this research has burgeoned in recent years. Because smoking initiation among, maintenance and cessation among, and tobacco marketing to women have been studied by investigators using a variety of disciplinary perspectives and approaches, no single organizing framework exists for addressing the question of why women smoke. The research has shown that like most behaviors, tobacco use or nonuse results from a complex mix of influences that range from factors that are directly tied to tobacco use (e.g., beliefs about the consequences of smoking) to those that appear to have little to do with tobacco use (e.g., parenting styles and school characteristics).

# Factors Influencing Initiation of Smoking

## Overview of Studies Examined

Nearly all first use of tobacco occurs before high school graduation, and because nicotine is addictive, adolescents who smoke regularly are likely to become adult smokers (U.S. Department of Health and Human Services [USDHHS] 1994). Research on smoking initiation has, therefore, focused on adolescents and has been informed by a wealth of behavioral studies. Predictors of use of tobacco and other substances (Conrad et al. 1992; Hawkins et al. 1992; USDHHS 1994) and theories of adolescents' use of such substances (Petraitis et al. 1995) point to a complex set of interrelated factors.

Many efforts have been made to provide either a theoretical basis or an integrated framework for examining influences on smoking initiation. As a step toward an integrated approach, Petraitis and colleagues (1995) suggested that factors affecting tobacco use can be classified along two dimensions—type of influence and level of influence. These authors suggested that three distinct types of influence underlie existing theories of tobacco use—social, cultural, and personal. Social influences include the characteristics, beliefs, attitudes, and behaviors of the persons who make up the more intimate support system of adolescents, such as family and friends. Cultural influences include the practices and norms of the broader social environment of adolescents, such as the community, neighborhood, and school. Personal influences include individual biological characteristics, personality traits, affective states, and behavioral skills. For each type of influence, three levels of influence—ultimate, distal, and proximal—have been defined by work in evolutionary biology (Alcock 1989), cognitive science (Massaro 1991), and personality theory (Marshall 1991). McKinlay and Marceau (2000a,b) have emphasized the importance of a broad new integration of approaches and multilevel explanations. The levels of influence affect the nature and strength of the type of influence. Ultimate influences are broad, exogenous factors that gradually direct persons toward a behavior but are not strongly predictive. Distal influences are intermediate or indirect factors that may be more predictive. Proximal influences, which are the most immediate precursors of a behavior, are most predictive. The study of social, cultural, and personal domains among adolescents and the various levels of influence has undergone considerable theoretical development. This review of smoking initiation examined more than 100 studies in which tobacco use was an outcome variable. Selected characteristics and major gender-specific findings of the longitudinal studies are shown in Table 4.1.

The primary dependent variables analyzed in the studies differed greatly, ranging from initiation of smoking to amount smoked. The studies most relevant to this report were longitudinal investigations that examined gender-specific results related to smoking initiation among adolescents, including predictors of smoking initiation (Ahlgren et al. 1982; Brunswick and Messeri 1983–84; Skinner et al. 1985; Charlton and Blair 1989; McNeill et al. 1989; Simon et al. 1995), pathways leading to smoking initiation (Flay et al. 1994; Pierce et al. 1996; Pallonen et al. 1998), and predictors of both initiation of and escalation to regular smoking (Chassin et al. 1984, 1986; Santi et al. 1990–91). A few longitudinal studies addressed only escalation to regular smoking (Semmer et al. 1987; Urberg et al. 1991; Hu et al. 1995a). Some cross-sectional studies that compared students who had tried smoking with those who had never tried smoking are also discussed in this text because adolescent smokers are usually recent beginners (USDHHS 1994).

Many of the predictor variables were not defined comparably across studies. Even variables with the same labels may have actually been assessed with different measures. For example, some researchers who studied "school bonding" used attitudinal measures (e.g., attitudes toward school), whereas others used behavioral measures (e.g., truancy). Many studies also examined gender-specific differences in risk factors that predict the frequency or amount of cigarette smoking, not just the initiation of smoking (Kellam et al. 1980; Ensminger et al. 1982; Krohn et al. 1986; Lawrance and Rubinson 1986; Akers et al. 1987; Wills and Vaughan 1989; Waldron and Lye 1990; Bauman et al. 1992; Botvin et al. 1992; Rowe et al. 1992; Winefield et al. 1992; Kandel et al. 1994; Schifano et al. 1994; Sussman et al. 1994).

## Social and Environmental Factors

### Accessibility of Tobacco Products

Accessibility of tobacco products is an important environmental factor that influences smoking initiation by adolescents (Lynch and Bonnie 1994; USDHHS 1994; Forster and Wolfson 1998). In numerous surveys conducted since the late 1980s, youth often self-reported that their most common source of cigarettes was purchase from retail stores (Lynch and Bonnie 1994; USDHHS 1994; Centers for Disease Control and Prevention [CDC] 1996a,b; Forster and Wolfson 1998). Since the early 1990s, noncommercial or social sources (other minors, parents, older friends) have also been studied (Cummings et al. 1992; CDC 1996b; Forster et al. 1997). Evidence suggested, however, that much of the tobacco provided by minors to other minors was initially purchased from commercial sources by the adolescent donor (Wolfson et al. 1997). Some of these self-report surveys have found that adolescent girls may be less likely than boys to report usually purchasing their own cigarettes (CDC 1996b; Kann et al. 1998). Additionally, results from the Memphis Health Project (Robinson and Klesges 1997) indicated that girls were less likely than boys to view cigarettes as affordable and easy to obtain. Field research concerning minors' access began in the late 1980s and has generally concentrated on assessing rates of illegal sales of tobacco to minors from retail stores during compliance checks in which underage youth attempt to purchase tobacco products (DiFranza et al. 1987; USDHHS 1994; Forster and Wolfson 1998; Forster et al. 1998). Compliance check studies in which both girls and boys participated generally found that retailers were more likely to sell cigarettes to girls than to boys of the same age (Forster and Wolfson 1998).

### Pricing of Tobacco Products

Although considerable research has been done on the effect of price on smoking among smokers (Wasserman et al. 1991; Hu et al. 1995b; Chaloupka and Grossman 1996; CDC 1998), little empirical research exists on the effect of price on smoking initiation. Lewit and Coate (1982) used cross-sectional survey data and found that a price increase appeared to affect the decision to become a smoker rather than the decision to smoke less frequently. They also found that the smoking behavior among young adults (20 through 25 years old) was more sensitive to price changes than that among older persons and that male smokers, particularly those aged 20 through 35 years, were quite responsive to price, whereas female smokers were essentially unaffected by price. Chaloupka (1990, 1991a,b) also found that women were much less responsive to price than were men, but, in contrast with the findings of Lewit and Coate (1982), Chaloupka found that adolescents and young adults (aged 17 through 24 years) were less responsive to price than were older age groups. In a CDC (1998) study, data analyzed from 14 years of the National Health Interview Survey showed that a 10-percent increase in price led to a 2.6-percent reduction in the demand for cigarettes among males and a 1.9-percent reduction among females. Thus, females were less responsive to price, as other studies have also found.

Mullahy (1985) found that both the decision to smoke and the quantity of cigarettes consumed by smokers were negatively related to cigarette prices among both men and women. As in the Lewit and Coate (1982) study, Mullahy (1985) found that cigarette prices had a greater effect on the decision to smoke than they did on cigarette consumption. Similarly, he found that men were somewhat more responsive to price than were women (average elasticities of -0.56 and -0.39, respectively). Of the studies that examined price in relation to initiation, two (Lewit et al. 1997; Dee and Evans 1998) found a significant inverse relationship between price and smoking initiation, and one (DeCicca et al. 1998) found no significant relationship. Dee and Evans (1998) estimated the price elasticity of smoking initiation to be in the range of -0.63 to -0.77. This finding implied that for every 10-percent increase in the price of cigarettes, a 6.6- to 7.7-percent reduction in the onset of smoking would be expected. Lewit and colleagues (1997) found that a 10-percent increase in price reduced the onset of smoking by 9.5 percent.

Chaloupka (1992) explored whether differences existed in the impact of clean indoor air laws on cigarette demand among women and men. The results for women and men showed dramatic differences in their response to both clean indoor air laws and cigarette prices. Men living in states with clean indoor air laws were found to smoke significantly less, on average, than their counterparts living in states with no restrictions on smoking. The smoking behavior among women, however, was found to be virtually unaffected by restrictions on cigarette smoking. Increased cigarette prices were found to lower the average cigarette consumption among men, whereas cigarette prices had no impact on smoking among women.

### Advertising and Promotion of Tobacco Products

Defining a self-image is an important developmental task during adolescence (French and Perry 1996). Attractive images of young smokers displayed in tobacco advertisements are likely to "implant" the idea of initiation of smoking behavior in adolescent minds as a means to achieve the desired self-image. Therefore, it is not surprising that adolescents generally notice and respond to messages in tobacco advertising and promotion. A study by Pollay and colleagues (1996) found that brand choices among adolescents were significantly related to cigarette advertising and that the relationship between brand choices and brand advertising was stronger among adolescents than among adults.

Gilpin and Pierce (1997) suggested that the tobacco industry's expanded budget for marketing and increased emphasis on marketing tactics that may be particularly pertinent to young people influenced rates of smoking initiation among adolescents. Results from the statewide California Tobacco Survey led Evans and associates (1995) to conclude that tobacco advertising and marketing may have a stronger effect on smoking initiation among adolescents than does exposure to peers and family members who smoke. On the basis of a study of 7th and 8th graders, Botvin and colleagues (1993) reported that exposure to tobacco advertising was predictive of current smoking status. A study performed in rural New England showed that one-third of 6th through 12th graders possessed cigarette promotional items (e.g., T-shirts, hats, and backpacks) (Sargent et al. 1997). Students who owned such items were 4.1 times as likely to be smokers as students who did not own these items. One study revealed that ownership of and willingness to use cigarette promotional items were less common among girls than among boys (Gilpin et al. 1997).

Although advertising is thought to influence smoking initiation, information about differential gender effects of tobacco advertising and promotion on smoking initiation is limited. For a more detailed discussion of the relationship between historic trends in tobacco marketing targeted to women and time trends in smoking among girls and young women, see "Influence of Tobacco Marketing on Smoking Initiation by Females" later in this chapter.

### Parental Hostility, Strictness, and Family Conflict

Study results on the effect of parental strictness on smoking initiation among adolescents have been conflicting. Some studies found that strictness and hostility of parents toward their children increased the risk for smoking initiation among adolescent boys (e.g., Chassin et al. 1984). However, other studies concluded that perception of parental strictness by adolescent children did not contribute to smoking initiation (e.g., McNeill et al. 1989).

**Table 4.1. Longitudinal studies with gender-specific findings on beliefs, experiences, and behaviors related to smoking initiation**

| Study | Location | Study period | Study type or source | Population: Age/grade at study entry | Population: Racial or ethnic origin | Population: Sample size* |
|---|---|---|---|---|---|---|
| Aaron et al. 1995 | Pittsburgh, Pennsylvania | 3 years | School | 12–16 years | 73% white, 24% black, 3% Hispanic or Asian | 1,245 |
| Abernathy et al. 1995 | Calgary, Alberta | 4 years | School | Grade 6 | Not specified | 3,567 |
| Ahlgren et al. 1982 | Suburban Minneapolis, Minnesota | 1 year | School | 10–13 years (grades 5 and 6) | "Mostly white" | ≤ 625 |
| Akers et al. 1987 | Midwestern United States | 5 years | School | 12–13 years and 16–17 years (grades 7 and 12) | Not specified | ≤ 454 |
| Aloise-Young et al. 1994 | Los Angeles County and Orange County, California | 1 year | School | Grade 7 | Not specified | 1,512 |
| Ary and Biglan 1998 | Lane County, Oregon | 1 year | School | 12–17 years (grades 7–10) | 92% white, 1% black, 1% Asian, 3.5% American Indian | ≤ 801 |
| Best et al. 1995[†] | Southeastern Ontario | 4 years | School | 12–14 years (grade 6) | Not specified | ≤ 3,566 |
| Biglan et al. 1995 | Northwestern United States | 18 months | Home | 14–17 years | 91% white, 3% black, <2% Hispanic, 2% Asian, 2% American Indian | 593 |
| Botvin et al. 1992 | New York State | 2 years | School | Grades 7–9 | 91% white, 2% black, 2% Hispanic, 1% American Indian | ~460 |
| Brunswick and Messeri 1983–84 | New York City | 6–8 years | Not specified | 12–17 years | 100% black | 283–380 |

*Note:* Studies that examined differences in tobacco-related messages in male- and female-oriented magazines are not included.

*Ranges are given for sample sizes that varied from analysis to analysis in the study. Upper limits indicate that it was unclear whether the reported number reflected the number of subjects in the study or the subset of subjects with sufficient data for analysis.

[†]Study was based on the same sample as Santi et al. 1990–91.

| Dependent variables | Major gender-specific findings |
|---|---|
| Smoking behavior (six choices) | Females who were less physically active were more likely to initiate smoking. No relationship was found between physical activity and smoking initiation among males. |
| Never smoked vs. ever smoked | For females, smoking and reported self-esteem were strongly associated. No association was found between smoking and self-esteem for males. |
| Having ever smoked, smoking during 6-month period (new smoker, continuing smoker, former smoker) | No significant gender-specific differences were found for former or current smokers, parental smoking, self-esteem, or attitudes toward school. |
| Lifetime smoking status (1 = never, 6 = daily) | Adolescent girls were more influenced in their smoking behavior by boyfriends than adolescent boys were by girlfriends. |
| Role of group membership in peer influence on smoking behavior | No significant gender-specific differences were found in the comparison of group members' and group outsiders' susceptibility to peer influence on smoking behavior. |
| Number of cigarettes smoked in last week | No significant gender-specific differences in predictor variables were found. Predictor variables included pretest smoking rate; level of addiction to cigarettes; level of experience with cigarettes; socioeconomic status; parent, sibling, and peer smoking behavior; use of alcohol and marijuana; number of offers to smoke received; and intention to smoke. |
| Never smoked, tried once, smoked more than once during 12 months | For females, a higher score on the following factors was related to higher risk of smoking initiation: rebelliousness, rejection of adult authority, personal dissatisfaction, and peer approval. For males, only rebelliousness and rejection of adult authority were associated with higher risk of smoking initiation. Within the same rebelliousness score, females were significantly more likely than males to make the transition from nonsmoking to smoking. |
| Smoking frequency during last 24 hours and last month, number of years of smoking, average number of cigarettes/day | No significant gender-specific differences were found in adolescent problem behavior, the social context of the family environment, and the peer social context, as predictor variables. |
| Lifetime smoking status (1 = never, 10 = >1 pack/day) | Girls in grade 7 who perceived that one-half of persons their age smoked were more likely to be smokers in grade 9 than were boys in grade 7 who reported the same perception. |
| Initiation of smoking over 6–8 years | Five domains of predictors (personal background, school achievement, family-peer orientations, psychogenic orientations, and health attitudes and behaviors) were examined. Overall, the studied adolescent behaviors and attitudes better predicted smoking among females than among males. |

**Table 4.1. Continued**

| Study | Location | Study period | Study type or source | Population: Age/grade at study entry | Population: Racial or ethnic origin | Population: Sample size* |
|---|---|---|---|---|---|---|
| Brunswick and Messeri 1984 | New York City | 6–8 years | Population | 12–17 years | 100% black | 283–380 |
| Burke et al. 1997 | Australia | 9 years | School-based | 9 years at study entry | Not specified | 583–1,565 |
| Charlton and Blair 1989 | Northern England | 4 months | School | 12–13 years | Not specified | 1,390 |
| Chassin et al. 1984‡ | Midwestern United States | 1 year | School | 12–17 years (grades 6–11) | 96% white | 2,818 |
| Chassin et al. 1986‡ | Midwestern United States | 1 year | School | 12–17 years (grades 6–11) | 96% white | ≤ 2,155 |
| Chassin et al. 1990‡ | Midwestern United States | 4 years | Mail | 12–17 years | 96% white | 1,844–3,238 |
| Chassin et al. 1992‡ | Midwestern United States | 8 years | School or mail | 12–17 years (grades 6–11) | 97% white | 765 |
| Cohen et al. 1994 | Los Angeles, California (metropolitan area) | 3 years | School | Cohort 1: 13 years (grade 5)<br>Cohort 2: 15 years (grade 7) | Cohort 1: 39% white, 4% black, 30% Hispanic, 15% Asian<br>Cohort 2: 40% white, 4% black, 28% Hispanic, 15% Asian | 1,376 |

*Ranges are given for sample sizes that varied from analysis to analysis in the study. Upper limits indicate that it was unclear whether the reported number reflected the number of subjects in the study or the subset of subjects with sufficient data for analysis.
‡Studies were based on the same sample.

| Dependent variables | Major gender-specific findings |
| --- | --- |
| Initiation of smoking over 6–8 years | Psychogenic factors and differential socialization influences were analyzed to determine their role in the observed link between school achievement and smoking: smoking was mediated by psychogenic factors only for girls. Males who expressed lower social expectancy were more likely to initiate smoking, but this relationship was not a mediating factor for school achievement and smoking. |
| Never smoked vs. ever smoked | Clustering of adverse health behaviors among young female and male smokers was observed. For females, smoking, unsafe drinking, low physical activity, and lower fiber intake showed clustering. For males, smoking, unsafe drinking, and higher fat intake showed clustering, but physical activity and fiber intake did not. |
| Initiation of at least trial smoking during 4-month period (no, yes) | Four variables were significantly related to smoking initiation for females: having at least one parent who smoked, holding positive views on smoking, being aware of at least one cigarette brand, and having a best friend who smoked. None of the variables was consistently related to smoking initiation for males. |
| Initiation of at least trial smoking over 1 year, transition over 1 year from having tried smoking to smoking regularly (no, yes) | Male experimenters who were at risk of becoming regular smokers were more prone to deviance than girls were. |
| Initiation of at least trial smoking over 1 year, transition over 1 year from having tried smoking to smoking regularly (no, yes) | For persons who had never smoked at baseline, the effects of parental smoking were significant only for girls. Among experimenters at baseline, girls who perceived their friends as having positive attitudes about smoking were more likely to become regular smokers. For initial experimenters, girls whose friends had lower expectations of them were more likely to become regular smokers, whereas boys whose friends had higher expectations of them were more likely to become regular smokers. |
| Current smoking status (0 = nonsmoker, 1 = weekly smoker) | No significant gender-specific differences were found in the assessment of adolescent smoking increasing the risk for adult smoking. |
| Initiation and increase in smoking during 6-year period | Low socioeconomic status places girls at higher risk for smoking than boys. |
| Initiation of smoking over 4 years (cohort 1) and 3 years (cohort 2) of follow-up | Perceptions of risk factors for alcohol and tobacco use and parenting behaviors were compared in girls and boys. Children who reported more time spent with parents and who communicated more frequently with parents had lower initiation rates for alcohol and tobacco use in the last month. Disruptive behavior increased the chances of tobacco use in the last month. Boys reported higher levels of disruptive behavior. Girls reported being monitored more by parents and having higher levels of communication with parents. |

**Table 4.1. Continued**

| Study | Location | Study period | Study type or source | Population: Age/grade at study entry | Population: Racial or ethnic origin | Population: Sample size* |
|---|---|---|---|---|---|---|
| Dinh et al. 1995 | Washington State | 4 years | School | Grade 5 | 87% white, 5% mixed | ≤ 1,593 |
| Distefan et al. 1998 | United States | 4 years | Population Telephone and mail | 12–18 years | Not specified | 4,149 |
| Ensminger et al. 1982 | Chicago, Illinois | 10 years | School | Grade 1 | 100% black | ≤ 705 |
| French et al. 1994 | Minnesota | 4 years | School | Grades 7–10 | 87% white | 1,705 |
| Green et al. 1991 | Glasgow, Scotland | 20 years | Home and mail | 15, 35, and 55 years | Not specified | 722–846 |
| Hibbett and Fogelman 1990 | England | 23 years | Not specified | Newborn and 7, 11, 16, and 23 years | Not specified | ≤ 5,663 |
| Hu et al. 1995a | San Diego and Los Angeles, California | 2 years | School | Grade 7 | 32.5% white, 15.5% black, 35.5% Hispanic, 16.5% Asian or other | 2,433 |
| Hunter et al. 1987 | Bogalusa, Louisiana | 2 years | School | 8–17 years | 67% white, 33% black | ≤ 2,380 |
| Kandel et al. 1994 | New York State | 19 years | In-home interviews | Cohort 1: Grades 10 and 11 | Not specified | 192 |
| | United States | 19 years | In-home interviews | Cohort 2: 10–18 years | Not specified | 796 |
| Kellam et al. 1980 | Chicago, Illinois | 10 years | School | Grade 10 | 100% black | ≤ 705 |

*Ranges are given for sample sizes that varied from analysis to analysis in the study. Upper limits indicate that it was unclear whether the reported number reflected the number of subjects in the study or the subset of subjects with sufficient data for analysis.

| Dependent variables | Major gender-specific findings |
|---|---|
| Weekly smoking (no, yes) | Compared with girls, boys in grade 5 who perceived smokers as leaders were more likely to report weekly smoking in grade 9. In grade 5, boys who perceived smokers as dirty and "uncool" were less likely to report weekly smoking in grade 9 than were girls. |
| Progression from never smoked to experimenter or from experimenter to current smoker | No significant gender-specific differences in parental influences on adolescent smoking initiation were found. |
| Daily smoking (0 = less than daily, 1 = daily) | No significant gender-specific differences were found in frequency of cigarette use, and only slight differences were found in the relationship between the independent variables and cigarette use. For males, early shyness and aggressiveness related to later cigarette use. |
| Transition from nonsmoking to regular smoking at 1-year follow-up | Girls who dieted or who were worried about their weight were more likely to initiate smoking than were girls who did not have these concerns. For boys, weight concerns and dieting were not significantly related to smoking initiation. |
| Daily smoking (no, yes) | Average weekly smoking was higher among male smokers than among female smokers. |
| Daily smoking status (0 = nonsmoker, 4 = >30 cigarettes/day) | Compared with nontruants, truants of both genders were more likely to be smokers. This trend appeared to be more pronounced for females. |
| Smoking frequency (0 = never, 3 = regular smoking) over four waves | The effects of friends' smoking were more pronounced for females than for males. An increase in the influence of friends was more pronounced for females than for males. |
| Ever tried smoking (no, yes) | Gender and racial groups had different responses for the influence of friends and family on smoking behavior. Black females seemed to be less influenced by the smoking behavior of their female siblings, mother, and father than were white females. Black males seemed to be less influenced by the smoking behavior of their fathers and sisters than were white males. |
| Cohort 1: ever smoked (no, yes), smoked in last year (no, yes)<br>Cohort 2: ever smoked (no, yes), smoked in last 3 months (no, yes) | Maternal smoking during pregnancy was significantly related to the child's smoking 13 years later. Maternal smoking during pregnancy had a stronger influence on daughters than on sons. |
| Lifetime smoking status (1 = never, 5 = ≥ 1 pack/day) | A strong association was found between teenage social involvement and drug use, including cigarette smoking, for males. This association was not found for females. |

**Table 4.1. Continued**

| Study | Location | Study period | Study type or source | Population: Age/grade at study entry | Population: Racial or ethnic origin | Population: Sample size* |
|---|---|---|---|---|---|---|
| Killen et al. 1997 | Northern California | 3–4 years | School | 15 years (mean) (grade 9) | 45% white, 3% black, 15% Hispanic, 23% Asian, 3% Pacific Islander, 2% American Indian, 6% other | 1,026 |
| Lawrance and Rubinson 1986 | Midwestern United States | ≤ 8 months | School | Grades 6–8 | Not specified | ≤ 554 |
| McCaul et al. 1982 | Moorhead, Minnesota | 1 year | Clinic, home | Grades 7 and 8 | White | 297 |
| McGee and Stanton 1993§ | Dunedin, New Zealand | 15 years | Clinic, home | 9 years | Not specified | 719 |
| McNeill et al. 1989 | Bristol, England | 30 months | Clinic, home, or school | 11–13 years | Not specified | 1,574 |
| Mittelmark et al. 1987 | Minneapolis and St. Paul, Minnesota (metropolitan area) | 2 years | School | Grades 7–11 | Not specified | 462 |
| Pederson et al. 1998 | Scarborough, Ontario | 2 years | School | Grade 8 | Not specified | 1,533 |
| Pierce et al. 1996 | United States | 4 years | Teenage Attitudes and Practices Surveys I and II | 12–18 years | 71% white, 17% black, 8% Hispanic, 4% Asian or other | 4,500 |
| Pulkkinen 1982 | Finland | 12 years | School | 8 years | Not specified | ≤ 135 |
| Reynolds and Nichols 1976 | United States | 1 year | Mailed questionnaire | Grade 12 | Not specified | 712–852 |
| Rowe et al. 1992 | Midwestern United States | 8 years | School, mail, or telephone | Grades 6–12 | 96% white | ≤ 4,156 |

*Ranges are given for sample sizes that varied from analysis to analysis in the study. Upper limits indicate that it was unclear whether the reported number reflected the number of subjects in the study or the subset of subjects with sufficient data for analysis.

§Study was based on the same sample as the studies by Stanton and Silva 1991, 1992 and Stanton et al. 1995.

| Dependent variables | Major gender-specific findings |
|---|---|
| Smoking (lifetime exposure) | Among nonsmokers at baseline, girls and boys who had more friends who smoked were more likely to try smoking. Girls who had higher sociability scores were more likely to try smoking, whereas boys with higher levels of depression were more likely to try smoking. |
| Lifetime smoking status (never smoked, trial smoking, current smoker) | No significant gender-specific differences in social and emotional variables were found. |
| Smoking (at least once a week) vs. nonsmoking (all others) | No significant gender-specific differences were found in the predictor variables studied, including the smoking behaviors of students' friends and family and students' school behavior, beliefs about smoking, and intentions to smoke in the future. |
| At least trial smoking by age 13 years (no, yes), continued smoking between ages 13 and 15 years (no, yes) | Compared with boys, girls were 1.5 times more likely to continue smoking from age 13 to 15 years. Girls who reported no smoking at age 13 years were more likely than boys to smoke at age 15 years. |
| Initiation of at least trial smoking over 30-month period (no, yes) | Being a female was the second strongest predictor of smoking initiation after previous experimentation with cigarettes. |
| Initiation of more than experimental smoking over 2-year period (no, yes) | Females who began to smoke were more likely to have siblings who smoked, have a positive image of smokers, believe less that adults should be role models regarding smoking, and have less-educated parents. Males who began to smoke were more independent, less worried about health risks, and less involved in decision making in their families. |
| Current smoker, experimental smoker, former smoker, nonsmoker | For females, higher levels of depression were associated with greater use of tobacco. |
| Experimentation with smoking, established smoking | Boys were more likely than girls to experiment with cigarettes. |
| Current smoking status (never smoked, experimental smoker, former smoker, occasional smoker, regular smoker) | Girls tended to be more susceptible to the modeling effects of sisters, peers, and parents in smoking and drinking. |
| Smoking frequency (from 0 to >2 packs/day) | Smokers were less well adjusted than nonsmokers and tended to be more involved in antisocial activities. These relationships were stronger for females than for males. |
| Lifetime smoking status (1 = never smoked, 2 = trial smoking, 3 = smoked at least monthly, 4 = former smoker) | In the prevalence-driven model, the rate of transition from experimenter to regular smoker was higher for females than for males. |

**Table 4.1. Continued**

| Study | Location | Study period | Study type or source | Population: Age/grade at study entry | Population: Racial or ethnic origin | Population: Sample size* |
|---|---|---|---|---|---|---|
| Santi et al. 1990–91[Δ] | Southwestern Ontario | 6 years | School | Grade 6 | Not specified | 1,614 |
| Santi et al. 1994 | Southwestern Ontario | 3 years | School | 11.5 years (mean) (grade 6) | Not specified | ≤ 3,884 |
| Semmer et al. 1987 | Berlin and Bremen, Germany | 2 years | School | 13.5 years (mean) (grades 7 and 8) | Not specified | 712–760 |
| Simon et al. 1995 | San Diego and Los Angeles, California | 1 year | School | 13 years (grade 7) | 57% white, 3% black, 24% Hispanic, 9% Asian, 7% other | 836 |
| Skinner and Krohn 1992[¶] | Midwestern United States | 5 years | School | 13–18 years (grades 7–12) | Not specified | 172–182 |
| Skinner et al. 1985[¶] | Midwestern United States | 3 years | School | grades 7–12 | Not specified | ≤ 426 |
| Stanton and Silva 1991** | Dunedin, New Zealand | 6 years | Clinic, school, or home | 9 years | 5.4% Maori or Polynesian origin | 734–779 |
| Stanton and Silva 1992** | Dunedin, New Zealand | 6 years | Clinic, school, or home | 9 years | 5.4% Maori or Polynesian origin | 734–779 |
| Stanton et al. 1995** | Dunedin, New Zealand | 18 years | Clinic, school, or home | 9 years | 3% Maori or Polynesian origin | 546–705 |

*Ranges are given for sample sizes that varied from analysis to analysis in the study. Upper limits indicate that it was unclear whether the reported number reflected the number of subjects in the study or the subset of subjects with sufficient data for analysis.
[Δ]Study was based on the same sample as Best et al. 1995.
[¶]Studies were based on the same sample.
**Studies were based on the same sample as McGee and Stanton 1993.

| Dependent variables | Major gender-specific findings |
|---|---|
| Initiation of at least experimental smoking over 2-year period (no, yes) | Males started smoking earlier than females, but females reported higher rates of initiation from grade 7 to the end of grade 9 than did males. |
| Transition to more smoking over 1-year period (no, yes) | No significant gender-specific differences were found in the adolescent dispositions of self-definition, social compliance, and affect regulation facilitating transitions in stages of smoking. |
| Initiation of at least experimental smoking over 6-month period (no, yes) | Females were more likely than males to be influenced by their friends' smoking. |
| Initiation of at least experimental smoking over 1-year period (no, yes) | High scores on risk taking had a stronger relationship to smoking for females than for males. |
| Lifetime smoking status (1 = never, 6 = daily) | The social process model was more useful in accounting for the dynamics associated with cigarette use for females than for males. Lack of commitment to education and activities were associated more with female deviance than with male deviance. |
| Initiation of at least experimental smoking over 2-year period (no, yes) | Females who associated with female peers who smoked were more likely to start smoking than were females who had less association with female peers who smoked. |
| Smoked in last 2 years (no, yes) | Effect of friends smoking was more related to boys' smoking than girls' smoking in the previous 2 years at ages 9 and 15 years. At age 15 years, girls were more likely than boys to be daily smokers if they observed friends smoking, if their brothers smoked, or if they had no preference for nonsmoking friends. |
| Smoked in last 2 years (no, yes) | Results concerning the influence of parents and friends were very similar for girls and boys. Recent smoking cessation by mothers seemed to delay smoking among daughters but not among sons. |
| Smoked in last 2 years (no, yes) | Delinquency was associated with a higher risk for girls. Aggressive behavior in girls may put them at a higher risk for succumbing to the peer pressure to smoke. For boys, having a lower socioeconomic status, receiving low social support from the family, having an older father, and obtaining higher scores for inattention were associated with a higher risk for smoking initiation. |

**Table 4.1. Continued**

| Study | Location | Study period | Study type or source | Population: Age/grade at study entry | Population: Racial or ethnic origin | Population: Sample size* |
|---|---|---|---|---|---|---|
| Sussman et al. 1987 | Los Angeles, California (metropolitan area) | 1 year | School | 13 years (grades 7 and 8) | 57% white, 9% black, 24% Hispanic, 9% Asian | ≤ 874 |
| Sussman et al. 1994 | San Diego and Los Angeles, California | 1 year | School | 13 years (mean) (grade 7) | 60% white, 7% black, 27% Hispanic, 6% Asian or other | 931 |
| Swan et al. 1990 | Derbyshire, England | 10 years | School | 11.7–12.7 years | Not specified | 6,000 |
| Urberg 1992†† | Midwestern United States | 1 year | School | 17 years (mean) (grade 11) | 96% white | ≤ 324 |
| Urberg et al. 1991†† | Midwestern United States | 1 year | School | 14 and 17 years (mean) (grades 8 and 11) | 96% white | 309 |
| Wills 1986‡‡ | New York City | 2 years | School | 12–14 years (grades 7 and 8) | 46% white, 23% Hispanic | 300–600 |
| Wills and Vaughan 1989‡‡ | New York City | 2 years | School | 12–14 years (grades 7 and 8) | 50% white, 20% black, 20% Hispanic | ≤ 1,576 |
| Winefield et al. 1992, 1993 | Australia | 9 years | Mailed questionnaire | 15.6 years (average) (grades 10–12) | Not specified | ≤ 478 |
| Wu and Anthony 1999 | Atlanta, Georgia | Up to 5 years | School | Ages 8–14 | 24% white, 75% black, 1% Hispanic, American Indian, or Asian | 1,731 |

*Ranges are given for sample sizes that varied from analysis to analysis in the study. Upper limits indicate that it was unclear whether the reported number reflected the number of subjects in the study or the subset of subjects with sufficient data for analysis.
††Studies were based on the same sample.
‡‡Studies were based on the same sample.

| Dependent variables | Major gender-specific findings |
|---|---|
| Initiation of at least experimental smoking over 1-year period (no, yes) | Females were not as influenced as males by adult approval of smoking and by risk-taking preferences. Females were more aware of health consequences than males. Among white females, availability of cigarettes was a predictor of smoking initiation. For Hispanic females, low achievement in school was a strong predictor. For black males, peer pressure was a predictor, and for Asian males, difficulty refusing offers of cigarettes and intentions to smoke in the future were predictors. |
| Lifetime smoking status (1 = never, 8 = heavy daily) | No significant gender-specific differences for the predictor of group self-identification were found. |
| Experimental smoking, regular smoking | Maternal smoking was associated with a higher rate of smoking initiation for females. Females who were involved in organized sports were less likely to start smoking, whereas involvement in sports did not affect smoking initiation in males. Females who were involved in organized social activities were more likely to start smoking than were males. |
| Number of cigarettes smoked in last week | Males were more influenced than females by peer smoking behavior. |
| Differences between number of cigarettes smoked weekly in year 1 and year 2 | No significant gender-specific differences in the influence of best friends and social crowd on smoking were found. |
| Smoking summary score (1–5) | Socially related measures had a higher association with substance use for females than for males. |
| Lifetime smoking status (1 = never, 5 = weekly) | The association between peer support and smoking was strong for females but weak for males. |
| Current smoking status (nonsmoker, light smoker, heavy smoker) | No significant gender-specific differences in the psychological aspects of smoking (self-esteem, depressive affect, negative mood, hopelessness, psychological disturbance, locus of control, social alienation) were found. |
| Initiation of smoking | Antecedent smoking was associated with increased risk of depressed mood but not vice versa. Gender-specific findings were not presented, but gender was not an independent prediction of initiation in multivariate analyses. |

Biglan and coworkers (1995) studied a sample of 643 adolescents at three time intervals. Family conflict at time 1 predicted inadequate parental monitoring at time 2, and inadequate parental monitoring, association with deviant peers, parental smoking, and peer smoking at time 2 predicted smoking at time 3. The model was the same for girls and boys, and no significant differences were found in the path coefficients. These findings suggested that family conflict influences tobacco use indirectly and that the mechanism among girls and boys is similar.

**Level of Parental Supervision, Involvement, or Attachment**

Parents who closely supervise their children know where their children are and monitor what they are doing. Results of some studies suggested that close supervision deters smoking among adolescents (Chassin et al. 1986; Mittelmark et al. 1987; Radziszewska et al. 1996; Jackson et al. 1997), and findings in two studies suggested that parental supervision may be a greater deterrent among girls than among boys (Skinner et al. 1985; Krohn et al. 1986). This pattern might be explained by the finding that girls are generally monitored more closely than are boys (Cohen et al. 1994). One study revealed that authoritative parenting styles influenced children's smoking initiation independently of parental smoking status (Jackson et al. 1994). However, other studies showed no link between parental supervision and adolescent smoking (e.g., Krohn et al. 1983).

Parental involvement implies the active participation of parents in their children's lives. A longitudinal study of fifth and seventh graders found lower rates of smoking initiation among children who reported that their parents spent more time with them and communicated with them more frequently (Cohen et al. 1994). Girls tended to have better communication with their parents than did boys, but the relationship between interaction with parents and smoking initiation was not reported separately by gender. In one study, parental involvement in their children's school, religious, and athletic activities decreased the risk for smoking among both girls and boys (Krohn et al. 1986). In another study, children who perceived their parents as generally unconcerned about their social activities were slightly more likely to increase their smoking over a one-year period (Murray et al. 1983). The results of two other studies suggested, however, that this relationship may exist for boys only (Mittelmark et al. 1987; Stanton et al. 1995).

Longitudinal studies have reported that the risk for smoking among adolescents increases as their emotional bonds and sense of attachment to parents weaken (Conrad et al. 1992). Findings in several studies suggested that weak attachment to parents and risk for smoking do not differ by gender (Ensminger et al. 1982; Krohn et al. 1986; Kumpfer and Turner 1990–91). One study of female college students found that poor father-daughter relationships (e.g., spending little time together or poor communication) correlated with the daughters' smoking (Brook et al. 1987).

**Parental Smoking**

Parents who smoke are more likely than those who do not to have children who smoke (Conrad et al. 1992; Jackson et al. 1997). Studies found that children in grades four through six (mean age, 11 years) were almost three times as likely to have smoked cigarettes in the past 30 days if they lived with an adult smoker (Morris et al. 1993) and that adolescents were about two times as likely to have smoked daily if one or both parents smoked (Green et al. 1991). One study found that adolescents whose parents had stopped smoking were about one-third less likely to have ever smoked than were those with parents who still smoked (Farkas et al. 1999). Several studies reported that girls and boys are equally susceptible to the effects of parental smoking (Chassin et al. 1984; Santi et al. 1990–91; Green et al. 1991; Glendinning et al. 1994) and to parental attitudes toward smoking (Ary and Biglan 1988). However, some researchers found differences in receptivity to parental smoking among girls and boys. One study showed that boys were more influenced by parental smoking than were girls (Sussman et al. 1987), but most of the studies suggested that girls may be more influenced than boys (Chassin et al. 1986; Charlton and Blair 1989; Swan et al. 1990; van Roosmalen and McDaniel 1992; Flay et al. 1994; Kandel et al. 1994; Hu et al. 1995a; Robinson et al. 1997).

The effects of maternal smoking may differ among girls and boys. In three studies, maternal smoking tended to have a slightly greater effect on subsequent smoking among girls than among boys (Ahlgren et al. 1982; Pulkkinen 1982; Bauman et al. 1992). This finding was confirmed in a study of 201 parent-child triads that used independent reporting of smoking status from each member of the domestic group (Kandel and Wu 1995), unlike the majority of studies, which used the child's report about parents' smoking. Stanton and Silva (1992) reported that recent smoking cessation among mothers apparently helped to delay and perhaps deter smoking among daughters but not among sons. Thus, adolescent girls may be more likely than adolescent boys to model their smoking on their mothers' smoking behavior. In one study, however, maternal smoking significantly predicted smoking among sons but not among daughters (Skinner et al. 1985).

**Sibling Smoking**

One study reported that smoking among older siblings had little or no influence on smoking among their younger sisters and brothers (Ary and Biglan 1988), but other evidence suggested that young siblings are influenced by sibling smoking (Swan et al. 1990; Conrad et al. 1992; Daly et al. 1993). The effect was equal among girls and boys in one study (Santi et al. 1990–91). In other studies, the effect was stronger among girls (Chassin et al. 1984; Mittelmark et al. 1987; van Roosmalen and McDaniel 1992; Pierce et al. 1993) or among boys (Brunswick and Messeri 1983–84; Stanton and Silva 1991). The pattern may vary by race or ethnicity (Hunter et al. 1987); in particular, African American girls appeared to be less susceptible than white girls to the influence of siblings, other family members, and peers who smoked. At present, no conclusion can be drawn about the comparative susceptibility of girls and boys to sibling smoking.

**Peer Smoking**

In many studies, one of the strongest risk factors for smoking is exposure to peers, especially close friends, who smoke (USDHHS 1994; Meijer et al. 1996; Gritz et al. 1998). Friends' smoking was predictive of some phase of smoking in all but 1 (Newcomb et al. 1989) of 16 longitudinal studies reviewed by Conrad and associates (1992). Results of many studies suggested that involvement with peers who smoke has a similar effect among girls and boys (Palmer 1970; McCaul et al. 1982; Pulkkinen 1982; Chassin et al. 1984, 1986; Gottlieb and Baker 1986; Krohn et al. 1986; Mittelmark et al. 1987; Sussman et al. 1987; Santi et al. 1990–91; Stanton and Silva 1992; Urberg 1992; van Roosmalen and McDaniel 1992; McGee and Stanton 1993; Pierce et al. 1993; Glendinning et al. 1994). Findings in other studies suggested that peer smoking affects adolescent girls and boys somewhat differently. In a few studies, boys who smoked had more friends who were smokers (Morris et al. 1993) and were more influenced by the smoking-related attitudes (Chassin et al. 1984) and behaviors of their peers than were girls who smoked (Urberg et al. 1991). However, most of the studies that reported gender-specific differences suggested that girls are more influenced by peer smoking than are boys (Semmer et al. 1987; Charlton and Blair 1989; Pirie et al. 1991; Waldron et al. 1991; Rowe et al. 1992; Sarason et al. 1992; Skinner and Krohn 1992; Hu et al. 1995a). Akers and colleagues (1987) reported that adolescent girls were more influenced in their smoking behavior by their boyfriends than adolescent boys were influenced by their girlfriends. However, Skinner and associates (1985) found that the initiation of smoking among girls tended to coincide with increasing involvement with other girls who smoked but not with boys who smoked.

Bauman and Ennett (1994) contended that the examination of simple peer associations may be less revealing than the exploration of social networks among peers. These researchers and their colleagues pointed to the homogeneity of adolescent friendship cliques with regard to smoking and noted that, in a formal network analysis of 87 such cliques, most were composed entirely of nonsmokers (Ennett et al. 1994). The study results suggested that cliques may contribute more to the maintenance of nonsmoking status than to the initiation of smoking. These findings were strongest among all-female and among all-white cliques. In another analysis of the same data, the authors pointed out that adolescents who did not belong to a clique had a higher probability of smoking than did adolescents who belonged to a clique (Ennett and Bauman 1993).

**Perceived Norms and Prevalence of Smoking**

Adolescents whose close peers smoke tend to perceive that smoking is far more normative than it actually is (Conrad et al. 1992; USDHHS 1994). One study revealed that seventh-grade girls estimated the overall incidence of smoking among their peers at significantly higher levels than did seventh-grade boys (Robinson and Klesges 1997). At least three studies have examined gender-specific differences in perceived social norms of adolescent smoking and smoking initiation. In two studies, significantly more females than males reported social norms as a reason for experimenting with cigarettes or beginning to smoke (Botvin et al. 1992; Sarason et al. 1992). In the third study, the opposite gender-specific effect was observed (Chassin et al. 1984).

### Perceived Peer Attitudes Toward Smoking

In one study of a multiethnic sample of adolescents, perceived approval of smoking by one's three best friends was significantly associated with susceptibility to smoking and ever smoking (Gritz et al. 1998). In other studies, even though boys reported more often than girls that their friends' approval of smoking was an important influence on their smoking, peer smoking appeared to be an equally strong risk factor for smoking among girls and boys (Pierce et al. 1993; Flay et al. 1994).

### Strong Attachment to Peers

Among adolescents, strong bonds with parents tend to deter smoking, and strong bonds with peers tend to promote smoking. Indeed, Conrad and colleagues (1992) found that in nine longitudinal studies, adolescents were more likely to experiment with cigarettes or to start smoking regularly if they had developed close emotional attachments to other adolescents, spent more and more time with friends, had a large number of close friends, reported that agreement with peers was increasingly important, or had a boyfriend or girlfriend (Kellam et al. 1980; Ahlgren et al. 1982; Krohn et al. 1983; Murray et al. 1983; Chassin et al. 1984; Skinner et al. 1985; Semmer et al. 1987; Sussman et al. 1987; McNeill et al. 1989). Several studies have reported no gender-specific differences in the effects of peer bonds on smoking (McNeill et al. 1989; Swan et al. 1990; Sussman et al. 1994). One study among African Americans, however, showed that the number of close friends an adolescent reported having was a predictor of smoking initiation for boys only (Brunswick and Messeri 1983–84). In another study, positive social events and peer support increased the likelihood of smoking among more girls than boys (Wills 1986), and Best and colleagues (1995) suggested that among adolescents for whom peer approval is especially important, girls may be more likely than boys to smoke.

### Interaction of Social Influences

Flay and associates (1994) tested a model that examined how the following factors interact to influence smoking initiation among adolescents: (1) friends' smoking, (2) parental smoking, (3) expectation of negative outcome from smoking, (4) perceived friends' approval of smoking, (5) perceived parental approval of smoking, (6) refusal self-efficacy (i.e., confidence in one's ability to resist temptations to try smoking), and (7) intention to smoke or not to smoke. The findings showed that friends' smoking influenced smoking initiation both directly and indirectly and that friends' smoking was a stronger influence than parental smoking. Parental smoking had a stronger effect among girls than among boys, but this gender-specific influence was tempered by parental approval or disapproval of smoking. Disapproval mediated the influence of parental smoking among girls but not among boys, and parental approval was an important predictor that girls would start to smoke. These results are consistent with other findings that girls may be more susceptible than boys to social influences, especially parental influences (see "Parental Smoking" earlier in this chapter). No significant gender-specific differences were observed in how the pathways from self-efficacy and expectations of negative outcome affected smoking initiation.

Previous research suggested that parental influence, in general, remains constant or decreases but that the influence of peers increases as adolescents develop (e.g., Krosnick and Judd 1982). A more recent study indicated that the pattern of change in parental and peer influences on smoking may differ among girls and boys (Hu et al. 1995a). In this longitudinal study, data were collected at four time points from grades seven through nine. Smoking status was predicted by using previous smoking status and the effects of time, friends' smoking, and parental smoking. In general, the effects of friends' smoking were stronger than the influence of parental smoking, and the effects of friends' smoking appeared to increase over time, whereas the influence of parental smoking remained fairly constant. Although parental smoking predicted initiation and escalation of smoking equally, friends' smoking was more predictive of initiation than of escalation. The effects of friends' smoking were stronger among girls than among boys, and the tendency for the influence of friends to increase with time was also more noticeable among girls.

Pederson and colleagues (1998) examined the dose-response relationships between various social variables (e.g., maternal smoking, parental approval of smoking, sibling smoking, and friends' smoking) and smoking status among eighth-grade students. The study revealed strong dose-response relationships between these social variables and smoking status for the entire group and, in most cases, among females and males when data were analyzed separately.

## Personal Characteristics

### Socioeconomic Status and Parental Education

Several studies have shown that low socioeconomic status puts adolescents at higher risk for smoking (Conrad et al. 1992; USDHHS 1994). At least three studies have examined whether the risk for smoking among daughters and sons is affected differently by the socioeconomic status of their parents. Findings in two studies suggested that low socioeconomic status places girls at higher risk than boys (Chassin et al. 1992; Glendinning et al. 1994). The third study produced a contrary finding, but it was conducted among college students, a group in which low socioeconomic status may have been underrepresented (Gottlieb and Baker 1986).

National surveys consistently showed that education (number of years of schooling) is inversely related to cigarette smoking among women and men (see Chapter 2). However, data from the Monitoring the Future Surveys provided little evidence of a gender-specific effect of parental education on risk for smoking among high school seniors for the period 1994–1998. Among seniors whose parents had not graduated from high school, females were more likely than males to smoke, but in general the prevalence of current smoking among both females and males differed little across level of parental education (see "Relationship of Smoking to Sociodemographic Factors" in Chapter 2 and Table 2.11).

Ferrence (1988) proposed a model of diffusion of innovations (Rogers and Shoemaker 1971) to help elucidate gender-specific differences in relation to initiation and cessation of smoking. In general, persons with better economic resources, more education, and greater power adopt new ideas and behaviors and accumulate material goods earlier than those with fewer such resources. This fact may explain why men historically started smoking before women did. Gender-specific differences in relation to economic resources, education, and power have changed over time in concert with changes in the roles of women in society. The first women to smoke were those who, by virtue of their resources, were considered avant-garde. Similarly, in recent decades, the reduction in smoking prevalence occurred first among persons having greater resources. This explanation is supported by theories on social roles (Dicken 1978, 1982; Deaux and Major 1987; Eagly 1987; Waldron 1991).

### Behavioral Control

Theories on smoking and drug use (Petraitis et al. 1995) contend that persons may be unable to resist temptations to smoke if they are unable to control certain other behaviors, including tendencies to be impulsive, easily distracted, or aggressive or to exhibit type A behavior. Studies have shown that smoking was more common among (1) adolescents who reported getting into trouble at school (Krohn et al. 1986); (2) young adults who had been aggressive, quarrelsome, and impatient at age 8 years (Pulkkinen 1982); (3) young adults who as children did not solve problems reasonably, did not negotiate with others, and were not conciliatory toward others (Pulkkinen 1982); and (4) adults who demonstrated type A behavior (Forgays et al. 1993).

Results in several studies suggested that a lack of behavioral control plays a larger role in smoking among girls than among boys. Aggressive behavior may put girls at significantly higher risk than boys for succumbing to peer pressures to smoke (Stanton et al. 1995). In one study, young women, but not young men, were more likely to initiate smoking as adolescents if they focused more on short-term goals than on long-term goals (Brunswick and Messeri 1983–84).

### Sociability

Adolescents who are shy or lack social skills may find it especially difficult to resist peer pressure to smoke. Studies indicated that adolescents may view smoking as a vehicle for entering a desired friendship group (e.g., Aloise-Young et al. 1994), but two studies suggested that this is true only among boys (Gottlieb and Green 1984; Allen et al. 1994). In a study of girl and boy smokers and nonsmokers, Allen and coworkers (1994) concluded that adolescent boys may have used smoking to cope with social insecurity, whereas adolescent girls who smoked were more socially competent and self-confident than were girls who did not smoke. Killen and colleagues (1997) also found that sociability was related to smoking initiation among adolescent girls.

### Fatalism and External Locus of Control

Persons who have an external locus of control generally believe that their lives are controlled by external forces (e.g., fate or God) and may believe that they can do little to prevent negative events from affecting them. In one study, investigators found no link between locus of control during adolescence and smoking during adulthood (Winefield et al. 1992). Other studies, however, suggested that fatalism and an external locus of control are associated with smoking initiation (Brunswick and Messeri 1984; Chassin et al. 1984).

**Intelligence, Academic Performance, and Commitment to School**

In their analysis of data from the 1990 California Youth Tobacco Survey, Hu and colleagues (1998) found that students who reported their performance in school as below average were more likely than better-than-average students to be current or former smokers. They found no gender-specific differences in the likelihood of being a former smoker or in attempts to stop smoking. An earlier study found that scores on tests of intelligence and readiness for school during first grade were not related to smoking among 16- and 17-year-old African American girls or boys (Kellam et al. 1980). Another study of adolescents reported that poorer academic achievement increased the risk for smoking among girls and boys, but that the importance of two achievement measures differed; reading test scores were stronger predictors among girls, whereas grade point average better predicted smoking among boys (Brunswick and Messeri 1983–84, 1984).

Weak commitment to school consistently predicts the initiation and progression of smoking among adolescents (Conrad et al. 1992). In one longitudinal study, investigators found no gender-specific difference in the effect of weak school bonds on subsequent smoking (Ensminger et al. 1982). However, three other studies suggested that commitment to school affects girls more strongly than it affects boys (Hibbett and Fogelman 1990; Waldron et al. 1991; Skinner and Krohn 1992), and one study reported the reverse (Chassin et al. 1984). Because of these conflicting findings, no conclusion can be drawn about gender-specific differences in relation to school bonds and adolescent smoking.

**Rebelliousness, Risk Taking, and Other Health-Related Behaviors**

Longitudinal studies of smoking consistently have shown that adolescents are at risk for smoking if they previously rebelled against rules, teachers, or adults in general (Mittelmark et al. 1987); opposed disciplinary rules at school (Murray et al. 1983); or tolerated deviant behavior in others (Chassin et al. 1984). Although adolescent rebelliousness appears to be less common among girls than among boys (Robinson and Klesges 1997), findings in some longitudinal studies suggested that rebelliousness and tolerance for unconventional behavior may affect smoking initiation among girls and boys equally (Skinner and Krohn 1992; Simon et al. 1995). However, several studies have shown that smoking was more highly correlated among girls than among boys in regard to the following characteristics: rebelliousness (Pierce et al. 1993), feelings of being decreasingly bound by laws and parental rules (Skinner et al. 1985), higher levels of both rebelliousness and rejection of adult authority (Best et al. 1995), and tolerance of deviant behavior (Chassin et al. 1984). Stanton and colleagues (1995) found that delinquency significantly increased the risk for smoking among girls but was not related to smoking among boys. One study found that 17-year-old girls were more likely than boys the same age to smoke experimentally if they went to bars, taverns, or nightclubs; had been in trouble with the police; or had been involved in fights (Waldron et al. 1991). Findings from this study paralleled earlier reports about rebelliousness (Sussman et al. 1987).

Sensation seeking has been defined as willingness to take risks for the sake of stimulation and arousal (Zuckerman et al. 1987). Sensation seeking and risk taking appear to be related to smoking among adolescents (Simon et al. 1995; Petridou et al. 1997; Wahlgren et al. 1997; Coogan et al. 1998).

Clustering of smoking and other unhealthy behaviors suggested the formation of a "risk behavior syndrome" during adolescence (Escobedo et al. 1997). This syndrome may emerge as early as elementary school (Coogan et al. 1998). Data from the National Health Interview Survey indicated that smoking aggregates with marijuana use, binge drinking, and fighting among African Americans, Hispanics, and whites of both genders (Escobedo et al. 1997). Other U.S. national survey data also showed a strong relationship between smoking and use of other substances, including alcohol, among girls and young women (see Chapter 2). A British study examined smoking status, exercise, and dietary behaviors among 14- and 15-year-old adolescents (Coulson et al. 1997). Smoking was associated with lower levels of exercise, lower consumption of fruits and vegetables, and greater consumption of high-fat foods. In addition, evidence from the Youth Risk Behavior Survey suggested that participating in interscholastic sports inhibits the development of regular and heavy smoking among adolescents (Escobedo et al. 1993). Furthermore, some studies reported that the more physically active and fit adolescent girls were, the less likely they were to initiate smoking (e.g., Waldron et al. 1991; Aaron et al. 1995). A British study found that girls who had a teenage pregnancy were more likely to smoke cigarettes than were girls who had not been pregnant (Seamark and Gray 1998).

Results from the longitudinal Minnesota Heart Health Program provided evidence that smoking, physical inactivity, and poor dietary preferences cluster in childhood and tend to endure through adolescence (Kelder et al. 1994; Lytle et al. 1995). Similar clustering of smoking and other unhealthy behaviors were reported in an Australian study with follow-up on a cohort of persons aged 9 years through early adulthood (Burke et al. 1997). At age 18 years, smoking, excessive alcohol use, and poor dietary preferences were clustered among both women and men; physical inactivity was also part of the cluster among women.

### Religiousness

Most studies on the relationship between religiousness and smoking suggested that religious beliefs are important in the decision of some persons not to smoke. After age 17 years, young women who attended church only occasionally were more than twice as likely to start smoking as were those who attended regularly (Daly et al. 1993). In general, more women than men report religious commitment, which appears to be associated with a lower rate of smoking among women (Reynolds and Nichols 1976; Brook et al. 1987; Grunberg et al. 1991; Waldron 1991). Study data indicated that among high school seniors of both genders, the prevalence of smoking is inversely related to the self-reported importance of religion (see "Relationship of Smoking to Sociodemographic Factors" in Chapter 2). In three studies that examined gender-specific differences in religious attitudes among adolescents, religion deterred smoking among females more than it did among males, and a lack of religious commitment contributed to smoking among females more than it did among males (Gottlieb and Green 1984; Krohn et al. 1986; Waldron et al. 1991). In contrast, Skinner and colleagues (1985) found that religiousness had no effect on smoking by either gender.

### Self-Esteem

Adolescents who have poor self-esteem may have difficulty resisting pressures to smoke, especially if they believe that smoking will enhance their image. In some longitudinal studies, adolescents with low self-esteem were significantly more likely than those with high self-esteem to start smoking within the next year (Ahlgren et al. 1982; Simon et al. 1995). Other longitudinal studies, however, detected no link between self-esteem and subsequent smoking (Brunswick and Messeri 1983–84; Winefield et al. 1992). One study showed that girls who scored high on personal dissatisfaction (e.g., desire to have more friends, be thinner, or be less socially anxious) were more likely to smoke than were girls who appeared to be more personally satisfied (Best et al. 1995). This relationship between personal dissatisfaction and smoking was not observed among boys. Similar findings from another study suggested that self-esteem may be a factor in the smoking behavior among girls in grades six through eight but not among males in any grade (Abernathy et al. 1995).

### Emotional Distress

Theories of smoking and drug use have suggested that persons may have difficulty resisting temptations to smoke if they are anxious, hostile, irritable, depressed, or psychologically distressed (Petraitis et al. 1995). Evidence of a link between emotional distress and smoking is mixed, however. Many of the studies have focused on adults, so it is not clear to what extent the findings can be extrapolated to smoking initiation, which generally occurs among adolescents. Some investigators have found no association between smoking, hopelessness, stress, nervousness, negative mood, psychological disturbances, or level of anxiety (Winefield et al. 1992; Simon et al. 1995). Others have found links between smoking and anger (Modrcin-McCarthy and Tollett 1993); stress (Wills 1986); stressful life events (Frone et al. 1994); depression (Pederson et al. 1998); and anxiety levels, physical complaints, and hostility (Forgays et al. 1993; Schifano et al. 1994). A study by Johnson and Gilbert (1991) reported that the intense feelings of anger and irritability were related to both smoking initiation and maintenance among African American adolescents, whereas among white adolescents these emotions were associated only with smoking initiation. One qualitative investigation reported that the most frequent reasons for smoking among girls in grades 10 and 11 were stress reduction and relaxation (Nichter et al. 1997). Although exceptions have been reported (Oleckno and Blacconiere 1990; Allen et al. 1994; Frone et al. 1994), findings in several studies suggested that symptoms of distress are more strongly associated with smoking among females than among males (Brunswick and Messeri 1984; Gottlieb and Green 1984; Knott 1984; Semmer et al. 1987; Lee et al. 1988; Waldron et al. 1991; Pierce et al. 1993).

### Coping Styles

Two studies have examined whether there are gender-specific differences in the link between smoking levels and the way persons cope with their problems, but such differences do not appear to exist. In one study, MacLean and coworkers (1996) found no connection between smoking level during the past month and the frequency with which 17-year-old girls and boys used various strategies (e.g., getting angry) to cope with problems. In a study of 12-year-olds, Wills and Vaughan (1989) examined the relationship between current smoking and earlier tendencies to seek adult or parental help with problems, but they found no differences by gender in this relationship. These researchers did find that, among adolescents who had previously relied on peers for help with problems, girls were far more likely than boys to smoke, but it is unclear whether this effect related primarily to coping styles or to peer attachments.

### Perceived Refusal Skills

Adolescents who are confident of their ability to resist pressures to smoke may be better able to avoid smoking than those who are not confident. Although girls may have stronger doubts about avoiding cigarette smoking in the future than do boys (van Roosmalen and McDaniel 1992), attempts to reduce those doubts appear to have the same effect among girls and boys. Findings in experimental studies suggested that refusal skills can be taught effectively to both girls and boys (Sallis et al. 1990), and results of longitudinal studies suggested that self-doubts about the ability to refuse offers to smoke affect girls and boys equally (Lawrance and Rubinson 1986; Flay et al. 1994). In one study, however, this finding was not true among all racial and ethnic groups; for 13-year-old Asian children who one year earlier had doubted their ability to refuse an offer of a cigarette, the prevalence of smoking was higher among boys than among girls (Sussman et al. 1987).

### Previous Experimentation with Tobacco and Intention to Smoke

Findings in three longitudinal studies suggested that girls and boys who experiment with cigarettes during adolescence are at generally similar risk for progression from experimentation to regular smoking. In two of these studies, the investigators found no gender-specific differences in the link between experimental smoking during adolescence and regular smoking during early adulthood (Chassin et al. 1990; McGee and Stanton 1993). In the third study, the researchers found that the amount smoked at ages 10 through 13 years was strongly related to the amount smoked at ages 14 through 17 years and that the link between previous and current smoking may have been stronger among boys than among girls (Skinner and Krohn 1992). Two studies showed that girls and boys were equally likely to smoke if at least one year earlier they had thought they might smoke in the future (Ary and Biglan 1988; McNeill et al. 1989). In a large study of 4,500 adolescents, the lack of a firm decision not to smoke was a strong baseline predictor of both experimentation and progression to regular smoking (Pierce et al. 1996). However, intention was not as important as exposure to other smokers in influencing the transition from experimentation to regular smoking. No gender differences were found.

### Susceptibility to Smoking

As smoking prevention moves toward use of more tailored and individualized programs, identifying precursors of smoking initiation becomes increasingly important. The ability to classify adolescents as being at higher or at lower risk for smoking initiation is critical to the development of appropriate intervention techniques.

Two theoretical concepts appear to be particularly useful for identifying adolescents at risk for smoking initiation: the transtheoretical model of change (Prochaska et al. 1992; Pallonen 1998; Pallonen et al. 1998) and susceptibility to smoking (Pierce et al. 1996). The transtheoretical model of change postulates gradual progression through a series of discrete stages of cognitive and behavioral change, simultaneously integrating constructs such as stages of change, decisional balance (pros and cons of smoking behavior), situational temptations to try smoking (Hudmon et al. 1997), and self-efficacy. Pallonen and colleagues (1998) proposed integration of the stages of adolescent smoking initiation and cessation. The four stages of smoking initiation are (1) acquisition-precontemplation, (2) acquisition-contemplation, (3) acquisition-preparation, and (4) recent acquisition. These stages have been validated in a sample of high school students. The scores for perceived advantages (pros) of smoking and temptations to try smoking were closely related to the stages of smoking initiation. The continuum based on the four stages of change appears to provide a concise and theoretically sound approach to smoking initiation in adolescent populations.

Susceptibility to smoking is a measure of intention to smoke. According to this concept, "susceptible" adolescents exhibit a lack of firm commitment not to smoke in the future. The construct of susceptibility to smoking has been used in the California Tobacco Survey and other studies; its rationale and validation have been extensively presented in the literature (Pierce et al. 1995, 1996; Unger et al. 1997; Jackson 1998). Adolescents are susceptible to smoking if they have made no determined decision not to smoke in the next year or if offered a cigarette by a friend. The susceptibility measure integrates intentions and expectations of future behavior; therefore, it identifies persons with a cognitive predisposition to smoking. Longitudinal studies have demonstrated that susceptibility is a stronger predictor of smoking experimentation among both females and males than are other well-established predictors, such as exposure to smokers in the immediate social environment (Pierce et al. 1996; Jackson 1998). A recent study reported that the susceptibility construct can predict who among adolescent experimental smokers will become established smokers (Distefan et al. 1998).

## Expectations of Personal Effects of Smoking

### Beliefs About Effects on Image and Health

In several longitudinal studies of smoking among adolescents, smoking was more common among persons who lacked knowledge of the health consequences of smoking, doubted that nicotine is addictive, and had mostly positive beliefs about smoking (Conrad et al. 1992). Attitudes that put adolescents at risk for smoking included (1) having tolerance for smoking by others, (2) believing that smoking makes people look good and enhances their image, (3) having the opinion that smoking is fun or pleasant, (4) expecting generally positive consequences from smoking, and (5) placing more value on the perceived positive results of smoking than on the negative consequences. The belief that smoking makes people have an unpleasant smell, look silly, or feel sick reduced the risk for smoking.

Evidence suggested that some attitudes about smoking are especially important among girls. In some studies, girls were found to be at higher risk than boys for smoking if they thought the harmful effects of smoking had been exaggerated (Waldron et al. 1991) or if they dismissed the health hazards of smoking (Swan et al. 1990). In a study of persons 18 through 23 years old, thoughts about health were an important deterrent to smoking among women but not among men (Brunswick and Messeri 1983–84). However, another study showed that boys expected more benefits from smoking than did girls and that the relationship between the expected number of benefits and susceptibility to smoking was stronger among boys than among girls (Pierce et al. 1993).

Findings have been inconclusive on gender-specific differences in whether smokers are perceived to be mature, confident, and self-reliant. In one study, this image was positively associated with smoking among both girls and boys (McGee and Stanton 1993), but in two other studies, such an image was more important among girls than among boys (Mittelmark et al. 1987; Waldron et al. 1991), while in another study such an image was more important among boys than among girls (Dinh et al. 1995).

### Concerns About Weight Control

Many girls believe that smoking helps to control weight by suppressing appetite (USDHHS 1980; Klesges et al. 1989, 1997). Findings in several cross-sectional studies suggested that concerns about body weight and dieting are related to smoking status among adolescent girls (Charlton 1984; Gritz and Crane 1991; Pirie et al. 1991). Among 1,915 students in grades 10 through 12 in one school district in Mississippi, girls who smoked were more likely than girls who did not smoke to perceive themselves as fat (Page et al. 1993). This association was not found among boys. Both girls and boys who smoked were less satisfied with their weight than were nonsmokers. A study of Catholic high school students in Memphis, Tennessee, found that among white students who smoked more than once a week, girls (39 percent) were significantly more likely than boys (12 percent) to use smoking in an attempt to control weight (Camp et al. 1993). A longitudinal study of 1,705 students in grades 7 through 10 indicated that concerns about weight and dieting behaviors (e.g., constant thoughts about weight and trying to lose weight) were positively related to smoking initiation among girls but not among boys (French et al. 1994). At baseline, fear of gaining weight, the desire to be thin, and trying to lose weight were also positively related to current smoking among girls.

Although most of these studies reported a relationship between smoking status and concerns about weight, investigators in only one study (Camp et al. 1993) controlled for many other known correlates of smoking: age, race and ethnicity, number of smoking models (e.g., peers who smoke), perceived value of smoking, degree of social support, risk-taking behavior, rebelliousness, and pharmacologic and emotional reactions to early experimentation with smoking. In that study, being female predicted smoking for weight control reasons.

Most of these studies on adolescents' beliefs about smoking and weight control were conducted primarily or exclusively among white study participants. The processes of smoking initiation may be different across racial and ethnic groups (Flay et al. 1994; Klesges and Robinson 1995). For example, according to a school-based survey conducted in the early 1980s, concerns about weight and dieting may have been less important among African American girls than among white girls (Sussman et al. 1987). In a survey of 6,967 seventh-grade adolescents in an urban school system, Robinson and colleagues (1997) found that African American adolescents who knew about the weight-suppressing effect of smoking were less likely to experiment with cigarettes than were those who believed that smoking had no effect on weight. Among white adolescents, weight control beliefs were not associated with cigarette experimentation. No gender differences were reported.

#### Beliefs About Mood Control and Depression

The belief that smoking can control negative moods and produce positive moods is important among many girls. One study showed that girls were no more likely than boys to smoke for relaxation or relief from problems or anxieties (McGee and Stanton 1993). However, at least two studies showed that females were more likely than males to say that they smoked to control negative emotions (Semmer et al. 1987; Novacek et al. 1991). Pirie and associates (1991) also found that young women who smoked were significantly more likely than young men who smoked to say that they would be tense and irritable if they stopped smoking.

Depression in adolescence predicts depression in young adulthood (Kandel and Davies 1986) and may have an important interrelationship with smoking. Among adults, major depression is strongly related to smoking (Anda et al. 1990; Glassman et al. 1990; Kendler et al. 1993), although neither the directionality of the association nor its gender-specific effect is completely understood. Findings in a large cross-sectional study suggested that depression and anxiety were associated with smoking among teenage girls of all ages but only among younger teenage boys (Patton et al. 1996). A study in Atlanta of 1,731 youths aged 8 through 14 years who were assessed at least twice from 1989 through 1994 found that antecedent tobacco smoking was associated with an increased risk for subsequent depressed mood but that antecedent depressed mood was not associated with risk for subsequently initiating smoking (Wu and Anthony 1999). Findings were not presented separately by gender, but gender was included in multivariate analyses and was not an independent predictor of smoking initiation. (See "Depression and Other Psychiatric Disorders" in Chapter 3.)

### Biological Factors

A growing body of research has explored the interaction between genetic and environmental influences on both initiation and maintenance of smoking (reviewed by Heath and Madden 1995); this work has often been based on complex statistical and genetic models. Studies of monozygotic and dizygotic twins (Boomsa et al. 1994; Maes et al. 1999) or of twins reared apart and reared together (Kendler et al. 2000) suggested that heritable factors account for a substantial proportion of the observed variation in tobacco use, although the range of estimates across studies is wide.

Epidemiologic studies among adults provided additional evidence of genetic predisposition to cigarette smoking. For example, Spitz and associates (1998) reported that patients with lung cancer who had genetic polymorphism at the locus for the $D_2$ dopamine receptor were more likely to have started smoking at an earlier age and to have smoked more heavily than those without the polymorphism. Lerman and colleagues (1999) reported that the dopamine transporter gene, *SLC6A3-9*, may influence smoking initiation before the age of 16 years, but gender-specific results were not reported. Currently this is an active area of investigation, and further exploration of genetic factors, particularly in racially and ethnically diverse populations, is warranted.

Some studies suggested gender differences in nicotine metabolism (Grunberg et al. 1991) or suggested that women trying to quit are more likely to report withdrawal symptoms than are men (Gritz et al. 1996) or are likely to recall their withdrawal symptoms as more severe than do men (Pomerleau et al. 1994). However, it appears that differences in metabolism may not exist once amount of smoking is controlled for (see "Nicotine Pharmacology and Addiction" in Chapter 3), and it is unclear whether differences in withdrawal responses are subjective or physiologic (Niaura et al. 1998; Eissenberg et al. 1999). Sussman and colleagues (1998) reported that adolescent female smokers were more likely than their male counterparts to report having difficulty going a day without smoking, but it is not known whether any gender differences related to nicotine metabolism or sensitivity exist that affect initiation.

Little is known about whether endogenous hormones affect the likelihood of smoking initiation among females. The findings of Bauman and colleagues (1992) suggested that testosterone levels among girls but not among boys increase receptivity to the influence of maternal smoking—girls with relatively high testosterone levels may be more likely than girls with low testosterone levels to model their mothers' smoking behavior. Using blood samples obtained from a cohort of pregnant women in the 1960s, Kandel and Udry (1999) reported a positive correlation between maternal prenatal testosterone levels and subsequent smoking among female offspring at adolescence. Also, early onset of puberty may prompt girls to smoke (Wilson et al. 1994); this phenomenon may reflect either hormonal levels or social pressures associated with early puberty. Further research is needed to determine whether hormones influence smoking initiation.

### Summary

This qualitative assessment revealed a considerable degree of inconsistency in research findings across studies that have examined gender-specific differences in smoking initiation. Some of the inconsistency resulted from differences in the study populations examined and from differences in study design and quality. However, considering the literature as a whole, certain conclusions seem warranted. Most risk factors for smoking initiation appear to be similar among girls and boys. Evidence indicated that strength of attachment to family and friends and smoking by parents and peers have considerable influence on smoking initiation, but study results were inconsistent, which makes it not possible to conclude that girls and boys are differentially affected by such factors. Likewise, perceptions about norms, prevalence of smoking, and attitudes of peers toward smoking, as well as commitment to school, are strong predictors of smoking initiation; whether they affect girls and boys differently is unclear. Some studies suggested that girls are more likely than boys to smoke if they are rebellious, reject conventional values, or lack commitment to religion. Others suggested that poor self-esteem and emotional distress are more strongly associated with smoking initiation among girls than among boys. Among girls, however, those who are more sociable appear to be at higher risk for smoking initiation than are less socially confident girls. Girls also appear to be especially affected by a positive image of smoking, desire for weight control, and the perception that smoking controls negative moods. Both genders appear similarly affected by coping style, poor refusal skills, low self-efficacy, previous use of tobacco, and intention to smoke. Studies of genetic and hormonal factors in relation to smoking initiation have only recently begun, and it is premature to draw conclusions regarding gender-specific differences related to such factors. Advertising and promotion of tobacco products also affect the likelihood of initiation (see "Influence of Tobacco Marketing on Smoking Initiation by Females" later in this chapter).

## Factors Influencing Maintenance or Cessation of Smoking

### Overview of the Studies Examined

Factors that influence continuation of smoking exert an effect throughout the lives of smokers. The interrelationship of these factors is complex, but the data on maintenance or cessation of smoking have not been as extensive as the data on smoking initiation. Although considerable effort has been invested in studies to assess therapeutic methods of achieving smoking cessation (Fiore et al. 2000), few longitudinal studies have examined predictors of continued smoking, attempts to stop smoking, short- or long-term cessation, or relapse to smoking among women who smoke regularly and are not enrolled in smoking cessation programs.

To assess studies of smoking maintenance and cessation, a general-purpose framework was used in the 1989 Surgeon General's report on the health consequences of smoking (USDHHS 1989, Chapter 5, Part II). The report discussed three general types of predictors of maintenance or cessation of smoking:

(1) pharmacologic processes and conditions, which are basic factors that interact to produce addiction and to support continued smoking (e.g., number of cigarettes smoked, number of previous attempts to stop smoking, and number of years of smoking);

(2) cognition and decision-making ability (e.g., knowledge about the effects of smoking on health, motivation to continue or to stop smoking, and confidence in one's ability to stop smoking); and

(3) personal characteristics and social context (personality, demographic factors, and environmental influences).

The "transtheoretical model" of Prochaska and colleagues (1992) posits a sequence of five stages in the process of smoking cessation: precontemplation, contemplation, preparation, action, and maintenance of cessation. This model, often referred to as the stages of change model, provides a template for evaluating willingness to change. It has been used in many studies of smoking cessation and as an adjunct to clinical and public health smoking cessation programs.

A major conclusion of the 1980 Surgeon General's report on the health consequences of smoking among women was that "Women at higher education and income levels are more likely to succeed in quitting" (USDHHS 1980, p. 347). The report also noted that successful smoking cessation is associated with a strong commitment to change, involvement in programs that use behavioral techniques, and social support for smoking cessation. These conclusions were based on information about persons who sought treatment to stop smoking; the conclusions revealed little about successful efforts by persons who did not seek treatment. Furthermore, the report recommended development of intervention strategies to target social norms and the particular needs and concerns among women, such as social support and weight gain. According to the report, the longitudinal data available were insufficient to address the factors that influence the cessation process among active smokers. Before 1980, only one longitudinal study of the psychosocial and behavioral aspects of smoking among women had been conducted (Cherry and Kiernan 1976).

Because most smokers, both women and men, stop smoking without formal cessation programs (Schwartz and Dubitzky 1967; Fiore et al. 1990; Yankelovich Partners 1998), understanding the factors that contribute to their attempts to stop smoking and their success in doing so would be helpful in the planning of public health efforts and smoking cessation programs. Both cross-sectional and longitudinal designs have been used to investigate factors related to changes in smoking status among adults who smoke regularly. Cross-sectional study designs have well-recognized limitations, most notably that the temporal relationship between smoking outcomes and predictor variables cannot be satisfactorily assessed (Flay et al. 1983; Chassin et al. 1986; Collins et al. 1987; Conrad et al. 1992). In contrast, even though longitudinal studies do not prove causation, they can be used to place potential predictors and outcomes in temporal sequence and, thus, to suggest possible cause-and-effect relationships (Conrad et al. 1992). Thousands of studies of smoking and its determinants have been conducted, but despite the plea of the Surgeon General's report in 1980, very few longitudinal studies have investigated factors related to changes in the smoking behavior among women who have not enrolled in cessation programs or who have not participated in laboratory studies.

This review includes longitudinal observational studies in which female smokers were surveyed and were followed up over time. Studies that provided results for female smokers and male smokers separately also were included in this review to examine differences in predictors of smoking status between females and males. Studies were excluded for one or more of the following reasons: (1) Results were based on data from smokers exposed to an intervention. (2) Results were based on cross-sectional data, even though the data were collected as part of a longitudinal study. (3) Data analyses did not examine factors related to smoking outcome, did not stratify by gender, or did not examine changes in smoking behavior over time. (4) The primary focus of the study was smoking initiation or transition to regular smoking among adolescents or adults who had previously stopped smoking. (5) The research addressed validity and feasibility of study designs, smoking prevalence, or effects on health rather than smoking maintenance and cessation.

With the use of these guidelines, only 13 studies were selected after review of 2,552 abstracts of research published between 1966 and May 1999; they are available in the MEDLINE, PsycINFO, and Psychlit databases. One unpublished study was also identified through consultation with experts in the field of smoking and health.

Of the 13 studies of smoking maintenance or cessation reviewed here (Table 4.2), 6 included women only, and 7 included both women and men. Study populations ranged from children and adolescents who were followed up into young adulthood to persons aged 65 years or older at enrollment in the study. Four studies were part of national surveys, and 1 study focused on data from a registry of twins. Seven studies were conducted in the United States; the remaining 6 were performed in Denmark, England, Finland, Norway, and Sweden. Most of the studies involved urban populations.

Eight studies used self-administered questionnaires to determine smoking status; five used either telephone or household in-person interviews. Although retrospective data on smoking status during pregnancy were included in two studies, they are likely to be accurate. The information for one of these studies was obtained just two weeks after childbirth and information for the other at the time of delivery, with data on smoking during early pregnancy having been obtained by a nurse or physician at the first routine prenatal visit with a standardized form used in Norway. In two studies, biochemical validation of smoking cessation was performed. Several of the studies were not conducted explicitly to study smoking but included smoking in investigations of other health behaviors or outcomes, such as psychosocial factors affecting infant feeding practices. In the study by O'Campo and colleagues (1992), extensive information on smoking patterns was obtained because it was assumed to be relevant to breastfeeding, but attitudinal and cognitive factors related to smoking behavior were not goals of the study and, thus, were not examined.

Most of the 13 studies focused on a narrow group of predictor variables, which limited the conclusions that could be drawn about the interaction of female gender and other variables. Only two studies (Garvey et al. 1992; Rose et al. 1996) included variables from all three of the domains set forth in the 1989 Surgeon General's report (pharmacologic processes and conditions, cognition and decision-making ability, and personal characteristics and social context). The specific variables and populations in these two studies differed. In all 13 studies, logistic regression, discriminate analysis, or proportional hazard models were used to discriminate between regular smokers at baseline assessment who had stopped smoking by the time of follow-up and those who had not stopped smoking.

A range of criteria was used to define smoking status, and several studies did not clearly define or limit those criteria. For example, one study (Cnattingius et al. 1992) compared continuing smokers with those who had stopped smoking during pregnancy. However, the group of continuing smokers included both women who had stopped smoking and subsequently started again and those who had never stopped smoking during pregnancy. As a result, the differences between smokers and those who had stopped smoking may have been diluted. Only one study (Garvey et al. 1992) involved separate consideration of predictors of early relapse and late relapse to smoking. The time between the first and final follow-up visits ranged from approximately nine months to 15 years in the 13 studies, but changes in baseline characteristics were not taken into account in the presentation of follow-up results. Consequently, if a baseline factor such as depression was measured when a woman was 20 years old but changed over time, conclusions about its relationship to smoking status years later may have been incorrect.

The percentage of women who were regular smokers at the beginning of the studies and for whom complete data were available at two or more follow-up periods ranged from 50 to 98 percent. High attrition is particularly problematic because it is likely not to be random (Ockene et al. 1982).

## Transitions from Regular Smoking

### Attempts to Stop Smoking

In 1987, among those who have ever smoked, only 18.5 percent of men and 19.5 percent of women in the United States reported they had never tried to quit (USDHHS 1990). In 1998, an estimated 39.2 percent of current daily smokers had stopped smoking for at least a day during the preceding 12 months because they were trying to quit (CDC 2000). However, only a small percentage of persons who try to quit in any given year remain abstinent.

Rose and colleagues (1996) examined the natural history of smoking from adolescence to adulthood and evaluated predictors of attempts to stop smoking in the previous five years. The category "quit attempt" included two groups: those who had stopped smoking but started again within six months or fewer, and those who abstained for more than six months. The study participants, females and males in grades 6 through 12 in a midwestern county school

**Table 4.2. Characteristics of 13 longitudinal studies of smoking maintenance and cessation among women who smoked regularly**

| Demographic group/study | Population | End point | Study period | Sample size | Final response rate (%) |
|---|---|---|---|---|---|
| **Young persons** | | | | | |
| Cherry and Kiernan 1976 | Female and male respondents to National Survey of Health and Development who completed the Maudsley Personality Inventory at age 16 years and had follow-up at ages 20 and 25 years<br>England | Relationship of personality scores to changes in smoking behavior | 9 years (1962–1971) | 2,753 | 73 |
| Rose et al. 1996 | Girls and boys in grades 6–12 who were evaluated for psychosocial factors<br>Midwestern United States | Psychosocial measures as predictors of attempts to stop smoking and of smoking cessation in adult regular smokers | Follow-up at 3 and 11 years (1984–1994) | 8,556 | 73 |
| **Pregnant women** | | | | | |
| Cnattingius et al. 1992 | Women registered at prenatal clinic<br>Uppsala, Sweden | Differences in predictors during pregnancy in women who stop smoking and those who continue to smoke | 24–26 and 34–36 weeks' gestation | 1,104 | 98 |
| O'Campo et al. 1992 | Women recruited in third trimester of pregnancy<br>48% white, 52% black<br>Maryland | Sociodemographic factors related to continued smoking during pregnancy; to early postpartum relapse to smoking; and to practices in infant feeding | 1–3 and 6–12 weeks after childbirth | 1,900 | 90 |
| Dejin-Karlsson et al. 1996 | Primigravidas registered at four antenatal clinics over a 1-year period who reported smoking at conception<br>83% Swedish, 17% non-Swedish<br>Malmö, Sweden | Psychosocial factors related to continued smoking during pregnancy | 12 weeks' gestation | 404 | 88 |
| Nafstad et al. 1996 | Mothers of children participating in the Oslo Birth Cohort who had completed information on smoking habits at all three assessments (early pregnancy, delivery, 1 year after childbirth)<br>Norway | Determinants for changes in maternal smoking behavior during and after pregnancy[†] | Early pregnancy, delivery, and 1 year after childbirth | 3,207* | 75 |

*Multivariate analysis conducted on subgroup of 3,039 cohabitating women only.
[†]Cessation attempt: smokers who reported cessation at delivery. Cessation: smokers who reported stopping smoking during 1st year after delivery.

**Table 4.2. Continued**

| Demographic group/study | Population | End point | Study period | Sample size | Final response rate (%) |
|---|---|---|---|---|---|
| **Young and middle-aged adults** | | | | | |
| Colditz et al., unpublished data | National sample of female nurses in Nurses' Health Study<br>United States | Factors affecting smoking and smoking cessation, as determined in a long-term longitudinal study | Follow-up every 2 years for 10 years (1976–1986) | 121,700 | 85 |
| Kaprio and Koskenvuo 1988 | Women and men with a twin<br>~40% smokers<br>Finland | Psychological, socioeconomic, and medical preditors of smoking cessation, continuation of smoking, or never smoking | Follow-up at 6 years | 2,620 | 89 |
| Williamson et al. 1991 | Noninstitutionalized civilian population of women and men from First National Health and Nutrition Examination Study<br>Women: 81% white, 18% black, 0.4% other<br>Men: 85% white, 15% black, 0.4% other<br>United States | Accurate estimates of weight gain related to cessation of smoking in general population | 6.7–12.5 years for women<br>6.7–12.6 years for men | 2,653 | 93 |
| Garvey et al. 1992 | Female and male volunteers who had recently stopped smoking<br>Boston, Massachusetts | Predictors of early and late relapse to smoking in those who tried to stop smoking | Bimonthly follow-up for 1 year | 235 | 90 |
| Hibbard 1993 | Female members of health maintenance organization who smoked and had long-term follow-up<br>United States | Societal factors predicting smoking cessation | ≤ 15 years of follow-up | 168 | 50 |
| Osler 1993 | Random sample of women and men in National Central Person Registry<br>Denmark | Social and individual factors associated with differences in smoking, physical activity, and consumption of fruits and vegetables, as determined in a longitudinal study | Follow-up at 5 years (1982–1987) | 1,675 | 83 |
| **Older adults** | | | | | |
| Salive and Blazer 1993 | Older adult women and men in a large population in Established Populations for the Epidemiologic Studies of the Elderly Trial<br>46% white, 54% black<br>North Carolina | Relationship of smoking cessation and depression in a sample of older adults | 3 years | 677 | 80 |

system, were first surveyed during a three-year period (1980–1983) and again for follow-up periods in 1987 and 1994. The study assessed changes in smoking status as of 1994 among participants who were smokers in 1987. The primary focus was on cognitive factors (e.g., confidence, health beliefs and values, and motivations for smoking) and personal characteristics (e.g., demographics, parental smoking status and education, employment status, social role, and negative affect).

In analyses based on the combined data for females and males, Rose and colleagues (1996) determined that smokers who reported an attempt to stop smoking were more likely to be women, to be married, to have more social roles, and to use smoking to control negative affect. Smokers who reported an attempt to stop smoking also gave higher ratings to the value of health and the perceived likelihood of not smoking in one year than did those who had made no attempt to stop smoking. Female smokers with lower sensory motivation (e.g., less enjoyment in handling a cigarette) were more likely to have attempted to stop smoking, whereas the opposite was true among male smokers. The view that smoking has a negative effect on personal health was related to attempts to stop smoking among heavy smokers but not among light smokers.

Although females were more likely than males to attempt to stop smoking, no gender-specific differences were observed in the success of these attempts (Rose et al. 1996). Because study participants were of childbearing age, pregnancy may have increased the number of attempts among women to stop smoking. The number of cigarettes smoked daily did not affect attempts to stop smoking when other factors were controlled for, but it did affect the success of these attempts. In general, both females and males who attempt to stop smoking may be cognitively more ready to stop (i.e., have higher perceived likelihood of not smoking and higher perceived value of health) than do smokers who do not attempt to stop (Rose et al. 1996). These findings are difficult to generalize, however, because the study population was relatively well educated, white, young, and from the Midwest. In addition, some potentially relevant predictors among women (e.g., motives to control weight and spousal support) were not assessed.

### Smoking Cessation

Because all 13 studies in this overview (Table 4.2) investigated predictors of smoking cessation, considering smoking cessation among young persons, pregnant women, young and middle-aged adults, and older adults separately is possible.

#### *Young Persons*

Two studies focused on smoking cessation among young persons (Cherry and Kiernan 1976; Rose et al. 1996). Cherry and Kiernan examined the relationship between personality scores and smoking behavior in a cohort of respondents to the National Survey of Health and Development, which was conducted in England. A geographically diverse sample of young persons was surveyed at age 16 years in 1962, age 20 years in 1966, and age 25 years in 1971. At baseline, participants completed the Maudsley Personality Inventory (Eysenck 1958), and information about smoking behavior was obtained at the follow-up intervals. By age 25 years, complete information on both cigarette smoking and personality was available for 2,753 of the 5,362 persons included in the baseline survey, excluding cigar and pipe smokers. The definition of smoking cessation did not specify a period of abstinence, but smokers who had "given up smoking" by age 25 years were considered "quitters" (Cherry and Kiernan 1976).

Variables studied by Cherry and Kiernan (1976) included some measures of pharmacologic and conditioning processes (e.g., age at smoking initiation, smoking rate, and degree of inhalation) as well as personal characteristics (e.g., personality traits of neuroticism or extroversion). Basic differences in personality traits were found among current smokers, former smokers, and nonsmokers. Separate assessments were made for females and males. Among both genders, smokers had higher scores for extroversion than did nonsmokers and former smokers had the highest mean score, but this score was not significantly higher than that among current smokers. Scores on the extroversion scale predicted smoking cessation by age 25 years, and extroverts were more likely than introverts to stop smoking. The number of cigarettes smoked also predicted smoking cessation by age 25 years; smokers who consumed fewer than 10 cigarettes per day were more likely to stop smoking. Higher scores for neuroticism predicted smoking cessation among males but not among females.

The study by Rose and colleagues (1996), described earlier, examined psychosocial predictors of attempts to stop smoking and of successful attempts. More females than males attempted to stop smoking, but gender was not related to successful smoking cessation. These findings differed from results of the cross-sectional component of the Community

Intervention Trial for Smoking Cessation. In that trial, investigators studied 3,553 adults (51 percent women) in 20 U.S. communities. They found that women were as likely as men to attempt to stop smoking but were less likely to remain abstinent (Royce et al. 1997).

Rose and associates (1996) found that the following factors were predictors of success in attempts to stop smoking: achieving higher educational level, consuming fewer cigarettes, having greater expectation of not smoking in one year, valuing health, reporting less social pressure to stop smoking, and not living with children. Gender was included as a covariate, but none of these variables interacted significantly with gender. Except for not living with children, these factors also were related to smoking cessation in a prospective intervention study of men only (e.g., Ockene et al. 1982). Prospective studies of women and men that did not stratify results by gender found that factors related to smoking cessation were lower level of depression (Anda et al. 1990; Breslau et al. 1993), incompatibility of social role with smoking (Hellman et al. 1991), and higher level of social support for not smoking (Sorensen and Pechacek 1987; Ockene 1993; Royce et al. 1997).

Both studies reviewed here (Cherry and Kiernan 1976; Rose et al. 1996) suggested that low cigarette consumption at baseline predicted smoking cessation; findings were similar by gender. Other variables in the pharmacologic and conditioning domain were not predictive. (Rose and colleagues [1996] defined early initiation as the start of smoking in grades 6 through 12 and late initiation as the start of smoking after high school. Cherry and Kiernan [1976], on the other hand, used smoking by age 16 years as the cutoff for early initiation.) Rose and colleagues (1996) found that participants' self-ratings of their likelihood of not smoking in one year predicted smoking cessation in the total sample but not among females or males separately. Longitudinal studies that did not report results specifically for women showed that positive self-efficacy and confidence in one's ability to stop smoking predicted abstinence (Ockene et al. 1981; Yates and Thain 1985; Gritz et al. 1988; Wojcik 1988; Haaga 1990; Ockene et al. 1992; Schmitz et al. 1993; de Vries and Backbier 1994; Gulliver et al. 1995). In one study (Wojcik 1988), self-efficacy was a strong predictor of abstinence among smokers who tried to stop smoking on their own but not among those who attended a smoking cessation program.

The relationship between negative affect and smoking outcomes varied. Young persons in the study by Rose and coworkers (1996) who reported that they smoked to control negative affect, and who thus may have had relatively poor coping skills, were more likely to attempt cessation but less likely to succeed than were those who did not use cigarettes to control affect. This finding was consistent with results in other studies linking ability to cope with negative situations to successful smoking cessation and prolonged abstinence (Shiffman 1982; Abrams et al. 1987; Breslau et al. 1993). The only difference in the results for females and males in the study by Rose and associates (1996) was the relationship between having motives to smoke for stimulation (e.g., smoking "to perk self up") and making a successful effort to stop smoking. Lower levels of motives for stimulation were related to successful smoking cessation among females, whereas higher levels were related to cessation among males.

*Pregnant Women*

Four studies investigated the predictors of smoking cessation among pregnant women. In a study of 1,104 smokers registered at prenatal clinics in Uppsala, Sweden, Cnattingius and colleagues (1992) investigated the predictors of continued smoking and the predictors of cessation through 36 weeks' gestation. Smoking cessation was defined as having stopped smoking sometime before each assessment. Of the smokers, 29 percent reported having stopped smoking at some time during pregnancy; most of them had stopped smoking before registering for prenatal care. Women who had stopped smoking were compared with those who continued to smoke and with those who relapsed to smoking. Predictors of smoking cessation included having fewer children, living with the baby's father, not being a heavy smoker, and not having other smokers in the home. High level of education and older age at smoking initiation increased the likelihood of smoking cessation. Somatic symptoms (e.g., chest pain, back pain, insomnia, and anxiety) early in pregnancy were not related to changes in smoking status. The investigators did not evaluate the effect of symptoms specific to pregnancy, such as morning sickness and fatigue, on smoking cessation.

In the second study of pregnant women, O'Campo and coworkers (1992) examined the predictors of smoking cessation during pregnancy among urban women in the United States; about equal numbers of white and African American women were studied. The women were interviewed once during weeks 1 through 3 after childbirth and once during weeks 6 through 12 after childbirth.

Disproportionate sampling was used to include a large number of women who were breastfeeding their infants. Prenatal smoking status was determined retrospectively, at the first postpartum interview, and smoking cessation was defined as cessation of smoking before pregnancy or when pregnancy was confirmed during the first trimester. Smoking prevalence before pregnancy was 32 percent, which was consistent with the prevalence reported in two other studies (Kleinman et al. 1988; Fingerhut et al. 1990). Of the women who smoked before pregnancy, 41 percent had stopped smoking during the prenatal period (O'Campo et al. 1992). Among white women, personal characteristics, including younger age, higher education, and whether the birth was the woman's first, were predictors of smoking cessation, whereas among African American women, intention to breastfeed was the only predictor of cessation. These results were consistent with findings in other studies of former smokers (Kleinman and Madans 1985; Fingerhut et al. 1990; Milham and Davis 1991; Ockene 1993; Wakefield et al. 1993).

A third study of pregnant women conducted in Malmö, Sweden, by Dejin-Karlsson and colleagues (1996) examined psychosocial factors related to continued smoking during early pregnancy. Four hundred and four women who were pregnant for the first time and who smoked at the time of conception completed a self-administered questionnaire at the first prenatal visit and on the postnatal ward after delivery. The study focused on demographic factors; psychosocial factors such as social network, social support, and control in daily life; psychosocial characteristics in the workplace; and lifestyle factors such as smoking and alcohol habits. Smoking categories were loosely defined. Prepregnancy smokers were pregnant women who reported at the time of their first prenatal visit that they had smoked around the time of conception. Prenatal smokers were women who at the first prenatal visit reported they were currently smoking regularly or irregularly. Prenatal "quitters" were women who at their first prenatal visit reported that they had stopped smoking because of pregnancy. Information in the medical records was used to validate smoking data collected in the study, and a high degree of agreement was found (kappa = 0.091). Factors related to persistent smoking in early pregnancy were reported, but persistent smoking was not clearly defined. Moreover, the report focuses only on factors related to change in smoking behavior during the brief period from conception (retrospective report) to 8 through 12 weeks' gestation.

After adjustment for age, educational level, nationality, cohabiting status, passive smoking, and years of smoking, findings in this study showed that unmarried women, women whose pregnancies were unplanned, and women with higher job strain (i.e., high job demands and low control) and low psychosocial resources (e.g., low social participation, low instrumental support, and low support from the child's father) were most likely to continue smoking after learning of their pregnancy. Women with lower education and younger women also were more likely to continue smoking. Women who were exposed to passive smoking were more likely to continue to smoke, a finding consistent with other studies that showed that support from one's partner (Nafstad et al. 1996) and smoking status of the partner (Coppotelli and Orleans 1985; McBride et al. 1992) can influence a woman's ability to stop smoking. Lower physical activity was related to continued smoking, but alcohol consumption was not.

Another study of pregnant women examined predictors of attempts to stop smoking and of renewed smoking among cohabiting women in Oslo, Norway (Nafstad et al. 1996). This study was intended to estimate whether changes in women's smoking behavior during and after pregnancy were related to the smoking habits of their cohabitants. Data from early pregnancy were gathered from a standardized registration form filled out by a nurse or midwife at the prenatal visit of 8 through 12 weeks' gestation. A self-administered questionnaire was filled in by the mother (if possible, together with the father) at the maternity ward. The women were categorized as nonsmokers or smokers (occasional smokers and daily smokers). Mothers with complete information on smoking habits at all three data points (early pregnancy, delivery, and 1 year after delivery) were included in the study.

Among 940 cohabiting smokers, having a higher educational level, being primiparous, and having a nonsmoking cohabitant were positively related to smoking cessation during pregnancy (Nafstad et al. 1996). Although cessation during the first year after delivery among women who smoked in late pregnancy was low (13 percent), breastfeeding longer than six months, being primiparous, and not having smoked in early pregnancy were related to cessation. All of the women selected for this study were simultaneously participating in a project on risk factors for obstructive lung disease in early childhood, which may have contributed to an unusually high cessation rate during pregnancy in this study compared with other studies. In addition, the use of self-reports at follow-up visits and medical records (information obtained from health care providers) at baseline may have created a misclassification of women who had stopped smoking and new smokers. Women may have been less likely to reveal their smoking status to a health care provider during pregnancy but more willing to reveal their smoking status at delivery when they were asked to fill out a questionnaire. Despite these measurement issues, this study supports the growing literature suggesting that partners' smoking status can influence women's ability to stop smoking and not to start again.

All of these studies of pregnant women used different definitions of cessation and were conducted in different countries (Norway, Sweden, and the United States), which makes comparisons difficult. In addition, no study evaluated variables related to cognition and decision making. Nevertheless, findings suggested that lower level of education, higher parity, a less supportive environment or social network, a higher number of cigarettes smoked per day, and longer duration of previous smoking are important determinants of continued smoking among pregnant women. Similarly, attempts to stop smoking are increased by living with a nonsmoker, having low parity, having a higher education, and breastfeeding for at least six months.

Studies of women in smoking cessation programs (Coppotelli and Orleans 1985), women who had already stopped smoking (McBride et al. 1992), and women invited to participate in focus groups on smoking cessation (Lacey et al. 1993) have demonstrated that support from a partner predicts smoking cessation and maintenance of cessation among women. Having partners who were former smokers or who successfully stopped smoking at the same time increased maintenance of cessation in a population of employed women (Coppotelli and Orleans 1985). In a longitudinal study of women who had stopped smoking during pregnancy, those who were married to or lived with a smoker were more likely to relapse by week 6 after childbirth than were those who lived with a nonsmoker (McBride et al. 1992).

*Young and Middle-Aged Adults*

Six studies reviewed here (Kaprio and Koskenvuo 1988; Williamson et al. 1991; Garvey et al. 1992; Hibbard 1993; Osler 1993; Graham A. Colditz et al., unpublished data) addressed smoking cessation among young and middle-aged adults, but study populations and definitions of smoking cessation varied considerably. The U.S. Nurses' Health Study examined trends in smoking and predictors of cessation among 121,700 female nurses; more than 80 percent of the study population were followed up (Graham A. Colditz et al., unpublished data). Over a 10-year period (1976–1986), the prevalence of smoking decreased by approximately 10 percent. Smoking cessation was defined as having been a smoker at one follow-up time and not smoking at the subsequent assessment; the length of the cessation period was not specified. Pharmacologic variables and personal characteristics were examined as predictors of smoking status. Predictors of smoking cessation included older age at smoking initiation, fewer cigarettes smoked per day, younger age at smoking cessation, and past attempts to stop smoking. The techniques that participants used to stop smoking were not evaluated. Some nurses who had stopped smoking may have enrolled in smoking cessation programs, but because relatively few people in the United States use these programs (Fiore et al. 1990; Yankelovich Partners 1998), their influence on the study results is likely to be small.

Because of their occupational and educational status, participants in the U.S. Nurses' Health Study may not be representative of women in the general population. During the study period, social norms changed in regard to smoking by health care professionals and in health care settings. For example, by 1986, an increasing number of hospitals and physicians' offices had adopted smoking restrictions (Pappenhagen and Weil 1988). Thus, working in a health care setting may have affected smoking cessation among the study participants.

Garvey and colleagues (1992) studied predictors of early relapse to smoking (within 7 days of smoking cessation) and late relapse (31 through 364 days after cessation) among 235 community volunteers. Although the focus of this study was on relapse, the results indicated that longer abstinence during a previous attempt to stop smoking, higher motivation to stop, higher confidence in the ability to abstain for three months, and lower alcohol consumption were related to sustained abstinence from smoking. These results were consistent with research findings on the relationship of self-efficacy and confidence to successful smoking cessation (Yates and Thain 1985). In the study of Garvey and associates (1992), none of the smokers who were successful in attempts to stop smoking had both a spouse who smoked and more than 50 percent of friends who smoked.

Hibbard (1993) examined the predictors of smoking cessation in a cohort of women enrolled in a 15-year follow-up study of members of a U.S. health maintenance organization. Of 168 women identified as smokers at baseline, 33 percent had stopped smoking before the follow-up visit. Assessment of smoking cessation was based on self-report, and no period for abstinence was specified. Pharmacologic, personal, and social variables were included in the study. After adjustment for age, education, and lower number of cigarettes smoked, the only variables that predicted smoking status were occupation and control over one's job. Women with higher occupational status, regardless of level of education, were more likely to stop smoking, as were women who reported having more control over their work. These results were consistent with research findings that suggested that greater control over work leads to less stress for workers (Karasek 1998) and that women with high job-related stress are more likely to smoke than are those with low job-related stress (Ikard and Tomkins 1973; Abrams et al. 1987; Sorensen and Pechacek 1987; Livson and Leino 1988; USDHHS 1989). Hibbard's study (1993) has limitations that raise concerns about the generalizability of the results. The small proportion of women who were married (13 percent) hampered assessment of the effect of marital variables, and the study did not examine psychological variables such as depression and anxiety. Moreover, 50 percent of the original cohort was lost to follow-up.

A study of twins in Finland examined the psychological, socioeconomic, and medical predictors of smoking cessation (Kaprio and Koskenvuo 1988). To prevent correlations between twins from affecting the analysis, only one twin from each pair was included in this study. Smoking cessation was defined as having been a current smoker at baseline and a former smoker at the six-year follow-up; the period of abstinence was not defined. Because the age ranges for women and men differed (20 through 39 years for women; 20 through 54 years for men), the men were divided into two groups for the analyses (20 through 34 years and 35 through 54 years). Only the younger male cohort is discussed here. Pharmacologic, personal, and social variables were examined in relation to smoking cessation. Predictors of cessation among women were higher level of education, lower number of cigarettes smoked daily, and fewer years of smoking. Predictors of smoking cessation among men were higher level of education, lower number of cigarettes smoked daily, frequent alcohol use, and greater number of periods of unemployment. Although several of the personal and social variables (e.g., duration of sleep, daily coffee consumption, and symptoms of breathlessness) were univariate predictors of smoking cessation, they were not significant in a comprehensive multivariate model. Furthermore, the amount of variance accounted for by the predictors was quite small (6 to 11 percent).

Osler (1993) studied the interrelationships of smoking, physical activity during leisure time, fruit and vegetable consumption, and social class over a five-year period among adults in Denmark. Smoking cessation was defined as having stopped smoking during the previous five years, but duration of cessation was not specified. At baseline in 1982, 52 percent of the women and 60 percent of the men were current smokers; at follow-up in 1987, the prevalence of smoking had dropped to 45 percent among women and 51 percent among men. Among both genders, predictors of smoking cessation included being in the highest social strata, being older, and having higher intake of vegetables. Increased physical activity was associated with smoking cessation among men but not among women.

The effect of smoking cessation on weight gain was examined in a national cohort of women and men aged 25 through 74 years from the Epidemiologic Followup Study of the First National Health and Nutrition Examination Survey (Williamson et al. 1991). The cohort included 1,885 continuing smokers and 768 former smokers who continued to abstain from smoking; the follow-up period was 6 through 13 years. Only personal characteristics (demographics, medical condition, reproductive history, and physical activity) were investigated as predictors of smoking cessation. Smoking cessation was defined as success in efforts to stop smoking, within one year of follow-up, after reported smoking at baseline. Compared with continuing smokers, persons who continued to abstain from smoking were older, better educated, more likely to be white, and more likely to have been light smokers.

*Older Adults*

Only one study (Salive and Blazer 1993) investigated predictors of smoking cessation among older adults. As part of the Established Populations for Epidemiologic Studies of the Elderly, 287 women and 390 men aged 65 years or older were followed up for three years. The researchers examined the relationship between smoking cessation and depression (as measured by the Center for Epidemiological Studies Depression Scale), pharmacologic processes (number of cigarettes per day and number of years of smoking), and personal characteristics (demographic variables, medical history, and disease during study interval). Smoking cessation was defined as reported success in efforts to stop smoking before follow-up, after reported smoking at baseline. The smoking prevalence was 15.4 percent at baseline and 13.0 percent at the third annual follow-up. Women smokers who were depressed were more likely than those who were not depressed to stop smoking; smoking fewer cigarettes at baseline also predicted smoking cessation among women. Among men, neither depression nor amount smoked was related to change in smoking status. Older age, the only predictor of smoking cessation among men, was not a predictor among women.

Some studies found that depression reduced the likelihood of smoking cessation (Glassman et al. 1990; Hall et al. 1993), and in some studies this effect was more pronounced among women than among men (Anda et al. 1990; Glassman et al. 1990). The latter studies included primarily middle-aged smokers, however, and the relationship between smoking and depression may be different among older adults. Longitudinal studies are needed to examine this relationship across the life span.

## Relapse to Smoking

Variables related to relapse to smoking were investigated in studies of pregnant women (O'Campo et al. 1992), female nurses (Williamson et al. 1989; Graham A. Colditz et al., unpublished data), and women and men who attempted to stop smoking (Garvey et al. 1992). In a fourth study, relapse was identified as an outcome variable, but only a few participants relapsed, which precluded multivariate analysis of predictors of relapse (Salive and Blazer 1993).

O'Campo and colleagues (1992) examined the relationship between early relapse and personal characteristics (race, education, age, martial status, and method of infant feeding) during and after pregnancy. Relapse was defined as having stopped smoking just before pregnancy or during the first trimester, remaining abstinent throughout pregnancy, and resuming smoking by the second interview at weeks 6 through 12 after childbirth. Overall, 46 percent of pregnant African American women and 28 percent of pregnant white women relapsed; 70 percent of those who relapsed resumed smoking by week 3 after childbirth. It is highly likely that even more women relapsed after the second interview. Other studies suggested that relapse continues past the initial postpartum period but at a lower rate (National Center for Health Statistics 1988a,b; Fingerhut et al. 1990; Mullen et al. 1990; Windsor et al. 1993). The high incidence of relapse during the postpartum period in the general population suggested that concern for health of the fetus is a strong deterrent to smoking during pregnancy but that women may be less aware of, or less concerned about, the risks from environmental tobacco smoke on the health of infants and children (USDHHS 1986; Fingerhut et al. 1990). Women may find little personal benefit and may lack support for continued abstinence from smoking after delivery as they face the demands of a new infant, return to work, and other postpartum changes.

O'Campo and associates (1992) found that, although the proportion of women who relapsed differed among African Americans and whites, when all factors were examined together, race was not a predictor of relapse, nor was age, marital status, or parity. The only predictor of relapse was the use of formula instead of breast milk for infant feeding, a finding consistent with results of a longitudinal study of women after childbirth (McBride et al. 1992). The finding that other personal characteristics were not independent predictors of relapse was consistent with survey data based on recall (Fingerhut et al. 1990). Even though studies of smokers enrolled in cessation programs (Coppotelli and Orleans 1985) have shown that spousal support influences a woman's ability to remain abstinent, no measures of spousal smoking habits or spousal support for smoking cessation were examined in the study by O'Campo and associates (1992).

In the U.S. Nurses' Health Study, women were considered to have relapsed if they were former smokers at one assessment period but reported current smoking at a later 2-year follow-up (Graham A. Colditz et al., unpublished data). This definition classified women who relapsed in a group with widely varying durations of abstinence. The likelihood of relapse was strongly inversely related to duration of abstinence from smoking. On average, 20.4 percent of women who had abstained for less than 2 years but only 1.4 percent of women who had abstained for 10 years or more were current smokers 2 years later.

Garvey and colleagues (1992) examined predictors of early relapse (within 7 days of smoking cessation) and late relapse (31 through 364 days after cessation) among 235 adults who were followed up after a self-initiated attempt to stop smoking. The investigators found that 62 percent of women and men combined had relapsed within two weeks of smoking cessation, 76 percent had relapsed by one month, and 87 percent had relapsed within one year. Shorter periods of abstinence from smoking during previous attempts to stop smoking, lower motivation to stop smoking, lower confidence in the ability to abstain from smoking for three months, and higher alcohol consumption were all associated with relapse by one year, but demographic variables, including gender as well as age and education level, did not predict relapse. When the relationship of predictor variables to smoking cessation was analyzed separately for women and for men, the only variable with a significant influence was weight control. Women who were more likely to smoke to control weight were less likely to relapse early than were women with lower ratings on this motive. The opposite was true among men. In a comparison of women who relapsed within seven days with those who abstained from smoking for one year, two significant predictor variables were found: confidence in abstaining for three months and duration of the longest previous abstinence.

The finding that women who smoked to control weight were less likely to relapse early (Garvey et al. 1992) was unexpected, because evidence from other studies suggested that concern about weight gain deters more women than men from smoking cessation (Hall et al. 1986; Sorensen and Pechacek 1987; Klesges et al. 1989; Pirie et al. 1991, 1992; French et al. 1995). Furthermore, many people, particularly women, report that they are concerned about weight gain after they stop smoking (Sorensen and Pechacek 1987; USDHHS 1988; Klesges et al. 1989; Gomberg and Nirenberg 1991; Pirie et al. 1991). Longitudinal studies are needed to investigate the temporal relationship between smoking to control weight and changes in smoking behavior.

Other studies also have demonstrated that short duration of a previous attempt to stop smoking is related to relapse (Ockene et al. 1981; Curry and McBride 1994). Many studies showed that a low degree of commitment, motivation, and confidence in the ability to stop smoking was associated with relapse (e.g., Ockene et al. 1981; Baer et al. 1986; Hall et al. 1990; Ockene et al. 1992; de Vries and Backbier 1994; Gulliver et al. 1995). These findings may reflect the role of self-efficacy in preventing relapse. In one study, former smokers who abstained for three months were more likely than those who relapsed to attribute success in smoking cessation to internal factors under their control and to their own actions (Schmitz et al. 1993). Former smokers who remained abstinent also reported greater self-efficacy in relation to smoking. High self-efficacy has been consistently associated with abstinence from smoking (Yates and Thain 1985).

The findings that lack of confidence and shorter duration of previous abstinence from smoking are related to relapse are particularly relevant among women. Some evidence from laboratory studies (Abrams et al. 1987) and cross-sectional survey data (Waldron 1991) suggested that women may be less confident of their ability to control negative moods without smoking cigarettes, which puts them at higher risk for relapse. One study showed that women were more likely to relapse because of internal pressures during negative emotional situations, whereas men were more likely to relapse because of external pressures (e.g., work-related stress) (Borland 1990). The investigator suggested that men may be more likely to blame others for relapse and, thus, to sustain the feeling of self-efficacy, which facilitates sustained resumption of abstinence. However, women may be more likely to blame themselves, which can lead to lack of confidence, low self-efficacy, and continued smoking.

## Summary

The longitudinal studies presented here, even when supplemented by other types of studies that explore the predictors of smoking maintenance or cessation among women, did not provide as rich a view of factors as did the research on smoking initiation. Nonetheless, factors identified in the 13 studies reviewed (Table 4.3) supported several conclusions that inform our understanding of the behavior of women who smoke. One predictor of attempts to stop smoking appears to be cognitive readiness—the belief that stopping will confer health benefits and the expectation of not smoking in the next year. Good predictors of success in smoking cessation among women are higher education, social support, and fewer cigarettes smoked per day. Women who relapse to smoking are more likely than those who remain abstinent to have shorter previous intervals of smoking cessation and lower self-efficacy with regard to the likelihood of success in smoking cessation. Little is known about the predictors of relapse among women during pregnancy or after childbirth, but it appears that women who stop smoking during pregnancy are less likely to relapse if they breastfeed their babies.

**Table 4.3. Factors found to predict attempts to stop smoking, smoking cessation, and relapse to smoking among women who were current smokers in the 13 longitudinal studies reviewed**

| Stage of smoking/ demographic group | Factors | |
|---|---|---|
| | **Personal** | **Social or cultural** |
| **Attempted cessation** | | |
| Young persons | High perceived likelihood of not smoking in 1 year<br>High value on health<br>Perception of personally relevant health consequences of smoking cessation<br>Female gender<br>Control of negative affect<br>College education<br>Low-sensory motivation | Married<br>More social roles |
| Pregnant women | Not having smoked at conception<br>Low parity<br>High level of education<br>Breastfeeding >6 months | Living with nonsmoker |
| **Cessation** | | |
| Young persons | Extroversion<br>Low consumption of cigarettes<br>High perceived likelihood of not smoking in 1 year<br>High value on health<br>High-sensory motivation | Low social pressure to stop smoking<br>Employment<br>No children at home<br>More-educated parents<br>Some college education<br>High-sensory motivation and heavy smoking |
| Pregnant women | Low parity<br>Light smoking<br>High level of education<br>Young age<br>Older age at initiation of smoking<br>Intent to breastfeed<br>Shorter duration of smoking | Living with infant's father<br>No other smokers in home<br>Married<br>Planned pregnancy<br>No exposure to passive smoking<br>High social participation<br>Higher support from child's father<br>Low job strain |
| Young and middle-aged adults | Previous attempts to stop smoking<br>Confidence in ability to stop smoking in 3 months<br>Number of days abstinent on longest previous attempt to stop smoking<br>Job contentment<br>Level of education<br>Number of cigarettes smoked<br>Highest social group<br>Self-rated good health<br>Increased vegetable intake | |
| Older adults | Depressive symptoms<br>Fewer cigarettes smoked at baseline | |
| **Relapse** | | |
| Pregnant women | Formula feeding of infant<br>Shorter duration of previous abstinence | |

*Notes:* (a) The 13 studies reviewed as described in Table 4.2.
(b) Except where noted, these factors are important for women but apply equally to both sexes.

# Marketing Cigarettes to Women

This section presents general data on tobacco marketing and data on the influence of marketing on attitudes and behavior both in the United States and abroad. Modern marketing works best when companies use a coordinated and multifaceted approach that includes advertising, promotion, public relations, and sales strategies (Kotler 1991). Cigarette promotions targeted to women carry through the themes, packaging, and colors used in magazine ads and thus produce a product message that is pervasive and coherent.

Researchers of tobacco marketing to women have adopted an empirical approach that uses the description of actual marketing events to elucidate their impact. They have examined the major forms of marketing and have tried to define the related commitment of resources and specific techniques used. This research has resulted in an accumulated understanding of the marketing process through observation of historical trends and the in-depth analyses of landmark marketing campaigns. In 1993, the tobacco industry spent a record $6.2 billion to advertise and promote cigarettes and smokeless tobacco; 91 percent of this amount was spent on promotions (Federal Trade Commission [FTC] 2000). In 1998, the total expenditure was $6.73 billion, a 19.0-percent increase over the previous year and a 37.6-percent increase from 1995, with a similar proportional distribution of expenditures for advertising and promotion (Table 4.4). Marketing expenditures increased 150 percent from 1986 through 1993, with a 15-percent increase from 1992 through 1993 alone (FTC 2000). As of 1995, expenditures had increased more than 11 times from the $491 million spent in 1975. Marketing expenditures for long cigarettes (94 to 101 mm) and ultralong cigarettes (110 to 121 mm), which are primarily targeted to women, increased from 29 percent of total spending in 1975 to 43 percent in 1994, then declined slightly to 40 percent through 1998. The market share for these long cigarettes increased from 25 percent in 1975 to 40 percent in 1998 (FTC 2000).

Sponsorship of cigarette marketing (e.g., programs such as sports events; entertainment tours and attractions; festivals, fairs, and annual events; and the arts) is used by companies as a central platform for directing other marketing activities (IEG 1995a). Tobacco sponsorships peaked in 1993 at $165 million and declined to $139 million in 1995. Tobacco accounted for 4.0 percent of total expenditures for all consumer product sponsorships in North America in 1995. The top three tobacco sponsors in 1995 were Philip Morris Companies, Inc., RJR Nabisco (parent company of R.J. Reynolds), and the United States Tobacco Company. Of the 3,000 sponsorship opportunities available in 1995, approximately one-fourth had restrictions on tobacco sponsorship, and 93 percent of these excluded tobacco sponsorship (IEG 1995b).

## Marketing Techniques

### Advertising

The considerable resources devoted to advertising and promotion are placed in the service of techniques with extraordinary power to sell products. Advertising builds a brand's image (Kotler 1991; Mark and Silverman 1992; Bissell 1994), raises the salience of a brand, and conditions consumers to form the attitudes needed to purchase the product (Percy and Rossiter 1992). Attitudes include a cognitive or logical component (e.g., beliefs about benefit) and an affective component (e.g., emotions that energize behavior) (Percy and Rossiter 1992). Consumers often buy products because of the psychological and social meaning the products represent to them (Kindra et al. 1994). Advertising of cigarette brands uses specific themes to suggest distinctive identities (Chapman and Fitzgerald 1982). A classic example is the Marlboro man, who projects a sense of adventure, freedom, and being in charge of his own destiny (Trachtenberg 1987). Smokers and potential smokers may identify with the projected images and purchase the brand as a surrogate for adopting the portrayed behavior (Solomon 1983; Botvin et al. 1993). Brand images may pose solutions to identity problems and appeal to persons who are socially insecure (Chapman and Fitzgerald 1982; Trachtenberg 1987). The theme of a cigarette advertisement (e.g., adventure, glamour, and independence) evokes an enhanced self-image (Solomon 1983), and consumers may feel they are purchasing enhancement along with the product. Typically, the ads use attractive, youthful models and portray smoking in socially pleasing circumstances and surroundings. Repeated exposure to such ads may have a strong influence on the brand

**Table 4.4. Expenditures for domestic cigarette advertising and promotion, 1995–1998**

| | 1995 | | 1996 | | 1997 | | 1998 | |
|---|---|---|---|---|---|---|---|---|
| | Total dollars | % of total | Total dollars | % of total | Total dollars | % of total | Total dollars* | % of total |
| **Advertising** | | | | | | | | |
| Newspapers | 19,122 | 0.4 | 14,067 | 0.3 | 16,980 | 0.3 | 29,444 | 0.4 |
| Magazines | 248,848 | 5.1 | 243,046 | 4.8 | 236,950 | 4.2 | 281,296 | 4.2 |
| Outdoor | 273,664 | 5.6 | 292,261 | 5.7 | 295,334 | 5.2 | 294,721 | 4.4 |
| Transit | 22,543 | 0.5 | 28,865 | 0.6 | 26,407 | 0.5 | 40,158 | 0.6 |
| Total | 564,177 | 11 | 578,239 | 11 | 575,671 | 10 | 645,619 | 9.6 |
| **Promotion** | | | | | | | | |
| Point of sale | 259,035 | 5.3 | 252,619 | 4.9 | 305,360 | 5.4 | 290,739 | 4.3 |
| Promotional allowances | 1,865,657 | 38.1 | 2,150,838 | 42.1 | 2,438,468 | 43.1 | 2,878,919 | 42.8 |
| Sampling distribution | 13,836 | 0.3 | 15,945 | 0.3 | 22,065 | 0.4 | 14,436 | 0.2 |
| Specialty item distribution | 665,173 | 13.6 | 544,345 | 10.7 | 512,602 | 9.6 | 355,835 | 5.3 |
| Public entertainment | 110,669 | 2.3 | 171,177 | 3.4 | 195,203 | 3.4 | 248,536 | 3.7 |
| Direct mail | 34,618 | 0.7 | 38,703 | 0.8 | 37,310 | 0.7 | 57,772 | 0.9 |
| Endorsements and testimonials | 0 | 0 | 0 | 0 | 0 | 0 | 0 | 0 |
| Coupons and retail value added[†] | 1,348,378 | 27.5 | 1,308,708 | 25.6 | 1,522,913 | 26.9 | 2,179,590 | 32.4 |
| Internet[‡] | NA | NA | 432 | 0.0 | 215 | 0.0 | 125 | 0.0 |
| Other[Δ] | 33,680 | 0.7 | 46,264 | 0.9 | 50,207 | 1.0 | 61,584 | 0.9 |
| Total | 4,331,046 | 89 | 4,529,031 | 89 | 5,084,343 | 90 | 6,087,536 | 90.5 |
| **Grand total** | 4,895,223 | 100[¶] | 5,107,270 | 100 | 5,660,014 | 100 | 6,733,155** | 100 |

*In thousands of U.S. dollars.
[†]1997 was the first year the Federal Trade Commission required the cigarette companies to report separately their expenditures for coupons and for retail value added.
[‡]1996 was the first year the Federal Trade Commission identified the Internet as a separate category of expenditures.
[§]NA = Not available.
[Δ]Expenditures for audiovisual promotion are included in "Other" to avoid disclosure of data for individual companies.
[¶]Because of rounding, sums of percentages may not equal 100%.
**Total dollar value as published in the printed report.
Source: Federal Trade Commission 2000.

selection of consumers who identify with the lifestyles and images used (Bearden and Etzel 1982). For some consumers, cigarette smoking may actually contribute to their structuring of social reality, self-concept, and behavior (Solomon 1983).

Advertising is also used to reduce fear of the health risks from smoking (Botvin et al. 1993) by presenting facts and figures (e.g., information on nicotine and tar content) or by using positive imagery (e.g., clear blue skies and white-capped mountain peaks). For example, many modern ads have shown models engaged in exercise (Pollay and Lavack 1993). In addition, advertising is used to encourage brand loyalty by reinforcing preferences rather than encouraging brand switching (Raj 1985; Tellis 1988). Image reinforcement attracts repeat purchasers. In one market research study, Marlboro customers were offered half-priced Marlboro cigarettes packaged in generic brown boxes; only 21 percent of customers were attracted to the offer (Trachtenberg 1987).

### Promotions

An effective marketing strategy uses both advertising and promotions. Promotions are typically used to convince people to try a product, to increase purchase volume, to encourage brand switching, to win customer loyalty, and to enhance corporate image (Gagnon and Osterhaus 1985; Warner et al. 1986; Levin 1988; Tellis 1988; Kotler 1991; Mark and Silverman 1992; Zinn 1994). Retail value-added promotions stimulate short-term sales (Kotler 1991). Because women and youth are sensitive to low prices, reduced prices may be an especially effective tool for reaching them (Lynch and Bonnie 1994; Townsend et al. 1994; Chaloupka and Warner 1999). Promotional allowances paid to retailers help to ensure prominent placement of a product in high-volume areas or near products such as candy or liquor (Kotler 1991; Lynch and Bonnie 1994).

Point-of-sale promotions influence consumers when they are making purchase decisions and, thus, also build support among retailers (Gagnon and Osterhaus 1985; Lynch and Bonnie 1994). Such promotions allow targeted marketing, are easy to evaluate with sales data, and are relatively inexpensive (Gagnon and Osterhaus 1985). Women are an especially lucrative target for promotions because they make about 80 percent of the purchase decisions in the marketplace (E. Janice Leeming, Executive Director, Marketing to Women, letter to Sharon Dean, Corporate Fact Finders, April 12, 1993).

Specialty items that contain brand names or logos, such as clothing and accessories, often serve as walking ads and enhance the perception that tobacco use is the norm (Lynch and Bonnie 1994). For cigarettes, these items do not carry the health warning required for other forms of advertising and promotion (Slade et al. 1995). Coupon redemption helps to create databases of millions of smokers for further promotions (Lynch and Bonnie 1994; Zinn 1994), and these databases also provide demographic information for marketing and for encouraging smokers to become politically involved in issues related to tobacco policy.

Tobacco companies have also used innovative promotional campaigns by offering discounts on common household items unrelated to tobacco. For example, Philip Morris has offered discounts on turkeys, milk, soft drinks, and washer detergent with the purchase of tobacco products (Slade 1994). If tighter restrictions on tobacco advertising and promotion were implemented, more of this type of marketing may occur. Consumer products that women are more likely than men to purchase will be prime candidates for such an approach to product promotion.

**Sponsorship**

Brand or corporate sponsorship of public entertainment, sporting events, or organizations that promote specific causes provides multiple benefits to the corporations. Sponsors spend money to achieve commercial objectives; sponsorship is economical because it allows a company to reach a niche market without wasting resources and provides "embedded advertising," which links product attributes or lifestyle images to an active event (IEG 1995a, p. 5). Sponsorship also promotes audience loyalty. For example, for the cost of a 30-second spot during a Super Bowl broadcast, a company can sponsor a team in the NASCAR Winston Cup series and receive more than 30 hours of television coverage. Companies also use sponsorship to drive sales, through discounted tickets and point-of-purchase display ads (IEG 1995a).

Sponsorship associates a brand with prestigious events and may make the brand appear more credible than its competitors (Kotler 1991; IEG 1995a). Tobacco industry sponsorship may also lend an aura of social legitimacy to smoking, create gratitude from the recipient institutions, gain allies, or encourage neutrality toward industry activities and thereby soften public criticism of the industry (Elkind 1985; Ernster 1986; Levin 1988; Williams 1991).

**Product Packaging**

The packaging of a brand of cigarettes, including name, logo, and colors, presents an image that cues attitudes toward the brand and affects its attractiveness (Britt 1978; Beede and Lawson 1992; Health Canada 1995). When repeated in advertising copy, the attributes of the brand become familiar stimuli that enhance recall and retention (Beede and Lawson 1992). Brand images may be used to attract women and men or to counteract negative stereotypes, such as the idea that smoking is inappropriate for women (Elkind 1985). These images may be particularly important among young female smokers. Brand is an important component of consumer decisions among children (Ward et al. 1977), and minors can successfully recall tobacco brand images and slogans (USDHHS 1994). Cigarette advertising may have predisposing and reinforcing effects among children (Aitken et al. 1991).

Tobacco is the ultimate "badge product" (Bissell 1994, p. 16) for tobacco marketing generally and for product packaging specifically. For product packaging, it is a badge product because it is used frequently, is displayed in social settings, and shows its package design and brand every time it is used (Trachtenberg

1987; Bissell 1994; Pollay 1994). Color, design, and shape symbolically convey the image of the brand. Because visual image alone often stimulates the purchase of a brand (Percy and Rossiter 1992), consumer recall of the brand name at the time of purchase is not necessary.

Packaging influences the attitude of a consumer toward a product and the choice of a brand (Opatow 1984; Gordon et al. 1994). Graphics and color convey nonverbal messages. For example, blue and white signify cleanliness and purity and are frequently used for health products (Opatow 1984). Light blue signifies calm and coolness. Red connotes excitement, passion, strength, wealth, and power (Gordon et al. 1994; Kindra et al. 1994) and is frequently used for male-oriented products. Red is a popular color for tobacco packaging because it demonstrably aids recall of the product (Beede and Lawson 1992; Health Canada 1995). Green suggests coolness, restfulness, nature, cleanliness, and youthfulness. Pastels are associated with femininity: light purple suggests freshness, springtime, and flowers; pink suggests innocence and relaxation; and light yellow suggests freshness and intelligence (Gordon et al. 1994; Kindra et al. 1994).

In recent years, internal tobacco industry documents have become available and are easily retrievable from various Web sites. A good inventory of tobacco industry Web sites is available through the CDC's Office on Smoking and Health Web site at http://www.cdc.gov/tobacco. A few examples from tobacco industry documents are provided below to illustrate how the tobacco companies have viewed women. These excerpts were obtained from the report "Big Tobacco and Women," available at the following Web site: http://www.ash.org.uk.

An RJR document titled "Women's Response to Advertising Imagery" noted: "With the exceptions of career women and single women who work to support themselves, all female segments in the present study reacted positively to advertising imagery associated with the following dimensions: intimacy and closeness, tenderness and gentleness, loving, caring, and sharing."

An RJR document from 1983, summarizing focus groups held with women, noted: "There is greater agreement as to how and why women began smoking in the first place. Beyond the easily recognized pressure of peers, women smoke to indicate passage into adulthood and as part of this transitional period, to exhibit anti-authoritarian behavior."

The internal tobacco industry documents also contain evidence that children were explicitly targeted with promotional campaigns. For example, a handwritten letter from a parent sent to RJR in 1981 noted: "Dear Sirs, You are sending Christmas Cards and Coupons to encourage my 15-year-old daughter to smoke. Please remove my daughter from your mailing list."

In a 1981 report titled "Social Trends Among Female Smokers," British American Tobacco commented on women's attitudes toward smoking: "(1) concern about smoking too much, (2) actively looking for new brands of cigarettes to smoke, (3) believe there should be different cigarettes for men and women, (4) report using, at least occasionally, cigarettes for enjoyment, (5) acceptable if used moderately, cigarettes for enjoyment, (6) low tar and nicotine cigarette represent a major step in the direction of making smoking less harmful to the health" (http://www.ash.org.uk).

## Historical Antecedents

Modern concepts of cigarette marketing had their genesis about 80 years ago, as the industry first developed its techniques in national campaign efforts for mass markets. Early in this century, major cigarette brands did not explicitly target women for "fear that they may draw the lightning of the busybody element that brought about prohibition" (Bonner 1926, p. 21). During the 1920s, however, this restraint was cast aside. Marlboro, for example, was positioned in the mid-1920s as a premium-priced brand of cigarettes advertised to women as being "Mild as May" (Bonner 1926, p. 21). A billboard campaign for Chesterfield in 1926 showed a woman seated next to a male companion who was smoking; she asks him to "Blow Some [smoke] My Way" (Bonner 1926, p. 46). This request was described nearly four decades later as one of the great ads of all time (*Printers' Ink* 1963). The scene was originally cast in a moonlit setting, but variations portrayed the couple on or in "couches, porch swings, roadsters, and rumble seats" (Goodrum and Dalrymple 1990, p. 196). This campaign precipitated public expressions of moral outrage, because smoking was considered audacious behavior for a woman, symbolizing a rebellious, libertine lifestyle. Most women who smoked, for example, were free of family restraints—college girls, city sophisticates, and flappers (Schudson 1984; Ernster 1985).

George Washington Hill, of the American Tobacco Company, the manufacturer of Lucky Strike cigarettes, was described as "obsessed" by the yet-to-be-tapped potential of the female market. He was quoted by his own public relations consultant as saying, "It will be like opening a new gold mine right in our front yard" (Bernays 1965, p. 383). Hill hired advertising agent A.D. Lasker because of his success with the delicate task of using national magazines to sell sanitary napkins to women (Gunther 1960). Lasker and Hill paid European actresses and opera stars to give testimonials for the Lucky Strike brand and, for a while, cited a survey of physicians claiming that "Luckies" were less irritating than other brands.

To combat these promotional efforts, Edward Bernays, a public relations specialist, was hired by Liggett & Myers for its Chesterfield brand of cigarettes. Bernays ridiculed the opera star campaign by creating the Tobacco Society for Voice Culture, an organization with the aim "to establish a home for singers and actors whose voices have cracked under the strain of their cigarette testimonials" (Bernays 1965, p. 374). In response to the survey of physicians, 5,000 copies of an article entitled "Cigarette Copy Bunk, Physicians Declare Blanket Endorsement Used in Ads Unwarranted" were distributed to influential persons (Bernays 1965, p. 375). When the American Tobacco Company lured Bernays away from the makers of Chesterfield, he consulted A.A. Brill, a famous psychoanalyst who interpreted cigarettes as "symbols of freedom" (Bernays 1965, p. 386). Subsequently, Bernays mounted publicity stunts, such as hiring women to smoke in New York City's Easter Parade and to wear placards identifying their cigarettes as "torches of freedom" (Bernays 1965, p. 387).

By the late 1920s, ads for Old Gold, Camel, and other brands were featuring women (Figure 4.1). Cigarette ads began appearing in magazines with large female readerships, including *True Story, Picture-Play, Junior League Magazine, Delineator, Pictorial Review, Modern Priscilla, House & Garden, Vogue, Harper's Bazaar, Vanity Fair,* and fiction magazines (Tilley 1985). By the mid-1930s, cigarette ads targeting women were so commonplace that one ad for the mentholated Spud brand had the caption "To read the ads these days, a fellow'd think the pretty girls do all the smoking" (*The Saturday Evening Post* 1935, p. 42). Another ad appealed to women with "Doesn't irritate my girlish throat either" (*Tide* 1936, p. 11). In 1938, a Camel ad featured a young woman identified as a successful business "girl" who chose Camels because "they never bother my throat" (*Life* 1938) (Figure 4.2). At the same time, an ad for the Tareyton brand of the American Tobacco Company targeted women with the slogan "Moist lips are thrilling lips! Keep them soft, alluring" (*Tide* 1936, p. 12). Marlboro, still positioned as a woman's cigarette in 1943, was advertised in *Mademoiselle, Charm, Glamour, Vogue, House & Garden,* and *Cosmopolitan* and was available with both an ivory tip and a red "beauty tip" to mask lipstick stains (Sobczynski 1983, p. M-14) (Figure 4.3). During World War II, cigarette ads showed women in either uniform or war-industry garb, touting the mildness of the product (Figure 4.2).

**Figure 4.1. By the late 1920s, women were appearing in ads for Old Gold and other cigarette brands**

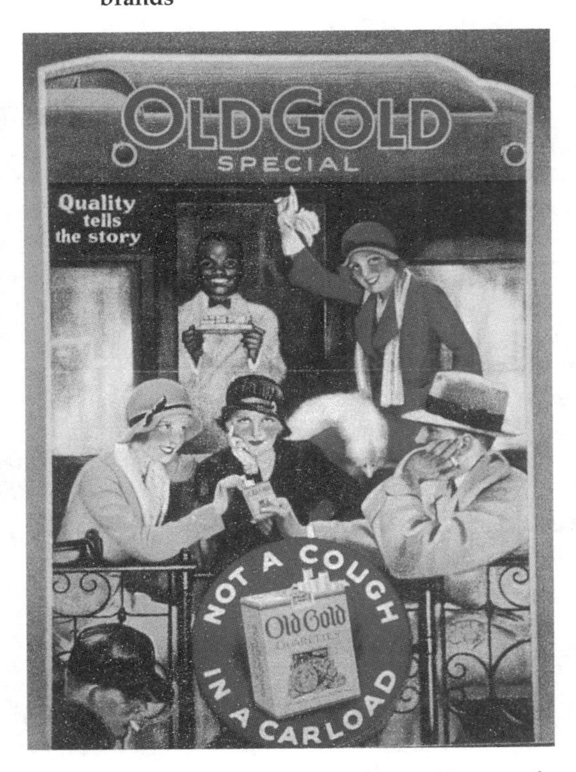


Source: Tobacco Industry Promotion Series, History of Advertising Archives, Faculty of Commerce, University of British Columbia, Vancouver, Canada.

### Making Cigarettes Glamorous

The best known advertising campaign of the American Tobacco Company urged women to "Reach for a Lucky Instead of a Sweet" (Wagner 1929, p. 344; Wallace 1929; *Journal of the American Medical Association* [*JAMA*] 1930) (Figure 4.4). Once the association of smoking with slimness was well established, the ads counseled women to "avoid that future shadow" and featured silhouettes of women with large double chins or fat ankles behind images of svelte young women (*JAMA* 1930; Tyler 1964, p. 100) (Figure 4.4). This positioning of Lucky Strike as an aid to weight control led to a 312-percent increase in sales for this

**Figure 4.2. In 1938, a Camel ad featured a business "girl," and in the World War II era, Chesterfield and Camel ads showed women in war industry garb and military uniform, respectively—all touting the mildness of cigarettes**

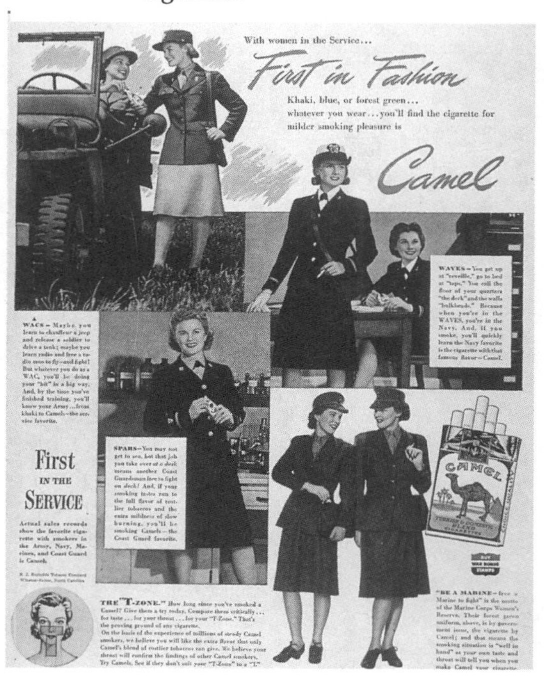


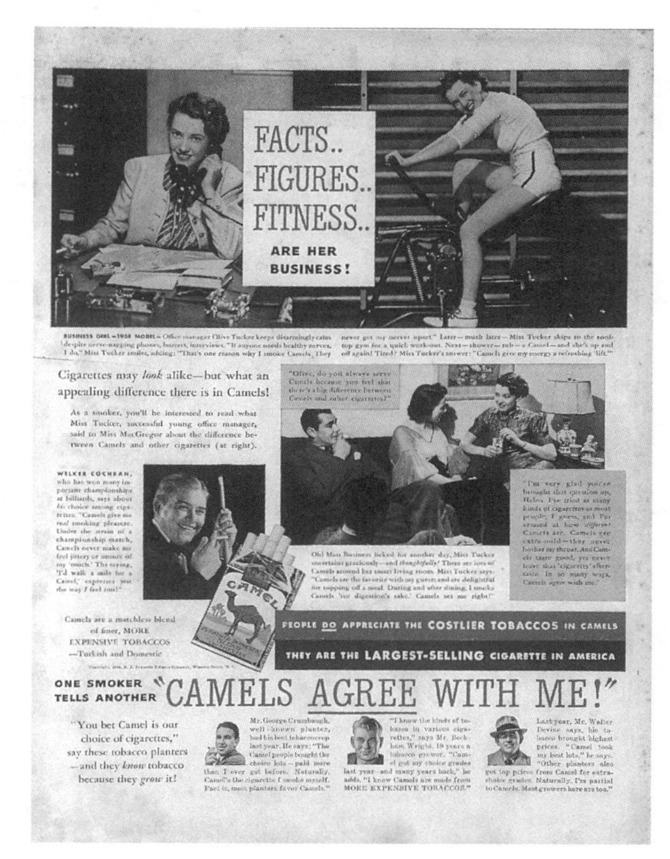


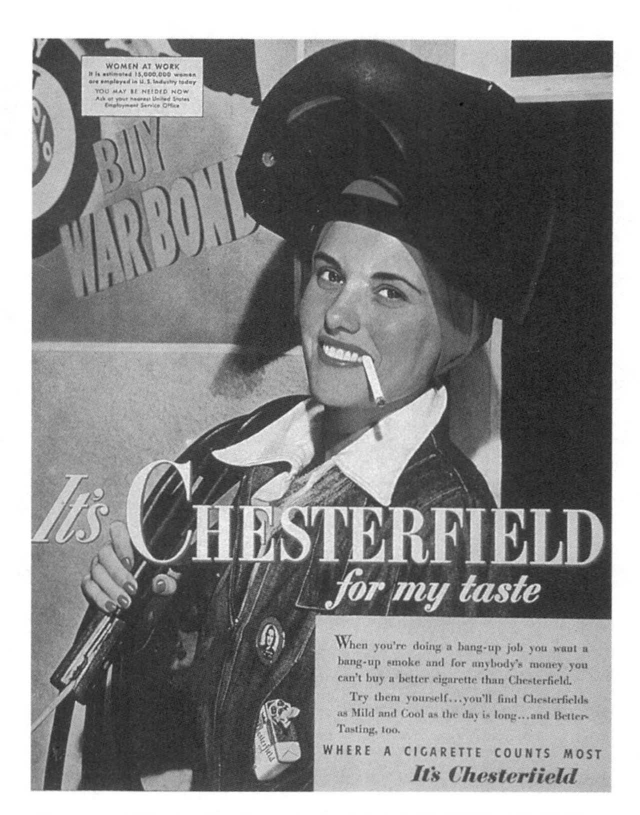


Sources: Clockwise from top right: *Life* 1938; *Life* 1943a; *Life* 1943b.

brand in the very first year of the advertising campaign, despite the protests of sugar and candy interests (Gunther 1960).

During this time, Bernays (1965) pursued the emphasis on slimness for the American Tobacco Company by "flooding fashion editors with photographs of thin Parisian models in haute couture dresses" (Bernays 1965, p. 383). After research showed the green Lucky Strike package was unpopular with some women because it clashed with clothing, Bernays worked with clothing manufacturers, department stores, magazine fashion editors, and interior decorators and sent out press releases describing the psychological benefits of the color green as "the color of spring, an emblem of hope, victory (over depression) and plenty" (Bernays 1965, p. 390).

In the late 1930s, testimonials claiming benefits of cigarettes to the throat were reinstated. Ads describing Lucky Strike cigarettes as a light, gentle smoke that offered "throat protection" included testimonials from "leading artists of radio, stage, screen and opera,

**Figure 4.3. A 1943 Marlboro ad in six women's magazines promoted a red beauty tip to hide lipstick stains**

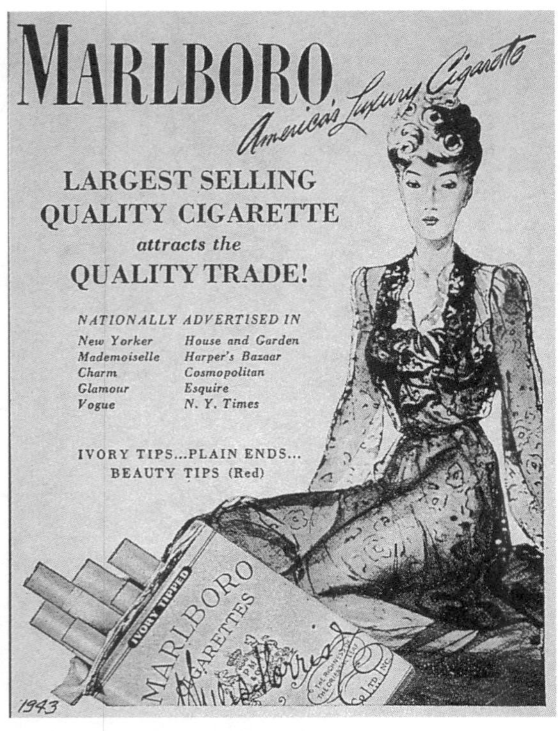


Source: Tobacco Industry Promotion Series, History of Advertising Archives, Faculty of Commerce, University of British Columbia, Vancouver, Canada.

whose voices are their fortune" (Pollay 1993, p. 5), including Miriam Hopkins, Carole Lombard, Joan Crawford, Myrna Loy, Dolores Del Rio, and Claudette Colbert. By 1940 and continuing through the years of World War II, Chesterfield ads regularly featured glamour photographs of a Chesterfield girl of the month, primarily from the world of fashion models and Hollywood starlets. Some endorsers were famous stars, including Rita Hayworth, Rosalind Russell, and Betty Grable (Pollay 1993). From 1943 through 1946, ads for the Regent brand of cigarettes featured drawings of celebrities, including Diana Barrymore, Joan Blondell, Jinx Falkenberg, Merle Oberon, Jane Wyatt, Arlene Francis, Celeste Holm, and June Havoc (Pollay 1993). The trend continued after World War II, with Chesterfield endorsements from women show business celebrities, such as Jo Stafford, Ann Sheridan, Virginia Mayo, Ethel Merman, and Dorothy Lamour (Pollay 1993). In 1946, one of the now famous "More doctors smoke Camels..."

**Figure 4.4. The best known advertising campaign of the American Tobacco Company appealed to the desire of women to be slim, as shown by 1920s and 1930s Lucky Strike ads**

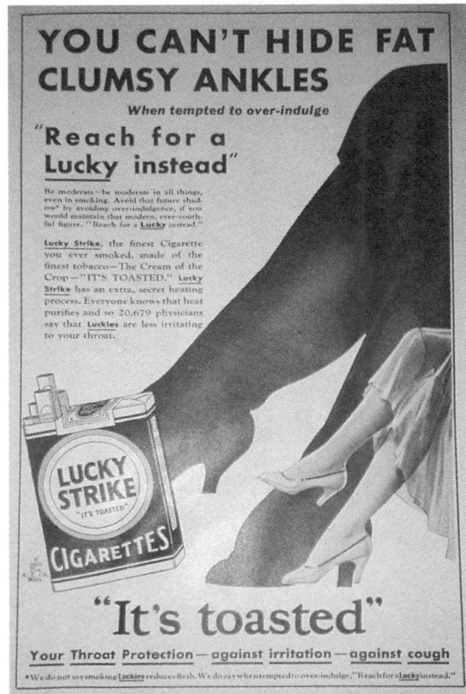


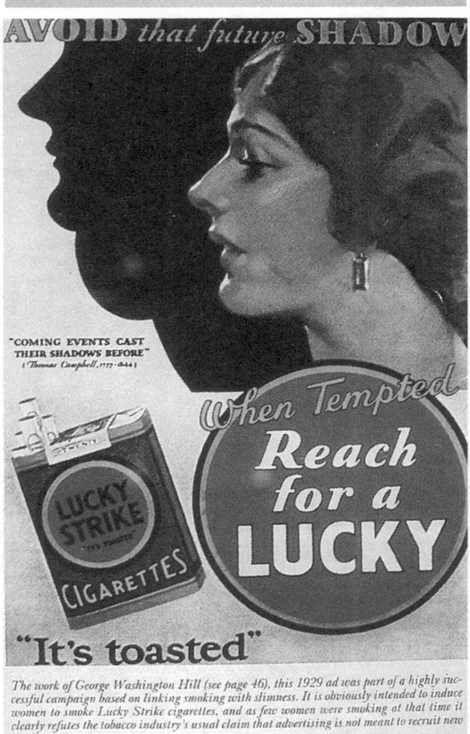


Source: Tobacco Industry Promotion Series, History of Advertising Archives, Faculty of Commerce, University of British Columbia, Vancouver, Canada.

ads featured a female physician, who is identified as the 1946 version of the "Lady with a Lamp" (Figure 4.5). In the early 1950s, Camel cigarettes, too, were endorsed by celebrities, including opera star Nadine O'Connor and movie star Joan Crawford, in ads claiming "Not one single case of throat irritation due to smoking Camels" (Starch 1951; Starch 1953, p. 73).

**Recognition of Power of Advertising**

The trade presses of both the advertising and tobacco industries were unequivocal in giving credit to advertising for the growth of cigarette sales, especially among women. "The growth of cigarette consumption has, itself, been due largely to heavy advertising expenditure.... It would be hard to find an industry that better illustrates the economic value of advertising in increasing consumption of a commodity" (Weld 1937, p. 70). Advertising was viewed not only as a vehicle for increased sales, but also "as an educator of public opinion.... The cigarette companies were instrumental in destroying the fetters of an outmoded convention [against women smoking].... The advertising appropriations of the cigarette companies have been truly large and truly productive...." (*Tobacco Retailers' Almanac* 1938, p. 18).

**Figure 4.5. A 1946 Camel ad featured a female physician—one of the testimonials claiming benefits of cigarettes and the throat**

Lady with a Lamp
(1946 Version)
According to a recent Nationwide survey:
MORE DOCTORS SMOKE CAMELS THAN ANY OTHER CIGARETTE
TRY CAMELS ON YOUR "T-ZONE"
CAMEL
CAMELS
Costlier Tobaccos

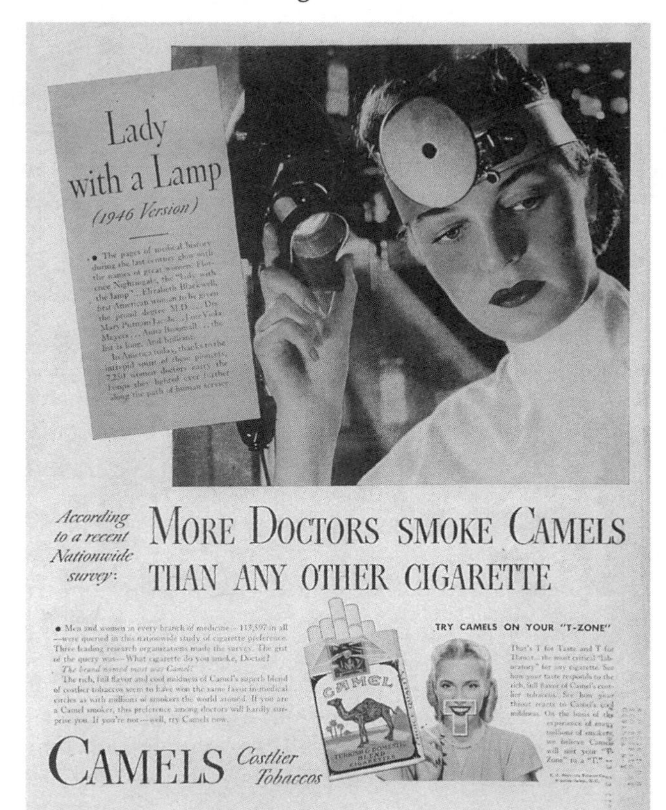

Source: *Life* 1946.

Fueled by past successes in encouraging ever more women to take up cigarette smoking, industry insiders remained confident that the post-World War II period offered even more untapped potential. "Women can be converted and there are a lot of them—particularly through the Middle and Far Western States—that have not had that comforting experience of smoking a cigarette" (Dunhill 1949, p. 32). Responding to a survey, cigarette industry leaders agreed that "a massive potential market still exists among women and young adults" and acknowledged that recruitment of these millions of prospective smokers was "the major objective for the immediate future and on a long-term basis as well" (*United States Tobacco Journal* 1950, p. 3). Even after the health scare that started in December 1952 with the publication in *Reader's Digest* of a brief article entitled "Cancer by the Carton" (*Reader's Digest* 1952), optimism about recruiting female nonsmokers was publicly expressed. In 1953, an article in the *United States Tobacco Journal* (1953) claimed that "more than three-fifths of the nation's women comprise a potential new market for the cigarette industry" (*United States Tobacco Journal* 1953, p. 3). This estimate was based on a survey of 16 cities where only "40.53 percent of the women in these markets now smoke cigarettes" (*United States Tobacco Journal* 1953, p. 3).

**Links of Fashion to Advertising**

Fashion was prominent in cigarette advertising during the 1950s. R.J. Reynolds' "elegant swashbuckling" Cavalier (*Tide* 1950, p. 53), a brand and trade character, was used for many fashion tie-ins in 1950. The Cavalier lapel pin was acquired by thousands of women, and adaptations of his hat and shoes were sold in women's clothing stores. Cavalier was also connected with a new women's raincoat, a housecoat, a fall suit, and a sleeve cuff. A milliner sold a Cavalier hat in 24 colors and gave buyers free packs of Cavalier cigarettes. Sample packs of cigarettes had long been distributed to hotel fashion shows, women's society meetings, bridge clubs, airlines, secretarial schools, and companies with employee lounges (*Tide* 1950).

Ads for the Parliament brand were "drenched in fashion appeal," by using "a haut [sic] monde tone" (*Printers' Ink* 1955, p. 87). Another ad, showing a woman wearing gloves and placing L&M cigarettes in her purse, declared, "Just Where You'd Expect to Find

L&M" (Gerry 1956, p. 23). Lorillard developed nationwide promotional campaigns that linked the company's Kent and Newport brands with such fashion magazines as *Vogue* and *Mademoiselle,* department stores, specialty stores, and several prominent fashion houses. Six dresses were designed exclusively for the Kent brand. Meanwhile, Newport's "Refreshing Change" promotional drive featured chemise dresses, sportswear, and swimsuits created by a range of designers to appeal to young women (*United States Tobacco Journal* 1958, p. 20). In announcing these campaigns, Lorillard's vice president and director of advertising commented, "It will enable us to reach the fashion pace-setters in many important communities, and psychologically, we think our use of this special avenue for women's attention—an indirect sell—will be appreciated by the more fashion-conscious sex" (*United States Tobacco Journal* 1958, p. 20). In addition, 200 of the department stores involved in this promotion used point-of-sale merchandising to promote Kent and Newport cigarettes (*Printers' Ink* 1958). Also targeting fashion-conscious women, Liggett & Myers developed designer packaging for king-sized Lark, L&M, and Chesterfield (*Advertising Age* 1968b). Even some ads having a health protection theme used fashion variants, such as Pall Mall's 1952 "Guard Against Throat-Scratch" ad featuring a fashionable woman (Figure 4.6).

**Figure 4.6. In a 1952 ad, Pall Mall used the image of a fashionable woman as part of a health protection theme**

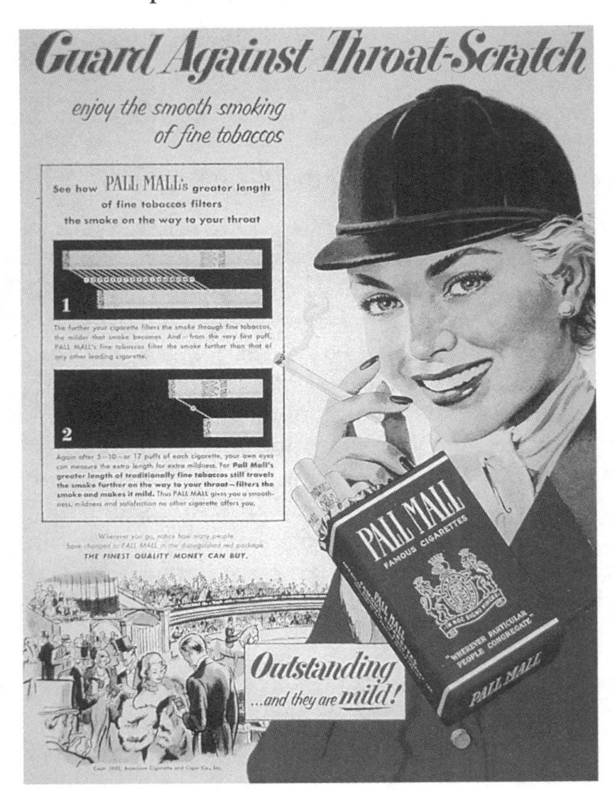


Source: *Life* 1952.

In the early 1950s, the *Chicago Tribune* hired the firm Social Research, Inc. to study the habits and attitudes of cigarette purchasers. The findings indicated that people had brand preferences even though they could not differentiate among cigarettes when they were blindfolded. Participants believed that each brand had certain qualities and that some brands were more or less appropriate for either men or women. In particular, the novel king-sized and cork- and filter-tipped brands were considered feminine at that time. A motivation researcher in the 1950s described smoking as an expression of freedom and worldliness among women, an idea he believed could be exploited and reinforced by advertising (Martineau 1957).

James Bowling of Philip Morris USA (subsidiary of Philip Morris Companies, Inc.) commented, "The ladies have led every major cigarette trend in the past 15 years.... Our studies show that they were the first to embrace king-sized cigarettes, menthol, charcoal, and recessed filters" (Sanchagrin 1968, p. 26). By 1953, the wave of new product introductions for king-sized and filter-tipped versions of both traditional and new brands had begun, and women smokers accepted the "new and improved" products (*Advertising Age* 1953). Sellers of traditional brands also continued to target their advertising to women.

### Influence of Tobacco Marketing on Smoking Initiation Among Females

This section reviews the evidence linking tobacco marketing to smoking initiation. Because not all studies have focused on females, this topic is reviewed rather broadly here, including tobacco marketing that specifically targeted girls and women and marketing that was not necessarily gender specific. When comparisons between females and males are available, they are reported.

As described earlier in this chapter, the tobacco industry changed its marketing strategy over the years to build and maintain its customer base. Marketing efforts were directed particularly to women in the 1920s and 1930s and again in the late 1960s, when niche brands were introduced. In this section, temporal trends in smoking initiation among females, compared with trends among males, are examined with respect to marketing campaigns. (For in-depth discussion of trends among females, see "Trends in Current Smoking Among Women" in Chapter 2.) The focus is on adolescents and young adults, because most people begin smoking before they reach mature adulthood (USDHHS 1994).

The earliest nationally representative U.S. data on smoking initiation were from the 1955 Current Population Survey (Haenszel et al. 1956). In this survey, respondents were asked about smoking history, and those who had ever smoked were asked the age at which they started to smoke regularly (Haenszel et al. 1956). Very few females born between 1890 and 1899 had ever smoked (Figure 4.7). Only 7.5 percent of the females in the cohort born in 1900–1909 had started to smoke regularly by age 21 years, and 14.9 percent had by age 30 years—the midpoint age of that cohort when the tobacco industry campaign to recruit female smokers was in full swing. However, 19.6 percent of the females in the cohort born in 1910–1919, who were teenagers during at least the early part of the campaign, began smoking by age 21 years. By comparison, 51.2 percent of males in the cohort born in 1900–1909 started smoking by age 21 years, and 61.3 percent of them had begun by age 30 years. A slight increase was noted in the proportion of males who smoked by age 21 (to 56.9 percent) for the cohort born in 1910–1919.

Data collected as part of the National Health Interview Survey beginning in 1970 presented a similar picture. In each of six surveys (1970, 1978, 1979, 1980, 1987, and 1988), respondents who had ever smoked were asked the age at which they started to smoke regularly. Data for adults aged 20 years or older were combined to analyze smoking initiation patterns over time among females and males at ages 14 through 17, 18 through 21, and 22 through 25 years for the periods 1910–1925 and 1926–1939 (Pierce and Gilpin 1995). Smoking initiation among women aged 18 through 25 years began to increase significantly in the mid-1920s, the same time that the tobacco industry mounted the Chesterfield and Lucky Strike campaigns directed at females. The trend was most striking among women aged 18 through 21 years; smoking initiation increased from 0.5 percent in 1910–1911 to more than 1.5 percent in 1924–1925, and reached nearly 5 percent in 1938–1939. Among women aged 22

**Figure 4.7. Cumulative percentage of females who had become regular smokers, by birth cohort**

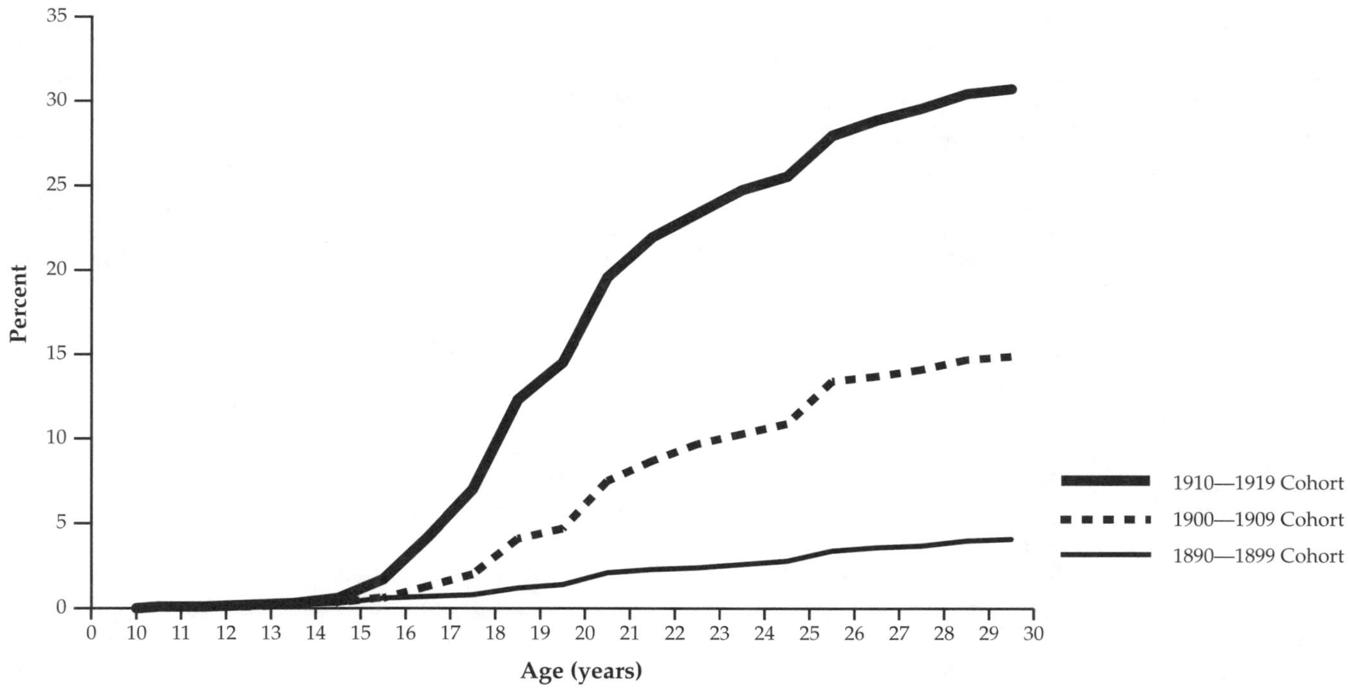

Source: Haenszel et al. 1956.

through 25 years, smoking initiation was near zero in 1910–1911, then increased to about 0.5 percent in 1924–1925 and to 1.8 percent in 1938–1939. Among girls aged 14 through 17 years, smoking initiation was low in 1910–1925 (<1 percent), increased after 1925, and reached about 2.5 percent by 1938–1939. It is unlikely that smoking initiation among females would have increased during that time had the tobacco industry not stimulated the demand. The two brands of cigarettes most heavily pitched to women during the campaign were Lucky Strike and Chesterfield. The Lucky Strike campaign of the mid-1920s that encouraged women to "Reach for a Lucky Instead of a Sweet" resulted in a dramatic increase in sales; Lucky Strike went from being the third-ranked brand in 1925, with sales of 13.7 billion cigarettes, to the first-ranked brand in 1930, with sales of more than 40 billion (Pierce and Gilpin 1995).

Patterns of smoking initiation from the post-World War II period through the mid-1980s were examined in relation to the introduction of brands targeted primarily to females (Pierce et al. 1994). The results indicated that incidence of smoking initiation among girls aged 17 years or younger was stable or declined slightly from the mid-1950s through the mid-1960s. After 1967, initiation of smoking among girls climbed dramatically, especially for girls aged 14 through 17 years, although increases were apparent even for girls as young as 11 years old. This upward trend in smoking initiation among adolescent girls continued until the mid-1970s. The increases from 1967 to the peak observed in the 1970s were approximately 110 percent for age 12 years, 55 percent for age 13 years, 70 percent for age 14 years, 75 percent for age 15 years, 55 percent for age 16 years, and 35 percent for age 17 years. Initiation rates among girls aged 14 through 17 years rapidly increased in parallel with the combined sales of the leading women's niche brands during this period (Virginia Slims, Silva Thins, and Eve) (Figure 4.8) (see text box "Virginia Slims: A Case Study in Marketing Success"). In contrast, smoking initiation among men aged 18 through 20 years declined abruptly after World War II, plateaued during the 1950s and early 1960s, then fell sharply. Among boys 16 and 17 years of age, initiation of smoking showed a steady downward trend throughout the study period, and for those 15 years of age or younger, it either decreased slightly or remained fairly constant.

By the early 1980s, smoking initiation among both male and female adolescents aged 14 through 17 years was decreasing significantly (Gilpin and Pierce 1997). This downward trend was also observed among young adults aged 18 through 21 years. Although the decline in initiation of smoking continued among young adults, a parallel decline was not observed among adolescents aged 14 through 17 years. Smoking initiation among adolescents decreased from 5.4 percent in 1980 to 4.7 percent in 1984, then increased to 5.5 percent in 1989, possibly reflecting increased tobacco marketing expenditures between 1984 and 1989 (CDC 1995). The incidence of smoking initiation and the prevalence of smoking among adolescents continued to increase during a time of increased expenditures on new marketing strategies for promoting tobacco use. The prevalence of current smoking among female high school seniors increased from 25.8 percent in 1992 to 32.4 percent in 1996. The proportional increase among boys was similar (Johnston et al. 1996; University of Michigan 1996). This period includes the observed peak (1993) of advertising and promotion by the tobacco industry. (See Table 2.9 in Chapter 2 for prevalence rates of smoking among high school seniors, 1976–2000.)

The Joe Camel character debuted in January 1988, before the marked rise in the initiation of smoking among adolescents that occurred in 1993. The Teenage Attitudes and Practices Surveys indicated that brand preference for Camel increased from 8.1 percent in 1989 to 13.3 percent in 1993 (CDC 1994). Among adolescents who purchased their own cigarettes in 1993, 10.3 percent of girls and 16.1 percent of boys bought Camel cigarettes. During the same period, Marlboro cigarettes decreased in popularity (from 68.7 to 60.0 percent) but nonetheless continued to be the market share leader among adolescents; nearly the same percentages of girls and boys bought Marlboro (60.7 and 59.2 percent, respectively). It is possible that the Joe Camel campaign affected the popularity of Marlboro.

The trends in smoking initiation among adolescents suggested a relationship between tobacco marketing campaigns and smoking initiation but were not direct proof of cause and effect. One Australian survey of 5,686 schoolchildren aged 10 through 12 years used a "semantic differential" measure of approval or disapproval of cigarette advertising in general (Alexander et al. 1983). Children who approved of cigarette ads were more than twice as likely to adopt smoking at a follow-up of 12 months. In another Australian study of 2,366 children and adolescents (modal age, 12 years), respondents were asked whether cigarette ads made them think that they would like to smoke a cigarette (Armstrong et al.

**Figure 4.8. Smoking initiation rates for 14- to 17-year-old girls, 1966–1979,* and expenditures for three cigarette brands† targeted to women, 1967–1978**

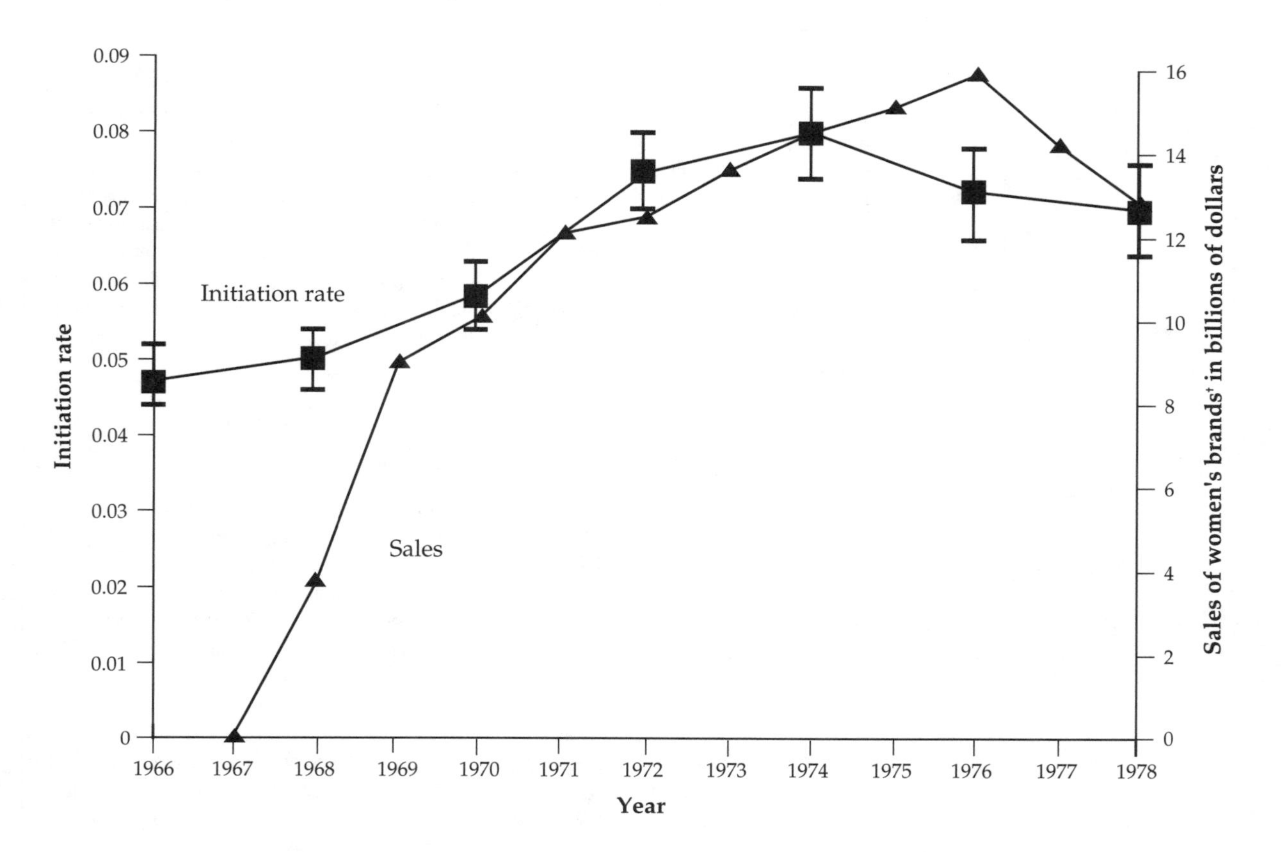


*The initiation data were aggregated in two-year intervals. Therefore, the data point for 1978, for example, is actually for 1978–1979.
†Virginia Slims, Silva Thins, and Eve cigarettes.
Sources: Pierce et al. 1994; Pierce and Gilpin 1995.

1990). Youth indicating that the ad had some influence on them were about three times as likely to use cigarettes at the 2-year follow-up as were those who indicated that the ad had no influence. The magnitude of the effect was nearly the same among girls and boys and about the same as having a sibling of the same sex who smoked.

A study conducted in schools in England and Wales in 1986–1988 among 3,694 children aged 11 through 15 years sought detailed information on recall of common cigarette ads in magazines (Goddard 1990). Students were shown ads without any print identifying the brand and were asked to rate them as beautiful, quite nice, not very nice, or disgusting. Scores were constructed for recognition (number correct) and for liking (number called beautiful or quite nice). Although girls generally scored lower than boys on both measures, baseline scores were significantly higher among girls who smoked at the time of follow-up than among girls who did not; this difference was not apparent among boys.

In another British study, 2,338 boys and girls aged 12 and 13 years who had never smoked were surveyed and then surveyed again four months later, with similar results (Charlton and Blair 1989). The participants were asked to name a cigarette brand and whether they had a favorite brand. For girls, being able to name a cigarette brand was among the four factors, of nine possible factors, significantly related to smoking during the period between the surveys; none of the factors was significant for boys. Another British study, a longitudinal study of 9- and 10-year-old

**Figure 4.9. Philip Morris launched advertising of Virginia Slims in 1968 with the slogan "You've come a long way, baby" and switched in the 1990s to "It's a woman thing"**

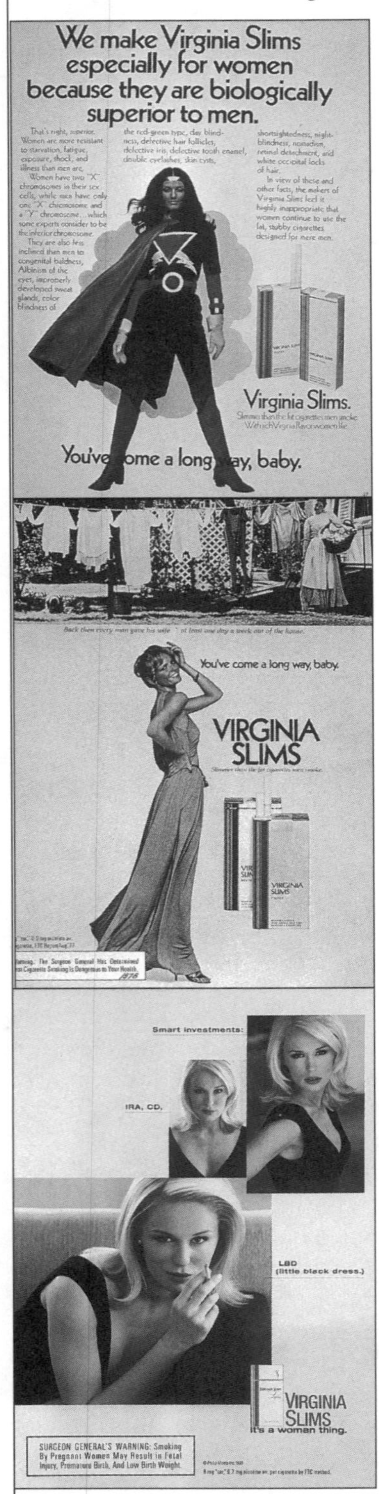


Sources: From top to bottom: *Playboy* 1971; *Time* 1978; *Glamour* 1999.

## Virginia Slims: A Case Study in Marketing Success

In the late 1960s, after more than a decade of substantial success with repositioning Marlboro as a masculine brand, Philip Morris decided to appeal to women through a new brand of cigarettes. Spurning strategies based on traditional feminine imagery, the tobacco company launched advertising for Virginia Slims in 1968, touting the 100-mm "slimmer than the usual" cigarette with the slogan "You've come a long way, baby" (*Advertising Age* 1968a, p. 33; *Advertising Age* 1968c, p. 2) (Figure 4.9). This advertising strategy showed canny insight into the importance of the emerging women's movement and enlisted several themes of that movement in its approach. The success of Virginia Slims and its advertising relative to competitive products and their advertising demonstrated the importance of image-based advertising in establishing an attitude and persona for the brand. It also made clear the greater appeal of ads that suggest attitudes of independence over those that emphasize frilly fashionability. The switch in the mid-1990s to the slogan "It's a woman thing" in ads for Virginia Slims cigarettes is a logical marketing response to the evolution of the women's movement—a theme the brand has always attempted to use to its advantage (Figure 4.9). In 1999, Philip Morris launched the Virginia Slims "Find Your Voice" campaign featuring women of diverse racial and ethnic backgrounds, including African Americans, Asians, Hispanics, and whites (Figure 4.10). The appearance of the models in the advertisements and the accompanying copy suggested that women in different ethnic and cultural groups have unique needs for self-expression, and the ads' slogan attempted to associate the Virginia Slims brand with fulfilling such needs: "Virginia Slims/ Find Your Voice."

Underlying the initial advertising campaign to launch the brand was the finding of motivation research that "cigarettes are either masculine or feminine but never successfully neuter" (Weinstein 1970, p. 4). After toying with several combinations of names and product variations, the advertisers focused on variants of "Virginia," because it was the home state of Philip Morris, the name of the marketing director's wife, and a "great name for a cigarette with a feminine personality. It not only has traditional tobacco overtones, but it romantically suggests moonlight, gentle breezes, and green hills" (Weinstein 1970, p. 4). The creation of brand personality would be achieved by using aspects of style, tone, music, and visuals, rather than information, because the advertising team believed that "in cigarette advertising... 90 percent of what you communicate is non-verbal" (Weinstein 1970, p. 13). This task, pursued by a staff that was initially all male, was described as "15 Guys in Search of a Feminine Identity" (Weinstein 1970, p. 1).

The advertising agency sought to capitalize on the product's distinctive thinness, which provided "visual intrigue," "tactile distinctiveness," and "style and grace" (Weinstein 1970, p. 2). The team also believed that the success of the pioneering king-sized Pall Mall cigarettes was due in part to how it flattered women—that is, "the extra length made their noses look shorter. Maybe this thin cigarette similarly could be liked because it makes your hand look slimmer and more graceful" (Weinstein 1970, p. 2).

However, the team rejected an overtly cosmetic appeal, such as a gold package or naming the product Vanity or Tiffany and promoting it in *Vogue,* for fear that this approach would make the brand a novelty product and appeal to too few women. They finally settled on a "fun personality for the brand—a lively, sparkly, happy cigarette" (Weinstein 1970, p. 13). They described the brand as "The first cigarette for women only,... designed slimmer for a woman's slimmer hands and lips; designed with the kind of flavor women like; and packaged in a slim purse pack" (Weinstein 1970, p. 7).

The advertising team created the concept of exploiting the issue of women's rights, which had reemerged in the late 1960s. They used the slogan "You've come a long way, baby" and ran copy that contrasted women's historical lack of rights with the modern situation in which women could have everything, even "a cigarette brand for [their] very own" (Weinstein 1970, p. 16). "Congratulations on your success" (Weinstein 1970, p. 20). The year that Virginia Slims was launched, its advertising was carried on 9 network television programs, on local television and radio, and in 16 women's publications and Sunday supplements (Sanchagrin 1968). Television programs that carried Virginia Slims ads included *Mission: Impossible, Family Affair, Hogan's Heroes, Mayberry R.F.D., The Red Skelton Show, Green Acres,* Thursday and Friday night movies, and the *CBS Evening News.* Print ads to launch Virginia Slims appeared in *American Home, Cosmopolitan, Ebony, Family Circle, Glamour, Harper's Bazaar, Ladies' Home Journal, Life, Look, Mademoiselle, McCall's,* the *True Story* group, *TV Guide, Woman's Day, Vogue,* and *Women's Wear Daily* (*Advertising Age* 1968c).

The Virginia Slims campaign was very successful (*Advertising Age* 1970), and its slogan may have resonated with the rhetoric of the burgeoning women's movement of the late 1960s. However, one advertising trade column described the campaign as featuring a "rebellious but unliberated woman"

**Figure 4.10. Ads from the multicultural "Find Your Voice" campaign**

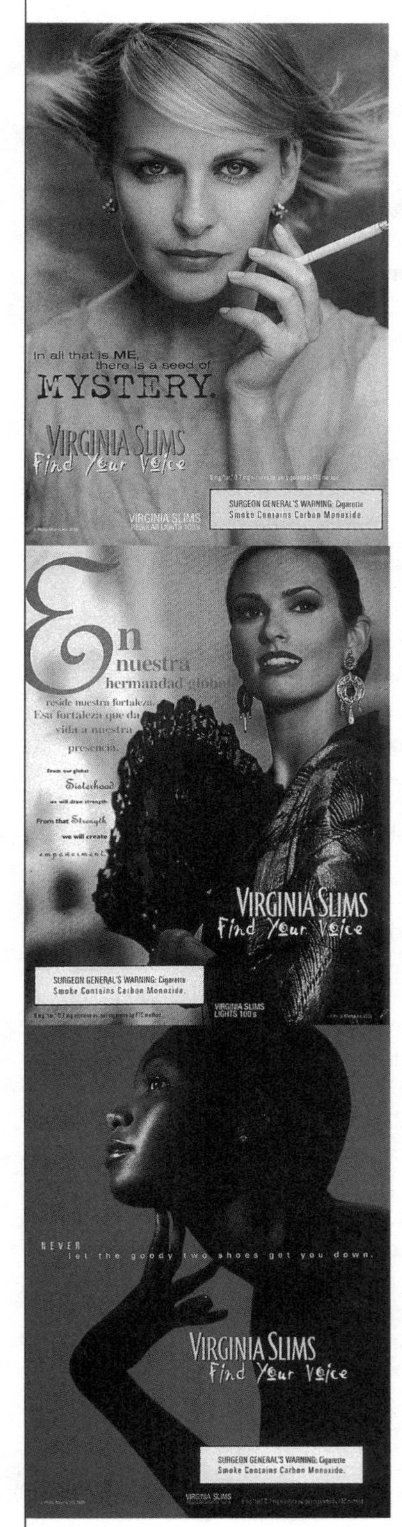


Sources: From top to bottom: *Glamour* 2000b; *Ladies' Home Journal* 2000a; *Glamour* 2000a.

(*Advertising Age* 1973, p. N8), and the inclusion of the word "baby" in the slogan resulted in some criticism from feminists (Kluger 1996). For more than two decades, ads in the campaign showed variations on the theme of a strikingly dressed, contemporary woman contrasted with unappealing background images of women in the past. But rarely, if ever, were the contemporary women portrayed as carrying out responsibilities; they were portrayed merely as very slim models wearing trendy styles. The ads mocked the older generation's experience, attitudes, and behavioral constraints, in part by contrasting new fashions with the old fashioned. Advertising agency personnel later explained that the agency wanted to avoid "the obvious trap of being too feminine" (*Advertising Age* 1968d, p. 2), but fashion was an important element in this campaign. In fact, Philip Morris placed an ad in *Women's Wear Daily* to thank the fashion trade for providing designs for its 1973 Virginia Slims campaign. The list of contributors included top designers Bill Blass, Pierre Cardin, and Halston (*Advertising Age* 1974a).

After January 2, 1971, when cigarette advertising was no longer permitted on broadcast media, the volume of advertising in women's magazines increased dramatically—threefold to fourfold from the first quarter of 1970 through 1971. For example, the number of pages devoted to cigarette advertising rose from 5 to 22 pages per quarter in *Ladies' Home Journal,* from 7 to 21 pages in *Redbook,* from 5 to 19 pages in *Woman's Day,* from 6 to 24 pages in *Cosmopolitan,* and from 7 to 21 pages in *Family Circle* (Revett 1971). This intensity of advertising in women's magazines continued into the 1980s. Regular readers of *Glamour, House & Garden, Ladies' Home Journal, Mademoiselle, McCall's, Metropolitan Home, Vogue,* and *Woman's Day* were exposed to about 100 cigarette ads annually in each magazine (Whelan 1984). Readers of *Better Homes and Gardens, Cosmopolitan, Family Circle,* and *Redbook* were exposed to 200 cigarette ads annually in each magazine, and reading *Newsweek, People, TV Guide,* or *Time* meant exposure to more than 400 ads per year. In 1974, Virginia Slims alone was supported by $8.3 million in advertising in magazines, newspapers, and Sunday supplements (*Advertising Age* 1974b).

Virginia Slims ran an award-winning premium promotion in 1977—the Ginny Jogger jogging suit. Persons who wanted to obtain the outfit were required to submit cash receipts and proof of Virginia Slims purchase (Robinson 1979). Some 30,000 sweat suits were distributed, 50 percent more than expected. In the mid-1970s, about 400,000 additional items were distributed, including 200,000 T-shirts bearing the slogan "You've come a long way, baby," 110,000 jerseys, and 70,000 sweaters. By the mid-1980s, the mix of promotional items had changed. The items were more likely to contrast the "then-and-now" choices of women and to highlight the availability of previously all-male goods (e.g., a little black book for telephone numbers, jogging suits, rugby shirts, and boxing shorts). A promotional history was introduced, the Book of Days, a hardbound appointment calendar noting dates in history, including the date when Virginia Slims were launched in 1968; historical anecdotes; and sexist quotations. It was reported that one million books were printed annually (Robinson 1985).

Virginia Slims started sponsoring women's professional tennis in 1970, and a full season of tournaments was played in 1971. That year, events were held in 20 cities and featured eight professionals, including Billie Jean King and Rosemary Casals (Brinkman 1976). Free samples of Virginia Slims were given away at stadium entrances (Ernster 1985), and contract players were not allowed to take public positions against cigarette sponsorship (Brinkman 1976). The brand's public relations firm developed a program for reaching the media with "stories and angles of interest that extended far beyond match results and sports pages.... The Virginia Slims media guide, published annually... became the encyclopedia of women's tennis" (Harris 1991, p. 208). Media luncheons were held at the start of the season in New York and before each event in every tournament city, where charity tie-ins created more publicity. Although cigarette advertising was banned from television, the Virginia Slims Tournament was covered by the networks (Harris 1991). A Philip Morris marketing vice president explained, "Virginia Slims gets worldwide publicity and an opportunity to sample adult audiences and to spin off retail promotions" (Harris 1991, p. 209). The company also gained grateful allies: in 1990, when the U.S. Secretary of Health and Human Services, Louis Sullivan, M.D., called for an end to sports sponsorships by cigarette firms, Zina Garrison and Billie Jean King supported the industry in press interviews (Harris 1991). In 1995–1996, Philip Morris ended its $5 million annual sponsorship of the Virginia Slims professional women's tennis tour, replacing it with the annual Virginia Slims Legends Tour, at a cost of approximately $3 million. This six-stop event combined a tournament of former tennis greats (e.g., Billie Jean King, Chris Evert, and Martina Navratilova) and a concert featuring prominent female singers (e.g., Barbara Mandrell and Gladys Knight). The stated intention of the new tour was to reach older women (IEG 1995b).

children followed for several years, found that among girls, those aware of the most heavily advertised cigarette brands (Benson and Hedges, Silk Cut) were significantly more likely to start smoking than were those who named other brands (While et al. 1996). A longitudinal study of more than 1,000 Massachusetts youth found that exposure to brand-specific cigarette advertising in magazines was associated with later smoking initiation of these brands (Pucci and Siegel 1999). Among girls, the top seven brands were Marlboro, Camel, Newport, Winston, Capri, Virginia Slims, and Kool.

A number of other studies have investigated advertising awareness, self-image, and perceived attributes of smokers (USDHHS 1994). One of these studies showed that more than 90 percent of 6-year-olds tested in day-care settings in Atlanta and Augusta, Georgia, were able to match the Old Joe (Camel) logo to cigarettes, about the same percentage that could link Mickey Mouse to the Disney channel (Fischer et al. 1991). The tobacco industry attacked this study and funded research in Australia designed to replicate the study and to eliminate some of its alleged shortcomings (Mizerski 1995). Study results confirmed that, in Australia too, recognition of Old Joe was high and increased with age (72 percent of 6-year-olds). The study also assessed, in a matching exercise, the children's liking for products by having them point to a picture of a smiling or frowning face. Forty percent of 3-year-olds but fewer than 5 percent of 5-year-olds demonstrated a liking for cigarettes. The author concluded that, because a high level of recognition was not associated with positive affect, advertising did not encourage children to smoke. This study, however, like the others cited, was not designed to examine the association between early recognition of a cigarette brand logo and later initiation of smoking. Perhaps the more significant observation in all these studies was the high level of recognition of the Joe Camel icon and its association with cigarettes, even among young children.

Whatever children's view of smoking may be, as they approach the middle-school years, they become increasingly concerned with self-image, and messages contained in tobacco advertising and promotions likely play a role in changing their attitudes and behaviors (Arnett and Terhanian 1998; Feighery et al. 1998). Using data from the youth portion of the 1993 California Tobacco Survey, a study from California (Evans et al. 1995) identified an association between receptivity to tobacco marketing and susceptibility to smoking. (A separate longitudinal study identified susceptibility to smoking at baseline as being predictive of future cigarette use [Pierce et al. 1996]). Beside naming a favorite tobacco ad or believing in the benefits of smoking promoted by tobacco advertising, the index of receptivity to tobacco marketing in the California study included possession of a tobacco promotional item, such as a key chain, lighter, or T-shirt with a tobacco brand logo on it. The association between possession of a tobacco promotional item and susceptibility to smoking (Evans et al. 1995) was verified in two other cross-sectional studies, one that involved a national sample of adolescents (Altman et al. 1996) and one that included students in rural New England (Sargent et al. 1997).

Promotional items are typically obtained at the point of sale as a premium or from coupon redemption. However, many adolescents also obtain them as gifts from family or friends (Gilpin et al. 1997; Sargent et al. 1997). In 1993, a national study of U.S. girls and boys aged 12 through 17 years showed that 35 percent had collected tobacco coupons (e.g., Camel Cash and Marlboro Adventure Miles), had a promotional catalog, or owned a promotional item (Coeytaux et al. 1995). More than 1 in 10 of the girls and boys (10.6 percent) reported having owned at least one tobacco promotional item. Extrapolating to the entire population of U.S. girls and boys aged 12 through 17 years, the authors estimated that 7.4 million had participated in a tobacco promotional campaign. The amount of the tobacco marketing budget devoted to promotions of this sort, in contrast to traditional print advertising, has increased substantially since 1985 (Gilpin et al. 1997; Redmond 1999). The deviation from observed prevalence and prevalence predicted by a diffusion model of daily smoking among ninth graders nationwide (based on a series of cross-sectional surveys) was correlated with the upswing in tobacco promotional expenditures (Redmond 1999).

A recent longitudinal study further demonstrated the relationship between tobacco promotional items and smoking initiation among youth. In 1996, youth who participated in the 1993 California Tobacco Survey were contacted again for a study funded by The Robert Wood Johnson Foundation. Among those who were not susceptible to smoking and who had never smoked in 1993, receptivity to tobacco marketing predicted those who became susceptible to smoking or who smoked by 1996 (Pierce et al. 1998). Receptivity to tobacco promotional items (having a promotional item or being willing to use one) carried 2.89 times the risk for progression toward smoking than did minimal receptivity. Receptivity to tobacco advertising (having a favorite tobacco ad, but not owning or being willing to use a promotional item) carried a 1.82 increased risk. Minimally receptive adolescents had no promotional items, would not be willing to use one, had no favorite cigarette ad, and could or would not name a brand as being the most advertised. No interaction of advertising receptivity with gender was observed, and the analysis adjusted for demographics, school performance, and parental and peer smoking. From this study, it was estimated that 34 percent of adolescent experimentation with cigarettes can be attributed to tobacco advertising and promotions. Another longitudinal study of 529 Massachusetts teens aged 12 through 15 years, interviewed in 1993 and again in 1997, produced very similar findings (Biener and Siegel 2000).

## Themes in Tobacco Marketing Targeted to Women

As noted, tobacco marketers target particular brands and messages to women (Ernster 1985; Amos 1992; Amos and Bostock 1992a; USDHHS 1994). The brand image of some cigarettes is unmistakably feminine, and most of their consumers are women. The fact that smoking among women in North America has become so widely acceptable, if not desirable, is a remarkable cultural shift that has its roots in the effective promotion of smoking as a symbol of freedom and emancipation (Amos and Haglund 2000). However, brands developed exclusively for women (e.g., Virginia Slims, Eve, Misty, and Capri) account for only 5 to 10 percent of the total cigarette market (*Marketing to Women* 1991). Because women represent nearly one-half of all smokers, many women are obviously attracted to brands that appear gender neutral or overtly targeted to men.

Warner and Goldenhar (1992) examined the advertising revenues of 92 magazines published in 1959–1986. The relative share of cigarette advertising revenues by magazine category over these 28 years was determined. Magazines were coded in categories as women's, sports, news, highbrow, professional, crafts and trade magazines, or other. Relative share was defined as a "category's percentage of cigarette advertising revenues in the sample of 92 magazines divided by its percentage of total advertising revenues" (Warner and Goldenhar 1992, p. 25). Relative share during 1983–1986 was highest among crafts and trade magazines (1.78) and sports magazines (1.76). However, the relative share of cigarette advertising revenues increased from 0.14 to 1.11 among women's magazines over the 28 years covered by the study, and between 1983 and 1986 it grew faster among women's magazines than for any other category of magazines. Included among the 18 publications in the women's magazines category were *Better Homes and Gardens, Cosmopolitan, Ladies' Home Journal,* and *Working Woman.*

That tobacco marketing targeted to women emphasizes themes such as slimness, women's equality, freedom of choice, independence, glamour, and romance is widely acknowledged (Altman et al. 1987; Albright et al. 1988; Guinan 1988; Krupka et al. 1990; Krupka and Vener 1992; Covell et al. 1994; Califano 1995). A number of empirical studies supported this view. An analysis of 1,827 ads in five popular magazines (*Good Housekeeping, Look, Newsweek, Sports Illustrated,* and *TV Guide*) across three time spans (1950–1951, 1960–1961, and 1970–1971) examined ads for tobacco, nonalcoholic beverages, automobiles, home appliances, office equipment, and airline travel (Sexton and Haberman 1974). Tobacco ads accounted for 24 percent of all ads. In the 1950s, ads typically portrayed women as models or public personalities, rather than as social companions, employees, or consumers, and women were generally presented in the background rather than as central figures. In the 1960s and 1970s, women were portrayed primarily as social companions or dates, not as employees, housewives, or mothers (Sexton and Haberman 1974).

In a content analysis of 778 tobacco ads in eight popular magazines (*Rolling Stone, Cycle World, Mademoiselle, Ladies' Home Journal, Time, Popular Science, TV Guide,* and *Ebony*) published in 1960–1985, Altman and colleagues examined the extent of segmentation and the themes of ads (Altman et al. 1987; Albright et al. 1988; Basil et al. 1991). The percentage of tobacco ads in women's magazines increased substantially over time. By 1985, cigarette ads in women's magazines comprised 34 percent of all cigarette ads across the eight magazines, up from about 10 percent in 1960. A study of magazines for youth published in 1972–1985 showed a similar trend (Albright et al. 1988). In all magazines, ads that showed the act of smoking or visible smoke decreased over the study period (Altman et al. 1987). In contrast, the association of smoking with health and vitality and with images of risk, adventure, recreation, and eroticism increased. Compared with other magazines, women's magazines were more likely to have ads for low-tar, low-nicotine brands of cigarettes and ads featuring sexual images and were less likely to have ads featuring adventure or risk themes (Altman et al. 1987). In a follow-up study that added *Jet* and *Essence* to the database and extended the years of study to 1989, models in cigarette ads in women's magazines were more likely than models in men's magazines to be portrayed as coy or seductive or to be engaged in horseplay or romantic situations (Basil et al. 1991). Covell and colleagues (1994) found that among adolescents, girls had a stronger preference than boys for image-oriented ads.

An analysis of 74 popular magazines published in 1988, one-half of which were women's magazines, showed that 63 percent of 241 tobacco ads were in women's magazines (Krupka et al. 1990). Statistical tests were not used, but tobacco advertising in women's magazines was reported to be more likely than that in men's magazines to feature low-tar, low-nicotine cigarettes (13.7 vs. 6.6 percent) and themes of social success (10.2 vs. 7.2 percent), refreshment or pleasure (8.4 vs. 6.6 percent), or independence or self-reliance (7.1 vs. 1.1 percent) and to use models with attractive and lean silhouettes (13.5 vs. 0.6 percent). Tobacco ads in men's magazines were more likely than those in women's magazines to focus on taste, flavor, or quality (24.3 vs. 16.4 percent); masculine activities (25.4 vs. 6.7 percent); prize giveaways (8.3 vs. 3.9 percent); and leisure, excitement, or thrill (6.1 vs. 1.8 percent). In a content analysis of 352 tobacco ads in 18 popular magazines in 1945, 1955, 1965, 1972, and 1985, England and coworkers (1987) demonstrated that advertising themes changed substantially over time; only the theme of taste endured. By 1985, ads using testimonials and emphasizing the quality of the tobacco no longer appeared, and portrayal of models holding cigarettes dropped by one-third. Instead, ads focused on attributes such as low tar content, filters, and the cigarette length. The gender and activity of models differed across magazine types. Ads that showed women engaged in activities were more likely to appear in women's magazines (25.3 percent) than in general or news magazines (6.5 percent) or men's magazines (1.9 percent). Ads that showed men engaged in activities were more likely to appear in men's magazines (52.3 percent) than in general or news magazines (40.0 percent) or women's magazines (18.7 percent). The proportion of ads that showed both women and men engaged in activities did not differ markedly by magazine type (33.3 percent in women's magazines, 23.4 percent in men's magazines, and 30 percent in general or news magazines).

Cigarette advertising targeted to women has long been characterized by themes such as thinness, style, glamour, sophistication, sexual attractiveness, social inclusion, athleticism, liberation, freedom, and independence (Howe 1984; Elkind 1985; Ernster 1985, 1986; Kilbourne 1989). Through the years, ads have depicted these themes in a variety of ways. Salem used a romantic appeal of "springtime, green fields, and soft summer dresses" (Weinstein 1970, p. 10). In 1970, Brown & Williamson introduced Flair, a fashion cigarette for women, in test markets (O'Connor 1970). The next year, Liggett & Myers introduced Eve, which had a feminine floral design on the filter (*Advertising Age* 1970) (Figure 4.11). Because of the impending ban on broadcast advertising, Eve's introduction was backed by a flood of print advertising, and successful test marketing was conducted in four cities. The national campaign included ads in *TV Guide*, women's magazines (including *Ebony*, *Essence*, and *Tuesday* for black women), and periodicals devoted to house and gardens topics. Other venues were entertainment programs such as *Playbill*, full-color newspaper ads, Sunday supplements, and outdoor advertising in the top 25 markets. The ultrafeminine floral design of Eve, however, did not prove as popular in its appeal as the pseudoliberated appeal of Virginia Slims. In 1974, Eve was repackaged and repositioned to "free the brand from total domination by its packaging," because executives believed it was not "perceived as a real cigaret" (O'Connor 1974, p. 8). The new ad copy read "We asked her if she wanted a ladylike cigaret. She said, 'Hell, no'" (O'Connor 1974, p. 8).

In the 1980s, women's brands remained an important element in cigarette advertising. Lorillard's ads for the Satin brand appealed to self-indulgence—"Spoil Yourself with Satin"—and targeted the woman who was "self-confident, relaxed, realizing her goals" (Sobczynski 1983, p. M-15) (Figure 4.11). The More brand offered a long, thin cigarette to women, "especially the 18 to 34 year old female who considers herself to be sophisticated" (Sobczynski 1983, p. M-15) (Figure 4.11). The director of marketing for More said, "Cigarets are a product people first wear, then smoke" (Masloski 1981, p. S-7). The extra-long brown More 120s "appeal to older more sophisticated women—women who are stylish, assertive, [and] want to call attention to themselves" (Masloski 1981, p. S-7). The premium-priced Ritz, a name suggesting an "opulent life style" (Hollie 1985, p. 29), was designed by Yves Saint Laurent and sold by R.J. Reynolds. It was intended to set a "new standard of stylishness" and targeted "the fashion-conscious woman... probably single, owns a designer handbag, reads *Vogue* and spends a high percentage of her

**Figure 4.11. Tobacco marketers targeted particular brands to women—Eve, Style, Satin, and More**

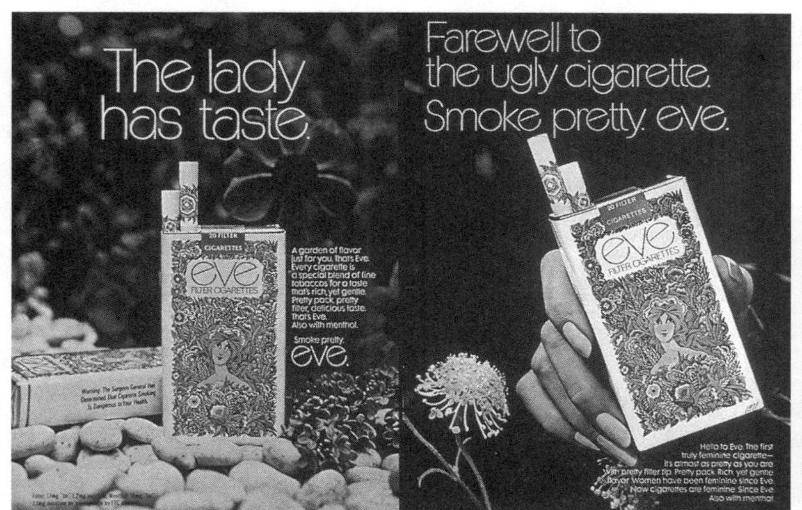


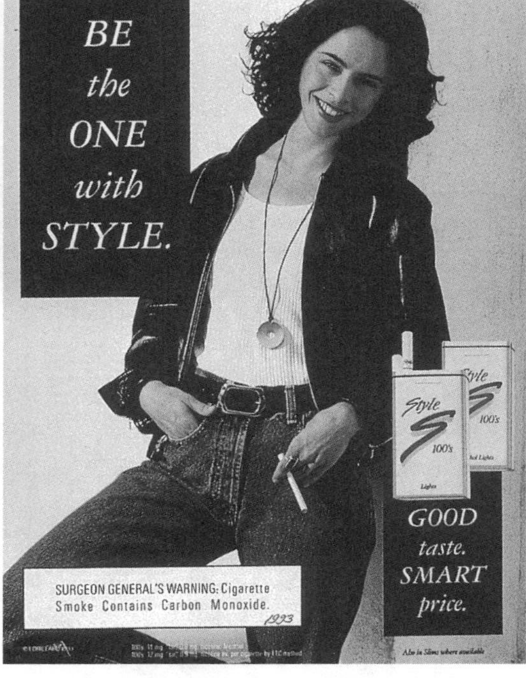


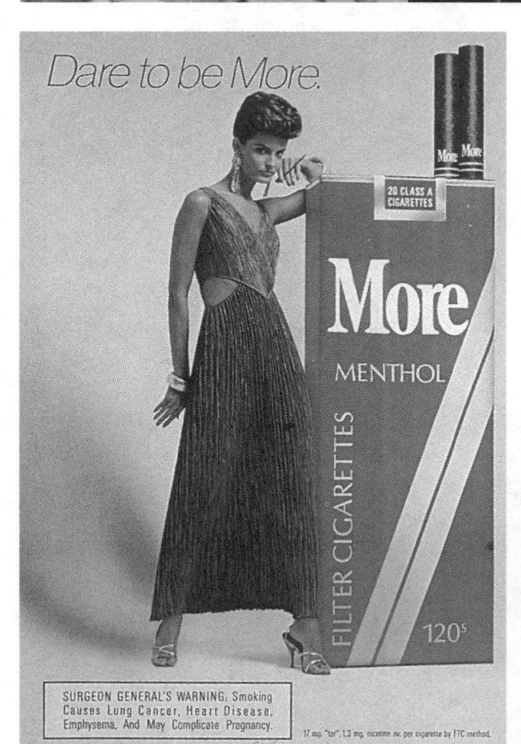


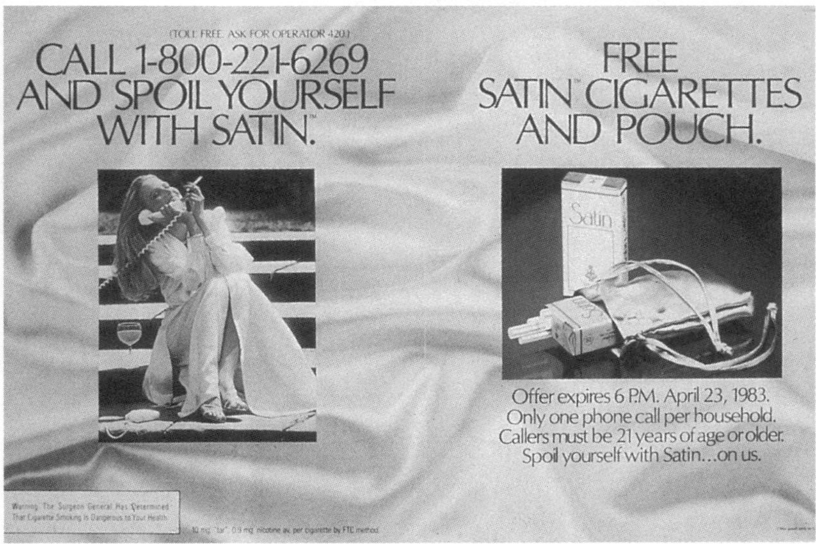


Sources: Clockwise from top left: (Eve, Style, and Satin) Tobacco Industry Promotion Series, Faculty of Commerce, History of Advertising Archives, University of British Columbia, History of Advertising Archives, Vancouver, Canada; (More) *Ladies' Home Journal* 1986.

income on clothes" (Hollie 1985, p. 29). A Lorillard brand was bluntly labeled Style (Figure 4.11).

By the end of the 1980s and into the 1990s, cigarette manufacturers were using various technologies to make products that would appeal to women. Virginia Slims offered a variant called Superslims (Figure 4.12) that was not only even thinner than the original cigarette but was also claimed to reduce sidestream smoke, and Capri offered "the slimmest slim" (Figure 4.12).

R.J. Reynolds placed four-page ads in women's magazines for the novel Chelsea brand, which had a vanilla-like scent. This campaign included the industry's first "scratch-and-sniff" ad. New paper technology allowed release of a similar aroma while the cigarette was lit, thus masking the smell of ambient smoke (Dagnoli 1989). Chelsea was promoted with a compact lighter featuring a small mirror, coupons for free packs of cigarettes, and in-store, buy-one-get-one-free offers. In the fall of 1995, ads for Capri

**Figure 4.12. By the late 1980s and into the 1990s, cigarette manufacturers were trying to make products more appealing to women: Superslims, with the claim of reduced sidestream smoke; "slim 'n sassy" Misty; and Capri, "the slimmest slim"**

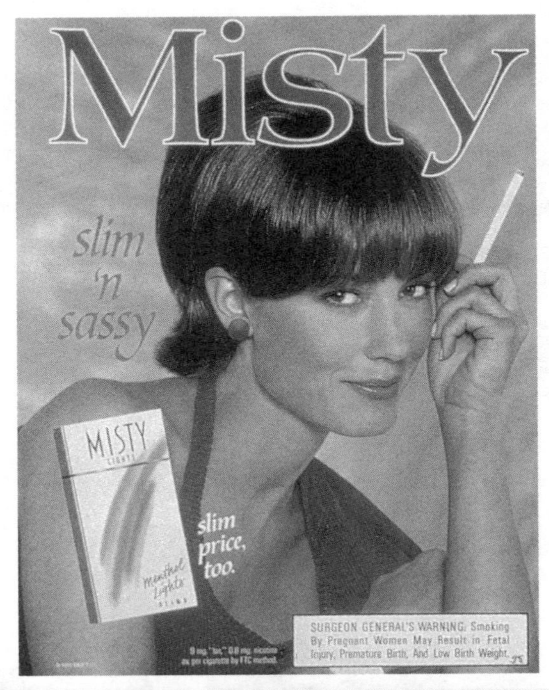


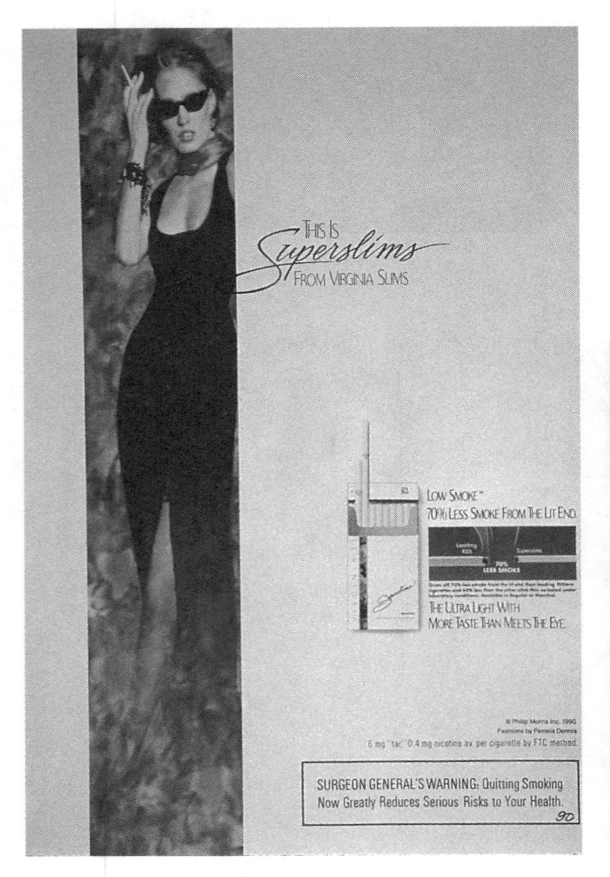


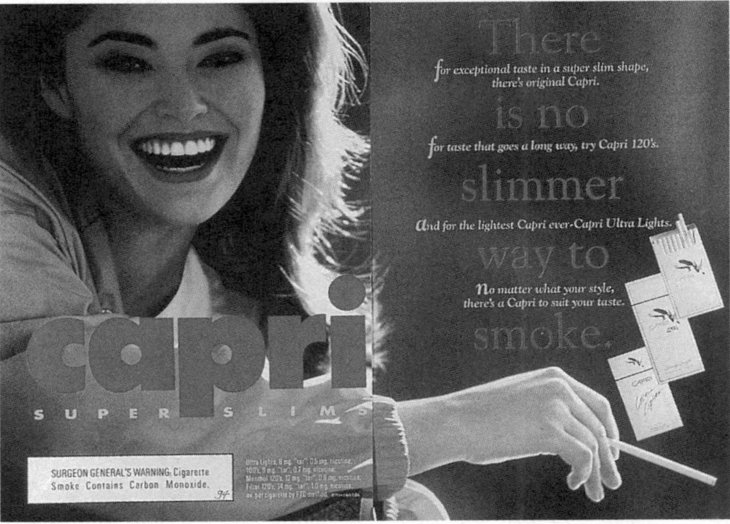


Sources: Clockwise from bottom left: Tobacco Industry Promotion Series, History of Advertising Archives, Faculty of Commerce, University of British Columbia, Vancouver, Canada; *Marie Claire* 1995; *Allure* 1995a.

Superslims appeared in women's magazines with the slogan "She's gone to Capri and she's not coming back" (*Allure* 1995a). These ads featured thin models, glamorously or romantically dressed, posed in a European isle setting and holding the ultraslim cigarette (*Allure* 1995a; *Cosmopolitan* 1995a).

One ad that featured women, but presumably was not targeted to women, deserves mention because negative press and opposition by women's groups, as well as health advocacy organizations and members of Congress, led to its eventually being pulled by the manufacturer. It was a four-page ad for Camel cigarettes placed by R.J. Reynolds in 1989, as part of its "Smooth moves" campaign (*Health Letter* 1989, cover; *Time* 1989). The first page of the ad pictured an alluring blonde woman with the caption "Bored? Lonely? Restless? What You Need Is...." The middle two pages provided "foolproof dating advice" (e.g., "always break the ice by offering her a Camel") and tips on how to impress someone at the beach (e.g., "Run into the water, grab someone and drag her back to the shore as if you've saved her from drowning. The more she kicks and screams, the better"). The final page instructed readers on "how to get a FREE pack even if you don't like to redeem coupons" (e.g., "ask your best friend to redeem it or ask a kind-looking stranger to redeem it") (*Health Letter* 1989, cover).

## Contemporary Cigarette Advertisements and Promotions

A variety of approaches were used to promote the Virginia Slims brand in the 1990s. One ad for Virginia Slims Lights showed a young couple dressed casually in blue and white who were playing backgammon outdoors. The copy read "Who says you can't make the first move?" and "You've come a long way, baby" (*Harper's Bazaar* 1995). A more suggestive ad showed a model posing under a palm tree clad in animal-print clothing that matched the red and black copy, "Tame and timid? That goes against my instincts" (*Cosmopolitan* 1995c). Other Virginia Slims ads promoted merchandise. One, in pinks and whites with copy that read "Glamour... Gotta have it," portrayed a glamorous blonde woman and offered the latest V-Wear (clothing and accessories) catalog (*People* 1995d). In another ad, an alluring blonde woman dressed in a satiny white suit offered the Virginia Slims calendar with a white, black, and red color scheme (*Vanity Fair* 1995b). Beginning in late 1999, Philip Morris promoted Virginia Slims in a multicultural campaign with the tagline, "Find Your Voice" (Figure 4.10). The underlying message of this campaign was freedom, emancipation, and empowerment. In a harsh critique of this campaign, the editors of *Ms.* magazine wrote in the June/July 2000 issue: "In their relentless quest to get and keep women hooked on smoking, the Virginia Slims folks give the term 'pimp' new meaning. They've long hitched their cancer sticks to women's liberation with smarmy pitches like 'You've come a long way, baby.' Now Virginia Slims has set its sights on globalizing addiction and equalizing smoking-related illnesses. In their latest campaign, which debuted in the fall of 1999, they issue a cynical, multicultural call to women to 'find your voice.'"

Misty, also heavily advertised in women's magazines, used head shots of attractive women holding the slim cigarette. The copy read "Slim 'n sassy... slim price too" (*Marie Claire* 1995). The colors in the Misty brush-stroke logo (pink, blue, green, and yellow) were repeated in the copy, background, clothing, and accessories (Figure 4.12).

Ads targeted to gays and lesbians for major tobacco brands have appeared since at least the early 1990s (Goebel 1994). For example, a Virginia Slims ad featured a man and woman walking together, with the woman smiling over her shoulder at another woman and a caption that read, "If you always follow the straight and narrow, you'll never know what's around the corner."

Gender-neutral brands often feature young couples. A Merit ad, for example, showed a couple embracing, each in a leather jacket, with the slogan "You've got Merit" (*New Woman* 1995b). Parliament ads showed casually dressed couples, sometimes in swimwear, in a pristine setting of crystal-clear skies and blue water (*People* 1995a). Either the woman or man held the cigarette, and the slogan "The perfect recess" was the only copy, along with the blue and white Parliament package.

Ads for brands seemingly targeted to men (e.g., Marlboro) but popular too among women have also appeared in women's magazines. Marlboro ads featured cowboys in outdoor pursuits, often under deep blue skies and beside or in very blue water (*Glamour* 1995a; *Vogue* 1995c). White, gold, blue, and red were the key colors used, with slogans such as "Come to Marlboro country" and "Some mornings, it's quiet enough to hear the break of day."

Rarely, an ad focuses on the product itself. For example, Carlton ads displayed only the package, a woman's hand against a blue satin background, and copy that read "Carlton is lowest" (*Ladies' Home Journal*

1995; McCall's 1995). Fine print claimed that Carlton was the lowest in tar and nicotine of the king-sized, soft-pack cigarettes.

Some research suggested that women of all ages are more responsive than men to the price of tobacco (Townsend et al. 1994), and discount brands such as Basic and Doral are heavily advertised in women's publications. Ads for Basic showed a red-and-white cigarette pack against a white background and objects with corresponding copy, such as a white sun lounge with "Your basic smoking lounge" (*New Woman* 1995a, p. 131) or T-shirts, jeans, and sneakers bearing the message "Your basic 3-piece suit" (*Entertainment Weekly* 1995, p. 33). Ads included the slogan "It tastes good. It costs less" (*New Woman* 1995a).

Camel ads featuring the macho cartoon character Joe Camel were first introduced in 1987 (*Mademoiselle* 1995). In 1994, Camel ads debuted Joe's female counterpart, Josephine, who was featured in four-page foldout ads that showed female and male camel characters drinking, smoking, shooting pool, and socializing at Joe's Place. The slogan was "There's something for everyone at Joe's Place" (Goldman 1994; *Redbook* 1994). The Josephine ads soon disappeared, but a Camel collector's pack was introduced in magazine ads in 1995. These ads, which showed a glamorous starlet as she appeared on the package in 1934, carried the slogan "This woman has a past" (*Vogue* 1995b).

Advocacy ads sponsored by tobacco companies also appeared in magazines with predominantly female audiences. Philip Morris placed a series of ads with the theme "We want you to know where we stand," ridiculing attacks on smokers, supporting freedom of choice, or explaining the company's new program to limit youth access to cigarettes (*Allure* 1995b; *Glamour* 1995b; *Vanity Fair* 1995a). Ads for Philip Morris' Benson & Hedges cigarettes spoofed nonsmoking restrictions in public places in a series of ads on the theme "The length you go for pleasure." Ads (*Cosmopolitan* 1995b) showed smokers eating in an open-air restaurant atop a pole several stories aboveground, business persons smoking while perched on carved figures along a public building's roofline (*Vanity Fair* 1995c), and commuters smoking atop a speeding train (People 1995e).

R.J. Reynolds' "Survival Guide for the 90's" ad offered a cartoon-illustrated "common sense guide to life in the nineties" (*People* 1995b). It depicted situations in which smoking is awkward, alongside other modern frustrations such as long lines at automated tellers, sweaty gym equipment, and violators in supermarket express lanes. The ad noted that "Together, we can work it out," that "Most smoking issues can be resolved through dialogue," and that "Discussion will help solve the issues without further Government intervention."

The most successful women's brand, Virginia Slims, has offered a yearly engagement calendar and the V-Wear catalog featuring clothing, jewelry, and accessories coordinated with the themes and colors of the print advertising and product packaging. The theme of the fall 1995 advertising campaign was glamour, and the catalog offered a purple satin charmeuse blouse (with proof of purchase of 125 packs of cigarettes), rhinestone bangles (55 packs), a camel coat trimmed in faux leopard (325 packs), a classic sweater set in the raspberry color of the advertising copy and product packaging (200 packs), makeup brushes wrapped in a raspberry satin pouch (65 packs), a black coat lined in raspberry (325 packs), and other accessory items. Marketing themes were carried through in stores, where small plastic shopping baskets and checkout lane markers featured ads for Virginia Slims and purchases were slipped into plastic drawstring bags bearing the Virginia Slims logo and colors (*People* 1995d).

To promote Capri Superslims, Brown & Williamson used point-of-sale displays and value-added gifts. Multiple-pack boxes contained premium items such as mugs and caps bearing the Capri label in colors coordinated with the ad and package. A single-pack package contained a Capri lighter. Underscoring the long length of Capri Superslims, a free umbrella and two packs of cigarettes were sold in a tall box. The American Tobacco Company's Misty Slims also offered color-coordinated items in multiple-pack containers. An address book, cigarette lighter, T-shirt, fashion booklet, and Rand McNally guide to factory outlet shopping malls carried through the Misty advertising "look" (Trinkets and Trash: A Collection of Tobacco Product Advertising and Promotion, 1999, personal collection of John Slade, University of Medicine and Dentistry of New Jersey, New Brunswick, NJ).

R.J. Reynolds' catalogs offered items that could be redeemed by using the Camel Cash notes (C-notes) in cigarette packs. Items included a Midnight Oasis leather lipstick holder (40 C-notes), ladies' nightshirt (60 C-notes), camel necklace (20 C-notes) and earrings (21 C-notes) and many items of clothing and sporting gear, as well as lighters, barware, and accessories (*Redbook* 1994). Philip Morris offered the Marlboro Country Store: empty packs could be exchanged for clothing bearing the Marlboro logo. In addition, the campaign helped the company to develop a database of smokers and provided millions of Americans with logo-bearing items to wear or use (Zinn 1994). Philip Morris also spent $200 million on its Marlboro Adventure Team catalog, which featured outdoor equipment and clothing (Zinn 1994). R.J. Reynolds has invested resources in so-called "relationship marketing." For example, in 1999 in Tobaccoville, North Carolina, where R.J. Reynolds' largest tobacco plant is located, the company held a party with music, blackjack, and free cigarettes for 3,700 of its customers (Doral Brand smokers) (Fairclough 1999).

Another form of promotion combined giveaways with advocacy advertising. Themes such as freedom and liberty were used to promote smokers' rights. For example, Brown & Williamson mailed its customers a crystal Christmas tree ornament etched with the image of the Liberty Bell and the B&W logo. The ornament came in a pouch inside a gilt-engraved display carton that bore a quote from the chief executive officer emphasizing the importance of Americans having the freedom to make informed choices. Philip Morris enclosed a two-pack box of Benson & Hedges with a deck of playing cards imprinted with a photograph of tourists climbing the head of the Statue of Liberty. These promotions were not specific to one gender or the other, but they may have had considerable appeal to women (Trinkets and Trash: A Collection of Tobacco Product Advertising and Promotion, 1999, personal collection of John Slade, University of Medicine and Dentistry of New Jersey, New Brunswick, NJ).

The tobacco industry is not uniformly successful in its efforts to tailor smoking messages to target audiences. Although the campaigns for Virginia Slims and several other brands targeted to women struck a responsive chord, the campaign to promote Dakota, a cigarette that targeted the "virile female," did not (Specter 1990, p. A-1). After a complex series of marketing events, in which antitobacco advocacy played a considerable role, the product was eventually withdrawn (see text box "Dakota: A Case Study in Marketing Failure").

In June 2000, during the time when chief executives of tobacco companies were testifying during the Florida class-action suit against them, Philip Morris announced that it was removing tobacco advertisements from 42 magazines because it was concerned about the teen readership of these magazines (*Advertising Age* 2000). Whether this was true or not, this step indicated that in recent years, concern over teen exposure to tobacco advertisements has become part of the public dialogue.

## Sponsorship

Tobacco company sponsorship has included sporting events; women's fashion and cultural events; and women's political, ethnic, and research activities. The preeminent example of sponsorships targeted to women is women's tennis, an activity that capitalizes on the attributes of independence, assertiveness, and success. Virginia Slims and Kim, its British counterpart (Elkind 1985), have used television coverage and other media outlets to promote their brand names and logos (Ernster 1985). At one Wimbledon match, Martina Navratilova wore a tennis outfit in the colors of Kim packaging and bearing the Kim logo (Ernster 1986).

R.J. Reynolds' More brand sponsored a series of fashion shows in shopping malls that were tied to advertising in fashion magazines. Designers in the fashion industry received More Fashion Awards (Ernster 1988). Tobacco companies have also sponsored rock concerts and other music concerts with high appeal to female audiences.

Tobacco company sponsorships have benefited the arts as well. For example, tobacco companies sponsored a national tour of The Joffrey Ballet, performances of the Alvin Ailey American Dance Theater, an exhibit featuring photographs of Dr. Martin Luther King, Jr., the Arts Festival of Atlanta (Georgia) (a family event with more than 10 million attendees), and the Vatican Art Exhibit at The Metropolitan Museum of Art (New York, New York) (Ernster 1988; Lynch and Bonnie 1994; IEG 1995b). In 1995, Philip Morris spent $1.2 million to sponsor 15 dance companies (e.g., American Ballet Theatre, Dance Theatre of Harlem, and The Joffrey Ballet) and two dance events (IEG 1995b).

Sponsorships of festivals and fairs, such as the Kool Jazz Festival and Hispanic Cinco de Mayo street fairs, create dependence on the tobacco industry for community cultural events (Lynch and Bonnie 1994). Marlboro (Philip Morris) sponsored 18 major fairs in 1995 (e.g., state fairs in Illinois, Ohio, and Texas) and spent $850,000 to reach 20 million family members. In 1996, Lorillard's Newport brand sponsored 31 New York City family and children's events at a cost of $155,000 to reach more than 15 million attendees. These events included the Second Avenue Family Festival, the Great July 4th Festival, the Avenue of the Americas Family Expo, and, in collaboration with the Sierra Club, Earth Day (IEG 1995b).

Civic improvement has also received tobacco sponsorship. Brown & Williamson supported the Kool Achiever Awards to recognize persons who

## Dakota: A Case Study in Marketing Failure

Loss of broadcast media outlets and recognition of the heterogeneity of current and potential women smokers have led to two important trends in cigarette marketing: an increasingly high degree of specificity in the psychological research on and definition of the target consumer, and the increasing and now dominant use of promotions, sponsorships, and public relations instead of conventional media advertising. These trends are illustrated by R.J. Reynolds' promotional plan for the Dakota brand (Freedman and McCarthy 1990; Trueheart 1991). Information on this plan came to light after an anonymous insider sent information to advocacy groups (USDHHS 2000).

Market research had shown the potential to influence poorly educated, young, blue-collar women, some of whom were described as "virile females" (Specter 1990, p. A-1). Documents on the promotional plan for Dakota cigarettes described the consumers targeted by the company as women who appreciated traditional "masculine" values—particularly being "independent, in control, self-confident"—and who might otherwise smoke Marlboro cigarettes (Project VF Recommended Next Steps, unpublished data). The targeted women were 18 through 24 years old, with no education beyond high school. They held entry-level service or factory jobs, had no career prospects, and had a high probability of being unemployed or employed only part time. Their clothes were casual (e.g., jeans, knit tops, sweaters, shorts, warm-up suits, and sweatshirts and sweatpants), and they wore little makeup. Their taste in television programs included evening soap operas and situation comedies with working-class heroines, such as Roseanne, and their music tastes centered on all-male, classic rock bands. According to the promotional plan, the virile female spent her free time with her boyfriend, "doing whatever he is doing" (*Trone Advertising* 1989, p. 5) and aspired to getting married in her early twenties and having a family. She and her friends pursued interests such as "cruising" (*Trone Advertising* 1989, p. 5), partying, listening to classic rock and roll, attending various motor sports (e.g., drag races, hot-rod shows, tractor pulls, and motorcycle races), playing softball and bowling, watching wrestling and "Tough Man" (*Trone Advertising* 1989, p. 6) competitions, and attending fairs and carnivals. These characteristics were described as "hot buttons" for appealing to the virile female and her friends (*Trone Advertising* 1989, p. 7).

Forty package backgrounds and 40 names for the new brand were tested in Philadelphia, Pennsylvania. Several variations in packaging and product were considered, including a slide box, a foil inner seal, a wider cigarette, and a slower burning cigarette with a higher puff count. Research explored the packaging colors blue, brown, and burgundy. The women in the focus group preferred burgundy, rating the color as "unique/different, attractive, friends would carry, high quality, modern/contemporary" (Project VF Packaging Test, unpublished data). Consumers in Atlanta were the test group for 120 ad concepts for this new brand of cigarettes, and evaluations by consumers in Baltimore, Maryland, were subsequently used to refine 50 ad concepts. The selected set of advertising images was tested with five focus groups of Marlboro smokers in Chicago, Illinois, who were 18 through 20 years old (Gene Shore, President, Gene Shore Associates, letter to Penny Cohen, Marketing Research Manager, R.J. Reynolds Company, September 5, 1989).

The tested ads seemed successful in conveying the desired imagery of "independent yet approachable, sociable yet also enjoying her own company, feeling equal to men yet enjoying a warm fun relationship with a man," without alienating younger males (Gene Shore, President, Gene Shore Associates, letter to Penny Cohen, Marketing Research Manager, R.J. Reynolds Company, September 5, 1989) (Figure 4.13). Negative reactions to the tested ads occurred either among women with "traditional values" who did not aspire to the "Dakota woman's independence, assertiveness and control" or among the "more conservative/introverted respondents [who] may have felt somewhat threatened by the strong personalities conveyed" (Gene Shore, President, Gene Shore Associates, letter to Penny Cohen, Marketing Research Manager, R.J. Reynolds Company, September 5, 1989). Several slogans using "smooth" were tested, including "Smooth. Streetwise," "Smooth revolution," and "Smooth action. Slow burn." "Where smooth comes easy" was preferred for its consistency with the "attitude/personality" of the Dakota woman (Gene Shore, President, Gene Shore Associates, letter to Penny Cohen, Marketing Research Manager, R.J. Reynolds Company, September 5, 1989). Marketing choices emphasized point-of-sale merchandising and materials usable in promotional venues, such as bars. Promotional items considered were "door decals, in/out stickers, floormats, change cups, banners, neon signs, counter mats, 3-D (three-dimensional) motion signs, clock[s], gas pump toppers, and store hour signs" (*Trone Advertising* 1989, p. 36).

Promotional activities for the Dakota brand were intended to be "tightly targeted [and] extremely impactful and [to use] innovative communication techniques" (Promotional Marketing, Inc. 1989, p. 2). Many promotional concepts were developed, corresponding to the many hot buttons and interests of the targeted women. One

**Figure 4.13. Dakota ad conveys the image of women enjoying warm, fun relationships with men**

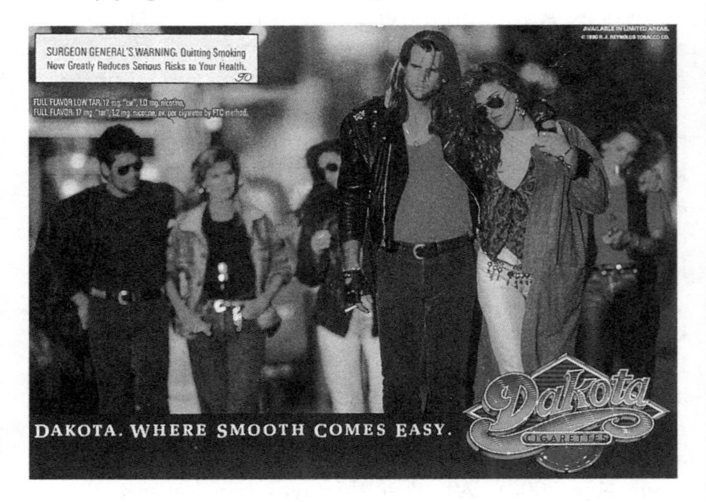


Source: Tobacco Industry Promotion Series, History of Advertising Archives, Faculty of Commerce, University of British Columbia, Vancouver, Canada.

proposal was a "Night of the Living Hunks" contest, for which the prize was a date with a male stripper. The targeted women's interest in romance suggested a soap opera trivia contest and free copies of a customized Dakota romance novel in exchange for redeemable one-pack coupons. Other ideas included limousine parties, vouchers for car shows, and parties in large parking lots where participants could pose against a Dakota backdrop while a camera generated poster-sized pictures. "Party packages" custom designed for women's "hot spots" (e.g., bowling alleys, bars, apartments, and company picnics) (*Trone Advertising* 1989, p. 31) were also proposed. Packages would include decorations, games, prizes, supplies, and samples of Dakota cigarettes (*Trone Advertising* 1989).

Detailed tactical plans and budgets were developed for several promotions related to the targeted women's inclination to patronize bars with rock and roll music. Participating bars and clubs would receive a video jukebox featuring the Dakota colors and logo. An all-male rock band would be named Dakota and perform at local clubs surrounded by a large Dakota banner. The band's clothing, stage materials, and limousine all would bear the Dakota logo. Women in the audience could receive, in a special Dakota folder, instant photographs of themselves with the band. Cassettes of the Dakota band would be handed out with a sweepstakes form to collect names for a direct-mail list; winners would have pictures taken with the band, would be given clothing with the Dakota logo, and would be "official Dakota Groupies for a night" (Promotional Marketing, Inc. 1989, p. 6). Auditions would be held for a girl singer to perform as guest artist; posters in clubs, newspaper ads, and direct mail would publicize this competition. Dakota would conduct screen tests for five finalists to appear in a "feature role" in a music video of the band. Registration, which would be conducted in clubs, required that another person, such as a friend, sign up screen test participants so that both names could be captured for mailing lists. A "Rock Until You Drop" event was to be publicized by a local radio station and hosted by its disc jockey. Two stages would allow for continuous music, and Dakota samples would be distributed during the event. Before this mega Battle of the Bands event (Promotional Marketing, Inc. 1989, p. 8), Dakota parties in nightclubs would award free tickets, limousines, and drinks to selected entrants. All entries would provide names and addresses for the mailing list. Implementation in test markets called for weekly distribution of 500 T-shirts, 30 jackets, 1,000 Polaroid photographs and folders, 250 cassettes, 200 sweepstakes forms, and 250 posters to support the planned events. Implementation also called for neon bar signs, as well as Dakota logos on napkins, coasters, stirrers, table tents, ashtrays, and mirrors (Promotional Marketing, Inc. 1989).

The total development costs were considerable. Even six months before the scheduled spring 1990 test marketing and before costs were incurred for ads or promotions, the cost of the project had exceeded $1.4 million (Natalie Perkins, memorandum to Laura Bender, September 20, 1989). In addition, the campaign may have had some public relations costs for the industry. A sizable advocacy campaign was mounted to highlight the targeting and promotion efforts (USDHHS 2000). The effect of the advocacy effort is unclear, but the Dakota brand ultimately had little market impact, and it was withdrawn. The campaign illustrated that psychological subtleties and knowledge of lifestyle patterns were used to define women precisely and that risks from positioning the brand narrowly existed, in that it may have resulted in disinterest among consumers outside this narrow lifestyle segment.

improve life in inner-city communities. They honored five leaders annually and donated $50,000 to each of several nonprofit inner-city services chosen by the honorees (Levin 1988). The company involved the National Urban League, Inc., the National Association for the Advancement of Colored People, and the National Newspaper Publishers Association in the selection process (Lynch and Bonnie 1994).

In addition, the tobacco industry has provided financial support to women's organizations, especially those that promote women's leadership in business and politics (Williams 1991). These groups have included the National Women's Political Caucus, the Women's Campaign Fund, the Women's Research & Education Institute (an affiliate of the Congressional Caucus for Women's Issues), the League of Women Voters Education Fund, Women Executives in State Government, the Center for Women Policy Studies, the Center for the American Woman and Politics, the American Association of University Women, and the American Federation of Business and Professional Women's Clubs (Levin 1988; Williams 1991). In mid-1999, it was reported that Philip Morris, along with a few other large corporations and women's advocacy groups, formed the Safe@Work coalition, a group dedicated to protecting women who were stalked by their abusers in the workplace (Ellin 2000). Likewise, Philip Morris, through Doors of Hope, a partnership it entered into with the National Network to End Domestic Violence Fund, provided over $1 million in grants to 132 organizations around the country who were tackling domestic violence (Adams 1998).

In the past, Philip Morris funded printing of the program for a meeting of the National Organization for Women (Ernster 1985), but the organization later eschewed tobacco company funding (Williams 1991). The Center for American Women and Politics at Rutgers University (New Brunswick, New Jersey) accepted money from Philip Morris and R.J. Reynolds to hold a conference that drew one-half of the nation's female state legislators (Williams 1991). In 1987, the National Women's Political Caucus received $130,000 from R.J. Reynolds and Philip Morris, which accounted for 10 to 15 percent of the group's budget (Levin 1988). Former caucus advisory board member Patricia Schroeder (D-CO, U.S. House of Representatives, 1972–1996) provided positions to persons with fellowships funded by Philip Morris through the Women's Research & Education Institute and, in 1989, presented the Good Guy Award of the National Women's Political Caucus to a vice president of Philip Morris (Williams 1991). Philip Morris also sponsored a national directory of women elected officials (Levin 1988) and funded internships for the Center for Women Policy Studies. A compendium of organizations and events throughout the United States that received tobacco industry support during 1995–1999 lists 10 programs specifically for women and 2 additional sponsorships for addressing domestic violence (Siegel 2000).

Groups representing minority women have been the recipients of tobacco company funding. These groups include the National Coalition of 100 Black Women, the Mexican American National Women's Association, the U.S. Hispanic Women's Chamber of Commerce, the Asian Pacific American Women's Leadership Institute, and the National Association of Negro Business and Professional Women's Clubs (Williams 1991). Philip Morris sponsored leadership training programs in New York for Hispanic women and, in 1987, gave $150,000 to the U.S. Hispanic Chamber of Commerce (Levin 1988). Tobacco companies also supported the National Council of La Raza, the League of United Latin American Citizens, the National Hispanic Scholarship Fund, the National Association of Hispanic Journalists, the United Negro College Fund, the National Urban League, Inc., the National Newspaper Publishers' Association (a black publishers group), and the Black Journalist's Hall of Fame. In addition, they sponsored directories of national black, Hispanic, and Asian organizations (Ernster 1988; Levin 1988; Williams 1991).

In 1987, Philip Morris gave over $2.4 million to more than 180 black, Hispanic, and women's groups, and R.J. Reynolds gave $1.9 million to 49 women's and minority groups (Levin 1988). Such support buys visibility and credibility and may foster neutrality or support of tobacco industry positions (Warner 1986; Ernster 1988; Levin 1988; Williams 1991). As noted earlier, marketing that associates a consumer product with a cause is typically used to buy goodwill as the return on investment (IEG 1995a). The Women's Research & Education Institute fellowship director was quoted as saying, "I simply think it's part of their way to make themselves look better. They know that they're perceived negatively by representatives who are concerned with health issues. To tell you the truth, I'm not that interested. I'm just glad they fund us" (Levin 1988, p. 15). The executive director of the Women's Campaign Fund observed, "They were there for us when nobody else was. They legitimized corporate giving to political women's groups, from my perspective" (Williams 1991, p. A-16). An August 1986 Tobacco Institute memo stated, "We began intensive discussions with representatives of key women's organizations. Most have assured us that, for the time being, smoking is not a priority issue for them" (Levin 1988, p. 17).

Few women's groups that take tobacco money support campaigns against smoking (Williams 1991). In 1991, the Congressional Caucus on Women's Issues introduced the Women's Health Equity Act. Although it was a package of 22 bills including 6 covering disease prevention, none of the proposals addressed smoking (Williams 1991). Moreover, support for minority causes appears to have borne fruit for tobacco interests. *The National Black Monitor*, which is inserted monthly into 80 newspapers targeted to blacks, ran a three-part series on the tobacco industry. In one of the articles, blacks were called on to "oppose any proposed legislation that often serves as a vehicle for intensified discrimination against this industry which has befriended us, often far more than any other, in our hour of greatest need" (Levin 1988, p. 17). The February installment, ghostwritten by R.J. Reynolds, argued that "relentless discrimination still rages unabashedly on a cross-country scope against another group of targets—the tobacco industry and 50 million private citizens who smoke" (Levin 1988, p. 17).

Auto racing is another popular venue used by tobacco companies to market their products. Race car events are associated with courage, independence, adventure, and aggressiveness (Pollay and Lavack 1993). Although the stereotype is that men, not women, follow auto racing, the sport is of keen interest to many women, especially in the southeastern United States. Tobacco company sponsorship of motor racing events includes the NASCAR Winston Cup stock car race series, the Marlboro Grand Prix, the IndyCar World Series sponsored by Marlboro, and drag racing sponsored by Winston. Individual cars and drivers are also sponsored. A benefit of sponsorship is exposure of the brand and logo of cigarettes on television. In 1992, more than 350 motor sports broadcasts reached more than 915 million people (Slade 1995). On these broadcasts, tobacco brands received about

54 hours of television exposure and were mentioned more than 10,000 times—exposure with a value of approximately $41 million for Winston, $12 million for Marlboro, and $4 million for Camel.

## Provisions of the Master Settlement Agreement

In the historic agreement known as the Master Settlement Agreement (MSA), executed November 23, 1998, 11 tobacco companies agreed to pay $246 million to 46 states over 25 years. The MSA contained numerous provisions important to public health, among them an array of marketing and advertising restrictions (Wilson 1999).

### Restrictions on Brand Name Sponsorships

- Prohibits brand name sponsorship of concerts, events with a significant youth audience, and team sports (football, basketball, baseball, hockey, or soccer).
- Prohibits sponsorship of events where the paid participants or contestants are underage.
- Limits tobacco companies to one brand name sponsorship per year, after current contracts (in effect as of August 1, 1998) expire or after three years, whichever comes first.
- Provides a special exception to the prohibition of the sponsorship of concerts for the Brown & Williamson company by permitting it to sponsor either the GPC country music festival or the Kool jazz festival (formerly both were annual events). The agreement also permits the company to sponsor one other brand name event that was part of a contract in existence before August 1, 1998, for a period not to exceed three years.
- Allows corporate sponsorship of athletic, musical, cultural, artistic, or social events as long as the corporate name does not include the brand name of a domestic tobacco product.
- Bans the use of tobacco brand names in stadiums and arenas.
- Limits the duration and restricts the placement of advertising for sponsored events.

### General Advertising and Marketing Restrictions

- Bans use of cartoon characters, but not human subjects (e.g., the Marlboro Man), in the advertising, promotion, packaging, or labeling of tobacco products, effective May 22, 1999.
- Bans payments to promote tobacco products in movies, television shows, theater productions or live performances, videos, and video games.
- Bans distribution and sale of nontobacco merchandise with brand name logos (e.g., caps, T-shirts, backpacks), effective July 1, 1999.
- Prohibits tobacco companies from authorizing third parties to use or advertise brand names.
- Requires tobacco companies to designate a contact in each state that will respond to Attorney General complaints of prohibited third-party activity.
- Exempts licensing agreements or contracts in existence as of July 1, 1998, but does not permit the licensing agreements or contracts to be extended.
- Bans future cigarette brands from being named after recognized nontobacco brand or trade names (e.g., Harley-Davidson, Yves Saint Laurent, Cartier) or nationally recognized sports teams, entertainment groups, or individual celebrities.

### Restrictions on Outdoor Advertising

- Bans all transit and outdoor advertising (including billboards, signs, and placards larger than a poster) in arenas, stadiums, shopping malls, and video game arcades. Poster-sized signs and placards can be placed in arenas, stadiums, shopping malls, and video game arcades, but must conform to the overall agreement regarding the targeting of advertising to children.
- Requires tobacco billboards and transit ads to be removed by April 22, 1999.
- Allows states to substitute, at industry expense and for the duration of billboard lease periods, alternative advertising that discourages smoking among youth.
- Bans tobacco companies from entering into agreements that would prohibit advertising discouraging tobacco use.

These provisions of the MSA primarily addressed tobacco marketing to youth and have yet to be evaluated as to how they affect tobacco companies' patterns of marketing to women. The first study attempting to document the effect of the MSA marketing and advertising restrictions found that tobacco companies were shifting advertising dollars into point-of-sale promotions and advertising instead of billboards (University of Illinois at Chicago 2000).

## Marketing on the Internet

The future of tobacco advertising and promotion may lie in cyberspace. The World Wide Web on the Internet offers endless possibilities for promoting tobacco use and marketing tobacco products. For users of the Web, hundreds of smoking-related Web sites can be found. (No Web sites are listed here because addresses change so frequently.) These include sites selling smoking clothing and novelty items, such as *Smoke* magazine, and sites providing photographs of women smoking, some of which are pornographic. The Web also offers lists of and information about female celebrities who smoke, as well as photographs of celebrities smoking. Smoking chat rooms and even an interactive novel, *Jack Tar*, which features background photographs of women smoking, are available. There is a smokers' resource site, and many sites are supported by purveyors of cigarettes, cigars, and smokeless tobacco. Using the keywords "smoke," "smoking," "tobacco," and other related terms in any Web site browser will yield many Web site hits.

## Marketing of Smokeless Tobacco and Cigars

As described in "Other Tobacco Use" in Chapter 2, the prevalence of smokeless tobacco use remains low among women and girls in the United States, and advertising of smokeless tobacco products does not appear to be targeted to women.

However, the marketing of cigars to women is an innovation in tobacco advertising, and aggressive marketing to women can be expected to increase women's market share in the future. The Consolidated Cigar Corporation (manufacturers of Muriel, Dutch Masters, El Producto, and Backwoods) has developed new types of cigars for the women's market (Shanken 1996). A spokesperson for Davidoff of Geneva, a cigar store on Madison Avenue in New York City, said in 1995 that its share of women buyers had recently doubled to six percent (Besonen 1995).

Cigars are frequently promoted to women through advertising and special events, such as a $95 per seat dinner held in New York City that featured gourmet foods, champagne, wine, and cigars. The invitation read "An evening dedicated to the women of the 90's!" (Besonen 1995, p. 40). These food, wine, and cigar events—labeled by the industry as "smokers"—have been held throughout the country. Magazines such as *Cigar Aficionado* have prominently displayed photographs of women smoking cigars at these events. Of seven cigar smokers photographed at a March 1995 smoker held at the Walt Disney World Swan Hotel in Orlando, Florida, four were women. The same issue showed two women smoking cigars at a New Orleans (Louisiana) women's smoker held in April 1995, and a New Jersey bride, still in her gown and veil, was shown puffing on a stogie. Women and men could be seen smoking cigars at the April 1995 international cigar celebrations held in 31 Ritz-Carlton hotels around the world, which were sponsored by the General Cigar Company, Inc. and *Cigar Aficionado.* At the Los Angeles movie premiere of *Lord of Illusions,* Dutch actress Famke Janssen, who also costarred in the James Bond movie *Goldeneye,* smoked a cigar beside director Clive Barker (*People* 1995c). An ad in the autumn issue of *Cigar Aficionado* promoted Big Smoke evenings to be held at upscale hotels in San Francisco and Los Angeles, California; New York City; Miami, Florida; Boston, Massachusetts; Chicago, Illinois; and Dallas, Texas (*Cigar Aficionado* 1995b). These events featured handmade cigars from around the world, "the best" spirits and wines, and food from leading "cigar-friendly" restaurants; the cost was $150 per ticket.

Some ads for cigars (e.g., El Sublimado, C.A.O. Premium Cigars, and Don Diego) have featured women smoking them (*Cigar Aficionado* 1995c,d,e). One Don Diego ad showed a glamorous woman puffing a stogie and the phrase "Agnes, have you seen my Don Diegos?" Women smoking cigars have also been featured in ads for establishments such as Bally's Casino in Las Vegas, Nevada, and the Trump Plaza in Atlantic City, New Jersey (*Cigar Aficionado* 1995a,f), and for nontobacco products such as Buffalo jeans (*Vogue* 1995a).

*Cigar Aficionado* runs features on women celebrities, such as Whoopi Goldberg, who smoke cigars. The cover of the autumn 1995 issue showed supermodel Linda Evangelista, dressed in ivory satin, ostrich feathers, and diamonds, holding a cigar. The accompanying eight-page article touted her two-year history of cigar smoking and her favorite cigar. A full-page photograph showed her exhaling cigar smoke, another page reprinted her fashion magazine covers, and another showed her in various poses holding a cigar and wearing only a man's shirt and tie (Rothstein 1995). To promote the issue, *Cigar Aficionado* ran full-page newspaper ads of the cover photograph with copy reading, "Light up with Linda!" (*New York Times* 1995).

Widespread marketing of cigars on the Internet has featured young women modeling cigar-themed sportswear and content likely to appeal to youth of both sexes (Malone and Bero 2000). A Web site devoted to women and cigar smoking also exists (CigarWoman.com 2000). As of July 2000, the Web site defined its focus as follows: "A woman's online source to finding out the best information about cigars, accessories and more. Whoever said it was a man's tradition to enjoy a good stogie? We are working very hard to bring women cigar smokers a place they can feel comfortable and secure about smoking cigars" (CigarWoman.com 2000).

Marketing of cigars also occurs in more subtle ways through product placement in films. A recent study (Goldstein et al. 1999) found that 56 percent of 50 G-rated children's movies reviewed included tobacco use episodes and that of these, cigars were the preferred tobacco for more characters (59 percent) than were cigarettes (21 percent).

According to an FTC report (1999), unit sales of cigars increased by 15 percent between 1996 and 1997, from 3.8 billion to 4.4 billion cigars. During this period, the number of brands marketed increased by 54 percent, from 207 in 1996 to 319 in 1997. Likewise, the variety of cigars available to consumers increased from 1,437 in 1996 to 2,025 in 1997. Concomitant with this increase in sales and varieties of cigars, cigar advertising and promotion increased by 32 percent, from $30.9 million in 1996 to $41 million in 1997. In 1997, the largest proportion of advertising and promotional expenditures was allocated to promotional allowances (39.8 percent), magazines (24.1 percent), and point of sale (13 percent). Internet advertising, while small in actual dollars, rose 180 percent, from $78,000 in 1996 to over $218,000 in 1997. Among women college students, a 1999 survey found that 25 percent reported any lifetime use of cigars and 13.6 percent reported cigar use within the past year (Rigotti et al. 2000).

## Press Self-Censorship in Relation to Cigarette Advertising

Magazines that accept cigarette ads have been reported to be less likely to publish stories on the health effects of tobacco use than are those that do not accept such ads (Smith 1978; Whelan et al. 1981; Ernster 1985; Warner 1985; Weis and Burke 1986; White and Whelan 1986; Kessler 1989; Warner and Goldenhar 1989; Warner et al. 1992b). This finding raised the question of whether dependence on revenues derived from tobacco advertising influences the type and content of articles published. If media coverage of smoking and health in popular magazines is influenced by tobacco companies or their advertising agencies, then media self-censorship must be considered a factor contributing to the lack of public understanding of smoking as a health risk.

In a content analysis of 12 popular women's magazines (*Good Housekeeping, Seventeen, McCall's, Vogue, Harper's Bazaar, Cosmopolitan, Mademoiselle, Redbook, Family Circle, Ms., Ladies' Home Journal,* and *Woman's Day*) from 1967 through 1979, Whelan and colleagues (1981) found only 24 articles about smoking. Several of these articles discussed the unpleasantness of attempting to stop smoking. Eleven of the articles appeared in *Good Housekeeping,* which does not accept tobacco ads. In stark contrast, during the same period, these same 12 magazines contained 54 stories on stress, 103 on nutrition, 121 on contraceptives, and 258 on mental health. Some omissions were glaring. For example, in one article entitled "The ABC's of Preventive Medicine," many health topics were discussed without a single mention of smoking or tobacco (Whelan et al. 1981).

One investigator examined tobacco advertising and the editorial policies of three women's magazines (*Ms., Good Housekeeping,* and *Seventeen*) published in 1972–1979 (Hesterman 1987). The analysis showed that *Good Housekeeping,* which did not accept tobacco advertising, ran an average of 2.1 stories on smoking and health and 11.2 articles on all health topics each year. *Seventeen,* which also did not accept tobacco advertising, ran a smoking and health story only once every two years and 2.2 health articles each year. *Ms.,* which did accept tobacco advertising, ran 5.7 health stories every year, but none addressed the health risks from smoking. On the bases of the findings, extensive interviews with editorial staff of the three magazines, and a review of the literature, the investigator concluded that editorial autonomy on issues related to the health effects of smoking was compromised when a magazine accepted tobacco advertising.

In 1986, another content analysis of 19 popular magazines was published (White and Whelan 1986); 14 of the 19 were women's magazines. The report rated *Reader's Digest* as having the best coverage of the risks from smoking, and *Prevention, The Saturday Evening Post, Good Housekeeping,* and *Vogue,* in that order, were rated as having excellent coverage. Except for *Vogue,* magazines with the best coverage did not accept cigarette advertising. The researchers found that when *The Saturday Evening Post* stopped accepting tobacco ads in 1983, the magazine's coverage of smoking and health increased substantially. Of the 19 magazines, 12 were rated as having poor coverage of smoking and health; for 1 magazine (*McCall's*) the rating was "coverage may be improving." In 1986, *Cosmopolitan* printed one of the only articles it ever published on smoking, and it addressed the reduced risk for endometrial cancer among heavy smokers. The researchers in this study of 19 magazines concluded that magazines that accepted cigarette ads were less likely to publish articles about the health risks from smoking than were those that did not accept such ads.

Other researchers examined the cigarette and alcohol ads in *Ms.* magazine's annual "Beauty of Health" issues published in 1983–1986 (Minkler et al. 1987). The issues of "Beauty of Health" published over the four years contained an average of 5.4 tobacco ads, and cigarette companies often purchased the back outside cover of the magazine, which costs about one-third more than a full page in other parts of the magazine. The primary themes of the ads were related to the product (e.g., taste, tradition, or history), social status (e.g., wealth, prestige, and success), and health (e.g., fitness and exercise). The researchers also examined the titles of articles published in *Ms.* in 1972–1986; none of the 188 articles on health-related topics mentioned tobacco or smoking.

During a press luncheon in the Soviet Union in the late 1980s, Gloria Steinem, founding editor of *Ms.* magazine, was asked by a Soviet official how to subtly influence press coverage of Glasnost. She replied, "Advertising" (Steinem 1990, p. 18). Questioned later by a journalist disturbed by her response, which implied that freedom of the press could be compromised, she noted that the media influences what consumers read through "soft" stories, "advertorials," and self-censorship of topics that concern the largest advertisers. With respect to women's magazines, Steinem said, "There, it isn't just a little content that's devoted to attracting ads, it's almost all of it" (Steinem 1990, p. 18). Since 1990, *Ms.* magazine has not accepted advertising of any sort and has been fully supported by readers.

One investigator studied the types of issues addressed in 1983–1987 in five popular women's magazines that carried cigarette advertising (*Cosmopolitan, Mademoiselle, McCall's, Ms.,* and *Woman's Day*) and one that did not accept cigarette advertising (*Good Housekeeping*) (Kessler 1989). The study showed that women's health was a major topic in all these magazines; 694 editorial references were made to health in the 375 issues of magazines examined. In the five magazines that accepted tobacco advertising, cigarette ads constituted from 8.0 to 17.1 percent of all advertising pages but occupied between 18.3 percent and 85.0 percent of all of premium pages (front and back covers). During this five-year period, none of the magazines covered the health risks from smoking in a full-length feature, column, review, or editorial. When smoking was discussed, it was usually in a 50- to 100-word newsbrief or in statements of one or two sentences, including three mentions of the positive effects of smoking. Only eight newsbriefs in the six magazines over the five-year period focused on smoking-related health risks, and none of these mentioned lung cancer, heart disease, or pregnancy. During the same period, more than 1,300 articles on the health risks from smoking were published in the scientific literature. Furthermore, the references to smoking that did appear in the women's magazines were often very misleading, incomplete, or inaccurate. For example, a *Woman's Day* article on protecting children's health listed "not smoking" as number 14 in a list of 15 recommendations, and the only risk from smoking mentioned was house fires. Smoking during pregnancy or around children was not discussed. A *McCall's* article mentioned the risk from smoking during pregnancy but recommended only that women consider stopping one week before the due date. When news briefs and other stories were taken into account, *Good Housekeeping* accounted for one-third of a total of 40 references to cigarettes in the magazines and was the only magazine to mention the link to lung cancer, but it too gave minimal attention to the health hazards of smoking. Kessler (1989) suggested that magazine editors and publishers may fear that editorial matter offensive to tobacco producers might result in loss of advertising from the non-tobacco subsidiaries of parent tobacco companies.

In a large-scale, longitudinal study, Warner and colleagues analyzed the content of 99 popular U.S. magazines published during 1959–1969 and 1973–1986 to determine the probability of publication of articles on the risks from smoking as a function of revenue derived from cigarette advertising (Warner and Goldenhar 1989; Warner et al. 1992a). The probability of publishing an article on the risks from smoking was 11.9 percent among all magazines that did not carry cigarette advertising and 8.3 percent among those that did advertise cigarettes. Among women's magazines, the probabilities were 11.7 and 5.0

percent, respectively. Among women's magazines, each 1-percent increase in revenues derived from cigarette advertising resulted in a 1.9-percent decrease in the probability that the risk from smoking would be covered in magazine stories. The decrease found among women's magazines was three times that among all other magazines (Warner et al. 1992b). A similar study examined 13 magazines for 1997 and 1998 and found that women's magazines continue to downplay the hazards of cigarette smoking. During this period, only 1 of 519 health-related articles featured smoking. Articles about smoking-related diseases "de-emphasized or neglected" the role played by smoking (Lukachko and Whelan 1999, p. 6). In some cases, the magazines gave "inappropriate or unscientific recommendations" about tobacco (Lukachko and Whelan 1999, p. 6). These magazines carried slightly more than three ads on average per issue studied (Lukachko and Whelan 1999). An examination of the content of magazines targeting African American women found far more advertising than health information. *Jet*, *Ebony*, and *Essence* were studied from 1987 through 1994; 1,477 tobacco ads and only six articles on lung cancer were found (Hoffman-Goetz et al. 1997).

## International Marketing of Cigarettes to Women

Tobacco companies have been active in foreign countries, building overseas manufacturing facilities and purchasing local tobacco companies. The companies have entered into joint ventures, provided technical assistance and funding for foreign tobacco growers (e.g., in Africa, Asia, and South America), established public relations tobacco institutes in many countries, and entered into comprehensive bilateral agreements with national monopolies (e.g., in China) (Williams 1995a,b,c,d; Weldner 1996).

After the U.S. government applied pressure to open markets to trade, the market share of U.S. cigarettes in Asian countries such as Japan, Taiwan, South Korea, and Thailand, increased dramatically (Chaloupka 1996). This increase was associated with a sixfold increase from 1978 through 1994 in the number of cigarettes smoked by persons younger than age 20 years (*Japan Times* 1995). The prevalence of smoking also increased among students in Korea (Suh et al. 1997), and in Taiwan, experimental smoking by adolescents aged 15 through 17 years rose from 3.3 percent in 1985 to 20.5 percent in 1991 (John Tung Foundation 1994). The rise of smoking among women and children in Asia has coincided with aggressive Western-style advertising (Lam and Mackay 1995). Although firm evidence to support direct associations has been lacking, this preliminary evidence suggested a pattern of association similar to that seen in the United States and emphasizes the enormous potential of marketing to change social norms.

Around the world, transnational tobacco companies continue to deny evidence of the link between smoking and ill health. They have attempted to obstruct public health action on tobacco, influence trade agreements, verbally attack organizations and persons working on tobacco issues, and produce spurious arguments about freedom of choice and economic advantage. Governments in many developing countries are unfamiliar with these tactics and, in many cases, have not been able to counter them effectively (Mackay and Crofton 1996).

**Historical Overview**

It was not until about 1930 that ads targeting women were first published in Europe. Although women had appeared in British ads earlier, they were purely decorative, the aim being to attract the attention of male smokers. Only in the late 1920s and early 1930s, following changing social attitudes, was it acceptable for women to be seen smoking in public.

During the 1940s and 1950s, the images and messages used in ads aimed at women expanded. Smoking was promoted as enhancing relaxation. One example is a 1947 ad that read "Afternoon off. Is anything more pleasant or soothing than pottering in the garden on a fine afternoon?… And nothing completes your peace of mind more than an 'Embassy'" (*Woman's Own* 1947). Similarly, a Craven 'A' advertisement of 1951 stated that "One can let the world go by, as Craven 'A' smokers do" (*Sphere* 1951). Other themes reflected a woman's "flair for quality" (e.g., a Gold Flake ad in 1950) (*Woman's Own* 1950), her intelligence (e.g., in ads in *Minor* in 1952 and 1953; *Picture Post* 1952, 1953b), or the sporty life (e.g., a Kensitas ad in 1953) (*Illustrated* 1952) and outdoor pursuits (e.g., in ads for Players Navy Cut in 1953 and 1956) (*Woman and Home* 1953; *Picture Post* 1956). Cigarettes were also portrayed as a passport to sexual attractiveness and success. The copy for a 1952 Craven 'A' ad read "When two young people share the same taste, their hearts are one" (*Woman* 1952), and an advertisement for the same brand in 1953 stated that "When two's company and three is infinitely too many, the pleasure of Craven 'A' completes the perfect understanding between young people together" (*Picture Post* 1953a). Similar ads also started to appear in other

European countries, later than in the United Kingdom, reflecting a slower change in social and cultural attitudes toward women in these countries. For example, tobacco companies in Sweden did not start to advertise directly to women until the 1950s, when smoking was portrayed as glamorous and as a way for women to gain admission to the world of men. During the 1960s, ads in Sweden promoted smoking as a symbol of female liberation and equality (Haglund 1988).

The targeting of women in many Western countries entered a new phase in the 1970s and 1980s, after the 1968 launch of Virginia Slims in the United States. The number of women in the labor force had increased, a key factor in the decision of tobacco companies to develop a range of marketing strategies to appeal to women. The strategies included altering the product and its price, availability, and image through innovative packaging and promotion (Ernster 1986).

In the 1980s, concern over the large number of men who had stopped smoking may have played a part in prompting the tobacco industry to increase its emphasis on women. This phenomenon was reflected in the British trade journal *Tobacco*, which carried articles with such titles as "Suggesting that Retailers Should 'Look to the Ladies'" (Reisman 1983), "Women—A Separate Market" (Cole 1988b), and "Creating a Female Taste" (Gill and Garrett 1989).

Until the 1980s, little tobacco marketing took place in developing countries. National tobacco monopolies in these countries generally either did not promote their products or did so only minimally. Beginning in the 1980s, however, when young women in some countries were becoming more economically independent and began to copy Western fashion and trends, transnational tobacco companies introduced tobacco ads into developing countries. Many of the initial ads had a masculine focus (e.g., the Marlboro man), but gradually a range of ads was produced, including gender-neutral ads (e.g., a pleasant mountain scene or a blue lagoon), ads that showed both women and men (e.g., enjoying the outdoors in a group), and ads in which only women were shown (e.g., ads for Virginia Slims). Designer cigarettes then appeared. In 1989, the brand Yves Saint Laurent, its elegant package designed to appeal to women, was launched in Malaysia and other Asian countries. Some of the national tobacco monopolies and companies, such as those in Indonesia and Japan, began to copy this promotional targeting of women (Mackay and Crofton 1996).

The precise amount of money spent on advertising, sponsorship, and other promotion throughout the world is not known, but the fragmented information available suggested that the amount is considerable. In the mid-1980s, the combined annual tobacco advertising expenditures for 10 Latin American countries totaled $116.7 million (USDHHS 1992).

*Advertising Age* reported data for 1989 on advertising in 38 countries, based on media totals provided by research companies, media tracking services, marketing publications, and advertising agencies in each country. The reliability of available data varied by country, but Philip Morris ranked 1st in advertising in Argentina, Hong Kong (China), and Pan-Arabia (Bahrain, Kuwait, Oman, Qatar, Saudi Arabia, and the United Arab Emirates). It ranked 5th in Germany and the United Kingdom, 7th in Canada, and 10th in Mexico (*Advertising Age* 1990). Since that time, enormous increases in marketing expenditures by U.S. tobacco companies have occurred in China, the countries of Eastern Europe, and other developing countries (Amos 1992; Hille 1995).

In 1994, Marlboro was the biggest advertiser among cigarette brands in China (US$5.2 million), followed by State Express 555 (US$3.1 million) (Hille 1995). Expenditures were expected to continue to grow, and media directors predicted that any restrictions or bans on tobacco advertising in the electronic and print media would be unlikely to affect tobacco companies' expenditures because the companies could use other forms of advertising to which restrictions did not apply (Hille 1995).

### Marketing Strategies

The ways in which tobacco companies target women vary across countries. Factors that influence marketing strategies include (1) the current prevalence of smoking among women, (2) restrictions on tobacco marketing, which vary from no restrictions to complete bans, (3) cultural norms, and (4) women's access to different media. However, strategies generally mirror those used in the United Kingdom and the United States, which is not surprising, because British and U.S. companies are the main exporters of cigarettes and have become increasingly involved in new markets (Chapman and Wong 1990; Kholmogorova and Prokhorov 1994). When doing business abroad, tobacco companies often apply business standards different from and less stringent than those they use in their own country. Ads that are either not allowed or would be ethically or culturally unacceptable in the United States (e.g., religious images of the Madonna) are used in other countries (Chapman and Stanton 1994), and many countries do not require health warnings in ads.

*Types of Media*

Worldwide, all media are used for tobacco advertising—television, film, video, radio, print, billboard, Internet direct mailing, public transportation vehicles and facilities, bus stops, and point-of-sale displays. In countries that ban direct advertising, tobacco companies turn to indirect advertising and sponsorship (Naett and Pollitzer 1991b). The global expansion of mass media continues to provide new opportunities for advertisers. The development of satellite television means that even the most remote villages in developing countries can be reached by advertisers, and no international laws govern tobacco advertising on satellite broadcasts. Since the fall of communism, tobacco advertising has increased dramatically in both print and television in Central and Eastern Europe.

One of the most popular media for reaching women throughout the world, particularly where tobacco advertising is banned on television, is women's magazines (Amos and Bostock 1992a). In a study of the top-selling women's magazines in 13 European countries, more than two-thirds were found to accept cigarette ads (Amos and Bostock 1992b). A more recent study of the most popular women's magazines in 17 countries in Europe also found that the majority of these magazines accepted cigarette ads (Amos et al. 1998). Many of these ads appeared to be designed to appeal to women, particularly in countries that had few restrictions on tobacco advertising (e.g., the Netherlands and Germany). Women's magazines are regularly read by about one-half of all women in the United Kingdom (Amos et al. 1991) and more than 50 million women in the European Union (Amos and Bostock 1992a). Furthermore, these magazines are read by women of all ages and backgrounds. By careful selection, advertisers can target specific groups, such as young women, and trendsetters. Women's magazines have been launched in several Central and Eastern European countries, and some of the most successful publications (*Elle, Cosmopolitan,* and *Marie Claire*) are now published in several countries and sold throughout the world. Magazines can lend a presumed social acceptability or stylish image to smoking. The health editor of *British Vogue* stated that publication of an ad in the magazine was "as good as a stamp of acceptability" (Jacobson and Amos 1985, p. 13). This de facto approval may be particularly important in countries where smoking prevalence is low among women and where tobacco companies are attempting to associate smoking with Western values.

*Direct Advertising*

As in the United States, tobacco advertising in other countries portrays a variety of attractive images and themes that have been used to promote the social acceptability of smoking among women and to highlight attributes of particular brands. Smoking has been promoted as being glamorous, sophisticated, fun, romantic, sexually attractive, healthy, sporty, sociable, relaxing, calming, emancipating, feminine, and rebellious and as an aid to weight loss.

Depending on restrictions on cigarette advertising, these images and themes have been conveyed in different ways. In countries with few or unenforced restrictions, verbal and visual images are explicit. One ad featured an attractive young woman alone who was relaxing in a bath (Philip Morris). Another ad showed a sexually alluring young woman, with copy reading "La seduction pure et dure (Gitanes Blondes)." In countries where such explicit images are prohibited, subtle images are used. For example, luxury is represented by silk or satin and by symbols of success or style. Ads of this kind include photographs of designer clothes and expensive and exotic locations (European Bureau for Action on Smoking Prevention 1989; Karaoglou and Naett 1991; Naett and Pollitzer 1991a).

One of the most common themes for ads in developed countries is increasingly used in developing countries—that smoking is both a passport to and a symbol of a woman's emancipation, independence, and success. For example, Virginia Slims ads have urged women in Japan to "Be you" and have told Hong Kong women, "You're on your way." Capri ads have encouraged women to have their own opinions, as when a young woman is shown with the caption "It's so me." Gauloises Blondes cigarettes have been promoted as reflecting "L'esprit libre" (Free spirit) in the Netherlands and "Liberte, toujours" (Freedom, always) in Germany and South Africa. In Japan, Capri ads have featured European role models, such as a dress designer saying, "The dress I design represents my own way of life." Ads for Virginia Slims have shown a pair of white female and male rugby players with the tag line "The locker rooms are separate but the playground and the goal are common" (Chapman 1986). Chapman (1986) suggested that ads like these that show Western images of liberated women also represent a form of cultural imperialism by the tobacco companies.

In South Africa, where smoking by women of childbearing age has been socially taboo among blacks, ads for Benson & Hedges have begun to feature young black women. In one ad, a young woman wearing aerobics gear is smoking a cigarette with a young black man. In another ad, a black woman wearing traditional headgear is seated beside a black man and is shown accepting a cigarette from a white man. The copy, "Share the feeling, share the taste," echoes the African cultural value of "ubuntu" (communalism), by which people share whatever they have (Val Hooper, Graduate School of Business, University of Cape Town, fax to Amanda Amos, October 4, 1995).

An editorial in the June 1990 *Tobacco Reporter* noted the growth opportunities for sales to women in Asia. It suggested that as women become more independent, cigarette use may symbolize their newly acquired freedom (Zimmerman 1990). In responding to criticism of his company's targeting of women, a regional manager of corporate affairs for Philip Morris Asia, Inc., said that the company was only responding to an existing market: "You can't create markets. You can only create a product for which there is a demand" (Anderson 1993, p. 6).

*Products and Packaging Focused on Women*

Tobacco companies have produced many brands specifically for women, including Kim, Virginia Slims, Capri, Vogue, MS, and More. Although sales of these brands currently tend to be relatively low outside the United States, the advertising explicitly promotes smoking as a desirable and acceptable female habit, often in countries where the prevalence of smoking among women is very low. For example, in Hong Kong, where fewer than 2 percent of women younger than age 40 years smoked, Virginia Slims was launched in an apparent attempt to create a new female market (Anderson 1993).

Many companies have also developed long, extra-slim, and low-tar versions of popular brands of cigarettes in an attempt to appeal to women. Slender female models are often depicted smoking these "feminized" cigarettes, and the copy tends to emphasize words such as mild, light, slim, slender, and long. While supposedly describing the merits of the cigarettes, these copy lines associate the product with two key female aspirations—being slim and being attractive. In Europe, the journal *Tobacco* described the brand Vogue as a "stylish type of cigarette with obvious feminine appeal, being slim and therefore highly distinctive" (Cole 1988a, p. 15). Vogue has been advertised in South Africa with themes that associate Vogue with European style (Cole 1988a). One study, designed to identify factors related to the high prevalence of smoking among a sample of women airline employees of Asian origin, showed no significant difference in health knowledge between smokers and nonsmokers (Li et al. 1994). However, a greater percentage of smokers than nonsmokers believed that smoking would help control weight and tended to perceive women depicted in cigarette ads as attractive, elegant, fit, sociable, and adventurous.

Using strategies similar to the extensive promotions in the United States, companies in other countries have produced special gift packs and offers designed to appeal to women. In Taiwan, a luxurious Yves Saint Laurent gift pack that contained two cartons of cigarettes and one crystal item was launched to coincide with the Lunar New Year. In Hungary, the L&M brand of cigarettes has offered free holidays in the United States along the legendary Route 66 (Kiskegyed 1996, *Tina* 1996). In Germany, readers of women's magazines have been encouraged to send for free "test-set" packs of the low-tar brand Reemtsma R1 Minima (*Brigitte* 1998). In Japan, purchasers of Mila Schön cigarettes had the chance to win handbags and ladies' watches (*Asahi Shimbun Weekly Aera* 1995).

*Brand Stretching*

The use of brand or company names on nontobacco goods and services is now widespread in both developed and developing countries. Widely advertised travel agencies operating in Europe and Asia, as well as holiday travel packages, are named after tobacco brands such as Peter Stuyvesant, Camel, and Silk Cut. Holidays sponsored by Kent have been advertised on satellite transmissions. In 1995, 25 Marlboro Classics shops were located throughout the world, including China, Indonesia, Japan, Korea, the Philippines, Taiwan, and Thailand. The Fortuna brand name has appeared in ads for Spanish sportswear featuring tennis star Steffi Graf (Amos 1997).

*Sponsorship*

Throughout the world, tobacco companies sponsor sports events, the arts, pop and rock concerts, university departments, and even health organizations, again paralleling the use of sponsorship in the United States. Sports sponsorship is generally limited to exciting, popular national sports that are televised. Sponsorship can gain positive publicity for tobacco companies by linking them with internationally known women and female role models. For example, in 1995, Great Britain's late Princess Diana, who was known to be opposed to tobacco use, attended the Salem Open Tennis Tournament in Hong Kong and accepted a check from the sponsor, R.J. Reynolds, to benefit the Hong Kong Red Cross (Harper 1995).

Sports figures are also used in ads. In 1995, the makers of Benson & Hedges cigarettes ran whole-page ads featuring female climber Lum Yuet Mei in newspapers in Malaysia, where direct advertising is banned. She was suspended from a rock face and was quoted as saying, "Tonight cling on to me as I attempt to conquer the amazing Dolomite cliffs." The name Benson & Hedges was at the top of the page, and the brand's golden colors were featured in the ad, which was entitled "She took the challenge and realized her golden dream" (*New Straits Times* 1995, p. 5).

Tobacco sponsorship of the arts in Asia has included sponsorship for British entertainer Peter Ustinov (Hong Kong in 1992), Tony Bennett jazz concerts (Thailand in 1993), the Central Ballet of China (1994), Andrew Lloyd Webber's *The Phantom of the Opera* (Hong Kong in 1995), and ASEAN Arts Awards (Asia in 1994). The Benson & Hedges Fashion Design Awards are presented in New Zealand, and tobacco companies have donated sculptures to the National Congress building and provided scholarships for musical prodigies in Chile (Perl 1994).

Events and activities popular among young people are also sponsored by tobacco companies. Free tickets to films and to pop and rock concerts have been given in exchange for empty cigarette packets in Hong Kong and Taiwan. *The Marlboro Music Hour,* a program of American pop music, has been broadcast daily throughout China. The combination of Western pop music and bilingual presentation makes the program extremely popular among China's young people. U.S. singers, such as Paula Abdul (*Tin Tin Daily News* 1992) and Madonna (*South China Morning Post* 1990), who do not promote tobacco in the United States, have allowed their names to be associated with cigarettes in other countries. R.J. Reynolds has sponsored free music shows promoting Salem cigarettes at the Hong Kong Coliseum, and Philip Morris has offered discount coupons for music videodisks with purchase of its Special Lights brand. Both companies state that their promotions are targeted to smokers older than 18 years (*Hong Kong Economic Journal* 1990). Some of the Asian tobacco monopolies and companies, especially Japan Tobacco International, have copied this sponsorship through music festivals, such as Mild Seven, featuring Roberta Flack. Tobacco manufacturing machines and posters to "the future customers" were displayed at a promotional event by Japan Tobacco International, in which 5,000 toys were distributed and a doll show of television characters was featured (Asahi News Service 1993). In Sri Lanka, girls have been targeted at discotheques sponsored by Benson & Hedges, where Golden Girls offer them free cigarettes and ask them to light up while at the discotheque (Seimon and Mehl 1998).

In 1989, Philip Morris contributed US$50,000 toward training physicians to work with disabled persons in China (*World Tobacco* 1989). The tobacco companies have sponsored events for Asian journalists, including a conference on environmental tobacco smoke in Bali (1992) and free visits to the United States from Thailand (1993) and Hong Kong (1995).

The tobacco companies have also exported "antismoking" materials. For example, R.J. Reynolds has introduced a teaching kit into Hong Kong schools (R.J. Reynolds Tobacco Company 1993). This bright, colorful, trendy kit suggests to children that smoking is an adult habit, but the message may have the reverse effect. The kit does not seriously discuss the health effects of smoking or the addictive nature of tobacco, nor does it encourage parents and teachers to set an example by attempting to stop smoking. Indeed, the materials tell smokers that if they are like most other smokers, they smoke for enjoyment. Nonetheless, by distributing the kit, the tobacco industry may claim to be behaving responsibly, and governments may be given the impression that regulations to protect young people from smoking are unnecessary. In Chile, tobacco companies have demonstrated an interest in children by paying for television sets for rural schools (Perl 1994).

*Product Placement*

Product placement is typified by the paid insertion of brand name products in U.S. films, which are shown throughout the world. For example, Philip Morris paid $42,500 to have Lois Lane smoke Marlboro cigarettes in *Superman II* (*Berkeley Wellness Letter* 1990), and Liggett paid $30,000 to show Eve cigarettes in *Supergirl* (*Tobacco and Youth Reporter* 1989; *Berkeley Wellness Letter* 1990). In *Working Girl,* secretary Melanie Griffith conspicuously carried a carton of Lark cigarettes for boss Sigourney Weaver (*Tobacco and Youth Reporter* 1989). Product placement has also been documented in films produced in developing regions (Dykes 1989). This technique circumvents bans on direct advertising and is difficult to document and regulate.

*Promotion of Tobacco Industry*

Several companies use the media overseas to enhance the tobacco industry's image and to defend smokers and smoking, again paralleling U.S. practices. This type of promotion presents tobacco companies as good corporate citizens, thus potentially creating public support and reducing opposition to industry policy positions (Stubenvoll 1990). Newspaper ads in other countries have highlighted the export achievements of specific companies, challenged proposed bans on tobacco advertising and sponsorship, raised questions about the scientific evidence of the effects of passive smoking, and attempted to shift public attitudes toward opposition of tobacco control measures (Chapman 1992). Even though these ads are directed at both women and men, some have highlighted women's issues. For example, in Portugal, where tobacco advertising is banned, the National Public Tobacco Company launched a mass media campaign in 1995 to support privatization of the company. One theme of the campaign was that the company provided employment for Portuguese women and tried to improve their working conditions.

**Media Censorship**

Very few studies have examined the effect that advertising outside the United States may have on editorial policies. However, at least one British magazine that accepted cigarette ads admitted finding it difficult to endorse positions that contradicted its advertising (Jacobson and Amos 1985). In a study conducted during 1989–1990, investigators found that, of 71 women's magazines published in 13 European countries, 69 percent accepted cigarette ads and 54 percent allowed photographs of persons smoking (Amos and Bostock 1992a). Responses to a question on coverage of smoking and health were received from 63 of the magazines; only 22 percent had published an article of one page or more on the health effects of smoking, 37 percent had given more minor coverage to smoking and health, and 41 percent had not covered the topic at all. Magazines that accepted cigarette ads were less likely to have carried articles on smoking and health than were those that did not publish cigarette ads. A more recent study of 111 women's magazines in 17 European countries in 1996 and 1997 found that 55 percent of the magazines that responded accepted cigarette ads, but only 31 percent had published an article of one page or more on smoking and health in the previous 12 months; only 4 of the magazines had a policy of voluntarily refusing cigarette advertising (Amos et al. 1998). Magazines that accepted tobacco advertising seemed less likely to give coverage to smoking and health. Indeed, 1 German magazine stated that it informed tobacco companies if it was going to publish material on nonsmoking and that the companies could stop their ads for that issue. In a study of four popular women's magazines published in Ireland in 1989–1993, the proportion of space devoted to tobacco ads and articles that conveyed the positive attributes of smoking or that were critical of tobacco control interventions was 1.95 percent of total magazine space (Howell 1994). This amount of space was 14.5 times greater than the space devoted to articles about the risks from smoking. Many magazines throughout the world appear to promote smoking among women by showing fashion photographs of models smoking and photographs of well-known personalities smoking that accompany editorial articles. In South Africa, one tobacco company refused to pay for a cigarette ad in a women's magazine after the ad appeared opposite a letter criticizing articles that promoted smoking (Yussuf Saloojee, National Council Against Smoking, fax to Amanda Amos, October 11, 1995).

**Bans and Restrictions on Tobacco Advertising and Promotion**

Many countries have banned all tobacco advertising and promotion (e.g., Australia, Finland, France, Norway, Singapore, Sweden, and Thailand). In 1998, the European Union adopted a directive on tobacco promotion. This directive will ban most tobacco advertising and sponsorship in the 15 countries of the European Union by July 30, 2006. Other countries have banned direct advertising, and still others have instituted partial restraints. Such bans are often circumvented by tobacco companies through various promotional venues such as creation of retail stores named after cigarette brands or corporate sponsorship of sporting and other events. Moreover, national bans on tobacco advertising may be rendered ineffective by tobacco promotion on satellite television, by cable broadcasting, or via the Internet, because no international laws regulate these venues (Solberg and Blum 1995).

Even in countries with strong regulations restricting tobacco advertising, attempts are constantly made to bypass the spirit of these bans (Solberg and Blum 1995; Weir 1995). In 1994, after a ban on direct ads for tobacco on television in China, Reuters reported that Philip Morris had staged an "unprecedented marketing coup" by showing ads "dressed up as public affairs shows" (*Hong Kong Standard* 1994,

p. 94). Moreover, implementation of bans may be poor, despite the excellence of some bans on paper, as evidenced in Eastern European countries and Mongolia, or it may be undermined by cross-border advertising. For example, Singapore has a comprehensive ban on tobacco marketing, but tobacco-sponsored television programs reach Singapore from Malaysia.

Several countries, such as Japan and the United Kingdom, have generally adopted a nonlegislative approach to tobacco control in which marketing is governed by voluntary codes or agreements. (This position will change in the United Kingdom as it implements the European Union's directive on tobacco promotion described here.) These codes often contain specific regulations designed to reduce or prevent the targeting of women, especially young women. However, these voluntary agreements often fail to achieve their aims (Jacobson and Amos 1985; Amos et al. 1989; Toxic Substances Board 1989; Naett and Pollitzer 1991a; Mindell 1993). For example, the Tobacco Institute in Japan has advertising codes prohibiting the use of models younger than 25 years old, the promotion of sales to women, the depiction of women smoking in ads, and the placement of advertising in women's magazines. However, both Virginia Slims and Capri are advertised in Japan. Ads for Frontier Menthol Slims have featured young female models, and tobacco vending machines have shown Virginia Slims videotapes of young women dancing—all of which violate the codes. Indeed, the government of the United Kingdom concluded in its 1998 report "Smoking Kills—A White Paper on Tobacco" that little evidence existed that indicated previous voluntary agreements on tobacco advertising in the United Kingdom had worked (Secretary of State for Health et al. 1998, p. 47–48). The government therefore decided to enact legislation to implement the 1998 Directive of the European Union that will ban most tobacco advertising and promotion.

Members of the public health community argue that tobacco advertising and promotion activities increase consumption of tobacco products by increasing demand via new recruits. The tobacco industry, on the other hand, argues that advertising and promotional activities serve only to maintain consumer brand loyalty or cause current tobacco users to switch brands. Advertising and promotion activities, they contend, do not contribute to recruitment. Studies have generally shown a modest positive effect or no effect of advertising on consumption (Jha and Chaloupka 1999). These conclusions must be interpreted cautiously, because the studies have generally used highly aggregated data for all advertisers, in all media, and often over large populations. Use of such aggregated data hides small changes and thus minimizes the possible impact of an additional dollar of advertising expenditure on tobacco consumption (Jha and Chaloupka 1999). In other words, small changes that may be discernible in an analysis of less aggregated data would be lost or obscured in an analysis of aggregated data. Studies that use less aggregated data have shown larger positive effects of advertising on consumption; however, such studies are very costly (Jha and Chaloupka 1999) and therefore few, if any, have been conducted.

An indirect and less costly method of discerning the impact of tobacco advertising on consumption is examination of the effects of restrictions and bans on tobacco consumption (Saffer and Chaloupka 2000). The Toxic Substances Board of New Zealand, which examined the relationship between government policies on tobacco promotion and tobacco consumption trends in 33 countries between 1970 and 1986, concluded that the abolition of tobacco promotion was an essential part of a comprehensive policy to lower tobacco consumption (Toxic Substances Board 1989). The Regional Office for the Western Pacific World Health Organization called for a region free of tobacco advertising by the year 2000 to protect Asian children from commercial pressure to smoke (Warner 1986). The debate on the impact of such policy actions has been lively and partisan. Studies have examined the impact of partial cigarette advertising bans on consumption and the impact of total bans. The evidence suggested that partial bans have little or no effect on reducing tobacco consumption, whereas total advertising bans covering all media prove to be most effective in reducing tobacco consumption. Partial bans are ineffective because tobacco companies can substitute nonbanned media for banned media without reducing the amount of dollars spent on advertising. When advertising via all media is banned, the industry's opportunity to substitute among media is effectively constrained. Thus, advertising expenditure must be adjusted up or down. Using data from 1970 through 1992, a recent study of 22 high-income countries concluded that comprehensive bans on cigarette advertising and promotion can reduce smoking but that more limited partial bans have little or no effect (Saffer and Chaloupka 2000). The study concluded that if the most comprehensive advertising bans were in place, tobacco consumption would fall by more than 6 percent in high-income countries.

Another study (Jha and Chaloupka 1999) of 100 countries compared consumption trends over time among those with relatively complete bans on advertising and promotion and those with no such bans. In the countries with nearly complete bans, the downward trend in consumption was much steeper. Because it was not possible to control for all factors in every country, other factors could have contributed to the decline in consumption in some countries. In a review of the effects of various interventions on adolescent smoking, Willemsen and De Zwart (1999) concluded that advertising bans lead not only to decreased consumption among adults but also contribute to reductions in initiation among adolescents; gender-specific effects were not reported.

### Protests Against Targeting of Women

Until recently, most of the challenges to the tobacco industry's targeting of women have been restricted to countries with the longest history of widespread smoking among women, including Australia, Canada, Finland, Sweden, and the United Kingdom (Jacobson 1992; Canadian Ministry of Health 1993). However, organizations in both developed and developing countries are beginning to protest tactics used to target women. In 1990, the International Network of Women Against Tobacco was formed by women from about 60 countries. One of the organization's three main goals is to counter the marketing and promotion of tobacco to women throughout the world (see "Tobacco Control Advocacy Programs by and for Women" in Chapter 5). Women's Action on Smoking is now active in many nations, including Japan, where smoking prevalence has been low among women but high among men (*World Smoking and Health* 1994). Women's Action on Smoking in Japan instituted a hotline to provide health advice to workers, mostly women who are exposed to cigarette smoke, and sent to callers information on the health effects of environmental tobacco smoke, advice on how to avoid exposure, and suggestions on advocating for workplace restrictions on smoking. In India in 1990, when Golden Tobacco Company began targeting women with a new brand, MS Special Filter (Gupta and Ball 1990), protests quickly followed. Ads for the brand featured Indian women wearing Western clothing in affluent settings, which are symbols of liberation for Indian women who are gaining financial and professional independence. A group of medical school professors and health workers wrote to newspapers urging them not to accept advertising for the cigarette (Crossette 1990). Members of Bailancho Saad, a little-known group of women activists, objected to the brand name as an inappropriate use of the prefix Ms., called for bans on advertising and a boycott of the cigarette, and defaced billboards advertising the product (Alvares 1990).

## Summary

Tobacco marketing to women has emphasized themes such as slimness, social and physical attractiveness, style, romance, women's equality, independence, and even sassiness. Simply distilled, marketing has focused on self-image and the somewhat antithetical needs for social acceptance and independence. It is not known to what extent marketers have made use of the considerable body of published evidence on why women smoke, although tobacco marketing strategies echo a number of issues identified in the published research, including concerns about weight, tendencies toward risk taking and rebelliousness, and positive images of smokers.

# Conclusions

1. Girls who initiate smoking are more likely than those who do not smoke to have parents or friends who smoke. They also tend to have weaker attachments to parents and family and stronger attachments to peers and friends. They perceive smoking prevalence to be higher than it actually is, are inclined to risk taking and rebelliousness, have a weaker commitment to school or religion, have less knowledge of the adverse consequences of smoking and the addictiveness of nicotine, believe that smoking can control weight and negative moods, and have a positive image of smokers. Although the strength of the association by gender differs across studies, most of these factors are associated with an increased risk for smoking among both girls and boys.
2. Girls appear to be more affected than boys by the desire to smoke for weight control and by the perception that smoking controls negative moods; girls may also be more influenced than boys to smoke by rebelliousness or a rejection of conventional values.
3. Women who continue to smoke and those who fail at attempts to stop smoking tend to have lower education and employment levels than do women who quit smoking. They also tend to be more addicted to cigarettes as evidenced by the smoking of a higher number of cigarettes per day, to be cognitively less ready to stop smoking, to have less social support for stopping, and to be less confident in resisting temptations to smoke.
4. Women have been extensively targeted in tobacco marketing, and tobacco companies have produced brands specifically for women, both in the United States and overseas. Myriad examples of tobacco ads and promotions targeted to women indicate that such marketing is dominated by themes of both social desirability and independence, which are conveyed through ads featuring slim, attractive, athletic models. Between 1995 and 1998, expenditures for domestic cigarette advertising and promotion increased 37.3 percent, from $4.90 billion to $6.73 billion.
5. Tobacco industry marketing, including product design, advertising, and promotional activities, is a factor influencing susceptibility to and initiation of smoking.
6. The dependence of the media on revenues from tobacco advertising oriented to women, coupled with tobacco company sponsorship of women's fashions and of artistic, athletic, political, and other events, has tended to stifle media coverage of the health consequences of smoking among women and to mute criticism of the tobacco industry by women public figures.

# References


Aaron DJ, Dearwater SR, Anderson R, Olsen T, Kriska AM, Laporte RE. Physical activity and the initiation of high-risk health behaviors in adolescents. *Medicine and Science in Sports and Exercise* 1995; 27(12):1639–45.

Abernathy TJ, Massad L, Romano-Dwyer L. The relationship between smoking and self-esteem. *Adolescence* 1995;30(120):899–907.

Abrams DB, Monti PM, Pinto RP, Elder JP, Brown RA, Jacobus SI. Psychosocial stress and coping in smokers who relapse or quit. *Health Psychology* 1987; 6(4):289–303.

Adams SH. Philip Morris awards 132 abuse grants. *Richmond Times-Dispatch* 1998 Oct 31;B-6; city edition.

*Advertising Age.* King-size and special cigaret brands threaten leadership of regulars: Sweetser. *Advertising Age* 1953;24(13):38–9.

*Advertising Age.* Benson & Hedges introduces new cigaret for women. *Advertising Age* 1968a;39(31):33.

*Advertising Age.* Liggett & Myers designer packs get N.Y. distribution. *Advertising Age* 1968b;39(21):164.

*Advertising Age.* Virginia Slims goes national with heavy multi-media backing. *Advertising Age* 1968c; 39(39):2.

*Advertising Age.* Burnet again shifts cigaret's sex appeal; after making Marlboro male, shop found Slims ads had excess frou-frou. *Advertising Age* 1968d;39(52):2, 29.

*Advertising Age.* Women smokers prove fickle, as Embra bombs, Virginia Slims score. *Advertising Age* 1970;41(25):2.

*Advertising Age.* Latest rebellious but unliberated woman [picture caption]. *Advertising Age* 1973; 44(37):N8.

*Advertising Age.* Adbeat: Philip Morris Inc. *Advertising Age* 1974a;45(1):51.

*Advertising Age.* Big spender in print advertising is Philip Morris [picture caption]. *Advertising Age* 1974b;45(34):157.

*Advertising Age.* Top 10 advertisers in 38 countries. *Advertising Age* 1990 Nov 19:S-4, S-6, S-10, S-28.

*Advertising Age.* Philip Morris abandons more magazines. *Advertising Age* 2000 June 16; <http://adage.com/news_and_features/features/20000616/article2.html>; accessed: July 21, 2000.

Ahlgren A, Norem AA, Hochhauser M, Garvin J. Antecedents of smoking among pre-adolescents. *Journal of Drug Education* 1982;12(4):325–40.

Aitken PP, Eadie DR, Hastings GB, Haywood AJ. Predisposing effects of cigarette advertising on children's intentions to smoke when older. *British Journal of Addiction* 1991;86(4):383–90.

Akers RL, Skinner WF, Krohn MD, Lauer RM. Recent trends in teenage tobacco use: findings from a five-year longitudinal study. *Sociology and Social Research* 1987;71(2):110–4.

Albright CL, Altman DG, Slater MD, Maccoby N. Cigarette advertisements in magazines: evidence for a differential focus on women's and youth magazines. *Health Education Quarterly* 1988;15(2): 225–33.

Alcock J. *Animal Behavior: An Evolutionary Approach.* Sunderland (MA): Sinauer Associates, 1989.

Alexander HM, Callcott R, Dobson AJ, Hardes GR, Lloyd DM, O'Connell DL, Leeder SR. Cigarette smoking and drug use in schoolchildren: IV—factors associated with changes in smoking behaviour. *International Journal of Epidemiology* 1983;12(1): 59–66.

Allen O, Page RM, Moore L, Hewitt C. Gender differences in selected psychosocial characteristics of adolescent smokers and nonsmokers. *Health Values* 1994;18(2):34–9.

Aloise-Young PA, Graham JW, Hansen WB. Peer influence on smoking initiation during early adolescence: a comparison of group members and group outsiders. *Journal of Applied Psychology* 1994;79(2): 281–7.

*Allure.* [Capri advertisement]. *Allure* 1995a (Sept): 154–5.

*Allure.* [Philip Morris advertisement]. *Allure* 1995b (Sept):138.

Altman DG, Levine DW, Coeytaux R, Slade J, Jaffe R. Tobacco promotion and susceptibility to tobacco use among adolescents aged 12 through 17 years in a nationally representative sample. *American Journal of Public Health* 1996;86(11):1590–3.

Altman DG, Slater MD, Albright CL, Maccoby N. How an unhealthy product is sold: cigarette advertising in magazines, 1960–1985. *Journal of Communication* 1987;37(4):95–106.

Alvares N. Feminists fight against smoking ads. *Japan Times* 1990 Nov 4:10.

Amos A. Cigarette advertising and marketing strategies. *Tobacco Control* 1992;1(1):3–4.

Amos A. Creating a global tobacco culture among women. In: Waller M, Lipponen S, editors. *Smokefree Europe: A Forum for Networks.* Helsinki (Finland): Finnish Centre for Health Promotion 1997:110–7.

Amos A, Bostock Y. Policy on cigarette advertising and coverage of smoking and health in European women's magazines. *British Medical Journal* 1992a; 304(6819):99–101.

Amos A, Bostock Y. *Putting Women in the Picture: Cigarette Advertising Policy and Coverage of Smoking and Health in Women's Magazines in Europe.* London: British Medical Association, 1992b.

Amos A, Bostock C, Bostock Y. Women's magazines and tobacco in Europe. *Lancet* 1998;352(9130): 786–7.

Amos A, Haglund M. From social taboo to "torch of freedom": the marketing of cigarettes to women. *Tobacco Control* 2000;9(1):3–8.

Amos A, Hillhouse A, Robertson G. Tobacco advertising and children—the impact of the voluntary agreement. *Health Education Research* 1989;4(1): 51–7.

Amos A, Jacobson B, White P. Cigarette advertising policy and coverage of smoking and health in British women's magazines. *Lancet* 1991;337(8733): 93–6.

Anda RF, Williamson DF, Escobedo LG, Mast EE, Giovino GA, Remington PL. Depression and the dynamics of smoking. A national perspective. *Journal of the American Medical Association* 1990; 264(12):1541–5.

Anderson E. Health disaster warning. *South China Morning Post* 1993 Apr 3:6.

Armstrong BK, de Klerk NH, Shean RE, Dunn DA, Dolin PJ. Influence of education and advertising on the uptake of smoking by children. *Medical Journal of Australia* 1990;152(3):117–24.

Arnett JJ, Terhanian G. Adolescents' responses to cigarette advertisements: links between exposure, liking, and the appeal of smoking. *Tobacco Control* 1998;7(2):129–33.

Ary DV, Biglan A. Longitudinal changes in adolescent cigarette smoking behavior: onset and cessation. *Journal of Behavioral Medicine* 1988;11(4):361–82.

Asahi News Service. Japan: tobacco marketing strategies criticized [newswire]. Asahi News Service 1993 Jun 10.

*Asahi Shimbun Weekly Aera.* [Mila Schön advertisement]. *Asahi Shimbun Weekly Aera* 1995 Sept 4:37.

Baer JS, Holt CS, Lichtenstein E. Self-efficacy and smoking reexamined: construct validity and clinical utility. *Journal of Consulting and Clinical Psychology* 1986;54(6):846–52.

Bandura A. *Social Foundations of Thought and Action: A Social Cognitive Theory.* Englewood Cliffs (NJ): Prentice-Hall, 1986.

Basil MD, Schooler C, Altman DG, Slater M, Albright CL, Maccoby N. How cigarettes are advertised in magazines: special messages for special markets. *Health Communication* 1991;3(2):75–91.

Bauman KE, Ennett ST. Peer influence on adolescent drug use. *American Psychologist* 1994;49(9):820–2.

Bauman KE, Foshee VA, Haley NJ. The interaction of sociological and biological factors in adolescent cigarette smoking. *Addictive Behaviors* 1992;17(5): 459–67.

Bearden WO, Etzel MJ. Reference group influence on product and brand purchase decisions. *Journal of Consumer Research* 1982;9(2):183–94.

Beede P, Lawson R. The effect of plain packages on the perception of cigarette health warnings. *Public Health* 1992;106(4):315–22.

*Berkeley Wellness Letter.* Smoking in movies: license to kill. *Berkeley Wellness Letter* 1990;6(7):7.

Bernays EL. *Biography of an Idea: Memoirs of Public Relations Counsel Edward L. Bernays.* New York: Simon and Schuster, 1965.

Besonen J. Stogies, a gal's best friend. *New York Times* 1995 Aug 27;Sect 1:40 (col 4).

Best JA, Brown KS, Cameron R, Manske SM, Santi S. Gender and predisposing attributes as predictors of smoking onset: implications for theory and practice. *Journal of Health Education* 1995;26(Suppl 2): S52–S60.

Biener L, Siegel M. Tobacco marketing and adolescent smoking: more support for a causal inference. *American Journal of Public Health* 2000;90(3):407–11.

Biglan A, Duncan TE, Ary DV, Smolkowski K. Peer and parental influences on adolescent tobacco use. *Journal of Behavioral Medicine* 1995;18(4):315–30.

Bissell J. How do you market an image brand when the image falls out of favor? *Brandweek* 1994;35(23): 16.

Bonner L. Why cigarette makers don't advertise to women. *Advertising and Selling* 1926 Oct 20:21, 46, 48.

Boomsma DI, Koopmans JR, Van Doornen LJP, Orlebeke JF. Genetic and social influences on starting to smoke: a study of Dutch adolescent twins and their parents. *Addiction* 1994;89(2):219–26.

Borland R. Slip-ups and relapse in attempts to quit smoking. *Addictive Behaviors* 1990;15(3):235–45.

Botvin GJ, Botvin EM, Baker E, Dusenbury L, Goldberg CJ. The false consensus effect: predicting adolescents' tobacco use from normative expectations. *Psychological Reports* 1992;70(1):171–8.

Botvin GJ, Goldberg CJ, Botvin EM, Dusenbury L. Smoking behavior of adolescents exposed to cigarette advertising. *Public Health Reports* 1993;108(2): 217–24.

Breslau N, Kilbey MM, Andreski P. Nicotine dependence and major depression: new evidence from a prospective investigation. *Archives of General Psychiatry* 1993;50(1):31–5.

*Brigitte.* [R1 Minima advertisement]. *Brigitte* 1998 (Dec):1112–3.

Brinkman J. *Virginia Slims Circuit:* 1976 *Virginia Slims Tennis Media Guide.* New York: Philip Morris, 1976.

Britt SH. *Psychological Principles of Marketing and Consumer Behavior.* Lexington (MA): Lexington Books/ DC Heath and Co., 1978.

Brook JS, Gordon AS, Brook DW. Fathers and daughters: their relationship and personality characteristics associated with the daughter's smoking behavior. *Journal of Genetic Psychology* 1987;148(1): 31–44.

Brunswick AF, Messeri P. Causal factors in onset of adolescents' cigarette smoking: a prospective study of urban black youth. *Advances in Alcohol and Substance Abuse* 1983–84;3(1–2):35–52.

Brunswick AF, Messeri PA. Origins of cigarette smoking in academic achievement, stress and social expectations: does gender make a difference? *Journal of Early Adolescence* 1984;4(4):353–70.

Burke V, Milligan RAK, Beilin LJ, Dunbar D, Spencer M, Balde E, Gracey MP. Clustering of health-related behaviors among 18-year-old Australians. *Preventive Medicine* 1997;26(5 Pt 1):724–33.

Califano JA Jr. The wrong way to stay slim [letter]. *New England Journal of Medicine* 1995;333(18): 1214–6.

Camp DE, Klesges RC, Relyea G. The relationship between body weight concerns and adolescent smoking. *Health Psychology* 1993;12(1):24–32.

Canadian Ministry of Health. *Act Now: Women and Tobacco.* British Columbia (Canada): Ministry of Health, Office of Health Promotion, Steering Committee on the National Strategy to Reduce Tobacco Use in Canada, Working Group on Women and Tobacco, 1993.

Centers for Disease Control and Prevention. Changes in the cigarette brand preferences of adolescent smokers—United States, 1989–1993. *Morbidity and Mortality Weekly Report* 1994;43(32):577–81.

Centers for Disease Control and Prevention. Trends in smoking initiation among adolescents and young adults—United States, 1980–1989. *Morbidity and Mortality Weekly Report* 1995;44(28):521–5.

Centers for Disease Control and Prevention. Accessibility of tobacco products to youths aged 12–17 years—United States, 1989 and 1993. *Morbidity and Mortality Weekly Report* 1996a;45(6): 125–30.

Centers for Disease Control and Prevention. Tobacco use and usual source of cigarettes among high school students—United States, 1995. *Morbidity and Mortality Weekly Report* 1996b;45(20):413–8.

Centers for Disease Control and Prevention. Response to increases in cigarette prices by race/ ethnicity, income and age groups—United States, 1976–1993. *Morbidity and Mortality Weekly Report* 1998;47(29):605–9.

Centers for Disease Control and Prevention. Cigarette smoking among adults—United States, 1998. *Morbidity and Mortality Weekly Report* 2000;49(39):881–4.

Chaloupka F. Rational addictive behavior and cigarette smoking. *Journal of Political Economy* 1991a; 99(4):722–42.

Chaloupka F. Clean indoor air laws, addiction and cigarette smoking. *Applied Economics* 1992;24(2): 193–205.

Chaloupka FJ. *Men, women, and addiction: the case of cigarette smoking.* Working paper no. 3267. Cambridge (MA): National Bureau of Economic Research, 1990.

Chaloupka FJ. *Cigarette taxation, addiction, and smoking control. Final report.* Grant no. 5 RO2 CA48360. Rockville (MD): National Cancer Institute, 1991b.

Chaloupka FJ. *U.S. trade policy and cigarette smoking in Asia.* Working paper no. 5543. Cambridge (MA): National Bureau of Economic Research, 1996.

Chaloupka FJ, Grossman M. *Price, tobacco control policies and youth smoking.* Working paper no. 5740. Cambridge (MA): National Bureau of Economic Research, 1996.

Chaloupka FJ, Warner KE. *The economics of smoking.* Working paper no. 7047. Cambridge (MA): National Bureau of Economic Research, 1999.

Chapman S. *Great Expectorations: Advertising and the Tobacco Industry.* Comedia Series No. 35. London: Comedia Publishing Group, 1986.

Chapman S. Anatomy of a campaign: the attempt to defeat the New South Wales (Australia) tobacco advertising prohibition bill 1991. *Tobacco Control* 1992;1(1):50–6.

Chapman S, Fitzgerald B. Brand preference and advertising recall in adolescent smokers: some implications for health promotion. *American Journal of Public Health* 1982;72(5):491–4.

Chapman S, Stanton H. Philippines: poverty, powerlessness and Our Lady of Cigarettes. *Tobacco Control* 1994;3(3):200–1.

Chapman S, Wong WL. *Tobacco Control in the Third World: A Resource Atlas.* Penang (Malaysia): International Organization of Consumers Unions, 1990.

Charlton A. Smoking and weight control in teenagers. *Public Health, London* 1984;98(5):227–81.

Charlton A, Blair V. Predicting the onset of smoking in boys and girls. *Social Science and Medicine* 1989; 29(7):813–8.

Chassin L, Presson CC, Sherman SJ, Corty E, Olshavsky RW. Predicting the onset of cigarette smoking in adolescents: a longitudinal study. *Journal of Applied Social Psychology* 1984;14(3): 224–43.

Chassin L, Presson CC, Sherman SJ, Edwards DA. The natural history of cigarette smoking: predicting young-adult smoking outcomes from adolescent smoking patterns. *Health Psychology* 1990;9(6): 701–16.

Chassin L, Presson CC, Sherman SJ, Edwards DA. Parent educational attainment and adolescent cigarette smoking. *Journal of Substance Abuse* 1992; 4(3):219–34.

Chassin L, Presson CC, Sherman SJ, Montello D, McGrew J. Changes in peer and parent influence during adolescence: longitudinal versus cross-sectional perspectives on smoking initiation. *Developmental Psychology* 1986;22(3):327–34.

Cherry N, Kiernan KE. Personality scores and smoking behaviour: a longitudinal study. *British Journal of Preventive and Social Medicine* 1976;30(2):123–31.

*Cigar Aficionado.* [Ballys advertisement]. *Cigar Aficionado* 1995a;4(1):328.

*Cigar Aficionado.* [Big Smoke advertisement]. *Cigar Aficionado* 1995b;4(1):347.

*Cigar Aficionado.* [CAO advertisement]. *Cigar Aficionado* 1995c;4(1):302.

*Cigar Aficionado.* [Don Diegos advertisement]. *Cigar Aficionado* 1995d;4(1):209.

*Cigar Aficionado.* [El Sublimado advertisement]. *Cigar Aficionado* 1995e;4(1):264.

*Cigar Aficionado.* [Trump Plaza advertisement]. *Cigar Aficionado* 1995f;4(1):98.

CigarWoman.com. About Us; <http://www.cigarwoman.com/about.html>; accessed: July 21, 2000.

Cnattingius S, Lindmark G, Meirik O. Who continues to smoke while pregnant? *Journal of Epidemiology and Community Health* 1992;46(3):218–21.

Coeytaux RR, Altman DG, Slade J. Tobacco promotions in the hands of youth. *Tobacco Control* 1995; 4(3):253–7.

Cohen DA, Richardson J, LaBree L. Parenting behaviors and the onset of smoking and alcohol use: a longitudinal study. *Pediatrics* 1994;94(3):368–75.

Cole J. For a special occasion. *Tobacco* 1988a (Dec): 15–6.

Cole J. Women—a separate market? *Tobacco* 1988b (Mar):7–9.

Collins LM, Sussman S, Rauch JM, Dent CW, Johnson CA, Hansen WB, Flay BR. Psychosocial predictors of young adolescent cigarette smoking: a sixteen-month, three-wave longitudinal study. *Journal of Applied Social Psychology* 1987;17(6):554–73.

Conrad KM, Flay BR, Hill D. Why children start smoking cigarettes: predictors of onset. *British Journal of Addiction* 1992;87(12):1711–24.

Coogan PF, Adams M, Geller AC, Brooks D, Miller DR, Lew RA, Koh HK. Factors associated with smoking among children and adolescents in Connecticut. *American Journal of Preventive Medicine* 1998;15(1):17–24.

Coppotelli HC, Orleans CT. Partner support and other determinants of smoking cessation maintenance among women. *Journal of Consulting and Clinical Psychology* 1985;53(4):455–60.

*Cosmopolitan.* [Capri advertisement]. *Cosmopolitan* 1995a (Sept):86–7.

*Cosmopolitan.* [Benson & Hedges 100s advertisement]. *Cosmopolitan* 1995b (Sept):67.

*Cosmopolitan.* [Virginia Slims advertisement]. *Cosmopolitan* 1995c (Sept):105.

Coulson NS, Eiser C, Eiser JR. Diet, smoking and exercise: interrelationships between adolescent health behaviors. *Child: Care, Health and Development* 1997;23(3):207–16.

Covell K, Dion KL, Dion KK. Gender differences in evaluations of tobacco and alcohol advertisments. *Canadian Journal of Behavioural Science* 1994;26(3): 404–20.

Crossette B. Women in Delhi angered by smoking pitch. *New York Times* 1990 Mar 18;139(48178):A18 (col 1).

Cummings KM, Sciandra E, Pechacek TF, Orlandi M, Lynn WR for the COMMIT Research Group. Where teenagers get their cigarettes: a survey of the purchasing habits of 13–16 year olds in 12 US communities. *Tobacco Control* 1992;1(4):264–7.

Curry SJ, McBride CM. Relapse prevention for smoking cessation: review and evaluation of concepts and interventions. *Annual Review of Public Health* 1994;15:345–66.

Dagnoli J. Another RJR 'breakthrough': Chelsea cigarette touts fresh aroma. *Advertising Age* 1989;60(6): 3, 63.

Daly KA, Lund EM, Harty KC, Ersted SA. Factors associated with late smoking initiation in Minnesota women. *American Journal of Public Health* 1993; 83(9):1333–5.

de Vries H, Backbier E. Self-efficacy as an important determinant of quitting among pregnant women who smoke: the Φ-pattern. *Preventive Medicine* 1994; 23(2):167–74.

Deaux K, Major B. Putting gender into context: an interactive model of gender-related behavior. *Psychological Review* 1987;94(3):369–89.

DeCicca P, Kenkel D, Mathios A. Putting out the Fires: Will Higher Taxes Reduce Youth Smoking? Paper presented at the American Economics Association annual meeting, January 3–5, 1998, Chicago, Illinois.

Dee TS, Evans WN. *Putting out the fires or just fanning the flames? A comment on DeCicca, Kenkel and Mathios.* Working paper. Atlanta: Georgia Institute of Technology, School of Economics, 1998.

Dejin-Karlsson E, Hanson BS, Östergren PO, Ranstam J, Isacsson SO, Sjöberg NO. Psychosocial resources and persistent smoking in early pregnancy—a population study of women in their first pregnancy in Sweden. *Journal of Epidemiology and Community Health* 1996;50(1):33–9.

DeKay WT, Buss DM. Human nature, individual differences, and the importance of context: perspectives from evolutionary psychology. *Current Directions in Psychological Science* 1992;1(6):184–9.

Dicken C. Sex roles, smoking, and smoking cessation. *Journal of Health and Social Behavior* 1978;19(3): 324–34.

Dicken C. Sex-role orientation and smoking. *Psychological Reports* 1982;51(2):483–9.

DiFranza JR, Norwood BD, Garner DW, Tye JB. Legislative efforts to protect children from tobacco. *Journal of the American Medical Association* 1987; 257(24):3387–9.

Dinh KT, Sarason IG, Peterson AV, Onstad LE. Children's perceptions of smokers and nonsmokers: a longitudinal study. *Health Psychology* 1995; 14(1):32–40.

Distefan JM, Gilpin EA, Choi WS, Pierce JP. Parental influences predict adolescent smoking in the United States, 1989–1993. *Journal of Adolescent Health* 1998;22(6):466–74.

Dunhill GR. Cigarette sales at peak, 10 billion over 1947. *Advertising and Selling* 1949;42(1):31–2.

Dykes J. Taste of the future for tobacco men. *South China Morning Post* 1989 Aug 16:23.

Eagly AH. *Sex Differences in Social Behavior: A Social-Role Interpretation.* Hillsdale (NJ): Lawrence Erlbaum Associates, 1987.

Eissenberg T, Adams C, Riggins EC III, Likness M. Smokers' sex and the effects of tobacco cigarettes: subject-rated and physiological measures. *Nicotine and Tobacco Research* 1999;1(4):317–24.

Elkind AK. The social definition of women's smoking behaviour. *Social Science and Medicine* 1985;20(12): 1269–78.

Ellin A. Agony of domestic violence at the office. *New York Times* 2000 Mar 1;Section G:1 (col 1).

England B, Pasternack S, Utt SH. Cigarette advertising: my, how you've changed. Paper presented at the Annual Meeting of the Association for Education in Journalism and Mass Communication; 1987 Aug 1–4; San Antonio (TX).

Ennett ST, Bauman KE. Peer group structure and adolescent cigarette smoking: a social network analysis. *Journal of Health and Social Behavior* 1993;34(3): 226–36.

Ennett ST, Bauman KE, Koch GG. Variability in cigarette smoking within and between adolescent friendship cliques. *Addictive Behaviors* 1994;19(3): 295–305.

Ensminger ME, Brown CH, Kellam SG. Sex differences in antecedents of substance use among adolescents. *Journal of Social Issues* 1982;38(2):25–42.

*Entertainment Weekly.* [Basic advertisement]. *Entertainment Weekly* 1995 Sept 22:33.

Ernster VL. Mixed messages for women: a social history of cigarette smoking and advertising. *New York State Journal of Medicine* 1985;85(7):335–40.

Ernster VL. Women, smoking, cigarette advertising and cancer. *Women and Health* 1986;11(3–4):217–35.

Ernster VL. Trends in smoking, cancer risk, and cigarette promotion: current priorities for reducing tobacco exposure. *Cancer* 1988;62(8):1702–12.

Escobedo LG, Marcus SE, Holtzman D, Giovino GA. Sports participation, age at smoking initiation, and the risk of smoking among US high school students. *Journal of the American Medical Association* 1993;269(11):1391–5.

Escobedo LG, Reddy M, DuRant RH. Relationship between cigarette smoking and health risk and problem behaviors among US adolescents. *Archives of Pediatrics and Adolescent Medicine* 1997;151(1): 66–71.

European Bureau for Action on Smoking Prevention. The message behind the ads. *BASP Newsletter* 1989 (Oct-Nov-Dec);7:43–7.

Evans N, Farkas A, Gilpin E, Berry C, Pierce JP. Influence of tobacco marketing and exposure to smokers on adolescent susceptibility to smoking. *Journal of the National Cancer Institute* 1995;87(20): 1538–45.

Eysenck HJ. A short questionnaire for the measurement of two dimensions of personality. *Journal of Applied Psychology* 1958;42(1):14–7.

Fairclough G. Dancing, blackjack and free smokes: with parties and junkets, R.J. Reynolds nurtures brand loyalty for Doral. *The Wall Street Journal* 1999 Oct 26;B1.

Farkas AJ, Distefan JM, Choi WS, Gilpin EA, Pierce JP. Does parental smoking cessation discourage adolescent smoking? *Preventive Medicine* 1999;28(3): 213–8.

Federal Trade Commission. *Report to Congress: Cigar Sales and Advertising and Promotional Expenditures for Calendar Years 1996 and 1997.* Washington: Federal Trade Commisssion, 1999.

Federal Trade Commission. *Report to Congress for 1998: Pursuant to the Federal Cigarette Labeling and Advertising Act.* Washington: Federal Trade Commission, 2000.

Feighery E, Borzekowski DL, Schooler C, Flora J. Seeing, wanting, owning: the relationship between receptivity to tobacco marketing and smoking susceptibility in young people. *Tobacco Control* 1998;7(2):123–8.

Ferrence RG. Sex differences in cigarette smoking in Canada, 1900–1978: a reconstructed cohort study. *Canadian Journal of Public Health* 1988;79(3):160–5.

Fingerhut LA, Kleinman JC, Kendrick JS. Smoking before, during and after pregnancy. American *Journal of Public Health* 1990;80(5):541–4.

Fiore MC, Bailey WC, Cohen SJ, Dorfman SF, Goldstein MG, Gritz ER, Heyman RB, Jaén CR, Kottke TE, Lando HA, Mecklenburg R, Mullen PD, Nett LM, Robinson K, Stitzer ML, Tommasello AC, Villejo L, Wewers ME. *Treating Tobacco Use and Dependence.* Clinical Practice Guideline. Rockville (MD): U.S. Department of Health and Human Services, Public Health Service, 2000.

Fiore MC, Novotny TE, Pierce JP, Giovino GA, Hatziandreu EJ, Newcomb PA, Surawicz TS, Davis RM. Methods used to quit smoking in the United States: do cessation programs help? *Journal of the American Medical Association* 1990;263(20): 2760–5.

Fischer PM, Schwartz MP, Richards JW Jr, Goldstein AO, Rojas TH. Brand logo recognition by children aged 3 to 6 years: Mickey Mouse and Old Joe the Camel. *Journal of the American Medical Association* 1991;266(22):3145–8.

Flay BR, D'Avernas JR, Best JA, Kersell MW, Ryan KB. Cigarette smoking: why young people do it and ways of preventing it. In: McGrath PJ, Firestone P, editors. *Pediatric and Adolescent Behavioral Medicine.* Springer Series on Behavior Therapy and Behavioral Medicine, Vol. 10. New York: Springer Publishing, 1983:132–83.

Flay BR, Hu FB, Siddiqui O, Day LE, Hedeker D, Petraitis J, Richardson J, Sussman S. Differential influence of parental smoking and friends' smoking on adolescent initiation and escalation of smoking. *Journal of Health and Social Behavior* 1994;35(3): 248–65.

Forgays DG, Bonaiuto P, Wrzesniewski K, Forgays DK. Personality and cigarette smoking in Italy, Poland, and the United States. *International Journal of the Addictions* 1993;28(5):399–413.

Forster JL, Murray DM, Wolfson M, Blaine TM, Wagenaar AC, Hennrikus DJ. The effects of community policies to reduce youth access to tobacco. *American Journal of Public Health* 1998;88(8):1193–8.

Forster JL, Wolfson M. Youth access to tobacco: policies and politics. *Annual Review of Public Health* 1998;19:203–35.

Forster JL, Wolfson M, Murray DM, Wagenaar AC, Claxton AJ. Perceived and measured availability of tobacco to youths in 14 Minnesota communities: the TPOP study. *American Journal of Preventive Medicine* 1997;13(3):167–74.

Frankenhaeuser M. The psychophysiology of workload, stress, and health: comparison between the sexes. *Annals of Behavioral Medicine* 1991;13(4): 197–204.

Freedman AM, McCarthy MJ. New smoke from RJR under fire. *Wall Street Journal* 1990 Feb 20;Sect B:B1 (col 3), B7 (col 1).

French SA, Perry CL. Smoking among adolescent girls: prevalence and etiology. *Journal of the American Medical Women's Association* 1996;51(1–2): 25–8.

French SA, Perry CL, Leon GR, Fulkerson JA. Weight concerns, dieting behavior, and smoking initiation among adolescents: a prospective study. *American Journal of Public Health* 1994;84(11):1818–20.

French SA, Story M, Downes B, Resnick MD, Blum RW. Frequent dieting among adolescents: psychosocial and health behavior correlates. *American Journal of Public Health* 1995;85(5):695–701.

Frone MR, Cooper ML, Russell M. Stressful life events, gender, and substance use: an application of Tobit regression. *Psychology of Addictive Behaviors* 1994;8(2):59–69.

Gagnon JP, Osterhaus JT. Research note: effectiveness of floor displays on the sales of retail products. *Journal of Retailing* 1985;61(1):104–16.

Garvey AJ, Bliss RE, Hitchcock JL, Heinold JW, Rosner B. Predictors of smoking relapse among self-quitters: a report from the Normative Aging Study. *Addictive Behaviors* 1992;17(4):367–77.

Gerry R. How to persuade a lady. *Printers' Ink* 1956; 256(9):21–3.

Gill BR, Garrett SJ. Creating a female taste. *Tobacco* 1989(Mar):6–7.

Gilpin EA, Pierce JP. Trends in adolescent smoking initiation in the United States: is tobacco marketing an influence? *Tobacco Control* 1997;6(2):122–7.

Gilpin EA, Pierce JP, Rosbrook B. Are adolescents receptive to current sales promotion practices of the tobacco industry? *Preventive Medicine* 1997; 26(1):14–21.

*Glamour*. [Marlboro advertisement]. *Glamour* 1995a (Oct):128–9.

*Glamour*. [Philip Morris advertisement]. *Glamour* 1995b (Oct):150.

*Glamour*. [Virginia Slims advertisement]. *Glamour* 1999 (Jan):back cover.

*Glamour*. [Virginia Slims advertisement]. *Glamour* 2000a (Apr):307.

*Glamour*. [Virginia Slims advertisement]. *Glamour* 2000b (June):34.

Glassman AH, Helzer JE, Covey LS, Cottler LB, Stetner F, Tipp JE, Johnson J. Smoking, smoking cessation, and major depression. *Journal of the American Medical Association* 1990;264(12):1546–9.

Glendinning A, Shucksmith J, Hendry L. Social class and adolescent smoking behaviour. *Social Science and Medicine* 1994;38(10):1449–60.

Goddard E. *Why Children Start Smoking: An Enquiry Carried out by Social Survey Division of OPCS on Behalf of the Department of Health.* London: Office of Population Censuses and Surveys, Social Survey Division, 1990.

Goebel K. Lesbians and gays face tobacco targeting. *Tobacco Control* 1994;3(1):65–7.

Goldman K. A stable of females has joined Joe Camel in controversial cigarette ad campaign. *Wall Street Journal* 1994 Feb 18;Sect B:1.

Goldstein AO, Sobel RA, Newman GR. Tobacco and alcohol use in G-rated children's animated films. *Journal of the American Medical Association* 1999; 281(12):1131–6.

Gomberg ESL, Nirenberg TD. Women and substance abuse [commentary]. *Journal of Substance Abuse* 1991;3(2):255–67.

Goodrum C, Dalrymple H. *Advertising in America: The First 200 Years.* New York: Harry N. Abrams, 1990.

Gordon A, Finlay K, Watts T. The psychological effects of colour in consumer product packaging. *Canadian Journal of Marketing Research* 1994;13: 3–11.

Gottlieb NH, Baker JA. The relative influence of health beliefs, parental and peer behaviors and exercise program participation on smoking, alcohol use and physical activity. *Social Science and Medicine* 1986;22(9):915–27.

Gottlieb NH, Green LW. Life events, social network, life-style, and health: an analysis of the 1979 National Survey of Personal Health Practices and Consequences. *Health Education Quarterly* 1984; 11(1):91–105.

Green G, Macintyre S, West P, Ecob R. Like parent like child? Associations between drinking and smoking behaviour of parents and their children. *British Journal of Addiction* 1991;86(6):745–58.

Gritz ER, Carr CR, Marcus AC. Unaided smoking cessation: Great American Smokeout and New Year's Day quitters. *Journal of Psychosocial Oncology* 1988; 6(3–4):217–34.

Gritz ER, Crane LA. Use of diet pills and amphetamines to lose weight among smoking and nonsmoking high school seniors. *Health Psychology* 1991;10(5):330–5.

Gritz ER, Nielsen IR, Brooks LA. Smoking cessation and gender: the influence of physiological, psychological, and behavioral factors. *Journal of the American Medical Women's Association* 1996; 51(1–2):35–42.

Gritz ER, Prokhorov AV, Hudmon KS, Chamberlain RM, Taylor WC, DiClemente CC, Johnston DA, Hu S, Jones LA, Jones MM, Rosenblum CK, Ayars CL, Amos CI. Cigarette smoking in a multiethnic population of youth: methods and baseline findings. *Preventive Medicine* 1998;27(3):365–84.

Grunberg NE, Winders SE, Wewers ME. Gender differences in tobacco use. *Health Psychology* 1991; 10(2):143–53.

Guinan ME. Cigarette advertising to women: taking responsibility. *Journal of the American Medical Women's Association* 1988;43(4):123–4.

Gulliver SB, Hughes JR, Solomon LJ, Dey AN. An investigation of self-efficacy, partner support and daily stresses as predictors of relapse to smoking in self-quitters. *Addiction* 1995;90(6):767–72.

Gunther J. *Taken at the Flood: The Story of Albert D. Lasker.* New York: Harper and Brothers, 1960.

Gupta PC, Ball K. India: tobacco tragedy. *Lancet* 1990; 335(8689):594–5.

Haaga DA. Issues in relating self-efficacy to smoking relapse: importance of an Achilles' heel situation and of prior quitting experience. *Journal of Substance Abuse* 1990;2(2):191–200.

Haenszel W, Shimkin MB, Miller HP. *Tobacco Smoking Patterns in the United States.* Public Health Monograph 45. U.S. Department of Health, Education, and Welfare, Public Health Service, Office on Smoking and Health, 1956. DHEW Publication No. (PHS) 463.

Haglund M. Development trends in smoking among women in Sweden—an analysis. In: Aoki M, Hisamichi S, Tominage S, editors. *Smoking and Health 1987. Proceedings of the 6th World Conference on Smoking and Health; Tokyo;* 9–12 Nov 1987. International Congress Series 780. New York: Excerpta Medica, 1988:525–9.

Hall SM, Ginsberg D, Jones RT. Smoking cessation and weight gain. *Journal of Consulting and Clinical Psychology* 1986;54(3):342–6.

Hall SM, Havassy BE, Wasserman DA. Commitment to abstinence and acute stress in relapse to alcohol, opiates, and nicotine. *Journal of Consulting and Clinical Psychology* 1990;58(2):175–81.

Hall SM, Munoz RF, Reus VI, Sees KL. Nicotine, negative affect, and depression. *Journal of Consulting and Clinical Psychology* 1993;61(5):761–7.

Harper M. Di's big haul for charity. *Washington Post* 1995 Apr 24;Sect D:3.

*Harper's Bazaar.* [Virginia Slims advertisement]. *Harper's Bazaar* 1995 (Sept);(3406):328.

Harris TL. *The Marketers Guide to Public Relations: How Today's Top Companies Are Using the New PR to Gain a Competitive Edge.* New York: John Wiley and Sons, 1991.

Hawkins JD, Catalano RF, Miller JY. Risk and protective factors for alcohol and other drug problems in adolescence and early adulthood: implications for substance abuse prevention. *Psychological Bulletin* 1992;112(1):64–105.

Health Canada. *When Packages Can't Speak: Possible Impacts of Plain and Generic Packaging of Tobacco Products; Expert Panel Report.* Ottawa: Ministry of Health, Health Canada, 1995.

*Health Letter.* Camel ad: is male violence a "smooth move?" *Health Letter* 1989 Aug 12:cover.

Heath AC, Madden PAF. Genetic influences on smoking behavior. In: Turner JR, Cardon LR, Hewitt JK, editors. *Behavior Genetic Approaches in Behavioral Medicine.* New York: Plenum Press, 1995:45–66.

Hellman R, Cummings KM, Haughey BP, Zielezny MA, O'Shea RM. Predictors of attempting and succeeding at smoking cessation. *Health Education Research* 1991;6(1):77–86.

Hesterman V. You've come a long way, baby—or have you? Women's magazines, cigarette advertisements, health articles, and editorial autonomy. Paper presented at the Annual Meeting of the Association for Education in Journalism and Mass Communication; 1987 Aug 1–4; San Antonio (TX).

Hibbard JH. Social roles as predictors of cessation in a cohort of women smokers. *Women and Health* 1993; 20(4):71–80.

Hibbett A, Fogelman K. Future lives of truants: family formation and health-related behaviour. *British Journal of Educational Psychology* 1990;60(2):171–9.

Hille A. Major leap forecast in China adex. *Media* 1995 Mar 17:1.

Hoffman-Goetz L, Gerlach KK, Marino C, Mills SL. Cancer coverage and tobacco advertising in African-American women's popular magazines. *Journal of Community Health* 1997;22(4):261–70.

Hollie PG. Segmented cigarette market. *New York Times* 1985 Mar 23;Business Sect:29 (col 3), 31.

*Hong Kong Economic Journal.* HK: tobacco companies adopt free gift tactics. *Hong Kong Economic Journal* 1990 Dec 10:22.

*Hong Kong Standard.* U.S. firm stages marketing coup. *Hong Kong Standard* 1994 Feb 19:94.

Howe H. An historical review of women, smoking, and advertising. *Health Education* 1984;15(3):3–8.

Howell F. Tobacco advertising and coverage of smoking and health in women's magazines. *Irish Medical Journal* 1994;87(5):140–1.

Hu FB, Flay BR, Hedeker D, Siddiqui O, Day LE. The influences of friends' and parental smoking on adolescent smoking behavior: the effects of time and prior smoking. *Journal of Applied Social Psychology* 1995a;25(22):2018–47.

Hu T, Lin Z, Keeler TE. Teenage smoking, attempts to quit, and school performance. *American Journal of Public Health* 1998;88(6):940–3.

Hu TW, Ren QF, Keeler TE, Bartlett J. The demand for cigarettes in California and behavioural risk factors. *Health Economics* 1995b;4(1):7–14.

Hudmon KS, Prokhorov AV, Koehly LM, DiClemente CC, Gritz ER. Psychometric properties of the Decisional Balance Scale and the temptations to try smoking inventory in adolescents. *Journal of Child and Adolescent Substance Abuse* 1997;6(3):1–18.

Hunter SM, Croft JB, Vizelberg IA, Berenson GS. Psychosocial influences on cigarette smoking among youth in a southern community: the Bogalusa Heart Study. *Morbidity and Mortality Weekly Report* 1987;36(Suppl 4):17S–23S.

IEG. *IEG's Complete Guide to Sponsorship: Everything You Need to Know about Sports, Arts, Event, Entertainment and Cause Marketing*. Chicago: IEG, 1995a.

IEG. *IEG Intelligence Report on Tobacco Company Sponsorship for the Robert Wood Johnson Foundation:* 1995 Sponsorship. Chicago: IEG, 1995b.

Ikard FF, Tomkins S. The experience of affect as a determinant of smoking behavior: a series of validity studies. *Journal of Abnormal Psychology* 1973; 81(2):172–81.

*Illustrated*. [Kensitas advertisement]. *Illustrated* 1952 May 17:36.

Jackson C. Cognitive susceptibility to smoking and initiation of smoking during childhood: a longitudinal study. *Preventive Medicine* 1998;27(1):129–34.

Jackson C, Bee-Gates DJ, Henriksen L. Authoritative parenting, child competencies, and initiation of cigarette smoking. *Health Education Quarterly* 1994; 21(1):103–16.

Jackson C, Henriksen L, Dickinson D, Levine DW. The early use of alcohol and tobacco: its relation to children's competence and parents' behavior. *American Journal of Public Health* 1997;87(3):359–64.

Jacobson B. Putting women in the picture. *Tobacco Control* 1992;1(2):123–5.

Jacobson B, Amos A. *When Smoke Gets in Your Eyes: Cigarette Advertising Policy and Coverage of Smoking and Health in Women's Magazines*. London: British Medical Association, 1985.

*Japan Times*. Young people lighting up more often. *Japan Times* 1995 Sept 5.

Jessor R, Donovan JE, Costa FM. Beyond *Adolescence: Problem Behavior and Young Adult Development*. New York: Cambridge University Press, 1991.

Jha P, Chaloupka FJ. *Curbing the Epidemic: Governments and the Economics of Tobacco Control*. Washington: World Bank, 1999.

John Tung Foundation. *A Study on the Cognition, Attitudes, Behaviour and Psychological Traits Regarding Smoking, Drinking, and Betel Nut Chewing among Adolescents in Taiwan, Republic of China*. Health Care Work Research Unit Report. Taiwan (Republic of China): John Tung Foundation, 1994.

Johnson EH, Gilbert D. Familial and psychological correlates of smoking in black and white adolescents. *Ethnicity and Disease* 1991;1(4):320–4.

Johnston LD, O'Malley PM, Bachman JG. *National Survey Results on Drug Use from the Monitoring the Future Project, 1975–1995: Vol. I. Secondary School Students*. Rockville (MD): U.S. Department of Health and Human Services, Public Health Service, National Institutes of Health, National Institute on Drug Abuse, 1996.

*Journal of the American Medical Association*. Bureau of investigation: tobacco advertising gone mad. The health angle, as exploited by "Lucky Strike Cigarets" and "Cremo Cigars." *Journal of the American Medical Association* 1930;94(11):8–10.

Kandel DB, Davies M. Adult sequelae of adolescent depressive symptoms. *Archives of General Psychiatry* 1986;43(3):255–62.

Kandel DB, Udry JR. Prenatal effects of maternal smoking on daughters' smoking: nicotine or testosterone exposure? *American Journal of Public Health* 1999;89(9):1377–83.

Kandel DB, Wu P. The contributions of mothers and fathers to the intergenerational transmission of cigarette smoking in adolescence. *Journal of Research on Adolescence* 1995;5(2):225–52.

Kandel DB, Wu P, Davies M. Maternal smoking during pregnancy and smoking by adolescent daughters. *American Journal of Public Health* 1994;84(9): 1407–13.

Kann L, Kinchen SA, Williams BI, Ross JG, Lowry R, Hill CV, Grunbaum JA, Blumson PS, Collins JL, Kolbe LJ. Youth risk behavior surveillance—United States, 1997. *Morbidity and Mortality Weekly Report* 1998;47(SS-3):1–89.

Kaprio J, Koskenvuo M. A prospective study of psychological and socioeconomic characteristics, health behavior and morbidity in cigarette smokers prior to quitting compared to persistent smokers and non-smokers. *Journal of Clinical Epidemiology* 1988;41(2):139–50.

Karaoglou A, Naett C. *Report on Women and Tobacco: 'Is She Still a Smoker?'* Brussels: European Bureau for Action on Smoking Prevention, 1991.

Karasek R. The demand/control model: a social, emotional, and physiological approach to stress risk and active behaviour development. In: *Encyclopaedia of Occupational Health and Safety*. 4th ed. Geneva: International Labour Office, 1998.

Kelder SH, Perry CL, Klepp KI, Lytle LL. Longitudinal tracking of adolescent smoking, physical activity, and food choice behaviors. *American Journal of Public Health* 1994;84(7):1121–6.

Kellam SG, Ensminger ME, Simon MB. Mental health in first grade and teenage drug, alcohol, and cigarette use. *Drug and Alcohol Dependence* 1980;5(4): 273–304.

Kendler KS, Neale MC, MacLean CJ, Heath AC, Eaves LJ, Kessler RC. Smoking and major depression: a causal analysis. *Archives of General Psychiatry* 1993; 50(1):36–43.

Kendler KS, Thornton LM, Pedersen NL. Tobacco consumption in Swedish twins reared apart and reared together. *Archives of General Psychiatry* 2000; 57(9):886–92.

Kessler L. Women's magazines' coverage of smoking related health hazards. *Journalism Quarterly* 1989; 66(2):316–22, 445.

Kholmogorova GT, Prokhorov AV. West goes East: the new tobacco situation in Russia. *Tobacco Control* 1994;3(2):145–7.

Kilbourne J. Women and smoking: who needs equal rights? *Journal of the American Medical Women's Association* 1989;44(2):58.

Killen JD, Robinson TN, Haydel KF, Hayward C, Wilson DM, Hammer LD, Litt IF, Taylor CB. Prospective study of risk factors for the initiation of cigarette smoking. *Journal of Consulting and Clinical Psychology* 1997;65(6):1011–6.

Kindra GS, Laroche M, Muller TE. *Consumer Behavior: the Canadian Perspective.* 2nd ed. Scarborough (Canada): Nelson Canada, 1994.

*Kiskegyed.* [L&M advertisement]. *Kisekegyed* 1996 Aug 27:10.

Kleinman JC, Madans JH. The effects of maternal smoking, physical stature, and educational attainment on the incidence of low birth weight. *American Journal of Epidemiology* 1985;121(6):843–55.

Kleinman JC, Pierre MB Jr, Madans JH, Land GH, Schramm WF. The effects of maternal smoking on fetal and infant mortality. *American Journal of Epidemiology* 1988;127(2):274–82.

Klesges RC, Elliott VE, Robinson LA. Chronic dieting and the belief that smoking controls body weight in a biracial, population-based adolescent sample. *Tobacco Control* 1997;6(2):89–94.

Klesges RC, Meyers AW, Klesges LM, LaVasque ME. Smoking, body weight, and their effects on smoking behavior: a comprehensive review of the literature. *Psychological Bulletin* 1989;106(2):204–30.

Klesges RC, Robinson LA. Predictors of smoking onset in adolescent African American boys and girls. *Journal of Health Education* 1995;26(2):85–90.

Knott VJ. Electrodermal activity during aversive stimulation: sex differences in smokers and nonsmokers. *Addictive Behaviors* 1984;9(2):195–9.

Kotler P. *Marketing Management: Analysis, Planning, Implementation, and Control.* 7th ed. Englewood Cliffs (NJ): Prentice Hall, 1991.

Krohn MD, Massey JL, Skinner WF, Lauer RM. Social bonding theory and adolescent cigarette smoking: a longitudinal analysis. *Journal of Health and Social Behavior* 1983;24(4):337–49.

Krohn MD, Naughton MJ, Skinner WF, Becker SL, Lauer RM. Social disaffection, friendship patterns and adolescent cigarette use: the Muscatine Study. *Journal of School Health* 1986;56(4):146–50.

Krosnick JA, Judd CM. Transitions in social influence at adolescence: who induces cigarette smoking? *Developmental Psychology* 1982;18(3):359–68.

Krupka LR, Vener AM. Gender differences in drug (prescription, non-prescription, alcohol and tobacco) advertising: trends and implications. *Journal of Drug Issues* 1992;22(2):339–60.

Krupka LR, Vener AM, Richmond G. Tobacco advertising in gender-oriented popular magazines. *Journal of Drug Education* 1990;20(1):15–29.

Kumpfer KL, Turner CW. The social ecology model of adolescent substance abuse: implications for prevention. *International Journal of the Addictions* 1990–91;25(4A):435–63.

Lacey LP, Manfredi C, Balch G, Warnecke RB, Allen K, Edwards C. Social support in smoking cessation among black women in Chicago public housing. *Public Health Reports* 1993;108(3):387–94.

*Ladies' Home Journal* [More advertisement]. *Ladies' Home Journal* 1986;103(4):61.

*Ladies' Home Journal.* [Carlton advertisement]. *Ladies' Home Journal* 1995;112(10):53.

*Ladies' Home Journal.* [Virginia Slims advertisement]. *Ladies' Home Journal* 2000;117(6):9.

Lam TH, Mackay J. Asia: the new opium war. In: Slama K, editor. *Tobacco and Health.* New York: Plenum Press, 1995:251–3.

Lawrance L, Rubinson L. Self-efficacy as a predictor of smoking behavior in young adolescents. *Addictive Behaviors* 1986;11(4):367–82.

Lee DJ, Mendes de Leon CF, Markides KS. The relationship between hostility, smoking, and alcohol consumption in Mexican Americans. *International Journal of the Addictions* 1988;23(9):887–96.

Lerman C, Caporaso NE, Audrain J, Main D, Bowman ED, Lockshin B, Boyd NR, Shields PG. Evidence suggesting the role of specific genetic factors in cigarette smoking. *Health Psychology* 1999;18(1): 14–20.

Levin M. The tobacco industry's strange bedfellows. *Business and Society Review* 1988 (Spring):11–7.

Lewit EM, Coate D. The potential for using excise taxes to reduce smoking. *Journal of Health Economics* 1982;1(2):121–45.

Lewit EM, Hyland A, Kerrebrock N, Cummings KM. Price, public policy, and smoking in young people. *Tobacco Control* 1997;6(Suppl 2):S17–S24.

Li C, Fielding R, Marcoolyn G, Wong CM, Hedley A. Smoking behaviour among female airline cabin crew from ten Asian countries. *Tobacco Control* 1994; 3(1):21–9.

*Life*. [Camel advertisement]. *Life* June 20, 1938;4(25): back cover.

*Life*. [Chesterfield advertisement]. *Life* March 15, 1943a; 14(11):back cover.

*Life*. [Camel advertisement]. *Life* November 8, 1943b; 15(19):back cover.

*Life*. [Camel advertisement]. *Life* September 30, 1946; 21(14):back cover.

*Life*. [Pall Mall advertisement]. *Life* November 24, 1952; 33(21):109.

Livson N, Leino EV. Cigarette smoking motives: factorial structure and gender differences in a longitudinal study. *International Journal of the Addictions* 1988;23(6):535–44.

Lukachko A, Whelan EM. *You've Come a Long Way… or Have You? Popular Women's Magazines are Still Downplaying the Risks of Smoking*. New York: American Council on Science and Health, 1999.

Lynch BS, Bonnie RJ. *Growing Up Tobacco Free: Preventing Nicotine Addiction in Children and Youths*. Washington: National Academy Press, 1994.

Lytle LA, Kelder SH, Perry CL, Klepp KI. Covariance of adolescent health behaviors: the class of 1989 study. *Health Education Research* 1995;10(2):133–46.

Mackay J, Crofton J. Tobacco and the developing world. *British Medical Bulletin* 1996;52(1):206–21.

MacLean MG, MacKinnon DP, Pentz MA. Adolescent coping, cigarette use and alcohol use: a cross substance comparison. Paper presented at the 104th Convention of the American Psychological Association; 1996 Aug; Toronto.

*Mademoiselle*. [Camel Lights advertisement]. *Mademoiselle* 1995 (June):180–1.

Maes HH, Woodard CE, Murrelle L, Meyer JM, Silberg JL, Hewitt JK, Rutter M, Simonoff E, Pickles A, Carbonneau R, Neale MC, Eaves LJ. Tobacco, alcohol and drug use in eight- to sixteen-year-old twins: the Virginia Twin Study of Adolescent Behavioral Development. *Journal of Studies on Alcohol* 1999;60(3):293–305.

Magnusson D. Wanted: A psychology of situations. In: Magnusson D, editor. *Toward a Psychology of Situations: An International Perspective*. Hillsdale (NJ): Lawrence Erlbaum Associates, 1981:9–36.

Malone RE, Bero LA. Cigars, youth, and the Internet link. *American Journal of Public Health* 2000;90(5): 790–2.

*Marie Claire*. [Misty advertisement]. *Marie Claire* 1995 (Oct):165.

Mark JI, Silverman JH. How much is a loyal customer worth? *Across the Board* 1992 (May):36–9.

*Marketing to Women*. Breast cancer deaths and cigarette advertising dollars rise. *Marketing to Women* 1991;4(8):8.

Marshall GN. Levels of analysis and personality: lessons from the person-situation debate? *Psychological Science* 1991;2(6):427–8.

Martineau P. *Motivation in Advertising: Motives That Make People Buy*. New York: McGraw-Hill, 1957.

Masloski T. New design aims to get more out of less. *Advertising Age* 1981;52(54):S-6–S-7.

Massaro DW. Psychology as a cognitive science. *Psychological Science* 1991;2(5):302–7.

McBride CM, Pirie PL, Curry SJ. Postpartum relapse to smoking: a prospective study. *Health Education Research* 1992;7(3):381–90.

*McCall's*. [Carlton advertisement]. *McCall's* 1995; 123(1):135.

McCaul KD, Glasgow R, O'Neill HK, Freeborn V, Rump BS. Predicting adolescent smoking. *Journal of School Health* 1982;52(8):342–6.

McGee R, Stanton WR. A longitudinal study of reasons for smoking in adolescence. *Addictions* 1993; 88(2):265–71.

McKinlay JB, Marceau LD. To boldly go…. *American Journal of Public Health* 2000a;90(1):25–33.

McKinlay JB, Marceau LD. Upstream public health policy: lessons from the battle of tobacco. *International Journal of Health Services* 2000b;30(1):49–69.

McNeill AD, Jarvis MJ, Stapleton JA, Russell MAH, Eiser JR, Gammage P, Gray EM. Prospective study of factors predicting uptake of smoking in adolescents. *Journal of Epidemiology and Community Health* 1989;43(1):72–80.

Meijer B, Branski D, Knol K, Kerem E. Cigarette smoking habits among schoolchildren. *Chest* 1996;110(4): 921–6.

Milham S Jr, Davis RL. Cigarette smoking during pregnancy and mother's occupation. *Journal of Occupational Medicine* 1991;33(4):468–73.

Mindell JS. The UK voluntary agreement on tobacco advertising: a comatose policy? *Tobacco Control* 1993;2(3):209–14.

Minkler M, Wallack L, Madden P. Alcohol and cigarette advertising in Ms. magazine. *Journal of Public Health Policy* 1987;8(2):164–79.

Mittelmark MB, Murray DM, Luepker RV, Pechacek TF, Pirie PL, Pallonen UE. Predicting experimentation with cigarettes: the Childhood Antecedents of Smoking Study (CHSS). *American Journal of Public Health* 1987;77(2):206–8.

Mizerski R. The relationship between cartoon trade character recognition and attitude toward product category in young children. *Journal of Marketing* 1995;59(Oct):58–70.

Modrcin-McCarthy MA, Tollett J. Unhealthy, unfit, and too angry to care? In: Thomas SP, editor. *Women and Anger.* Focus on Women Series, Vol. 15. New York: Springer Publishing, 1993:154–69.

Morris GSD, Vo AN, Bassin S, Savaglio D, Wong ND. Prevalence and sociobehavioral correlates of tobacco use among Hispanic children: the Tobacco Resistance Activity Program. *Journal of School Health* 1993;63(9):391–6.

Mullahy J. Cigarette smoking: habits, health concerns, and heterogeneous unobservables in a microeconometric analysis of consumer demand [dissertation]. Charlottesville (VA): University of Virginia, 1985.

Mullen PD, Quinn VP, Ershoff DH. Maintenance of nonsmoking postpartum by women who stopped during pregnancy. *American Journal of Public Health* 1990;80(8):992–4.

Murray M, Swan AV, Johnson MRD, Bewley BR. Some factors associated with increased risk of smoking by children. *Journal of Child Psychology and Psychiatry and Allied Disciplines* 1983;24(2):223–32.

Naett C, Pollitzer A. Effectiveness of voluntary agreements. In: Joossens L, Karaoglou A, editors. *Tobacco Advertising "Give Children a Chance."* Brussels: European Bureau for Action on Smoking Prevention, 1991a:18–9.

Naett C, Pollitzer A. Issues related to indirect advertising. In: Joossens L, Karaoglou A, editors. *Tobacco Advertising "Give Children a Chance."* Brussels: European Bureau for Action on Smoking Prevention, 1991b:9–11.

Nafstad P, Botten G, Hagen J. Partner's smoking: a major determinant for changes in women's smoking behaviour during and after pregnancy. *Public Health* 1996;110:379–85.

National Center for Health Statistics, Mosher WD, Pratt WF. Fecundity, infertility, and reproductive health in the United States, 1982. *Vital and Health Statistics.* Series 2, No. 106. Hyattsville (MD): U.S. Department of Health and Human Services, Public Health Service, Centers for Disease Control, National Center for Health Statistics, 1988a.

National Center for Health Statistics, Schoenborn CA. Health promotion and disease prevention: United States, 1985. *Vital and Health Statistics.* Series 10, No. 163. Hyattsville (MD): U.S. Department of Health and Human Services, Public Health Service, Centers for Disease Control, National Center for Health Statistics, 1988b. DHHS Publication No. (PHS) 88-1591.

*New Straits Times.* [Benson & Hedges advertisement]. *New Straits Times* 1995 Aug 14:5.

*New Woman.* [Basic advertisement]. *New Woman* 1995a (Oct):131.

*New Woman.* [Merit advertisement]. *New Woman* 1995b (Oct):38–9.

*New York Times.* [Cigar Aficionado advertisement]. *New York Times* 1995 Sept 12;Sect A:A-11.

Newcomb MD, McCarthy WJ, Bentler PM. Cigarette smoking, academic lifestyle, and social impact efficacy: an eight-year study from early adolescence to young adulthood. *Journal of Applied Social Psychology* 1989;19(3 Pt 1):251–81.

Niaura R, Shadel WG, Abrams DB, Monti PM, Rohsenow DJ, Sirota A. Individual differences in cue reactivity among smokers trying to quit: effects of gender and cue type. *Addictive Behavior* 1998;23(2):209–24.

Nichter M, Nichter M, Vuckovic N, Quintero G, Ritenbaugh C. Smoking experimentation and initiation among adolescent girls: qualitative and quantitative findings. *Tobacco Control* 1997;6(4): 285–95.

Novacek J, Raskin R, Hogan R. Why do adolescents use drugs? Age, sex, and user differences. *Journal of Youth and Adolescence* 1991;20(5):475–92.

O'Campo P, Faden RR, Brown H, Gielen AC. The impact of pregnancy on women's prenatal and postpartum smoking behavior. *American Journal of Preventive Medicine* 1992;8(1):8–13.

Ockene JK. Smoking among women across the life span: prevalence, interventions, and implications for cessation research. *Annals of Behavioral Medicine* 1993;15(2–3):135–48.

Ockene JK, Hymowitz N, Sexton M, Broste SK. Comparison of patterns of smoking behavior change among smokers in the Multiple Risk Factor Intervention Trial (MRFIT). *Preventive Medicine* 1982;11(6):621–38.

Ockene JK, Kristeller JL, Goldberg R, Ockene I, Merriam P, Barrett S, Pekow P, Hosmer D, Gianelly R. Smoking cessation and severity of disease: the Coronary Artery Smoking Intervention Study. *Health Psychology* 1992;11(2):119–26.

Ockene JK, Nutall R, Benfari RC, Hurwitz I, Ockene IS. A psychosocial model of smoking cessation and maintenance of cessation. *Preventive Medicine* 1981;10(5):623–38.

O'Connor JJ. Special cigaret types make October new product news: some brands stress tar-nicotine content; others aim at femmes. *Advertising Age* 1970;41(43):12.

O'Connor JJ. Eve reposition designed to downplay packaging. *Advertising Age* 1974;45(36):8.

Oleckno WA, Blacconiere MJ. A multiple discriminant analysis of smoking status and health-related attitudes and behaviors. *American Journal of Preventive Medicine* 1990;6(6):323–9.

Opatow L. Packaging is most effective when it works in harmony with the positioning of a brand. *Marketing News* 1984 Feb 3:3–4.

Osler M. Social class and health behaviour in Danish adults: a longitudinal study. *Public Health* 1993; 107(4):251–60.

Page RM, Allen O, Moore L, Hewitt C. Co-occurrence of substance use and loneliness as a risk factor for adolescent hopelessness. *Journal of School Health* 1993;63(2):104–8.

Pallonen UE. Transtheoretical measures for adolescent and adult smokers: similarities and differences. *Preventive Medicine* 1998;27(5 Pt 3):A29–A38.

Pallonen UE, Prochaska JO, Velicer WF, Prokhorov AV, Smith NF. Stages of acquisition and cessation for adolescent smoking: an empirical integration. *Addictive Behaviors* 1998;23(3):303–24.

Palmer AB. Some variables contributing to the onset of cigarette smoking among junior high school students. *Social Science and Medicine* 1970;4(3): 359–66.

Pappenhagen JS, Weil PA. Does policy match practice? A new College survey shows where healthcare executives score hits and misses. *Healthcare Executive* 1988;3(3):32–5.

Patton GC, Hibbert M, Rosier MJ, Carlin JB, Caust J, Bowes G. Is smoking associated with depression and anxiety in teenagers? *American Journal of Public Health* 1996;86(2):225–30.

Pederson LL, Koval JJ, McGrady GA, Tyas SL. The degree and type of relationship between psychosocial variables and smoking status for students in grade 8: is there a dose-response relationship? *Preventive Medicine* 1998;27(3):337–47.

*People*. [Parliament advertisement]. *People* 1995a Sept 18:29.

*People*. [RJ Reynolds advertisement]. *People* 1995b Sept 18:54–5.

*People*. Star Tracks [photograph]. *People* 1995c Sept 11: 13.

*People*. [Virginia Slims advertisement]. *People* 1995d; 44(7):12.

*People*. [Benson & Hedges advertisement]. *People* 1995e Sept 18:93.

Percy L, Rossiter JR. A model of brand awareness and brand attitude advertising strategies. *Psychology and Marketing* 1992;9(4):263–74.

Perl R. Scenes from Chile. *Tobacco Control* 1994;3(2): 161–2.

Petraitis J, Flay BR, Miller TQ. Reviewing theories of adolescent substance use: organizing pieces in the puzzle. *Psychological Bulletin* 1995;117(1):67–86.

Petridou E, Zavitsanos X, Dessypris N, Frangakis C, Mandyla M, Doxiadis S, Trichopoulos D. Adolescents in high-risk trajectory: clustering of risky behavior and the origins of socioeconomic health differentials. *Preventive Medicine* 1997;26(2):215–9.

*Picture Post*. [Minor advertisement]. *Picture Post* 1952 July 5:back cover.

*Picture Post*. [Craven 'A' advertisement]. *Picture Post* 1953a Feb 14:2.

*Picture Post*. [Minor advertisement]. *Picture Post* 1953b Feb 21:back cover.

*Picture Post*. [Player's Navy Cut advertisement]. *Picture Post* 1956 June 23:18.

Pierce JP, Choi WS, Gilpin EA, Farkas AJ, Berry CC. Tobacco industry promotion of cigarettes and adolescent smoking. *Journal of the American Medical Association* 1998;279(7):511–5.

Pierce JP, Choi WS, Gilpin EA, Farkas AJ, Merritt RK. Validation of susceptibility as a predictor of which adolescents take up smoking in the United States. *Health Psychology* 1996;15(5):355–61.

Pierce JP, Farkas A, Evans N, Berry C, Choi W, Rosbrook B, Johnson M, Bal DG. *Tobacco Use in California 1992: A Focus on Preventing Uptake in Adolescents*. Sacramento (CA): California Department of Health Services, 1993.

Pierce JP, Farkas AJ, Evans N, Gilpin EA. An improved surveillance measure for adolescent smoking? *Tobacco Control* 1995;4(Suppl 1):S47–S56.

Pierce JP, Gilpin EA. A historical analysis of tobacco marketing and the uptake of smoking by youth in the United States: 1890–1977. *Health Psychology* 1995;14(6):500–8.

Pierce JP, Lee L, Gilpin EA. Smoking initiation by adolescent girls, 1944 through 1988: an association with targeted advertising. *Journal of the American Medical Association* 1994;271(8):608–11.

Pirie PL, McBride CM, Hellerstedt W, Jeffery RW, Hatsukami D, Allen S, Lando H. Smoking cessation in women concerned about weight. *American Journal of Public Health* 1992;82(9):1238–43.

Pirie PL, Murray DM, Luepker RV. Gender differences in cigarette smoking and quitting in a cohort of young adults. *American Journal of Public Health* 1991;81(3):324–7.

*Playboy.* [Virginia Slims advertisement]. *Playboy* 1971; 18(4):27.

Pollay RW. *Cigarette advertising and life* (1937–1947). Working paper. Vancouver (Canada): University of British Columbia, 1993.

Pollay RW. Exposure of U.S. youth to cigarette television advertising in the 1960's. *Tobacco Control* 1994; 3(2):130–3.

Pollay RW, Lavack AM. The targeting of youths by cigarette marketers: archival evidence on trial. *Advances in Consumer Research* 1993;20:266–71.

Pollay RW, Siddarth S, Siegel M, Haddix A, Merritt RK, Giovino GA, Eriksen MP. The last straw? Cigarette advertising and realized market shares among youths and adults, 1979–1993. *Journal of Marketing* 1996;60:1–16.

Pomerleau CS, Tate JC, Lumley MA, Pomerleau OF. Gender differences in prospectively versus retrospectively assessed smoking withdrawal symptoms. *Journal of Substance Abuse* 1994;6(4):433–40.

*Printers' Ink.* Fashion gets new emphasis as advertisers vie for females. *Printers' Ink* 1955;251(10):87.

*Printers' Ink.* Fashion and filters [photograph]. *Printers' Ink* 1958;263(4):13.

*Printers' Ink.* The great ads of all time. *Printers' Ink* 1963;283(11):14–7.

Prochaska JO, DiClemente CC, Norcross JC. In search of how people change: applications to addictive behaviors. *American Psychologist* 1992;47(9):1102–14.

Promotional Marketing, Inc. Dakota field marketing concepts presented to R.J. Reynolds Tobacco Co. Chicago: Promotional Marketing, Inc., 1989.

Pucci LG, Siegel M. Exposure to brand-specific cigarette advertising in magazines and its impact on youth smoking. *Preventive Medicine* 1999;29(5): 313–20.

Pulkkinen L. The onset and continuity of smoking and drinking in adolescence. *Acta Psychologica Fennica* 1982;9:11–30.

Radziszewska B, Richardson JL, Dent CW, Flay BR. Parenting style and adolescent depressive symptoms, smoking, and academic achievement: ethnic, gender, and SES differences. *Journal of Behavioral Medicine* 1996;19(3):289–305.

Raj SP. Striking a balance between brand "popularity" and brand loyalty. *Journal of Marketing* 1985;49 (Winter):53–9.

*Reader's Digest.* Cancer by the carton. *Reader's Digest* 1952;61(368):7–8.

*Redbook.* [Camel Special Lights advertisement]. *Redbook* 1994;182(5):74a–74b.

Redmond WH. Effects of sales promotion on smoking among U.S. ninth graders. *Preventive Medicine* 1999; 28(3):243–50.

Reisman E. Suggesting that retailers should: look to the ladies. *Tobacco* 1983 (Mar):17–9.

Revett J. Cigarets account for sizable part of women's magazine ad increases. *Advertising Age* 1971;42(9): 57.

Reynolds C, Nichols R. Personality and behavioral correlates of cigarette smoking: one-year follow-up. *Psychological Reports* 1976;38(1):251–8.

Rigotti NA, Lee JE, Wechsler H. US college students' use of tobacco products: results of a national survey. *Journal of the American Medical Association* 2000; 284(6):699–705.

R.J. Reynolds Tobacco Company. *Right decisions, right now* [booklet]. Winston-Salem (NC): R.J. Reynolds Tobacco Company, May 1993.

Robinson WA. *Best Sales Promotions of 1977/1978 (3rd Annual).* Chicago: Crain Books, 1979.

Robinson WA. Virginia Slims come a long way in 17 years. *Advertising Age* 1985;56(42):30.

Robinson LA, Klesges RC. Ethnic and gender differences in risk factors for smoking onset. *Health Psychology* 1997;16(6):499–505.

Robinson LA, Klesges RC, Zbikowski SM, Glaser R. Predictors of risk for different stages of adolescent smoking in a biracial sample. *Journal of Consulting and Clinical Psychology* 1997;65(4):653–62.

Rogers EM, Shoemaker FF. *Communication of Innovations: Cross-Cultural Approach.* 2nd ed. New York: Free Press, 1971.

Rose JS, Chassin L, Presson CC, Sherman SJ. Prospective predictors of quit attempts and smoking cessation in young adults. *Health Psychology* 1996;15(4): 261–8.

Rothstein M. A study in perfection: supermodel Linda Evangelista loves her job, a glass of wine, and a good cigar. *Cigar Aficionado* 1995;4(1):90–103.

Rowe DC, Chassin L, Presson CC, Edwards D, Sherman SJ. An "epidemic" model of adolescent cigarette smoking. *Journal of Applied Social Psychology* 1992;22(4):261–85.

Royce JM, Corbett K, Sorensen G, Ockene J. Gender, social pressure, and smoking cessations: the Community Intervention Trial for Smoking Cessation (COMMIT) at baseline. *Social Science and Medicine* 1997;44(3):359–70.

Sadava SW. Psychosocial interactionism and substance use. *Drugs and Society* 1987;2(1):1–30.

Saffer H, Chaloupka F. The effect of tobacco advertising bans on tobacco consumption. *Journal of Health Economics* 2000;19(6):1117–37.

Salive ME, Blazer DG. Depression and smoking cessation in older adults: a longitudinal study. *Journal of the American Geriatrics Society* 1993;41(12): 1313–6.

Sallis JF, Elder JP, Wildey MB, de Moor C, Young RL, Shulkin JJ, Helme JM. Assessing skills for refusing cigarettes and smokeless tobacco. *Journal of Behavioral Medicine* 1990;13(5):489–503.

Sanchagrin T. How have cigarette advertisers held the line? *Printers' Ink Marketing/Communications* 1968; 296(11):24–30.

Santi S, Best JA, Brown KS, Cargo M. Social environment and smoking initiation. *International Journal of the Addictions* 1990–91;25(7A–8A):881–903.

Santi SM, Cargo M, Brown KS, Best JA, Cameron R. Dispositional risk factors for smoking-stage transitions: a social influences program as an effect modifier. *Addictive Behaviors* 1994;19(3):269–85.

Sarason IG, Mankowski ES, Peterson AV Jr, Dinh KT. Adolescents' reasons for smoking. *Journal of School Health* 1992;62(5):185–90.

Sargent JD, Dalton MA, Beach M, Bernhardt A, Pullin D, Stevens M. Cigarette promotional items in public schools. *Archives of Pediatrics and Adolescent Medicine* 1997;151(12):1189–96.

*Saturday Evening Post*. [Spud advertisement]. *Saturday Evening Post* 1935;207(39):42.

Schifano F, Forza G, Gallimberti L. Smoking habit and psychological distress in adolescent female students. *American Journal on Addictions* 1994;3(2): 100–5.

Schmitz JM, Rosenfarb IS, Payne TJ. Cognitive and affective responses to successful coping during smoking cessation. *Journal of Substance Abuse* 1993; 5(1):61–72.

Schudson M. *Advertising, the Uneasy Persuasion: Its Dubious Impact on American Society.* New York: Basic Books, 1984.

Schwartz JL, Dubitzky M. Expressed willingness of smokers to try 10 smoking withdrawal methods. *Public Health Reports* 1967;82(10):855–61.

Seamark CJ, Gray DJ. Teenagers and risk-taking: pregnancy and smoking. *British Journal of General Practice* 1998;48(427):985–6.

Secretary of State for Health and the Secretaries of State for Scotland, Wales and Northern Ireland. *Smoking Kills. A White Paper on Tobacco.* The Stationery Office, 1998.

Seimon T, Mehl G. Strategic marketing of cigarettes to young people in Sri Lanka: "go ahead—I want to see you smoke it now." *Tobacco Control* 1998;7(4): 429–33.

Semmer NK, Cleary PD, Dwyer JH, Fuchs R, Lippert P. Psychosocial predictors of adolescent smoking in two German cities: the Berlin-Bremen Study. *Morbidity and Mortality Weekly Report* 1987;36 (Suppl 4):3S–10S.

Sexton DE, Haberman P. Women in magazine advertisements. *Journal of Advertising Research* 1974;14(4): 41–6.

Shanken MR. Interview: Richard DiMeola. *Cigar Aficionado* 1996;4:74–6, 80, 83, 85, 87, 90, 93–4, 97–8, 100, 102, 105.

Shiffman S. Relapse following smoking cessation: a situational analysis. *Journal of Consulting and Clinical Psychology* 1982;50(1):71–86.

Siegel M. Tobacco Industry Sponsorship in the United States, 1995–1999; <http://dcc2.bumc.bu.edu/tobacco/t1women.htm>; accessed: December 11, 2000.

Simon TR, Sussman S, Dent CW, Burton D, Flay BR. Prospective correlates of exclusive or combined adolescent use of cigarettes and smokeless tobacco: a replication-extension. *Addictive Behaviors* 1995; 20(4):517–24.

Skinner WF, Krohn MD. Age and gender differences in a social process model of adolescent cigarette use. *Sociological Inquiry* 1992;62(1):56–82.

Skinner WF, Massey JL, Krohn MD, Lauer RM. Social influences and constraints on the initiation and cessation of adolescent tobacco use. *Journal of Behavioral Medicine* 1985;8(4):353–76.

Slade J. Why unbranded promos? *Tobacco Control* 1994; 3(1):72.

Slade J. Tobacco product advertising during motorsports broadcasts: a quantitative assessment. In: Slama K, editor. *Tobacco and Health.* New York: Plenum Press, 1995:925–7.

Slade J, Altman D, Coeytaux R. Teenagers participate in tobacco promotions. In: Slama K, editor. *Tobacco and Health.* New York: Plenum Press, 1995:937–8.

Smith RC. The magazine's smoking habit. *Columbia Journalism Review* 1978;16(5):29–31.

Sobczynski A. Marketers clamor to offer a lady a cigarette. *Advertising Age* 1983;54(5):M14–M16.

Solberg E, Blum A. Guidelines for policy: is it really possible to eliminate tobacco advertising and promotion. In: Slama K, editor. *Tobacco and Health.* New York: Plenum Press, 1995:939–41.

Solomon MR. The role of products as social stimuli: a symbolic interactionism perspective. *Journal of Consumer Research* 1983;10(3):319–29.

Sorensen G, Pechacek TF. Attitudes toward smoking cessation among men and women. *Journal of Behavioral Medicine* 1987;10(2):129–37.

*South China Morning Post.* [Salem advertisement]. *South China Morning Post* 1990 Aug 2:19.

Specter M. Marketers target 'virile female': R.J. Reynolds plans to introduce cigarette. *Washington Post* 1990 Feb 17;Sect A:A1 (col 5), A8 (col 1).

*Sphere.* [Craven 'A' advertisement]. *Sphere* 1951 Jan 20:4.

Spitz MR, Shi H, Yang F, Hudmon KS, Jiang H, Chamberlain RM, Amos CI, Wan Y, Cinciripini P, Hong WK, Wu X. Case-control study of the D2 dopamine receptor gene and smoking status in lung cancer patients. *Journal of the National Cancer Institute* 1998;90(5):358–63.

Stanton WR, Lowe JB, Silva PA. Antecedents of vulnerability and resilience to smoking among adolescents. *Journal of Adolescent Health* 1995;16(1): 71–7.

Stanton WR, Silva PA. Children's exposure to smoking. *International Journal of Epidemiology* 1991;20(4): 933–7.

Stanton WR, Silva PA. A longitudinal study of the influence of parents and friends on children's initiation of smoking. *Journal of Applied Developmental Psychology* 1992;13(4):423–34.

Starch D. Starch reports best read advertisements. *Advertising Agency and Advertising and Selling* 1951; 44(5):74–5.

Starch D. Best-read magazine advertisements. *Advertising Agency and Advertising and Selling* 1953;46(2): 72–3.

Steinem G. Sex, lies, & advertising. *Ms.* 1990 (Jul–Aug): 18–28.

Stubenvoll R. Smoke signals from Eastern Europe. *Tobacco* 1990 (Dec):14–15.

Suh I, Kim IS, Jee SH, Lee KH. The changing pattern of cigarette smoking of students in junior and senior high schools in Korea (1988–1997). In: *Tobacco—The Growing Epidemic. 10th World Conference on Tobacco OR Health, Bejing, China; 1997 Aug 24–28.* Bejing, 1997:81.

Sussman S, Dent CW, Flay BR, Hansen WB, Johnson CA. Psychosocial predictors of cigarette smoking onset by white, black, Hispanic, and Asian adolescents in Southern California. *Morbidity and Mortality Weekly Report* 1987;36(Suppl 4):11S–16S.

Sussman S, Dent CW, McAdams LA, Stacy AW, Burton D, Flay BR. Group self-identification and adolescent cigarette smoking: a 1-year prospective study. *Journal of Abnormal Psychology* 1994;103(3): 576–80.

Sussman S, Dent CW, Nezami E, Stacy AW, Burton D, Flay BR. Reasons for quitting and smoking temptation among adolescent smokers: gender differences. *Substance Use and Misuse* 1998;33(14): 2703–20.

Swan AV, Creeser R, Murray M. When and why children first start to smoke. *International Journal of Epidemiology* 1990;19(2):323–30.

Tellis GJ. Advertising exposure, loyalty, and brand purchase: a two-stage model of choice. *Journal of Marketing Research* 1988;25(2):134–44.

*Tide.* Campaigns: cigarets. *Tide* 1936;10(10):11–12.

*Tide.* How Cavalier builds tie-ins. *Tide* 1950;24(46):53.

Tilley NM. *The R.J. Reynolds Tobacco Company.* Chapel Hill (NC): University of North Carolina Press, 1985.

*Time.* [Virginia Slims advertisement]. *Time* 1978 Mar 20:111(12):95.

*Time.* Is the Camel a sexist pig? *Time* 1989 Aug 7:41.

*Tin Tin Daily News.* [Salem advertisment]. *Tin Tin Daily News* 1992 Jan 22:21.

*Tina.* [L&M advertisement]. *Tina* 1996 Aug 29:32.

*Tobacco and Youth Reporter.* Cigarette ads in kids' movies. *Tobacco and Youth Reporter* 1989;4(1):1.

*Tobacco Retailers' Almanac.* Cigarette growth. *Tobacco Retailers' Almanac.* 3rd ed. New York: Retail Tobacco Dealers of America, 1938:18–9.

Townsend J, Roderick P, Cooper J. Cigarette smoking by socioeconomic group, sex, and age: effect of price, income, and health publicity. *British Medical Journal* 1994;309(6959):923–7.

Toxic Substances Board. *Health or Tobacco: An End to Tobacco Advertising and Promotion.* Wellington (New Zealand): Toxic Substances Board, 1989.

Trachtenberg JA. Here's one tough cowboy. *Forbes* 1987 Feb 9:108–10.

*Trone Advertising.* V.F. Year 1 Promotion Recommendations. *Trone Advertising,* 1989.

Trueheart C. Marketers test Dakota cigarettes. *Washington Post* 1991 Aug 14;Sect C:4 (col 1).

Tyler WD. A gallery of American advertising—100 years of creative progress reviewed. *Advertising Age* 1964;35(49):99–135.

Unger JB, Johnson CA, Stoddard JL, Nezami E, Chou CP. Identification of adolescents at risk for smoking initiation: validation of a measure of susceptibility. *Addictive Behavior* 1997;22(1):81–91.

*United States Tobacco Journal.* Every branch of industry girds to cope with growing crisis: cigarette executives expect added volume. *United States Tobacco Journal* 1950;154(26):3 (col 2).

*United States Tobacco Journal.* Huge female market seen: cigarettes face big new outlet. *United States Tobacco Journal* 1953;159(26):3 (col 4), 27.

*United States Tobacco Journal.* Lorillard uses fashion to push Kent, Newport. *United States Tobacco Journal* 1958;169(16):12 (col 3), 20.

University of Illinois at Chicago. Billboard ban having minimal effect on tobacco advertising: study shows tobacco industry finding other ways to market products [press release]. Chicago: University of Illinois at Chicago, Health Research and Policy Centers, July 19, 2000.

University of Michigan. *Cigarette smoking continues to rise among American teenagers in 1996* [press release]. Ann Arbor (MI): University of Michigan, News and Information Services, 1996 Dec 19.

Urberg KA. Locus of peer influence: social crowd and best friend. *Journal of Youth and Adolescence* 1992; 21(4):439–50.

Urberg KA, Cheng C-H, Shyu S-J. Grade changes in peer influence on adolescent cigarette smoking: a comparison of two measures. *Addictive Behaviors* 1991;16(1–2):21–8.

U.S. Department of Health and Human Services. *The Health Consequences of Smoking for Women. A Report of the Surgeon General.* Washington: U.S. Department of Health and Human Services, Public Health Service, Office of the Assistant Secretary for Health, Office on Smoking and Health, 1980.

U.S. Department of Health and Human Services. *The Health Consequences of Involuntary Smoking. A Report of the Surgeon General.* U.S. Department of Health and Human Services, Public Health Service, Centers for Disease Control, Center for Health Promotion and Education, Office on Smoking and Health, 1986. DHHS Publication No. (CDC) 87-8398.

U.S. Department of Health and Human Services. *The Health Consequences of Smoking: Nicotine Addiction. A Report of the Surgeon General.* Atlanta: U.S. Department of Health and Human Services, Public Health Service, Centers for Disease Control, Center for Health Promotion and Education, Office on Smoking and Health, 1988. DHHS Publication No. (CDC) 88-8406.

U.S. Department of Health and Human Services. *Reducing the Health Consequences of Smoking: 25 Years of Progress. A Report of the Surgeon General.* Rockville (MD): U.S. Department of Health and Human Services, Public Health Service, Centers for Disease Control, Center for Chronic Disease Prevention and Health Promotion, Office on Smoking and Health, 1989. DHHS Publication No. (CDC) 89-8411.

U.S. Department of Health and Human Services. *The Health Benefits of Smoking Cessation. A Report of the Surgeon General.* Atlanta: U.S. Department of Health and Human Services, Public Health Service, Centers for Disease Control, Center for Chronic Disease Prevention and Health Promotion, Office on Smoking and Health, 1990. DHHS Publication No. (CDC) 90-8416.

U.S. Department of Health and Human Services. *Smoking and Health in the Americas. A 1992 Report of the Surgeon General, in Collaboration with the Pan American Health Organization.* Atlanta: U.S. Department of Health and Human Services, Public Health Service, Centers for Disease Control, National Center for Chronic Disease Prevention and Health Promotion, Office on Smoking and Health, 1992. DHHS Publication No. (CDC) 92-8419.

U.S. Department of Health and Human Services. *Preventing Tobacco Use Among Young People. A Report of the Surgeon General.* Atlanta: U.S. Department of Health and Human Services, Public Health Service, Centers for Disease Control and Prevention, National Center for Chronic Disease Prevention and Health Promotion, Office on Smoking and Health, 1994.

U.S. Department of Health and Human Services. *Reducing Tobacco Use. A Report of the Surgeon General.* Atlanta: U.S. Department of Health and Human Services, Centers for Disease Control and Prevention, National Center for Chronic Disease Prevention and Health Promotion, Office on Smoking and Health, 2000.

van Roosmalen EH, McDaniel SA. Adolescent smoking intentions: gender differences in peer context. *Adolescence* 1992;27(105):87–105.

*Vanity Fair.* [Philip Morris advertisement]. *Vanity Fair* 1995a (Oct):197.

*Vanity Fair.* [Virginia Slims advertisement]. *Vanity Fair* 1995b (Oct):128–129.

*Vanity Fair.* [Benson & Hedges advertisement]. *Vanity Fair* 1995c (Oct):back cover.

*Vogue.* [Buffalo Jeans advertisement]. *Vogue* 1995a (Sept):303.

*Vogue.* [Camel advertisement]. *Vogue* 1995b (Aug):143.

*Vogue.* [Marlboro Lights advertisement]. *Vogue* 1995c (Sept):208–209.

Wagner P. Cigarettes vs. candy: war correspondence from a new battle front. *New Republic* 1929;57(741): 343–5.

Wahlgren DR, Hovell MF, Slymen DJ, Conway TL, Hofstetter CR, Jones JA. Predictors of tobacco use initiation in adolescents: a two-year prospective study and theoretical discussion. *Tobacco Control* 1997;6(2):95–103.

Wakefield M, Gillies P, Graham H, Madeley R, Symonds M. Characteristics associated with smoking cessation during pregnancy among working class women. *Addiction* 1993;88(10):1423–30.

Waldron I. Patterns and causes of gender differences in smoking. *Social Science and Medicine* 1991;32(9): 989–1005.

Waldron I, Lye D. Relationships between teenage smoking and attitudes toward women's rights, sex roles, marriage, sex and family. *Women and Health* 1990;16(3–4):23–46.

Waldron I, Lye D, Brandon A. Gender differences in teenage smoking. *Women and Health* 1991;17(2): 65–90.

Wallace R. A "Lucky" or a sweet—or both! *Nation* 1929;128(3323):305–7.

Ward S, Wackman DB, Wartella E. *How Children Learn to Buy: The Development of Consumer Information-Processing Skills.* People and Communications Series, Vol. 1. Beverly Hills (CA): Sage Publications, 1977.

Warner KE. Cigarette advertising and media coverage of smoking and health. *New England Journal of Medicine* 1985;312(6):384–8.

Warner KE. *Selling Smoke: Cigarette Advertising and Public Health.* Washington: American Public Health Association, 1986.

Warner KE, Butler J, Cummings KM, D'Onofrio C, Davis RM, Flay B, McKinney M, Myers ML, Pertschuk M, Robinson RG, Ryden L, Schudson M, Tye J, Wilkenfeld J. Report of the Tobacco Policy Research Study Group on tobacco marketing and promotion. *Tobacco Control* 1992a;1 (Suppl):S19–S23.

Warner KE, Ernster VL, Holbrook JH, Lewit EM, Pertschuk M, Steinfeld JL, Tye JB, Whelan EM. Promotion of tobacco products: issues and policy options. *Journal of Health Politics, Policy and Law* 1986;11(3):367–92.

Warner KE, Goldenhar LM. The cigarette advertising broadcast ban and magazine coverage of smoking and health. *Journal of Public Health Policy* 1989; 10(1):32–42.

Warner KE, Goldenhar LM. Targeting of cigarette advertising in U.S. magazines, 1959–1986. *Tobacco Control* 1992;1(1):25–30.

Warner KE, Goldenhar LM, McLaughlin CG. Cigarette advertising and magazine coverage of the hazards of smoking: a statistical analysis. *New England Journal of Medicine* 1992b;326(5):305–9.

Wasserman J, Manning WG, Newhouse JP, Winkler JD. The effects of excise taxes and regulations on cigarette smoking. *Journal of Health Economics* 1991; 10(1):43–64.

Weinstein H. How an agency builds a brand—the Virginia Slims story. Paper presented at the 1969 American Association of Advertising Agencies Eastern Annual Conference; 1970 Oct 28–29; New York.

Weir J. Tobacco advertising: the New Zealand experience. *Tobacco Control* 1995;4(1):90–1.

Weis WL, Burke C. Media content and tobacco advertising: an unhealthy addiction. *Journal of Communication* 1986;36(4):59–69.

Weld LDH. Advertising and tobacco. *Printers' Ink* 1937; 181(1):70–2, 76.

Weldner D. The real enemy. *Winston Salem Journal* 1996 Sept 2;Sect B:B1.

Whelan EM. *A Smoking Gun: How the Tobacco Industry Gets Away with Murder.* Philadelphia: George F. Stickley, 1984.

Whelan EM, Sheridan MJ, Meister KA, Mosher BA. Analysis of coverage of tobacco hazards in women's magazines. *Journal of Public Health Policy* 1981; 2(1):28–35.

While D, Kelly S, Huang W, Charlton A. Cigarette advertising and onset of smoking in children: questionnaire survey. *British Medical Journal* 1996; 313(7054):398–9.

White L, Whelan EM. How well do American magazines cover the health hazards of smoking? The 1986 survey. *American Council on Science and Health News and Views* 1986;7(3):1, 8–11.

Willemsen MC, De Zwart WM. The effectiveness of policy and health education strategies for reducing adolescent smoking: a review of the evidence. *Journal of Adolescence* 1999;22(5):587–99.

Williams B. Looking east for salvation. *Raleigh News and Observer* 1995a Apr 10:A1.

Williams B. New world order: North Carolina takes a back seat as tobacco thrives abroad. *Raleigh News and Observer* 1995b Apr 9:A1.

Williams B. U.S. tobacco firms invest heavily in China despite tight market: joint venture limited to 1 percent in nation of 300 million smokers. *Raleigh News and Observer* 1995c Apr 10:A6.

Williams B. As U.S. cigarette makers enter Eastern Europe, opponents aren't far behind. But war on smoking goes overseas. *Raleigh News and Observer* 1995d Apr 11:A1.

Williams M. Tobacco's hold on women's groups: anti-smokers charge leaders have sold out to industry money. *Washington Post* 1991 Nov 14; Sect A:1 (col 2), 16 (col 1).

Williamson DF, Madans J, Anda RF, Kleinman JC, Giovino GA, Byers T. Smoking cessation and severity of weight gain in a national cohort. *New England Journal of Medicine* 1991;324(11):739–45.

Williamson DF, Serdula MK, Kendrick JS, Binkin NJ. Comparing the prevalence of smoking in pregnant and nonpregnant women, 1985 to 1986. *Journal of the American Medical Association* 1989;261(1): 70–4.

Wills TA. Stress and coping in early adolescence: relationships to substance use in urban school samples. *Health Psychology* 1986;5(6):503–29.

Wills TA, Vaughan R. Social support and substance use in early adolescence. *Journal of Behavioral Medicine* 1989;12(4):321–39.

Wilson JJ. Summary of the Attorneys General Master Tobacco Settlement Agreement, March 1999; <http://www.ncsl.org/statefed/tmsasumm.htm>; accessed: December 14, 1999.

Wilson DM, Killen JD, Hayward C, Robinson TN, Hammer LD, Kraemer HC, Varady A, Taylor CB. Timing and rate of sexual maturation and the onset of cigarette and alcohol use among teenage girls. *Archives of Pediatric and Adolescent Medicine* 1994;148(8):789–95.

Windsor RA, Lowe JB, Perkins LL, Smith-Yoder D, Artz L, Crawford M, Amburgy K, Boyd NR. Health education for pregnant smokers: its behavioral impact and cost benefit. *American Journal of Public Health* 1993;83(2):201–6.

Winefield AH, Tiggemann M, Winefield HR, Goldney RD. *Growing Up with Unemployment: A Longitudinal Study of Its Psychological Impact.* New York: Routledge, 1993.

Winefield HR, Winefield AH, Tiggemann M. Psychological attributes of young adult smokers. *Psychological Reports* 1992;70(3 Pt 1):675–81.

Wojcik JV. Social learning predictors of the avoidance of smoking relapse. *Addictive Behaviors* 1988;13(2): 177–80.

Wolfson M, Forster JL, Claxton AJ, Murray DM. Adolescent smokers' provision of tobacco to other adolescents. *American Journal of Public Health* 1997; 87(4):649–51.

*Woman.* [Craven 'A' advertisement]. *Woman* 1952 Apr 5:36.

*Woman and Home.* [Player's Navy Cut advertisement]. *Woman and Home* 1953 Apr:59.

*Woman's Own.* [Embassy advertisement]. *Woman's Own* 1947 May 30:23.

*Woman's Own.* [Gold Flake advertisement]. *Woman's Own* 1950 Jan 5:18.

*World Smoking and Health.* Japan: calling women to action in Japan. *World Smoking and Health* 1994; 19(2):8–10.

*World Tobacco.* News. Views. Trends. China. *World Tobacco* 1989 Jan:8.

Wu L-T, Anthony JC. Tobacco smoking and depressed mood in late childhood and early adolescence. *American Journal of Public Health* 1999;89(12): 1837–40.

Yankelovich Partners. *Smoking Cessation Study.* Report prepared for Ketchum Public Relations and their client American Lung Association. Norwalk (CT): Yankelovich Partners, July 27, 1998; <http://www.lungusa.org/partner/yank/1.html>; accessed: August 15, 2000.

Yates AJ, Thain J. Self-efficacy as a predictor of relapse following voluntary cessation of smoking. *Addictive Behaviors* 1985;10(3):291–8.

Zimmerman C. Growth is watchword for Asian tobacco industry [editorial]. *Tobacco Reporter* 1990; 117(6):4.

Zinn L. The smoke clears at Marlboro. *Business Week* 1994 Jan 31:76–7.

Zuckerman M. Is sensation seeking a predisposing trait for alcoholism? In: Gottheil E, Druley KA, Pasko S, Weinstein SP, editors. *Stress and Addictions.* New York: Brunner/Mazel 1987:283–301.

# Chapter 5. Efforts to Reduce Tobacco Use Among Women

# Background and Overview of Smoking Cessation Methods

The 1980 Surgeon General's report, *The Health Consequences of Smoking for Women*, noted that women might start, continue, and fail to stop smoking for different reasons than do men (U.S. Department of Health and Human Services [USDHHS] 1980). The report concluded that "across all treatments, women have more difficulty giving up smoking than men, both at the end of treatment and at long-term points of measurement" (USDHHS 1980, p. 307). This conclusion was based on a simple analysis of self-reported smoking cessation in 14 studies that reported sufficient data for gender-specific comparisons. The report went on to recommend that further research was needed to identify factors that might contribute to observed outcome differences (e.g., women's greater worries about weight gain and greater putative reliance on smoking to regulate negative affect) and to explore possible interactions between treatment and gender. The report urged that research focus on identification of the differences between the smoking patterns among women and men so that optimal methods could be found to reduce smoking initiation and increase smoking cessation among women.

Much has happened in smoking cessation research since the 1980 report was released. Examination of some of the report's hypothesized differences in smoking cessation between women and men—social support, fear of weight gain, and commitment to health—has been the focus of research in the past 20 years. As several reviewers have noted (Berman and Gritz 1991; Clarke et al. 1993; Solomon and Flynn 1993; Gritz 1994; Marcus et al. 1994; Mermelstein and Borrelli 1995; Gritz et al. 1996; Lando and Gritz 1996), however, questions remain as to whether there are important differences by gender in smoking cessation, with some studies having pointed to differences and others to lack of differences.

During this same period, additional research has been conducted on issues thought to be specific to women (e.g., hormonal influences and depression), on gender-related differences in smoking cessation among specific subgroups of the population (e.g., smokers of low socioeconomic status [SES], those who smoke heavily, and minority group members), and on gender-related differences in response to smoking cessation programs (e.g., worksite programs, community-based programs, and policy changes).

In this chapter, an overview of smoking cessation research is presented. It emphasizes the challenges in understanding and addressing the special needs among women who smoke and in noting differences between women and men who achieve cessation. With the notable exception of cessation methods devised specifically for pregnant women, few approaches have focused expressly on women. Nevertheless, some investigators have occasionally examined and analyzed various treatment outcomes for possible differential effects of programs among women and men. This chapter addresses those differences. Even when gender-specific differences in treatment outcome have been reported, analyses to clarify the factors that might be responsible for the differences have rarely been described. Gender-specific differences in outcome might reflect differences in a wide array of smoking-related factors, including SES, social roles, concerns about weight, hormonal factors, smoking history, physical response to nicotine, motives for smoking cessation, and barriers to smoking cessation (Biener 1987; Clarke et al. 1993; Marcus et al. 1994). If substantive differences in smoking cessation outcomes exist between women and men, the underlying factors that contribute to gender-specific differences in treatment outcome are essential to understanding and identifying new and more successful ways to develop or tailor treatment for women (and men) who smoke. Where such information exists, it is also examined.

Although smoking cessation is the major emphasis of this chapter, little doubt exists that prevention of smoking initiation would be the most efficient way to reduce tobacco use among women. Smoking initiation typically begins in youth—more than 88 percent of smokers tried their first cigarette before age 18 years (USDHHS 1994). Thus, prevention efforts have focused primarily on young people, particularly adolescents. This chapter includes an examination of prevention research activities and their differential effects by gender.

Because women and girls make up only a very small fraction of the nation's smokeless tobacco users (Giovino et al. 1994; Centers for Disease Control and Prevention [CDC] 1995b) (see "Smokeless Tobacco" in Chapter 2) and very little has been done to assess methods to curtail smokeless tobacco use among women, this section focuses on strategies in cigarette smoking cessation research and treatment strategies. This is not to say that smokeless tobacco use is unimportant; rather, the data available have not provided information on gender-specific differences in cessation programs for smokeless tobacco users. Thus, conclusions cannot be drawn about gender-specific differences in smokeless tobacco use and cessation of use.

## Innovations in Smoking Cessation

The past two decades have seen a proliferation of methods of smoking cessation (USDHHS 1990, 2000). Among other developments, new emphasis was given to varied venues to reach women who smoke. Examples include the development and evaluation of innovative programs for prenatal, postpartum, and WIC (Special Supplemental Nutrition Program for Women, Infants, and Children) clinics (e.g., Windsor et al. 1993b; Keintz et al. 1994; Kendrick et al. 1995), worksites (Gritz et al. 1988), health maintenance organizations (HMOs) (Ershoff et al. 1989; Gritz et al. 1992), subsidized housing projects (Manfredi et al. 1992; Lacey et al. 1993), and mass-media messages aimed at women (e.g., Cummings et al. 1989; Davis et al. 1992; CDC 1995a; Mermelstein and Borrelli 1995). Some of this work also explored new avenues for reaching women in underserved minority populations (Manfredi et al. 1992; Lacey et al. 1993).

Other innovations in the past two decades include changes and advances in theoretical approaches to smoking cessation that resulted in new treatment approaches for women who wanted to stop smoking (Prochaska and DiClemente 1983; Popham et al. 1993; Prochaska 1994; Prochaska et al. 1992, 1993). The broad application of the principles of social marketing to population-based smoking cessation efforts (Black et al. 1993; Glanz and Rimer 1995) also led to a new focus on targeting and tailoring treatments, both for early-stage smokers (i.e., those not really thinking about stopping soon) (Lichtenstein 1997; Dijkstra et al. 1998, 1999) and for smokers within defined subgroups, such as minority or ethnic groups and elderly smokers at high risk for smoking or for diseases related to smoking (Dale et al. 1997; Orleans et al. 1998).

Initiatives included efforts to understand and target women in specific occupational, socioeconomic, and racial and ethnic subgroups (Gritz et al. 1988; Manfredi et al. 1992; Lacey et al. 1993; Crittenden et al. 1994) and women at different stages of the life cycle, from adolescence and young adulthood (Weissman et al. 1987; Pirie et al. 1991), to pregnancy and early parenthood (Mullen 1990), through old age (King et al. 1990). Efforts were also made to target women by appealing to their desires to protect children and family members from the effects of environmental tobacco smoke (ETS) (Cummings et al. 1989; Emmons et al. 1994). The initiatives also addressed gender-specific barriers, such as pervasive advertising targeted to women in general (Ernster 1993; Pierce et al. 1994b; CDC 1995a) or to subgroups of women with high stress and low SES (Manfredi et al. 1992; Crittenden et al. 1994), limited social support for stopping smoking (Coppotelli and Orleans 1985; Lacey et al. 1993), stress and negative affect (Biener 1987; Lacey et al. 1993), a need to control weight (Klesges et al. 1991; French et al. 1995; Meyers et al. 1997), or concerns about weight gain after smoking cessation (Sorensen and Pechacek 1987; Pirie et al. 1991; Marcus et al. 1994, 1999). From the recent innovations and the research conducted to date, we have learned much about the factors important to women and to successful smoking cessation. Nevertheless, more research is needed in some areas.

## Gender-Specific Similarities and Differences in Motives and Barriers to Stop Smoking

Studies to date have reported no major or consistent differences among women's and men's motivations for wanting to stop smoking, readiness to stop smoking, or general awareness of the harmful health effects of smoking. Nevertheless, current work has suggested that multiple gender-linked biopsychosocial factors that might influence motivation to smoke or that serve as barriers to smoking cessation be taken into account when a comprehensive approach toward tobacco control among women is developed (Waldron 1991; Marcus et al. 1994; Gritz et al. 1998). Further research is needed to increase our understanding of how gender-specific factors affect motivation for and the processes of smoking cessation.

Smokers have given a variety of reasons for wanting to stop smoking, but "health reasons" is the most frequently cited motivation for quitting. An analysis of data from the 1987 National Health Interview Survey (NHIS) Cancer Control Supplement found that the majority of both women and men smokers who tried to quit in the previous five years reported health motives for wanting to quit (both 62 percent) (Gilpin et al. 1992). Curry and associates (1990) reported no gender-related differences in health motives for smoking cessation in a large HMO population of adults. Orleans and associates (1990) found little relationship between gender and the perceived links between smoking and disease among respondents to the Adult Use of Tobacco Survey (AUTS) aged 50 through 74 years. More women than men, however, rated "future health" (77 vs. 69 percent), "present health" (62 vs. 52 percent), and "the effects of my smoking on others" (40 vs. 31 percent) to be important motives for smoking cessation. Similarly, Lando and associates (1991) found that women were more concerned than men about the health effects of their smoking on others. On the other hand, in a survey of 10 worksites, Sorensen and Pechacek (1987) reported that women smokers were less likely than men smokers to recognize the health benefits of smoking cessation. Also, Brownson and colleagues (1992) found that women (both smokers and nonsmokers) in a large Missouri sample were less likely than men to report awareness of the harmful health effects of smoking and exposure to ETS.

Previous Surgeon General's reports on smoking and health (USDHHS 1988, 1989) emphasized that many women may not be fully informed of important gender-specific health consequences of smoking and recommended educational campaigns publicizing the special health risks from smoking among women (see "Tobacco Control Advocacy Programs by and for Women" later in this chapter). The 1988 Surgeon General's report further noted that "reliance on cigarettes for bolstering an important, self-selected social image may make some women resistant to educational messages on the health consequences of smoking" (USDHHS 1988, p. 507). The lack of coverage about the harmful effects of smoking and pervasive tobacco advertising in women's print media (Ernster 1993) (see "Press Self-Censorship in Relation to Cigarette Advertising" in Chapter 4) and possible misconceptions about the relative "safety" of smoking low-tar and low-nicotine cigarettes (USDHHS 1989) may reinforce such an "optimistic bias" among women smokers, who are more likely than men to use such products (USDHHS 2000).

Findings have suggested that women may be particularly concerned about the dangers of their own smoking to children and family members. Cummings and colleagues (1989) developed a media campaign emphasizing the health dangers that a mother's smoking poses to her children. Smokers were encouraged to make a telephone call to the Cancer Information Service (CIS) of the National Cancer Institute (NCI) for help in stopping smoking. The campaign succeeded in boosting calls to CIS from smokers who were mothers of infants and young children. Gilpin and colleagues (1992) found that young women cited social reasons for smoking cessation slightly but significantly more often than did young men (23.9 vs. 19.3 percent). Reasons included pressure from family or friends (11 vs. 9 percent) and wanting to set a good example for children (4 vs. 2 percent). At both ends of the age spectrum, women reported stronger perceived social pressure to stop smoking than did men (Orleans et al. 1990; Pirie et al. 1991). Curry and colleagues (1990) found no gender-specific differences in cost or social motives for smoking cessation.

Motivating people to stop smoking also involves addressing smokers' concerns about the difficulties and negative consequences of smoking cessation and bolstering their confidence to stop (Miller and Rollnick 1991). Lando and colleagues (1991) found that women were significantly more likely than men to anticipate difficulty in quitting, to believe that they would still be smoking in five years, and to perceive more barriers to stopping smoking. Although women and men were equally likely to rate themselves as addicted to smoking, significantly more women than men said they would feel tense and irritable if they stopped (79 vs. 73 percent; $p < 0.05$); enjoyed smoking too much to stop (77 vs. 64 percent; $p < 0.001$); expected difficulty concentrating after stopping (45 vs. 36 percent; $p < 0.005$); and anticipated gaining considerable weight after stopping (69 vs. 40 percent; $p < 0.001$) (Lando et al. 1991). Similar patterns were seen among smokers aged 65 years or older in the 1986 AUTS who had tried to stop smoking in the past. Significantly more women than men noted weight gain when they had tried to stop (33 vs. 21 percent) and reported the following reasons for relapse to smoking: worry about weight gain (33 vs. 21 percent), headaches (9 vs. 4 percent), and family pressure to stop smoking (18 vs. 10 percent). In addition, significantly more women than men rated smoking as a valuable aid in weight control (54 vs. 48 percent) and in coping with stress (53 vs. 49 percent) (Orleans et al. 1990).

Few studies have explored possible gender-specific differences in the processes or pathways of smoking cessation (Blake et al. 1989). It may be that women and men smokers in the same study achieve similar outcomes by different routes, benefiting more or less from different treatment components or relying on different cognitive-behavioral and self-change processes. Swan and Denk (1987), for example, followed a sample of 209 women smokers and 172 men smokers who had achieved at least 3 months of abstinence after taking part in formal smoking cessation treatments. The investigators documented virtually identical rates of transition to relapse and subsequent recovery (return to abstinence) among women and men over the 12 months of follow-up. But they found quite different predictors of relapse among women who had stopped smoking (e.g., unemployment and heightened craving for nicotine) and men who had stopped smoking (e.g., having a father who smoked and the severity of "hassles") (Swan and Denk 1987, p. 544). Few studies have examined differences in preferences for treatment (Lando et al. 1991), or investigated interactions between treatment and gender, to understand whether women and men respond differently to the same treatment (Weissman et al. 1987; Curry et al. 1988; COMMIT Research Group 1995a; Ossip-Klein et al. 1997; Gritz et al. 1998).

A number of gender-linked biopsychosocial factors are potentially important motives for or barriers to smoking cessation among women who smoke. For example, the special medical risks from smoking among women, particularly those related to pregnancy, fertility, use of oral contraceptives, and age at menopause, have long been recognized as unique smoking cessation motives among women (USDHHS 1980, 1989). (See "Menstrual Function, Menopause, and Benign Gynecologic Conditions," "Smoking and Use of Oral Contraceptives" and "Reproductive Outcomes" in Chapter 3, and "Hormonal Influences" later in this chapter). Gender-specific differences in the mechanisms of nicotine addiction have received increasing attention. The results of laboratory studies that examined whether gender-specific differences in nicotine metabolism and sensitivity exist have been conflicting (see "Nicotine Pharmacology and Addiction" in Chapter 3). Data on whether the menstrual cycle phase affects nicotine intake also have been inconsistent, but some evidence has indicated exacerbated tobacco withdrawal symptoms during the premenstrual period (see "Hormonal Influences" later in this chapter).

All of the factors surrounding motivation for smoking cessation, taken collectively, dictate the use of a much wider lens when assessing the unique treatment needs and barriers among women who smoke. This assessment might involve routinely measuring potentially important psychosocial variables that are now seldom measured as covariates or predictors in intervention research, such as income level, number of dependent children and other household members, occupation, source of and access to primary health care, perceived value of health, physical self-esteem (e.g., attractiveness), perceived control over life events, perceived competence, concerns about weight, presence of eating disorders, personality and coping styles, perceived social support or isolation, perceived life stress and stressors (particularly those related to life-cycle changes and to stressful family and marital transitions and circumstances), job strain, demands of multiple roles, and strain related to particular roles (Cohen et al. 1983; Biener 1987; McGrath et al. 1990; Chesney 1991; Covey et al. 1992; Batten 1993). Whether addressing such factors would increase the likelihood of cessation requires more research.

## Smoking Cessation and Nicotine Addiction Treatment Methods

A vast variety of smoking cessation methods are available in the United States (USDHHS 1990, 1991b, 2000; Samet and Coultas 1991; Fiore et al. 2000). The methods range from self-help materials to very intensive clinical approaches to very broad community-based programs. Most women and men who attempt to stop smoking and those who do so successfully, do so on their own with little difference between women and men in long-term quit rates (6 to 12 months). Self-help approaches to cessation, minimal clinical assistance, and intensive clinical assistance also have shown few differences between women and men, although some studies reported that men are more likely to achieve long-term abstinence than are women (Research Committee of the British Thoracic Society 1990; Bjornson et al. 1995). Women are somewhat more likely than men to use formal smoking cessation programs (Fiore et al. 1990; Wagner et al. 1990; Glasgow et al. 1993; Yankelovich Partners 1998; Zhu et al. 2000). Substantial differences appear to exist between women and men in the processes of cessation, with women preferring a more gradual approach to cessation and using more cessation strategies than do men (Blake et al. 1989; Fiore et al. 1990; Lando et al. 1991; Whitlock et al. 1997). Women also reported having more withdrawal symptoms than did men (Pomerleau et al. 1994b; Gritz et al. 1996; Sussman et al. 1998a). One cessation method, use of nicotine replacement therapy, may be less effective among women than among men (Killen et al. 1990b; Hatsukami et al. 1995; Perkins 1996, 1999; Wetter et al. 1999a,b); however, other studies indicated no difference (Hughes 1993; Fiore et al. 1994; Jorenby et al. 1995).

### Unaided Smoking Cessation

Fiore and colleagues (1990) found that the vast majority of smokers who had tried to stop reported doing so on their own, although this has changed in recent years with increased use of pharmacologic aids (Yankelovich Partners 1998). The finding held among women as well as among men, although a slightly higher proportion of women than men (16.8 vs. 13.4 percent) reported using an assisted method to stop smoking (Fiore et al. 1990; Yankelovich Partners 1998). In a study of California smokers, women were 27 percent more likely than men to use assistance (self-help, counseling, nicotine replacement therapy) for smoking cessation. These gender differences remained after adjustment for age, education, ethnicity, and number of cigarettes smoked per day (Zhu et al. 2000). Univariate analysis of the 1986 AUTS data showed that more men than women were successful in smoking cessation. However, in a multivariate logistic regression analysis that controlled for variables of demography and smoking history, gender was not a significant predictor of successfully stopping smoking (Fiore et al. 1990).

Comparable results were seen in other large, population-based studies that used self-reports of smoking cessation. For example, the 1991 NHIS Health Promotion and Disease Prevention Supplement reported that although education, age, and race and ethnicity were significant predictors of adults' attempts to stop smoking and to maintain cessation, gender was not (CDC 1993b). Pirie and colleagues (1991) found that attempting to stop smoking and maintaining abstinence were equally common among women and men in a large Minnesota cohort of young adults, and Salive and colleagues (1992) reported that age-adjusted cessation and relapse rates differed little by gender among smokers aged 65 years or older in three large community cohorts. At variance with these findings, Ward and colleagues (1997) found that among adults who had stopped smoking without assistance, abstinence after one year was significantly greater among men than among women (8.6 vs. 0.0 percent). However, in another longitudinal analysis of smokers who attempted unaided smoking cessation, men who smoked were more likely than women who smoked to achieve initial cessation (1 month) (82 vs. 73 percent); no differences in long-term cessation were found (Marlatt et al. 1988).

In a descriptive comparison of 10 prospective studies of self-quitting, long-term abstinence was calculated among smokers who attempted to stop smoking on their own (Cohen et al. 1989). More than 5,000 smokers participated in the combined studies. Long-term cessation, relapse, and unsuccessful quit attempts were very similar among the studies. A formal meta-analysis of all of the studies did not show a gender effect on either 6-month or 12-month abstinence.

Differences are seen between women and men in the timing of smoking cessation. A higher proportion of women than men had stopped smoking at ages younger than 40 years, and a higher proportion of men than women had stopped smoking between 50 and 65 years of age. Jarvis (1994) postulated that gender-specific differences in life experiences, such as pregnancy and child rearing, may account for such trends. Alternatively, smoking uptake and quitting among U.S. men preceded that of U.S. women in this century. Thus, more men than women were likely to quit among older generations of smokers. Among recent birth cohorts, however, the patterns of uptake and quitting are more comparable among women and men. Gritz and colleagues (1996) suggested that menopause, with its attendant hormonal changes (leading to behavioral events such as fluctuations in affect or difficulty with weight control) and changes in social roles, provides a barrier to cessation.

Methods of smoking cessation vary somewhat by gender. In a survey of smokers at 10 worksites, Sorensen and Pechacek (1987) found that similar proportions of women smokers (70 percent) and men (73 percent) smokers were planning to change their smoking behavior (stop, cut down, or switch cigarette brand) in the next 12 months, but men were more likely to say they wanted to stop smoking entirely, and women were more likely to report wanting to reduce the number of cigarettes smoked. A similar pattern emerged in a larger Minnesota sample: women and men were equally likely to report intentions to change their smoking behavior in the next year, with men more often choosing to stop entirely and women more often choosing to cut down (Blake et al. 1989). Although women and men reported a similar number of previous attempts to stop smoking, women were also less successful in sustaining their attempts for longer than one week. These investigators concluded that women were more tentative and less committed to stopping smoking entirely and postulated that women may be less confident than men in their ability to stop, as well as less persistent in their efforts.

### Self-Help Programs

Numerous self-help interventions have been developed for smoking cessation, including manuals, videotapes, and mass-media programs designed to help smokers stop smoking on their own. Although the effects of self-help programs appear to be small and inconsistent (Fiore et al. 2000), they are appealing because they can be easily disseminated to the vast population of smokers who try to stop on their own each year (Fiore et al. 1990; Curry 1993).

Beginning in the mid-1980s, NCI funded seven large-scale controlled trials to develop and assess maximally effective self-help programs and materials.

These trials reached more than 200,000 smokers directly or indirectly in communities, worksites, hospitals, HMOs, and voluntary associations (Glynn et al. 1990). A summary of the results of the self-help trials (Cohen et al. 1989) indicated that a higher proportion of women smokers than men smokers enrolled, but no gender-specific differences in outcome were found. To date, little is known about the relationship between smokers' use of self-help materials and the outcomes of self-help treatment or about the impact of various treatment formats on program reach or efficacy (Curry 1993).

Few studies have explored gender-specific differences in self-help treatment methods or adjuncts (i.e., brief telephone counseling, tailored feedback, physician advice). Fewer have explored interactions between treatment and gender. A study of two interventions that used self-help materials targeted to older smokers (≥ 60 years old) (Ossip-Klein et al. 1997) found an interaction between treatment and gender. Among women, cessation levels were higher among those who received two proactive telephone calls. Among men, however, cessation levels were higher for those who received two mailed prompts to call a stop-smoking hotline. This result suggested that women may be more responsive to personal interaction.

A survey by Lando and associates (1991) also suggested that smoking cessation strategies should be different among women smokers and men smokers. In a study based in one of the Minnesota Heart Health Programs, they reported that women smokers were more interested than men smokers in using filters that successively reduced the amount of nicotine inhaled from a cigarette to help them prepare for smoking cessation.

Several self-help guides and programs have been developed exclusively for women smokers, including pregnant women (Windsor et al. 1985; Ershoff et al. 1989; Mayer et al. 1990), mothers of young children (Cummings et al. 1989; Davis et al. 1992), registered nurses (Gritz et al. 1988), HMO enrollees (Gritz et al. 1992), and women living in a low-SES urban area (Mermelstein and Borrelli 1995). Materials developed for pregnant women have been found to outperform generic materials (Windsor et al. 1985). One self-help study with pregnant smokers suggested that supplying smokers with repeated "cues to action" over time, by mail or phone, would itself have benefit (Ershoff et al. 1989). In a study of nonpregnant mothers of young children, however, cessation levels were similar among young women who used a specially developed tailored guide and among a similar group who used generic materials (both 12.5 percent) (Cummings et al. 1989; Davis et al. 1992).

Gritz and colleagues (1992) evaluated an intervention for women smokers (identified by survey, not volunteers) in a large HMO population who were mailed a six-week series of self-help booklets on smoking cessation. A comparison group of women smokers did not receive self-help material. The overall point prevalence abstinence (at least 48 hours) among all participants was 19 percent at 18 months, with no difference seen between the treatment group, which received an unsolicited, mailed self-help cessation program, and the control group. A more recent study provided support for using personalized messages with self-help material. In this study (Strecher et al. 1994), 359 adult smokers from a large family practice were interviewed briefly, then randomly assigned to receive either a generic letter on smoking cessation or a tailored letter containing advice geared to the smoker's individual health-related beliefs about the benefits of and barriers to smoking cessation, stage of change, and reasons for past failures to stop smoking. Tailoring health letters to the characteristics of each patient allowed the investigators to focus, in clear detail, only on the information most relevant to each smoker. Among light or moderate smokers, self-reported cessation at four months (adjusted for age, education, and gender) was significantly higher for those receiving tailored information than for those receiving generic letters. No significant differences in intervention effects were found between women and men.

#### Minimal Clinical Interventions

In the past decade or so, efforts have been made to increase the proportion of primary care providers who routinely advise their patients to stop smoking and assist them in that effort (Ockene 1987; USDHHS 1991a; Fiore et al. 1996, 2000; National Committee for Quality Assurance 1997). The 1991 NHIS Health Promotion and Disease Prevention Supplement found that 70 percent of adult smokers reported at least one visit to a physician in the preceding 12 months, with more than two-thirds reporting more than one visit (CDC 1993a). These statistics led to the projection that an additional one million smokers could be helped to stop smoking each year if primary care providers offered brief counseling to all of their patients who smoke (CDC 1993a).

The proportion of adult smokers who reported ever having been advised by a health care professional to stop smoking increased from 26 percent in 1976 to 56 percent in 1991 (CDC 1993a). In 1992, 52 percent of smokers who had seen a physician in the previous year reported receiving advice to stop smoking (Tomar et al. 1996). The likelihood of having been counseled to stop smoking was directly related to the number of health care visits reported and was slightly higher among women, who reported slightly more visits to a physician than did men (39 vs. 35 percent). Among smokers who had seen a dentist in the previous year, 24 percent reported they had received advice to stop smoking (Tomar et al. 1996). As was observed for counseling from a physician, the percentage receiving counseling by a dentist was slightly higher among women (27 vs. 22 percent). Tomar and colleagues (1996) noted that either smokers are less likely to remember the advice received from dentists than from physicians, or dentists are less likely to advise their patients to quit smoking. Additionally, the researchers concluded that dentists and physicians may not be maximizing their opportunities to advise patients who use tobacco to quit or may not be adequately communicating to their patients the importance of quitting.

Numerous controlled trials were launched in the mid-1980s to test the efficacy of "minimal contact" medical interventions, which relied on techniques that could easily be integrated into routine care and delivered to all smokers, regardless of their interest in smoking cessation. The emphasis was on brief counseling by a health care provider, supported by self-help materials on smoking cessation and, if appropriate, nicotine replacement therapy. Results of these trials showed that even brief interventions significantly improved patient outcomes (Glynn 1988; Kottke et al. 1988; Fiore et al. 1996, 2000). No gender-related differences were observed in attempts to stop smoking, cessation, or relapse, by 12-month cessation rates among HMO patients exposed to brief physician advice plus a nurse-assisted intervention (Whitlock et al. 1997). Women who tried to stop smoking used more cessation strategies than did men. This finding suggested that the processes of smoking cessation may differ by gender.

Two studies by the British Thoracic Society examined the effects of cessation advice from physicians, with or without other levels of encouragement, among adult patients (mean age, 51 years for women and 50 years for men) with smoking-related symptoms who were referred to either study by their physicians (Research Committee of the British Thoracic Society 1990). No significant interactions between type of intervention and gender were observed in either of the two studies, although one found significantly higher abstinence at 12-month follow-up among men than among women.

The 1996 publication, *Smoking Cessation, Clinical Practice Guideline* of the Agency for Health Care Policy and Research (AHCPR), and the 2000 U.S. Public Health Service (PHS) update, recommended that tobacco use be treated as a vital sign with no differential treatment guidelines by gender, except for treatment during pregnancy (Fiore et al. 1996, 2000). The PHS guideline states, "Many women are motivated to quit during pregnancy, and health care professionals can take advantage of this motivation by reinforcing the knowledge that cessation will reduce health risks to the fetus and that there are postpartum benefits for both the mother and the child" (Fiore et al. 2000, p. 93). It goes on to state, "Postpartum relapse may be decreased by continued emphasis on the relationship between maternal smoking and poor health outcomes in infants and children" (Fiore et al. 2000, p. 93). Findings from the Lung Health Study suggested that women with smoking-related disease may benefit from specific treatment (Bjornson et al. 1995); however, few minimal clinical interventions have been designed for women smokers in high-risk medical groups, such as women who use oral contraceptives or those with diabetes, heart disease, smoking-related cancer, osteoporosis, obesity, eating disorder, depression, or chemical dependence (Fisher et al. 1990a; Gritz et al. 1993).

**Intensive Clinical Interventions**

Intensive clinical interventions involve individual or group treatment in multiple sessions. The most successful treatments have been multicomponent cognitive-behavioral programs that incorporate strategies to prepare and motivate smokers to stop smoking (USDHHS 1988, 1989; Lando 1993; Fiore et al. 1996, 2000). Effective strategies vary in their long-term efficacy, from 14.4 percent for social support delivered in the clinical setting to 19.9 percent for rapid smoking, an aversive conditioning technique (Fiore et al. 1996, 2000).

Women are somewhat more likely than men to use intensive treatment programs (Fiore et al. 1990; Yankelovich Partners 1998). Similarly, women have a stronger interest than men in smoking cessation groups that offer mutual support through a buddy system and in treatment meetings over a long period (Lando et al. 1991). A few studies of formal treatment have examined interactions between treatment and gender. Flaxman (1978) found that women fared better with a delayed date to stop smoking than with immediate cessation, whereas the reverse was true among men. Curry and colleagues (1988) compared two theoretical approaches to smoking cessation: a traditional treatment program that emphasized absolute abstinence, enforced with a contingency contract that required those who smoked after their smoking cessation date to send a check for at least $15 to an organization or person they disliked, and a relapse prevention program that focused on the gradual acquisition of skills needed to abstain from smoking. Men had greater success with absolute abstinence and contingency contracting, whereas women were more successful in the relapse prevention program. In a small pilot study, Weissman and colleagues (1987) reported similar findings among adolescent smokers. The majority of the boys who took part in a program awarding money for achieving target (nonsmoking) levels of carbon monoxide stopped smoking, but all the girls who were enrolled dropped out and were unsuccessful. These results agreed with other evidence that women prefer a more gradual approach to smoking cessation (Sorensen and Pechacek 1987; Blake et al. 1989; Lando et al. 1991).

**Pharmacologic Adjuncts**

Pharmacologic approaches to smoking cessation raise a number of issues specific to women (Pomerleau 1996). As outlined in detail in the Surgeon General's report *Reducing Tobacco Use* (USDHHS 2000) and confirmed by the AHCPR and PHS cessation guidelines (Fiore et al. 1996, 2000), a number of effective and promising pharmacotherapies for nicotine addiction have emerged in the past decade: nicotine gum (polacrilex), transdermal nicotine patches, nicotine nasal spray, and oral nicotine inhalers (Hughes 1993; Henningfield 1995; Fiore et al. 1996, 2000; Hughes et al. 1999). Nicotine gum and the patch are approved for over-the-counter use (Hughes et al. 1999). Bupropion, a nonnicotine pharmaceutical, showed success in smoking cessation and was approved by the U.S. Food and Drug Administration (FDA) for smoking cessation (Ferry et al. 1992; Ferris and Cooper 1993; Hurt et al. 1997; Jorenby et al. 1999) (see also "Depression" later in this chapter). Two other formulations, clonidine and the antidepressant nortriptyline, have been recommended as second-line pharmacotherapies, but have not yet been approved by the FDA specifically for this purpose (Fiore et al. 2000). Anxiolytics, benzodiazepines, other antidepressants, beta-blockers, silver acetate, and mecamylamine have been studied but are not recommended for tobacco use treatment (Fiore et al. 2000).

Nicotine gum and patches are the best-studied nicotine replacement medications. Surgeon General's reports on smoking and health (USDHHS 1988, 1989, 2000) and several meta-analyses and reviews have concluded that nicotine gum boosts smoking cessation in minimal contact and intensive treatment programs by as much as 50 to 100 percent (Lam et al. 1987; Cepeda-Benito 1993; Hughes 1993; Tang et al. 1994; Fiore et al. 1996, 2000). Use of the gum alone or with brief medical interventions is beneficial (Fiore et al. 1996, 2000), but the gum probably works best with counseling to guide in proper use and chewing technique (Hughes 1993, 1995). Transdermal nicotine patches are easier to use than nicotine gum, cause fewer side effects that might disrupt appropriate use, and result in higher blood levels of nicotine and more stable replacement of nicotine (Killen et al. 1990b; Fiore et al. 1992; Hughes 1993). Moreover, dosing and weaning schedules are better defined and easier to follow with the patch (Fiore et al. 1992; Henningfield 1995). Both nicotine gum and nicotine patches have been found to reduce withdrawal discomfort after smoking is stopped. Some data suggested that nicotine gum (Killen et al. 1990b; Hatsukami et al. 1995; Perkins 1999) and the nicotine patch (Perkins 1996; Wetter et al. 1999a) may be less effective among women than among men, but other research has not reported differences by gender in their effectiveness (Hughes 1993; Fiore et al. 1994; Jorenby et al. 1995). Nevertheless, nicotine replacement has been shown to have value over placebo among women smokers and thus remains recommended for use (Fiore et al. 2000).

On average, women smoke less than do men, but some studies suggested women are more dependent on nicotine than are men smokers. Women's lower body weight and possibly greater sensitivity to nicotine have been proposed to explain comparable levels of repeated samples of plasma nicotine (Grunberg et al. 1991; Pomerleau et al. 1991a). Other studies reported no gender difference in nicotine dependency after adjustment for the intensity of smoking (Gunn 1986; Svikis et al. 1986; Pirie et al. 1991). Perkins and colleagues (1999) noted that women smokers are less dependent on nicotine than are men and suggested that women's smoking is reinforced by factors other than nicotine. Data from the 1991–1992 National Household Survey on Drug Abuse showed that 81 percent of younger female smokers (aged 12 through 24 years) and 79 percent of older female smokers (aged $\geq$ 25 years) rated themselves as addicted to tobacco on at least one of four different indices of nicotine addiction, including an inability to cut down on their smoking (CDC 1995a). (See "Nicotine Dependence Among Women and Girls" in Chapter 2 for more data on indicators of nicotine addiction.) The Lung Health Study suggested that men smokers may be less aware than women smokers of nicotine dependence and nicotine deprivation or less willing to admit their dependence (Bjornson et al. 1995). Accordingly, women may be more likely to use nicotine replacement therapies (Fiore et al. 1990; Orleans et al. 1994b; Bjornson et al. 1995; Lando and Gritz 1996).

One intervention study of women found that transdermal nicotine replacement therapy or placebo nicotine replacement therapy was less effective in controlling objective withdrawal symptoms among women than among men (Wetter et al. 1999b). However, self-reports of withdrawal symptoms did not reveal any gender-specific differences.

Other evidence suggested that women remember their withdrawal symptoms as being more severe than do men (Pomerleau et al. 1994b). In a randomized trial of women and men smokers, participants were asked to rate withdrawal symptoms during previous quit attempts and during a current quit attempt. Although no differences were observed between women and men for any current withdrawal symptoms reported, three of four retrospectively assessed withdrawal symptoms (irritability, difficulty concentrating, and increased appetite) were reported significantly more often among women than among men. Gritz and colleagues (1996), in a review of the withdrawal distress literature, noted that women are more likely to report withdrawal symptoms than are men when attempting cessation. They also noted that the relapse rate was higher among women who reported intense withdrawal symptoms than among those who reported fewer withdrawal symptoms. That pattern was not found among men.

Sussman and colleagues (1998a) found that adolescent females were more likely than adolescent males to report having difficulty going a day without smoking and to report relying on cigarettes to improve daily functioning. In another study, physiologic differences between women and men who had recently stopped smoking and were exposed to cues to smoke were examined; women had a higher reactivity to cues than did men (Niaura et al. 1998). In a laboratory study that compared responses to smoking among women and men, Eissenberg and colleagues (1999) reported similar physiologic effects by gender but more sensitivity among women than men to some of the subjective effects of smoking.

Because of uncertainties over the safety of nicotine replacement during pregnancy, FDA has assigned a Pregnancy Category C warning to nicotine gum ("risk cannot be ruled out") and a Pregnancy Category D warning to transdermal nicotine ("positive evidence of risk") (Henningfield 1995). Hence, these aids are not routinely prescribed for pregnant or breastfeeding smokers. However, the benefits of nicotine replacement medication may outweigh the risks from smoking among pregnant and lactating mothers (Benowitz 1991; Oncken et al. 1996; Jorenby 1998). Caution is advised because nicotine itself poses risks to the fetus, including neurotoxicity (Slotkin 1998). Therefore, pregnant women should first be encouraged to quit without pharmacotherapy. However, nicotine replacement therapy may be indicated for pregnant women who are unable to quit smoking. If used, doses should be delivered at the lowest effective range, blood levels of nicotine should be monitored, and an intermittent delivery system (such as gum) should be used. More research is needed to determine the effects of nicotine replacement therapy among pregnant women and women using oral contraceptives or estrogen replacement therapy (Pomerleau et al. 1991a).

The action of bupropion (Zyban) is not well understood. Smokers who plan to stop smoking start treatment with bupropion at least 1 week before cessation and take the drug for up to 12 weeks (Hughes et al. 1999). Like nicotine replacement therapy, bupropion doubles smoking cessation rates compared with placebo alone, and one study suggested that a combination of bupropion and the nicotine patch produced cessation rates higher than did either treatment alone (Jorenby et al. 1999). Bupropion works well among smokers with or without a history of depression (see "Depression" later in this chapter), which suggested that its antidepressant effect does not account for its success in smoking cessation. No studies have been published in which the gender-specific effects of bupropion were examined.

Other pharmacologic adjuncts for treatment of tobacco dependence include therapies to block the reinforcing actions of nicotine (e.g., mecamylamine), nonspecific pharmacotherapies aimed at lowering cessation-related stress or depression (e.g., anxiolytics and antidepressants), and therapies for tobacco withdrawal symptoms (e.g., clonidine) (Jarvik and Henningfield 1993; Henningfield 1995; USDHHS 2000). Except for one antidepressant (nortriptyline) and clonidine (Hurt et al. 1997; Hall et al. 1998; Fiore et al. 2000), these approaches have not yet been established as effective adjuncts to standard behavioral treatments. Gender differences have not been examined.

### Population-Based Interventions

A number of population-based intervention programs have been developed and tested. Such programs focus on involving an entire population or subgroup of the population in intervention activities. Worksite programs, for example, seek to involve all worksite smokers in cessation activities, and evaluation is based on the entire worksite population (see "Worksite Programs to Reduce Smoking Among Women" later in this chapter). Interventions in religious organizations use the religious community to foster smoking cessation (see "Minority Women" later in this chapter). Community intervention programs such as the Community Intervention Trial for Smoking Cessation (COMMIT) seek to provide constant, inescapable messages about the value of smoking cessation (see "Community-Based Efforts to Reduce Smoking Among Women" later in this chapter). Telephone quit lines provide intensive counseling in a format that is easily accessible by smokers. Unlike many of the individual-oriented approaches discussed in this background section, population-based approaches are still somewhat immature. Generalization between programs and between venues is difficult. Nevertheless, as later sections of this chapter show, some promise exists for such population-based approaches for smoking cessation.

# Smoking Cessation Issues Unique Among Women

Recent studies have identified numerous gender-related factors and mechanisms that should be studied as predictors of smoking cessation, as well as risk factors for continued smoking or relapse. These factors include issues that are of unique concern among women, such as hormonal influences and pregnancy, as well as barriers to cessation, such as fear of weight gain, lack of social support, and depression. Future research must take into account the entire biopsychosocial domain of factors important in women's smoking and smoking cessation.

## Hormonal Influences

Women's lives are biologically punctuated by menarche and menopause, by the monthly cycle of ovulation and bleeding, and by pregnancy and childbirth. These events are accompanied by striking hormonal changes and fluctuations. Many women use exogenous hormones to control their fertility and to modulate the effects of menopause. Furthermore, a minority of women engage in abnormal eating and dieting practices that profoundly dysregulate hormonal patterns (Hetherington and Burnett 1994).

Because nicotine is known to alter mood, cognitive function, and performance, nicotine intake and effects, withdrawal symptoms, and the ability to stop smoking and stay abstinent may all reasonably vary in response to hormonal fluctuations that also affect mood, cognitive function, and performance. For this reason, looking at women as a single group may obscure differences in women's smoking across the life cycle.

Studies of hormonal influences on smoking are relatively new. Whether nicotine intake varies according to phase of menstrual cycle is unclear; some studies have found no difference by menstrual phase (Pomerleau et al. 1994a; Allen et al. 1996), others have found increased smoking during the premenstruum (Steinberg and Chereck 1989), and others have noted decreased smoking during ovulation (DeBon et al. 1995). Studies that examined the menstrual cycle and effects on smoking withdrawal symptoms are more consistent. On the basis of a small number of studies, women, including those with premenstrual dysphoric disorder, appear to do better in quitting during the luteal phase than in the follicular phase, and withdrawal symptoms appear to be less intense during the luteal phase (O'Hara et al. 1989; Perkins et al. 2000). The effects of hormone replacement therapy (HRT) on smoking are still being investigated.

### Smoking and Menstrual Cycle

To date, most studies of the endocrine effects on nicotine addiction and withdrawal have focused on the female smoker with regular menstrual cycles. Important questions about the possible mediating role of menstrual phase-related changes in energy regulation, appetite, and weight; depression; and vulnerability or resistance to stress among smokers remain largely unexplored.

*Nicotine Intake During Menstrual Cycle*

Studies of the effects of menstrual phase on smoking have been conducted, under both field and laboratory conditions, and have produced conflicting results. Two investigations conducted under field conditions showed smoking, as measured by number of cigarettes smoked, to be highly stable across the phases of the menstrual cycle (Pomerleau et al. 1994a; Allen et al. 1996); in another study, one-third of the women showed decreased smoking on the day of ovulation (DeBon et al. 1995).

Laboratory studies are less representative of actual smoking than field studies. The laboratory studies conducted to date tend to complicate rather than resolve the issue of nicotine intake during the menstrual cycle. Mello and colleagues (1987) studied women in an inpatient setting for 21 days and reported increased smoking during the premenstruum among 70 percent of participants. In a laboratory study, however, Steinberg and Cherek (1989) found an increase in the number of puffs, total puff duration, or both per session during menses compared with the premenstruum and with all other days combined, with no further phase-related distinctions. Pomerleau and colleagues (1992) conducted a laboratory study in which they measured increments in plasma levels of nicotine after participants smoked a single cigarette, in the context of smoking ad libitum. They found a trend toward increased nicotine intake in the mid-to-late follicular phase.

An interesting finding by Allen and colleagues (1996) is that despite the lack of phase-related differences in nicotine intake during the phases of the menstrual cycle, as evidenced by the record of smoking, 58 percent of the participants believed that they smoked more before menses and only 3 percent believed that they smoked less. Such perceptions may play an important role in planning cessation attempts. Furthermore, to the extent that such expectancies contribute to resistance to treatment, investigations that address this cognitive error may enhance the efficacy of strategies to prevent relapse.

Some of the inconsistencies regarding findings around nicotine intake during the menstrual cycle may be attributable to design limitations, discrepancies in methods and definition of the phases, differences in sample selection, or failure to control for psychopathology. Although more rigorously controlled studies may eventually introduce order into the current confusing picture, it is reasonably safe to conclude that if phase-related differences in smoking exist among smokers with no psychopathology, they are small and subtle (Pomerleau et al. 1994a). Studies of smoking and the menstrual cycle fall short of the exacting standards recommended. Future studies should include biological verification of menstrual phase and testing over two months or more because of high intercycle variability for many parameters, which may be even greater among smokers than among nonsmokers (Halbreich and Endicott 1985; American Psychiatric Association [APA] 1994; Hornsby et al. 1998; Windham et al. 1999).

*Effects of Menstrual Cycle Phase on Tolerance and Sensitivity to Nicotine*

Masson (1995) studied cardiovascular effects of controlled doses of nicotine or tobacco smoke as well as acute tolerance (reduced response to a subsequent administration of the same dose) and found no differences among normally menstruating smokers as a function of menstrual phase. Because the primary focus of the study was on users of oral contraceptives, participants were tested during menses and during the premenstruum but not at midcycle. A more recent study (Marks et al. 1999), in which women were tested in four hormonally verified menstrual phases, also showed no significant differences in menstrual phase for physiologic, biochemical, or subjective response to administration of a fixed dose of nicotine. These findings suggested that differential sensitivity to nicotine on the basis of phase is not likely to complicate attempts to stop smoking.

*Withdrawal and Abstinence Symptoms During Menstrual Cycle*

Although the effects of menstrual phase on actual smoking are negligible, the evidence for effects on withdrawal symptoms has been somewhat more convincing. O'Hara and colleagues (1989) examined withdrawal symptoms among persons who stopped smoking and found that women who stopped during the luteal phase rated their withdrawal symptoms significantly higher than did those who stopped during the follicular phase. In the group overall, highly significant correlations were found between withdrawal scores and ratings of menstrual distress. Although this study used a relatively crude definition of phase, designating the 15 days before onset of bleeding as "luteal" and the remainder of the cycle as "follicular," a subsequent laboratory study replicated this finding (Pomerleau et al. 1992). Similarly, on the basis of a larger study, Perkins and colleagues (2000) found that the 37 women who quit smoking during the luteal phase were significantly more likely than the 41 women who quit during the follicular phase to experience withdrawal symptoms and to self-report depressive symptoms during their quit week. No differences were observed between the groups during the two-week pre-quit baseline.

Allen and colleagues (1999) failed to detect phase-related differences in withdrawal symptoms. The setting of this study was an inpatient unit, which may have lessened the impact of environmental cues for the withdrawal symptoms. In a study of 166 women smokers who had no history of psychiatric disorders and who reported negative experiences during previous smoking cessation attempts, women with depressive mood as a withdrawal symptom were significantly more likely than women without depressive mood to report changes in mood related to menstrual phase (Pomerleau and Pomerleau 1994). These findings raised the possibility that a history of depressive mood as a withdrawal symptom constitutes a risk factor for menstrual phase-related problems during smoking cessation (see "Depression" later in this chapter).

Withdrawal has also been assessed under conditions of smoking ad libitum (spontaneous, discretionary smoking). One study (Allen et al. 1996) found evidence of withdrawal symptoms peaking in the premenstruum, but at least two other studies showed that withdrawal and menstrual symptoms, although elevated in the premenstruum, are even higher during menses (Pomerleau et al. 1992; DeBon et al. 1995). Until knowledge of smoking during the menstrual cycle is further refined, it is probably most useful to think of the perimenstrual period, including actual bleeding days and the days before the onset of bleeding, as the critical time for exacerbation of withdrawal symptoms.

Beside studies of standard measures of nicotine withdrawal, at least three studies have investigated the possibility that menstrual phase, alone and in interaction with smoking abstinence, affects other potentially relevant variables of behavior. Eck and colleagues (1997) compared food intake and weight changes among women smokers randomly assigned to smoking cessation for 10 days during either the follicular phase or the luteal phase. Food intake increased among both groups of participants during smoking cessation but was unaffected by phase. Weight, however, increased by 1.8 kg in the luteal phase group but remained stable in the follicular phase group. Pomerleau and colleagues (1994c) administered a battery of tests of motor performance (e.g., finger tapping) and of focused attention to women smokers during menses and during the midluteal phase, under conditions of smoking or overnight abstinence. To evaluate focused attention, the Stroop test was used to examine the ability to remember discordant information about the written name of a color and the color in which the name is written. On the basis of findings in the literature, the investigators hypothesized that superior performance would be seen during the midluteal phase, as observed by Hampson and Kimura (1988). Although the expected performance decrement on the Stroop test was observed after overnight abstinence from smoking, neither menstrual phase nor interaction effects emerged. This finding raised the possibility that the antiestrogenic effects of smoking (Michnovicz et al. 1986; Baron et al. 1990) may attenuate the phase-related differences in performance observed by Hampson and Kimura (1988).

*Effects of Menstrual Cycle Phase on Ability to Stop Smoking and Likelihood of Relapse*

Although often assumed, the link between the withdrawal experience and the ability to achieve and maintain abstinence from smoking has not been unequivocally established (Hughes and Hatsukami 1986; Kenford et al. 1994). Little is known about whether heightened symptoms in the premenstruum increase the difficulty of maintaining smoking cessation during this time. One study found that women in the premenstrual phase were significantly less successful than either women at midcycle or men in maintaining abstinence for two consecutive days (Craig et al. 1992). Klesges (unpublished data, 1994; see review by Gritz et al. 1996) found that among women who were paid $150 to stop smoking, 70 percent of those randomly assigned to stop smoking in the follicular phase but only 52 percent in the luteal phase were successful. Duration of abstinence was not reported. Moreover, among women who attempted to stop in the luteal phase, those who succeeded had lower baseline levels of premenstrual distress than those who did not succeed. Other studies, however, found that women were most likely to relapse to smoking during menses, regardless of the phase of the menstrual cycle in which they stopped smoking (Frye et al. 1992; Perkins et al. 2000). Thus, whether women should time smoking cessation attempts so that they do not coincide with the perimenstrual phase is unclear (O'Hara et al. 1989; Perkins et al.

2000). More data on outcome are needed before it can be concluded that starting a cessation attempt during the perimenstruum truly compromises chances of success. Moreover, the value of timing a cessation attempt to avoid the perimenstruum may vary because of individual biological variation in the experience of perimenstrual symptoms.

It has been proposed that endocrine dysregulation induced by smoking and the attendant discomfort might help motivate women to stop smoking (Jensen and Coambs 1994; Charlton and While 1996). Reported effects of smoking that suggested dysregulation of the hypothalamic-pituitary axis include dysmenorrhea among adolescents (Procopé and Timonen 1971; Jensen and Coambs 1994) and among adults (Wood et al. 1979; Sloss and Frerichs 1983; Brown et al. 1988; Hornsby et al. 1998), nausea and vomiting during pregnancy (Gulick et al. 1989), and perimenopausal symptoms, including "hot flashes" (Greenberg et al. 1987; Shaw 1997). Some of these studies relied on retrospective rather than prospective data, and inconsistencies in the literature (e.g., Andersch and Milsom 1982; Gannon et al. 1987) suggested the need for further research. If increased endocrine-related discomfort among women smokers is confirmed, this message should be part of educational efforts aimed at women.

*Premenstrual Dysphoric Disorder*

Premenstrual dysphoria is a cluster of transient psychological changes consisting of mood swings, anxiety, anger, and depression-like symptoms. Marks and colleagues (1994) examined data from smokers who met the criteria of the *Diagnostic and Statistical Manual of Mental Disorders,* third edition, revised, for late luteal phase dysphoric disorder (APA 1987), which was renamed premenstrual dysphoric disorder in the *Diagnostic and Statistical Manual of Mental Disorders,* fourth edition (APA 1994). These smokers were asked to keep daily diaries rating menstrual symptoms, smoking, and use of drugs other than nicotine. Significant increases in smoking were observed during menses, with lesser, nonsignificant elevations during the premenstrual phase.

A limitation of the study by Marks and colleagues (1994) was that reports of amount of smoking were collected once at the end of the day by using a relational Likert-type scale rather than a quantitative measure. Moreover, the actual magnitude of the differences in nicotine intake could not be determined and may be quite small in clinical terms. If the findings of this study are confirmed, however, they may point to strategies that may be particularly helpful among women with premenstrual dysphoria who smoke. For example, severely affected persons may be told that the chances of success may be enhanced by properly timed dietary, pharmacologic, and behavioral interventions (Gonsalves et al. 1991).

Comorbidity of premenstrual dysphoric disorder and depression is considerable (Endicott and Halbreich 1988), and the dysphoric disorder may constitute a subtype of depression (Marks 1992). In view of the well-documented association between depression and smoking (Glassman et al. 1990; Glassman 1993; Kendler et al. 1993) (see "Depression and Other Psychiatric Disorders" in Chapter 3), smoking among women with other forms of depression may also be keyed to the menstrual phase. Among women with a history of depression, the possible role of menstrual phase in precipitating relapse to smoking or depressive episodes after smoking cessation (Covey et al. 1990; Glassman 1993; Dalack et al. 1995) deserves consideration. If this association proves to be valid, recommendations to begin cessation attempts during the follicular phase also may be applicable to women with a history of depression.

**Effects of Oral Contraceptives**

In 1982–1988, nearly one-fourth of users of oral contraceptives were smokers (Barrett et al. 1994). Cardiovascular responses of oral contraceptive users (Emmons and Weidner 1988; Davis and Matthews 1990) suggested that oral contraceptive use may enhance the reactivity of blood pressure, though not heart rate, to cognitive stress but that its use does not affect reactivity to nicotine. Another study of oral contraceptive users and nonusers, on the other hand, found that the users had larger nicotine-induced increases in heart rate than did nonusers (Masson 1995). These studies suggested differential endocrine-mediated sympathetic activation by nicotine. Masson further observed that oral contraceptive use attenuated the reductions in anxiety after smoking among women who menstruated regularly. Lack of random assignment to oral contraceptive use or nonuse, however, complicates interpretation of all these findings, because self-selection into either category may be associated with personality differences that would also affect reactivity or anxiety. Moreover, a consensus panel recently reviewed the evidence on the health effects of oral contraceptive use and smoking and recommended that women older than 35 years who smoke more than 15 cigarettes per day should not be using oral contraceptives (Schiff et al. 1999).

Furthermore, to minimize as much as possible the risks for stroke and acute myocardial infarction, the panel suggested that oral contraceptives containing very low doses of ethinyl estradiol be given to smokers, especially women smokers older than 35 years of age.

**Effects of Menopause and Aging on Smoking**

Most, although not all, studies have shown an earlier age at menopause among women who smoke (see "Menstrual Function, Menopause, and Benign Gynecologic Conditions" in Chapter 3). Menopause, on the other hand, may be an obstacle to stopping smoking. Using data collected in Great Britain, Jarvis (1994) argued that although the percentage of persons who have ever smoked and who became former smokers was higher among men than among women, the difference was accounted for almost entirely by differences in the age distribution in the population that had stopped smoking. For ages 16 through 42 years, the relative risk (RR) for smoking cessation was higher among women than among men. Among women and men aged 43 through 50 years, the RR was about equal, and at ages 51 through 57 years, the RR among women compared with men dropped dramatically, rising somewhat at ages 58 through 64 years and at 65 through 70 years and still further at ages 71 years or older, but not reaching equality. The differences were attenuated slightly by adjustment for sociodemographic variables. However, other investigators have suggested that these findings are a "cohort effect" related to historical gender-specific differences in smoking prevalence and quitting (see "Current Prevalence of Smoking" in Chapter 2).

The effect of HRT may be related to menopausal effects on smoking cessation. Greenberg and colleagues (1987) found an excess of smokers among new HRT users and, among smokers, a relationship between the number of cigarettes smoked and the likelihood of HRT use. Because HRT is often prescribed for the symptoms of menopause, the authors speculated that smoking may initiate or aggravate the symptoms for which HRT is prescribed but conceded that several alternative explanations were possible. Possible alternatives include the effect of weight, affect, osteoporosis, SES, and family on the likelihood that HRT will be prescribed; all of these factors also influence or are influenced by smoking (Matthews et al. 1990). Thus, it seems unlikely that this question can be resolved without studies that include random assignment to receive HRT or placebo.

The Women's Health Initiative is a long-term study that will provide opportunities to address these questions. This study has collected and continues to collect information on ever smoking, current smoking, age at smoking initiation, amount smoked, and other smoking-related variables that can be correlated with the study arm to which women are randomly assigned. The arms include HRT in various formulations (e.g., estrogen alone or estrogen and progestin) versus placebo, offering the opportunity to understand the role of HRT in smoking (Women's Health Initiative Protocol for Clinical Trial and Observational Study Components 1998).

## Pregnancy

The first published report (Baric et al. 1976) of a smoking cessation program for pregnant women appeared in 1976, 19 years after the first epidemiologic study that linked maternal cigarette smoking and low birth weight (Simpson 1957). The intervention, which consisted of brief advice from a physician to stop smoking, increased self-reported smoking cessation. Since then, numerous intervention trials conducted in diverse populations of pregnant women have been reported; generally, a positive treatment effect is seen (Ershoff et al. 1989; Windsor et al. 1993b; Secker-Walker et al. 1995). The majority of pregnant women (up to 67 percent at 12 months after delivery) begin smoking again after delivery (Sexton et al. 1987; Fingerhut et al. 1990; McBride and Pirie 1990; Mullen et al. 1990; McBride et al. 1992). This finding indicated a need for further research to reduce postpartum relapse.

Previous reviewers who used qualitative and quantitative methods and varying criteria for choosing studies have concluded that prenatal smoking cessation programs are effective (Lumley and Astbury 1989; Mullen 1990; Floyd et al. 1993; Ockene 1993; Dolan-Mullen et al. 1994; O'Campo et al. 1995; Fiore et al. 1996; Windsor et al. 1998). The AHCPR Smoking Cessation Clinical Practice Guideline Panel (Fiore et al. 1996) used its own meta-analysis and a previous meta-analysis (Dolan-Mullen et al. 1994) and concluded that compared with no interventions, intervention during pregnancy increases smoking cessation. A PHS update of the cessation guideline meta-analysis (Fiore et al. 2000) indicated that extended or augmented psychosocial interventions that exceeded minimal physician advice to quit smoking nearly tripled cessation rates among pregnant women.

### Smoking Cessation

For this review, studies published in English were identified through bibliographies in reviews of the literature, by experts, and in online databases. Trials were excluded unless they were randomized, controlled trials published between 1976 and 1998 and had biochemically confirmed abstinence. The strong "demand" for pregnant women to "not smoke" may compromise the validity of self-report. For example, two trials found high percentages of deception (28 and 35 percent) in late pregnancy (Windsor et al. 1993b; Kendrick et al. 1995) and differential deception between treatment groups (32 vs. 17 percent) and control groups (49 vs. 32 percent).

Multivariate analyses of the effect of participants' baseline characteristics on smoking during late pregnancy were conducted in two trials. Findings from the two studies that used relatively intensive treatment and produced a large overall effect suggested that women who had experienced problems during pregnancy (e.g., vomiting or high blood pressure) had lower saliva levels of thiocyanate in their eighth month, indicating a lower level of smoking (Hebel et al. 1985; Ershoff et al. 1989). Such problems may have increased the women's sense of susceptibility to health effects and may have increased their motivation to stop smoking. Women with more education also had lower levels of thiocyanate during pregnancy. Indicators of higher levels of smoking before and early in pregnancy were related to higher eight-month thiocyanate levels.

Windsor and colleagues (1993b) examined smoking cessation among African American women and among low-income women by using univariate tests. Cessation was significantly higher among African American women in treatment groups than in control groups (18.1 vs. 10.7 percent; $p = 0.03$) and was lower but not significantly different among white women in treatment groups than in control groups (5.2 vs. 10.0 percent; $p = 0.08$). A separate analysis of a subsample, with baseline measures of cotinine level, revealed that virtually all women who stopped smoking were those whose saliva samples contained less than 100 ng of cotinine/mL at the first prenatal visit. Thus, the major effect of programs tested to date appears to be among lighter smokers. This finding was replicated in subsequent studies (Hartmann et al. 1996; Woodby et al. 1999).

Estimates of overall effectiveness of cessation programs for pregnant women may underrepresent the impact of these programs. On the basis of a study with multiple validated measures beginning in the 20th week of pregnancy (Ershoff et al. 1989), the difference between treatment and control groups appeared larger in the second trimester (RR, 2.6) than in the eighth and ninth months (RR, 1.5). Although some relapse occurred among women in the treatment group, the chief reason for the smaller difference in the eighth and ninth months was late smoking cessation in the control group. Thus, one effect of intervention may be to advance cessation that might have occurred later in the pregnancy.

In four trials that reported biochemically verified measures (Sexton and Hebel 1984; Windsor et al. 1985, 1993a; Secker-Walker et al. 1994; Hartmann et al. 1996), the number of cigarettes smoked in the eighth and ninth months of pregnancy was significantly reduced. Evidence has shown that reduction confers some protection for the fetus, whether the reduction is defined as a change in mean level of thiocyanate in the treatment group (Hebel et al. 1988) or as a decrease in cotinine level of 50 percent or more from baseline (Li et al. 1993). Hebel and colleagues (1988), however, found that the benefit was almost entirely restricted to those who achieved total abstinence, were smoking less than one cigarette per day, or were smoking one to five cigarettes per day at eight months' gestation.

### Preventing Relapse Before Delivery

In 1990, Fingerhut and coworkers (1990) reported that across studies, approximately one-fourth of pregnant smokers had stopped smoking before their first prenatal visit. Published estimates have ranged from 15 percent in a largely African American public maternity clinic population (Windsor et al. 1993b) to 42 percent in a primarily white HMO population (Petersen et al. 1992). Although the majority of these "spontaneous quitters" remained free of smoking throughout pregnancy, as many as 33 percent relapsed before delivery, as evidenced by biochemical confirmation in a population receiving no intervention (Lowe et al. 1997).

To date, five randomized trials with biochemical confirmation of nonsmoking in late pregnancy have tested interventions to prevent relapse among persons who had stopped spontaneously. The RRs were all close to 1.0 and were not significant.

Several of these trials have produced a profile of women at high risk for relapse. The risk factors include stopping smoking only within one or two weeks of beginning prenatal care as opposed to earlier, having low confidence in maintaining cessation, being younger, being a heavier smoker before pregnancy, experiencing less nausea during pregnancy, and having previous children (Quinn et al. 1991; Secker-Walker et al. 1995).

### Effectiveness in Improving Birth Outcomes and Associated Economic Benefits

Four studies of whether an intervention during pregnancy increases smoking cessation also evaluated the effect of the cessation intervention on birth outcomes. Although three studies found a lower risk for low birth weight associated with intervention (Sexton and Hebel 1984; Ershoff et al. 1990; Hjalmarson et al. 1991), none of the findings was statistically significant. A fourth study (Secker-Walker et al. 1994) found no lower risks, but it also found no effect of the intervention on smoking cessation. The only study to evaluate the effect of a prenatal smoking cessation program on interuterine growth retardation (Ershoff et al. 1990) found a protective effect that was of borderline statistical significance (RR, 0.2; 95 percent confidence interval [CI], 0.0 to 1.1). Although evaluation of individual cessation programs has not shown a statistically significant reduction in birth outcomes, the relationship between maternal cessation and reduction in low birth weight has been well documented (USDHHS 1990).

The economic benefits of smoking cessation during pregnancy have been estimated in relation to birth outcomes. One analysis, based on a RR of 2.6 for sustained cessation beginning by the 20th week of pregnancy (Ershoff et al. 1989), found a benefit-to-cost ratio of 3:1 (a savings of $300 in costs for the neonates' initial hospital episode for every $100 spent on smoking cessation) (Ershoff et al. 1990). A second analysis was based on a RR of 1.7 for smoking cessation, hospital and physician costs at birth, rehospitalization costs in the first year of life, and long-term health care costs, as estimated by the Office of Technology Assessment (Windsor et al. 1993b). In this analysis, the low estimate of the benefit-to-cost ratio was 18:1, and the high estimate was 46:1. A more recent simulation analysis estimated savings that would derive from reductions in the number of low birth weight babies in the United States if smoking prevalence were reduced before or during the first trimester of pregnancy. It found that an annual decline in smoking prevalence of one percentage point would prevent 1,300 low birth weight babies and save $21 million (in 1995 dollars) in direct medical costs in the first year alone (Lightwood et al. 1999). These analyses suggested that prenatal smoking cessation interventions can provide short-term economic benefit to the sponsoring health care provider.

### Postpartum Smoking

Despite successful abstinence for 5 months or more, many women who stop smoking during pregnancy return to smoking within 6 months after the birth. Postpartum relapse has been reported at 32 to 54 percent at six weeks after delivery (Ershoff et al. 1983; Mullen et al. 1990), 45 percent at 3 months (Sexton et al. 1987), 56 to 65 percent at 6 months (Fingerhut et al. 1990; McBride and Pirie 1990; Mullen et al. 1990; McBride et al. 1992), and 67 percent at 12 months (Fingerhut et al. 1990). Most of these studies confirmed cessation biochemically at least once during pregnancy (Ershoff et al. 1983; Sexton et al. 1987; Mullen et al. 1990; McBride et al. 1992).

Conversion of a greater proportion of prenatal abstainers to long-term abstainers is needed. In a test of different ways to prevent women who had abstained from smoking during pregnancy from taking up smoking again in postpartum, 897 pregnant women from two HMOs were enrolled in a study (McBride et al. 1999). Participants received one of three interventions: self-help booklets only, booklet plus prepartum intervention, or booklet plus prepartum and postpartum intervention. All interventions were delivered by mail and telephone. Relapse to smoking at eight weeks postpartum was slightly lower, though not significantly so, among women in the prepartum group (33 percent) and the postpartum group (35 percent) than among women in the self-help booklet only group (44 percent, $p = 0.09$). Among women who received the postpartum intervention, rate of relapse to smoking was slower; however, at 12 months postpartum the three groups had the same rate of abstinence from smoking. Similarly, little success in long-term abstinence has been reported from cessation programs for mothers of young children (Greenberg et al. 1994; Wall et al. 1995). Wall and colleagues (1995), however, reported that a pediatrician-based program increased self-reported continued abstinence at 6 months after delivery among women who had stopped smoking during pregnancy.

Predictors of postpartum relapse may provide clues for developing smoking cessation programs. Some risk factors include having a partner who smokes, having friends who smoke, lack of confidence at midpregnancy regarding continued nonsmoking, and concern about weight (McBride and Pirie 1990; McBride et al. 1992; Severson et al. 1995; Mullen et al. 1997).

# Factors of Special Importance Among Women and to Smoking Cessation

## Weight Control

Smoking is related to body mass index (BMI), with smokers having lower BMI than do nonsmokers; this finding holds among both women and men (Rásky et al. 1996). Women are more likely than men to express concern about gaining weight when quitting smoking; however, few studies have found a relationship between weight concerns and smoking cessation among either women or men. Similarly, actual weight gain during cessation does not appear to predict relapse (Gritz et al. 1990; Killen et al. 1990a; Gourlay et al. 1994). Behavioral weight control programs have limited success in controlling weight gain during cessation, and generally no differences exist between women and men (Hall et al. 1992; Pirie et al. 1992). Exercise programs for weight control appear to have some benefit among women but have not been tested among men (Marcus et al. 1999). Pharmacologic approaches to weight control accompanying cessation include nicotine gum and bupropion. Such approaches appear to be useful as long as the quitter continues to take the drug; however, studies have indicated no difference in weight gain between treatment and control groups after the drug is withdrawn (Fiore et al. 2000). Other pharmacologic agents are only beginning to be explored.

Some smokers are concerned about gaining weight if they stop smoking. This concern is particularly common among women who smoke. In a survey of college students, Klesges and Klesges (1988) found that 39 percent of female students and 25 percent of male students reported that smoking was a dieting strategy. Among those who had attempted to stop smoking, 20 percent of female students and 7 percent of male students cited weight gain as the reason for relapse. Similarly, in a survey of young adults, Pirie and colleagues (1991) found the item "If I quit smoking, I would probably gain a lot of weight" to be endorsed by significantly more women who smoked (57.9 percent) than men who smoked (26.3 percent). Among current smokers who had attempted to stop smoking, weight gain was cited as a withdrawal symptom by 26.1 percent of women and 14.5 percent of men; among former smokers, it was cited by 29.5 percent of women and 19.2 percent of men.

In a prospective study of smokers identified in worksites, however, the belief that one would gain weight after smoking cessation was not related to participation in the cessation program (Klesges et al. 1988). Similarly, Jeffery and colleagues (1997) found no relationship between weight concerns and serious attempts to quit smoking. McGovern and colleagues (1994) found that women who participated in a cessation program weighed less than their smoking counterparts in the general population, which perhaps indicated that participants had less concern about weight. No difference in weight was observed between men smokers who participated in the program and those in the general population.

Smokers who are concerned about weight gain are thought to be less successful in smoking cessation treatment; this theory has been the focus of much research. Despite cross-sectional survey results indicating that weight gain is frequently cited as a reason for relapse (Klesges and Klesges 1988), prospective studies have had mixed results. In a study of 417 women, French and coworkers (1992) found that concern about weight was unrelated to successful smoking cessation. In a prospective study conducted at a worksite, dieting behaviors at baseline were found, in univariate analysis, to be unrelated to smoking cessation at the two-year follow-up; multivariate analyses showed that women smokers who had previously participated in weight loss programs, and who therefore were thought to be more concerned about weight, were more rather than less likely to stop smoking during the two years of follow-up (French et al. 1995). In a study of registered nurses in a smoking cessation program based at worksites (Gritz et al. 1990), neither weight gain during a previous cessation attempt nor fear of gaining weight as a deterrent in the past differentiated nurses who were abstinent at all follow-up points from nurses who were not continuously abstinent or from those who never stopped smoking. In a cohort of women and men smokers, Jeffery and colleagues (1997) found no relationship between weight concerns and smoking cessation. Furthermore, no differences were noted between women and men in concerns about weight or BMI and smoking outcomes. Gourlay and colleagues (1994) found a higher percentage of cessation at 26 weeks among those more concerned about weight gain at baseline. On the other hand, Klesges and colleagues (1988) reported that those who stopped smoking were less likely at baseline to believe that they would gain weight after cessation than were those who did not stop. Streater and colleagues (1989) found that persons successful in maintaining abstinence from smoking during a 12-week study had lower levels of concern about weight gain before the study than did study participants who relapsed during the trial, but this difference was not significant. In another study, women in a smoking cessation intervention who reported at baseline that they would resume smoking if they gained weight were more likely to have relapsed at all follow-up points (Meyers et al. 1997).

Actual weight gain during initial periods of abstinence from smoking has not been shown to be a predictor of relapse in prospective studies. Killen and colleagues (1990a), in a study of 630 women and 588 men, found no relationship overall between early weight gain and abstinence at the six-month follow-up. Hall and colleagues (1986), however, in a study of 133 women smokers and 122 men smokers, found that persons who gained more weight in the initial stages of abstinence were more likely to remain abstinent at longer term follow-ups than were those who gained less weight. A similar finding was reported by Gourlay and colleagues (1994) in a study of 823 women smokers and 658 men smokers. None of those studies found a gender difference in weight gain and abstinence. Persons who continue to abstain may abandon their concern about weight in favor of the "higher good" of cessation (Hall et al. 1986; Gritz et al. 1990). Nevertheless, the concern about weight gain has led researchers to devise strategies to control weight gain after smoking cessation, hypothesizing that these strategies will result in better smoking cessation outcomes.

### Behavioral Weight Management Programs

Two small intervention studies that combined behavioral weight control and smoking cessation interventions (Grinstead 1981; Mermelstein 1987) have been summarized in a previous report (USDHHS 1990). Neither of those programs succeeded in affecting smoking cessation, although one of them (Mermelstein 1987) succeeded in reducing weight gain after smoking cessation.

More recently, two large clinical trials tested the use of behavioral weight management programs as an adjunct to standard smoking cessation programs. Hall and colleagues (1992) reported on a trial that randomly assigned 131 female smokers and 49 male smokers to one of three groups: (1) an innovative intervention that combined a smoking cessation program with daily monitoring of weight and contingent caloric reduction, an individual exercise plan, and behavioral self-management principles; (2) a nonspecific weight control program oriented toward providing insight into eating styles through discussion groups, nutrition and exercise information, group support, and therapeutic attention; and (3) a standard treatment program consisting of an information packet on good nutrition and exercise. All three groups received a smoking cessation program that combined aversive smoking and relapse prevention skills training in seven sessions. Contrary to the hypothesis, the group receiving only the information packet had significantly better smoking cessation outcomes than did either of the active weight control groups. Validated seven-day abstinence rates were 35 percent in the standard treatment group, 22 percent in the nonspecific treatment group, and 21 percent in the innovative treatment group. At 52 weeks, participants who stopped smoking had gained 3.61, 3.35, and 0.86 kg, respectively. No differences were found by gender. The authors offered two possible explanations for their findings: either the complexity of weight control interventions detracted from simultaneous efforts to stop smoking, or the caloric reduction prescribed in the active weight treatment programs actually encouraged smoking. The second explanation is consistent with the literature on animal studies and the reinforcing value of psychoactive drugs under conditions of caloric deprivation (Perkins 1994).

In the largest trial to date using random assignment (Pirie et al. 1992), 417 women smokers were assigned to (1) a standard smoking cessation program (*Freedom From Smoking® for You and Your Family,* an American Lung Association program), (2) the standard program plus nicotine gum, (3) the standard program plus a behavioral weight management program, or (4) the standard program plus both nicotine gum and the behavioral weight management program. Both nicotine gum and the weight management program were hypothesized to have effects on controlling weight. The standard program plus nicotine gum produced significantly better smoking cessation outcomes (both point prevalence and continuous abstinence at one-year follow-up) than did the standard program alone. The standard program plus the weight management program did not produce better smoking cessation outcomes than did the standard program alone. When both weight management and nicotine gum were added to the standard program, the combination produced significantly poorer outcomes than did the standard treatment plus nicotine gum. Contrary to the hypothesis, no difference was noted in weight gain across treatments among persons who had abstained from smoking continuously for 12 months. The reasons for the lack of effectiveness of the weight control components are unclear. Compliance with aspects of the weight control programs, such as keeping food records, fell to low levels by the end of the intervention.

**Exercise Programs**

Exercise programs have been proposed as possible adjuncts to smoking cessation programs, in part because of their effects on weight control (Russell et al. 1988). A large observational study of U.S. nurses found that smoking cessation was associated with weight gain but that this relationship was diminished by spontaneous exercise, with a dose-response effect (Kawachi et al. 1996). Because calorie reduction may enhance the reinforcing value of smoking, exercise programs may be more successful than programs that focus on control of eating. Several reports have described exercise interventions in groups of women, but all these studies were small and short term. Russell and colleagues (1988) found no effect of the exercise intervention on either smoking cessation or weight outcomes in a study of 42 women randomly assigned to three treatment groups (exercise, general support, and a brief-contact control group).

Marcus and colleagues (1991) described an exercise intervention in a study of 20 women randomly assigned to one of two programs: 10 received a smoking cessation program only, and 10 received the smoking cessation program plus a supervised exercise program. At the end of treatment (4 weeks after smoking cessation), five of the exercise participants and none of the other participants were abstinent from smoking; the difference was significant. A second study controlled for the extra time exercise participants spent with counselors by having the nonexercise group spend an equal amount of time with health educators (Marcus et al. 1995). Twenty women were randomized to each of the two groups, but neither weight change nor smoking cessation was significantly different between groups. However, the exercise group had slightly higher rates of abstinence and lost a small amount of weight. A larger study (Marcus et al. 1999) randomly assigned 281 women smokers to a cognitive-behavioral program with exercise or the same program without exercise, but with equal contact time with staff. Compared with smokers in the control group, those in the exercise arm of the study had higher smoking cessation rates immediately after the program (19.4 vs. 10.2 percent; $p = 0.03$), at 3 months after the program (16.4 vs. 8.2 percent; $p = 0.03$), and at 12 months (11.9 vs. 5.4 percent; $p = 0.05$). Furthermore, the exercise group had gained less weight than the control group (3.1 vs. 5.4 kg; $p = 0.03$). To ascertain whether there are differential effects on weight gain among women compared with men, trials that include a weight management component should be conducted among women and men and results analyzed by gender.

**Pharmacologic Approaches in Relation to Weight Control**

Pharmacologic approaches hold some promise for controlling the weight gain that often accompanies smoking cessation. These approaches are less complex than behavioral weight management programs and can thus more easily be incorporated into smoking cessation programs.

*Nicotine Replacement*

Perhaps the most widely studied pharmacologic agent for weight control after smoking cessation is nicotine itself, which is generally thought to be the agent responsible for the effects of cigarette smoking on controlling weight. The effects of nicotine on smoking cessation and weight gain have been assessed through the use of various delivery systems: nicotine polacrilex gum, transdermal nicotine, nasal spray, and inhalers (see "Pharmacologic Adjuncts" earlier in this chapter).

Since the 1970s, the research literature has hinted that nicotine polacrilex gum may reduce the amount of weight gain after smoking cessation. In 1987, Fagerström (1987) reviewed the existing studies and noted that, in the five published studies that compared nicotine gum and placebo, the placebo users in each study gained slightly more weight or were slightly more likely to gain weight. In each of these studies, however, the effects were small and nonsignificant.

Research published since Fagerström's review has been divided on the issue of whether nicotine gum contributes to weight control after smoking cessation. In an observational analysis, Emont and Cummings (1987) found a significant inverse correlation between the dose of nicotine gum and weight gain among persons who smoked more than 26 cigarettes per day at baseline. In other observational analyses, long-term users of nicotine gum had gained significantly less weight at the one-year follow-up than had nonusers (3.1 vs. 5.2 kg) (Hajek et al. 1988; Killen et al. 1990a), and similar observations were made at the six-month follow-up (1.1 vs. 1.8 kg). Trials of nicotine polacrilex in which participants were randomly assigned to a condition, however, have reported mixed findings with respect to weight gain. In at least two trials with long-term follow-up, persons randomly assigned to receive nicotine gum did not gain less weight than those not receiving the gum (Hall et al. 1986; Pirie et al. 1992). In another trial in which participants were randomly assigned to different recommended dosages of nicotine gum (Gross et al. 1995), no relationship between treatment group and weight gain was found at 12 weeks after smoking cessation, but a significant inverse relationship was observed between weight gain and level of cotinine (a measure of actual exposure to nicotine). Leischow and colleagues (1992) reported a significant inverse dose-response effect on weight change among women but not among men in a trial in which participants were randomly assigned to placebo, 2-mg gum, or 4-mg gum, but follow-up was very short (4 weeks).

Several randomized trials found that nicotine gum delays, rather than prevents, weight gain after smoking cessation. Gross and coworkers (1989) reported significant differences in weight gain at 10 weeks of abstinence among smokers randomly assigned to receive either nicotine gum or placebo. By 3 months of abstinence, however, when most participants had discontinued gum use, the difference in weight was no longer significant. Nides and colleagues (1994) found an inverse relationship between the number of pieces of nicotine gum used per day and the percentage of baseline weight gained through 4 and 12 months among both women and men who had maintained abstinence from smoking. Participants who stopped using nicotine gum gained more weight than those who continued to use the gum. Doherty and colleagues (1996) reported that nicotine gum suppressed weight gain linearly with increasing nicotine dose and that smokers who substituted a greater portion of their baseline cotinine level with nicotine replacement gained less weight.

Much less information is available about the effects of other methods of nicotine delivery on weight control. Several studies found no weight control effects of the transdermal nicotine patch (Tønnesen et al. 1991; Transdermal Nicotine Study Group 1991) or a nicotine inhaler (Tønnesen et al. 1993) among persons who successfully stopped smoking by these methods. However, a study by Dale and associates (1998) of the nicotine patch reported that amount of weight gained was inversely related to the proportion of baseline cotinine level that was replaced by nicotine patches. However, the weight gain was delayed, not prevented. At the one-year follow-up, weight change was not associated with the total dose of transdermal nicotine used or the average proportion of cotinine replaced during treatment. Weight changes at one year were not associated with gender. In another study, weight gain was reduced among those who stopped smoking with the use of nicotine nasal spray (Sutherland et al. 1992), but no apparent lasting effect on weight was observed among those who discontinued the nasal spray. The explanation for these differences in effect on weight by nicotine delivered in various ways is unclear.

#### *Other Pharmacologic Agents*

Several other pharmacologic agents have been assessed for their effect on weight gain after smoking cessation. Pomerleau and colleagues (1991b) studied the effects of fluoxetine hydrochloride (Prozac), which had previously been observed to produce weight loss, possibly by reducing cravings for carbohydrate, in a group of participants who had stopped or stringently reduced smoking. Results were reported for 21 persons (14 women and 7 men); of these, 11 received placebo and 10 received the active drug (60 mg/day). Ten weeks after the smoking cessation date, significantly more weight gain was reported by the placebo group than by the fluoxetine hydrochloride group (3.3 vs. -0.6 kg). Gender effects were not reported.

Spring and colleagues (1991) compared *d*-fenfluramine, an appetite suppressant, and placebo in a double-blind trial among obese females who smoked. *d*-Fenfluramine is hypothesized to release serotonin and thereby improve mood and to reduce carbohydrate consumption and weight gain. Four weeks after the smoking cessation date, 50 percent of 16 participants who received *d*-fenfluramine and 33 percent of 15 participants who received placebo were abstinent from smoking, but this difference was not statistically significant. The *d*-fenfluramine group had lost an average of 0.82 kg, and the placebo group had gained an average of 1.59 kg, a significant difference. When only those who had stopped smoking were compared, the difference in weight change remained significant (-0.82 kg in the *d*-fenfluramine group vs. 1.31 kg in the placebo group) (Spring et al. 1992). The observed weight change was correlated with greater increases in caloric intake in the placebo group than in the *d*-fenfluramine group, particularly in intake of carbohydrate-rich foods. After smoking cessation, *d*-fenfluramine appeared to help control appetite and weight gain, but it did not demonstrate an important effect on smoking cessation. In view of recent findings of serious medical complications resulting from use of this pharmacologic agent, the role of *d*-fenfluramine products in smoking cessation may be controversial (Connolly et al. 1997; Mark et al. 1997).

Klesges and colleagues (1990) studied the effects of phenylpropanolamine, an over-the-counter weight control product, on the weight gain associated with smoking cessation. The study population consisted of women smokers who were asked to stop smoking for two weeks. They were randomly assigned to receive phenylpropanolamine gum, placebo gum, or no gum. Weight gain at the end of two weeks was 0.04 kg in the phenylpropanolamine group, 0.72 kg in the placebo gum group, and 0.88 kg in the no gum group. Fifteen of the 16 women assigned to the phenylpropanolamine group succeeded in stopping, significantly more than in the group assigned to placebo gum (12 of 21) or the group assigned to no gum (14 of 20).

Studies have examined weight changes among smokers who took bupropion (150 to 300 mg/day), which is sold for smoking cessation under the trade name Zyban. In such studies, smokers who took bupropion gained less weight initially. When the drug was stopped, however, no significant differences existed in weight gain (Hurt et al. 1997; Jorenby et al. 1999).

## Depression

Many studies have confirmed that smoking is perceived to reduce negative affect, reduce stress, enhance positive affect, and provide a means to distract attention from disturbing stimuli. Studies of antidepressant therapy in smoking cessation have shown that antidepressants may effect changes in brain chemistry that are beneficial for cessation, whether or not a smoker is depressed (Edwards et al. 1989; Hall et al. 1998; Prochazka et al. 1998). Few studies have addressed gender-specific differences. Some evidence has suggested that smokers who have depressive symptoms at the time of a cessation attempt or who have a prior history of depressive symptoms are more likely than those with no such symptoms to benefit from antidepressant therapy (Niaura et al. 1995; Hall et al. 1998). Behavioral interventions for smokers with mood disorders appear to be more successful when social support is provided (Hall et al. 1996; Muñoz et al. 1997; Hall et al. 1998).

### Pathways Linking Depression and Smoking

Overrepresentation of persons with major depressive disorder (MDD) among patients of smoking cessation clinics has been noted (see "Depression and Other Psychiatric Disorders" in Chapter 3). Lifetime rates of MDD in cessation studies conducted at the University of California, San Francisco, have been reported at 46 percent (Ginsberg et al. 1995), 31 percent (Hall et al. 1994), and 22 percent (Hall et al. 1996). In all three of the university samples, women were more likely than men to report a history of depression.

Depression has complex relationships with other behaviors. Cigarette smoking may serve many needs among persons who tend toward depression or who are currently depressed. Among those addicted to nicotine, smoking is reinforcing and produces quick and direct reinforcement intrinsically. Pharmacologically, smoking has a stimulating effect that may indirectly increase one's chance of receiving positive reinforcement for continuing to smoke (Hall et al. 1993).

Studies of the effects of nicotine on mood were summarized in the 1988 Surgeon General's report on nicotine addiction (USDHHS 1988). Depressive mood, anxiety, nervousness, restlessness, irritability, impatience, anger, aggression, fatigue, and drowsiness have all been reported after smoking cessation (Hughes and Hatsukami 1986). Most of these symptoms appear to peak at one to two weeks after smoking cessation and return to baseline after one month (USDHHS 1988).

Theoretically, nicotine replacement therapies for nicotine withdrawal should eliminate these negative affect states; however, not all nicotine withdrawal symptoms are relieved with nicotine replacement. Irritability appears to be the only symptom that is uniformly alleviated; anger, anxiety, and impatience are frequently relieved (Hughes et al. 1991). Less consistently relieved are depressive mood, restlessness, annoyance, and hostility (Hughes et al. 1991).

### Antidepressant Interventions in Smoking Treatment

Most studies of antidepressant treatment in smoking cessation have either not addressed gender-specific differences or have found none. In a male-only study using an antidepressant (imipramine hydrochloride, 75 mg) in smoking cessation treatment, Jacobs and colleagues (1971) found no benefit; however, smokers were encouraged to stop smoking within the first two weeks of treatment, before the usual onset of antidepressant efficacy. In a small trial, Edwards and associates (1989) found that patients who received three weeks of doxepin treatment (150 mg) were more likely to be abstinent at two months than were patients who received placebo. No gender-specific differences were reported.

Recent studies of antidepressants in smoking treatment have been motivated by the putative effect of nicotine on neurotransmitters and by the effect of antidepressants on these same neurotransmitters. Hall and colleagues (1998) described the effects of nortriptyline among smokers (110 women and 89 men) with or without a history of MDD. Nortriptyline dose began at 50 mg for all patients; attempts were made to adjust levels to the therapeutic range for MDD (50 to 150 ng/mL). Independent of depression history, the percentage of participants who remained abstinent from smoking was higher among those who received nortriptyline than among those who received placebo, and overall results did not differ significantly by gender. Post hoc analyses found that women with a history of MDD were less likely than women with no such history to be abstinent on follow-up, but this relationship was not found among men. A study by Prochazka and colleagues (1998) also reported that nortriptyline increased cessation among smokers not currently suffering from depression. Although women were included in the study, results were not reported by gender.

Several studies that used bupropion have been reported (Ferry et al. 1992; Ferris and Cooper 1993; Hurt et al. 1997; Jorenby et al. 1999). Although the mechanism of bupropion is unknown, one hypothesis suggested it is primarily noradrenergic (Ferris and Cooper 1993). The majority of the studies found significantly higher smoking cessation rates among those who used bupropion.

### Behavioral Interventions Targeted to Smokers with Mood Disorders

Five clinical trials have used behavioral interventions to treat smokers with mood disorders. They either did not report gender-specific differences or did not find such differences.

In the first trial (Zelman et al. 1992), 126 smokers were randomly assigned to one of two psychosocial strategies for smoking cessation, either skills training or support, and one of two "nicotine exposure" categories, either 2-mg nicotine gum or rapid smoking, in which a puff is inhaled from a cigarette every six seconds over a predetermined time period (e.g., 15 or 30 minutes). No differences were found among the four treatment groups at the one-year follow-up. These investigators did not report gender-specific differences.

Hall and associates (1996) classified patients by the presence or absence of a history of MDD. Patients were randomly assigned to either placebo or 2-mg nicotine gum and to either the cognitive-behavioral mood management treatment or an expanded health education program equivalent in time and therapeutic contact. A history of depression was not found to be associated with differences in treatment outcomes. The studies by Hall's group examined the data for gender-specific differences and found none. This result may be because of the level of social support provided (see "Social Support" later in this chapter). Repeating the study, but comparing the 10-session cognitive-behavioral mood management intervention with a 5-session health education control, Hall and associates (1998) showed the cognitive-behavioral intervention to be superior to the control intervention among smokers with a history of depression—a finding consistent with earlier work (Hall et al. 1994).

Another recent study suggested that cognitive-behavioral intervention may have effects among smokers with a history of depression (Muñoz et al. 1997). A self-administered mood management program for smoking cessation was provided to Spanish-speaking Latinos. The intervention resulted in a higher abstinence rate (23 percent) than a smoking cessation guide alone (11 percent). Participants who had a history of MDD but who were not currently depressed reported an even higher abstinence rate in the self-administered mood management program (31 percent). Gender-specific differences were not reported.

The pattern of results noted across the published studies tentatively suggested that increased emotional support may be useful among smokers who want to stop smoking and who have a history of mood disorder or who enter treatment with mood that is poorer relative to other smokers.

## Social Support

Both social support during smoking cessation treatment and social support derived from family and friends have been shown to improve cessation rates (Fiore et al. 2000). Whether gender differences exist in the role of social support on long-term smoking cessation remains inconclusive. Some smoking cessation studies reported a greater effect of social support among women (Fisher et al. 1991, 1993; Pirie et al.

1997), while others reported a greater effect among men (Murray et al. 1995). More studies are needed to examine the role of social support by gender and to determine whether it exerts an effect independent of other factors (e.g., depression and possible hormonal influences) thought to influence successful cessation among women.

**Gender and Social Support**

On average, women appear to be more responsive to social events in their environment and to be more skillful at developing a range of satisfying and supportive social relationships than are men. However, the substantial responsibility that social networks carry may also increase stress, which in turn may increase the likelihood of smoking and decrease the likelihood of cessation. Perhaps as a result of this susceptibility to social influence, women who live with a smoker are less likely to stop smoking than are men who live with a smoker (Gritz et al. 1996). Cessation efforts may also be compromised by gender-specific stereotypes that discourage women from acting assertively on their own behalf (Blechman 1981). On the other hand, findings have suggested that women are more likely than men to believe that prevention and treatment of substance abuse, including smoking, is effective (Kauffman et al. 1997).

The multiple obligations created by women's social roles also appear to influence smoking cessation. For example, stopping smoking for the sake of a child or newborn is less likely among mothers with many caretaking responsibilities than among mothers with fewer responsibilities (Graham 1992). In qualitative research interviews with women who had smoked throughout pregnancy, Graham (1976) found that continued smoking was frequently attributed to anticipated negative emotional side effects of smoking cessation and to the likely impacts of these side effects on husbands and children.

Several studies indicated that women tend to be more attuned to their social surroundings than are men (Belle 1987; Acitelli and Antonucci 1994). Women are more likely than men to rate highly the importance of social support in stopping smoking (Cormier et al. 1990; DiLorenzo et al. 1990; Gritz et al. 1996), are somewhat more likely to join smoking cessation groups (Shiffman 1982; Fiore et al. 1990; Yankelovich Partners 1998), give higher ratings to the importance of emotional support (e.g., listening, encouragement, and understanding) than to more concrete assistance to reduce stressors and other temptations to relapse, and when successful, are more likely to report having received social support to stop smoking (Cormier et al. 1990; DiLorenzo et al. 1990).

Ratings of social support received from family and friends have been found to predict smoking cessation (Mermelstein et al. 1986; Morgan et al. 1988; Murray et al. 1995; Gritz et al. 1996). Coppotelli and Orleans (1985) studied women's reports of support from their spouses for stopping smoking. Questionnaires were completed an average of 6.4 days after smoking cessation. Supportive acts predicted continued cessation at six to eight weeks after smoking cessation. These acts included response to the woman's request for help, support while she was stopping, and tolerance for the woman's struggles with smoking cessation and with her edginess, mood swings, and anxiety. In another study, women attempting to stop smoking reported both expecting and receiving a higher ratio of positive-to-negative behaviors compared with women not attempting to stop (Cohen and Lichtenstein 1990). This ratio was also predictive of continuous abstinence at 12 months.

Several other relationships make social support important among women who attempt to stop smoking. Depression is related to greater likelihood of smoking and complicates cessation (Glassman et al. 1990) (see "Depression" earlier in this chapter and "Depression and Other Psychiatric Disorders" in Chapter 3). Depression is more prevalent among women than among men, and social support appears to be related to level of depression (McGrath et al. 1990). Women are more likely than men to report smoking to reduce negative affect and stress (Gritz et al. 1996; Secker-Walker et al. 1996; Ward et al. 1997). Women trying to stop smoking have rated emotional or empathic support as more beneficial than instrumental support (Fisher et al. 1993).

Despite the convergence of data that have suggested that social support should be useful in helping women to stop smoking, evaluations of the relationship have remained inconclusive. Murray and colleagues (1995) found that the presence of a support person in cessation attempts had a greater effect among men than among women. Others also reported greater benefits of support among men than among women (Pirie et al. 1997). Other studies, however, suggested that women may benefit from social support more than do men, at least in the short term. In a program that emphasized small-group discussion, buddy systems, and exchange of perceptions and experiences, 71 percent of women were abstinent at the end of the program; only 26 percent in a comparison group were abstinent at the end of a program that emphasized self-management ($p < 0.02$). Among men in the same study, 47 and 43 percent, respectively, were abstinent at the end of the program (Fisher et al. 1991, 1993). Those findings replicated an earlier study that suggested that programs emphasizing social support might have a short-term advantage for women (Fisher and Bishop 1986). Unfortunately, the greater cessation rate among women was not reflected in follow-up assessments. The fact that such striking changes do not persist over time may not necessarily mean that support is unimportant, but that, as with many important determinants of behavior, its influence is maintained only if it continues to be available (Fisher 1997).

# Smoking Cessation in Specific Groups of Women and Girls

## Adolescent Girls

A number of programs and materials for adolescent smoking cessation have been developed and implemented, but typically evaluation has been anecdotal or descriptive (USDHHS 1994). Evidence has indicated that the proportion of adolescent smokers who participate in smoking cessation programs is low, attrition is high, and few participants quit smoking (USDHHS 1994; Moolchan et al. 2000). Few of the studies have reported data by gender. At present, data are insufficient to draw strong conclusions about gender-specific differences in smoking cessation interventions for adolescents. Overall, the findings suggested that adolescent girls might be more responsive than boys to social support, such as family or peer encouragement. Because regular smoking typically begins in the teenage years, effective smoking cessation messages and methods for adolescent girls who smoke are greatly needed, as are smoking prevention programs targeted to young nonsmokers.

### School-Based Smoking Cessation Programs

School-based smoking cessation programs have been evaluated in several studies, with varying degrees of rigor and success. In an early study, St. Pierre and colleagues (1983) trained peer leaders to conduct a six-session program for high school students. The program content reflected standard cognitive-behavioral methods used in adult programs. Intensive recruitment yielded only six girls and six boys (smokers of 6 to 30 cigarettes per day) who completed the program. At the end of the program, none of the participants had stopped smoking, and the five girls for whom data were available tended to reduce their smoking less than the boys did.

The largest and most systematic school-based smoking cessation study (Sussman et al. 1995, 1998a,b) involved rural and suburban high schools in two states. Within each of the 16 schools in the study, students who volunteered to participate in a smoking cessation clinic were randomly assigned to a clinic group or to a wait-list control group. No gender-specific data were reported for cessation outcomes; the percentage who stopped smoking was very low for the total sample.

Participants were asked about 22 possible reasons for wanting to quit smoking. Only four significant gender-specific differences were found (Sussman et al. 1998a). These reasons were "if my girlfriend/boyfriend asked me to quit" (51 percent of girls vs. 57 percent of boys), "if someone close to me died because of smoking" (42 percent of girls vs. 49 percent of boys), "to look calmer" (14 percent of girls vs. 9 percent of boys), and "to have more endurance" (22 percent of girls vs. 18 percent of boys). Among girls, the four most frequently endorsed reasons for stopping were that a boyfriend asked (51 percent), a significant other had died (42 percent), the girl had a desire to live longer (42 percent), and a physician told her to stop (40 percent).

No gender-specific differences were found in the self-reported stage of readiness to stop smoking or in answers to the questions, "Do you think you will ever quit smoking?" and "Would you be able to quit on your own?" (Sussman et al. 1998a). Girls were more likely than boys to report being tempted to smoke in 9 out of 16 hypothetical circumstances, including circumstances indicating nicotine dependence, and girls were less likely than boys to answer yes to the question, "Have you really tried to quit smoking before?" (65 vs. 59 percent; $p < 0.03$). Boys were more likely than girls to report that they might participate in a cessation program at school.

Another study by Sussman and colleagues (1998b) assessed self-initiated smoking cessation among adolescents. In the follow-up of a large sample of adolescents in alternative schools, gender did not predict cessation. Similarly, Hu and colleagues (1998) did not find gender to be a predictor of cessation. In an assessment of predictors of smoking cessation among adolescents in New Hampshire high schools, Sargent and colleagues (1998) found a weak association between gender and cessation, with boys more likely to stop smoking than were girls (adjusted RR, 1.3; 95 percent CI, 0.7 to 2.5). When all the predictive factors were entered into a logistic regression, gender no longer was predictive.

A few studies evaluated smoking cessation strategies for adolescents in vocational high schools, settings likely to have a high proportion of smokers (Pallonen et al. 1994, 1998; Smith et al. 1994). The interventions were delivered by computer and featured the expert system adapted from a program used with adult smokers (Velicer et al. 1993). The expert system elicited relevant information from the student (e.g., smoking history and interest in smoking cessation) and delivered feedback and suggestions tailored to this information. Data from 10th- and 11th-grade vocational students indicated that girls rated the computerized intervention program significantly more positively than did boys (Smith et al. 1994). No gender-specific data were reported for cessation.

Balch (1998) conducted focus groups with high school smokers in three states and observed that girls expressed more interest in participating in group programs than did boys. The authors interpreted this observation as a reflection of girls' greater concern about the opinions of others.

### Other Smoking Cessation Programs

Biglan and colleagues (summarized in Hollis et al. 1994) used an HMO to identify youth smokers. Adolescents who met the eligibility criteria were randomly assigned to a smoking cessation intervention or to a control group that received no treatment. The focus of the intervention was a 60-minute consultation with a nurse practitioner at a convenient HMO clinic. Incentives were offered for attending these sessions. A lottery with the chance to win $100 was established, and abstinence from smoking was required to win. There was no effect of the intervention overall, and differences by gender were not reported.

Adolescents who received treatment for substance abuse have high smoking rates, and the treatment setting provides an opportunity for smoking intervention (Myers 1999). In a small study, 6 of 35 adolescents were abstinent at the three-month post-intervention follow-up. Gender was not a predictor of response to treatment.

Weissman and colleagues (1987) recruited 11 "hard core" smokers (5 girls and 6 boys) aged 13 through 18 years who were attending an alternative school. The participants were selected from smokers who auditioned for parts in a smoking prevention videotape or who were identified by those who auditioned. Their average age was 15.6 years, they had smoked for an average of 2.5 years, and they smoked an average of 18 cigarettes per day. Monetary rewards were based on achieving target levels of carbon monoxide in expired air samples. Five of the six boys successfully reduced smoking and carbon monoxide levels each month during the reduction and cessation phases. Unannounced probes for four months after the cessation date indicated continued abstinence by two boys, sporadic smoking by two, and low-level daily smoking by one. In contrast, all five girls dropped out during the program and continued smoking.

Hurt and colleagues (2000) tested the efficacy of the nicotine patch in 101 adolescent smokers, of whom 41 percent were female. The nonrandomized trial drew volunteers whose median smoking was 20 cigarettes per day (range, 10 to 40). At the end of therapy (6 weeks), 10.9 percent of participants were abstinent, as verified by expired carbon monoxide and plasma cotinine. At six months, however, only 5.0 percent were abstinent, a rate that appears lower than the secular trend for cessation among adolescents (Sussman et al. 1995, 1998b). Gender differences were not reported.

## Women Who Smoke Heavily

Among persons who smoke heavily, women are more likely than men to join smoking cessation programs (Cohen et al. 1989; Wagner et al. 1990; Orleans et al. 1991b; Thompson et al. 1998). In cessation studies, a number of researchers have found that women who smoke heavily are less likely to achieve long-term cessation than are men (Bjornson et al. 1995; Nides et al. 1995), but others have found no difference in quitting between women and men who smoke heavily (Goldberg et al. 1993; Fortmann and Killen 1995).

### Characteristics Related to Heavy Smoking

Persons who smoke heavily account for a disproportionately high share of mortality related to smoking (USDHHS 1984). To ensure that the classification of heavy smokers does not include moderate smokers who round up their daily smoking to 20 cigarettes (1 pack) per day, 25 cigarettes per day has been adopted by many researchers as the point at which smokers are considered heavy smokers (Sorensen et al. 1992b; COMMIT Research Group 1995a,b); however, some researchers have used 20 or more cigarettes per day as a definition of heavy smoking (Glassman et al. 1988; Serxner et al. 1992; Thornton et al. 1994).

Research has suggested that those who smoke heavily display characteristics of nicotine addiction that distinguish them from lighter smokers (USDHHS 1988). Using the Fagerström Tolerance Questionnaire, investigators have demonstrated that heavy smokers are more dependent on nicotine than are light or moderate smokers. Heavy smokers also have internal cues that trigger smoking, have more difficulty stopping, and have more withdrawal symptoms (e.g., anxiety and fatigue) during smoking cessation (Killen et al. 1988; Goldberg et al. 1993). Among heavy smokers, females are more likely than males to report feeling dependent on cigarettes and feeling unable to cut down (CDC 1995a), to have lower expectations of stopping in the near future, to report their last attempt to stop as difficult, to want assistance in stopping, and to be more concerned with weight gain (Sorensen et al. 1992b). Women who are heavy smokers may be more likely than men who are heavy smokers to view a reduction in the amount smoked as preferable to smoking cessation (Blake et al. 1989).

Although heavy smoking is inversely related to smoking cessation (Cohen et al. 1989; Wagner et al. 1990; Orleans et al. 1991b; Kozlowski et al. 1994), heavy smokers are more likely than light or moderate smokers to join smoking cessation activities (Cohen et al. 1989; Wagner et al. 1990; Orleans et al. 1991b; O'Loughlin et al. 1997; Thompson et al. 1998). Wagner and colleagues (1990) used a large, defined population of 50,000 smokers in an HMO database to examine rates of participation in self-help activities for smoking cessation. Comparing a 10-percent random sample of smokers drawn 10 months before the project began with smokers who volunteered to participate in the project, they found that heavy smokers were more likely to participate than were lighter smokers (RR, 2.8; 95 percent CI, 1.9 to 3.8). Moreover, women were significantly more likely than men (63 vs. 48 percent) to participate. Women were especially more likely than men to participate if they had symptoms related to smoking (e.g., a cough or shortness of breath) (RR, 5.6; 95 percent CI, 3.01 to 10.4). The authors did not report the proportions who stopped smoking. Sorensen and colleagues (1992b) also found that among women, those who smoked heavily were significantly more likely than light or moderate smokers (64 vs. 47 percent) to state that they wanted assistance to stop smoking.

### Unassisted Smoking Cessation Among Women Who Smoke Heavily

Little is known about the natural history of smoking cessation among women who are heavy smokers or about the gender-specific differences in smoking cessation among heavy smokers. The COMMIT study followed cohorts of heavy smokers and light or moderate smokers for five years (COMMIT Research Group, unpublished data). The cohorts in the comparison communities provided data on unassisted smoking cessation among both women and men who smoked heavily. More than one-half of the women (55.6 percent) and men (53.9 percent) who smoked heavily reported decreasing the number of cigarettes they smoked per day during the five years of the study. Men reported slightly more attempts to stop smoking for at least 24 hours (2.9) than did women (2.2). Among persons who sustained cessation for six months or more at the end of the five years, cessation was slightly higher among men than women who smoked heavily (19.6 vs. 17.2 percent). Among heavy smokers, the RR for smoking cessation was 0.6 (95 percent CI, 0.4 to 0.9) among women compared with men after adjustment for age, ethnicity, and education.

### Cessation Programs for Women Who Smoke Heavily

As part of a smoking cessation intervention delivered by physicians, women and men who smoked heavily were compared with women and men who were lighter smokers (Goldberg et al. 1993). Among women at baseline, heavy smokers had higher levels of addiction than did lighter smokers. They had also smoked longer, had made fewer attempts to stop smoking, were less confident of their ability to stop smoking, had higher perceptions that others wanted them to stop smoking, and had previous physical symptoms related to smoking (e.g., lung disease and asthma). Interventions consisted of physician advice, counseling specific to the patient, and counseling plus nicotine gum. At the end of six months, continuous cessation for one week was achieved by 10 percent of women who were heavy smokers and 15 percent of women who were light smokers. Among heavy smokers, a comparable percentage of women (10 percent) and men (11 percent) stopped smoking.

The Lung Health Study, an ongoing randomized study of more than 3,900 smokers, examined long-term cessation at 12 and 36 months (Bjornson et al. 1995). Participants received intervention consisting of a message from a physician, a 12-week behavioral change program, nicotine gum, and a maintenance program; 91 percent of participants attended at least one class of the cessation program. For analysis, participants were classified as heavy smokers (≥ 30 cigarettes per day) or lighter smokers (<30 cigarettes per day). Cessation among women who were heavy smokers was 21 percent at 12 months and 14 percent at 36 months; among men, the quit rate was 28 percent at 12 months and 22 percent at 36 months.

The Lung Health Study also reported that women initially found it more difficult than men to stop smoking. Smoking cessation history, such as previous long-term cessation (6 months), identification of any cigarette other than the first cigarette of the day as being the most difficult to give up, better long-term health (e.g., no asthma or breathlessness), and support for stopping were all predictive of initial cessation. Both women and men were more likely to have an early relapse (within 4 to 12 months) if they reported smoking at all since the cessation day. No other factor was predictive of early relapse among women. Predictors of late relapse (at 12 to 24 months) among women included nicotine gum use at 12 months and having other smokers in the house at 12 months. Predictors for early relapse among men were any smoking since the cessation day and use of nicotine gum at 4 months; men were less likely to relapse if they had a support person at the orientation and lower dependence on nicotine at baseline (Nides et al. 1995). The study also found that women with higher dependence on nicotine, as assessed by smoking when emotionally triggered, feeling deprived when not smoking, being physiologically dependent, and waiting a low number of minutes to the first cigarette of the day, found it harder to stop smoking than did men with similar ratings of nicotine dependence (Bjornson et al. 1995).

In contrast to the Lung Health Study, in a study of 1,044 persons who used nicotine gum for cessation, data were stratified by both gender and amount smoked. This study found no difference in cessation between heavy and light smokers or between women and men (Fortmann and Killen 1995). The researchers also found that persons who smoked heavily were more likely to relapse, but found no gender-specific differences.

## Women of Low Socioeconomic Status

Smoking prevalence is inversely related to SES, regardless of the indicator(s) used and regardless of gender (see Chapter 2). Similarly, women of low SES have lower rates of smoking cessation than do women of higher SES. On a population level, the less educated and those living below poverty level have been reported to be less likely to achieve smoking cessation (Novotny et al. 1988), a finding confirmed by others (Fiore et al. 1990; Hatziandreu et al. 1990; Winkleby et al. 1992). Mass-media attempts to reach women smokers of low SES have had some effect, with women more likely than men to watch televised programs and read materials; however, the cessation rates among women tend to be lower than those among men except in the long term (24 months) (Warnecke et al. 1992). A number of studies have examined quit rates among pregnant women of low SES. Spontaneous cessation rates appear to be lower than those among pregnant women of higher SES (Cnattingius et al. 1992; O'Campo et al. 1992). Cessation programs directed at pregnant women of low SES appear to increase quit rates over control programs that provide usual care such as distribution of brochures and lists of local cessation programs; quit rates appear to be directly related to the intensity of the intervention (Windsor et al. 1993b; Albrecht et al. 1994; Lillington et al. 1995). The effect of worksite programs for low-SES women smokers is a new area of exploration, but at least one study suggested that worksites may be good venues for reaching these women (Gritz et al. 1998).

### Measures of Low Socioeconomic Status

SES is assessed in many ways, most often by using measures of income, education, or occupation. The three factors are strongly correlated, and each has been used separately as a proxy for SES. Income is a good indicator of overall SES, and studies have defined female smokers with low income as those living below the poverty level (Novotny et al. 1988), living below a specified income (Warnecke et al. 1991; Manfredi et al. 1992; Kendrick et al. 1995), or eligible for public housing (Manfredi et al. 1992) or other public services (Albrecht et al. 1994; Brayden and Christensen 1994; Keintz et al. 1994; Rafuse 1994; Lillington et al. 1995). Years of education is the most commonly reported measure of SES (Macaskill et al. 1992; Winkleby et al. 1992; Windsor et al. 1993b; Albrecht et al. 1994; Kendrick et al. 1995), and it appears to be the measure most strongly related to smoking cessation (Pierce et al. 1989; Hatziandreu et al. 1990). Occupational status is also used as an indicator of SES, with blue-collar occupations indicating lower SES than do white-collar occupations (USDHHS 1985; Jeffery et al. 1993; Gritz et al. 1998).

### Cessation Programs in Public Health Settings

Smoking cessation programs for low-income women have been instituted in public health clinics and community health centers. Recognizing that women of low SES have severe economic problems that may result in significant stress and that may be partially relieved by smoking, some cessation programs have included a wide range of topics that address stress management, self-esteem, group support, and general activities that improve quality of life (Rafuse 1994). This intensive intervention resulted in a 20- to 25-percent cessation rate. Other efforts have encouraged women of low SES to participate in group classes on smoking cessation and in counseling with a physician (Macken et al. 1991) or in clinic-reinforced, self-help cessation activities (Keintz et al. 1994). Unfortunately, only a small proportion of women of low SES appear to take advantage of these programs. A clinic serving a primarily female, low-income, urban population found that 24 percent of women who smoked were interested in a smoking cessation class with a physician, but only 36 percent of those interested (8.6 percent of all the women who smoked) actually kept their appointments (Macken et al. 1991). Another study in a community primary care health clinic found that half of 55 women smokers surveyed indicated on an initial questionnaire that they would be willing to participate in a smoking cessation program (Pohl et al. 1998). However, only 20 percent of the original group showed up for the first class.

Manfredi and colleagues (1998) identified and surveyed low-income women about a number of issues they thought might be related to motivation to stop smoking. Of all the potential predictors studied, only health effects, not wanting to be addicted, and the expense of cigarettes were related to wanting to stop.

Keintz and colleagues (1994) performed follow-up on more than 1,200 women in a public health setting in which the women smokers received advice and a self-help guide on cessation. In a retrospective survey administered before the intervention, a random sample of 3,260 women attending the clinics was drawn. Of the survey participants, 5.2 percent of clients who smoked at the beginning of the prior 12-month period were estimated as having been abstinent from smoking for 90 or more days during those 12 months. After one year of exposure to the intervention program, 9.1 percent of women smokers in the clinics had stopped smoking for at least 90 days, a statistically significant difference. An examination of the characteristics of women successful in achieving cessation included those who were lighter smokers (<25 cigarettes per day), were more educated (high school or more), were less addicted (smoked the first cigarette >30 minutes after awaking), and were more confident in their ability to stop smoking. Logistic regression analyses identified three factors related to cessation: confidence in ability to stop smoking, the interaction of lower addiction (Fagerström score) and age, and the interaction of addiction and education—which was the strongest of the multivariate factors.

A Canadian smoking cessation program targeting low-income women was available through local community groups and was delivered free of charge by trained facilitators (O'Loughlin et al. 1997). The materials and content were developed to be specifically relevant to low-income women. Although the cessation program was targeted to women and attracted mostly women (n = 83, 73.5 percent), men (n = 30, 26.5 percent) were also allowed to participate. Despite being targeted to women, cessation rates were higher among men (40.0 percent at 1 month, 26.1 percent at 6 months) than among women (28.2 percent at 1 month, 21.1 percent at 6 months). The statistical significance of these findings was not reported.

### Effects of Mass Media

Studies of the mass media suggested that smokers of low SES, especially women, are more likely than smokers of higher SES to seek information from visual sources, especially television, and that such campaigns can be targeted to specific groups. For example, a seven-month media campaign in San Francisco, California, which was designed to change people's level of information, showed that a culturally appropriate, multichannel campaign can improve community knowledge (Marín et al. 1990a).

In a large, televised cessation intervention in the Chicago, Illinois, area, Warnecke and colleagues (1991) found that, overall, women were more likely than men to watch televised smoking cessation programs, attend group sessions, and refer daily to the self-help cessation manual. A multiple regression model of participation in the program showed that gender and income were the only significant variables in predicting whether televised segments would be watched. Women, African Americans, and persons with low income were the most likely to watch the televised segments. Overall, women with low income (<$13,000 per year) were more likely than men with low income to view and recall the televised segments. Gender and education were significant in predicting the frequency with which smokers referred to the self-help manual and the level of recall of the manual. Among those with more than a high school education, women were more likely than men to refer to the manual daily and to recall parts of the manual. Regardless of SES, women smokers were more responsive than men smokers to the media. Cessation rates were high in the intervention group at 12 months after treatment (14 vs. 6 percent) and at 24 months (6 vs. 2 percent). Significantly more men than women had quit at all follow-up points, except at 24 months (Warnecke et al. 1992).

As part of the Chicago televised project, women with very low income (median, $5,000 per year) who lived in subsidized public housing were asked about their smoking behavior six months before the intervention for smoking cessation began (Manfredi et al. 1992). Compared with the general population of smokers who were not residents of public housing, the women residents had a lower desire to stop smoking, reported fewer previous attempts to stop, perceived fewer risks from smoking, had more smokers among their friends, and were less knowledgeable about where to receive information about or assistance with smoking cessation. As in other studies of low-income populations (Rafuse 1994), respondents in eight focus groups reported they had highly stressful lives that they perceived as partially assuaged by smoking (Lacey et al. 1993). Women also reported little social support for stopping, saw smoking as a pleasure, saw few risks from smoking, reported that "everyone" in their environment smoked, had no information about how to stop smoking, and perceived that enough willpower would lead to cessation.

A large mass-media campaign in Sydney and Melbourne, Australia, also concluded that television was a good way to present antismoking messages to smokers of low SES (Macaskill et al. 1992). The researchers assessed smoking prevalence during the first year of the campaign and five years after it, and they used the rate ratio (prevalence after intervention relative to prevalence before intervention) adjusted for age. Among women in Sydney and among men in both Sydney and Melbourne, the rate ratio by educational level was consistently lower after than before the intervention, and no linear trend with increasing education was apparent. Among women in Melbourne, those with some university education had a lower rate ratio than did women with less education.

#### Cessation Programs for Pregnant Women of Low Socioeconomic Status

A few studies have examined natural smoking cessation patterns among pregnant women of low SES. In a prospective study of approximately 1,900 pregnant women who were smokers just before becoming pregnant or during pregnancy or who had relapsed after giving birth, 41 percent who had smoked before pregnancy stopped during pregnancy (O'Campo et al. 1992). Cessation rates during pregnancy increased substantially with level of education among white women: 13 percent of those with less than 12 years of education but 67 percent of those with more than 12 years of education stopped smoking. Among African American women, 35 percent of those with less than 12 years of education but 49 percent of those with more than 12 years of education stopped. Logistic regression, adjusted for the effects of education, age, parity, marital status, and intention to breastfeed an infant, indicated that white women who had stopped smoking were more likely to be younger than 25 years of age (RR, 3.4; 90 percent CI, 1.3 to 9.0), to have more than 12 years of education (RR, 21.8; 90 percent CI, 5.1 to 92.5), to have no other children (RR, 2.9; 90 percent CI, 1.3 to 9.0), to be married (RR, 2.3; 90 percent CI, 0.8 to 6.3), and to intend to breastfeed (RR, 1.2; 90 percent CI, 0.5 to 2.9). Among African American women, only intent to breastfeed was significantly associated with smoking cessation during pregnancy (RR, 2.7; 90 percent CI, 1.2 to 6.0). A similar study in Sweden that examined all women users of prenatal care clinics in one county (3,678 participants) found that pregnant women with low education were less likely to stop smoking during pregnancy (RR, 1.2 for 9 years of education; 90 percent CI, 1.0 to 1.5) (RR, 0.7 for 12 years of education; 95 percent CI, 0.5 to 0.9) (Cnattingius et al. 1992). Furthermore, spontaneous smoking cessation during pregnancy appears to be lower among women of low SES than among women of higher SES. Two studies that involved pregnant women of higher SES showed that 41 percent had stopped smoking spontaneously (Messimer et al. 1989; Mullen et al. 1990); an earlier study showed that 22 percent of pregnant women of low SES had stopped smoking spontaneously (Windsor et al. 1985).

A review of five randomized, controlled trials on smoking cessation conducted between 1983 and 1993 with a total of 4,277 low-income pregnant women indicated that low-level, minimal contact interventions had some effect in this population. Cessation rates ranged from 3 to 18 percent (Albrecht et al. 1994). The most intensive interventions had much better results (quit rates of 11 to 18 percent) than did low-intensity interventions. In one study, for example, 11 percent of women who received one-to-one counseling and instructions in behavioral change had stopped smoking, whereas only 3 percent of women in the control group did so (Albrecht et al. 1994). A Los Angeles, California, study of low-income pregnant women in four WIC sites (155 intervention women and 400 control women) found that 43 percent of women in the intervention group but 25 percent of women in the control group achieved cessation (Lillington et al. 1995). The proportion of women who maintained cessation after childbirth was 25.3 percent among the treated women and 11.6 percent among the control women.

An intensive intervention program that depended heavily on one-to-one counseling in a clinical setting achieved 30.8 percent smoking cessation among counseled low-income pregnant women; uncounseled control women achieved a 15.4-percent cessation rate (not confirmed by urine testing) (Brayden and Christensen 1994). A study that used only minimal intervention was conducted among low-income pregnant women at WIC sites in three states (Kendrick et al. 1995). Self-reported cessation was significantly higher among women in the intervention group than in the control group (13.0 vs. 9.0 percent). However, when cotinine level was used, the results differed for the subset of participants who provided urine samples for verification (51 vs. 68 percent) and no significant difference was found in cessation (6.1 vs. 5.9 percent). Windsor and colleagues (1993b) reported a study in which 814 low-income pregnant women were randomly assigned to a smoking cessation intervention that consisted of a short counseling session, self-help cessation materials, clinic reinforcement, and social support or to a control group. Cessation was 14.3 percent in the intervention group and 8.5 percent in the control group.

#### Cessation Activities in Occupational Settings for Women of Low Socioeconomic Status

Currently, women make up 37.7 percent of the workforce in manufacturing companies (Tom Nardone, U.S. Bureau of Labor Statistics, fax to Beti Thompson, November 4, 1997). Although it is not known precisely how many of those women hold blue-collar occupations, a study of 114 manufacturing worksites identified 76.4 percent of their female employees as holding blue-collar jobs (Gritz et al. 1998). Smoking cessation activities in occupational settings attract more women than men in general, but participation by blue-collar workers, regardless of gender, is very low (Schilling et al. 1985; Sorensen et al. 1986; Jeffery et al. 1993). Cessation rates by gender have rarely been reported (Jeffery et al. 1993; Gritz et al. 1998). A recent trial that involved 114 worksites and more than 28,000 workers sought to increase rates of smoking cessation among the employees (Gritz et al. 1998). Comprehensive activities to foster smoking cessation took place in intervention worksites (Abrams et al. 1994a; Sorensen et al. 1996). Although the proportion of employees who stopped smoking was similar overall in the intervention worksites and control worksites, a significantly higher proportion of women in intervention worksites than in control worksites stopped for six months or longer (15.0 vs. 10.6 percent; $p = 0.03$) (Gritz et al. 1998). When age and occupational status (white collar vs. blue collar) were held constant, the RR for smoking cessation among women in the intervention group was greater than that among women in the comparison group (RR, 1.5; 95 percent CI, 1.01 to 2.2) in worksites where more than 75 percent of the women employees held blue-collar occupations.

### Minority Women

To date, little research has been conducted to assess the effectiveness of various smoking cessation interventions among minority women in the United States (King et al. 1997; USDHHS 1998). Research among racial and ethnic groups, particularly behavioral research, is complex because accessing the target populations is difficult and because minority groups do not trust researchers (USDHHS 1998). In general, African American, Hispanic, and American Indian or Alaska Native women want to stop smoking at rates similar to those of non-Hispanic whites, and want to stop smoking more than do men in their racial or ethnic group. Mixed results have been observed in studies that have examined differences in quit rates between African American women and non-Hispanic white women. Overall, research has suggested that more African American men achieve cessation than do African American women (Royce et al. 1995; Fisher et al. 1998). Studies targeting pregnant African American and Hispanic women have been inconsistent, with some studies finding a difference between non-Hispanic whites and other racial and ethnic groups (Gebauer et al. 1998) and other studies finding no difference (Windsor et al. 1985, 1993b; O'Campo et al. 1992).

### African American Women

Data from the 1993 NHIS showed that 74.9 percent of African American women smokers would like to stop smoking (68.9 percent of African American men and 72.4 percent of white women who smoke would like to stop) (USDHHS 1998) (see also Chapter 2). Several studies have attempted to determine psychosocial and environmental factors that may identify an African American woman's degree of readiness to stop smoking, as well as the predictors of readiness, for use in developing cessation programs for this population.

Ahijevych and Wewers (1993) surveyed 187 African American women smokers aged 18 through 69 years in a metropolitan area in Columbus, Ohio, to describe determinants of smoking and smoking cessation. Cessation attempts had been made by 83 percent of these women: 22 percent of the women had tried five or more times to stop smoking, 21 percent three or four times, and 41 percent one or two times.

The Minnesota Heart Survey, a 1985–1986 cross-sectional study, described the smoking and cessation behaviors of urban African Americans and whites, aged 35 through 74 years, in Minneapolis-St. Paul, Minnesota (Hahn et al. 1990). Of the 593 African American women in the survey, 18 percent were former smokers and 33 percent were current smokers. No significant differences were found between the African American women and white women regarding intentions to change smoking behaviors in the next year. Crittenden and colleagues (1994) administered a questionnaire on readiness to quit to 495 women who smoked (55 percent African Americans, 42 percent non-Hispanic whites) at four public health clinics in the Chicago area. Race was not related to readiness to change.

#### *Self-Help Attempts Among African American Women*

Resnicow and colleagues (1997) tested a self-help smoking cessation program that included a printed guide, a videotape, and a booster telephone call to a cohort of 650 inner-city African Americans (377 women and 273 men) in Harlem, New York. No significant differences were observed between intervention and control groups. Further, results were not different by gender.

A targeted media campaign designed to motivate African Americans to call NCI's CIS line for smoking cessation assistance randomly assigned 14 communities to intervention or control (Boyd et al. 1998). After a media campaign that lasted approximately one year (with time off between media spots), the volume of calls from African Americans was significantly higher in the intervention than control communities ($p < 0.008$). More calls came from African American women (55 percent) than from African American men (45 percent). Cessation rates were not reported.

#### *Cessation Programs for Pregnant African American Women*

Much of the research that has been reported on cessation programs for African American women has focused on pregnant women. Pregnancy is an opportune time in a woman's life for a smoking cessation program (see "Pregnancy" earlier in this chapter). Several approaches have been tested in prenatal smoking cessation programs for low-income African American women.

In a prospective interview survey in Baltimore, Maryland, of 1,900 pregnant women (52 percent African Americans, 48 percent whites), O'Campo and colleagues (1992) found that intention to breastfeed was the only predictor for smoking cessation during pregnancy among African American women, whereas among white women predictors included educational level, age, and parity (see "Women of Low Socioeconomic Status" earlier in this chapter). No significant difference was observed between African Americans and whites in cessation. Relapse to smoking after delivery was high: 46 percent of African American women and 28 percent of white women who had stopped smoking during pregnancy relapsed within 6 to 12 weeks after delivery. The best predictor of early relapse after delivery among African American and white mothers alike was formula feeding of the infant.

Byrd and Meade (1993) examined the effect of a brief-contact smoking cessation program among 57 pregnant women at two Milwaukee clinics, of whom 79 percent were African American. After receiving educational materials, study participants were randomly assigned to receive usual care (e.g., advice on smoking) provided by clinic physicians or to receive counseling from a nurse who used a systematic, tailored approach based on the protocol developed by NCI (the Four A's: Ask, Advise, Assist, Arrange). No statistically significant difference was noted in smoking status among those who received the usual care and those who received the nurse counseling intervention.

In another study that used NCI's Four A's protocol, nurses delivered the intervention to pregnant women in a primary care prenatal clinic (Gebauer et al. 1998). A control group was assessed one year before recruitment of the intervention group. The 84 women in the intervention arm (50 percent African Americans) received individualized counseling delivered by an advanced-practice nurse, combined with a telephone contact 7 to 10 days after the initial clinic visit. The three-month cotinine-validated abstinence rate was 15.5 percent among the intervention group and 0.0 percent among the control group, a statistically significant difference ($p < 0.001$). Among women abstinent at the follow-up visit, a significantly greater percentage were African American (84.6 percent) than white (15.4 percent).

Lillington and colleagues (1995) designed a culturally appropriate program for low-income African American women and Hispanic women who were pregnant or who had recently given birth. The study enrolled 768 women from four WIC clinics in south and central Los Angeles and obtained follow-up data for 555 women (155 in the intervention group, 400 in the control group). Of the 555 participants, 53 percent were African American and 43 percent were Hispanic; 41 percent were current smokers and 59 percent were former smokers. Women in the control group received usual care, printed information about the risks from smoking, and a group message on smoking cessation. Of the women who were smokers at baseline, 44 percent of those at the intervention clinics and 23 percent of those at the control clinics were abstinent at nine months' gestation ($p = 0.004$), and 27 percent of those at the intervention sites and 8.5 percent at the control sites were abstinent at six weeks after delivery ($p = 0.002$). Among African American women who were former smokers at baseline, significantly lower relapse rates were reported in the intervention group than in the control group at nine months' gestation and at six weeks after delivery. (See "Hispanic Women" later in this chapter for results for Hispanic women in the study.)

Windsor and colleagues (1985) compared the effectiveness of two self-help interventions with the standard smoking cessation information given to pregnant women at three public health maternity clinics in Birmingham, Alabama. Of the 309 study participants, 62 percent were African American. The women were randomly assigned to one of three groups (two intervention and one control). Cessation was determined by self-report at midpregnancy and at the end of pregnancy, with confirmation by testing salivary thiocyanate. Six percent of women who received the first self-help intervention and 14 percent who received the second self-help intervention stopped smoking, whereas only 2 percent in the control group stopped smoking. Race was not a predictor of cessation.

In a later study, a three-component health education intervention for low-income pregnant women at four public health maternity clinics was compared with routine care and information on the risks from smoking (Windsor et al. 1993b). Of the 814 women in this study, 52 percent were African American. Only patients who reported having stopped smoking at their first and follow-up clinic visits and who had a cotinine level of 30 ng/mL or less were considered to have stopped smoking. Study results indicated that the multistep intervention was effective in changing smoking behavior. The proportions who stopped were similar among African American women and white women.

When the methods of the Birmingham trial (Windsor et al. 1993b) were replicated in a large prenatal clinic in Baltimore, Maryland, that served predominantly low-income, African American women, the intervention was not effective (Gielen et al. 1997). At their first prenatal visit, 391 smokers were randomly assigned to an intervention group to receive usual clinic information plus a prenatal and postpartum intervention or to a control group that received only usual clinic information. Almost 85 percent of the patients in both the intervention ($n = 193$) and control ($n = 198$) groups continued the preconception smoking pattern throughout pregnancy. Of the 13 women who had stopped smoking and who were followed up to six months after delivery, 85 percent relapsed.

*Other Cessation Programs for African American Women*

Royce and colleagues (1995) examined the usefulness of NCI's Four A's approach in smoking cessation counseling delivered by a health care clinician in conjunction with socioculturally appropriate self-help materials on smoking cessation and relapse prevention for low-income African Americans. At baseline, 153 African American smokers (96 women and 57 men) in a neighborhood clinic in Harlem (New York City, New York) were interviewed briefly as they waited for their clinic appointment. At the end of the interview, patients in the study received a copy of the project-designed KICKIT! guidebook, the KICKIT! videotape, and a tracking form to give the clinician. They subsequently received newsletters that contained tips on smoking prevention and monthly mailings with information about smoking cessation contests and prizes. Of the 117 patients (77 women and 40 men) who completed follow-up surveys approximately seven months after the intervention, 14 percent of the women and 35 percent of the men reported that they had stopped smoking.

In a randomized, controlled trial to increase smoking cessation rates among African American clients of a community health center, smokers were randomly assigned to one of three conditions: prompting by a health care provider only, health care provider prompt plus tailored print communication, or health care provider prompt plus tailored print communication plus tailored telephone counseling (Lipkus et al. 1999). At follow-up, a significant difference was found in the cessation rate among those who received provider prompt plus tailored print media (32.7 percent) compared with those who received the health care provider prompt alone (13.2 percent) or the health care provider prompt plus tailored print communication plus tailored telephone counseling (19.2 percent) ($p < 0.05$).

A smoking cessation intervention program in a nontraditional venue was a program for mothers of children in the Head Start Program (Jones et al. 1994). In a population with a baseline smoking prevalence of 43 percent, abstinence was 11 percent immediately after the intervention and 12 percent at the six-month follow-up in the intervention group and only 3 and 6 percent, respectively, in the control group.

Fisher and colleagues (1998) evaluated a community organization approach in predominantly African American communities. Using a quasi-experimental design, this 24-month study involved three low-income, mainly African American, St. Louis (Missouri) neighborhoods in planning and implementing activities to promote nonsmoking. Intervention neighborhoods were compared with comparable control neighborhoods in Kansas City (Missouri). At least two-thirds of the neighborhood residents in both the intervention and control neighborhoods were women. Changes in prevalence of smoking were evaluated through random telephone surveys of the neighborhoods in 1990 and two years later. There were 504 respondents in St. Louis, the intervention site, and 1,040 in Kansas City, the control site, at baseline. The cross-sectional survey two years later, in 1992, questioned 547 individuals in St. Louis and 1,034 in Kansas City. Although smoking prevalence decreased overall among respondents in the intervention versus comparison communities (7 vs. 1 percent; $p = 0.028$), the reduction in prevalence was not statistically significant among African Americans (5 vs. 1 percent; $p = 0.20$). An examination of smoking cessation rates by gender indicated that men were more likely to stop smoking than were women (RR, 1.6; 95 percent CI, 1.3 to 1.9).

A trial of smoking cessation through church-based programs among rural African Americans was conducted in two Virginia counties (Schorling et al. 1997). The intervention combined one-on-one counseling with self-help and community-wide activities. Population-based cohorts of smokers were contacted at baseline and at 18 months. At follow-up, the smoking cessation rate in the intervention county was 9.6 and 5.4 percent in the control county ($p = 0.18$). No difference was found by gender in smoking cessation rate.

Another study that targeted African Americans randomly assigned 22 churches predominantly attended by African Americans in Baltimore, Maryland, to an intensive intervention that included pastoral sermons, testimonies during church services, lay counselors, access to support, guides to cessation, and other materials or to a minimal self-help intervention (Voorhees et al. 1996). No significant differences in smoking cessation were observed between the trial arms. Gender was not a predictor of progress along the stages of change.

In a study of 410 inner-city African American cigarette smokers (61 percent females) who were interested in stopping smoking, Ahluwalia and colleagues (1998) enrolled participants in a randomized trial of the transdermal nicotine patch. No significant effects by gender were found in relation to abstinence at 10 weeks or at six months.

### Hispanic Women

Little work has been published on smoking cessation among Hispanic women in the United States. NHIS data for 1993 showed that a high percentage of Hispanic smokers wanted to stop smoking—79.3 percent of Hispanic women and 63.8 percent of Hispanic men (USDHHS 1998). Reports have shown smoking among Hispanics in the United States to be positively associated with acculturation (Sabogal et al. 1989; Otero-Sabogal et al. 1995). On the basis of a telephone survey of Hispanics aged 15 through 64 years who were living in the San Francisco, California, metropolitan area, Marín and colleagues (1989) found a gender-specific difference in the relationship of acculturation to smoking: men who were less acculturated and women who were more acculturated were more likely to smoke. Other investigators found that among smokers, more acculturated Hispanics had higher levels of addiction and lower levels of self-efficacy in smoking cessation than did less acculturated Hispanics (Sabogal et al. 1989). The Hispanic population in the United States represents a diverse group of subcultures and stages of immigration and acculturation, all of which should be taken into account in smoking cessation research.

In a study of cultural attitudes and expectations regarding smoking, Marín and colleagues (1990b) found no significant gender-specific differences among Hispanics, except that more women than men reported enjoyment in continued smoking. The study of 263 Hispanic smokers and 150 non-Hispanic white smokers in San Francisco found that Hispanic smokers and non-Hispanic white smokers held some different attitudes and expectations about smoking and cessation. Hispanics were significantly more certain than non-Hispanic whites that stopping smoking would provide a better example to their children, improve family relations, make breathing easier, and result in having a better taste in one's mouth. Hispanics were less likely than whites to smoke at home for relaxation or with meals. Also, fewer Hispanic smokers were certain that smoking cessation would bring withdrawal symptoms.

These findings have been incorporated into a self-help manual. Evaluation of the *Rompa con el Vicio: Una Guía para Dejar de Fumar* (USDHHS 1993c) self-help manual, which incorporated the findings described above, has shown that it was well received by Hispanic smokers. More than 20 percent of a sample of volunteers who picked up the manual at community stores or clinics reported having stopped smoking at 2.5 months after reading it, but this proportion declined to 13.7 percent after 14 months (Pérez-Stable et al. 1991). Telephone surveys conducted after implementation of a culturally appropriate, community-based smoking cessation program in the Latino community of San Francisco (Programa Latina para Dejar de Fumar) found that women were more likely than men to report awareness of the program and of the availability of printed information (Marín and Pérez-Stable 1995).

Lillington and colleagues (1995) published a report of a smoking cessation intervention for pregnant women that included 234 Hispanics among the 555 enrollees. Contrary to the study's results for African American women, this program did not significantly affect smoking cessation among Hispanic women, either at nine months' gestation or at six weeks after delivery.

A smoking cessation study that involved 93 Hispanic women and men in Queens, New York, found no difference in cessation at 12 months between a multicomponent, culturally specific intervention and a minimal-contact self-help program (Nevid and Javier 1997). Results were not significantly different by gender.

**American Indian or Alaska Native Women**

A number of factors not only complicate research on smoking patterns among American Indians and Alaska Natives but also seem to preclude generalization from one population to another. Specifically, reported smoking rates have varied widely among American Indian tribal affiliations and by geographic location, from as low as 13 percent among Navajos to as high as 70 percent among Indians outside the Southwest (Lando et al. 1992). Additionally, the type of cigarettes, manner of inhaling, and number of cigarettes smoked vary widely. Moreover, 54 percent of American Indians live in urban settings, and another large percentage live on rural reservations. No studies have addressed factors that may influence smoking cessation among American Indian or Alaska Native women specifically. A few studies that combined results for women and men have been reported.

NHIS data showed interest in smoking cessation among American Indians and Alaska Natives who smoked. In 1993, 70.3 percent of American Indian or Alaska Native women and 57.3 percent of men who smoked indicated that they would like to stop (USDHHS 1998).

A smoking cessation project in four urban Indian Health clinics enrolled 601 Native American smokers; they were randomly assigned to participate in a Doctors Helping Smokers model to increase smoking cessation (Johnson et al. 1997). After one year of treatment, the investigators found a higher rate of self-reported cessation in the treatment group than in the control group (7.1 vs. 4.9 percent), but cotinine levels indicated that cessation rates were comparable for both study arms. Rates were not reported separately by gender.

Recent work with the Lumbee Indians in North Carolina has explored the prevalence and predictors of tobacco use among Lumbee women (Spangler et al. 1997). Data have suggested that a church intervention would be a good approach for Lumbee women who have high rates of tobacco use. In a survey of 400 adult Lumbee Indians, 63 percent were church members, and a dose-response relationship was observed between church attendance and the number of cigarettes smoked per day (Spangler et al. 1998).

### Asian or Pacific Islander Women

Because of the small sample sizes of Asians and Pacific Islanders who have participated in epidemiologic surveys and smoking cessation programs, little information has been available on cessation rates and associated factors (King et al. 1997). In one of the few studies that examined racial and ethnic differences in smoking behavior and attitudes among patients at physician practices, Asian smokers (women and men) reported significantly more pressure from friends to stop smoking than did white, African American, or Hispanic smokers. Asians and Hispanics were significantly more likely than the other racial and ethnic groups to report that not exposing their children to smoking was an important reason for quitting (Vander Martin et al. 1990). No studies of smoking cessation interventions among Asian or Pacific Islander women have been reported.

## Older Women

### Special Health Concerns and Smoking Cessation Needs Among Older Women Who Smoke

Older women have some unique smoking risks, including increased risk for postmenopausal osteoporosis (see "Menstrual Function, Menopause, and Benign Gynecologic Conditions" in Chapter 3). Although no studies have focused specifically on smoking cessation among older women, some studies have been able to analyze data for this group, with mixed results. Rimer and colleagues (1994) found that older men were more likely to quit than older women. On the other hand, Hill and colleagues (1993) found that older women were more likely to quit than older men. Yet another study found no differences in quitting between older women and older men (Ossip-Klein et al. 1997). More research is needed for this group.

Older women who smoke are less likely than older men who smoke to be married, to have at least a high school education, or to belong to community organizations and are more likely to be widowed, to live alone, to be unemployed, and to report an annual household income of less than $25,000 (King et al. 1990; Orleans et al. 1990, 1991a; Bjornson et al. 1995). King and associates (1990) found that disparities between women and men aged 50 through 64 years in educational level and marital status were associated with continued smoking versus smoking cessation. Bjornson and colleagues (1995) reported similar results for participants in the Lung Health Study (mean age at entry into the study, 49 years).

The age gap in awareness of the health effects of smoking is just as apparent among women as it is among men (Orleans et al. 1990, 1994a), but some gender-specific differences have implications for treatment. In one study, older women aged 50 through 74 years who smoked were significantly less likely than their male counterparts to report that they had ever received advice from a physician to stop smoking (53 vs. 58 percent) (Orleans et al. 1994a). Nonetheless, significantly more of these women than men rated concerns about their future health (77 vs. 69 percent), their present health (62 vs. 52 percent), the effects of their smoking on others (40 vs. 31 percent), and the cost of smoking (38 vs. 26 percent) as important motives to stop smoking. Older women also were significantly more likely than older men who smoked to report weight gain (33 vs. 21 percent) or possible weight gain (30 vs. 18 percent) as important barriers to smoking cessation. As Gritz (1994) pointed out, women's greater difficulty in controlling their weight in the perimenopausal and postmenopausal periods may prove to be an additional barrier to smoking cessation.

### Promising Treatment Approaches for Older Women Who Smoke

The 1990 Surgeon General's report on the health benefits of smoking cessation (USDHHS 1990) declared older adults in the United States to be an important target for national smoking cessation initiatives. These initiatives spurred new efforts to develop and evaluate smoking cessation treatments for this population. Several studies have indicated that older adults, both women and men, benefit from a variety of smoking cessation treatments and are at least as likely as younger smokers to succeed in stopping smoking, either on their own or with the aid of a formal clinic, self-help, or pharmacologic treatment (Vetter and Ford 1990; Hill et al. 1993; Orleans et al. 1994b; Rimer et al. 1994; Morgan et al. 1996; Ossip-Klein et al. 1997). No studies have examined treatments specifically tailored for older women, but one study found that *Clear Horizons*, a self-help guide tailored for all older adults, proved more effective at a 12-month follow-up than did a generic smoking cessation guide designed for smokers of all ages (Rimer et al. 1994).

Evidence of gender-specific differences in smoking cessation outcomes among older smokers has not been consistent. Hill and colleagues (1993) reported a higher percentage of biochemically verified or informant-verified cessation among older women than among older men after an intensive three-month group treatment program that involved behavioral training alone, behavioral training with nicotine gum, behavioral training with physical exercise, or physical exercise only. Participants were aged 50 years or older and had smoked for at least 30 years. Rimer and colleagues (1994) assigned persons aged 50 through 74 years to three study groups: those who received the *Clear Horizons* guide plus two reinforcing telephone calls, those who received the guide alone, and those who received the generic NCI smoking cessation guide, *Clearing the Air* (control group). In all three groups combined, the investigators found that the three-month, self-reported cessation was significantly higher among men than among women (13 vs. 8 percent). In a recent study of smokers aged 60 years or older using the *Clear Horizons* guide, Ossip-Klein and colleagues (1997) found that a higher percentage of women stopped smoking if they received two proactive telephone calls along with the guide, whereas the percentage of men who stopped was higher if they received the guide with two mailed prompts to call a smoking cessation helpline. Orleans and colleagues (1994b) found no gender-specific differences at six-month follow-up in the percentage of smokers aged 65 through 74 years who filled prescriptions for transdermal nicotine.

Two randomized controlled trials of older adults seen in primary care settings found that brief intervention doubled the number of persons who stopped smoking (Vetter and Ford 1990; Morgan et al. 1996). Neither Morgan and colleagues (1996) nor Vetter and Ford (1990) reported gender-specific differences.

Dale and colleagues (1997) found a 24.8-percent six-month cessation rate among 615 women and men patients aged 65 through 82 years who received brief smoking cessation consultation that combined behavioral counseling with recommended pharmacologic aids. Orleans and colleagues (1994b) found a self-reported six-month cessation rate of 29 percent among low-income women and men smokers aged 65 through 74 years who had received transdermal nicotine with minimal smoking cessation advice or who had received help from their health care providers. More frequent contact with physicians or pharmacists was associated with more appropriate use of the patch (e.g., less concomitant smoking) and a higher percentage of cessation. Neither study reported results by gender.

# Programmatic and Policy Approaches to Smoking Cessation

## Worksite Programs to Reduce Smoking Among Women

Almost two-thirds of women between 20 and 65 years of age are in the labor force in the United States (U.S. Department of Commerce 1993). Consequently, workplace programs to reduce smoking can reach a large segment of women who smoke. A review of quitting among those who participate in smoking cessation programs conducted in worksites suggested that women and men are equally likely to stop smoking in programs conducted at the site. Mixed results have been found, however, for the effect of worksite-wide cessation activities among all smokers at the site. Of three studies, one had an overall effect and two did not. However, only one study analyzed data by gender (Gritz et al. 1998); an effect was found among women in the treatment arm compared with women in the control arm. More studies need to conduct separate analysis by gender. Similarly, examination of the effects of restrictive worksite smoking policies on cessation indicated an overall effect; however, few studies reported the data by gender.

### Prevalence of Worksite Smoking Control Interventions

*On-Site Smoking Cessation Activities*

On-site smoking cessation activities include intensive multisession groups similar to clinic programs, self-help individual or group programs, stop-smoking contests, and learning opportunities such as lung function tests and alveolar carbon monoxide readings. At the less intensive end of the spectrum are activities such as distributing literature on smoking cessation or on risks from smoking. The Office of Disease Prevention and Health Promotion of USDHHS sponsored two national surveys (in 1985 and 1992) that assessed the prevalence of a variety of worksite health promotion activities. (See Fielding and Piserchia 1989 and USDHHS 1993a for a description of the methods and basic findings of the 1985 and 1992 surveys, respectively.) Each survey included a probability sample of about 1,500 private worksites that employed 50 or more workers. In 1985, about 14 percent of worksites offered some sort of "participatory" smoking cessation activity (counseling, classes, or special events) and about 19 percent offered information in the form of brochures, cessation manuals, and posters. In 1992, approximately 22 percent of all worksites offered participatory activities and approximately 36 percent offered informational resources (USDHHS 1993b). Both surveys found that cessation activities were substantially more prevalent among the larger worksites than among the smaller worksites. Worksite resources also varied according to industry (Table 5.1). Worksites in the utilities, transportation, and communication industries were most likely to offer on-site activities, and those in the wholesale and retail industries were least likely to do so.

*Restrictive Smoking Policies*

Restrictive smoking policies are often seen as a facilitator of smoking cessation. The growth of worksite smoking restrictions has been dramatic (Fielding and Piserchia 1989; USDHHS 1993a). In 1985, 27 percent of the worksites sampled reported having a "formal policy restricting smoking." At that time, any policy that limited smoking to particular areas or times (e.g., only during breaks or lunch) was considered a formal smoking policy. The 1992 survey, which posed the question more explicitly, found that 59 percent of worksites either banned indoor smoking entirely or restricted it to separately ventilated areas. Another 28 percent restricted smoking to designated areas without separate ventilation.

As with on-site smoking cessation activities, restrictive smoking policies are more common in larger worksites. Among the smallest sites surveyed in 1992, 32 percent reported being smoke-free; among the largest sites, 55 percent were smoke-free. Restrictive policies were most prevalent in the service and

**Table 5.1. Women's access to worksite tobacco control resources in various industries during the 1990s**

| | Industry | | | | | |
|---|---|---|---|---|---|---|
| | Manufacturing | Wholesale and retail | Services | Utilities, transportation, communication | Finance, insurance, real estate | Other |
| Percentage of private worksites with smoking cessation activities, 1992* | 44.6 | 33.1 | 40.8 | 49.0 | 40.4 | 36.7 |
| Percentage of private worksites with ban on indoor smoking, 1992* | 28.3 | 26.5 | 41.7 | 34.5 | 42.0 | 35.3 |
| Percentage of women reporting smoke-free worksites | | | | | | |
| 1993† | 36.9 | 31.8 | 63.1 | 52.4 | 56.1 | 33.5 |
| 1996‡ | 55.7 | 52.7 | 77.5 | 71.9 | 73.5 | 60.2 |
| Percentage of current smokers among women, 1996‡ § | 27.1 | 29.1 | 18.8 | 22.5 | 19.5 | 21.1 |

*U.S. Department of Health and Human Services 1993b.

†U.S. Bureau of the Census, National Cancer Institute Tobacco Use Supplement, public use data tape, 1992–1993.

‡U.S. Bureau of the Census, National Cancer Institute Tobacco Use Supplement, public use data tape, 1995–1996.

§In 1996, 12.5% of employed women worked in manufacturing; 21.8% in wholesale and retail; 46.4% in services; 4.1% in utilities, transportation, communication; 8.4% in finance, insurance, real estate; and 6.8% in other industries.

financial industries and least prevalent in the wholesale and retail industry. Surveys of women workers about worksite smoking policies in 1993 and 1996 reflected the same industry differences that emerged from the national worksite surveys in 1985 and 1992 (Table 5.1).

*Women's Access to Worksite Smoking Control Resources*

Women tend to be segregated into particular industries, and smoking prevalence varies markedly by industry. For example, in 1996, 46.4 percent of employed women were working in the service industry (Table 5.1). Of those women, 37.6 percent were employed in professional services such as health and education, and a subset (8.7 percent) were employed in business or personal services such as advertising, data processing, hotels, and entertainment. The prevalence of smoking among women in these service industries was lower (18.8 percent) than that among women in other industries. The service industry ranked first of five major industries in the prevalence of women who reported smoke-free worksites and third in the prevalence of smoking cessation activities. The next largest employer of women was the wholesale and retail industry, which included 21.8 percent of working women in the United States. The smoking prevalence among women was much higher in this industry (29.1 percent) than in the service industry, and this industry ranked lowest in the prevalence of smoke-free worksites and in the prevalence of worksite smoking cessation activities.

**Efficacy of Worksite Interventions for Women Who Smoke**

*On-Site Smoking Cessation Activities*

To ascertain the efficacy of on-site worksite smoking cessation programs, Fisher and associates (1990b) performed a meta-analysis. The analysis included 20 controlled studies of worksite smoking cessation programs conducted between 1984 and 1990. For 18 of the 20 studies, the cessation proportion was defined as the percentage of program participants who stopped smoking. For the remaining two studies, the cessation proportion was based on smokers in the worksite as a whole. The authors determined that participating in an intervention worksite smoking cessation program increased the likelihood of smoking cessation by 58 percent over being in the control group or comparison group. The percentage of women versus men in the treatment conditions did not appear to be associated with the proportion who stopped smoking, a finding that suggested that women and men who participated were equally likely to stop smoking.

The effect of worksite smoking cessation activities on the smoking behavior among all smokers at the worksite has been investigated in three multisite, randomized trials with multiple risk factors; each of these trials involved sustained interventions over several years (Jeffery et al. 1993; Glasgow et al. 1995; Sorensen et al. 1996). In each case, the outcome variable was either the change in smoking prevalence in the participating worksites from baseline to the end of the intervention period or the difference in the proportion of those who stopped smoking in intervention versus comparison sites. Before-and-after surveys were conducted on cross-sectional and cohort samples of entire worksite populations. Only one study (Jeffery et al. 1993) demonstrated a significant reduction in smoking prevalence among both women and men combined in intervention versus comparison sites.

The Healthy Worker Project (Jeffery et al. 1993) randomly assigned 32 worksites to a group that received two-year smoking cessation treatment or to a control group that received no treatment. In the treatment group, 11-session classes given by professional health educators were repeatedly offered to all smokers. Smoking prevalence at the treatment sites decreased by 2 to 4 percentage points among women and men combined, whereas it increased by 1 percentage point at the comparison sites, a statistically significant effect. Slightly more than one-half of the employees and approximately two-thirds of program participants were women, but differences in the effect of the program were not reported by gender.

The Take Heart Project (Glasgow et al. 1995) randomly assigned 26 sites to an 18-month, multifaceted tobacco control and nutrition intervention or to a control condition. Results indicated that smoking prevalence dropped by 3 to 5 percentage points in both the intervention and control conditions, and no significant benefit of the intervention was discernible. A replication of the Take Heart trial suggested that smoking prevalence decreased at the intervention worksites, but the differences were not significant (Glasgow et al. 1997b). The data were not reported by gender.

The Working Well Trial (Sorensen et al. 1996) tested the effectiveness of a worksite smoking cessation intervention at 84 worksites. The sites were randomly assigned to an intervention program or to a comparison program. Intervention sites received an intensive series of programs that was geared for all levels of readiness to stop smoking and that was directed both at individual workers and the worksite environment. Comparison sites received either no intervention or a minimal intervention consisting of posters and self-help manuals. Results indicated a decline in smoking prevalence of 3 to 4 percentage points among both the intervention and comparison sites. Although the proportion of smokers who stopped smoking was slightly higher in the intervention sites than in the comparison sites (13.8 vs. 12.3 percent), the difference was not statistically significant. A subsequent analysis of data from the Working Well Trial examined smoking cessation results among women and men separately (Gritz et al. 1998). Results demonstrated a significant effect among women but not among men. Women at the intervention worksites were 1.5 times as likely to stop smoking as women at the comparison worksites (see "Cessation Activities in Occupational Settings for Women of Low Socioeconomic Status" earlier in this chapter).

*Restrictive Smoking Policies*

There is reason to expect that a restrictive smoking policy would contribute to heightened cessation among smokers because of its effect on motivation and on reducing cues that could trigger relapse (Walsh and Gordon 1986; Biener et al. 1989a). Although consistent evidence has indicated that restrictive policies reduce the number of cigarettes consumed daily (Biener et al. 1989b; Borland et al. 1990; Brigham et al. 1994), evidence for increased cessation has been more ambiguous. In a study in which data were gathered on employed women and men who were current or former smokers, multivariate analyses were used to examine associations between worksite smoking policies and cessation, with smoking status the response variable in logistic regression (Brenner and Mielck 1992). The study included 98 women smokers, of whom 66 were allowed to smoke at the workplace and 31 were not; 45 percent of the women not allowed to smoke at the workplace stopped smoking, whereas 18 percent of women allowed to smoke at the workplace stopped (RR, 0.2; 95 percent CI, 0.1 to 0.5). This result suggested that, at least among women, restrictive worksite policies were useful for encouraging cessation. Patten and colleagues (1995a) analyzed the cessation proportion in a representative sample of California workers who were followed up over two years as a function of the worksite smoking policy they reported at each assessment. The cessation rate for smokers continuously employed at a smoke-free site was more than double the rate for those continuously employed at a non-smoke-free site (21.7 vs. 9.2 percent). In a separate analysis of the 1990–1992 longitudinal sample of the California Tobacco Survey, Pierce and colleagues (1994a) provided additional evidence for the efficacy of worksite smoking bans. Using an index of progress toward smoking cessation that has been shown to have predictive validity and controlling for demographic characteristics, they demonstrated that workers employed at smoke-free sites in 1992 were significantly more likely than those not employed at smoke-free sites to have made progress toward smoking cessation. Similarly, a longitudinal analysis of data collected for COMMIT found that among persons who were smokers in 1988, those who reported working in a smoke-free worksite in 1993 were 25 percent more likely to have stopped smoking during the intervening period than those employed in sites with less restrictive policies (Glasgow et al. 1997a).

Analyses of the Massachusetts Tobacco Survey, a telephone survey of a representative sample of adults in Massachusetts conducted by the Center for Survey Research at the University of Massachusetts (Boston) in 1994, indicated that restrictive policies may be particularly beneficial for women who smoke (Lois Biener, unpublished data). Controlling for daily smoking rate, the researchers found that both women smokers and men smokers employed at smoke-free worksites reported smoking significantly fewer cigarettes during working hours than did their counterparts employed at sites where some smoking was permitted. When asked whether they smoked less at work because of the worksite policy, women were more likely than men to answer in the affirmative (85 vs. 66 percent). Women were also significantly more likely than men to attribute a reduced overall rate of daily smoking to their worksite policy (73 vs. 54 percent).

## Community-Based Efforts to Reduce Smoking Among Women

Community studies offer opportunities for all smokers in a community to receive messages and assistance in smoking cessation. In the dozen or so community studies that have been conducted, the results have been mixed. Recent outcomes of community studies in the United States have tended to show few, if any, differences in smoking cessation between women and men (Fortmann et al. 1993; Commit Research Group 1995a,b; Lando et al. 1995; Winkleby et al. 1997). Some studies in other countries (e.g., Africa, India) have shown differences in cessation between women and men. In these studies, women were more likely to quit (Steenkamp et al. 1991; Anantha et al. 1995). It is unclear why such differences exist.

**Community Studies of Smoking Cessation**

Several community studies have been conducted to investigate behavioral risk factors related to cardiovascular disease (Farquhar et al. 1977; Maccoby et al. 1977; Farquhar 1978; McAlister et al. 1982). Smoking cessation was one of the behavior changes addressed. Only one randomized study in the United States, COMMIT, focused exclusively on smoking cessation (COMMIT Research Group 1991, 1995a).

Table 5.2 summarizes the community studies. The types of smoking changes reported in community studies have varied widely. Some studies reported net differences in changes from baseline prevalence between intervention and comparison communities. Others reported before-and-after changes in prevalence for intervention communities only. Still others reported on smoking cessation in a cohort of smokers followed up over time or in a group of smokers asked retrospectively about their smoking behavior. Finally, some studies reported changes in the number of cigarettes smoked. Not all studies reported on smoking cessation or prevalence among women and men separately. The cessation proportion is presented as the percentage of the cohort (intervention or control) that stopped smoking. Significance tests are based on comparisons between intervention communities and control communities in the change in smoking prevalence or cessation proportion.

The Community, Hypertension, Atherosclerosis, and Diabetes Program (CHAD) was initiated in Israel in 1970. It was a community-based program directed at reducing cardiovascular risk factors among residents of four adjacent housing projects (Abramson et al. 1981). Survey assessment at baseline (1970) and 5 years later (1975) showed a net decrease in smoking prevalence among women that was far less than that among men and was not significantly different from that in the control community. By 10 years after intervention, however, net decreases in smoking prevalence were significantly greater in the intervention sites than in the control sites among both women and men, and the declines were greater than those seen in the rest of Israel for the same period (Gofin et al. 1986).

Both the Stanford Three-Community Study and the Finnish North Karelia Project commenced in 1972. Both projects used mass media; Stanford also used intensive face-to-face intervention for persons at high risk for smoking-related diseases (Farquhar et al. 1977; Maccoby et al. 1977), and the North Karelia Project used community organization, environmental modification, and educational programs (Salonen et al. 1981; McAlister et al. 1982; Puska et al. 1983b). The Stanford study did not report overall results among women and men separately. In the North Karelia Project, significant differences between the intervention and control counties in smoking prevalence occurred among men but not among women (Salonen et al. 1981; Puska et al. 1983b).

A series of community-based antismoking campaigns in Australia that began in 1978 used mass-media and community programs to encourage smoking cessation. Significant differences in the change in smoking prevalence among women were found in the North Coast study (Egger et al. 1983) and the Sydney study (Dwyer et al. 1986), but the results for the Melbourne study (Pierce et al. 1990) were less clear. In the North Coast study, women and men aged 18 through 25 years had lower smoking prevalence in both intervention communities than did women and men aged 65 years or older (Egger et al. 1983). The reductions in prevalence in all age groups were more pronounced in the media plus community programs' town than in the media only town. In Melbourne, the prevalence of smoking among women with at least some university education declined by 23 percent, the largest rate of decline among all the groups in either the intervention city or control city (Macaskill et al. 1992).

The Coronary Risk Factor Study (CORIS) conducted in three rural South African cities with both white and black Afrikaner residents used small media (posters, billboards, newspapers, and direct mail) to encourage persons to lower their risk factors for coronary artery disease, including smoking (Steenkamp et al. 1991). The media campaign was supplemented in one of the cities with an interpersonal intervention for high-risk persons. This intervention included an intensive smoking cessation program. Net decreases in the prevalence of smoking among women ranged from 3.0 to 4.0 percentage points in the two intervention communities. Among men, the net difference between the intervention and control cities was an increase in smoking prevalence of 0.9 percentage points in the city with only a media campaign and a decrease of 3.7 percentage points in the city with media plus intervention. The percentage of women who stopped smoking was significantly higher in the intervention cities than in the control city and was also higher than that among men.

Three community-based projects to reduce coronary heart disease were the Stanford Five-City Project, the Minnesota Heart Health Program, and the

Pawtucket Heart Health Program (Winkleby et al. 1992, 1997; Fortmann et al. 1993). Each had intervention and control cities and used a variety of community-based programs, such as mass media, community education, and multiple education channels. In the Stanford Five-City Project, smoking cessation increased in cohorts of women and men in both the intervention and control cities, but the difference between cessation rates in these cities was significant only among men. Cross-sectional surveys also found that the prevalence of smoking decreased significantly among men, but not among women. The Minnesota Heart Health Program reported no significant differences in the prevalence of smoking cessation between cohorts in the intervention and control cities. However, cross-sectional surveys conducted annually showed an intervention effect among women of 1.3 percent overall above the secular trend ($p < 0.05$), but no significant effect among men (Lando et al. 1995; Winkleby et al. 1997). The Pawtucket Heart Health Program found no significant differences in the prevalence of smoking cessation between cohorts in the intervention and control cities followed up over time, but it did not report results of the cohort by gender (Carleton et al. 1995). A joint analysis of the cross-sectional data from these three studies found no significant decreases in smoking prevalence or increases in smoking cessation associated with the intervention among either women or men (Winkleby et al. 1997).

A six-year, three-community study (one intervention community and two control communities), initiated in India in 1986, focused solely on tobacco use. It sought to prevent initiation of tobacco use among nonusers and to encourage cessation among users. Prevalence of tobacco use was higher among women than among men at baseline, but 99 percent of the women tobacco users chewed tobacco or used snuff instead of smoking tobacco. The total prevalence of tobacco use decreased significantly more in the intervention community than in the control communities, and the differences were greater among women than among men (Anantha et al. 1995).

COMMIT recruited 11 pairs of communities, focused exclusively on smoking cessation, and used the community as the unit of both randomization and analysis (COMMIT Research Group 1995a). Cohorts of heavy smokers ($\geq$ 25 cigarettes per day) and light or moderate smokers (<25 cigarettes per day) were followed up annually. A cross-sectional survey also was conducted at baseline and again at the end of the study. In the cohort of heavy smokers, no significant intervention effect on the proportion who had stopped smoking was found. Although men were significantly more likely than women to stop smoking, this difference disappeared when treatment condition, age, and education were controlled for. In the cohort of light or moderate smokers, smokers in the intervention cities stopped smoking in significantly higher proportions than did smokers in the control cities, but fewer women than men stopped. No significant interaction of gender by treatment was observed (COMMIT Research Group 1995b).

A number of smaller, nonrandomized community studies have been conducted in recent years. In a quasi-experimental design, Fisher and colleagues (1998) organized three low-income, predominantly African American neighborhoods in St. Louis, Missouri, to promote nonsmoking, and compared the outcomes with those in three similar neighborhoods in Kansas City, Missouri (see "Other Cessation Programs for African American Women" earlier in this chapter). The investigators found significant treatment effects, and men were significantly more likely than women to stop smoking (RR, 1.6; 95 percent CI, 1.3 to 1.9).

A community-wide cable program used a time-series design to assess the effectiveness of cable television in promoting smoking cessation (Valois et al. 1996). At one year, the cessation rate was 17 percent. This percentage compared favorably with other televised cessation programs.

A number of other community smoking cessation intervention programs are in progress. These include the American Stop Smoking Intervention Study (ASSIST), which was initially funded by NCI and the American Cancer Society and has now been transferred to CDC; the SmokeLess States program funded by the Robert Wood Johnson Foundation; and Initiatives to Mobilize for the Prevention and Control of Tobacco Use (IMPACT), another CDC-funded program. In combination with concurrent activities at the federal, state, and local levels, these efforts to control tobacco use hold considerable promise for reducing smoking among women. An interim analysis found that by 1996, per capita tobacco consumption was 7 percent lower in the 17 states participating in the ASSIST program than in the 32 non-ASSIST states (Manley et al. 1997). However, results by gender have not yet been published.

**Table 5.2. Changes in smoking behavior reported in studies of community-based smoking cessation programs**

| Project | Community | | Percentage point change in smoking prevalence of intervention vs. control community | | Percentage of intervention cohort or control cohort that quit smoking | |
|---|---|---|---|---|---|---|
| | Intervention | Control | Women | Men | Women | Men |
| Israel Community, Hypertension, Atherosclerosis and Diabetes Program (1971–1981) | 4 housing projects | | -0.5 (at 5 years) | -5.9* (at 5 years) | NA[†] | NA |
| | | | -4.1* (at 10 years) | -7.2* (at 10 years) | NA | NA |
| | | 1 adjacent neighborhood | | | NA | NA |
| Stanford Three-Community Study (1972–1975) | | | Gender not reported | | | |
| | 1 city with mass media only | | 3.6 | | NA | NA |
| | 1 city with mass media plus individual intervention | | -35.1* | | 47.0* | 52.0* |
| | | 1 city | | | | |
| Finland North Karelia Project (1973–1983) | 1 rural county | | -0.1 (at 5 years) | -1.3* (at 5 years) | NA | NA |
| | | | -0.1 (at 10 years) | -2.7* (at 10 years) | NA | NA |
| | | 1 matched neighboring county | | | NA | NA |
| Australia | | | | | | |
| North Coast (1978–1980) | 1 city with mass media | | -6.3 to 3.9*[‡] | -6.2 to -3.0*[‡] | NR[§] | NR |
| | 1 city with mass media plus community programs | | -10.5 to -4.0* | -10.7 to -4.8*[‡] | NR | NR |
| | | 1 city | | | NR | NR |
| Sydney (1983–1984) | 1 city | | -0.9* | -1.4* | NR | NR |
| | | rest of Australia | | | NR | NR |
| Melbourne (1983–1988) | 1 city | | -5.0 to +5.0[Δ] | -3.0 to +1.0[Δ] | NA | NA |
| | | 1 city | | | NA | NA |

*p <0.05 vs. control community.
[†]NA = Not applicable; no cohort tracked.
[‡]Depending on age.
[§]NR = Not reported.
[Δ]Depending on education.
Sources: **Community Hypertension, Atherosclerosis and Diabetic Program:** Abramson et al. 1981. **Stanford Three-Community Study:** Maccoby et al. 1977; Meyer et al. 1980. **North Karelia Project:** Puska et al. 1979, 1983a,b; Salonen et al. 1981. **North Coast study:** Egger et al. 1983. **Sydney study:** Dwyer et al. 1986. **Melbourne study:** Pierce et al. 1990. **Coronary Risk Factor Study:** Steenkamp et al. 1991. **Stanford Five-City Project:** Fortmann et al. 1993. **Minnesota Heart Health Program:** Lando et al. 1995. **Pawtucket Heart Health Program:** Carleton et al. 1995. **Anti-tobacco Community Education:** Anatha et al. 1995. **COMMIT:** COMMIT Research Group 1995a,b.

**Table 5.2. Continued**

| Project | Community | | Percentage point change in smoking prevalence of intervention vs. control community | | Percentage of intervention cohort or control cohort that quit smoking | |
|---|---|---|---|---|---|---|
| | Intervention | Control | Women | Men | Women | Men |
| Africa Coronary Risk Factor Study (1979–1984) | 1 high-intensity city | | -4.0* | -3.7 | 31.4* | 22.8 |
| | 1 low-intensity city | | -3.0 | 0.9 | 28.3* | 16.9 |
| | | 1 city | | | 15.5 | 20.1 |
| Stanford Five-City Project (1979–1985) | 2 cities | | -0.6 | 1.02 | 4.8 | 10.9 |
| | | 3 cities | | | 5.6 | 2.3 |
| Minnesota Heart Health Program (1980–1990) | 3 cities | 3 cities | -1.3* | 0.01 | Differences reported to be not significant | |
| Pawtucket Heart Health Program (1981–1993) | | | Gender not reported | | Gender not reported | |
| | 1 city | | 2.6 | | -8.9 | |
| | | 1 city | | | -8.2 | |
| India Anti-tobacco Community Education[¶] | 1 area of 117 villages | | -13.4* | -8.1* | 36.7* | 26.5* |
| | | 1 area of 126 villages | | | 1.5 | 1.1 |
| | | 1 area of 120 villages | | | 0.5 | 1.1 |
| Community Intervention Trial for Smoking Cessation (COMMIT) (1988–1993) | | | Gender not reported | | | 19.2[††] |
| | 11 cities** | | -0.3 | | 17.6[††] | 31.4*[‡‡] |
| | | | | | 30.6*[‡‡] | 20.1[††] |
| | | 11 cities** | | | 17.6[††] | 28.4[‡‡] |
| | | | | | 27.7[‡‡] | |

*$p < 0.05$ vs. control community.
[¶]Data reflect all tobacco use (i.e., cigarettes, oral tobacco). Only 1% of women smoked tobacco; most chewed or used snuff.
**Randomized.
[††]Heavy smokers only.
[‡‡]Light/moderate smokers only.

## Tobacco-Related Policies: Attitudes and Effects

Since the first Surgeon General's report in 1964 on the health consequences of cigarette smoking, tobacco control policies have been an important component of the campaign to reduce tobacco use. Public attitudes toward these policies have been closely monitored through an array of public opinion surveys. Overall, few differences seem to exist between women and men and their attitudes toward tobacco-related policies. Women, however, are more likely than men to believe that second-hand smoke is very harmful (Saad 1997), to support tax increases if they benefit the community (Gallup Organization 1993), to restrict areas where youth can purchase tobacco products (Strouse and Hall 1994), and to support restrictions on the advertising and marketing of tobacco (Biener et al. 1994; Pierce et al. 1994a; Strouse and Hall 1994). Findings on the effects of tobacco use policies have been more mixed. In policies restricting smoking in public places, few gender differences appear to exist. The impact of taxation policies on women and men is mixed. Some studies indicated that women are less responsive than men to such policies (Chaloupka 1990, 1992; Chaloupka and Wechsler 1995), and others indicated that women are more responsive than men (Lewit et al. 1997; Chaloupka and Pacula 1998). Little information has been available about the effects of advertising and marketing restrictions on smoking onset or smoking cessation.

### Monitoring Public Tobacco-Related Attitudes

Federal, state, and local governments have introduced policies that range from federally mandated health warnings on all cigarette packaging and a ban on smoking on all domestic airline flights, to increases in state tobacco taxes and local ordinances restricting smoking in restaurants. Some organizations and accrediting bodies have instituted tobacco control policies for their members. For example, since 1991 the Joint Commission on Accreditation of Healthcare Organizations has required hospitals to be smoke-free as a condition of their accreditation. Even in the absence of legislation or accreditation requirements, an increasing number of employers are instituting policies restricting or banning smoking at the workplace.

Several caveats must be noted in the interpretation of these studies. Surveys assessing attitudes toward smoking policies have seldom been based on national random samples, thus limiting the generalizability of the findings. The few surveys that have included national random samples (Gallup Organization 1993; Strouse and Hall 1994) are generally of limited scope. In contrast, two surveys in Massachusetts (Biener et al. 1994) and California (California Department of Health Services, public use data tape, 1994) assessed a wide array of attitudes. These are states with progressive legislation supporting tobacco control, and the results of these surveys may not be representative of national opinions. The COMMIT project, representing a diverse set of communities, found little variation across communities in attitudes toward tobacco control policies (CDC 1991). Any differences in attitudes toward such policies among women and men may be related to differential smoking prevalence, which is a confounder that may not be measured in opinion surveys.

### Policies Restricting or Prohibiting Smoking

With increasing evidence of the health effects of exposure to ETS, policies prohibiting smoking in public places have multiplied. Restrictions on smoking have been legislated by state and local clean indoor air laws and have been adopted in worksites through the initiatives of individual employers or managers (see "Worksite Programs to Reduce Smoking Among Women" earlier in this chapter). Several studies have reported that women are more likely than men to work in places where smoking is restricted (Borland et al. 1992; Patten et al. 1995b; Gerlach et al. 1997; Royce et al. 1997) and that women report lower levels of workplace exposure to ETS (Borland et al. 1992; Patten et al. 1995b) and higher levels of compliance with smoking policies in their places of employment (Sorensen et al. 1992a).

#### *Attitudes Toward Restrictions and Prohibitions on Smoking*

A 1997 poll showed that a majority of women and men in the United States believed that second-hand smoke is very harmful to adults and that this perception differs by gender (61 percent of women and 49 percent of men) (Saad 1997). These prevalences are substantial increases from a 1994 poll in which only 45 percent of women and 27 percent of men thought that second-hand smoke was very harmful to adults (Saad 1997).

In surveys conducted in the early to mid-1990s, only small gender-specific differences were observed in attitudes toward banning smoking in indoor work areas, restaurants, shopping malls, public buildings, and indoor sports or concert arenas (Table 5.3). Other surveys have assessed employee attitudes toward policies restricting or prohibiting smoking in their own worksite. Support for such policies is generally high, and the few studies that have included gender in their analyses have found no differences in women's and men's attitudes toward these policies (Borland et al. 1989).

#### *Effects of Policies Restricting or Prohibiting Smoking*

A few studies have evaluated how legislation restricting or banning smoking affects smoking behavior. Chaloupka (1992) assessed the effect of clean indoor air laws on average cigarette consumption, by participants' state of residence. The laws were associated with significantly diminished average cigarette consumption. However, the effect of these laws differed by gender: average consumption among men was reduced after passage of these laws, whereas women's consumption was unaffected.

Two studies have focused on the effect of restrictions on smoking among young people. By using data from a nationally representative survey of students in

**Table 5.3. Support for policies that prohibit smoking in public places, by gender**

| Study | Location | Gender | Location of ban (% supporting policy) | | | | |
|---|---|---|---|---|---|---|---|
| | | | Indoor work areas | Restaurants | Shopping malls | Public buildings | Indoor sports or concert arenas |
| Forster et al. 1991 | 7 Minnesota communities | Women | | | | 49 | |
| | | Men | | | | 46 | |
| California Tobacco Survey 1993* | California | Women | | 41 | | | |
| | | Men | | 37 | | | |
| Massachusetts Tobacco Survey 1993† | Massachusetts | Women | | 49 | | 49 | 64 |
| | | Men | | 46 | | 43 | 52 |
| Shopland et al. 1995 | Maryland | Women | 62 | 47 | 54 | | 66 |
| | | Men | 57 | 46 | 50 | | 62 |

*Technical Report on Analytic Methods and Approaches Used in the 1993 California Tobacco Survey Analysis (Pierce et al. 1994a).

†1993 Massachusetts Tobacco Survey—Tobacco Use and Attitudes at the Start of the Massachusetts Control Program (Biener et al. 1994).

U.S. colleges and universities, Chaloupka and Wechsler (1995) estimated the effects of smoking restrictions among adolescents and young adults. Relatively stringent restrictions on smoking in public places were associated with lower prevalences of smoking, and any restrictions on smoking in public places were associated with smoking fewer cigarettes by smokers. School-based restrictions were associated with lower smoking prevalence among male students but were unrelated to smoking among female students. In contrast, the presence of smoking restrictions in restaurants was associated with lower smoking prevalence among female but not male students. Chaloupka and Pacula (1998) found that restrictions on smoking in public places significantly reduced smoking among male but not female students.

Several studies have examined the effect of restrictions on smoking in the workplace that were implemented independently of legislation (see "Worksite Programs to Reduce Smoking Among Women" earlier in this chapter). One policy analysis suggested that the proportion of women in a workplace had a positive effect on the imposition of smoking restrictions, but no significant effect was found on whether the worksite had a formal, written smoking policy (Gurdon and Flynn 1996). Most studies that have included gender-specific comparisons in their analyses, however, found no significant differences in the effect of these policies on smoking cessation (Millar 1988; Biener et al. 1989b; Stillman et al. 1990; Borland et al. 1991). One larger study assessed perceptions of smokiness and reactions to ETS exposure in 114 worksites in the Working Well Trial and found that although gender-specific differences were small, women were significantly more likely than men to perceive their worksite as smoky (Thompson et al. 1995). However, women were no more likely than men to report being bothered by ETS in the workplace. On the other hand, 1992 NHIS data showed that women exposed to smoking in their immediate work area were more likely than men exposed to ETS to report being bothered by cigarette smoke (see "Exposure to Environmental Tobacco Smoke" in Chapter 2). One assessment of the relationship between worksite smoking prohibitions and smoking cessation, based on a German national sample (Brenner and Mielck 1992), found that cessation, as measured by the percentage of persons who had ever smoked who were currently former smokers, was significantly higher among women who worked where smoking was banned than among those who worked where smoking was permitted. A similar trend was noted among men, but it was not statistically significant.

## Pricing and Taxation Policies

Cigarette price is a major determinant of cigarette consumption and one that can be influenced by tobacco tax policy (Lewit and Coate 1982; Wasserman et al. 1991; Peterson et al. 1992; Emont et al. 1993; Keeler et al. 1993; Meier and Licari 1997; Biener et al. 1998; CDC 1999). After the 1964 Surgeon General's report on the health consequences of smoking was published, states began to increase the tax on cigarettes as a means of discouraging smoking (Warner 1981). In recent years, some states have used revenues from tobacco taxes toward promotion of tobacco control.

### *Attitudes Toward Taxation Policies*

Most surveys that assessed overall public support for tax increases on tobacco observed small or no differences by gender. The 1993 California Tobacco Survey (California Department of Health Services, public use data tape, 1994) found that comparable percentages of women and men wanted to see an increase in the tobacco tax (52 vs. 49 percent). With one exception, related to the amount of the increase, little evidence indicated that women and men differed in their support for increased taxes (Forster et al. 1991; California Department of Health Services, public use data tape, 1994). The Massachusetts Tobacco Survey (Biener et al. 1994) found that women endorsed somewhat smaller cigarette tax increases per pack on average than did men ($1.47 vs. $1.81).

Women and men tend to differ in their support for tax increases, depending on the proposed use of the funds generated. A Gallup Organization poll (1993) of U.S. adults found that women were somewhat more likely than men to support an increased tobacco tax if they knew the funds would be used for community benefits such as supporting national health care (76 vs. 66 percent), rebuilding inner cities (52 vs. 45 percent), encouraging smokers to stop smoking (64 vs. 56 percent), and preventing smoking initiation among youth (76 vs. 71 percent). Similarly, a survey of Minnesota residents (Forster et al. 1991) found that women were significantly more likely than men to strongly support tax incentives to employers for smoking cessation programs at work (43 vs. 33 percent). The Massachusetts Tobacco Survey (Biener et al. 1994) found only small differences between women and men in support for additional tobacco taxation if the funds would be used for smoking reduction (80 vs. 76 percent), smoking and health programs (76 vs. 70 percent), or general government purposes (31 vs. 32 percent).

### *Effects of Taxation Policies*

The effects of taxation policies on smoking consumption has been assessed by using the standard economic estimate of the price elasticity of demand, which is the percentage change in quantity of cigarettes demanded resulting from a 1-percent change in price. Estimates of the price elasticity of demand for cigarettes vary with the methods used and the populations studied. The 1989 Surgeon General's report on the health consequences of smoking (USDHHS 1989) estimated it to be -0.47, meaning that a 10-percent increase in cigarette prices would result in an overall drop of 4.7 percent in the number of cigarettes demanded (Peterson et al. 1992). Estimated reductions in demand then result in increased smoking cessation, reductions in the number of cigarettes smoked, and prevention of smoking initiation among adolescents and children.

At least eight studies have assessed gender-specific differences in the effect of cigarette pricing on consumption, with inconsistent results. Four studies of U.S. adults concluded that women's cigarette consumption is less responsive to changes in cigarette prices than is men's (Lewit and Coate 1982; Mullahy 1985; Chaloupka 1990, 1992). A fifth study focused on the effect of cigarette pricing on smoking among U.S. college-age young adults. It found that the prevalence of smoking was more sensitive to price among the female students than among the male students but that the average cigarette consumption was more sensitive to price among the male students than among the female students (Chaloupka and Wechsler 1995). In contrast, several studies of U.S. high school students found that price had a larger effect on smoking prevalence among boys but a larger effect on average consumption among girls (Lewit et al. 1997; Chaloupka and Pacula 1998). Finally, one U.S. study and two British studies found that women's cigarette consumption was more responsive to price than men's and that women older than 45 years were more likely to buy generic brand cigarettes in response to price increases (Atkinson and Skegg 1973; Townsend et al. 1994; Cavin and Pierce 1996).

The effect of pricing on cigarette consumption is likely to be greatest among those with fewer economic resources, including adolescents and persons with low income. Several studies have found that cigarette pricing has larger effects among young people than among adults and that pricing changes are more likely to affect adolescents' decisions to smoke than the amount they smoke (Lewit and Coate 1982; Chaloupka and Pacula 1998). Other investigators have reported that smokers of low SES are especially responsive to price changes (Townsend 1987; Biener et al. 1998; CDC 1998c). Proposals to increase cigarette taxes to promote tobacco control among low-SES groups have raised some objections. The economic pressures of low-income families may directly contribute to their high smoking prevalences (Graham 1984, 1990; Marsh and McKay 1994). Reducing smoking in these population groups may require broader social policies that address underlying economic discrepancies.

### Policies Restricting Youth Access to Tobacco

Smoking is typically initiated during adolescence. Results of the 1991 National Household Surveys on Drug Abuse indicated that among persons who had ever tried a cigarette, 88 percent had tried their first cigarette by 18 years of age. Of those who had ever smoked daily, 71 percent did so by age 18 years (USDHHS 1994).

#### *Attitudes Toward Restrictions on Youth Access*

In general, adults strongly and consistently support curbs on minors' access to tobacco products, including access through vending machines. Women are generally more supportive of eliminating vending machines than are men, especially where the machines are accessible to youth (Table 5.4).

Public opinions toward other restrictions on youth access were assessed in the Robert Wood Johnson Youth Access Survey, a national opinion poll conducted in 1994 (Strouse and Hall 1994). Significantly more women than men supported requiring retailers to keep tobacco products behind the counter to prevent shoplifting by minors (83 vs. 71 percent) and supported allowing sale of cigarettes only in certain stores, as with alcohol (53 vs. 39 percent). No differences by gender were noted in support for requiring clerks to check identification of persons who appear underage or for increasing the legal age for sale of cigarettes to either age 19 years or age 21 years.

#### *Effects of Restrictions on Youth Access*

The effect of increased restrictions on use of tobacco among youths is not yet clear. Chaloupka and Pacula (1998) reported that the minimum age for legal purchase of cigarettes was significantly associated with reduced smoking prevalence and lower average consumption among boys, but not among girls. Even in the presence of such laws, girls may have more access to tobacco than do boys. Four studies have reported that girls were able to purchase tobacco with greater ease than were boys (Altman et al. 1989; Forster et al. 1992; Commonwealth of Massachusetts 1994; DiFranza et al. 1996). One of these studies reported that girls and boys were equally likely to be

**Table 5.4. Support for restrictions on vending machines, by gender**

| | | | Type of restriction (% supporting policy) | |
|---|---|---|---|---|
| Study | Location | Gender | Eliminate all vending machines | Eliminate vending machines where teenagers have access |
| Forster et al. 1991 | Minnesota | Women | 39 | 62 |
| | | Men | 32 | 56 |
| California Tobacco Survey 1993* | California | Women | | 89 |
| | | Men | | 85 |
| Massachusetts Tobacco Survey 1993† | Massachusetts | Women | 56 | 91 |
| | | Men | 53 | 94 |
| Mathematica 1994‡ | United States | Women | 79 | 94 |
| | | Men | 68 | 88 |

*Technical Report on Analytic Methods and Approaches Used in the 1993 California Tobacco Survey Analysis (Pierce et al. 1994a).

†1993 Massachusetts Tobacco Survey—Tobacco Use and Attitudes at the Start of the Massachusetts Control Program (Biener et al. 1994).

‡Robert Wood Johnson Foundation Youth Access Survey, December 1994 (Strouse and Hall 1994).

asked for proof of age when attempting to purchase cigarettes (DiFranza et al. 1996). A separate study by Altman and colleagues (1999) found that community interventions aimed at enforcement of restrictions on youth access resulted in a drop in the proportion of stores selling tobacco to minors from 75 percent to 0 percent at the final postintervention test in treatment communities. A significant intervention effect was found for gender in that females in the intervention communities were less likely to use tobacco after the intervention (which informed merchants of restrictions on youth access) than were females in the comparison communities; that association was not found among males.

### Policies Restricting Advertising and Marketing of Tobacco Products

*Attitudes Toward Restrictions on Tobacco Advertising and Marketing*

In response to growing concern about the effect of tobacco advertising among children and adolescents and in the face of tightening restrictions on tobacco advertising, several surveys have been conducted to assess public attitudes toward marketing restrictions. Five studies have indicated that women are more likely than men to support restrictions on marketing and advertising of tobacco (Table 5.5). An additional study similarly reported higher support from women than from men for other actions to restrict advertising that are designed to make cigarettes less appealing to children and adolescents, including support for "tombstone advertising" that would prohibit the use of visual appeals (77 vs. 69 percent), mandate plain packaging of cigarettes (51 vs. 42 percent), ban coupons for obtaining promotional items (79 vs. 61 percent), and eliminate the sale of single cigarettes (87 vs. 76 percent) (Strouse and Hall 1994).

In contrast, two studies have shown similarities in women's and men's support for advertising restrictions. A 1995 poll (Associated Press 1995) that assessed public support for President Bill Clinton's efforts to limit tobacco advertising and promotion

**Table 5.5. Support for restrictions on marketing and advertising of tobacco products, by gender**

| | | | Type of restriction (% supporting policy) | | | | |
|---|---|---|---|---|---|---|---|
| Study | Location | Gender | Ban on all ads | Ban on billboard ads | Ban on tobacco ads in newspapers and magazines | Ban on sponsoring events | Ban on free cigarette samples in public places |
| Forster et al. 1991 | Minnesota | Women | | 48 | 45 | | |
| | | Men | | 42 | 37 | | |
| California Tobacco Survey 1993* | California | Women | 59 | 66 | 60 | 63 | 85 |
| | | Men | 50 | 56 | 50 | 50 | 76 |
| Gallup Organization 1993 | United States | Women | 62 | | | | |
| | | Men | 43 | | | | |
| Massachusetts Tobacco Survey 1993† | Massachusetts | Women | | 56 | 47 | 68 | 84 |
| | | Men | | 43 | 39 | 49 | 76 |
| Mathematica 1994‡ | United States | Women | | 66 | 57 | 63 | 94 |
| | | Men | | 52 | 45 | 47 | 81 |

*Technical Report on Analytic Methods and Approaches Used in the 1993 California Tobacco Survey Analysis (Pierce et al. 1994a).

†1993 Massachusetts Tobacco Survey—Tobacco Use and Attitudes at the Start of the Massachusetts Control Program (Biener et al. 1994).

‡The Robert Wood Johnson Foundation Youth Access Survey, December 1994 (Strouse and Hall 1994).

aimed at girls and boys found no gender-specific differences in the proportion of respondents who would support tombstone advertising or a ban on "masked" tobacco promotions such as sportswear or event sponsorships. A 1993 poll (Gallup Organization 1993) found negligible differences between women and men in the proportions who thought that tobacco advertising was designed to appeal to children (75 vs. 78 percent), make smoking seem glamorous (65 vs. 63 percent), or encourage young people to smoke (69 vs. 63 percent).

*Effects of Restrictions on Tobacco Advertising and Marketing*

In recent years, many countries have imposed strict restrictions or bans on tobacco advertising and marketing (Mahood 1990; Mackay and Hedley 1997; Fraser 1998; Seffrin 1998; Watts 1998). In the United States, the attorneys-general settlement with the tobacco industry imposed substantial restrictions on advertising and marketing of tobacco products (Wilson 1999). Little information is available about the effects of these policies on smoking onset or smoking cessation. Laugesen and Meads (1991) analyzed 1960–1986 data from 22 countries of the Organisation for Economic Co-operation and Development and found that the severity of tobacco restrictions was associated with lower tobacco consumption. On the basis of the data they examined, the authors concluded that an increase in price and a ban in tobacco promotion would have resulted in a 40-percent reduction in tobacco consumption among adults in 1986. In a study that examined risk factors for smoking (including knowledge and attitudes about smoking, smoking status of family members, self-confidence, and exposure to tobacco advertising) in Hong Kong, Lam and colleagues (1998) found that tobacco advertising had the strongest association with smoking status (RR, 2.68; 95 percent CI, 2.33 to 3.07).

In a review of the effects of tobacco advertising bans, Willemsen and De Zwart (1999) concluded that advertising bans lead not only to decreased tobacco consumption among adults but also to reductions in onset among adolescents. To date, information has not been published on the effects of advertising restrictions among women compared with men. (See also "Bans and Restrictions on Tobacco Advertising and Promotion" in Chapter 4.)

# Smoking Prevention

Research on the prevention of smoking has been extensive over the past 20 years. Few of the prevention studies have stratified by gender; however, where they have, the results have been conflicting. In school-based programs, at least one study found an effect among girls compared with boys in the same program (Graham et al. 1990), and two others found effects among boys compared with girls in the same program (Klepp et al. 1993; Davis et al. 1995). Nonschool-based interventions also have had mixed results that showed no gender differences (Pentz et al. 1989a,b) or an effect among girls compared with boys (Kelder et al. 1995). A mass-media intervention targeted to girls was successful in reducing smoking prevalence among girls (Flynn et al. 1995; Worden et al. 1996). Overall, it is unclear why some programs appeal to girls and others to boys. Additional research is needed.

## Current Status of Prevention Research

The extant literature on gender-specific factors associated with initiation of cigarette use is reviewed elsewhere in this report (see "Factors Influencing Initiation of Smoking" in Chapter 4). Most reviews of studies of smoking prevention programs have not focused on assessing the effects of programs for adolescent females, but rather have attempted to determine the overall effectiveness of the programs and to identify key successful components of the programs (Rundall and Bruvold 1988; Glynn 1989; Bruvold 1993; Rooney and Murray 1996). Little systematic effort has been made to develop and evaluate preventive interventions specifically for girls.

### School-Based Interventions

Most intervention studies with adolescents have taken place in schools, which afford easy access to adolescent peer groups. School-based programs offer the opportunity to expose almost all children to the program and to evaluate the program's effects by assessing students over time. The impetus for these programs has been largely external to school systems and driven by federally funded research (Lynch and Bonnie 1994). Studies have focused on demonstrating the effectiveness of a program to reduce both initiation of tobacco use (primary prevention) and movement from experimental to regular use (secondary or tertiary prevention).

Several well-known projects did not report on gender-specific effects. These projects include the Life Skills Training Project (Botvin et al. 1990, 1995), the Midwestern Prevention Project (Pentz et al. 1989a,b), the Minnesota Smoking Prevention Program (Murray et al. 1987, 1988, 1989), Project ALERT (Ellickson et al. 1993), Project SHOUT (Elder et al. 1993), Project Towards No Tobacco Use (Sussman et al. 1993), and the Waterloo Smoking Prevention Project (Flay et al. 1985, 1989).

Graham and colleagues (1990) reported one-year follow-up results of Project SMART, which was designed to evaluate the effects of two programs based on social psychology. The study involved three seventh-grade cohorts (5,070 students) in the 1982–1983, 1983–1984, and 1984–1985 school years. Results were examined for six subgroups: male, female, white, African American, Hispanic, and Asian. The program was significantly effective in reducing cigarette smoking among girls ($p < 0.0001$) but not among boys.

The Oslo (Norway) Youth Study Smoking Prevention Program (Klepp et al. 1993) provided a 10-session smoking prevention program to students in fifth through seventh grades who were enrolled in Oslo schools in 1979 and 1980. The program, which was partly led by older students, encompassed education about the social, political, and health aspects of smoking; skill building to resist social pressures to smoke; and public commitment to remaining nonsmokers. The study included 1,013 students. The 10-year follow-up revealed significant effects of intervention among boys who had never smoked at baseline: 41.6 percent of the boys in the intervention group and 55.8 percent of the boys in the control group had ever smoked since baseline. No intervention effects were found among girls who had never smoked at baseline or among students of either gender who had experimented with smoking or who had smoked regularly (at least once a week) at baseline.

Gilchrist and colleagues (1989) reported on the combined results of two school-based interventions that emphasized skill building and were delivered by health educators in 10 sessions to 1,281 sixth graders in western Washington state between 1981 and 1984. The outcome measure was weekly smoking at the 24-month follow-up. Baseline risk for smoking was determined by previous smoking experience or by intention to smoke in the near future; girls and boys were classified as being at high or low risk. The intervention had a positive effect on each of the four risk-by-gender groups but was least effective among girls at high risk for smoking. Gilchrist and colleagues observed that the "developmental and social dynamics that propel female adolescents into smoking may differ from those operating on young males" (Gilchrist et al. 1989, p. 241). Their conclusions were somewhat at variance with the results of Project SMART discussed above, which was designed to develop social skills for refusing drug use; that program significantly reduced cigarette smoking among girls but not boys (Graham et al. 1990).

In the Southwest Cardiovascular Curriculum Project (Davis et al. 1995), tobacco use prevention was one of five components of a 13-week curriculum taught to Navajo and Pueblo fifth graders at rural elementary schools in New Mexico. Baseline questionnaires were completed by 2,018 students. Follow-up questionnaires that were administered within 3 weeks of the end of the curriculum were completed by 1,766 students (1,352 who had received the curriculum and 414 control students). Students were asked whether they had changed the amount of tobacco they smoked or chewed since baseline. Boys who participated in the curriculum were significantly more likely than those in the control group to report reducing the amount of tobacco they used (41.2 vs. 22.0 percent). The difference was not significant among girls (25.2 vs. 23.2 percent). Long-term effects of the curriculum cannot be determined from this study.

#### Community-Based Interventions

Several research programs have supplemented school-based programs with broader community efforts to create an environment that discourages smoking initiation. Such community efforts typically include media components and may also include community organization to support nonsmoking, greater enforcement of laws restricting access of minors to tobacco products, and efforts to educate adults. The North Karelia Youth Project relied on mass media in conjunction with a school-based program geared to dissuade youth from smoking. Vartiainen and associates (1990) found a preventive effect

8 years after the program ended, but at 15 years after intervention, differences between intervention and control schools were no longer statistically significant (Vartiainen et al. 1998). The preventive effect was more pronounced among young men (27 percent) than among young women (24 percent). However, the interaction between study arm and gender was not statistically significant.

A comprehensve community-based smoking prevention program, the Midwestern Prevention Project (Pentz et al. 1989a,b), randomized eight schools in Kansas City to receive an intervention program or a control program. The intervention program provided students with skills to resist social pressures to use tobacco and provided models intended to support the non-use of tobacco. Within all eight schools, a longitudinal sample of sixth- and seventh-grade students was followed for two years. At the end of six months, the prevalence of smoking was significantly lower in the intervention schools than in the control schools for lifetime smoking, smoking in the past month, and smoking in the past week. At the end of two years, a significant difference only in lifetime smoking was found between intervention and control schools. Significant program effects were noted within grade and racial categories, but not by gender.

A smoking prevention component of the Minnesota Heart Health Program (Perry et al. 1992; Kelder et al. 1995) was delivered to 7th-grade students. This six-session program relied on peer leaders to transmit new information, norms, and skills to their fellow students. Each year through 12th grade, students who had been assessed at baseline (6th grade) were reassessed for change in smoking status by self-report (never smoked, experimental smoker, former smoker, or weekly smoker). They were compared with a control cohort in a reference community, also in Minnesota. The survey of 12th graders included 45 percent of the original cohort of 2,401 6th graders. Cross-sectional analysis included all students who participated in each survey. Throughout the follow-up period, smoking rates were significantly lower among the intervention students than among the control cohort ($p < 0.04$ for grades 7 through 12). When the data were stratified by gender, the intervention effects were somewhat stronger among girls. The differences in smoking rates were significant in grades 7 through 11 among girls. Among boys the differences were significant in grades 7, 8, and 10; marginally significant in grades 9 and 12 ($p = 0.06$); and nonsignificant in grade 11. The authors hypothesized that "girls may be more receptive than boys to social influences models of health education" (Kelder et al. 1995, p. 5-42).

An innovative mass-media intervention for smoking prevention (Flynn et al. 1995; Worden et al. 1996) targeted girls. Participants were fourth-through sixth-grade students in two pairs of communities, one pair in the northeast United States and one pair in Montana. Students in two communities (one from each pair) received a modest school-based intervention (three or four class periods per year over four years). In the other two communities, the school-based intervention was supplemented with a four-year media campaign using paid and donated advertising time on broadcast and cable television programs and on radio stations. The media spots were designed to appeal to high-risk girls and boys at three developmental levels (grades 5 and 6, prepuberty; grades 7 and 8, puberty; and grades 9 and 10, adolescence). The researchers made a special effort to target high-risk girls when purchasing time in the media campaign, which resulted in more media spots targeting girls. Media spots were changed regularly to keep up with changing tastes and styles. The initial cohort of 5,458 students was surveyed annually for four years, then two years later to assess long-term impact. At each assessment point, students were asked the number of cigarettes they had smoked in the past week. Although saliva samples were not analyzed, they were collected from all students in an attempt to increase the accuracy of self-reports.

In grades 8 through 10, the weekly smoking prevalence was 40 percent lower among girls who had received the media-plus-school intervention than among girls who had received the school-only intervention. The difference in smoking prevalence persisted two years later when the students were surveyed in grades 10 through 12: 15.6 percent of girls in communities with the media-plus-school intervention but 29.4 percent in communities with the school-only intervention smoked weekly. Girls receiving the media-plus-school intervention also had lower increases in beliefs in the advantages of smoking, positive attitudes toward smoking, perceptions of peer smoking, and intentions to smoke. The differences in weekly smoking were not significant among boys.

### Public Health Initiatives

Few tobacco prevention programs or strategies, particularly those developed around sports and athletics, are designed specifically for girls. Although most tobacco prevention sports strategies appear gender neutral, they historically emphasize male-dominated sports such as baseball or football. This historic bias changed in 1996 with the introduction in the United States of the SmokeFree Kids & Soccer Campaign, a tobacco prevention strategy targeted to adolescent girls. This program is unique for its emphasis on the sport of soccer and, more significantly, for its emphasis on an increasingly popular women's sport in the United States and throughout the world.

Through a public health partnership between the U.S. Women's National Soccer team, CDC, and NCI, SmokeFree Kids & Soccer encourages girls to participate in soccer to maintain fitness, make friends, have fun, and resist the pressure to smoke. In appearances at local schools, youth soccer tournaments, and media interviews, members of the U.S. Women's National Soccer team underscore the negative effect of tobacco use on athletic performance and promote participation in soccer as an alternative to smoking. Donna Shalala, then USDHHS Secretary, launched the campaign in advance of the 1996 Olympics in Atlanta by saying,

> This campaign communicates not only the negative effects of tobacco use on athletic performance, but also promotes participation in sports as a positive alternative to smoking. [The campaign] is an excellent vehicle for reaching young people with the smoke-free message. Athletics give young people the very benefits they often seek from smoking: independence, status with their peers, a chance to make friends and a positive sense of self (Forbes 1996, p. 105).

The campaign also uses health sponsorship, a strategy that has been commonly used by commercial sponsors, including tobacco companies (Corti et al. 1997). By participating in physically strenuous sports like soccer, adolescent girls can reduce their risk of smoking while enhancing self-esteem and helping to broaden community support for a smoke-free society (USDHHS 1997). Work by the Canadian Association for the Advancement of Women and Sport and Physical Activity has underscored the important physical and emotional benefits that being part of an athletic team can play in reducing an adolescent girl's risk for smoking (Canadian Association for the Advancement of Women and Sport and Physical Activity 2001).

In the first year, Smoke-Free Kids & Soccer was introduced to more than one million children and adults through a combination of television, radio, posters, public events, and an interactive Web site (http://www.smokefree.gov). One of the most prominent components of the program was a series of six posters of the U.S. Women's National Soccer team, which were produced and distributed nationwide from 1996 through 2000 to hundreds of thousands of fans, both girls and boys. The posters encouraged girls to participate in soccer and to make "Smoke-Free" an integral part of their personal lifestyle. Messages such as "You don't get to be a champion by taking cigarette breaks," "Keep your engine running clean," "Smoke a defender... not a cigarette," and "My only addiction is the game" resonate with children and the adults who care about them. Program messages were promoted widely during the 1999 Women's World Cup in the United States, and through grants to state health departments for community-based health promotion activities.

At the 11th World Conference on Tobacco OR Health in August 2000, USDHHS and the World Health Organization joined the Federation Internationale de Football Association, the international governing body of soccer, to announce an international SmokeFree Soccer campaign to discourage tobacco use and to promote smoke-free and physically active lifestyles worldwide (11th World Conference on Tobacco OR Health 2000). Australian Health Minister Michael Wooldridge committed soccer players in his country to the initiative, saying it would be helpful in "promoting the benefits of being smoke-free"(Commonwealth of Australia 2000).

## Tobacco Control Advocacy Programs by and for Women

Apart from women's health groups and a handful of women's and girls' organizations, the tobacco control movement has not had great success involving women's organizations in women's tobacco control. Although women play important roles in the tobacco control movement, few have held top leadership positions (Mackay 1990; McLellan 1990; Greaves 1996). The public commitments made by the leaders of women's organizations from around the world at the 1999 Kobe Conference suggested that they are willing to play an important role in tobacco control advocacy (World Health Organization 1999a). New ways of working with women's groups are needed, such as having traditional tobacco control agencies show support for women and for women's issues broader than just smoking (Greaves 1996).

Historically, women's organizations that take on tobacco control have been oriented to education of their constituencies; however, some groups have mobilized themselves for action (e.g., flight attendant associations to ban smoking on airplane flights). Activities directed toward reducing advertising to women, as in magazines, have largely been unsuccessful. Similarly, countering tobacco sponsorship of women's sports events has been somewhat unsuccessful.

## Education and Mobilization

### Efforts to Raise Awareness and Encourage Action

For many women's and girls' organizations, educating their constituencies about how tobacco affects their lives is the first step to involvement in women's tobacco control. As a result of such education, women and girls may be motivated to participate in further activities to reduce tobacco use among women and girls. Education and mobilization activities vary but generally emphasize health-related issues, prevention of smoking, countering tobacco industry advertising targeted at women, financial sponsorship of women's groups, and legislation.

*Girls' Organizations*

Because most girls start smoking in early adolescence (see "Cigarette Smoking Among Girls" and "Smoking Initiation" in Chapter 2), many girls' organizations involved in tobacco control focus on prevention programs. The Girl Scouts of the USA has publications and programs that teach girls about the hazards of tobacco use and targeted tobacco advertising, as well as how to avoid tobacco use (Simpkins 1985; Eubanks 1992; Eubanks et al. 1995; Girl Scouts of the USA 1995). "Girl Scouts Against Smoking" includes antismoking patches and age-appropriate booklets containing information, activities, and resources (Girl Scouts of the USA 1996).

Girls Incorporated of Alameda County, California, designed the Jasira Warriors program to educate young African American girls about the tobacco industry's influence in their communities (Girls Incorporated of Alameda County 1995). The program was designed to empower the girls by building their self-esteem and decision-making skills through education on tobacco use.

*Women's Organizations*

Health organizations have led the way in health and prevention efforts related to tobacco use by women. The Strategic Coalition of Girls and Women United Against Tobacco, of the American Medical Women's Association (AMWA), is dedicated to reducing tobacco-related death and disease among women (Strategic Coalition of Girls and Women United Against Tobacco 1995). Organizations that participate in the coalition receive mailings on tobacco-related issues and are encouraged to involve their members in tobacco control efforts.

The Task Force on Women & Girls, Tobacco & Lung Cancer, of the American College of Chest Physicians (ACCP), has developed a comprehensive speaker's kit entitled Women and Girls, Tobacco and Cancer. The kit includes slides with extensive speaker notes as well as resource lists and materials (e.g., articles, brochures). For professional audiences, the goal of the materials is to inform colleagues (e.g., physicians, nurses, pulmonary rehabilitation specialists, and health educators) who can influence others and effect change. A section on public policy also is included for influencing legislators and the media (ACCP Task Force 1998).

Among other organizations dedicated to the health and well-being of women and girls and that have policies or programs on women and tobacco issues are the American College of Obstetricians and Gynecologists (American College of Obstetricians and Gynecologists 1990), ACCP (ACCP Task Force 1998), the American Nurses Association (American Nurses Association 1995), the Minnesota Nursing Network for Tobacco Control (American Cancer Society 1994), the National Organization for Women (NOW 1991), the National Organization of School Nurses (Grande et al. 1995), the American Indian Women's Health Education Resource Center (Christine David, unpublished data), the Swedish Nurses Against Tobacco (Swedish Nurses Against Tobacco 1994), the Young Women's Christian Association (Grande et al. 1995), and the National Association for Public Health Policy (National Association for Public Health Policy 1996). The policies of most of these organizations focus on the health effects of tobacco use and the education of members, and some include prevention messages or call attention to the targeting of women and girls by the tobacco industry (Grande et al. 1995).

*Other Organized Efforts*

A successful example of women mobilizing for tobacco control was the passage in October 1989 of landmark legislation to ban smoking on domestic airline flights of six hours or fewer (Morgan 1989). The most numerous voices in favor of this legislation came from various flight attendant associations, whose memberships were predominantly women. The Association of Professional Flight Attendants, the Flight Attendant Non-Smokers, the Association of Flight Attendants, AFL-CIO, and the National Association of Flight Attendants mobilized 100,000 flight attendants to support the legislation (Congressional Record 1989a,b). Flight attendants were concerned about adverse health effects, including lung cancer, resulting from their exposure to tobacco smoke in airline cabins.

The Office on Smoking and Health at CDC funds several organizations to work specifically on issues related to tobacco use among women. These organizations include AMWA, the International Network of Women Against Tobacco (INWAT), NOW, the National Association of African Americans for Positive Imagery, and the Northwest Portland Area Indian Health Board; all of these organizations include issues related to tobacco use among women in some of their activities (CDC 1998a,b).

The Maternal and Child Health Bureau of the Health Resources and Services Administration (HRSA) has worked with multiple states (Alaska, Delaware, Florida, Louisiana, Maryland, Massachusetts, Minnesota, Missouri, Montana, Nebraska, Nevada, New York, North Carolina, Ohio, South Dakota, Washington, West Virginia, and Wisconsin) and the District of Columbia, Puerto Rico, and Guam to incorporate performance measures on reducing cigarette smoking during pregnancy into the Title V, Maternal and Child Health Block Grant programs. Through this interstate network of performance measures, HRSA's Maternal and Child Health Bureau will be monitoring health care providers as they implement smoking cessation interventions for pregnant women. Details about this effort are available on their Web site at http://www.mchdata.net. Additionally, the HRSA-funded Healthy Start programs include smoking cessation for pregnant women as a major component of the initiative to reduce infant mortality.

The National Smoking Cessation Campaign for African American Women reached out to African American women's organizations and individuals to educate them about smoking cessation, to prevent nonsmokers from starting to smoke, and to advocate for smoke-free environments and divestiture from sponsorship by the tobacco industry (Morse Enterprises 1992). This focus transcended most smoking cessation programs by promoting changes in public policy that could reduce the environmental exposure to tobacco among African American women.

Some women's tobacco control groups have conducted qualitative research on what tobacco use and exposure means to women. INWAT commissioned some of its members to interview women around the world about how tobacco growing, manufacturing, and consumption affect women and girls (Greaves et al. 1994). Interviews were conducted in Brazil, Estonia, India, Indonesia, Japan, New Zealand, Northern Ireland, Spain, Tanzania, and the United States (Kentucky) (*World Smoking and Health* 1994). Beside health concerns, tobacco use and exposure were found to have significant economic, social, environmental, and cultural implications for the lives of women and girls. INWAT compiled the stories and published them in an edition of *World Smoking and Health* entitled "Herstories" (*World Smoking and Health* 1994). INWAT's goals were to encourage the global tobacco control movement to listen and react to the multifaceted aspects of how tobacco affects women's lives, and to inspire new approaches to tobacco control among women and girls (Greaves et al. 1994).

In 1994, the Commission for a Healthy New York established a special task force on women and tobacco to investigate the "tobacco problem from a woman's perspective and [develop] women-centered responses to it" (Commission for a Healthy New York 1995, p. 2). The task force found that few researchers had actually talked with women, either smokers or nonsmokers, about tobacco issues (Commission for a Healthy New York 1995). The task force conducted 30 roundtable discussions to learn why women and girls smoke and what they think of cigarette marketing campaigns. This qualitative research study, Women Talk to Women About Smoking, found that women still need to be educated on the deleterious effects of tobacco use and exposure on their lives. The women and girls interviewed linked gender-related factors such as low self-esteem, the stress of multiple roles, concern with body image, and social isolation to tobacco use among women and girls.

## Activities to Counter Tobacco Advertising and Sponsorship

Many of the campaigns that have been conducted on issues related to tobacco use among women have focused on the targeting of women by tobacco companies' advertising and sponsorship (see "Influence of Tobacco Marketing on Smoking Initiation by Females" in Chapter 4). Organizations have conducted counteradvertising and mass-media campaigns, attempted to persuade women's magazines to refrain from accepting tobacco ads, encouraged women's sporting groups to reject funding from the tobacco industry, and lobbied for clean air legislation.

### Counteradvertising and Mass-Media Campaigns

The Women vs. Smoking Network, a project funded by NCI and based at the Advocacy Institute in Washington, D.C., involved women's organizations, leaders, and publications in tobacco control efforts, especially efforts against tobacco advertising and promotion that target women (Women vs. Smoking Network 1990). The network catapulted the issue of targeted marketing to the national consciousness by strategically calling attention to the "Dakota Papers" (see text box 2 in "Contemporary Cigarette Advertisements and Promotions" in Chapter 4). These documents, sent anonymously to the network, contained a marketing strategy aimed at the "virile" female, described as a white female 18 through 20 years of age with no more than a high school education and minimal career opportunities and aspirations (Butler 1990). The network granted exclusive stories to certain television networks and newspapers, its members appeared on television with the Secretary of Health and Human Services, and it petitioned R.J. Reynolds to cease marketing the Dakota brand cigarette. As a result of strategies used by the network, the marketing plan for Dakota was changed and had limited test markets (Butler 1990). Unable to market Dakota under the original plan that called for targeting women with low educational levels, R.J. Reynolds ultimately pulled Dakota off the market because of low sales (*American Medical News* 1992).

Women And Girls Against Tobacco (WAGAT), which was funded by the California Department of Health Services, used the issue of advertising targeted to women and girls to educate and mobilize them (WAGAT 1993). One way WAGAT raised awareness was through purchasing kiosk space in shopping malls that attracted high concentrations of young people. The kiosks featured counterads on the tobacco industry's targeting of women as well as educational information (Regina Penna, Director, WAGAT, memorandum to WAGAT Advisory Board, May 6, 1994).

During the summer of 1998, NOW promoted the "We Have Come a Long Way, So Don't Call Me Baby" campaign at 58 Lilith Fair concerts. T-shirts, postcards, and a display were created to disseminate information about women and tobacco at these women-oriented concerts. Additionally, in September 1998, 1,000 new volunteers promoted the "Love Your Body Day" campaign. This campaign raised awareness about how the tobacco industry manipulates women into using tobacco by playing with popular notions of body image (CDC 1998b).

### Women's Magazine Projects

One of the major ways tobacco companies try to reach women is through women's magazines (Amos and Bostock 1992). Research has shown that women's magazines that accept tobacco advertising are significantly less likely to publish articles critical of women and smoking than are magazines that do not accept such ads (Warner et al. 1992) (see "Press Self-Censorship in Relation to Cigarette Advertising" in Chapter 4). The American Public Health Association conducted one of the first campaigns to uncover and attempt to change advertising policies of women's magazines (Johnson 1987). It requested that editors and publishers of 21 popular women's magazines include articles on the health hazards of smoking and wean their publications from tobacco industry advertising accounts. More than 50 women's, girls', and health organizations participated in the campaign. Eleven magazines responded, but none committed to change their advertising policy. Generally, the editors responded that the choice to run tobacco ads was based on the revenues received from the ad and that adult readers have the "freedom to choose" whether to buy a product (Johnson 1987).

As a result of a survey of cigarette advertising and health coverage in British women's magazines in 1984, the British government introduced voluntary advertising restrictions that prohibited magazines with a female readership of more than 200,000 and at least one-third of their readership aged 15 through 24 years from accepting cigarette ads (Action on Smoking and Health [ASH] Working Group on Women and Smoking 1990). A follow-up survey conducted by the ASH Working Group on Women and Smoking in 1989 documented whether the voluntary restrictions in Great Britain had affected cigarette advertising and health coverage in women's magazines. Coverage of smoking and health issues remained largely unchanged between the two surveys (ASH Working Group on Women and Smoking 1990).

In California, WAGAT sponsored the "Golden Handcuffs Challenge" (1993) to reduce the quantity of tobacco ads in national magazines with a large proportion of women readers (Ferris 1994). WAGAT asked the editors of *Essence, Glamour,* and *People* to write articles on the effects of tobacco advertising on editorial practice. *Glamour* and *People* declined the request after six months, and *Essence* never responded (Ferris 1994). During this time, the California Department of Health Services tried to place a paid antismoking ad in *Essence*. Even though the ad was paid for, it was deemed "too controversial" and never appeared (Ferris 1994). As *Essence* editor Linda Villarosa stated in an article in the *Harvard Public Health Review,* "alienating a tobacco company means more than kissing off just cigarettes; it may mean alienating a conglomerate" (Villarosa 1991, p. 20). WAGAT's campaign was illuminating in that, even if the tobacco control movement had substantial funds to attempt to "buy out" tobacco ads in magazines, such efforts might be met with resistance.

The Australian National Women's Magazine Project was run by the Quit Victoria project of the Victorian Smoking and Health Program (1991–1992). The objective was to increase the amount and quality of reporting on the health effects of smoking by using paid "advertorials" in a number of popular young women's magazines (Davidson 1991). In the midst of the campaign, legislation to ban tobacco ads in the print media was enacted. The Quit Victoria project surveyed magazines for smoking-related articles six months before and after the ban went into effect. Coverage of the health effects of smoking appeared to increase after Quit Victoria started advertising (before the ad ban went into effect), but little difference in specific editorials was found before and after the ban itself. Quit Victoria noted that magazines contained more photographs of celebrities smoking after the ban than previously (Michelle Scollo, Executive Director, Victorian Smoking and Health Program, letter to Deborah McLellan, September 11, 1992).

The placement of images in women's magazines of models smoking may increase as countries pass advertising bans. For example, although Italy has a ban on tobacco advertising, an issue of an Italian *Vogue* contained numerous pages of models smoking in ads for non-tobacco products; a cover showcased a world-famous model, Linda Evangelista, smoking (Amos and Bostock 1992; Amos 1993). The Italian case suggested that simply removing paid cigarette ads from magazines may not have the intended effect of entirely eliminating images of persons smoking or increasing coverage of issues related to smoking and health among women (Amos and Bostock 1992).

### Countering Tobacco Sponsorship of Women's Tennis

For many years, starting in 1971, Philip Morris sponsored professional women's tennis (Robinson et al. 1992). Public figures who have expressed gratitude for the tobacco industry's sponsorship include Martina Navratilova, perhaps the best known woman tennis player in the world. The loyalty of women's tennis to its tobacco industry sponsor was so great that Proctor and Gamble's offer to support a women's tennis tournament was refused in 1988.

Many communities have held counterevents. Doctors Ought to Care organized a series of Emphysema Slims tennis tournaments as counterevents to the Virginia Slims tournaments (USDHHS 1991b). In 1990, the District of Columbia Interagency Council on Smoking and Health organized a media event to bring attention to the tobacco industry's sponsorship of the Virginia Slims tennis tournament. The event was held at The George Washington University, Washington, D.C. (District of Columbia Interagency Council on Smoking and Health 1990). The highlight of the event was a statement by Secretary of Health and Human Services Dr. Louis W. Sullivan, who urged the tobacco industry to end its sponsorship of sports events (Broder 1990).

The next year (1991), the Virginia Slims tennis tournament returned to Washington, D.C., where it was to be held at an amphitheater on property of the National Park Service. National and local organizations combined efforts to halt the tobacco industry's sponsorship of the tournament on public property. As a result of a lawsuit, local protests, and media attention, the National Park Service agreed to ban tobacco industry-sponsored tennis tournaments on its property (Spolar 1991). As of 1994, Virginia Slims no longer sponsored the major national women's tennis events, although individual events in several cities and the Tennis Legends Tour are still sponsored by Virginia Slims (IEG 1995).

In Australia, sports have not exhibited the same loyalty to the tobacco industry. The Victorian Health Promotion Foundation in Australia has used money raised by taxes on tobacco products to replace tobacco industry sponsorship of sports and arts organizations (Daube 1992; Galbally 1994). Australia's success may reflect economics, because more than five times the budget necessary to replace tobacco sponsorship is available through the foundation (Daube 1992).

## Women's Leadership Development and Training

### Development of Women's Leadership in Tobacco Control

The desire for women to communicate and network on a global level was the foundation on which INWAT was built (McLellan 1990). Because one of the objectives of INWAT is to promote women's leadership in the tobacco control movement (INWAT 1994), it developed a training workshop that focused on tools for building such leadership: assessing knowledge, defining roles, enhancing skills, and building networks (McLellan et al. 1992). As a result of INWAT's efforts, the proportion of invited women speakers increased from 8 percent at the 1990 Seventh World Conference on Tobacco OR Health to 30 percent at the Eighth World Conference on Tobacco OR Health in 1992 (Jordan 1992; Gritz 1993). INWAT also succeeded in having world conferences adopt its resolutions on equity in representation and on funding for women at tobacco control conferences (*Tobacco Control* 1992).

INWAT has regional networks that focus on the needs of women in different parts of the world. The Latin American Women Association on Smoking Control (Associação de Mulheres da América Latina para o Controle do Tabagismo [AMALTA] 1994), the Canadian Network of Women Against Tobacco, INWAT-Europe, and WAGAT have been particularly active regional networks with funds committed to them (INWAT 1995). Other regional networks of INWAT exist in Africa, Asia, and Australia (INWAT 1999).

As a result of a resolution passed at the 1990 World Conference on Smoking and Health in Perth, Australia, the International Union Against Cancer organized the First International Conference on Women and Smoking, which took place in Northern Ireland in October 1992. This landmark event produced a series of recommendations that focused on raising awareness about women and tobacco, countering pressures on women to use tobacco, and organizing women for action in tobacco control (Health Promotion Agency of Northern Ireland and Ulster Cancer Foundation 1993).

In June 1994, the Women United Against Tobacco Workshop was convened by the American Public Health Association to develop a comprehensive national plan to reduce women's use of and exposure to tobacco (McLellan and Wright 1996). The resultant national consensus document included a goal to increase the number and power of women leaders in tobacco control by convening a summit on women and tobacco, promoting women spokespersons, and encouraging women's leadership within tobacco control organizations.

Most recently, in November of 1999, the World Health Organization sponsored an International Conference on Tobacco and Health in Kobe, Japan. It was titled, "Making a Difference to Tobacco and Health: Avoiding the Tobacco Epidemic in Women and Youth." The conference was attended by several hundred leaders of women's organizations and of other governmental and nongovernmental organizations from around the world, as well as by the media, health scientists, and public health advocates. Formal presentations addressed the worldwide prevalence and effects on women's health of active smoking and of ETS exposure, the economic costs of tobacco use, the international marketing of tobacco products to women, and other topics. The resultant Kobe Declaration included a number of strong resolutions, such as a call for a global ban on tobacco advertising, funding for counteradvertising that disconnects women's liberation and tobacco use, and mobilization of many segments of society in the fight against tobacco use (World Health Organization 1999b).

### Development of Tobacco Control Advocates in Women's Organizations

The California chapter of NOW launched the "Redefining Liberation" campaign to educate its members about issues related to tobacco use among women and to develop leadership on the subject within NOW's ranks (California NOW 1994). The California chapter used community-based strategies and developed an action guide and training videotape for its campaign to develop young leaders (Elizabeth Toledo, NOW, letter to Deborah McLellan, September 8, 1995). Early in 1998, the videotape was distributed to 40 states and every region throughout the United States (CDC 1998a).

The Strategic Coalition of Girls and Women United Against Tobacco, a project of AMWA with funding from CDC, also has trained leaders in women's organizations on tobacco control issues (AMWA 1995). In particular, AMWA trains women physicians and medical students in tobacco control and media advocacy to be spokespersons for tobacco control (AMWA 1995).

The Swedish National Institute of Public Health sponsors an innovative program with the Miss Sweden beauty pageant, requiring all Miss Sweden candidates since 1996 to be nonsmokers (Steimle 1999). The candidates are also required to work as tobacco educators in their local school districts for at least four to six weeks. One of the purposes of the project is to provide Swedish girls with fashionable role models who do not smoke. By 1997, more than 30,000 students in grades four through six had met a Miss Sweden candidate. The project has been well received by the schools and the media.

# Conclusions

1. Using evidence from studies that vary in design, sample characteristics, and intensity of the interventions studied, researchers to date have not found consistent gender-specific differences in the effectiveness of intervention programs for tobacco use. Some clinical studies have shown lower cessation rates among women than among men, but others have not. Many studies have not reported cessation results by gender.
2. Among women, biopsychosocial factors such as pregnancy, fear of weight gain, depression, and the need for social support appear to be associated with smoking maintenance, cessation, or relapse.
3. A higher percentage of women stop smoking during pregnancy, both spontaneously and with assistance, than at other times in their lives. Using pregnancy-specific programs can increase smoking cessation rates, which benefits infant health and is cost-effective. Only about one-third of women who stop smoking during pregnancy are still abstinent one year after the delivery.
4. Women fear weight gain during smoking cessation more than do men. However, few studies have found a relationship between weight concerns and smoking cessation among either women or men. Further, actual weight gain during cessation does not predict relapse to smoking.
5. Adolescent girls are more likely than adolescent boys to respond to smoking cessation programs that include social support from the family or their peer group.
6. Among persons who smoke heavily, women are more likely than men to report being dependent on cigarettes and to have lower expectations about stopping smoking, but it is not clear if such women are less likely to quit smoking.
7. Currently, no tobacco cessation method has proved to be any more or less successful among minority women than among white women in the same study, but research on smoking cessation among women of most racial and ethnic minorities has been scarce.
8. Women are more likely than men to affirm that they smoke less at work because of a worksite policy and are significantly more likely than men to attribute reduced amount of daily smoking to their worksite policy. Women also are more likely than men to support policies designed to prevent smoking initiation among adolescents, restrictions on youth access to tobacco products, and limits on tobacco advertising and promotion.
9. Successful interventions have been developed to prevent smoking among young people, but little systematic effort has been focused on developing and evaluating prevention interventions specifically for girls.

# References


11th World Conference on Tobacco OR Health. FIFA joins world health leaders to give tobacco the boot! *SmokeFree Soccer* campaign goes global. Chicago: 11th World Conference on Tobacco OR Health, 2000 Aug 11.

Abrams DB, Boutwell WB, Grizzle J, Heimendinger J, Sorensen G, Varnes J. Cancer control at the workplace: the Working Well Trial. *Preventive Medicine* 1994;23(1):15–27.

Abramson JH, Gofin R, Hopp C, Gofin J, Donchin M, Habib J. Evaluation of a community program for the control of cardiovascular risk factors: the CHAD program in Jerusalem. *Israel Journal of Medical Sciences* 1981;17(2–3):201–12.

Acitelli LK, Antonucci TC. Gender differences in the link between marital support and satisfaction in older couples. *Journal of Personality and Social Psychology* 1994;67(4):688–98.

Action on Smoking and Health Working Group on Women and Smoking. *Smoke Still Gets in Her Eyes. A Report on Cigarette Advertising in British Women's Magazines.* Dewsbury (UK): Action on Smoking and Health, 1990.

Ahijevych K, Wewers ME. Factors associated with nicotine dependence among African American women cigarette smokers. *Research in Nursing and Health* 1993;16(4):283–92.

Ahluwalia JS, Resnicow K, Clark WS. Knowledge about smoking, reasons for smoking, and reasons for wishing to quit in inner-city African Americans. *Ethnicity and Disease* 1998;8(3):385–93.

Albrecht SA, Rosella JD, Patrick T. Smoking among low-income, pregnant women: prevalence rates, cessation interventions, and clinical implications. *Birth* 1994;21(3):155–62.

Allen SS, Hatsukami D, Christianson D, Nelson D. Symptomatology and energy intake during the menstrual cycle in smoking women. *Journal of Substance Abuse* 1996;8(3):303–19.

Allen SS, Hatsukami D, Christianson D, Nelson D. Withdrawal and pre-menstrual symptomatology during the menstrual cycle in short-term smoking abstinence: effects of menstrual cycle on smoking abstinence. *Nicotine and Tobacco Research* 1999;1(2):129–42.

Altman DG, Foster V, Rasenick-Douss L, Tye JB. Reducing the illegal sale of cigarettes to minors. *Journal of the American Medical Association* 1989;261(1):80–3.

Altman DG, Wheelis AY, McFarlane M, Lee H-R, Fortmann SP. The relationship between tobacco access and use among adolescents: a four community study. *Social Science and Medicine* 1999;48(6):759–75.

American Cancer Society. *Minnesota ASSIST: Nurses & Tobacco Control*. Minneapolis (MN): American Cancer Society, Minnesota Division, 1994.

American College of Chest Physicians Task Force: Women, Tobacco and Lung Cancer. *Women & Girls, Tobacco and Cancer.* Innovations in Medical Education Consortium. Vancouver (Canada): American College of Chest Physicians, 1998.

American College of Obstetricians and Gynecologists. Tobacco industry criticized for ads aimed at women [press release]. Washington: American College of Obstetricians and Gynecologists, 1990 Oct 3.

*American Medical News*. No more Dakotas. *American Medical News* 1992 Apr 13:18.

American Medical Women's Association. *Progress Report for the Year 01 of the Strategic Coalition of Girls and Women United Against Tobacco.* Alexandria (VA): American Medical Women's Association, 1995.

American Nurses Association. Position statement on cessation of tobacco use. Washington: American Nurses Association, 1995.

American Psychiatric Association. *Diagnostic and Statistical Manual of Mental Disorders*. 3rd rev. ed. Washington: American Psychiatric Association, 1987.

American Psychiatric Association. *Diagnostic and Statistical Manual of Mental Disorders.* 4th ed. Washington: American Psychiatric Association, 1994.

Amos A. How women are exploited by the tobacco industry. In: *First International Conference on Women and Smoking. Conference proceedings and recommendations for action; 1992 Oct 5–7; Newcastle (Northern Ireland).* Health Promotion Agency of Northern Ireland and the Ulster Cancer Foundation, 1993:38–40.

Amos A, Bostock Y. Policy on cigarette advertising and coverage of smoking and health in European women's magazines. *British Medical Journal* 1992;304(6819):99–101.

Anantha N, Nandakumar A, Vishwanath N, Venkatesh T, Pallad YG, Manjunath P, Kumar DR, Murthy SGS, Shivashankariah, Dayananda CS. Efficacy of an anti-tobacco community education program in India. *Cancer Causes and Control* 1995;6(2):119–29.

Andersch B, Milsom I. An epidemiologic study of young women with dysmenorrhea. *American Journal of Obstetrics and Gynecology* 1982;144(6): 655–60.

Associação de Mulheres da América Latina para o Controle do Tabagismo (Latin American Women Association on Smoking Control). *AMALTA 1994: Activities Report.* Rio de Janeiro: Associação de Mulheres da América Latina para o Controle do Tabagismo, 1994.

Associated Press. Antismoking bid by Clinton finds opposition in poll. *Boston Globe* 1995 Aug 23:3 (col 5).

Atkinson AB, Skegg JL. Anti-smoking publicity and the demand for tobacco in the UK. *Manchester School of Economic and Social Studies* 1973;41(3): 265–82.

Balch GI. Exploring perceptions of smoking cessation among high school smokers: input and feedback from focus groups. *Preventive Medicine* 1998;27(5 Pt 3):A55–A63.

Baric L, MacArthur C, Sherwood M. A study of health education aspects of smoking in pregnancy. *International Journal of Health Education* 1976;19(Suppl 2):1–17.

Baron JA, La Vecchia C, Levi F. The antiestrogenic effect of cigarette smoking in women. *American Journal of Obstetrics and Gynecology* 1990;162(2): 502–14.

Barrett DH, Anda RF, Escobedo LG, Croft JB, Williamson DF, Marks JS. Trends in oral contraceptive use and cigarette smoking: Behavioral Risk Factor Surveillance System, 1982 and 1988. *Archives of Family Medicine* 1994;3(5):438–43.

Batten L. Respecting sameness and difference: taking account of gender in research on smoking. *Tobacco Control* 1993;2(3):185–6.

Belle D. Gender differences in the social moderators of stress. In: Barnett RC, Biener L, Baruch GK, editors. *Gender and Stress.* New York: Free Press, 1987: 257–77.

Benowitz NL. Nicotine replacement therapy during pregnancy. *Journal of the American Medical Association* 1991;266(22):3174–7.

Berman BA, Gritz ER. Women and smoking: current trends and issues for the 1990s. *Journal of Substance Abuse* 1991;3(2):221–38.

Biener L. Gender differences in the use of substances for coping. In: Barnett RC, Biener L, Baruch GK, editors. *Gender and Stress.* New York: Free Press, 1987:330–49.

Biener L, Abrams DB, Emmons K, Follick MJ. Evaluating worksite smoking policies: methodologic issues. *New York State Journal of Medicine* 1989a; 89(1):5–10.

Biener L, Abrams DB, Follick MJ, Dean L. A comparative evaluation of a restrictive smoking policy in a general hospital. *American Journal of Public Health* 1989b;79(2):192–5.

Biener L, Aseltine RH, Cohen B, Anderka M. Reactions of adult and teenaged smokers to the Massachusetts Tobacco Tax. *American Journal of Public Health* 1998;88(9):1389–91.

Biener L, Fowler FJ, Roman AM. 1993 Massachusetts Tobacco Survey: *Tobacco Use and Attitudes at the Start of the Massachusetts Tobacco Control Program.* Boston: University of Massachusetts, Center for Survey Research, 1994.

Bjornson W, Rand C, Connett JE, Lindgren P, Nides M, Pope F, Buist AS, Hoppe-Ryan C, O'Hara P. Gender differences in smoking cessation after 3 years in the Lung Health Study. *American Journal of Public Health* 1995;85(2):223–30.

Black DR, Loftus EA, Chatterjee R, Tiffany S, Babrow AS. Smoking cessation interventions for university students: recruitment and program design considerations based on social marketing theory. *Preventive Medicine* 1993;22(3):388–99.

Blake SM, Klepp K-I, Pechacek TF, Folsom AR, Luepker RV, Jacobs DR, Mittelmark MB. Differences in smoking cessation strategies between men and women. *Addictive Behaviors* 1989;14(4):409–18.

Blechman EA. Competence, depression, and behavior modification with women. In: Hersen M, Eisler RM, Miller PM, editors. *Progress in Behavior Modification.* Vol. 12. New York: Academic Press, 1981: 227–63.

Borland R, Chapman S, Owen N, Hill D. Effects of workplace smoking bans on cigarette consumption. *American Journal of Public Health* 1990;80(2): 178–80.

Borland R, Owen N, Hill D, Chapman S. Staff members' acceptance of the introduction of workplace smoking bans in the Australian public service. *Medical Journal of Australia* 1989;151(9):525–8.

Borland R, Owen N, Hill D, Schofield P. Predicting attempts and sustained cessation of smoking after the introduction of workplace smoking bans. *Health Psychology* 1991;10(5):336–42.

Borland R, Pierce JP, Burns DM, Gilpin E, Johnson M, Bal D. Protection from environmental tobacco smoke in California: the case for a smoke-free workplace. *Journal of the American Medical Association* 1992;268(6):749–52.

Botvin GJ, Baker E, Dusenbury L, Botvin EM, Diaz T. Long-term follow-up results of a randomized drug abuse prevention trial in a white middle-class population. *Journal of the American Medical Association* 1995;273(14):1106–12.

Botvin GJ, Baker E, Dusenbury L, Tortu S, Botvin EM. Preventing adolescent drug abuse through a multimodal cognitive-behavioral approach: results of a 3-year study. *Journal of Consulting and Clinical Psychology* 1990;58(4):437–46.

Boyd NR, Sutton C, Orleans CT, McClatchey MW, Bingler R, Fleisher L, Heller D, Baum S, Graves C, Ward J. Quit Today! A targeted communications campaign to increase use of the cancer information service by African American smokers. *Preventive Medicine* 1998;27(5 Pt 2):S50–S60.

Brayden RM, Christensen M. Smoking cessation counseling with low-income prenatal patients [letter]. *Southern Medical Journal* 1994;87(12):1288–9.

Brenner H, Mielck A. Smoking prohibition in the workplace and smoking cessation in the Federal Republic of Germany. *Preventive Medicine* 1992; 21(2):252–61.

Brigham J, Gross J, Stitzer ML, Felch LJ. Effects of a restricted work-site smoking policy on employees who smoke. *American Journal of Public Health* 1994; 84(5):773–8.

Broder K. Sullivan criticizes company for courting smokers at tennis matches. *Journal of the National Cancer Institute* 1990;82(7):551–2.

Brown S, Vessey M, Stratton I. The influence of method of contraception and cigarette smoking on menstrual patterns. *British Journal of Obstetrics and Gynaecology* 1988;95(9):905–10.

Brownson RC, Jackson-Thompson J, Wilkerson JC, Davis JR, Owens NW, Fisher EB Jr. Demographic and socioeconomic differences in beliefs about the health effects of smoking. *American Journal of Public Health* 1992;82(1):99–103.

Bruvold WH. A meta-analysis of adolescent smoking prevention programs. *American Journal of Public Health* 1993;83(6):872–80.

Butler J. The "Dakota Papers." Paper presented at the Women, Tobacco and Health pre-conference workshop at the Seventh World Conference on Tobacco and Health; 1990 Mar 30; Perth (Australia).

Byrd JC, Meade CD. Smoking cessation among pregnant women in an urban setting. *Wisconsin Medical Journal* 1993;92(11):609–12.

California NOW. The politics of women and smoking [fact sheet]. Sacramento (CA): California NOW, 1994.

Canadian Association for the Advancement of Women and Sport and Physical Activity. Evening the Odds: Adolescent Women, Tobacco and Physical Activity; <http://www.caaws.ca/Girls/eveningodds.htm>; accessed: January 26, 2001.

Carleton RA, Lasater TM, Assaf AR, Feldman HA, McKinlay S. The Pawtucket Heart Health Program: community changes in cardiovascular risk factors and projected disease risk. *American Journal of Public Health* 1995;85(6):777–85.

Cavin SW, Pierce JP. Low-cost cigarettes and smoking behavior in California, 1990–1993. *American Journal of Preventive Medicine* 1996;12(1):17–21.

Centers for Disease Control. Public attitudes regarding limits on public smoking and regulation of tobacco sales and advertising—10 U.S. communities, 1989. *Morbidity and Mortality Weekly Report* 1991;40(21):344–5,351–3.

Centers for Disease Control and Prevention. Physician and other health-care professional counseling of smokers to quit—United States, 1991. *Morbidity and Mortality Weekly Report* 1993a;42(44):854–7.

Centers for Disease Control and Prevention. Smoking cessation during previous year among adults—United States, 1990 and 1991. *Morbidity and Mortality Weekly Report* 1993b;42(26):504–7.

Centers for Disease Control and Prevention. Indicators of nicotine addiction among women—United States, 1991–1992. *Morbidity and Mortality Weekly Report* 1995a;44(6):102–5.

Centers for Disease Control and Prevention. Smokeless tobacco use among American Indian women—Southeastern North Carolina, 1991. *Morbidity and Mortality Weekly Report* 1995b;44(6):113–7.

Centers for Disease Control and Prevention. Initiative by organizations: tobacco control activities for February, 1998 [progress report]. Atlanta: Centers for Disease Control and Prevention, Center for Health Promotion and Disease Prevention, Office on Smoking and Health, 1998a.

Centers for Disease Control and Prevention. Monthly tobacco control activities for national organizations: May/June 1998 [progress report]. Atlanta: Centers for Disease Control and Prevention, Center for Health Promotion and Disease Prevention, Office on Smoking and Health, 1998b.

Centers for Disease Control and Prevention. Response to increases in cigarette prices by race/ethnicity, income, and age groups—United States,

1976–1993. *Morbidity and Mortality Weekly Report* 1998c;47(29):605–9.

Centers for Disease Control and Prevention. Decline in cigarette consumption following implementation of a comprehensive tobacco prevention and education program—Oregon, 1996–1998. *Morbidity and Mortality Weekly Report* 1999;48(7):140–3.

Cepeda-Benito A. Meta-analytical review of the efficacy of nicotine chewing gum in smoking treatment programs. *Journal of Consulting and Clinical Psychology* 1993;61(5):822–30.

Chaloupka F. Clean indoor air laws, addiction and cigarette smoking. *Applied Economics* 1992;24(2): 193–205.

Chaloupka FJ. *Men, women, and addiction: the case of cigarette smoking.* Working paper no. 3267. Cambridge (MA): National Bureau of Economic Research, 1990.

Chaloupka FJ, Pacula RL. *An examination of gender and race differences in youth smoking: responsiveness to price and tobacco control policies.* Working paper no. 6541. Cambridge (MA): National Bureau of Economic Research, 1998.

Chaloupka FJ, Wechsler H. *Price, tobacco control policies and smoking among young adults.* Working paper no. 5012. Cambridge (MA): National Bureau of Economic Research, 1995.

Charlton A, While D. Smoking and menstrual problems in 16-year-olds. *Journal of the Royal Society of Medicine* 1996;89(4):1935.

Chesney MA. Women, work-related stress, and smoking. In: Frankenhaeuser M, Lundberg U, Chesney M, editors. *Women, Work, and Health: Stress and Opportunities.* New York: Plenum Press, 1991: 139–55.

Clarke V, White V, Beckwith J, Borland R, Hill D. Are attitudes towards smoking different for males and females? *Tobacco Control* 1993;2(3):201–8.

Cnattingius S, Lindmark G, Meirik O. Who continues to smoke while pregnant? *Journal of Epidemiology and Community Health* 1992;46(3):218–21.

Cohen S, Kamarck T, Mermelstein R. A global measure of perceived stress. *Journal of Health and Social Behavior* 1983;24(4):385–96.

Cohen S, Lichtenstein E. Partner behaviors that support quitting smoking. *Journal of Consulting and Clinical Psychology* 1990;58(3):304–9.

Cohen S, Lichtenstein E, Prochaska JO, Rossi JS, Gritz ER, Carr CR, Orleans CT, Schoenbach VJ, Biener L, Abrams D, DiClemente C, Curry S, Marlatt GA, Cummings KM, Emont SL, Giovino G, Ossip-Klein D. Debunking myths about self-quitting: evidence from 10 prospective studies of persons who attempt to quit smoking by themselves. *American Psychologist* 1989;44(11):1355–65.

Commission for a Healthy New York. *Women Talk to Women about Smoking: A Report of the Women and Tobacco Task Force.* Albany (NY): Commission for a Healthy New York, 1995.

COMMIT Research Group. Community Intervention Trial for Smoking Cessation (COMMIT): summary of design and intervention. *Journal of the National Cancer Institute* 1991;83(22):1620–8.

COMMIT Research Group. Community Intervention Trial for Smoking Cessation (COMMIT): I. Cohort results from a four-year community intervention. *American Journal of Public Health* 1995a;85(2): 183–92.

COMMIT Research Group. Community Intervention Trial for Smoking Cessation (COMMIT): II. Changes in adult cigarette smoking prevalence. *American Journal of Public Health* 1995b;85(2): 193–200.

Commonwealth of Australia. Australia's women soccer team to send global anti-tobacco message [media release]. Canberra City (Australia): Commonwealth of Australia, Commonwealth Department of Health and Aged Care, 2000 Aug 13.

Commonwealth of Massachusetts. *Report on the Sale of Tobacco to Minors in Massachusetts.* Boston: Commonwealth of Massachusetts, Office of the Attorney General, 1994.

*Congressional Record.* Association of Professional Flight Attendants support for legislation to ban smoking on domestic flights [letter]. *Congressional Record,* 101st Congress, 1st session. 1989a;135 (Pt 14):20006.

*Congressional Record.* Flight Attendant Non-Smokers support for legislation to ban smoking on domestic airline flights [letter]. *Congressional Record,* 101st Congress, 1st session. 1989b;135(Pt 14): 20005–6.

Connolly HM, Crary JL, McGoon MD, Hensrud DD, Edwards BS, Edwards WD, Schaff HV. Valvular heart disease associated with fenfluramine-phentermine. *New England Journal of Medicine* 1997;337(9):581–8.

Coppotelli HC, Orleans CT. Partner support and other determinants of smoking cessation maintenance among women. *Journal of Consulting and Clinical Psychology* 1985;53(4):455–60.

Cormier J, Herbig LJ, DiLorenzo TM, Frensch P, Fisher EB Jr. Effects of social support, perceived competence, and partner smoking status in successful smoking quit attempts. Paper presented at the Association for Advancement of Behavior Therapy; 1990 Nov; San Francisco.

Corti B, Donovan RJ, Holman CDJ, Coten N, Jones SJ. Using sponsorship to promote health messages to children. *Health Education and Behavior* 1997;24(3): 276–86.

Covey LS, Glassman AH, Stetner F. Depression and depressive symptoms in smoking cessation. *Comprehensive Psychiatry* 1990;31(4):350–4.

Covey LS, Zang EA, Wynder EL. Cigarette smoking and occupational status: 1977 to 1990. *American Journal of Public Health* 1992;82(9):1230–4.

Craig D, Parrott A, Coomber J-A. Smoking cessation in women: effects of the menstrual cycle. *International Journal of the Addictions* 1992;27(6):697–706.

Crittenden KS, Manfredi C, Lacey L, Warnecke R, Parsons J. Measuring readiness and motivation to quit smoking among women in public health clinics. *Addictive Behaviors* 1994;19(5):497–507.

Cummings KM, Sciandra R, Davis S, Rimer B. Response to anti-smoking campaign aimed at mothers with young children. *Health Education Research* 1989;4(4):429–37.

Curry SJ. Self-help interventions for smoking cessation. *Journal of Consulting and Clinical Psychology* 1993;61(5):790–803.

Curry S, Wagner EH, Grothaus LC. Intrinsic and extrinsic motivation for smoking cessation. *Journal of Consulting and Clinical Psychology* 1990;58(3): 310–6.

Curry SJ, Marlatt GA, Gordon J, Baer JS. A comparison of alternative theoretical approaches to smoking cessation and relapse. *Health Psychology* 1988; 7(6):545–56.

Dalack GW, Glassman AH, Rivelli S, Covey L, Stetner F. Mood, major depression and fluoxetine response in cigarette smokers. *American Journal of Psychiatry* 1995;152(3):398–403.

Dale LC, Olsen DA, Patten CA, Schroeder DR, Croghan IT, Hurt RD, Offord KP, Wolter TD. Predictors of smoking cessation among elderly smokers treated for nicotine dependence. *Tobacco Control* 1997;6(3):181–7.

Dale LC, Schroeder DR, Wolter TD, Croghan IT, Hurt RD, Offord KP. Weight change after smoking cessation using variable doses of transdermal nicotine replacement. *Journal of General Internal Medicine* 1998;13(1):9–15.

Daube MM. Building on success: from Buenos Aires to Paris. *Tobacco Control* 1992;1(3):198–204.

Davidson M. National Womens Magazine Project outline [project report]. Victoria (Australia): Quit Victoria, 1991.

Davis MC, Matthews KA. Cigarette smoking and oral contraceptive use influence women's lipid, lipoprotein, and cardiovascular responses during stress. *Health Psychology* 1990;9(6):717–36.

Davis SM, Lambert LC, Gomez Y, Skipper B. Southwest Cardiovascular Curriculum Project: study findings for American Indian elementary students. *Journal of Health Education* 1995;26(Suppl 2): S-72–S-81.

Davis SW, Cummings KM, Rimer BK, Sciandra R, Stone JC. The impact of tailored self-help smoking cessation guides on young mothers. *Health Education Quarterly* 1992;19(4):495–504.

DeBon M, Klesges RC, Klesges LM. Symptomatology across the menstrual cycle in smoking and nonsmoking women. *Addictive Behaviors* 1995;20(3): 335–43.

DiFranza JR, Savageau JA, Aisquith BF. Youth access to tobacco: the effects of age, gender, vending machine locks, and "It's the Law" programs. *American Journal of Public Health* 1996;86(2):221–4.

Dijkstra A, De Vries H, Roijackers J. Targeting smokers with low readiness to change with tailored and nontailored self-help materials. *Preventive Medicine* 1999;28(2):203–11.

Dijkstra A, De Vries H, Roijackers J, van Breukelen G. Tailoring information to enhance quitting in smokers with low motivation to quit: three basic efficacy questions. *Health Psychology* 1998;17(6): 513–9.

DiLorenzo TM, Powers RW, Cormier JF, Herbig LJ, Fisher EB Jr. The role of social support and competence skills in smoking cessation among women. Paper presented at the 1990 World Conference on Lung Health, American Lung Association and International Union against Tuberculosis and Lung Disease; 1990 May; Boston.

District of Columbia Interagency Council on Smoking and Health. Protest of the 1990 Virginia Slims Tennis Tournament: summary of activities [report]. Washington: District of Columbia Interagency Council on Smoking and Health, 1990.

Doherty K, Militello FS, Kinnunen T, Garvey AJ. Nicotine gum dose and weight gain after smoking cessation. *Journal of Consulting and Clinical Psychology* 1996;64(4):799–807.

Dolan-Mullen P, Ramirez G, Groff JY. A meta-analysis of randomized trials of prenatal smoking cessation interventions. *American Journal of Obstetrics and Gynecology* 1994;171(5):1328–34.

Dwyer T, Pierce JP, Hannam CD, Burke N. Evaluation of the Sydney "Quit. For Life" anti-smoking campaign. Part 2. Changes in smoking prevalence. *Medical Journal of Australia* 1986;144(7):344–7.

Eck LH, Kleges RC, Meyers AW, Slawson DL, Winders SA. Changes in food consumption and body weight associated with smoking cessation across menstrual cycle phase. *Addictive Behaviors* 1997;22(6):775–82.

Edwards NB, Murphy JK, Downs AD, Ackerman BJ, Rosenthal TL. Doxepin as an adjunct to smoking cessation: a double-blind pilot study. *American Journal of Psychiatry* 1989;146(3):373–6.

Egger G, Fitzgerald W, Frape G, Monaem A, Rubinstein P, Tyler C, McKay B. Results of large scale media antismoking campaign in Australia: North Coast "Quit for Life" programme. *British Medical Journal* 1983;287(6399):1125–8.

Eissenberg T, Adams C, Riggins EC III, Likness M. Smokers' sex and the effects of tobacco cigarettes: subject-rated and physiological measures. *Nicotine and Tobacco Research* 1999;1(4):317–24.

Elder JP, Wildey M, de Moor C, Sallis JF Jr, Eckhardt L, Edwards C, Erickson A, Golbeck A, Hovell M, Johnston D, Levitz MD, Molgaard C, Young R, Vito D, Woodruff SI. The long-term prevention of tobacco use among junior high school students: classroom and telephone interventions. *American Journal of Public Health* 1993;83(9):1239–44.

Ellickson PL, Bell RM, Harrison ER. Changing adolescent propensities to use drugs: results from Project ALERT. *Health Education Quarterly* 1993;20(2): 227–42.

Emmons KM, Hammond SK, Abrams DB. Smoking at home: the impact of smoking cessation on nonsmokers' exposure to environmental tobacco smoke. *Health Psychology* 1994;13(6):516–20.

Emmons KM, Weidner G. The effects of cognitive and physical stress on cardiovascular reactivity among smokers and oral contraceptive users. *Psychophysiology* 1988;25(2):166–71.

Emont SL, Choi WS, Novotny TE, Giovino GA. Clean indoor air legislation, taxation, and smoking behaviour in the United States: an ecological analysis. *Tobacco Control* 1993;2(1):13–7.

Emont SL, Cummings KM. Weight gain following smoking cessation: a possible role for nicotine replacement in weight management. *Addictive Behaviors* 1987;12(2):151–5.

Endicott J, Halbreich U. Clinical significance of premenstrual dysphoric changes. *Journal of Clinical Psychiatry* 1988;49(12):486–9.

Ernster VL. Women and smoking [editorial]. *American Journal of Public Health* 1993;83(9):1202–3.

Ershoff DH, Aaronson NK, Danaher BG, Wasserman FW. Behavioral, health, and cost outcomes of an HMO-based prenatal health education program. *Public Health Reports* 1983;98(6):536–47.

Ershoff DH, Mullen PD, Quinn VP. A randomized trial of a serialized self-help smoking cessation program for pregnant women in an HMO. *American Journal of Public Health* 1989;79(2):182–7.

Ershoff DH, Quinn VP, Mullen PD, Lairson DR. Pregnancy and medical cost outcomes of a self-help prenatal smoking cessation program in a HMO. *Public Health Reports* 1990;105(4):340–7.

Eubanks T. *Developing Health and Fitness: Be Your Best!* New York: Girl Scouts of the United States of America, 1992.

Eubanks T, Mosatche HS, Cryan R, Bergerson C. *Cadette Girl Scout Handbook*. New York: Girl Scouts of the United States of America, 1995.

Fagerström K-O. Reducing the weight gain after stopping smoking. *Addictive Behaviors* 1987;12(1):91–3.

Farquhar JW. The community-based model of life style intervention trials. *American Journal of Epidemiology* 1978;108(2):103–11.

Farquhar JW, Maccoby N, Wood PD, Alexander JK, Breitrose H, Brown BW Jr, Haskell WL, McAlister AL, Meyer AJ, Nash JD, Stern MP. Community education for cardiovascular health. *Lancet* 1977; 1(8023):1192–5.

Ferris J. Butt out: publishers and their tobacco habit. *Columbia Journalism Review* 1994;Jan–Feb:16–8.

Ferris RM, Cooper BR. Mechanism of antidepressant activity of bupropion. *Journal of Clinical Psychiatry Monograph* 1993;11(1):2–14.

Ferry LH, Robbins AS, Scariati PD, Masterson A, Abbey DE, Burchette RJ. Enhancement of smoking cessation using the antidepressant bupropion hydrochloride. *Circulation* 1992;86(4 Suppl I):I-671.

Fielding JE, Piserchia PV. Frequency of worksite health promotion activities. *American Journal of Public Health* 1989;79(1):16–20.

Fingerhut LA, Kleinman JC, Kendrick JS. Smoking before, during, and after pregnancy. *American Journal of Public Health* 1990;80(5):541–4.

Fiore MC, Bailey WC, Cohen SJ, Dorfman SF, Goldstein MG, Gritz ER, Heyman RB, Holbrook J, Jaen CR, Kottke TE, Lando HA, Mecklenburg R, Mullen PD, Nett LM, Robinson K, Stitzer ML, Tommasello AC, Villejo L, Wewers ME. *Smoking Cessation*. Clinical Practice Guideline No. 18. Rockville (MD): U.S. Department of Health and Human Services, Public Health Service, Agency for Health Care Policy and Research, 1996. AHCPR Publication No. 96-0692.

Fiore MC, Bailey WC, Cohen SJ, Dorfman SF, Goldstein MG, Gritz ER, Heyman RB, Jaén CR, Kottke TE, Lando HA, Mecklenburg R, Mullen PD, Nett LM, Robinson K, Stitzer ML, Tommasello AC, Villejo L, Wewers ME. *Treating Tobacco Use and Dependence.* Clinical Practice Guideline. U.S. Department of Health and Human Services, Public Health Service, 2000.

Fiore MC, Jorenby DE, Baker TB, Kenford SL. Tobacco dependence and the nicotine patch: clinical guidelines for effective use. *Journal of the American Medical Association* 1992;268(19):2687–94.

Fiore MC, Novotny TE, Pierce JP, Giovino GA, Hatziandreu EJ, Newcomb PA, Surawicz TS, Davis RM. Methods used to quit smoking in the United States: do cessation programs help? *Journal of the American Medical Association* 1990;263(20): 2760–5.

Fiore MC, Smith SS, Jorenby DE, Baker TB. The effectiveness of the nicotine patch for smoking cessation: a meta-analysis. *Journal of the American Medical Association* 1994;271(24):1940–7.

Fisher EB Jr. Two approaches to social support in smoking cessation: commodity model and nondirective support. *Addictive Behaviors* 1997;22(6): 819–33.

Fisher EB, Auslander WF, Munro JF, Arfken CL, Brownson RC, Owens NW. Neighbors for a smoke free north side: evaluation of a community organization approach to promoting smoking cessation among African Americans. *American Journal of Public Health* 1998;88(11):1658–63.

Fisher EB Jr, Auslander WF, Sussman LJ, Arfken CL, Munro JR, Sykes RK, Sylvia SC, Strunk RC, Owens N, Harrison D, Jackson-Thompson J. Community organization and social support among African American women. Paper presented at the Office of Research on Women's Health Workshop on Recruitment and Retention of Women in Clinical Studies; 1993 July; Bethesda (MD).

Fisher EB Jr, Bishop DB. Sex roles, social support, and smoking cessation. Paper presented at the Society of Behavioral Medicine; 1986 Mar; San Francisco.

Fisher EB Jr, Haire-Joshu D, Morgan GD, Rehberg H, Rost K. Smoking and smoking cessation. *American Review of Respiratory Disease* 1990a;142(3):702–20.

Fisher EB Jr, Rehberg HR, Beaupre PM, Hughes CR, Levitt-Gilmour T, Davis JR, DiLorenzo TM. Gender differences in response to social support in smoking cessation. Paper presented at the Association for Advancement of Behavior Therapy; 1991 Nov; New York.

Fisher KJ, Glasgow RE, Terborg JR. Work site smoking cessation: a meta-analysis of long-term quit rates from controlled studies. *Journal of Occupational Medicine* 1990b;32(5):429–39.

Flaxman J. Quitting smoking now or later: gradual, abrupt, immediate, and delayed quitting. *Behavior Therapy* 1978;9(2):260–70.

Flay BR, Koepke D, Thomson SJ, Santi S, Best JA, Brown KS. Six-year follow-up of the first Waterloo School Smoking Prevention Trial. *American Journal of Public Health* 1989;79(10):1371–6.

Flay BR, Ryan KB, Best JA, Brown KS, Kersell MW, d'Avernas JR, Zanna MP. Are social-psychological smoking prevention programs effective? The Waterloo Study. *Journal of Behavioral Medicine* 1985; 8(1):37–59.

Floyd RL, Rimer BK, Giovino GA, Mullen PD, Sullivan SE. A review of smoking in pregnancy: effects on pregnancy outcomes and cessation efforts. *Annual Review of Public Health* 1993;14:379–411.

Flynn BS, Worden JK, Secker-Walker RH, Badger GJ, Geller BM. Cigarette smoking prevention effects of mass media and school interventions targeted to gender and age groups. *Journal of Health Education* 1995;26(Suppl 2):S-45–S-51.

Forbes R. Smoke-free soccer: US women take the lead. *Tobacco Control* 1996;5(2):105–6.

Forster JL, Hourigan M, McGovern P. Availability of cigarettes to underage youth in three communities. *Preventive Medicine* 1992;21(3):320–8.

Forster JL, McBride C, Jeffery R, Schmid TL, Pirie PL. Support for restrictive tobacco policies among residents of selected Minnesota communities. *American Journal of Health Promotion* 1991;6(2):99–104.

Fortmann SP, Killen JD. Nicotine gum and self-help behavioral treatment for smoking relapse prevention: results from a trial using population-based recruitment. *Journal of Consulting and Clinical Psychology* 1995;63(3):460–8.

Fortmann SP, Taylor CB, Flora JA, Jatulis DE. Changes in adult cigarette smoking prevalence after 5 years of community health education: the Stanford Five-City Project. *American Journal of Epidemiology* 1993; 137(1):82–96.

Fraser T. Phasing out of point-of-sale tobacco advertising in New Zealand. *Tobacco Control* 1998;7(1): 82–4.

French SA, Jeffery RW, Klesges LM, Forster JL. Weight concerns and change in smoking behavior over two years in a working population. *American Journal of Public Health* 1995;85(5):720–2.

French SA, Jeffery RW, Pirie PL, McBride CM. Do weight concerns hinder smoking cessation efforts? *Addictive Behaviors* 1992;17(3):219–26.

Frye CA, Ward KD, Bliss RE, Garvey AJ. Influence of the menstrual cycle on smoking relapse and withdrawal symptoms. In: Keefe FJ, editor. *Society of Behavioral Medicine. Thirteenth Annual Scientific Sessions; 1992 Mar 25–28; New York.* Rockville (MD): Society of Behavioral Medicine, 1992:107.

Galbally R. Using the money generated by increased tobacco taxation. Paper presented at the 9th World Conference on Tobacco and Health; 1994 Oct 10–14; Paris.

Gallup Organization. *The Public's Attitudes Toward Cigarette Advertising and Cigarette Tax Increase.* Princeton (NJ): Gallup Organization, 1993.

Gannon L, Hansel S, Goodwin J. Correlates of menopausal hot flashes. *Journal of Behavioral Medicine* 1987;10(3):277–85.

Gebauer C, Kwo CY, Haynes EF, Wewers ME. A nurse-managed smoking cessation intervention during pregnancy. *Journal of Obstetric, Gynecologic, and Neonatal Nursing* 1998;27(1):47–53.

Gerlach KK, Shopland DR, Hartman AM, Gibson JT, Pechacek TF. Workplace smoking policies in the United States: results from a national study of more than 100,000 workers. *Tobacco Control* 1997; 6(3):199–206.

Gielen AC, Windsor R, Faden RR, O'Campo P, Repke J, Davis M. Evaluation of a smoking cessation intervention for pregnant women in an urban prenatal clinic. *Health Education Research: Theory and Practice* 1997;12(2):247–54.

Gilchrist LD, Schinke SP, Nurius P. Reducing onset of habitual smoking among women. *Preventive Medicine* 1989;18(2):235–48.

Gilpin E, Pierce JP, Goodman J, Burns D, Shopland D. Reasons smokers give for stopping smoking: do they relate to success in stopping? *Tobacco Control* 1992;1(4):256–63.

Ginsberg D, Hall SM, Reus VI, Muñoz RF. Mood and depression diagnosis in smoking cessation. *Experimental and Clinical Psychopharmacology* 1995;3(4): 389–95.

Giovino GA, Schooley MW, Zhu B-P, Chrismon JH, Tomar SL, Peddicord JP, Merritt RK, Husten CG, Eriksen MP. Surveillance for selected tobacco-use behaviors—United States, 1900–1994. *Morbidity and Mortality Weekly Report* 1994;43(SS-3):1–43.

Girl Scouts of the United States of America. *A Resource Book for Senior Girl Scouts.* New York: Girl Scouts of the United States of America, 1995.

Girl Scouts of the United States of America. Girl Scouts against smoking [announcement]. New York: Girl Scouts of the United States of America, Membership and Programs, 1996.

Girls Incorporated of Alameda County. Report submitted for the outstanding program award: leadership and community action. San Leandro (CA): Girls Incorporated of Alameda County, 1995.

Glanz K, Rimer BK. *Theory at a Glance: A Guide for Health Promotion Practice.* U.S. Department of Health and Human Services, Public Health Service, National Institutes of Health, 1995. NIH Publication No. 95-3896.

Glasgow RE, Cummings KM, Hyland A. Relationship of worksite smoking policy to changes in employee tobacco use: findings from COMMIT. *Tobacco Control* 1997a;6(Suppl 2):S44–8.

Glasgow RE, McCaul KD, Fisher KJ. Participation in worksite health promotion: a critique of the literature and recommendations for future practice. *Health Education Quarterly* 1993;20(3):391–408.

Glasgow RE, Terborg JR, Hollis JF, Severson HH, Boles SM. Take heart: results from the initial phase of a work-site wellness program. *American Journal of Public Health* 1995;85(2):209–16.

Glasgow RE, Terborg JR, Strycker LA, Boles SM, Hollis JF. Take Heart II: replication of a worksite health promotion trial. *Journal of Behavioral Medicine* 1997b;20(2):143–61.

Glassman AH. Cigarette smoking: implications for psychiatric illness. *American Journal of Psychiatry* 1993;150(4):546–53.

Glassman AH, Helzer JE, Covey LS, Cottler LB, Stetner F, Tipp JE, Johnson J. Smoking, smoking cessation, and major depression. *Journal of the American Medical Association* 1990;264(12):1546–9.

Glassman AH, Stetner F, Walsh BT, Raizman PS, Fleiss JL, Cooper TB, Covey LS. Heavy smokers, smoking cessation, and clonidine: results of a double-blind, randomized trial. *Journal of the American Medical Association* 1988;259(19):2863–6.

Glynn TJ. Relative effectiveness of physician-initiated smoking cessation programs. *Cancer Bulletin* 1988; 40(6):359–64.

Glynn TJ. Essential elements of school-based smoking prevention programs. *Journal of School Health* 1989; 59(5):181–8.

Glynn TJ, Boyd GM, Gruman JC. *Self-Guided Strategies for Smoking Cessation: A Program Planner's Guide.* U.S. Department of Health and Human Services,

Public Health Service, National Institutes of Health, 1990. NIH Publication No. 91-3104.

Gofin J, Gofin R, Abramson JH, Ban R. Ten-year evaluation of hypertension, overweight, cholesterol, and smoking control: the CHAD program in Jerusalem. *Preventive Medicine* 1986;15(3):304–12.

Goldberg RJ, Ockene JK, Kristeller J, Kalan K, Landon J, Hosmer DW Jr. Factors associated with heavy smoking among men and women: the physician-delivered smoking intervention project. *American Heart Journal* 1993;125(3):818–23.

Gonsalves L, Domb J, Gidwani G. Depression, chronic fatigue, and the premenstrual syndrome. *Primary Care* 1991;18(2):369–80.

Gourlay SG, Forbes A, Marriner T, Pethica D, McNeil JJ. Prospective study of factors predicting outcome of transdermal nicotine treatment in smoking cessation. *British Medical Journal* 1994;309(6958): 842–6.

Graham H. Smoking in pregnancy: the attitudes of expectant mothers. *Social Science and Medicine* 1976; 10(7–8):399–405.

Graham H. *Women, Health and the Family.* Brighton (UK): Wheatsheaf Books, 1984.

Graham H. Behaving well: women's health behaviour in context. In: Roberts H, editor. *Women's Health Counts.* London: Routledge, 1990:195–219.

Graham H. *Smoking Among Working Class Mothers with Children: A Final Report.* Coventry (UK): University of Warwick, Department of Applied Social Studies, 1992.

Graham JW, Johnson CA, Hansen WB, Flay BR, Gee M. Drug use prevention programs, gender, and ethnicity: evaluation of three seventh-grade Project SMART cohorts. *Preventive Medicine* 1990; 19(3):305–13.

Grande D, Muller M, Radcliffe T, Cho C, Lynn W. Women's organizations and the control of smoking among women. Paper presented at the American Stop Smoking Intervention Study for Cancer Prevention (ASSIST) Information Exchange Conference; 1995 Oct 17–18; Washington.

Greaves L. *Smoke Screen: Women's Smoking and Social Control.* Halifax (Canada): Fernwood Publishing, 1996.

Greaves L, Jordan J, McLellan D. How tobacco touches women's lives. *World Smoking and Health* 1994; 19(2):2–3.

Greenberg G, Thompson SG, Meade TW. Relation between cigarette smoking and use of hormonal replacement therapy for menopausal symptoms. *Journal of Epidemiology and Community Health* 1987; 41(1):26–9.

Greenberg RA, Strecher VJ, Bauman KE, Boat BW, Fowler MG, Keyes LL, Denny FW, Chapman RS, Stedman HC, LaVange LM, Glover LH, Haley NJ, Loda FA. Evaluation of a home-based intervention program to reduce infant passive smoking and lower respiratory illness. *Journal of Behavioral Medicine* 1994;17(3):273–90.

Grinstead OA. Preventing weight gain following smoking cessation: a comparison of behavioral treatment approaches [dissertation]. Los Angeles: University of California, 1981.

Gritz ER. Lung cancer: now, more than ever, a feminist issue [editorial]. *Cancer* 1993;43(4):197–9.

Gritz ER. Biobehavioral factors in smoking and smoking cessation in women. In: Czajkowski SM, Hill DR, Clarkson TB, editors. *Women, Behavior, and Cardiovascular Disease. Proceedings of a Conference Sponsored by the Heart, Lung, and Blood Institute.* U.S. Department of Health and Human Services, Public Health Service, National Institutes of Health, 1994:53–67. NIH Publication No. 94-3309.

Gritz ER, Berman BA, Bastani R, Wu M. A randomized trial of a self-help smoking cessation intervention in a nonvolunteer female population: testing the limits of the public health model. *Health Psychology* 1992;11(5):280–9.

Gritz ER, Berman BA, Read LL, Marcus AC, Siau J. Weight change among registered nurses in a self-help smoking cessation program. *American Journal of Health Promotion* 1990;5(2):115–21.

Gritz ER, Kristeller JL, Burns DM. Treating nicotine addiction in high-risk groups and patients with medical co-morbidity. In: Orleans CT, Slade J, editors. *Nicotine Addiction: Principles and Management.* New York: Oxford University Press, 1993:279–309.

Gritz ER, Marcus AC, Berman BA, Read LL, Kanim LEA, Reeder SJ. Evaluation of a worksite self-help smoking cessation program for registered nurses. *American Journal of Health Promotion* 1988;3(2):2–35.

Gritz ER, Nielsen IR, Brooks LA. Smoking cessation and gender: the influence of physiological, psychological, and behavioral factors. *Journal of the American Medical Women's Association* 1996;51(1–2): 35–42.

Gritz ER, Thompson B, Emmons K, Ockene JK, McLerran DF, Nielsen IR. Gender differences among smokers and quitters in the Working Well Trial. *Preventive Medicine* 1998;27(4):553–61.

Gross J, Johnson J, Sigler L, Stitzer ML. Dose effects of nicotine gum. *Addictive Behaviors* 1995;20(3): 371–81.

Gross J, Stitzer ML, Maldonado J. Nicotine replacement: effects on postcessation weight gain. *Journal of Consulting and Clinical Psychology* 1989;57(1):87–92.

Grunberg NE, Winders SE, Wewers ME. Gender differences in tobacco use. *Health Psychology* 1991;10(2):143–53.

Gulick EE, Shaw V, Allison M. Dietary practices and pregnancy discomforts among urban Blacks. *Journal of Perinatology* 1989;9(3):271–80.

Gunn RC. Reactions to withdrawal symptoms and success in smoking cessation clinics. *Addictive Behaviors* 1986;11(1):49–53.

Gurdon MA, Flynn BS. Smoking policies in the workplace—the impact of gender. *Social Science Quarterly* 1996;77(3):674–84.

Hahn LP, Folsom AR, Sprafka JM, Norsted SW. Cigarette smoking and cessation behaviors among urban Blacks and Whites. *Public Health Reports* 1990;105(3):290–5.

Hajek P, Jackson P, Belcher M. Long-term use of nicotine chewing gum: occurrence, determinants, and effect on weight gain. *Journal of the American Medical Association* 1988;260(11):1593–6.

Halbreich U, Endicott J. Methodological issues in studies of premenstrual changes. *Psychoneuroendocrinology* 1985;10(1):15–32.

Hall SM, Ginsberg D, Jones RT. Smoking cessation and weight gain. *Journal of Consulting and Clinical Psychology* 1986;54(3):342–6.

Hall SM, Muñoz RF, Reus VI. Cognitive-behavioral intervention increases abstinence rates for depressive-history smokers. *Journal of Consulting and Clinical Psychology* 1994;62(1):141–6.

Hall SM, Muñoz RF, Reus VI, Sees KL. Nicotine, negative affect, and depression. *Journal of Consulting and Clinical Psychology* 1993;61(5):761–7.

Hall SM, Muñoz RF, Reus VI, Sees KL, Duncan C, Humfleet GL, Hartz DT. Mood management and nicotine gum in smoking treatment: a therapeutic contact and placebo controlled study. *Journal of Consulting and Clinical Psychology* 1996;64(5):1003–9.

Hall SM, Reus VI, Muñoz RF, Sees KL, Humfleet G, Hartz DT, Frederick S, Triffleman E. Nortriptyline and cognitive-behavioral therapy in the treatment of cigarette smoking. *Archives of General Psychiatry* 1998;55(8):683–90.

Hall SM, Tunstall CD, Vila KL, Duffy J. Weight gain prevention and smoking cessation: cautionary findings. *American Journal of Public Health* 1992;82(6):799–803.

Hampson E, Kimura D. Reciprocal effects of hormonal fluctuations on human motor and perceptual-spatial skills. *Behavioral Neuroscience* 1988;102(3):456–9.

Hartmann KE, Thorp JM Jr, Pahel-Short L, Koch MA. A randomized controlled trial of smoking cessation intervention in pregnancy in an academic clinic. *Obstetrics and Gynecology* 1996;87(4):621–6.

Hatsukami D, Skoog K, Allen S, Bliss R. Gender and the effects of different doses of nicotine gum on tobacco withdrawal symptoms. *Experimental and Clinical Psychopharmacology* 1995;3(2):163–73.

Hatziandreu EJ, Pierce JP, Lefkopoulou M, Fiore MC, Mills SL, Novotny TE, Giovino GA, Davis RM. Quitting smoking in the United States in 1986. *Journal of the National Cancer Institute* 1990;82(17):1402–6.

Health Promotion Agency of Northern Ireland and Ulster Cancer Foundation. *First International Conference on Women and Smoking. Conference Proceedings and Recommendations for Action; 1992 Oct 5–7; Newcastle, Northern Ireland.* Geneva: International Union Against Cancer, 1993.

Hebel JR, Fox NL, Sexton M. Dose-response of birth weight to various measures of maternal smoking during pregnancy. *Journal of Clinical Epidemiology* 1988;41(5):483–9.

Hebel JR, Nowicki P, Sexton M. The effect of antismoking intervention during pregnancy: an assessment of interactions with maternal characteristics. *American Journal of Epidemiology* 1985;122(1):135–48.

Henningfield JE. Nicotine medications for smoking cessation. *New England Journal of Medicine* 1995;333(18):1196–203.

Hetherington MM, Burnett L. Ageing and the pursuit of slimness: dietary restraint and weight satisfaction in elderly women. *British Journal of Clinical Psychology* 1994;33(Pt 3):391–400.

Hill RD, Rigdon M, Johnson S. Behavioral smoking cessation treatment for older chronic smokers. *Behavior Therapy* 1993;24(2):321–9.

Hjalmarson AIM, Hahn L, Svanberg B. Stopping smoking in pregnancy: effect of a self-help manual in controlled trial. *British Journal of Obstetrics and Gynaecology* 1991;98(3):260–4.

Hollis JF, Vogt TM, Stevens V, Biglan A, Severson H, Lichtenstein E. The Tobacco Reduction and Cancer Control (TRACC) program: team approaches to counseling in medical and dental settings. In: *Tobacco and the Clinician: Interventions for Medical and Dental Practice.* Smoking and Tobacco Control

Monograph 5. U.S. Department of Health and Human Services, Public Health Service, National Institutes of Health, National Cancer Institute, 1994:143–68. NIH Publication No. 94-3693.

Hornsby PP, Wilcox AJ, Weinberg CR. Cigarette smoking and disturbance of menstrual function. *Epidemiology* 1998;9(2):193–8.

Hu TW, Lin Z, Keeler TE. Teenage smoking, attempts to quit, and school performance. *American Journal of Public Health* 1998;88(6):940–3.

Hughes JR. Pharmacotherapy for smoking cessation: unvalidated assumptions, anomalies, and suggestions for future research. *Journal of Consulting and Clinical Psychology* 1993;61(5):751–60.

Hughes JR. Treatment of nicotine dependence: is more better? [editorial] *Journal of the American Medical Association* 1995;274(17):1390–1.

Hughes JR, Goldstein MG, Hurt RD, Shiffman S. Recent advances in the pharmacotherapy of smoking. *Journal of the American Medical Association* 1999;281(1):72–6.

Hughes JR, Gust SW, Skoog K, Keenan RM, Fenwick JW. Symptoms of tobacco withdrawal: a replication and extension. *Archives of General Psychiatry* 1991;48(1):52–9.

Hughes JR, Hatsukami D. Signs and symptoms of tobacco withdrawal. *Archives of General Psychiatry* 1986;43(3):289–94.

Hurt RD, Croghan GA, Beede SD, Wolter TD, Croghan IT, Patten CA. Nicotine patch therapy in 101 adolescent smokers: efficacy, withdrawal symptom relief, and carbon monoxide and plasma cotinine levels. *Archives of Pediatric and Adolescent Medicine* 2000;154(1):31–7.

Hurt RD, Sachs DP, Glover ED, Offord KP, Johnston JA, Dale LC, Khayrallah MA, Schroeder DR, Glover PN, Sullivan CR, Croghan IT, Sullivan PM. A comparison of sustained-release bupropion and placebo for smoking cessation [see comments]. *New England Journal of Medicine* 1997;337(17): 1195–202.

IEG. IEG intelligence report on tobacco company sponsorship for the Robert Wood Johnson Foundation: 1995 Sponsorships. Chicago: IEG, 1995.

International Network of Women Against Tobacco. INWAT Constitution: draft as of 14 Mar 1994. Washington: American Public Health Association, 1994.

International Network of Women Against Tobacco. *The Net* [newsletter]. 1995 Sept.

International Network of Women Against Tobacco. *The Net* [newsletter]. 1999 Summer.

Jacobs MA, Spilken AZ, Norman MM, Wohlberg GW, Knapp PH. Interaction of personality and treatment conditions associated with success in a smoking control program. *Psychosomatic Medicine* 1971;33(6):545–56.

Jarvik ME, Henningfield JE. Pharmacological adjuncts for the treatment of tobacco dependence. In: Orleans CT, Slade J, editors. *Nicotine Addiction: Principles and Management.* New York: Oxford University Press, 1993:245–61.

Jarvis MJ. Gender differences in smoking cessation: real or myth? *Tobacco Control* 1994;3(4):324–8.

Jeffery RW, Boles SM, Strycker LA, Glasgow RE. Smoking-specific weight gain concerns and smoking cessation in a working population. *Health Psychology* 1997;16(5):487–9.

Jeffery RW, Forster JL, French SA, Kelder SH, Lando HA, McGovern PG, Jacobs DR Jr, Baxter JE. The Healthy Worker Project: a work-site intervention for weight control and smoking cessation. *American Journal of Public Health* 1993;83(3):395–401.

Jensen PM, Coambs RB. Cigarette smoking and adolescent menstrual disorders. *Canadian Woman Studies* 1994;14(3):57–60.

Johnson L. A case study of changing advertising policies in women's magazines. Paper presented at the 115th Annual Meeting of the American Public Health Association and Related Organizations; 1987 Oct 18–Oct 22; New Orleans.

Johnson KM, Lando HA, Schmid LS, Solberg LI. The GAINS project: outcome of smoking cessation strategies in four urban Native American clinics. *Addictive Behaviors* 1997;22(2):207–18.

Jones R, Manfredi C, Mermelstein R, Raju N, Thomas V. The Head Start parent involvement program as a vehicle for smoking reduction intervention. *Journal of Family and Community Health* 1994;17:1–12.

Jordan J. Introduction. *World Smoking and Health* 1992; 17(1):2–4.

Jorenby DE. New developments in approaches to smoking cessation. *Current Opinion in Pulmonary Medicine* 1998;4(2):103–6.

Jorenby DE, Leischow SJ, Nides MA, Rennard SI, Johnston JA, Hughes AR, Smith SS, Muramoto ML, Daughton DM, Doan K, Fiore MC, Baker TB. A controlled trial of sustained-release bupropion, a nicotine patch, or both for smoking cessation [see comments]. *New England Journal of Medicine* 1999;340(9):685–91.

Jorenby DE, Smith SS, Fiore MC, Hurt RD, Offord KP, Croghan IT, Hays JT, Lewis SF, Baker TB. Varying nicotine patch dose and type of smoking cessation counseling. *Journal of the American Medical Association* 1995;274(17):1347–52.

Kauffman SE, Silver P, Poulin J. Gender differences in attitudes toward alcohol, tobacco, and other drugs. *Social Work* 1997;42(3):231–41.

Kawachi I, Troisi RJ, Rotnitzky AG, Coakley EH, Colditz GA. Can physical activity minimize weight gain in women after smoking cessation? *American Journal of Public Health* 1996;86(7): 999–1004.

Keeler TE, Hu T-W, Barnett PG, Manning WG. Taxation, regulation, and addiction: a demand function for cigarettes based on time-series evidence. *Journal of Health Economics* 1993;12(1):1–18.

Keintz MK, Fleisher L, Rimer BK. Reaching mothers of preschool-aged children with a targeted quit smoking intervention. *Journal of Community Health* 1994;19(1):25–40.

Kelder SH, Perry CL, Peters RJ Jr, Lytle LL, Klepp K-I. Gender differences in the Class of 1989 study: the school component of the Minnesota Heart Health Program. *Journal of Health Education* 1995; 26(Suppl 2):S-36–S-44.

Kendler KS, Neale MC, MacLean CJ, Heath AC, Eaves LJ, Kessler RC. Smoking and major depression: a causal analysis. *Archives of General Psychiatry* 1993; 50(1):36–43.

Kendrick JS, Zahniser SC, Miller N, Salas N, Stine J, Gargiullo PM, Floyd RL, Spierto FW, Sexton M, Metzger RW, Stockbauer JW, Hannon WH, Dalmat ME. Integrating smoking cessation into routine public prenatal care: the Smoking Cessation in Pregnancy project. *American Journal of Public Health* 1995;85(2):217–22.

Kenford SL, Fiore MC, Jorenby DE, Smith SS, Wetter D, Baker TB. Predicting smoking cessation: who will quit with and without the nicotine patch. *Journal of the American Medical Association* 1994; 271(8):589–94.

Killen JD, Fortmann SP, Newman B. Weight change among participants in a large sample minimal contact smoking relapse prevention trial. *Addictive Behaviors* 1990a;15(4):323–32.

Killen JD, Fortmann SP, Newman B, Varady A. Evaluation of a treatment approach combining nicotine gum with self-guided behavioral treatments for smoking relapse prevention. *Journal of Consulting and Clinical Psychology* 1990b;58(1):85–92.

Killen JD, Fortmann SP, Telch MJ, Newman B. Are heavy smokers different from light smokers? A comparison after 48 hours without cigarettes. *Journal of the American Medical Association* 1988;260(11): 1581–5.

King AC, Taylor CB, Haskell WL. Smoking in older women: is being female a 'risk factor' for continued cigarette use? *Archives of Internal Medicine* 1990;150(9):1841–6.

King TK, Borrelli B, Black C, Pinto BM, Marcus BH. Minority women and tobacco: implications for smoking cessation interventions. *Annals of Behavioral Medicine* 1997;19(3):301–13.

Klepp K-I, Tell GS, Vellar OD. Ten-year follow-up of the Oslo Youth Study Smoking Prevention Program. *Preventive Medicine* 1993;22(4):453–62.

Klesges RC, Brown K, Pascale RW, Murphy M, Williams E, Cigrang JA. Factors associated with participation, attrition, and outcome in a smoking cessation program at the workplace. *Health Psychology* 1988;7(6):575–89.

Klesges RC, Klesges LM. Cigarette smoking as a dieting strategy in a university population. *International Journal of Eating Disorders* 1988;7(3):413–9.

Klesges RC, Klesges LM, Meyers AW. Relationship of smoking status, energy balance, and body weight: analysis of the second National Health and Nutrition Examination Survey. *Journal of Consulting and Clinical Psychology* 1991;59(6):899–905.

Klesges RC, Klesges LM, Meyers AW, Klem ML, Isbell T. The effects of phenylpropanolamine on dietary intake, physical activity, and body weight after smoking cessation. *Clinical Pharmacology and Therapeutics* 1990;47(6):747–54.

Kluger R. *Ashes to Ashes: America's Hundred-Year Cigarette War, the Public Health, and the Unabashed Triumph of Philip Morris.* New York: Knopf, 1996.

Kottke TE, Battista RN, DeFriese GH, Brekke ML. Attributes of successful smoking cessation interventions in medical practice: a meta-analysis of 39 controlled trials. *Journal of the American Medical Association* 1988;259(19):2882–9.

Kozlowski LT, Porter CQ, Orleans CT, Pope MA, Heatherton T. Predicting smoking cessation with self-reported measures of nicotine dependence: FTQ, FTND, and HSI. *Drug and Alcohol Dependence* 1994;34(3):211–6.

Lacey LP, Manfredi C, Balch G, Warnecke RB, Allen K, Edwards C. Social support in smoking cessation among black women in Chicago public housing. *Public Health Reports* 1993;108(3):387–94.

Lam TH, Chung SF, Betson CL, Wong CM, Hedley AJ. Tobacco advertisements: one of the strongest risk factors for smoking in Hong Kong students. *American Journal of Preventive Medicine* 1998;14(3): 217–23.

Lam W, Sze PC, Sacks HS, Chalmers TC. Meta-analysis of randomized controlled trials of nicotine chewing-gum. *Lancet* 1987;2(8549):27–30.

Lando HA. Formal quit smoking treatments. In: Orleans CT, Slade J, editors. *Nicotine Addiction: Principles and Management*. New York: Oxford University Press, 1993:221–44.

Lando HA, Gritz ER. Smoking cessation techniques. *Journal of the American Medical Women's Association* 1996;51(1–2):31–4, 47.

Lando HA, Johnson KM, Graham-Tomasi RP, McGovern PG, Solberg L. Urban Indians' smoking patterns and interest in quitting. *Public Health Reports* 1992:107(3):340–4.

Lando HA, Pechacek TF, Pirie PL, Murray DM, Mittelmark MB, Lichtenstein E, Nothwehr F, Gray C. Changes in adult cigarette smoking in the Minnesota Heart Health Program. *American Journal of Public Health* 1995;85(2):201–8.

Lando HA, Pirie PL, Hellerstedt WL, McGovern PG. Survey of smoking patterns, attitudes, and interest in quitting. *American Journal of Preventive Medicine* 1991;7(1):18–23.

Laugesen M, Meads C. Tobacco advertising restrictions, price, income and tobacco consumption in OECD countries, 1960–1986. *British Journal of Addiction* 1991;86(10):1343–54.

Leischow SJ, Sachs DPL, Bostrom AG, Hansen MD. Effects of differing nicotine-replacement doses on weight gain after smoking cessation. *Archives of Family Medicine* 1992;1(2):233–7.

Lewit EM, Coate D. The potential for using excise taxes to reduce smoking. *Journal of Health Economics* 1982;1(2):121–45.

Lewit EM, Hyland A, Kerrebrock N, Cummings KM. Price, public policy, and smoking in young people. *Tobacco Control* 1997;6(Suppl 2):S17–S24.

Li CQ, Windsor RA, Perkins L, Goldenberg RL, Lowe JB. The impact on infant birth weight and gestational age of cotinine-validated smoking reduction during pregnancy. *Journal of the American Medical Association* 1993;269(12):1519–24.

Lichtenstein E. Behavioral research contributions and needs in cancer prevention and control: tobacco use prevention and cessation. *Preventive Medicine* 1997;26(5 Pt 2):S57–S63.

Lightwood JM, Phibbs CS, Glantz SA. Short-term health and economic benefits of smoking cessation: low birth weight. *Pediatrics* 1999;104(6):1312–20.

Lillington L, Royce J, Novak D, Ruvalcaba M, Chlebowski R. Evaluation of a smoking cessation program for pregnant minority women. *Cancer Practice* 1995;3(3):157–63.

Lipkus IM, Lyna PR, Rimer BK. Using tailored messages to enhance smoking cessation among African-Americans at a community health center. *Nicotine and Tobacco Research* 1999;1(1):77–85.

Lowe JB, Windsor R, Balanda KP, Woodby L. Smoking relapse prevention methods for pregnant women: a formative evaluation. *American Journal of Health Promotion* 1997;11(4):244–6.

Lumley J, Astbury J. Advice for pregnancy. In: Chalmers I, Enkin M, Keirse MJNC, editors. *Effective Care in Pregnancy and Childbirth.* Vol. 1, Pregnancy. Pts 1–5. Oxford: Oxford University Press, 1989:237–54.

Lynch BS, Bonnie RJ, editors. *Growing Up Tobacco Free: Preventing Nicotine Addiction in Children and Youths.* Washington: National Academy Press, 1994.

Macaskill P, Pierce JP, Simpson JM, Lyle DM. Mass media-led antismoking campaign can remove the education gap in quitting behavior. *American Journal of Public Health* 1992;82(1):96–8.

Maccoby N, Farquhar JW, Wood PD, Alexander J. Reducing the risk of cardiovascular disease: effects of a community-based campaign on knowledge and behavior. *Journal of Community Health* 1977;3(2):100–14.

Mackay JM. Smoking and women. Paper presented at the 15th International Cancer Congress; 1990 Aug 16–22; Hamburg (Federal Republic of Germany).

Mackay JM, Hedley A. Hong Kong bans tobacco advertising. *British Medical Journal* 1997;315(7099):8.

Macken KM, Wilder D, Mersy DJ, Madlon-Kay DJ. Smoking patterns in a low-income urban population: a challenge to smoking cessation efforts. *Journal of Family Practice* 1991;31(6):93, 95–6.

Mahood G. Treating the tobacco epidemic like an epidemic: the road to effective tobacco control in Canada. In: Durston B, Jamrozik K, editors. *Tobacco and Health 1990: The Global War. Proceedings of the Seventh World Conference on Tobacco and Health, 1st–5th April 1990, Perth, Western Australia*. East Perth (Australia): Organising Committee of the Seventh World Conference on Tobacco and Health, 1990:88–97.

Manfredi C, Lacey L, Warnecke R, Buis M. Smoking-related behavior, beliefs, and social environment of young Black women in subsidized public housing in Chicago. *American Journal of Public Health* 1992;82(2):267–72.

Manfredi C, Lacey LP, Warnecke R, Petraitis J. Sociopsychological correlates of motivation to quit smoking among low-SES African American women. *Health Education and Behavior* 1998;25(3):304–18.

Manley MW, Pierce JP, Gilpin EA, Rosbrook B, Berry C, Wun L. Impact of the American Stop Smoking Intervention Study on cigarette consumption. *Tobacco Control* 1997;6(Suppl 2):S12–S16.

Marcus BH, Albrecht AE, King TK, Parisi AF, Pinto BM, Roberts M, Niaura RS, Abrams DB. The efficacy of exercise as an aid for smoking cessation in women: a randomized controlled trial. *Archives of Internal Medicine* 1999;159(11):1229–34.

Marcus BH, Albrecht AE, Niaura RS, Abrams DB, Thompson PD. Usefulness of physical exercise for maintaining smoking cessation in women. *American Journal of Cardiology* 1991;68(4):406–7.

Marcus BH, Albrecht AE, Niaura RS, Taylor ER, Simkin LR, Feder SI, Abrams DB, Thompson PD. Exercise enhances the maintenance of smoking cessation in women. *Addictive Behaviors* 1995;20(1): 87–92.

Marcus BH, Emmons KM, Simkin LR, Albrecht AE, Stoney CM, Abrams DB. Women and smoking cessation: current status and future directions. *Medicine, Exercise, Nutrition and Health* 1994;3(1):17–31.

Marín G, Marín BV, Pérez-Stable EJ, Sabogal F, Otero-Sabogal R. Changes in information as a function of a culturally appropriate smoking cessation community intervention for Hispanics. *American Journal of Community Psychology* 1990a;18(6):847–64.

Marín G, Marín BV, Pérez-Stable EJ, Sabogal F, Otero-Sabogal R. Cultural differences in attitudes and expectancies between Hispanic and non-Hispanic White smokers. *Hispanic Journal of Behavioral Sciences* 1990b;12(4):422–36.

Marín G, Pérez-Stable EJ. Effectiveness of disseminating culturally appropriate smoking-cessation information: Programa Latina para Dejar de Fumar. *Journal of the National Cancer Institute Monographs* 1995;18:155–63.

Marín G, Pérez-Stable EJ, Marín BV. Cigarette smoking among San Francisco Hispanics: the role of acculturation and gender. *American Journal of Public Health* 1989;79(2):196–8.

Mark EJ, Patalas ED, Chang HT, Evans RJ, Kessler SC. Fatal pulmonary hypertension associated with short-term use of fenfluramine and phentermine. *New England Journal of Medicine* 1997;337(9):602–6.

Marks JL. An evaluation of the proposed DSM-III-R criteria for late luteal phase dysphoric disorder based on personal and family-history characteristics of women perceiving themselves as having premenstrual syndrome [dissertation]. Storrs (CT): University of Connecticut, 1992.

Marks JL, Hair CS, Klock SC, Ginsburg BE, Pomerleau CS. Effects of menstrual phase on intake of nicotine, caffeine, and alcohol and nonprescribed drugs in women with late luteal phase dysphoric disorder. *Journal of Substance Abuse* 1994;6(2): 235–43.

Marks JL, Pomerleau CS, Pomerleau OF. Effects of menstrual phase on reactivity to nicotine. *Addictive Behaviors* 1999;24(1):127–34.

Marlatt GA, Curry S, Gordon JR. A longitudinal analysis of unaided smoking cessation. *Journal of Consulting and Clinical Psychology* 1988;56(5):715–20.

Marsh A, McKay S. *Poor Smokers.* London: Policy Studies Institute, 1994.

Masson CL. Cardiovascular and mood responses to a quantified dose of nicotine in oral contraceptive users and nonusers [dissertation]. Carbondale (IL): Southern Illinois University, 1995.

Matthews KA, Bromberger J, Egeland G. Behavioral antecedents and consequences of the menopause. In: Korenman SG, editor. *The Menopause. Biological and Clinical Consequences of Ovarian Failure: Evolution and Management.* Norwell (MA): Serono Symposia, 1990:1–15.

Mayer JP, Hawkins B, Todd R. A randomized evaluation of smoking cessation interventions for pregnant women at a WIC clinic. *American Journal of Public Health* 1990;80(1):76–8.

McAlister A, Puska P, Salonen JT, Tuomilehto J, Koskela K. Theory and action for health promotion: illustrations from the North Karelia Project. *American Journal of Public Health* 1982;72(1):43–50.

McBride CM, Curry SJ, Lando HA, Pirie PL, Grothaus LC, Nelson JC. Prevention of relapse in women who quit smoking during pregnancy. *American Journal of Public Health* 1999;89(5):706–11.

McBride CM, Pirie PL. Postpartum smoking relapse. *Addictive Behaviors* 1990;15(2):165–8.

McBride CM, Pirie PL, Curry SJ. Postpartum relapse to smoking: a prospective study. *Health Education Research* 1992;7(3):381–90.

McGovern PG, Lando HA, Roski J, Pirie PL, Sprafka JM. A comparison of smoking cessation clinic participants with smokers in the general population. *Tobacco Control* 1994;3(4):329–33.

McGrath E, Keita GP, Strickland BR, Russo NF, editors. *Women and Depression: Risk Factors and Treatment Issues. Final Report of the American Psychological Association's National Task Force on Women and Depression.* Washington: American Psychological Association, 1990.

McLellan DL. The International Network of Women Against Tobacco. Paper presented at the 118th Annual Meeting of the American Public Health Association; 1990 Oct 3; New York.

McLellan DL, da Costa e Silva VL, Chollat-Traquet C. Building women's leadership in tobacco control. *Tobacco Alert* 1992 July:3.

McLellan DL, Wright J. The National Women's Tobacco Control Plan. *Journal of Public Health Policy* 1996; 17(1):47–58.

Meier KJ, Licari MJ. The effect of cigarette taxes on cigarette consumption, 1955 through 1994. *American Journal of Public Health* 1997;87(7):1126–30.

Mello NK, Mendelson JH, Palmieri SL. Cigarette smoking by women: interactions with alcohol use. *Psychopharmacology* 1987;93(1):8–15.

Mermelstein R. Preventing weight gain following smoking cessation. Paper presented at the Society of Behavioral Medicine Eighth Annual Scientific Session; 1987 Mar; Washington.

Mermelstein R, Cohen S, Lichtenstein E, Baer JS, Kamarck T. Social support and smoking cessation and maintenance. *Journal of Consulting and Clinical Psychology* 1986;54(4):447–53.

Mermelstein RJ, Borrelli B. Women and smoking. In: Stanton AL, Gallant SJ, editors. *The Psychology of Women's Health: Progress and Challenges in Research and Application.* Washington: American Psychological Association, 1995:307–48.

Messimer SR, Hickner JM, Henry RC. A comparison of two antismoking interventions among pregnant women in eleven private primary care practices. *Journal of Family Practice* 1989;28(3):283–8.

Meyer AJ, Nash JD, McAlister AL, Maccoby N, Farquhar JW. Skills training in a cardiovascular health education campaign. *Journal of Consulting and Clinical Psychology* 1980;48(2):129–42.

Meyers AW, Klesges RC, Winders SE, Ward KD, Peterson BA, Eck LH. Are weight concerns predictive of smoking cessation? A prospective analysis. *Journal of Consulting and Clinical Psychology* 1997; 65(3):448–52.

Michnovicz JJ, Hershcopf RJ, Naganuma H, Bradlow HL, Fishman J. Increased 2-hydroxylation of estradiol as a possible mechanism for the anti-estrogenic effect of cigarette smoking. *New England Journal of Medicine* 1986;315(21):1305–9.

Millar WJ. Evaluation of the impact of smoking restrictions in a government work setting. *Canadian Journal of Public Health* 1988;79(5):379–82.

Miller WR, Rollnick S. *Motivational Interviewing: Preparing People to Change Addictive Behavior.* New York: Guilford Press, 1991.

Moolchan ET, Ernst M, Henningfield JE. A review of tobacco smoking in adolescents: treatment implications. *Journal of the American Academy of Child and Adolescent Psychiatry* 2000;39(6):682–93.

Morgan D. Panel bans smoking on most flights: hill conferees accept 'milestone' limits for commercial carriers. *Washington Post* 1989 Oct 17;Sect A:1 (col 1).

Morgan GD, Ashenberg ZS, Fisher EB Jr. Abstinence from smoking and the social environment. *Journal of Consulting and Clinical Psychology* 1988;56(2): 298–301.

Morgan GD, Noll EL, Orleans CT, Rimer BK, Amfoh K, Bonney G. Reaching midlife and older smokers: tailored interventions for routine medical care. *Preventive Medicine* 1996;25(3):346–54.

Morse Enterprises. The campaign. Paper prepared for the Capital City Chapter Links symposium to launch the pilot for the National Smoking Cessation Campaign for African American Women; 1992 Nov 21; Bethesda (MD). Silver Spring (MD): Morse Enterprises, 1992.

Mullahy J. Cigarette smoking: habits, health concerns, and heterogeneous unobservables in a microeconometric analysis of consumer demand [dissertation]. Arlington (VA): University of Virginia, 1985.

Mullen PD. Smoking cessation counseling in prenatal care. In: Merkatz IR, Thompson JE, Mullen PD, Goldenberg RL, editors. *New Perspectives on Prenatal Care.* New York: Elsevier Science Publishing, 1990:161–76.

Mullen PD, Quinn VP, Ershoff DH. Maintenance of nonsmoking postpartum by women who stopped smoking during pregnancy. *American Journal of Public Health* 1990;80(8):992–4.

Mullen PD, Richardson MA, Quinn VP, Ershoff DH. Postpartum return to smoking: who is at risk and when? *American Journal of Health Promotion* 1997; 11(5):323–30.

Muñoz RF, Marín BV, Posner SF, Pérez-Stable EJ. Mood management mail intervention increases abstinence rates for Spanish-speaking Latino smokers. *American Journal of Community Psychology* 1997;25(3):325–43.

Murray DM, Davis-Hearn M, Goldman AI, Pirie P, Luepker RV. Four- and five-year follow-up results from four seventh-grade smoking prevention strategies. *Journal of Behavioral Medicine* 1988;11(4): 395–405.

Murray DM, Pirie P, Luepker RV, Pallonen U. Five- and six-year follow-up results from four seventh-grade smoking prevention strategies. *Journal of Behavioral Medicine* 1989;12(2):207–18.

Murray DM, Richards PS, Luepker RV, Johnson CA. The prevention of cigarette smoking in children: two- and three-year follow-up comparisons of four prevention strategies. *Journal of Behavioral Medicine* 1987;10(6):595–611.

Murray RP, Johnston JJ, Dolce JJ, Lee WW, O'Hara P. Social support for smoking cessation and abstinence: the Lung Health Study. Lung Health Study Research Group. *Addictive Behaviors* 1995;20(2): 159–70.

Myers MG. Smoking intervention with adolescent substance abusers. Initial recommendations. *Journal of Substance Abuse and Treatment* 1999;16(4): 289–98.

National Association for Public Health Policy. Policy on women and smoking [position statement]. Reston (VA): National Association for Public Health Policy, 1996.

National Committee for Quality Assurance. *HEDIS 3.0. Vol. 2. Technical Specifications.* Washington, DC: National Committee for Quality Assurance, 1997.

National Organization for Women. Resolution on women and tobacco passed by the National Organization for Women Board of Directors, Jan 21, 1991. Washington: National Organization for Women, 1991.

Nevid J, Javier RA. Preliminary investigation of a culturally specific smoking cessation intervention for Hispanic smokers. *American Journal of Health Promotion* 1997(3);11:198–207.

Niaura R, Goldstein MG, Depue J, Keuthen N, Kristeller J, Abrams D. Fluoxetine, symptoms of depression, and smoking cessation. *Annals of Behavioral Medicine* 1995;17(Suppl):S061.

Niaura R, Shadel WG, Abrams DB, Monti PM, Rohsenow DJ, Sirota A. Individual differences in cue reactivity among smokers trying to quit: effects of gender and cue type. *Addictive Behaviors* 1998;23(2):209–24.

Nides M, Rand C, Dolce J, Murray R, O'Hara P, Voelker H, Connett J. Weight gain as a function of smoking cessation and 2-mg nicotine gum use among middle-aged smokers with mild lung impairment in the first 2 years of the Lung Health Study. *Health Psychology* 1994;13(4):354–61.

Nides MA, Rakos RF, Gonzales D, Murray RP, Tashkin DP, Bjornson-Benson WM, Lindgren P, Connett JE. Predictors of initial smoking cessation and relapse through the first 2 years of the Lung Health Study. *Journal of Consulting and Clinical Psychology* 1995;63(1):60–9.

Novotny TE, Warner KE, Kendrick JS, Remington PL. Smoking by Blacks and Whites: socioeconomic and demographic differences. *American Journal of Public Health* 1988;78(9):1187–9.

O'Campo P, Davis MV, Gielen AC. Smoking cessation interventions for pregnant women: review and future directions. *Seminars in Perinatology* 1995; 19(4):279–85.

O'Campo P, Faden RR, Brown H, Gielen AC. The impact of pregnancy on women's prenatal and postpartum smoking behavior. *American Journal of Preventive Medicine* 1992;8(1):8–13.

Ockene JK. Physician-delivered interventions for smoking cessation: strategies for increasing effectiveness. *Preventive Medicine* 1987;16(5):723–37.

Ockene JK. Smoking among women across the life span: prevalence, interventions, and implications for cessation research. *Annals of Behavioral Medicine* 1993;15(2–3):135–48.

O'Hara P, Portser SA, Anderson BP. The influence of menstrual cycle changes on the tobacco withdrawal syndrome in women. *Addictive Behaviors* 1989; 14(6):595–600.

O'Loughlin J, Paradis G, Renaud L, Meshefedjian G, Barnett T. The "Yes, I Quit" smoking cessation course: does it help women in a low income community quit? *Journal of Community Health* 1997; 22(6):451–68.

Oncken CA, Hatsukami DK, Lupo VR, Lando HA, Gibeau LM, Hansen RJ. Effects of short-term use of nicotine gum in pregnant smokers. *Clinical Pharmacology and Therapeutics* 1996;59(6):654–61.

Orleans CT, Boyd NR, Bingler R, Sutton C, Fairclough D, Heller D, McClatchey M, Ward JA, Graves C, Fleisher L, Baum S. A self-help intervention for African American smokers: tailoring cancer information service counseling for a special population. *Preventive Medicine* 1998;27(5 Pt 2):S61–S70.

Orleans CT, Jepson C, Resch N, Rimer BK. Quitting motives and barriers among older smokers. The 1986 Adult Use of Tobacco Survey revisited. *Cancer* 1994a;74(7 Suppl):2055–61.

Orleans CT, Resch N, Noll E, Keintz MK, Rimer BK, Brown TV, Snedden TM. Use of transdermal nicotine in a state-level prescription plan for the elderly: a first look at 'real-world' patch users. *Journal of the American Medical Association* 1994b;271(8): 601–7.

Orleans CT, Rimer BK, Cristinzio S, Jepson C, Quade D, Porter CQ, Keintz MK, Fleisher L, Schoenbach VJ. *Smoking Patterns and Quitting Motives, Barriers and Strategies Among Older Smokers Aged 50–74: A Report for the American Association of Retired Persons.* Philadelphia: Fox Chase Cancer Center, 1990.

Orleans CT, Rimer BK, Cristinzio S, Keintz MK, Fleisher L. A national survey of older smokers: treatment needs of a growing population. *Health Psychology* 1991a;10(5):343–51.

Orleans CT, Schoenbach VJ, Wagner EH, Quade D, Salmon MA, Pearson DC, Fiedler J, Porter CQ, Kaplan BH. Self-help quit smoking interventions: effects of self-help materials, social support instructions, and telephone counseling. *Journal of Consulting and Clinical Psychology* 1991b;59(3): 439–48.

Ossip-Klein DJ, Carosella AM, Krusch DA. Self-help interventions for older smokers. *Tobacco Control* 1997;6(3):188–93.

Otero-Sabogal R, Sabogal F, Pérez-Stable E. Psychosocial correlates of smoking among immigrant Latina adolescents. *Journal of the National Cancer Institute Monographs* 1995;18:65–71.

Pallonen UE, Redding CA, Willey CJ, Prochaska JO. Gender differences in readiness to quit smoking among vocational students. Paper presented at the American Psychological Association Conference, Behavioral Factors in Women's Health: Creating an Agenda for the 21st Century; 1994 May 11–14; Washington.

Pallonen UE, Velicer WF, Prochaska JO, Rossi JS, Bellis JM, Tsoh JY, Migneault JP, Smith NF, Prokhorov AV. Computer-based smoking cessation interventions in adolescents: description, feasibility and six-month follow-up findings. *Substance Use and Misuse* 1998;3(4):935–65.

Patten CA, Gilpin E, Cavin SW, Pierce JP. Workplace smoking policy and changes in smoking behaviour in California: a suggested association. *Tobacco Control* 1995a;4(1):36–41.

Patten CA, Pierce JP, Cavin SW, Berry CC, Kaplan RM. Progress in protecting non-smokers from environmental tobacco smoke in California workplaces. *Tobacco Control* 1995b;4(2):139–44.

Pentz MA, MacKinnon DP, Dwyer JH, Wang EYI, Hansen WB, Flay BR, Johnson CA. Longitudinal effects of the Midwestern Prevention Project on regular and experimental smoking in adolescents. *Preventive Medicine* 1989a;18(2):304–21.

Pentz MA, MacKinnon DP, Flay BR, Hansen WB, Johnson CA, Dwyer JH. Primary prevention of chronic diseases in adolescence: effects of the Midwestern Prevention Project on tobacco use. *American Journal of Epidemiology* 1989b;130(4):713–24.

Pérez-Stable EJ, Sabogal F, Marín G, Marín BV, Otero-Sabogal R. Evaluation of "Guia para Dejar de Fumar," a self-help guide in Spanish to quit smoking. *Public Health Reports* 1991;106(5):564–70.

Perkins KA. Issues in the prevention of weight gain after smoking cessation. *Annals of Behavioral Medicine* 1994;16(1):46–52.

Perkins KA. Sex differences in nicotine versus nonnicotine reinforcement as determinants of tobacco smoking. *Experimental and Clinical Pyschopharmacology* 1996;4(2):166–77.

Perkins KA. Nicotine discrimination in men and women. *Pharmacology, Biochemistry and Behavior* 1999;64(2):295–9.

Perkins KA, Donny E, Caggiula AR. Sex differences in nicotine effects and self-administration: review of human and animal evidence. *Nicotine and Tobacco Research* 1999;1(4):301–15.

Perkins KA, Levine M, Marcus M, Shiffman S, D'Amico D, Miller A, Keins A, Ashcom J, Broge B. Tobacco withdrawal in women and menstrual cycle phase. *Journal of Consulting and Clinical Psychology* 2000:68(1):176–80.

Perry CL, Kelder SH, Murray DM, Klepp K-I. Communitywide smoking prevention: long-term outcomes of the Minnesota Heart Health Program and the Class of 1989 study. *American Journal of Public Health* 1992;82(9):1210–6.

Petersen L, Handel J, Kotch J, Podedworny T, Rosen A. Smoking reduction during pregnancy by a program of self-help and clinical support. *Obstetrics and Gynecology* 1992;79(6):924–30.

Peterson DE, Zeger SL, Remington PL, Anderson HA. The effect of state cigarette tax increases on cigarette sales, 1955 to 1988. *American Journal of Public Health* 1992;82(1):94–6.

Pierce JP, Evans N, Farkas AJ, Cavin SW, Berry C, Kramer M, Kealey S, Rosbrook B, Choi W, Kaplan RM. *Tobacco Use in California: An Evaluation of the Tobacco Control Program, 1989–1993.* La Jolla (CA): University of California, San Diego, 1994a.

Pierce JP, Fiore MC, Novotny TE, Hatziandreu EJ, Davis RM. Trends in cigarette smoking in the United States: educational differences are increasing. *Journal of the American Medical Association* 1989; 261(1):56–60.

Pierce JP, Lee L, Gilpin EA. Smoking initiation by adolescent girls, 1944 through 1988: an association with targeted advertising. *Journal of the American Medical Association* 1994b;271(8):608–11.

Pierce JP, Macaskill P, Hill D. Long-term effectiveness of mass media led antismoking campaigns in Australia. *American Journal of Public Health* 1990;80(5): 565–9.

Pirie PL, McBride CM, Hellerstedt W, Jeffery RW, Hatsukami D, Allen S, Lando H. Smoking cessation in women concerned about weight. *American Journal of Public Health* 1992;82(9):1238–43.

Pirie PL, Murray DM, Luepker RV. Gender differences in cigarette smoking and quitting in a cohort of young adults. *American Journal of Public Health* 1991;81(3):324–7.

Pirie PL, Rooney BL, Pechacek TF, Lando HA, Schmid LA. Incorporating social support into a community-wide smoking-cessation contest. *Addictive Behaviors* 1997;22(1):131–7.

Pohl JM, Martinelli A, Antonakos C. Predictors of participation in a smoking cessation intervention group among low-income women. *Addictive Behaviors* 1998;23(5):699–704.

Pomerleau CS. Smoking and nicotine replacement treatment issues specific to women. *American Journal of Health Behavior* 1996;20(5):291–9.

Pomerleau CS, Cole PA, Lumley MA, Marks JL, Pomerleau OF. Effects of menstrual phase on nicotine, alcohol, and caffeine intake in smokers. *Journal of Substance Abuse* 1994a;6(2):227–34.

Pomerleau CS, Garcia AW, Pomerleau OF, Cameron OG. The effects of menstrual phase and nicotine abstinence on nicotine intake and on biochemical and subjective measures in women smokers: a preliminary report. *Psychoneuroendocrinology* 1992; 17(6):627–38.

Pomerleau CS, Pomerleau OF. Gender differences in frequency of smoking withdrawal symptoms. *Annals of Behavioral Medicine* 1994;16(Suppl):S118.

Pomerleau CS, Pomerleau OF, Garcia AW. Biobehavioral research on nicotine use in women. *British Journal of Addiction* 1991a;86(5):527–31.

Pomerleau CS, Tate JC, Lumley MA, Pomerleau OF. Gender differences in prospectively versus retrospectively assessed smoking withdrawal symptoms. *Journal of Substance Abuse* 1994b;6(4):433–40.

Pomerleau CS, Teuscher F, Goeters S, Pomerleau OF. Effects of nicotine abstinence and menstrual phase on task performance. *Addictive Behaviors* 1994c; 19(4):357–62.

Pomerleau OF, Pomerleau CS, Morrell EM, Lowenbergh JM. Effects of fluoxetine on weight gain and food intake in smokers who reduce nicotine intake. *Psychoneuroendocrinology* 1991b;16(5):433–40.

Popham WJ, Potter LD, Bal DG, Johnson MD, Duerr JM, Quinn V. Do anti-smoking media campaigns help smokers quit? *Public Health Reports* 1993; 108(4):510–3.

Prochaska JO. Strong and weak principles for progressing from precontemplation to action on the basis of twelve problem behaviors. *Health Psychology* 1994;13(1):47–51.

Prochaska JO, DiClemente CC. Stages and processes of self-change of smoking: toward an integrative model of change. *Journal of Consulting and Clinical Psychology* 1983;51(3):390–5.

Prochaska JO, DiClemente CC, Norcross JC. In search of how people change: applications to addictive behaviors. *American Psychologist* 1992;47(9): 1102–14.

Prochaska JO, DiClemente CC, Velicer WF, Rossi JS. Standardized, individualized, interactive, and personalized self-help programs for smoking cessation. *Health Psychology* 1993;12(5):399–405.

Prochazka AV, Weaver MJ, Keller RT, Fryer GE, Licari PA, Lofaso D. A randomized trial of nortriptyline for smoking cessation. *Archives of Internal Medicine* 1998;158(18):1235–9.

Procopé B-J, Timonen S. The premenstrual syndrome in relation to sport, gymnastics and smoking. *Acta Obstetrica et Gynecologica Scandinavica* 1971;9 (Suppl 9):77.

Puska P, Nissinen A, Salonen JT, Toumilehto [sic] J. Ten years of the North Karelia Project: results with community-based prevention of coronary heart disease. *Scandinavian Journal of Social Medicine* 1983a;11(3):65–8.

Puska P, Salonen JT, Nissinen A, Tuomilehto J, Vartiainen E, Korhonen H, Tanskanen A, Rönnqvist P, Koskela K, Huttunen J. Change in risk factors for coronary heart disease during 10 years of a community intervention programme (North Karelia Project). *British Medical Journal* 1983b;287(6408): 1840–4.

Puska P, Tuomilehto J, Salonen J, Neittaanmäki L, Maki J, Virtamo J, Nissinen A, Koskela K, Takalo T. Changes in coronary risk factors during comprehensive five-year community programme to control cardiovascular diseases (North Karelia Project). *British Medical Journal* 1979;2(6199):1173–8.

Quinn VP, Mullen PD, Ershoff DH. Women who stop smoking spontaneously prior to prenatal care and predictors of relapse before delivery. *Addictive Behaviors* 1991;16(1–2):29–40.

Rafuse J. Smoking-cessation program targets low-income women. *Canadian Medical Association Journal* 1994;150(10):1683–4.

Rásky E, Stronegger WJ, Freidl W. The relationship between body weight and patterns of smoking in women and men. *International Journal of Epidemiology* 1996;25(6):1208–12.

Research Committee of the British Thoracic Society. Smoking cessation in patients: two further studies by the British Thoracic Society. *Thorax* 1990;45(11): 835–40.

Resnicow K, Vaughan R, Futterman R, Weston RE, Royce J, Parms C, Hearn MD, Smith M, Freeman HP, Orlandi MA. A self-help smoking cessation program for inner-city African Americans: results from the Harlem Health Connection Project. *Health Education and Behavior* 1997;24(2):201–17.

Rimer BK, Orleans CT, Fleisher L, Cristinzio S, Resch N, Telepchak J, Keintz MK. Does tailoring matter? The impact of a tailored guide on ratings and short-term smoking-related outcomes for older smokers. *Health Education Research* 1994;9(1):69–84.

Robinson RG, Barry M, Bloch M, Glantz S, Jordan J, Murray KB, Popper E, Sutton C, Tarr-Whelan K, Themba M, Younger S. Report of the Tobacco Policy Research Group on marketing and promotions targeted at African Americans, Latinos, and women. *Tobacco Control* 1992;1(Suppl):S24–S30.

Rooney BL, Murray DM. A meta-analysis of smoking-prevention programs after adjustment for errors in the unit of analysis. *Health Education Quarterly* 1996;23(1):48–64.

Royce JM, Ashford A, Resnicow K, Freeman HP, Caesar AA, Orlandi MA. Physician- and nurse-assisted smoking cessation in Harlem. *Journal of the National Medical Association* 1995;87(4):291–300.

Royce JM, Corbett K, Sorensen G, Ockene J. Gender, social pressure, and smoking cessations: the Community Intervention Trial for Smoking Cessation (COMMIT) at baseline. *Social Science and Medicine* 1997;44(3):359–70.

Rundall TG, Bruvold WH. A meta-analysis of school-based smoking and alcohol use prevention programs. *Health Education Quarterly* 1988;15(3): 317–34.

Russell PO, Epstein LH, Johnston JJ, Block DR, Blair E. The effects of physical activity as maintenance for smoking cessation. *Addictive Behaviors* 1988; 13(2):215–8.

Saad L. More Americans Fear Risk of Second-Hand Smoke. Princeton (NJ): Gallup Organization, 1997; <http://www.gallup.com/poll/releases/pr970718.asp>; accessed: November 29, 1999.

Sabogal F, Otero-Sabogal R, Pérez-Stable EJ, Marín BV-O, Marín G. Perceived self-efficacy to avoid cigarette smoking and addiction: differences between Hispanics and non-Hispanic Whites. Hispanic *Journal of Behavioral Sciences* 1989;11(2): 136–47.

Salive ME, Cornoni-Huntley J, LaCroix AZ, Ostfeld AM, Wallace RB, Hennekens CH. Predictors of smoking cessation and relapse in older adults. *American Journal of Public Health* 1992;82(9): 1268–71.

Salonen JT, Puska P, Kottke TE, Tuomilehto J. Changes in smoking, serum cholesterol and blood pressure levels during a community-based cardiovascular disease prevention program—the North Karelia Project. American *Journal of Epidemiology* 1981;114(1):81–94.

Samet JM, Coultas DB. *Clinics in Chest Medicine—Smoking Cessation.* Philadelphia: W.B. Saunders, 1991.

Sargent JD, Mott LA, Stevens M. Predictors of smoking cessation in adolescents. *Archives of Pediatrics and Adolescent Medicine* 1998;152(4):388–93.

Schiff I, Bell WR, Davis V, Kessler CM, Meyers C, Nakajima S, Sexton BJ. Oral contraceptives and smoking, current considerations: recommendations of a consensus panel. *American Journal of Obstetrics and Gynecology* 1999;180(6 Pt 2):S383–4.

Schilling RF, Gilchrist LD, Schinke SP. Smoking in the workplace: review of critical issues. *Public Health Reports* 1985;100(5):473–9.

Schorling JB, Roach J, Siegel M, Baturka N, Hunt DE, Guterbock TM, Stewart HL. A trial of church-based smoking cessation interventions for rural African Americans. *Preventive Medicine* 1997;26(1): 92–101.

Secker-Walker RH, Flynn BS, Solomon LJ, Vacek PM, Dorwaldt AL, Geller BM, Worden JK, Skelly JM. Helping women quit smoking: baseline observations for a community health education project. *American Journal of Preventive Medicine* 1996;12(5): 367–77.

Secker-Walker RH, Solomon LJ, Flynn BS, Skelly JM, Lepage SS, Goodwin GD, Mead PB. Individualized smoking cessation counseling during prenatal and early postnatal care. *American Journal of Obstetrics and Gynecology* 1994;171(5):1347–55.

Secker-Walker RH, Solomon LJ, Flynn BS, Skelly JM, Lepage SS, Goodwin GD, Mead PB. Smoking relapse prevention counseling during prenatal and early postnatal care. *American Journal of Preventive Medicine* 1995;11(2):86–93.

Seffrin JR. A European tobacco advertising ban. *Cancer Journal for Clinicians* 1998;48(4):254–6.

Serxner S, Catalano R, Dooley D, Mishra S. Influences on cigarette smoking quantity: selection, stress, or culture? *Journal of Occupational Medicine* 1992; 34(9):934–9.

Severson HH, Andrews JA, Lichtenstein E, Wall M, Zoref L. Predictors of smoking during and after pregnancy: a survey of mothers of newborns. *Preventive Medicine* 1995;24(1):23–8.

Sexton M, Hebel JR. A clinical trial of change in maternal smoking and its effect on birth weight. *Journal of the American Medical Association* 1984;251(7): 911–5.

Sexton M, Hebel JR, Fox NL. Postpartum smoking. In: Rosenberg MJ, editor. *Smoking and Reproductive Health.* Littleton (MA): PSG Publishing, 1987:222–6.

Shaw CR. The perimenopausal hot flash: epidemiology, physiology, and treatment. *Nurse Practitioner* 1997;22(3):55–6, 61–6.

Shiffman S. Relapse following smoking cessation: a situational analysis. *Journal of Consulting and Clinical Psychology* 1982;50(1):71–86.

Shopland DR, Hartman AM, Repace JL, Lynn WR. Smoking behavior, workplace policies, and public opinion regarding smoking restrictions in Maryland. *Maryland Medical Journal* 1995;44(2):99–104.

Simpkins VL. *Contemporary Issues: Tune In to Well-Being, Say No to Drugs.* New York: Girls Scouts of the United States of America, 1985.

Simpson WJ. A preliminary report on cigarette smoking and the incidence of prematurity. *American Journal of Obstetrics and Gynecology* 1957;73(4):808–15.

Sloss EM, Frerichs RR. Smoking and menstrual disorders. *International Journal of Epidemiology* 1983; 12(1):107–9.

Slotkin TA. Fetal nicotine or cocaine exposure: which one is worse? *Journal of Pharmacology and Experimental Therapeutics* 1998;285(3):931–45.

Smith NF, Migneault JP, Pirillo P, Pallonen UE, Prokhorov A, Prochaska JO. Anti-smoking programs that voc. tech. students like. Poster presented at the Society of Behavioral Medicine Meeting; 1994 Apr 14; Boston.

Solomon LJ, Flynn BS. Women who smoke. In: Orleans CT, Slade J, editors. *Nicotine Addiction: Principles and Management.* New York: Oxford University Press, 1993:339–49.

Sorensen G, Glasgow RE, Corbett K, Topor M. Compliance with worksite nonsmoking policies: baseline results from the COMMIT study of worksites. *American Journal of Health Promotion* 1992a;7(2): 103–9.

Sorensen G, Goldberg R, Ockene J, Klar J, Tannenbaum T, Lemeshow S. Heavy smoking among a sample of employed women. *American Journal of Preventive Medicine* 1992b;8(4):207–14.

Sorensen G, Pechacek T, Pallonen U. Occupational and worksite norms and attitudes about smoking cessation. *American Journal of Public Health* 1986; 76(5):544–9.

Sorensen G, Pechacek TF. Attitudes toward smoking cessation among men and women. *Journal of Behavioral Medicine* 1987;10(2):129–37.

Sorensen G, Thompson B, Glanz K, Feng Z, Kinne S, DiClemente C, Emmons K, Heimendinger J, Probart C, Lichtenstein E. Work site-based cancer prevention: primary results from the Working Well Trial. *American Journal of Public Health* 1996;86(7): 939–47.

Spangler JG, Bell RA, Dignan MB, Michielutte R. Prevalence and predictors of tobacco use among Lumbee Indian women in Robeson County, North Carolina. *Journal of Community Health* 1997;22(2): 115–25.

Spangler JG, Bell RA, Knick S, Michielutte R, Dignan MB, Summerson JH. Church-related correlates of tobacco use among Lumbee Indians in North Carolina. *Ethnicity and Disease* 1998;8(1):73–80.

Spolar C. Park Service bans tobacco sponsors: last tennis tourney for Virginia Slims. *Washington Post* 1991 Aug 16;Sect C:6 (col 1).

Spring B, Pingitore R, Kessler K. Strategies to minimize weight gain after smoking cessation: psycological [sic] and pharmacological intervention with specific reference to dexfenfluramine. *International Journal of Obesity* 1992;16(Suppl 3):S19–S23.

Spring B, Wurtman J, Gleason R, Wurtman R, Kessler K. Weight gain and withdrawal symptoms after smoking cessation: a preventive intervention using d-fenfluramine. *Health Psychology* 1991; 10(3):216–23.

St. Pierre RW, Shute RE, Jaycox S. Youth helping youth: a behavioral approach to the self-control of smoking. *Health Education* 1983;14(1):28–31.

Steenkamp HJ, Jooste PL, Jordaan PCJ, Swanepoel ASP, Rossouw JE. Changes in smoking during a community-based cardiovascular disease intervention programme: the Coronary Risk Factor Study. *South African Medical Journal* 1991;79(5):250–3.

Steimle S. New EU report: more women are smoking. *Journal of the National Cancer Institute* 1999;91(3): 212–3.

Steinberg JL, Cherek DR. Menstrual cycle and cigarette smoking behavior. *Addictive Behaviors* 1989; 14(2):173–9.

Stillman FA, Becker DM, Swank RT, Hantula D, Moses H, Glantz S, Waranch HR. Ending smoking at the Johns Hopkins Medical Institutions. *Journal of the American Medical Association* 1990;264(12): 1565–9.

Strategic Coalition of Girls and Women United Against Tobacco. Strategic Coalition of Girls and Women United Against Tobacco [fact sheet]. Alexandria (VA): American Medical Women's Association, 1995.

Streater JA Jr, Sargent RG, Ward DS. A study of factors associated with weight change in women who attempt smoking cessation. *Addictive Behaviors* 1989;14(5):523–30.

Strecher VJ, Kreuter M, Den Boer D-J, Kobrin S, Hospers HJ, Skinner CS. The effects of computer-tailored smoking cessation messages in family practice settings. *Journal of Family Practice* 1994; 39(3):262–70.

Strouse R, Hall J. *Robert Wood Johnson Foundation Youth Access Survey: Results of a National Household Survey to Assess Public Attitudes About Policy Alternatives for Limiting Minor's Access to Tobacco Products.* Princeton (NJ): Mathematica Policy Research, 1994. MPR Reference No. 8236.

Sussman S, Dent CW, Burton D, Stacy AW, Flay BR. *Developing School-Based Tobacco Use Prevention and Cessation Programs.* Thousand Oaks (CA): Sage Publications, 1995.

Sussman S, Dent CW, Nezami E, Stacy AW, Burton D, Flay BR. Reasons for quitting and smoking temptation among adolescent smokers: gender differences. *Substance Use and Misuse* 1998a;33(14): 2703–20.

Sussman S, Dent CW, Severson H, Burton D, Flay BR. Self-initiated quitting among adolescent smokers. *Preventive Medicine* 1998b;27(5 Pt 3):A19–A28.

Sussman S, Dent CW, Stacy AW, Sun P, Craig S, Simon TR, Burton D, Flay BR. Project Towards No Tobacco Use: 1-year behavior outcomes. *American Journal of Public Health* 1993;83(9):1245–50.

Sutherland G, Stapleton JA, Russell MAH, Jarvis MJ, Hajek P, Belcher M, Feyerabend C. Randomized controlled trial of nasal nicotine spray in smoking cessation. *Lancet* 1992;340(8815):324–9.

Svikis DS, Hatsukami DK, Hughes JR, Carroll KM, Pickens RW. Sex differences in tobacco withdrawal syndrome. *Addictive Behaviors* 1986;11(4):459–62.

Swan GE, Denk CE. Dynamic models for the maintenance of smoking cessation: event history analysis of late relapse. *Journal of Behavioral Medicine* 1987;10(6):527–54.

Swedish Nurses Against Tobacco. *Nurses! Organize Networks Against Tobacco.* Huddinge (Sweden): Huddinge University Hospital, 1994.

Tang JL, Law M, Wald N. How effective is nicotine replacement therapy in helping people to stop smoking? *British Medical Journal* 1994;308(6920): 21–6.

Thompson B, Emmons K, Abrams D, Ockene JK, Feng Z. ETS exposure in the workplace: perceptions and reactions by employees in 114 work sites. [published erratum in *Journal of Occupational and Environmental Medicine* 1995;37(12):1363]. *Journal of Occupational and Environmental Medicine* 1995; 37(9):1086–92.

Thompson B, Rich LE, Lynn WR, Shields R, Corle DK for the COMMIT Research Group. A voluntary smokers' registry: characteristics of joiners and non-joiners in the Community Intervention Trial for Smoking Cessation (COMMIT). *American Journal of Public Health* 1998;88(1):100–3.

Thornton A, Lee P, Fry J. Differences between smokers, ex-smokers, passive smokers and non-smokers. *Journal of Clinical Epidemiology* 1994; 47(10):1143–62.

*Tobacco Control.* Eighth World Conference on Tobacco or Health. Buenos Aires, Argentina, 30 March–3 April 1992. Conference resolutions: international support. *Tobacco Control* 1992;1(2):91–2.

Tomar SL, Husten CG, Manley MW. Do dentists and physicians advise tobacco users to quit? *Journal of the American Dental Association* 1996;127(2):259–65.

Tønnesen P, Nørregaard J, Mikkelsen K, Jørgensen S, Nilsson F. A double-blind trial of a nicotine inhaler for smoking cessation. *Journal of the American Medical Association* 1993;269(10):1268–71.

Tønnesen P, Nørregaard J, Simonsen K, Säwe U. A double-blind trial of a 16-hour transdermal nicotine patch in smoking cessation. *New England Journal of Medicine* 1991;325(5):311–5.

Townsend JL. Cigarette tax, economic welfare and social class patterns of smoking. *Applied Economics* 1987;19(3):355–65.

Townsend J, Roderick P, Cooper J. Cigarette smoking by socioeconomic group, sex, and age: effects of price, income, and health publicity. *British Medical Journal* 1994;309(6959):923–7.

Transdermal Nicotine Study Group. Transdermal nicotine for smoking cessation: six-month results from two multicenter controlled clinical trials. *Journal of the American Medical Association* 1991; 266(22):3133–8.

U.S. Department of Commerce. *1990 Census of Population: Social and Economic Characteristics. United States.* Washington: U.S. Department of Commerce, Economics and Statistics Administration, Bureau of the Census, 1993. 1990 CP-2-1.

U.S. Department of Health and Human Services. *The Health Consequences of Smoking for Women. A Report of the Surgeon General.* Washington: U.S. Department of Health and Human Services, Public Health Service, Office of the Assistant Secretary for Health, Office on Smoking and Health, 1980.

U.S. Department of Health and Human Services. *The Health Consequences of Smoking: Chronic Obstructive Lung Disease. A Report of the Surgeon General.* U.S. Department of Health and Human Services, Public Health Service, Office on Smoking and Health, 1984. DHHS Publication No. (PHS) 84-50205.

U.S. Department of Health and Human Services. *The Health Consequences of Smoking: Cancer and Chronic Lung Disease in the Workplace. A Report of the Surgeon General.* U.S. Department of Health and Human Services, Public Health Service, Office on Smoking and Health, 1985. DHHS Publication No. (PHS) 85-50207.

U.S. Department of Health and Human Services. *The Health Consequences of Smoking: Nicotine Addiction. A Report of the Surgeon General.* Atlanta: U.S. Department of Health and Human Services, Public Health Service, Centers for Disease Control, Center for Health Promotion and Education, Office on Smoking and Health, 1988. DHHS Publication No. (CDC) 88-8406.

U.S. Department of Health and Human Services. *Reducing the Health Consequences of Smoking: 25 Years of Progress. A Report of the Surgeon General.* Rockville (MD): U.S. Department of Health and Human Services, Public Health Service, Centers for Disease Control, Center for Chronic Disease Prevention and Health Promotion, Office on Smoking and Health, 1989. DHHS Publication No. (CDC) 89-8411.

U.S. Department of Health and Human Services. *The Health Benefits of Smoking Cessation. A Report of the Surgeon General.* Atlanta: U.S. Department of Health and Human Services, Public Health Service, Centers for Disease Control, Center for Chronic Disease Prevention and Health Promotion, Office on Smoking and Health, 1990. DHHS Publication No. (CDC) 90-8416.

U.S. Department of Health and Human Services. *Healthy People 2000. National Health Promotion and Disease Prevention Objectives.* U.S. Department of Health and Human Services, Public Health Service, 1991a. DHHS Publication No. (PHS) 91-50212.

U.S. Department of Health and Human Services. *Strategies to Control Tobacco Use in the United States: a Blueprint for Public Health Action in the 1990s.* Bethesda (MD): U.S. Department of Health and Human Services, Public Health Service, National Institutes of Health, National Cancer Institute, 1991b. NIH Publication No. 92-3316.

U.S. Department of Health and Human Services. *1992 National Survey of Worksite Health Promotion Activities: Final Report.* U.S. Department of Health and Human Services, Public Health Service, Office of the Assistant Secretary for Health, Office of Disease Prevention and Health Promotion, 1993a. NTIS Publication No. PB93-500023.

U.S. Department of Health and Human Services. 1992 National Survey of Worksite Health Promotion Activities: summary. *American Journal of Health Promotion* 1993b;7(6):452–64.

U.S. Department of Health and Human Services. *Rompa con el Vicio: Una Guía para Dejar de Fumar.* Washington: U.S. Department of Health and Human Services, Public Health Service, National Institutes of Health, National Cancer Institute, Programa Latino para Dejar de Fumar de San Francisco, 1993c. NIH Publication No. 94-3001.

U.S. Department of Health and Human Services. *Preventing Tobacco Use Among Young People. A Report of the Surgeon General.* Atlanta: U.S. Department of Health and Human Services, Public Health Service, Centers for Disease Control and Prevention, National Center for Chronic Disease Prevention and Health Promotion, Office on Smoking and Health, 1994.

U.S. Department of Health and Human Services. *The President's Council on Physical Fitness and Sports Report. Physical Activity & Sport in the Lives of Young Girls: Physical & Mental Health Dimensions from an Interdisciplinary Approach.* Washington: U.S. Department of Health and Human Services, Substance Abuse and Mental Health Services Administration, Center for Mental Health Services, 1997.

U.S. Department of Health and Human Services. *Tobacco Use Among U.S. Racial/Ethnic Minority Groups—African Americans, American Indians and Alaska Natives, Asian Americans and Pacific Islanders, and Hispanics. A Report of the Surgeon General.* Atlanta: U.S. Department of Health and Human Services, Centers for Disease Control and Prevention, National Center for Chronic Disease Prevention and Health Promotion, Office on Smoking and Health, 1998.

U.S. Department of Health and Human Services. *Reducing Tobacco Use. A Report of the Surgeon General.* Atlanta: U.S. Department of Health and Human Services, Centers for Disease Control and Prevention, National Center for Chronic Disease Prevention and Health Promotion, Office on Smoking and Health, 2000.

Valois RF, Adams KG, Kammermann SK. One-year evaluation results from CableQuit: a community cable television smoking cessation pilot program. *Journal of Behavioral Medicine* 1996;19(5):479–99.

Vander Martin R, Cummings SR, Coates TJ. Ethnicity and smoking: differences in white, black, Hispanic, and Asian medical patients who smoke. *American Journal of Preventive Medicine* 1990;6(4):194–9.

Vartiainen E, Paavola M, McAlister A, Puska P. Fifteen-year follow-up of smoking prevention effects in the North Karelia Youth Project. *American Journal of Public Health* 1998;88(1):81–5.

Vartiainen E, Pallonen U, McAlister AL, Puska P. Eight-year follow-up results of an adolescent smoking prevention program: the North Karelia Youth Project. *American Journal of Public Health* 1990;80(1):78–9.

Velicer WF, Prochaska JO, Bellis JM, DiClemente CC, Rossi JS, Fava JL, Steiger JH. An expert system intervention for smoking cessation. *Addictive Behaviors* 1993;18(3):269–90.

Vetter NJ, Ford D. Smoking prevention among people aged 60 and over: a randomized controlled trial. *Age and Ageing* 1990;19(3):164–8

Villarosa L. Caution: tobacco ads may be hazardous to your editorial freedom. *Harvard Public Health Review* 1991;2(3):18–21.

Voorhees CC, Stillman FA, Swank RT, Heagerty PJ, Levine DM, Becker DM. Heart, body, and soul: impact of church-based smoking cessation interventions on readiness to quit. *Preventive Medicine* 1996;25(3):277–85.

Wagner EH, Schoenbach VJ, Orleans CT, Grothaus LC, Saunders KW, Curry S, Pearson DC. Participation in a smoking cessation program: a population-based perspective. *American Journal of Preventive Medicine* 1990;6(5):258–66.

Waldron I. Patterns and causes of gender differences in smoking. *Social Science and Medicine* 1991;32(9): 989–1005.

Wall MA, Severson HH, Andrews JA, Lichtenstein E, Zoref L. Pediatric office-based smoking intervention: impact on maternal smoking and relapse. *Pediatrics* 1995;96(4):622–8.

Walsh DC, Gordon NP. Legal approaches to smoking deterrence. *Annual Review of Public Health* 1986; 7:127–49.

Ward KD, Klesges RC, Zbikowski SM, Bliss RE, Garvey AJ. Gender differences in the outcome of an unaided smoking cessation attempt. *Addictive Behaviors* 1997;22(4):521–33.

Warnecke RB, Flay BR, Kviz FJ, Gruder CL, Langenberg P, Crittenden KS, Mermelstein RJ, Aitken M, Wong SC, Cook TD. Characteristics of participants in a televised smoking cessation intervention. *Preventive Medicine* 1991;20(3):389–403.

Warnecke RB, Langenberg P, Wong SC, Flay BR, Cook TD. The second Chicago televised smoking cessation program: a 24-month follow-up. *American Journal of Public Health* 1992;82(6):835–40.

Warner KE. State legislation on smoking and health: a comparison of two policies. *Policy Sciences* 1981;13: 139–52.

Warner KE, Goldenhar LM, McLaughlin CG. Cigarette advertising and magazine coverage of the hazards of smoking: a statistical analysis. *New England Journal of Medicine* 1992;326(5):305–9.

Wasserman J, Manning WG, Newhouse JP, Winkler JD. The effects of excise taxes and regulations on cigarette smoking. *Journal of Health Economics* 1991; 10(1):43–64.

Watts J. Industry's voluntary tobacco-advertising ban to be tightened in Japan. *Lancet* 1998;351(9102):579.

Weissman W, Glasgow R, Biglan A, Lichtenstein E. Development and preliminary evaluation of a cessation program for adolescent smokers. *Psychology of Addictive Behaviors* 1987;1(2):84–91.

Wetter D, Kenford SL, Smith SS, Fiore MC, Jorenby DE, Baker TB. Gender differences in smoking cessation. *Journal of Consulting and Clinical Psychology* 1999a;67(4):555–62.

Wetter DW, Fiore MC, Young TB, McClure JB, de Moor CA, Baker T. Gender differences in response to nicotine replacement therapy: objective and subjective indexes of tobacco withdrawal. *Experimental and Clinical Psychopharmacology* 1999b; 7(2):135–44.

Whitlock EP, Vogt TM, Hollis JF, Lichtenstein E. Does gender affect response to a brief clinic-based smoking intervention? *American Journal of Preventive Medicine* 1997;13(3):159–66.

Willemsen MC, De Zwart WM. The effectiveness of policy and health education strategies for reducing adolescent smoking: a review of the evidence. *Journal of Adolescence* 1999;22(5):587–99.

Wilson JJ. Summary of the Attorneys General Master Tobacco Settlement Agreement, March 1999; <http://www.ncsl.org/statefed/tmsasumm.htm>; accessed: December 14, 1999.

Windham GC, Elkin EP, Swan SH, Waller KO, Fenster L. Cigarette smoking and effects on menstrual function. *Obstetrics and Gyneocology* 1999;93(1): 59–65.

Windsor RA, Boyd NR, Orleans CT. A meta-evaluation of smoking cessation intervention research among pregnant women: improving the science and art. *Health Education Research* 1998; 13(3):419–38.

Windsor RA, Cutter G, Morris J, Reese Y, Manzella B, Bartlett EE, Samuelson C, Spanos D. The effectiveness of smoking cessation methods for smokers in public health maternity clinics: a randomized trial. *American Journal of Public Health* 1985;75(12): 1389–92.

Windsor RA, Li CQ, Lowe JB, Perkins LL, Ershoff D, Glynn T. The dissemination of smoking cessation methods for pregnant women: achieving the year 2000 objectives. *American Journal of Public Health* 1993a;83(2):173–8.

Windsor RA, Lowe JB, Perkins LL, Smith-Yoder D, Artz L, Crawford M, Amburgy K, Boyd NR Jr. Health education for pregnant smokers: its behavioral impact and cost benefit. *American Journal of Public Health* 1993b;83(2):201–6.

Winkleby MA, Feldman HA, Murray DM. Joint analysis of three U.S. community intervention trials for reduction of cardiovascular disease risk. *Journal of Clinical Epidemiology* 1997;50(6):645–58.

Winkleby MA, Fortmann SP, Rockhill B. Trends in cardiovascular disease risk factors by educational level: the Stanford Five-City Project. *Preventive Medicine* 1992;21(5):592–601.

Women And Girls Against Tobacco. Women And Girls Against Tobacco mission statement. Berkeley (CA): Western Consortium for Public Health, Women And Girls Against Tobacco, 1993.

Women vs. Smoking Network. Mobilizing the women's community. Grant proposal prepared by the Women vs. Smoking Network. Washington: Advocacy Institute, 1990.

Women's Health Initiative Protocol for Clinical Trial and Observational Study Components. Seattle (WA): Fred Hutchinson Cancer Research Center, 1998.

Wood C, Larsen L, Williams R. Social and psychological factors in relation to premenstrual tension and menstrual pain. *Australian and New Zealand Journal of Obstetrics and Gynaecology* 1979;19(2):111–5.

Woodby LL, Windsor RA, Synder SW, Kohler CL, DiClemente CC. Predictors of smoking cessation during pregnancy. *Addiction* 1999;94(2):283–92.

Worden JK, Flynn BS, Solomon LJ, Secker-Walker RH, Badger GJ, Carpenter JH. Using mass media to prevent cigarette smoking among adolescent girls. *Health Education Quarterly* 1996;23(4):453–68.

World Health Organization. "Kobe Declaration" Calls for a Halt to the Tobacco Menace Among Women and Children [press release], Nov 18, 1999a; <http://www.who.int/inf-pr-1999/en/pr99-71.html>; accessed: September 12, 2000.

World Health Organization. WHO International Conference on Tobacco and Health, Kobe. "Making a Difference to Tobacco and Health: Avoiding the Tobacco Epidemic in Women and Youth." Kobe, Japan, Nov 14–18, 1999b; <http://tobacco.who.int/en/fctc/kobe/kobereport.asp>; accessed: September 6, 2000.

*World Smoking and Health*. Herstories. *World Smoking and Health* 1994;19(2):2–16.

Yankelovich Partners. *Smoking Cessation Study*. Report prepared for Ketchum Public Relations and their client American Lung Association. Norwalk (CT): Yankelovich Partners, July 27, 1998; <http://www.lungusa.org/partner/yank/1.html>; accessed: August 15, 2000.

Zelman DC, Brandon TH, Jorenby DE, Baker TB. Measures of affect and nicotine dependence predict differential response to smoking cessation treatments. *Journal of Consulting and Clinical Psychology* 1992;60(6):943–52.

Zhu S-H, Melcer T, Sun J, Rosbrook B, Pierce JP. Smoking cessation with and without assistance: a population-based analysis. *American Journal of Preventive Medicine* 2000;18(4):305–11.

# Chapter 6. A Vision for the Future: What Is Needed to Reduce Smoking Among Women

# Introduction

This report summarizes what is known about smoking among women, including patterns and trends in smoking prevalence, factors associated with smoking initiation and maintenance, the consequences of smoking for women's health, and interventions for smoking cessation and prevention. The report also describes historical and contemporary tobacco marketing targeted to women. Evidence of the health consequences of smoking, which had emerged somewhat earlier among men because of their earlier uptake of smoking, is now overwhelming among women. Tragically, in the face of continually mounting evidence of the enormous consequences of smoking for women's health, the tobacco industry continues to heavily target women in its advertising and promotional campaigns and is now attempting to export the epidemic of smoking to women in areas of the world where the smoking prevalence among females has traditionally been low. The single overarching theme emerging from this report is that ***smoking is a women's issue.*** What is needed to curb the epidemic of smoking and smoking-related diseases among women in the United States and throughout the world?

# Increase Awareness of the Impact of Smoking on Women's Health and Counter the Tobacco Industry's Targeting of Women

• ***Increase awareness of the devastating impact of smoking on women's health.*** Since 1980, when the first Surgeon General's report on women and smoking was published documenting the serious health consequences of smoking among women, the number of women affected by smoking-related diseases has increased dramatically. Smoking is now the leading known cause of preventable death and disease among women. Each year during the 1990s it accounted for more than 140,000 deaths among U.S. women. By 1987, lung cancer became the leading cause of cancer death among women, and in 2000 approximately 27,000 more women in the United States died of lung cancer (67,600) than of breast cancer (40,800). Smoking also claims women's lives through deaths due to other types of cancer as well as to cardiovascular, pulmonary, and other diseases—all risks shared with men who smoke. In addition, women experience unique health effects due to smoking, such as those related to pregnancy. In 1997, smoking accounted for an estimated 165,000 premature deaths among U.S. women. Exposure to environmental tobacco smoke also contributes to lung cancer and heart disease deaths among women and affects the health of their infants. The media, including women's magazines and broadcast programming, can play an important role in raising women's awareness of the magnitude of the impact of smoking on their health and in prioritizing the importance of smoking relative to the myriad other health-related topics covered.

• ***Expose and counter the tobacco industry's deliberate targeting of women and decry its efforts to link smoking, which is so harmful to women's health, with women's rights and progress in society.*** Even in the face of amassing evidence that a large percentage of women who smoke will die early, the tobacco industry has unabashedly exploited themes of liberation and success in its advertising—particularly in women's magazines—and promotions targeted to women. Through its sponsorship of women's sports, women's professional and leadership organizations, the arts, and so on, the industry has attempted to associate itself with things women most value (e.g., recent heavily advertised support from a major tobacco company for programs to curb domestic violence against women) (Levin 1999; Bischoff 2000–01). Such associations should be decried for what they are: attempts by the tobacco industry to position itself as an ally of women's causes and thereby to silence potential critics. Women should be appropriately outraged by and speak out against tobacco marketing campaigns that co-opt the language of women's empowerment, and they should recognize the irony of attempts by the tobacco industry to suggest that smoking—which leads to nicotine dependence and death among many women—is a form of independence. Such efforts on the part of women would be unnecessary if the tobacco industry would voluntarily desist with its ongoing efforts to target women and to associate tobacco use with women's freedom and progress.

## Support Women's Anti-Tobacco Advocacy Efforts and Publicize that Most Women Choose to Be Nonsmokers

• ***Encourage a more vocal constituency on issues related to women and smoking.*** Taking a lesson from the success of advocacy to reduce breast cancer, concerted efforts are needed to call public attention to the toll that lung cancer and other smoking-related diseases is exacting on women's health and to demand accountability on the part of the tobacco industry. Women affected by tobacco-related diseases and their families and friends can partner with women's and girls' organizations, women's magazines, female celebrities, and others—not only in an effort to raise awareness of tobacco-related disease as a women's issue, but also to call for policies and programs that deglamorize and discourage tobacco use. Some excellent but relatively small-scale efforts have already taken place in this area, but because of the magnitude of the problem, these efforts deserve much greater support.

• ***Recognize that nonsmoking is by far the norm among women.*** Although in recent years smoking prevalence has not declined as much as might be hoped, nearly four-fifths of U.S. women are nonsmokers. In some subgroups of the population, smoking is relatively rare (e.g., only 11.2 percent of women who have completed college are current smokers, and only 5.4 percent of black high school senior girls are daily smokers). Despite the positive images of women in tobacco advertisements, it is important to recognize that among adult women, those who are the most empowered, as measured by educational attainment, are the least likely to be smokers. Moreover, most women who do smoke say they would like to quit. The fact that almost all women have either rejected smoking for themselves or, if they do smoke now, wish to quit, should be promoted.

## Continue to Build the Science Base on Gender-Specific Outcomes and on How to Reduce Disparities Among Women

• ***Conduct further studies of the relationship between smoking and certain outcomes of importance to women's health.*** For example, does exposure to environmental tobacco smoke increase the risk for breast cancer? Some case-control studies suggested that possibility, but the link remains controversial, especially because relatively little evidence exists thus far supporting an association between active smoking and breast cancer. Any health effects of exposure to environmental tobacco smoke may be particularly important among women in developing countries, where the vast majority of women are nonsmokers but smoking prevalence among men is high. Tobacco products, particularly the cigarette brands that have been most heavily promoted to women smokers, may vary significantly in the levels of known carcinogens;

however, little data exist on how much brands vary in toxicity and whether any of these possible variations may be related to the changes in lung cancer histology over the last decades. More research is needed to evaluate whether changes in the tobacco product and increased exposure to tobacco-specific nitrosamines may be related to the increased incidence rates of adenocarcinoma of the lung. More data are also needed on the effects of employment in tobacco production on women's health, including data on reproductive outcomes among women who work with tobacco during pregnancy. This topic is not covered in the present report because of a paucity of information. In general, much better data are needed on the health effects of smoking among women in the developing world. Are the effects similar to those reported in the literature to date, which is based largely on studies of women smokers in the developed world, or are they modified by differences in lifestyle and environmental factors such as diet, viral exposures, or other sources of indoor air pollution?

• ***Encourage the reporting of gender-specific results from studies of factors influencing smoking behavior, smoking prevention and cessation interventions, and the health effects of tobacco use, including use of new tobacco products.*** The evidence to date has suggested that more similarities than differences exist between women and men in the factors that influence smoking initiation, addiction, and smoking cessation. When differences in smoking history are taken into account, health consequences also are generally similar. These conclusions are tempered by the fact that many research studies are not reporting gender-specific results. However, some studies do report gender differences in smoking cessation and the health effects of smoking; thus, issues regarding gender differences are not entirely resolved. For example, it is still not known whether susceptibility to lung cancer is greater among women smokers than among men smokers, or whether women are more likely than men to gain weight following smoking cessation. Researchers are strongly encouraged to use existing data sets to examine results by gender and to do so in future studies. Where these additional analyses suggest important gender differences, more research is needed to focus on the development of interventions tailored to the special needs of girls and women. As new "reduced-risk" tobacco products are marketed in the future, it will also be important to learn whether gender differences exist in the appeal and use of such products, as well as the health consequences of their use.

• ***Better understand how to reduce current disparities in smoking prevalence among women of different groups, as defined by socioeconomic status, race, ethnicity, and sexual orientation.*** Women with only 9 to 11 years of education are about three times as likely to be smokers as are women with a college education. American Indian or Alaska Native women are much more likely to smoke than are Hispanic women and Asian or Pacific Islander women. Limited data also suggest that lesbian women are more likely to smoke than are heterosexual women. Among teenage girls, whites are much more likely to smoke than are blacks. How can the decline in smoking among women who are less well educated be accelerated? Why are smoking rates so high among American Indian women? What contributes to the relatively low smoking prevalence among Hispanic women and Asian or Pacific Islander women, and what can be done to prevent smoking among them from rising in the future? What positive influences contributed to the vast majority of black teenage girls resisting smoking throughout the 1990s, in stark contrast to the relatively high smoking prevalence among white girls during the same period? The objective is to reduce smoking to the lowest possible level across all demographic groups. The answers to these questions will provide crucial information for intervention efforts.

• ***Determine why, during most of the 1990s, smoking prevalence declined so little among women and increased so markedly among teenage girls.*** This lack of progress is a major concern and threatens to prolong the epidemic of smoking-related disease among women. What are the influences that have kept smoking prevalence relatively stagnant among women and have contributed to the sharp increases in prevalence among teenage girls? Tobacco control policies are known to be effective in reducing smoking, and smoking prevalence tends to decline most where these policies are strongest. However, efforts to curb tobacco use do not operate in a vacuum, and powerful protobacco influences (ranging from tobacco advertising to the use of tobacco in movies) have promoted the social acceptability of smoking and thereby have dampened the effects of tobacco control programs. Moreover, ongoing monitoring of tobacco industry attempts to target women in this country and abroad are necessary for a comprehensive understanding of the influences that encourage women to smoke and for designing effective countermarketing campaigns. If, for example, smoking in movies by female celebrities promotes smoking, then discouraging such practices as well as engaging well-known actresses to be spokespersons on the issue of women and smoking should be a high priority.

• ***Develop a research and evaluation agenda related to women and smoking.*** As noted above, the impact of smoking and of exposure to environmental tobacco smoke on the risk of some disease outcomes has been inadequately studied for women. Determining whether gender-tailored interventions increase the effectiveness of various smoking prevention and cessation methods is important, as is documenting whether any gender differences exist in the effectiveness of pharmacologic treatments for tobacco cessation. A need also exists to determine which tobacco prevention and cessation interventions are most effective for specific subgroups of girls and women, especially those at highest risk for tobacco use (e.g., women with only 9 to 11 years of education, American Indian or Alaska Native women, and women with depression). The sparse data available on smoking among lesbian women suggest that prevalence exceeds that of U.S. women overall, but better data are clearly needed. Research designed to reduce disparities in smoking prevalence across all subgroups of the female population deserves high priority to help eliminate future disparities in smoking-related diseases. The components of programs and policies targeted to individual women, and those targeted to communities that produce the greatest reduction in smoking, need to be identified. Progress on these and other issues will be facilitated by the development of an agenda of research and evaluation priorities related to women and smoking.

## Act Now: We Know More than Enough

• ***Support efforts, at both individual and societal levels, to reduce smoking and exposure to environmental tobacco smoke among women.*** Proven smoking cessation methods are available for individual smokers, including behavioral and pharmacologic approaches that benefit women and men alike. Tobacco use treatments are among the most cost-effective of preventive health interventions; they should be part of all women's health care programs, and health insurance plans should cover such services. Efforts to maximize smoking cessation and maintenance of smoking cessation among women before, during, and after pregnancy deserve high priority, because pregnancy is a time of high motivation to quit and occurs when women have many years of potential life left. With respect to prevention, the knowledge that girls who are more academically inclined or who are more physically active are less likely to smoke suggests that supporting positive outlets for mental and physical development will contribute to reducing the tobacco epidemic as well. Because regular cigarette smoking typically is initiated early in the teenage years, effective smoking cessation and prevention programs for adolescent girls and young women are greatly needed. Societal-level efforts to reduce tobacco use and exposure to environmental tobacco smoke include media counteradvertising, increased tobacco taxes, laws to reduce youth access to tobacco products, and bans on smoking in public places.

• ***Enact comprehensive statewide tobacco control programs—because they work.*** There are known strategies for reducing the burden of smoking-related diseases, but making the investment in these proven strategies remains a challenge. Results from states such as Arizona, California, Florida, Maine, Massachusetts, and Oregon have demonstrated that smoking rates among both girls and women can be dramatically reduced. California was the first state to establish a comprehensive statewide tobacco control program in 1990, and it is now starting to observe the benefits of its sustained efforts: between 1988 and 1997, the incidence rate of lung cancer among women declined by 4.8 percent in California but increased by 13.2 percent in other regions of the United States (Centers for Disease Control and Prevention 2000). Another recent study concluded that the California program was associated with 33,300 fewer deaths from heart disease between 1989 and 1997 among women and men combined than would have been predicted if trends like those observed in the rest of the country had continued (Fichtenberg and

Glantz 2000). Enormous monetary settlement payments from state Medicaid lawsuits with the tobacco industry have provided the resources to fund major new comprehensive state-wide tobacco control efforts. However, a recent report found that only six states were meeting the minimum funding recommendations from the Centers for Disease Control and Prevention's *Best Practices for Comprehensive Tobacco Control Programs* (Campaign for Tobacco-Free Kids 2001).

## Stop the Epidemic of Smoking and Smoking-Related Diseases Among Women Globally

• ***Do everything possible to thwart the emerging epidemic of smoking among women in developing countries.*** Multinational policies that discourage spread of the epidemic of smoking and tobacco-related diseases among women in countries where smoking prevalence has traditionally been low should be strongly encouraged. Efforts to disassociate cigarette smoking from progress in achieving gender equity are particularly needed in the developing world (Magardie 2000). Because smoking prevalence among men is already high in many developing countries, even women who do not smoke themselves are already at risk because they are exposed to environmental tobacco smoke—and because they suffer the losses of male loved ones who are dying of tobacco-related diseases. It is urgent that what is already known about effective means of tobacco control at the societal level be disseminated as soon as possible throughout the world. A major measure of public health victory in the global war against smoking would be the arrest of smoking prevalence at its still generally low level among women in developing countries and a reversal of the now worrisome signs of increases in smoking among them. In November 1999, the World Health Organization (WHO) sponsored an international conference on smoking among women and youth which took place in Kobe, Japan. This conference resulted in the Kobe Declaration, which states that,

> The tobacco epidemic is an unrelenting public health disaster that spares no society. There are already over 200 million women smokers, and tobacco companies have launched aggressive campaigns to recruit women and girls worldwide.... It is urgent that we find comprehensive solutions to the danger of tobacco use and address the epidemic among women and girls (WHO 1999b).

• ***All national governments should strongly support WHO's Framework Convention for Tobacco Control.*** The Framework Convention for Tobacco Control is an international legal instrument designed to curb the global spread of tobacco use through specific protocols, currently being negotiated, that cover tobacco pricing, smuggling, advertising and sponsorship, and other activities (WHO 1999a). In the words of Dr. Gro Harlem Brundtland, director-general of WHO,

> If we do not act decisively, a hundred years from now our grandchildren and their children will look back and seriously question how people claiming to be committed to public health and social justice allowed the tobacco epidemic to unfold unchecked (Asma et al., in press).

# References


Asma S, Yang G, Samet J, Giovino G, Bettcher DW, Lopez A, Yach D. Tobacco. In: *Oxford Textbook of Public Health,* in press.

Bischoff D. Consuming passions. *Ms.* 2000–01 (Dec–Jan):60–5.

Campaign for Tobacco-Free Kids, American Cancer Society, American Heart Association, and American Lung Association. Show Us the Money: An Update on the States' Allocation of the Tobacco Settlement Dollars. Washington: Campaign for Tobacco-Free Kids, Jan 11, 2001; <http://tobaccofreekids.org/reports/settlements/settlement2001.pdf>; accessed: February 6, 2001.

Centers for Disease Control and Prevention. Declines in lung cancer rates—California, 1988–1997. *Morbidity and Mortality Weekly Report* 2000;49(47):1066–9.

Fichtenberg CM, Glantz SA. Association of the California Tobacco Control Program with declines in cigarette consumption and mortality from heart disease. *New England Journal of Medicine* 2000;343(24):1772–7.

Levin M. Philip Morris' new campaign echoes medical experts: tobacco company tries to rebuild its image on TV and online with frank health admissions about smoking and by publicizing its charitable causes. *Los Angeles Times* 1999 Oct 13; Business Sect (Pt C):1.

Magardie K. Tobacco groups target women. *Daily Mail and Guardian* 2000 Oct 26; <http://www.mg.co.za/mg/za/archive/2000oct/features/26oct-tobacco.html>; accessed: October 28, 2000.

World Health Organization. *Framework Convention on Tobacco Control.* Technical Briefing Series. Papers 1–5. Geneva: World Health Organization, 1999a.

World Health Organization. WHO International Conference on Tobacco and Health, Kobe, "Making a Difference in Tobacco and Health: Avoiding the Tobacco Epidemic in Women and Youth." Kobe, Japan, Nov 14–18, 1999b, Kobe Declaration; <http://tobacco.who.int/en/fctc/kobe/declaration.html>; accessed: February 5, 2001.

# Abbreviations

| | |
|---|---|
| **µg** | microgram |
| **AARP** | American Association of Retired Persons |
| **ABPI** | ankle brachial pressure index |
| **ACCP** | American College of Chest Physicians |
| **ACS** | American Cancer Society |
| **AD** | Alzheimer's disease |
| **ADD** | attention deficit disorder |
| **$AF_{exp}$** | attributable fraction among persons exposed |
| **AHCPR** | Agency for Health Care Policy and Research |
| **AIDS** | acquired immunodeficiency syndrome |
| **AMWA** | American Medical Women's Association |
| **APA** | American Psychiatric Association |
| **ASSIST** | American Stop Smoking Intervention Study |
| **AUTS** | Adult Use of Tobacco Survey |
| **BMI** | body mass index |
| **BRFS** | Behavioral Risk Factor Survey |
| **BRFSS** | Behavioral Risk Factor Surveillance System |
| **CASH** | Cancer and Steroid Hormone Study |
| **CDC** | Centers for Disease Control and Prevention |
| **CEPA** | California Environmental Protection Agency |
| **CHAD** | Community, Hypertension, Atherosclerosis, and Diabetes Program |
| **CHD** | coronary heart disease |
| **CI** | confidence interval |
| **CIN** | cervical intraepithelial neoplasia |
| **CIS** | Cancer Information Service |
| **CIS** | carcinoma in situ |
| **CNS** | central nervous system |
| **CO** | carbon monoxide |
| **COLD** | chronic obstructive lung disease |
| **COMMIT** | Community Intervention Trial for Smoking Cessation |
| **COPD** | chronic obstructive pulmonary disease |
| **CORIS** | Coronary Risk Factor Study |
| **CPS-I** | Cancer Prevention Study I |
| **CPS-II** | Cancer Prevention Study II |
| **CVD** | cardiovascular disease |
| **CYP1A1** | cytochrome P-450 1A1 |
| **DES** | diethylstilbestrol |
| **DHEAS** | dehydroepiandrosterone sulfate |
| **DNA** | deoxyribonucleic acid |
| **DRD4** | $D_4$ dopamine receptor |
| ***DSM-III-R*** | *Diagnostic and Statistical Manual of Mental Disorders*, third edition, revised |
| ***DSM-IV*** | *Diagnostic and Statistical Manual of Mental Disorders*, fourth edition |
| **EPA** | U.S. Environmental Protection Agency |
| **ER** | estrogen receptor |
| **ETS** | environmental tobacco smoke |
| **FCTC** | Framework Convention for Tobacco Control |
| **FDA** | U.S. Food and Drug Administration |
| **$FEF_{25-75}$** | forced expiratory flow between 25 and 75 percent of FVC |
| **$FEV_{0.75}$** | forced expiratory volume in 0.75 second |
| **$FEV_1$** | forced expiratory volume in 1 second |
| **FTC** | Federal Trade Commission |
| **FVC** | forced vital capacity |
| **g** | gram |
| **GSTM1** | glutathione *S*-transferase M1 |
| **HCFA** | Health Care Financing Administration |
| **HHANES** | Hispanic Health and Nutrition Examination Survey |
| **HIV** | human immunodeficiency virus |
| **HIV-1** | human immunodeficiency virus type 1 |
| **HMO** | health maintenance organization |
| **HPV** | human papillomavirus |
| **HRT** | hormone replacement therapy |
| **IARC** | International Agency for Research on Cancer |
| **IBD** | inflammatory bowel disease |
| ***ICD-9*** | *International Classification of Diseases*, ninth revision |
| **IMPACT** | Initiatives to Mobilize for the Prevention and Control of Tobacco Use |
| **INWAT** | International Network of Women Against Tobacco |
| **IUGR** | intrauterine growth retardation |
| ***JAMA*** | *Journal of the American Medical Association* |
| **kg** | kilogram |
| **L** | liter |
| **LBW** | low birth weight |

| | |
|---|---|
| **LPL** | lipoprotein lipase |
| **m** | meter |
| **MDD** | major depressive disorder |
| **mg** | milligram |
| **MI** | myocardial infarction |
| **mL** | milliliter |
| **mm** | millimeter |
| **mm Hg** | millimeter of mercury |
| **MSA** | Master Settlement Agreement |
| **MTF** | Monitoring the Future Survey |
| **NAB** | *N′*-nitrosoanabasine |
| **NAT** | *N′*-nitrosoanatabine |
| **NAT1** | *N*-acetyltransferase 1 |
| **NAT2** | *N*-acetyltransferase 2 |
| **NCHS** | National Center for Health Statistics |
| **NCI** | National Cancer Institute |
| **ng** | nanogram |
| **NHANES** | National Health and Nutrition Examination Survey |
| **NHANES II** | National Health and Nutrition Examination Survey II |
| **NHANES III** | National Health and Nutrition Examination Survey III |
| **NHIS** | National Health Interview Survey |
| **NHSDA** | National Household Survey on Drug Abuse |
| **NIDA** | National Institute on Drug Abuse |
| **NIOSH** | National Institute for Occupational Safety and Health |
| **NNK** | 4-(methylnitrosamino)-1-(3-pyridyl)-1-butanone |
| **NNN** | *N′*-nitrosonornicotine |
| **NOW** | National Organization for Women |
| **NRC** | National Research Council |
| **NTTS** | National Teenage Tobacco Survey |
| **NYTS** | National Youth Tobacco Survey |
| **OA** | osteoarthritis |
| **OC** | oral contraceptive |
| **OSH** | Office on Smoking and Health |
| **PAH** | polycyclic aromatic hydrocarbon |
| **PD** | Parkinson's disease |
| **PHS** | U.S. Public Health Service |
| **PID** | pelvic inflammatory disease |
| **PPROM** | preterm premature rupture of the membranes |
| **PROM** | premature rupture of the membranes |
| **RA** | rheumatoid arthritis |
| **RR** | relative risk |
| **SAMHSA** | Substance Abuse and Mental Health Services Administration |
| **SAMMEC** | Smoking Attributable Mortality, Morbidity, and Economic Costs |
| **SEER** | Surveillance, Epidemiology, and End Results Program |
| **SES** | socioeconomic status |
| **SGA** | small for gestational age |
| **SIDS** | sudden infant death syndrome |
| **SLE** | systemic lupus erythematosus |
| **SMR** | standardized mortality ratio |
| **STD** | sexually transmitted disease |
| **SUDAAN** | Survey Data Analysis |
| **TAPS I** | Teenage Attitudes and Practices Survey I |
| **TAPS II** | Teenage Attitudes and Practices Survey II |
| **TIA** | transient ischemic attack |
| **TSH** | thyroid-stimulating hormone |
| **TSNA** | tobacco-specific nitrosamine |
| **USDHEW** | U.S. Department of Health, Education, and Welfare |
| **USDHHS** | U.S. Department of Health and Human Services |
| **WAGAT** | Women and Girls Against Tobacco |
| **WHO** | World Health Organization |
| **WHR** | waist-to-hip ratio |
| **WIC** | Special Supplemental Nutrition Program for Women, Infants, and Children |
| **YPLL** | years of potential life lost |
| **YRBS** | Youth Risk Behavior Survey |
| **YRBSS** | Youth Risk Behavior Surveillance System |

# List of Tables and Figures

## Chapter 1. Introduction and Summary of Conclusions



## Chapter 2. Patterns of Tobacco Use Among Women and Girls

## Chapter 5. Efforts to Reduce Tobacco Use Among Women



## Chapter 6. A Vision for the Future: What Is Needed to Reduce Smoking Among Women

No tables or figures.

# Index

## A

## B

## C

## D

## E

## G

## H

## I



## J

## K



## L

## M

## N

## O

## P

## Q



## R

## S

## T

## U



## V



## W

## Y

## Z